a **LANGE** clinical manual

Ambulatory Medicine

The Primary Care of Families

third edition

D0971391

Edited by

Mark B. Mengel, MD, MPH
Professor and Chairman
Department of Community and Family Medicine
St. Louis University School of Medicine
St. Louis

L. Peter Schwiebert, MD
Associate Professor and Director
Predoctoral Division
Department of Family Medicine
University of Oklahoma College of Medicine
Oklahoma City

Lange Medical Books/McGraw-Hill
Medical Publishing Division

New York St. Louis San Francisco Auckland Bogotá Caracas Lisbon London
Madrid Mexico City Milan Montreal New Delhi San Juan
Singapore Sydney Tokyo Toronto

McGraw-Hill

A Division of The **McGraw·Hill** *Companies*

Ambulatory Medicine: The Primary Care of Families, Third Edition

Copyright © 2001 by The **McGraw-Hill Companies,** Inc. All rights reserved. Printed in the United States of America. Except as permitted under the United States Copyright Act of 1976, no part of this publication may be reproduced or distributed in any form or by any means, or stored in a data base or retrieval system, without the prior written permission of the publisher.

Copyright © 1996 by Appleton & Lange, A Simon & Schuster Company
Copyright © 1993 by Appleton & Lange

1234567890 DOC/DOC 09876543210

ISBN: 0-8385-0387-X

This book was set in Helvetica by Circle Graphics.
The editors were Janet Foltin, Harriet Lebowitz, and John M. Morriss.
The production supervisor was Philip Galea.

R.R. Donnelley & Sons Company was printer and binder.

This book is printed on acid-free paper.

Contents

Contributors

Louise S. Acheson, MD, MS
Associate Professor of Family Medicine, Case Western Reserve University School of Medicine, University Hospital of Cleveland, Cleveland

Aliza Acker-Bernstein, MD
Clinical Assistant Professor at Boston University Medical Center; Medical Director, Family Practice Residency Program, The Family Practice Center at the Hunt, Danvers, Massachusetts

Alan M. Adelman, MD, MS
Professor, Department of Family and Community Medicine, Hershey Medical Center, Pennsylvania State University College of Medicine, Hershey

Russell L. Anderson, MD
Professor and Head, Department of Family Medicine, Louisiana State University School of Medicine, New Orleans

Kenneth R. Bertka, MD
Director of Family Medicine Education, St. Vincent Mercy Medical Center, Toledo; Clinical Associate Professor, Department of Family Medicine, Medical College of Ohio, Toledo

Richard B. Birrer, MD
Associate Professor of Emergency Medicine, Albert Einstein College of Medicine; Associate Professor of Family Medicine, University of New York—Health Science Center at Brooklyn College of Medicine

Gregory H. Blake, MD, MPH
Professor and Chairman, Department of Family Medicine, University of Tennessee Medical Center, Knoxville

Richard J. Botelho, MD
Associate Professor of Family Medicine, Psychiatry, and Nursing; Director, Fellowship Training Program, Jacob Holler Family Medicine Center, Rochester, New York

Richard L. Brown, MD, MPH
Associate Professor, Department of Family Medicine, University of Wisconsin Medical School, Madison

Richard Brunader, MD
Associate Clinical Professor of Family and Community Medicine, University of California, San Francisco, School of Medicine

Wendy O. Buffet, MD
Assistant Clinical Professor, Department of Family and Community Medicine, University of California, San Francisco

Frank S. Celestino, MD
Associate Professor, Geriatrics Director, Wake Forest University School of Medicine, Health Promotion/Prevention, Winston-Salem, North Carolina

Jason Chao, MD, MS
Associate Professor of Family Medicine, Case Western Reserve University School of Medicine, University Hospital of Cleveland, Cleveland

Benjamin W. Chaska, MD, RPh
Medical Director, Oakwood Ambulatory Services Division, Oakwood Healthcare System, Dearbourn, Michigan

Neal D. Clemenson, MD
Director, Great Plains Family Practice Residency Program, Oklahoma City

Richard D. Clover, MD
Professor and Chairman, Department of Family and Community Medicine, University of Louisville, Louisville, Kentucky

John L. Coulehan, MD, MPH
Professor of Preventive Medicine, Health Sciences Center School of Medicine, State University of New York at Stony Brook; Director, Institute for Medicine in Contemporary Society

Michael A. Crouch, MD, MSPH
Associate Professor of Family and Community Medicine, Baylor College of Medicine, Houston

Brenda Powell Crownover, MD
Assistant Professor, Department of Family Medicine, Case Western Reserve University, University School of Medicine, Cleveland, Ohio

Mel P. Daly, MD
Director of Family Medicine, Subacute Unit, Greater Baltimore Medical Center, Baltimore, Maryland

Janice E. Daugherty, MD
Associate Professor of Family Medicine, East Carolina University School of Medicine, Greenville, North Carolina

Kent W. Davidson, MD
Associate Professor, Department of Family and Community Medicine, University of Arkansas College of Medicine, Little Rock

Marvin A. Dewar, MD, JD
Associate Professor of Community Health and Family Medicine, University of Florida College of Medicine, Gainesville

Pieter J. de Wet, MD
Medical Director, Tyler Total Wellness Center, Tyler; Associate Professor of Family Practice, University of Texas Health Center at Tyler

Larry L. Dickey, MD, MSW, MPH
Assistant Adjunct Professor, Department of Family and Community Medicine, University of California, San Francisco, School of Medicine; Chief, Office of Clinical Preventive Medicine, California Department of Health Services

Philip M. Diller, MD, PhD
Associate Professor of Clinical Family Medicine, University of Cincinnati Family Medical Program

Alison E. Dobbie, MB, ChB MRCGP
Assistant Professor and Director of Medical Student Education, Department of Family Medicine, University of Texas Heath Science Center at San Antonio

Mari E. Egan, MD
Instructor, PreClinical Curriculum Coordinator, Department of Family Medicine, Northwestern University

Ted D. Epperly, MD
Chairman, Department of Family and Community Medicine, Eisenhower Army Medical Center, Fort Gordon, Georgia

David W. Euans, MD
Clinical Associate Professor, Department of Family Medicine, Louisiana State University School of Medicine, New Orleans; Clinical Associate Professor, Department of Family and Community Medicine, Tulane University School of Medicine, New Orleans

Ellen R. Evans, MD
Assistant Clinical Professor, Department of Family Practice, Creighton University School of Medicine, Omaha; Medical Director, Restorative Care Unit, St. Joseph Hospital, Omaha; Director, Geriatric Consultation Services, Omaha

Scott A. Fields, MD
Vice Chair for Clinical Affairs, Department of Family Medicine; Associate Director, Integrated Primary Care Organization, Oregon Health Sciences University

James T. Flannick, PsyD
Assistant Professor, Franciscan University of Steubenville, Ohio; Partner, Clinical Psychologist, Parakleseos, LLC, Beaver, Pennsylvania

John P. Fogarty, MD
Professor, Chair and Physician Leader, Department of Family Practice, University of Vermont College of Medicine, Burlington

Laura B. Frankenstein, MD
Family Physician, Lynn Community Health Center, Lynn, Massachusetts

Keith A. Frey, MD, MBA
Chair, Department of Family Medicine, Mayo Clinic, Scottsdale, Arizona

Ronald H. Goldschmidt, MD
Professor and Vice Chairman, Department of Family and Community Medicine, University of California, San Francisco, School of Medicine; Director, Family Practice Inpatient Service, San Francisco General Hospital, San Francisco

James L. Greenwald, MD
Clinical Associate Professor, State University of New York Upstate Medical University

David R. Grube, MD
Clinical Associate Professor of Family Medicine, Department of Family Medicine, Oregon Health Sciences University School of Medicine, Portland

Cristina I. Gruta, PharmD
Assistant Clinical Professor of Pharmacy, University of California, San Francisco.

William J. Hall, MD
Chief, General Medicine, Geriatrics Unit, University of Rochester

John G. Halvorsen, MD, MS
Thomas and Ellen Foster Professor and Chair, Department of Family and Community Medicine, University of Illinois College of Medicine

Richard J. Ham, MD
SUNY Distinguished Chair in Geriatric Medicine; Professor of Medicine and Family Medicine, State University of New York Health Science Center at Syracuse

Cynthia L. Haq, MD
Associate Professor, Department of Family Medicine, University of Wisconsin-Madison; Director of Medical Student Education

Franklin Hargett, MD
Clinical Assistant Professor, Department of Family Medicine, University of North Carolina at Chapel Hill School of Medicine

Cathryn B. Heath, MD
Assistant Professor of Family Medicine, UMDNJ - Robert Wood Johnson Medical School

Caryl J. Heaton, DO
Associate Professor of Clinical Family Medicine, New Jersey Medical School—UMDNJ

Brian Hertz, MD
Program Director for Northern New Mexico Family Practice Residency, La Familia Medical Center

Allen Hixon, MD
Residency Program Director, University of Connecticut/St. Francis Hospital Family Medicine Residency Program

Joseph Hobbs, MD
Professor and Chairman, Department of Family Medicine, Medical College of Georgia School of Medicine, Augusta

Pamela Sue Horst, MD
Associate Professor of Family Medicine, State University of New York Upstate Medical University

Linda M. Ivy, MD
Private Practice, Family Medicine, San Antonio, Texas

Thomas M. Johnson, PhD
Clinical Professor, Family Medicine and Psychology, University of South Florida College of Medicine; Assistant Director, Family Practice Residency Program, Morton Plant Mease Healthcare Center

Mitchell A. Kaminski, MD
Clinical Assistant Professor, University of Maryland Medical School, Baltimore; Chairman, Department of Family Practice, Greater Baltimore Medical Center

Sanford R. Kimmel, MD
Associate Professor, Department of Family Medicine, Medical College of Ohio, Toledo

Evan W. Kligman, MD
Clinical Professor of Family Medicine, University of Iowa; Clinical Professor of Public Health, University of Arizona

Mark P. Knudson, MD, MSPH
Associate Professor and Director of Residency Training, Family Medicine, Wake Forest University School of Medicine, Winston-Salem, North Carolina

Christopher L. Krogh, MD, MPH†
Former Clinical Assistant Professor, University of Minnesota Medical School, Minneapolis

Mark A. Landis, MD
Private Practice, Hohenwald, Tennessee

David C. Lanier, MD
Acting Director, Center for Primary Care Research, Agency for Healthcare Research and Quality, Washington, DC

Denise LeBlanc-Ziegler, MD
Family Physician, Private Practice, Oklahoma City Clinic

Bruce M. LeClair, MD, MPH
Assistant Professor, Department of Family Medicine, Medical College of Georgia School of Medicine, Augusta

Martin S. Lipsky, MD
Professor and Chair, Department of Family Medicine, Northwestern University Medical School, Chicago

†Deceased

David P. Losh, MD
Associate Professor and Residency Program Director, Department of Family
Medicine, University of Washington School of Medicine, Seattle

Diane J. Madlon-Kay, MD
Associate Professor, Department of Family and Community Medicine, University of
Minnesota, St. Paul

Charles F. Margolis, MD
Professor of Clinical Family Medicine, Department of Family Medicine, University of
Cincinnati College of Medicine

James P. McKenna, MD
Clinical Assistant Professor of Family and Community Medicine, Pennsylvania State
University College of Medicine, Hershey; Director, Family Practice Residency
Program, The Medical Center, Beaver

Mark B. Mengel, MD, MPH
Professor and Chairman, Department of Community and Family Medicine, St. Louis
University School of Medicine, St. Louis, Missouri

Angela D. Mickalide, PhD, CHES
Adjunct Associate Professor of Prevention and Community Health, George
Washington University School of Medicine; Program Director, National Safe Kids
Campaign, Washington, DC

Donald B. Middleton, MD
Professor and Interim Chairman, Department of Family Medicine and Clinical
Epidemiology, University of Pittsburgh School of Medicine

Lynn V. Mitchell, MD, MPH
Adjunct Associate Professor, Public Health, University of Oklahoma College of
Medicine; Medical Director, Oklahoma Health Care Authority

Leonard W. Morgan, MD, PhD
Regional Chairman, Department of Family Medicine, Texas Tech University Health
Sciences Center, Odessa

Mary Kay Mroz, MD
Clinical Assistant Professor, Department of Family and Community Medicine,
University of Kansas School of Medicine, Wichita

George A. Nixon, MD
Associate Professor, Department of Family Medicine, Medical College of Georgia,
Augusta

Jim Nuovo, MD
Associate Professor, Department of Family and Community Medicine,
University of California School of Medicine, Davis

P. Richard Olson, MD*
Former Professor and Vice Chairman, Department of Family Medicine,
University of North Carolina School of Medicine, Chapel Hill

Tomás P. Owens, Jr., MD
Associate Director, Great Plains Family Practice Residency Program; Clinical
Associate Professor, Departments of Internal Medicine, Geriatric Medicine and
Family Preventive Medicine, University of Oklahoma Health Sciences Center,
Oklahoma City

Michael L. Parchman, MD
Associate Professor, Department of Family Medicine, Texas Tech University Health
Sciences Center, San Antonio, Texas

*Retired

Megeen Parker, MD
Clinical Assistant Professor, University of Wisconsin Health—Physicians Plus, University of Wisconsin Medical School, McFarland, Wisconsin

David Paul, MD, MPH
Assistant Professor, Department of Family Medicine, University of Oklahoma Health Sciences Center; Division Director of Occupational and Environmental Medicine, Oklahoma City

Dana W. Peterson, MD
Private Practice, Family Medicine, Southwest Medical Associates, Albuquerque, New Mexico

Marjorie Shaw Phillips, MS, RPh, FASHP
Adjunct Clinical Associate Professor of Pharmacy Practice, University of Georgia College of Pharmacy and Pharmacist, Medical College of Georgia Hospital and Clinics, Augusta

William G. Phillips, MD
Assistant Professor, Department of Family Medicine, Medical College of Georgia School of Medicine, Augusta

David V. Power, MB, BCh, BAO, MPH
Associate Director for Medical Student Education, Department of Family Practice and Community Health, University of Minnesota Medical School, Minneapolis

Martin Quan, MD
Professor of Clinical Family Medicine; Director of Residency Training, Department of Family Medicine, University of California School of Medicine, Los Angeles

Steven E. Reissman, DO
Chief, Department of Family Practice and Community Medicine, Martin Army Community Hospital, Fort Benning, Georgia

John C. Rogers, MD, MPH
Professor and Vice Chairman for Education, Department of Family and Community Medicine, Baylor College of Medicine, Houston, Texas

Paula Root, MD, MPH
Adjunct Assistant Professor, Department of Family and Preventive Medicine, University of Oklahoma College of Medicine, Oklahoma City

Ted C. Schaffer, MD
Assistant Professor, Department of Family Medicine, University of Pittsburgh School of Medicine; Director, Family Medicine Practice Residency Program, UMPM St. Margaret, Pittsburgh, Pennsylvania

William R. Scheibel, MD
Professor of Family Medicine, University of Wisconsin Medical School, Madison

F. David Schneider, MD, MSPH
Residency Program Director, Department of Family Practice, University of Texas Health Science Center at San Antonio

L. Peter Schwiebert, MD
Associate Professor and Director, Predoctoral Division, Department of Family Medicine, University of Oklahoma College of Medicine, Oklahoma City

William B. Shore, MD
Professor, Department of Family and Community Medicine, University of California, San Francisco

Clark B. Smith, MD
Associate Professor and Vice Chairman for Clinical Affairs, Department of Family Medicine, University of Tennessee, Memphis

Douglas R. Smucker, MD, MPH
Assistant Professor, Department of Family Medicine, University of Cincinnati, Ohio

Jeannette E. South-Paul, MD
Chair, Department of Family Medicine, Uniformed Services University of the Health Sciences, Bethesda, Maryland

Rhonda Agnes Sparks, MD
Assistant Professor, Department of Family and Preventive Medicine, Oklahoma University Health Science Center, Oklahoma City

Gerry A. Steiner, MD
Clinical Assistant Professor, Department of Family Medicine, Medical College of Ohio, Toledo

Jeffrey L. Susman, MD
Chairman, Department of Family Medicine, University of Cincinnati

Jay A. Swedberg, MD
Diplomate, American Board of Family Practice; Fellow, American Academy of Family Physicians, Casper, Wyoming

Melissa A. Talamantes, MS
Assistant Professor and Director of Community Medicine, Department of Family Practice, University of Texas Health Science Center at San Antonio

William L. Toffler, MD
Professor, Department of Family Medicine, Oregon Health Sciences University School of Medicine, Portland

Anthony F. Valdini, MD, MS
Research Director of Faculty Development; Fellowship Director, Greater Lawrence Family Health Center, Lawrence, Massachusetts

Richard Viken, MD
Chairman and Director, Department of Family Practice, University of Texas Health Center at Tyler

Linda L. Walker, MD
Associate Director, Family Practice Residency Program, The Medical Center, Columbus, Georgia

Barry D. Weiss, MD
Professor of Clinical Family and Community Medicine, University of Arizona College of Medicine, Tucson, Arizona

Stephen F. Wheeler, MEng, MD
Assistant Professor and Director of Residency Training, Department of Family and Community Medicine, University of Louisville, Louisville, Kentucky; Associate Dean for Admissions, University of Louisville School of Medicine

Jim L. Wilson, MD
Professor and Chairman, Department of Family Medicine, East Tennessee State University, James H. Quillen College of Medicine, Johnson City, Tennessee

Paul W. Wright, MD
Professor of Family Practice, University of Texas Health Center at Tyler

Jack A. Yanovski, MD, PhD
Chief, Unit on Growth and Obesity, Developmental Endocrinology Branch, National Institute of Child Health and Human Development, National Institutes of Health, Bethesda, Maryland

Susan Zelitch Yanovski, MD
Director, Obesity and Eating Disorders Program, National Institute of Diabetes and Digestive and Kidney Disease, Bethesda, Maryland

Mark W. Zilkoski, MD
Associate Professor of Clinical Family Medicine and Associate Director of Geriatric Education, Medical College of Ohio, Toledo

Foreword to the Second Edition

The primary care of families spans all age groups and crosses generations. Care for entire families has been the formal focus of family medicine clinicians, researchers, and educators around the world for more than 27 years—since family practice became recognized in the United States as a medical specialty in 1969. Managing such a broad clinical agenda has remained a worthy challenge, often hampered by the uncertainties of first contact, primary care in which the presenting symptom must be managed before it suggests an underlying diagnosis. Recognizing symptom patterns and managing early symptoms that may not progress to diagnosable disease are fundamental to this broad challenge unbounded by age and organ system. Brief and well-organized clinical references rarely address this challenge in readily accessible ways. The first edition of *Ambulatory Medicine: The Primary Care of Families*, however, did accomplish it well and became an international educational and clinical classic. The second edition improves this pocket reference, with new chapters and two new sections.*

Changes in the management of common complaints are addressed in updated chapters in the first section, complemented by such new chapters as "The Abnormal Pap Smear," by Neal D. Clemenson, MD, and "Genital Lesions," by Tomás P. Owens, Jr., MD. The efficiency of organizing this section alphabetically by presenting complaint or symptom is becoming even more useful as increasing time pressure affects our clinical interactions. Nearly all primary care clinicians must maintain a broad knowledge base while balancing other, nonclinical agendas each day. This manual demonstrates respect for this increasingly complex and demanding environment.

Section II, "Chronic Illnesses," has been updated and revised with a new chapter called "Cancer Pain Management," by David R. Grube, MD. Many family physicians and other primary care providers will appreciate this concise review of the basics of this time-honored physician's task.

Section VI, entirely new, is called "Special Populations" and includes such chapters as "The Adolescent Patient," by William B. Shore, MD, "The Care of the Patient with Disabilities," by Caryl J. Heaton, DO, and "The Elderly Patient," by Richard J. Ham, MD.

With all of these chapters, this handy manual bridges the gap between practice guidelines—filled with suggested therapy once the diagnosis is secure—and comprehensive textbooks—with definitive presentations on complex topics.

Busy clinicians, academic faculty, and administrative physicians with clinical roles will continue to need concise, well-organized pocket references. Drs Mengel and Schwiebert have brought together an esteemed group of contributors and have refined a quick-reference format to help all of us achieve our collective goal: the primary care of families.

Macaran A. Baird, MD, MS
President, Society of Teachers of Family Medicine, 1996–1997
Mayo Clinic

* In the third edition, new chapters on nose bleeds (epistaxis) and attention deficit/hyperactivity disorder have been added.

PURPOSE

This manual presents information on the most common complaints, problems, conditions, and diseases encountered by physicians who practice in the ambulatory primary care setting. These common conditions, which have been selected from surveys taken in family practice, internal medicine, and pediatric clinics, are arranged alphabetically in six sections. Evidenced-based information is presented in such a way that busy practitioners can access it rapidly. Practical, specific treatment information, including starting doses of medications, is offered. This manual also addresses preventive interventions commonly used in the primary care setting, and special patient populations encountered in the primary care setting.

ORGANIZATION AND SCOPE

Although most medical books are organized by organ system, we have structured this manual according to typical patient presentations in the primary care setting, for example, common symptoms and signs, follow-up needs for chronic physical or mental illnesses, and reproductive health concerns. In addition, we provide an evidenced-based approach to preventive health care and the needs of special patient populations.

Section I contains information on the most commonly encountered acute problems in the primary care setting. Information is presented in such a way that a busy practitioner can quickly form a list of diagnostic possibilities, perform a cost-effective diagnostic work-up, and prescribe therapy for the most common causes of these complaints.

Section II offers information on the treatment of patients with common chronic illnesses. Each chapter provides practical follow-up strategies for such patients, integrating cost-effective clinical management with important psychosocial issues.

Section III is important because many patients who are seen in primary care clinics have either a primary psychiatric disorder or a psychiatric disorder complicating the management of coexisting medical conditions. Strategies that effectively *identify* and *treat* patients with psychiatric disorders are presented clearly and succinctly.

Section IV addresses reproductive health issues, including contraception, infertility, and prenatal and postpartum care.

Section V will assist primary care physicians in the prevention of important diseases in their patients. Authors recommend interventions that can be easily applied in primary care clinics; areas addressed include counseling, immunizations, screening tests, and chemoprophylaxis.

Section VI outlines helpful approaches in caring for adolescents, seniors, and patients with disabilities.

In all chapters, authors have integrated principles of clinical decision-making and cost-effective clinical management and have considered psychosocial and contextual issues. When applicable, areas of controversy are identified. Where appropriate, alternative and complementary medicine interventions are discussed.

Other useful features of this manual include:

- A convenient outline format and selective use of boldface type to afford quick, easy access to key aspects of diagnosis and treatment.

- Flowcharts facilitating the diagnostic work-up or management of specific conditions.
- Emphasis on cost-effective, evidence-based strategies.

ACKNOWLEDGMENTS

First, we thank those of you who have used this manual. We received positive feedback from medical students and residents as well as from many practitioners who found the second edition to be a quick, practical reference text. We particularly appreciate those comments that have enabled us to strengthen many sections of the handbook and add new chapters and sections on topics that many readers considered important.

Second, we embarked on this third edition with some trepidation, as most of our authors are busy primary care physicians. We were pleasantly surprised to discover that many of these authors were eager to update their chapters and did so with great enthusiasm.

When time did not allow second edition authors to update their chapters, most were helpful in suggesting well-qualified authors willing to revise their work. We are delighted that all chapters have been updated and many have been totally rewritten, reflecting the rapid increase in information and changes in approach to therapy that have occurred in the mere 3 years since publication of the first edition.

Third, we thank the editors at McGraw-Hill for their encouragement and support. We had originally planned to revise this manual every 5 years; however, the editors were right in encouraging a shorter revision cycle. Also the outstanding editorial support of Linda Conheady, Diane Phillips, and Harriet Lebowitz has helped us express our ideas more clearly.

Last but far from least, we thank our spouses, Laura and Kathy, and our children, Sally, Kristen, and Matt, for their support and patience throughout this rapid editorial process. As we both had to take a great deal of work home, our families deserve special thanks and gratitude.

Mark B. Mengel, MD, MPH
L. Peter Schwiebert, MD
St. Louis, Missouri, and Oklahoma City, Oklahoma
September 2000

SECTION I. **Common Complaints**

1   Abdominal Pain

Alan M. Adelman, MD, MS

I. **Definition.** Abdominal pain is a subjective feeling of discomfort in the abdomen.
II. **Common diagnoses.** Nonspecific abdominal pain (NSAP) is the most frequent diagnosis of abdominal pain; 40–50% of final diagnoses are NSAP. NSAP, acute gastroenteritis, pelvic inflammatory disease (PID), and urinary tract infection (UTI) account for 60–70% of all diagnoses. Table 1–1 gives a complete listing of the most frequent diagnoses. Conditions causing abdominal pain that are discussed in this chapter include **irritable bowel syndrome (IBS), diverticulitis, cholecystitis, appendicitis, acute pancreatitis,** and **mesenteric ischemic disease.**

 Causes of abdominal pain that are discussed elsewhere in this book are PID (Chapter 55), UTI (Chapter 24), diarrheal syndromes (Chapter 19), peptic ulcer disease (Chapter 86), urinary tract stones (Chapter 37), and ectopic pregnancy (Chapter 55).
III. **Epidemiology.** Approximately 80% of patients with abdominal pain are seen three or fewer times for their pain. Almost half are seen only once for this problem. The lower abdomen is the most common region for pain, accounting for approximately two thirds of all medical visits for abdominal pain. Approximately 10% of patients are referred to a specialist. Surgical referrals predominate, general surgery being the most common (50%), followed by obstetrics and gynecology (33%). Approximately 10% of patients with abdominal pain are admitted to the hospital for evaluation and treatment.

   A. **Age.** Depending on the patient's age, abdominal pain is the 11th to 17th most common reason for visiting the family physician. Patients who seek medical attention for abdominal pain tend to be young; persons between the ages of 18 and 44 years seek attention most frequently. Certain diagnoses are more prevalent in certain age groups. Diverticulitis and mesenteric artery occlusion are found predominantly in the elderly, while IBS rarely presents initially in the elderly. Over 90% of children who have abdominal pain have NSAP. In one study, elderly patients presenting to an emergency room for evaluation of nontraumatic abdominal pain were more likely to have a surgical abdomen than were younger patients.
   B. **Gender.** Most patients who present with abdominal pain are female, even when gynecologic diagnoses are excluded.
IV. **Pathophysiology**
   A. **NSAP.** The exact cause of NSAP is unknown. It may represent a form of bowel motility disorder similar to IBS. The role of psychosocial factors is also not known, although some physicians feel that abdominal pain may be similar to tension headache as a somatic focus for stress.
   B. **IBS.** The exact cause of IBS is debated. IBS may represent a motility disorder of the gastrointestinal tract. Other causes, such as a gastrointestinal hormonal imbalance or a psychosocial cause such as depression or stress, have been postulated.
   C. **Diverticulitis.** Obstruction of a diverticulum leads to distention and subsequent inflammation of the peridiverticular tissue. Microperforation with localized spread to the peridiverticular area can also occur. Although not common, free perforation and intra-abdominal abscess formation can occur.
   D. **Cholecystitis.** Acute cholecystitis is caused by the stasis of bile in the gallbladder, resulting from blockage of the outlet of the gallbladder or the bile duct, usually by one or more gallstones, with subsequent inflammation. Gallstones are usually composed of cholesterol, and their formation is caused by changes in the composition of bile. Risk factors for formation of gallstones include obesity, use of oral contraceptive agents or clofibrate, and genetic factors.
   E. **Appendicitis.** Obstruction of the lumen of the appendix leads to distention and inflammation or infection. If the process progresses, infarction and rupture of the appendix occur, resulting in peritonitis.
   F. **Acute pancreatitis.** The exact cause of acute pancreatitis is unknown. It has been postulated that an initiating event, such as reflux of bile or duodenal juices

TABLE 1–1. FINAL DIAGNOSES FOR THE PRESENTING SYMPTOM OF ABDOMINAL PAIN

Diagnosis[1]	Percent[1]	Brewer et al Study Percent[2]
Abdominal pain, nonspecific	50.4	41.3
Acute gastroenteritis	9.2	6.9
Urinary tract infection	6.7	5.2
Irritable bowel syndrome	5.8	
Pelvic inflammatory disease	3.8	6.7
Hiatal hernia or reflux	2.3	
Diverticulosis	2.2	
Diarrhea, cause undetermined	1.6	
Cholelithiasis	1.6	3.7
Tumor, benign	1.4	
Duodenal ulcer	1.4	2.0
Urolithiasis	1.3	4.3
Appendicitis	1.1	4.3
Ulcerative colitis	0.9	
Muscular strain	0.9	
Other	9.5	

[1]Adapted from Adelman A: Abdominal pain in the primary care setting. J Fam Pract 1987;**25**:27.
[2]Adapted from Brewer RJ, et al: Abdominal pain: An analysis of 1,000 consecutive cases in a university emergency room. Am J Surg 1976;**131**:219.

or alcohol use, leads to leakage of pancreatic enzymes into the tissue of the pancreas. Subsequently, edema, fat necrosis, and tissue damage occur.

G. **Mesentric ischemic disease.** Occlusion is the result of blockage of arterial flow. This can occur as a result of either embolic obstruction or atherosclerotic vascular disease. Decreased cardiac output secondary to myocardial infarction or congestive heart failure can be a contributing factor. Ischemia and necrosis of the bowel follow.

V. **Symptoms.** The primary task for the physician is to differentiate a surgical problem that requires prompt attention from a self-limited, benign process. Although symptoms such as pain, anorexia, vomiting, diarrhea, and constipation alone often are not indicators of serious disease, and although the risk of a serious condition is relatively low, the physician must not dismiss the symptoms that follow as indications of a self-limited problem.

A. **Pain**
  1. **Pain that is capable of the actions listed below** can indicate serious disease.
     a. Awakens the patient from sleep.
     b. Continues for >6 hours.
     c. Changes in pattern (eg, appendicitis usually begins with epigastric or periumbilical pain and then localizes to the right lower quadrant).
     d. Is accompanied by syncope or fainting.
     e. Precedes vomiting (in one study, this occurred in 100% of patients with an abdomen requiring surgery, but in only 20% of those whose abdomen required medical treatment).
     f. Is worsened by breathing or a change in body position.
     g. Radiates, such as pain radiating to the shoulder in a patient with acute cholecystitis or to the back in a patient with acute pancreatitis or abdominal aneurysm.
  2. **Location of pain** can be helpful when coupled with other symptoms or signs. For example, right lower quadrant pain followed by emesis, fever, and leukocytosis is a classic presentation of appendicitis. However, location alone may not be a reliable indicator of the anatomic sites involved. For example, patients with IBS may present with pain anywhere in the abdomen.
  3. **Medications** such as erythromycin or tetracycline may cause abdominal discomfort. Other medications, such as corticosteroids, may mask or diminish pain. The patient's medication history should be examined.

B. **Persistent vomiting** may indicate a serious disease.

    C. Altered bowel function, such as diarrhea alternating with constipation, is characteristic in patients with IBS. These patients may also complain of abdominal distention, bloating, belching, excessive flatus, and mucus in the stool.

    D. Changes in mental status, appetite, functional abilities, energy levels, and sleep patterns may replace pain as the predominant symptoms. This is particularly true with elderly patients, who may present atypically. The age of the patient must be taken into consideration.

    E. The patient's **medical history** may suggest diagnoses. A history of atrial fibrillation, congestive heart failure, or recent myocardial infarction with periumbilical pain is suggestive of mesenteric artery occlusion. A history of abdominal surgery should alert the clinician to the possibility of obstruction secondary to adhesions. An appendectomy in a patient's history does not exclude the possibility of appendicitis, since the appendiceal stump may become inflamed with development of appendicitis. This is more prevalent in patients who have had a ruptured appendix in the past.

VI. Signs. The physician's major task is to identify any surgically correctable disease. A combination of symptoms and signs may help the physician to identify potentially life-threatening, surgically correctable disease.

    A. Rebound tenderness is frequently found in patients with a surgical abdomen. The location of pain and tenderness is not, in itself, very helpful; certain locations are fairly sensitive but not very specific. For appendicitis, right lower quadrant tenderness has a sensitivity of 0.81 and a specificity of 0.53. Similarly, only 5% of patients with right upper quadrant pain had cholecystitis.

    B. Bowel changes, particularly blood in the stool, demand attention. Serious conditions, such as peptic ulcer disease, tumors, or ulcerative colitis, must be ruled out.

    C. Abnormal bowel sounds occur more frequently in patients with a surgical abdomen than in those whose abdomen can be treated nonsurgically.

    D. An **abdominal mass** is found more frequently in patients with a surgical abdomen than in those not requiring surgery. A pulsatile abdominal mass accompanied by abdominal pain radiating to the back and diminished femoral pulses should arouse suspicion of a ruptured aortic aneurysm.

    E. Fever (sensitivity 0.67, specificity 0.79 for appendicitis) is more common in patients with a surgical abdomen than in their nonsurgical counterparts, although it may be absent in the elderly patient, even when the patient has a surgical abdomen.

    F. Rigidity (sensitivity 0.27, specificity 0.83 for appendicitis) and **guarding** (sensitivity 0.74, specificity 0.57 for appendicitis) are more frequently found in patients with a surgical abdomen than in those patients with a nonsurgical abdomen.

    G. Murphy's sign for gallbladder disease is helpful, if present, but is not sensitive.

    H. Iliopsoas sign (sensitivity 0.16, specificity 0.95 for appendicitis) is an indication of iliopsoas muscle irritation. This can be caused by an inflamed appendix. Again, it is not very sensitive or specific.

VII. Laboratory tests

    A. Blood leukocyte count (WBC). An elevated WBC (>12,000/µL) suggests inflammation or infection. Elderly patients with a surgical abdomen are less likely to have an elevated WBC. The presence of an elevated WBC and the trend of serial counts are more important than the actual WBC count.

    B. Abdominal series is often not helpful. The x-ray gives a specific diagnosis, such as free air or obstructive pattern, in <15% of patients. In most cases, the x-ray does not change the clinical diagnosis. **Chest x-ray** gives a specific diagnosis, such as free intra-abdominal air, in only 3% of examinations. Occasionally, pneumonia can cause abdominal pain.

    C. Serum lipase and **serum amylase** are the tests for acute pancreatitis. Although slight elevation of either amylase or lipase can occur with many abdominal conditions, an elevation three times above the normal range is rarely found in conditions other than acute pancreatitis. Lesser elevations can be found in perforated duodenal ulcer and mesenteric infarction.

    D. Ultrasonography or **computerized tomography (CT)** can be used to detect enlargement of the pancreas if the diagnosis of acute pancreatitis is in doubt. Ultrasonography is the test of choice for detection of gallstones. The sensitivity of this test is >90%. Ultrasonography (sensitivity 0.85, specificity 0.92) and CT (sensitivity 0.98, specificity 0.98) can also be used in the diagnosis of appendicitis.

E. Nuclear medicine hepatobiliary scanning (Choletec) is the test of choice in acute cholecystitis. Its accuracy is about 95% in patients with acute cholecystitis.

VIII. Treatment

A. NSAP

1. If a specific cause of the abdominal pain is not identified, watchful waiting with close follow-up is recommended. Most patients with NSAP have a benign, self-limited illness.

2. If the patient has cramping pain, suggestive of spasm, a short course of an antispasmodic such as **dicyclomine hydrochloride** (Bentyl), 20 mg four times daily, or **propantheline bromide** (Pro-Banthine), 15 mg before meals and at bedtime, can be given. Narcotic analgesics should be avoided.

3. Any foods that cause NSAP should be avoided.

B. IBS. The following treatments have been used successfully in IBS, but not all treatments are successful for every individual.

1. **Psychological management.** In some patients, stress management decreases anxiety and the frequency and severity of IBS. In selected patients, psychotherapy may be of benefit.

2. **High-fiber diet.** A high-fiber diet, supplemented at times with bulk agents such as **psyllium** (Metamucil), may be of benefit. Any specific foods that exacerbate or trigger IBS should be avoided.

3. **Antidiarrheal agents.** Patients with diarrhea may obtain symptomatic relief with an antidiarrheal agent such as **loperamide hydrochloride** (Imodium), 2–4 mg four times daily, or **diphenoxylate hydrochloride with atropine** (Lomotil), 10–20 mg four times daily.

4. **Antispasmodics.** Intermittent, limited courses of antispasmodics such as **dicyclomine hydrochloride** (Bentyl) may benefit patients with pain.

C. Diverticulitis. An individual over 40 years of age with left lower quadrant pain, an elevated temperature, and an elevated WBC must be suspected of having diverticulitis.

1. In mild cases in which the patient does not appear to be having a toxic reaction and has a normal temperature and WBC, the patient can be treated at home with a diet of clear liquids and broad-spectrum antibiotics such as **trimethoprim-sulfamethoxazole** (Bactrim) or **ciprofloxacin** (Cipro) and **metronidazole** (Flagyl).

2. If the patient appears to be toxic and has an elevated temperature and WBC, but exhibits no signs of obstruction or gross perforation, appropriate treatment includes hospitalization, clear fluids, and an intravenously administered broad-spectrum antibiotic such as **cefoxitin** (Mefoxin) or a combination of an **aminoglycoside** (gentamicin) and **clindamycin** (Cleocin).

3. If there is evidence of obstruction or perforation, surgical consultation should be obtained. The bowel should be rested, and the patient should take nothing by mouth and should receive intravenous hydration. If perforation is suspected, in addition to **cefoxitin**, an **aminoglycoside** and **clindamycin** should be added.

D. Cholecysitis

1. Patients should be hospitalized and treated with supportive measures, including intravenous hydration and pain management. Intravenous antibiotic therapy is appropriate if there is evidence of peritonitis, sepsis, or abscess formation. Surgical consultation should be obtained.

2. Once the acute process has "cooled down," elective cholecystectomy can be performed. The exact timing of the cholecystectomy is debated, with some physicians recommending surgery at least 2–3 days after the acute process has cooled down and others recommending surgery after 6 weeks.

3. Chemical dissolution of gallstones has been used successfully in some patients who cannot tolerate surgery.

E. Appendicitis. In an individual with fever and right lower quadrant pain, appendicitis must be suspected, and surgical evaluation should be obtained.

1. Surgery is the treatment of choice.

2. The use and choice of antibiotics are debated. Some practitioners recommend intravenous antibiotics once the diagnosis is suspected, while others administer antibiotics only if rupture is suspected or found.

F. Acute pancreatitis

1. Patients with acute pancreatitis are hospitalized and treated supportively with hydration, analgesia, nasogastric suction for vomiting or ileus, and monitor-

ing for respiratory distress, anemia, excessive bleeding, and hypocalcemia. Intravenous antibiotics are not of benefit in uncomplicated cases.

   2. Since alcohol is the leading cause of acute pancreatitis, alcohol use should be investigated. If alcoholism does exist, treatment should be encouraged (see Chapter 92).

G. **Mesenteric ischemic disease.** The early diagnosis of mesenteric ischemic disease is often difficult.

   1. The patient should be hospitalized for bowel rest, and intravenous fluids and antibiotics should be administered.
   2. Early surgical intervention can improve outcome if bowel necosis is present.
   3. Conservative therapy results in resolution of the ischemia in 50% of patients. Twenty percent of patients need resection of the bowel for total occlusion of the blood supply.

IX. Follow-up recommendations

   A. **NSAP** tends to be a self-limited illness. The patient needs reassurance and, at times, symptomatic treatment as outlined above. Follow-up evaluation is needed within 1–2 weeks to determine resolution. Failure to resolve or recurrence of the pain warrants further investigation.

   B. **IBS** is a chronic, recurring disease. Although it is chronic, patients should be reassured that IBS does not predispose the patient to a serious disease. Frequent follow-up may be needed until symptoms stabilize.

   C. **Diverticulitis.** Once the acute phase of the illness has resolved, the patient should begin a high-fiber diet. Long-term follow-up is needed. Fistula formation, obstruction, and perforations are complications of diverticulitis. Approximately 30% of patients eventually need surgery.

   D. **Cholecystitis.** In patients who have undergone cholecystectomy, right upper quadrant pain requires investigation to exclude retained common bile duct stones.

   E. **Appendicitis.** Once the appendix has been removed, no further problems should occur.

   F. **Acute pancreatitis.** The mortality rate is approximately 10%. The patient should be observed for the development of a pancreatic pseudocyst, which presents as an abdominal mass.

   G. **Mesenteric ischemic disease** may recur if the predisposing factors still exist or recur.

REFERENCES

Adelman A: Abdominal pain in the primary care setting. J Fam Pract 1987;**25**:27.

American College of Emergency Physicians: Clinical policy for the initial approach to patients presenting with a chief complaint of nontraumatic acute abdominal pain. Ann Emerg Med 1994;**23**:906.

Brewer RJ, et al: Abdominal pain: An analysis of 1,000 consecutive cases in a university emergency room. Am J Surg 1976;**131**:219.

Cope Z: *Cope's Early Diagnosis of the Acute Abdomen.* 19th ed, revised by Silen W. Oxford University Press; 1996.

Gilbert DN, et al (editors): *The Sanford Guide to Antimicrobial Therapy 1998.* 28th ed. Antimicrobial Therapy Inc; 1998.

Orr RK, et al: Ultrasonography to evaluate adults for appendicitis: Decision making based on meta-analysis and probabilistic reasoning. Acad Emerg Med 1995;**2**:644.

Rao PM, et al: Effect of computed tomography of the appendix on treatment of patients and use of hospital resources. N Engl J Med 1998;**338**:141.

Wagner JM, et al: Does this patient have appendicitis? JAMA 1996;**276**:1589.

---

2   The Abnormal Pap Smear

Neal D. Clemenson, MD

I. **Definition.** The Pap smear, a cytologic examination of exfoliated cervical and endocervical cells, was developed in the 1930s by Papanicolaou and is currently used as a screening tool for cervical neoplasia and carcinoma. Advances in our understanding of cervical disease, new reporting systems, and new diagnostic and treatment modalities make a systematic approach to the abnormal Pap smear very important. Recommendations for the frequency and method of the Pap smear may be found in Chapter 108.

Several systems are used for reporting the results of the Pap smear. The class system, which reported results of I (normal) through V (invasive cancer), provided inadequate information and has largely been replaced by newer systems. The Bethesda system provides the most complete information and has been widely adopted; its classification scheme is used in this chapter. Equivalent classifications in the World Health Organization (WHO) and cervical intraepithelial neoplasia (CIN) systems are provided. Since the systems are not interchangeable, it is essential that clinicians become familiar with the system used by their particular laboratory.

II. **Common diagnoses.** Many types of cervical and vaginal abnormalities can be detected by the Pap smear, including the following.

  A. **Atypical squamous cells of uncertain significance (ASCUS).** Inflammation may also be noted and a potential cause may be identified, including infection (see sections III,C and E). Hyperkeratosis or parakeratosis may be described, either of which usually indicates a reaction to trauma or inflammation.

  B. **Squamous intraepithelial lesions (SILs)** are graded as low-grade (LSIL), which corresponds to mild dysplasia or CIN 1, or high-grade (HSIL), which includes moderate and severe dysplasia (CINs 2 and 3) and carcinoma in situ (CIN 3).

  C. **Human papillomavirus (HPV) infection.**

  D. **Atypical glandular cells of undetermined significance (AGUS).**

  E. Other infections, including other **viruses, bacteria** (eg, *Chlamydia* or *Gardnerella*), **fungi** (eg, *Candida*), or **protozoa** (eg, *Trichomonas*).

  F. **Frank cervical carcinomas,** including squamous cell carcinomas and adenocarcinomas, as well as noncervical carcinomas, including endocervical carcinoma and vaginal carcinoma.

III. **Epidemiology**

  A. The epidemiology of **ASCUS** or **inflammation** in the absence of infection is unknown.

  B. The epidemiology of **squamous epithelial lesions** depends on the cause. HPV infection is discussed in section III,C; multiple causes are possible.

  C. **HPV infection** is generally contracted by sexual contact with an infected partner, who may be asymptomatic, although infection from nongenital lesions may occur as well. As with other sexually transmitted diseases, the risk increases with the number and risk status of sexual partners and may be reduced by the use of barrier contraception (eg, condoms). The prevalence of HPV infection has risen rapidly in recent years, although some of the increase may be due to increased recognition.

  D. The epidemiology of **AGUS** depends on the cause. It may represent endocervical, endometrial, or extrauterine disease, or its cause may be unknown.

  E. *Chlamydia* and *Trichomonas* infections are also sexually transmitted, and multiple sexually transmitted diseases may coexist. *Candida* infections are probably caused by alterations in the usual vaginal flora and may be triggered by antibiotics, altered host defenses, or other poorly understood causes. Frequent or severe *Candida* infections may occur in women with human immunodeficiency virus (HIV) infection or diabetes mellitus. Bacterial vaginosis is also caused by altered flora, but the cause of the alteration is not clear; it is generally believed not to be transmitted sexually.

  F. Cervical **carcinomas** (see sections III,B and C). Noncervical carcinomas are beyond the scope of this chapter.

IV. **Pathophysiology**

  A. **ASCUS** or **inflammation** may be caused by infection (see section III,E) but may also occur in the absence of infection; the pathophysiology in this situation is not well understood.

  B. Most **squamous epithelial lesions** are caused by HPV (see section III,C); others may be caused by carcinogens (eg, smoking) or other unknown factors. These lesions may spontaneously resolve, remain stable, or progress to higher-grade lesions or carcinoma. Patients with HIV infection may have a higher incidence of cervical neoplasia and may have a more rapid progression from precancerous cervical lesions to cancer.

   C. HPV is a small DNA virus that replicates in the nuclei of epithelial cells; some types may cause malignant transformation by incorporation into the host DNA. The infection may be subclinical or may cause condylomata or other lesions on the vulva, vagina, or cervix.

   D. AGUS may be caused by inflammation or neoplasia in the endocervix, endometrium, or extrauterine sites such as the ovaries, breast, or gastrointestinal tract.

   E. The vaginal or cervical epithelium can be infected by a variety of **bacteria, fungi, protozoans,** or **other microorganisms.** Colonization or disruption of the normal microbial environment may occur without altering the mucosa, or the infectious agent may elicit an inflammatory response and resultant cellular changes.

   F. Carcinomas (see section IV,B).

V. Symptoms and signs

   A. ASCUS and **inflammation** are usually asymptomatic unless associated with an infection (see sections III,C and E), although bleeding, especially after intercourse, may occur. Upon examination, the cervix may appear normal or may show redness, erosions, or friability, especially with more severe or widespread disease.

   B. SILs are usually asymptomatic but may be associated with bleeding; large lesions may cause vaginal discharge. The cervix may appear normal or may show redness, erosions, friability, or gross lesions. Acetic acid application (see section VI,B,1) may identify lesions that are not grossly visible.

   C. HPV infection may be subclinical or may cause condylomata, which can range in size from microscopic to several centimeters in diameter and can occur on the cervix, vagina, or vulva. Smaller lesions are usually asymptomatic, but large lesions can be associated with bleeding, discharge, and local irritation. Condylomata may be flat, raised, or filiform; their visibility can be enhanced by acetic acid application.

   D. AGUS may be asymptomatic or may have symptoms related to the underlying disease (eg, irregular bleeding with endometrial neoplasia).

   E. Other infections may be asymptomatic or may be associated with vaginal discharge, odor, or itching. Signs may include vaginal or cervical discharge or inflammation.

   F. Carcinomas may be asymptomatic or may cause bleeding or vaginal discharge. Metastatic disease may be associated with abdominal fullness, weight loss, or other symptoms related to the sites and nature of the metastases.

VI. Laboratory tests

   A. The **Pap smear** report should include the following information.

      1. Adequacy of the smear. An unsatisfactory smear should be repeated; a less than optimal smear may warrant repeat, treatment, or follow-up, depending on the specific findings and clinical situation. Many authorities no longer consider the absence of endocervical cells alone to be an indication of an inadequate smear, and the need to repeat smears without endocervical cells is a clinical judgment.

      2. The report should indicate a **specific diagnosis(es),** using the terminology of the particular reporting system, as well as any other findings, such as evidence of infection.

      3. The report may include a **pathologist's recommendation** regarding treatment and/or follow-up. This information may be helpful, but the clinician should determine the plans for the patient, depending on the situation and his or her clinical judgment.

   B. Additional tests

      1. Acetic acid application. Applying 5% acetic acid solution to the cervix for 1 minute will cause many condylomata or dyplastic areas to turn white (acetowhite lesions). These lesions should be evaluated by colposcopy and biopsy (see section VI,B,4).

      2. Biopsy. Prior to the widespread use of colposcopy, cervical biopsies of suspicious areas, or random biopsies if the areas were visually normal, were used to evaluate abnormal smears. With the availability of colposcopy, biopsy should be done only in conjunction with colposcopy.

      3. Cervicography (photographing the cervix for interpretation by a specially trained technician) and **speculoscopy** (examining the cervix under chemiluminescent illumination) have been described as intermediate triage methods, but their role in clinical practice requires further study.

4. **Colposcopy,** cervical examination under stereoscopic magnification by an experienced examiner along with biopsy of abnormal areas, is the definitive procedure for assessing many Pap smear abnormalities.
5. **HPV typing** can be done to determine whether a strain likely to cause malignancy is present, but its role in clinical practice requires further study.

C. **Diagnostic strategies.** Many strategies have been proposed to evaluate further specific Pap smear abnormalities and opinions vary widely, especially regarding ASCUS. The following strategies are based primarily on the 1992 National Cancer Institute Workshop guidelines. New information and local opinions, especially those of the clinician's consultants, should be considered in cases in which uncertainty exists.

1. **Inflammation with evidence of infection.** Infections should be appropriately treated (see Chapters 33 and 67). If the infection is sexually transmitted, the presence of other sexually transmitted diseases should be considered and appropriately evaluated as indicated.
2. **HPV infection.** Changes consistent with HPV infection warrant colposcopy, even in the absence of other findings. Other concomitant sexually transmitted diseases should also be considered.
3. **ASCUS or inflammation without evidence of infection.** The patient should be re-examined to identify a potential infection, since evidence of infection may not always be apparent on the Pap smear. During the examination, cultures or other diagnostic tests for infection should be performed based on clinical findings and risk factors (see Chapters 33 and 67). Empiric antibiotic or topical therapy should be avoided, as it may delay the diagnosis of an infection or persistent inflammation. If the patient is postmenopausal and is not receiving estrogen replacement, the smear can be repeated after a course of vaginal estrogen (eg, conjugated estrogen cream, 2 g every other day for 4 weeks); if the smear remains abnormal, colposcopy should be considered.
4. **SILs (dysplasia or CIN).** In the United States, many authorities recommend colposcopy for definitive diagnosis for all patients with SILs. In other countries, LSILs may be followed up with frequent Pap smears (see section VII,B). HSILs should always be evaluated by colposcopy.
5. **AGUS.** Endocervical AGUS should be evaluated by colposcopy with endocervical sampling, and endometrial AGUS should be evaluated by endometrial biopsy or other endometrial sampling. If a source is not found, an extrauterine source should be suspected; an expert in gynecologic cytopathology may be helpful in reviewing the smear.
6. **Other abnormalities.** If evidence of carcinoma is present, the patient should be referred for definitive evaluation and therapy. Endometrial cells may be found on a Pap taken during or shortly after menstruation, but if they are found in the second half of the menstrual cycle or in a postmenopausal woman, endometrial biopsy or other endometrial sampling should be considered.
7. **HIV.** Women with HIV may benefit from more aggressive management and follow-up, although definitive data are not yet available. Colposcopy may be appropriate for ASCUS and inflammation in these patients.

VII. **Treatment**

A. **ASCUS or inflammation.** If ASCUS is present without evidence of infection or persists after treatment and cure of an associated infection, the Pap smear should be repeated every 4–6 months for 2 years, followed by routine screening after three consecutive negative smears. If ASCUS is found during the 2-year follow-up period or patient compliance is questionable, colposcopy should be considered. Recent reports are yielding more information on the most efficient way to follow these patients; further studies of this issue are under way.

B. **SILs (dysplasia or CIN).** If colposcopy is performed, treatment will be dictated by specific findings. Close follow-up is another option in the patient in whom reliable follow-up can be assured, in which case the Pap smear should be repeated every 4–6 months for 2 years, with colposcopy for repeated abnormalities or routine screening after three consecutive negative smears.

C. **HPV** presents a great challenge in treatment, since the disease is multifocal and often subclinical. Gross lesions can be treated in various ways; see Chapter 33 for specific recommendations. The benefit of treating asymptomatic disease is

unclear, since complete eradication is usually not possible. HPV typing may identify those at high risk for carcinoma, but its role in clinical practice remains to be
defined. Helping the patient understand that the disease is not curable and that
it may increase her risk of cervical cancer is the most important component of
therapy. Annual Pap smears, or possibly annual colposcopy, is essential.
   D. **AGUS.** The treatment of AGUS depends on the source and is beyond the scope
      of this chapter.
   E. Specific **vaginal infections** should be treated as described in Chapters 33 and
      67. If the infection was sexually transmitted, the patient's partner(s) should be
      treated in order to prevent reinfection.
   F. **Carcinomas.** The treatment of carcinomas is generally surgical; referral to a
      physician experienced in oncology is indicated.
   G. **HIV.** Since women with HIV may be at higher risk for cervical neoplasia, some
      clinicians perform Pap smears twice a year. Annual colposcopy in place of Pap
      smears has also been recommended, but the practicality and cost-effectiveness
      of this approach are unclear.

REFERENCES

Alanen KW et al: Assessment of cytologic follow-up as the recommended Management for
   patients with atypical squamous cells of undetermined significance or low grade squamous
   intraepithelial lesions. Cancer 1998;**84:**5.
Brotzman GL, Julian TM: The minimally abnormal Papanicolaou smear. Am Fam Physician
   1996;**53:**1154.
Ferris DG et al: Triage of women with ASCUS and LSIL on Pap smear reports: Management by
   repeat Pap smear, HPV DNA testing, or colposcopy? J Fam Pract 1998;**46:**125.
Kurman RJ et al for the 1992 National Cancer Institute Workshop: Interim guidelines for man-
   agement of abnormal cervical cytology. JAMA 1994;**271:**1866.
National Cancer Institute Workshop: The 1988 Bethesda system for reporting cervical/vaginal
   cytological diagnoses. JAMA 1989;**262:**931.
Nuovo J et al: Management of patients with atypical and low-grade Pap smear abnormalities. Am
   Fam Physician 1995;**52:**2243.

---

3   Acute Scrotum

Ted D. Epperly, MD

I. **Definition.** *Acute scrotum* refers to scrotal pain caused typically within 48 hours by
   conditions either internal or external to the scrotum.
II. **Common diagnoses**
   A. **Inflammatory lesions,** such as epididymitis and orchitis.
   B. **Torsion** of the testicle itself or of the testicular or epididymal appendage.
   C. **Traumatic injuries,** such as testicular rupture.
   D. **Neoplasms,** particularly testicular tumors.
   E. **Extrascrotal causes,** such as inguinal hernia, prostatitis (see Chapter 64), and
      ureteral colic (see Chapter 37).
III. **Epidemiology.** Conditions causing acute scrotum affect approximately 0.1–0.3% of
   the male population each year.
   A. **Inflammatory lesions.** Populations at particular risk for acquiring **epididymitis**
      or **orchitis** include sexually active males, males with mumps infection, and
      males with underlying congenital urologic abnormalities. Viral orchitis (primarily
      mumps orchitis) occurs among nonimmunized children and young adults aged
      10–20 years. Approximately 20–35% of males who contract mumps develop
      orchitis, and approximately 35% of these cases involve both testes. Epididymitis
      is rare in boys and adolescents less than 18 years of age.
   B. **Testicular torsion** has a bimodal frequency of occurrence, with one peak in the
      perinatal period and another at age 13. Testicular torsion is rare in men over age
      30. The risk of a male's developing torsion of the testicle or its appendage by age
      25 is 1 in 160. Predisposing conditions other than age and sex include the "bell-

clapper" deformity (see section IV,B), excessive muscular exercise, straining, attempts at reduction of a hernia, sudden cremasteric spasm (eg, from cold water, a sudden scare, or intercourse), and trauma. The peak incidence of torsion of the testicular appendage is near age 10 and occurs almost always before puberty.

C. Traumatic injuries, including testicular ruptures, are rare and usually occur during sports-related accidents. Such injuries include straddle injuries and those caused by kicks and baseballs.

D. Testicular neoplasms are the third most frequently found tumor in men between the ages of 20 and 34, with an incidence of 2–3 per 100,000 men each year. A male with an undescended testicle, even if the testicle is surgically reduced, has a risk of cancer that is 2.5–20 times greater than that of a male with a descended testicle.

E. Extrascrotal causes

    1. Inguinal hernias are common and can occur in males of all ages. Congenital anatomic defects and excessive coughing or straining can predispose men to this condition.

    2. Ureteral colic from renal stones is found in approximately 1% of the population and is precipitated by conditions that supersaturate the urine with stone-forming salts or decrease the amount of urine production.

    3. Prostatitis is common in sexually active males. The incidence of this condition increases with age (see Chapter 64).

IV. Pathophysiology

A. Inflammatory lesions

    1. Epididymitis occurs via retrograde spread of infected prostatic and urethral secretions through the vas deferens. The bacteria in this material attack the cells of the epididymis, leading to the classic inflammatory response of swelling and pain.

        a. In men younger than 35 years of age, acute epididymitis is commonly associated with acute urethritis, usually caused by *Neisseria gonorrhoeae* or *Chlamydia trachomatis.*

        b. In men older than age 35, acute epididymitis is most often caused by enteric gram-negative rods in association with coexistent prostatitis or prostatism with cystitis.

        c. Ureteral stricture or congenital urologic abnormalities, such as ectopic ureters, may lead to genitourinary tract infection, including epididymitis.

    2. Orchitis is an inflammation that involves only the testes and is usually viral in origin. Viruses that have been associated with orchitis include influenza, Epstein-Barr, varicella, echo, and coxsackie. Orchitis can result from contiguous spread from the epididymis, leading to epididymo-orchitis; in this case, it may be bacterial in nature.

B. Torsion. Spontaneous **testicular torsion** is a sudden twisting of the spermatic cord in which the testicular mesentery anchors the testes to the scrotal wall. The mechanism of torsion of the testicular appendages is unknown.

    1. In some males, the tunica vaginalis inserts along the spermatic cord, rather than along the posterior aspect of the testis, as is usual, producing the classic bell-clapper deformity. This high insertion creates a narrower testicular mesentery that is more likely to twist; a spasm of the cremaster muscle can cause the testicle to twist as the testicle is drawn up toward the inguinal canal, leading to ischemia. An insufficient attachment of the testis to the scrotal sac underlies this abnormality and allows twisting and ischemia of the testicle to occur.

    2. Newborns can undergo torsion of the entire testicle and spermatic cord above the tunica vaginalis. The cause of torsion in newborns is unknown.

C. Testicular rupture occurs when the testicle is struck hard enough for the tunica albuginea to rupture. A hematocele (a hematoma within the tunica vaginalis) usually forms and can cause testicular hypoperfusion and necrosis.

D. Neoplasms can cause hemorrhage into the tumor, resulting in capsular distention and acute pain.

E. Extrascrotal causes

    1. A direct or indirect **inguinal hernia** often slides into the scrotal sac and may appear as a scrotal mass with accompanying pain secondary to distention and ischemia, especially if incarceration and strangulation result.

    2. The pain from **ureteral colic** and **prostatic inflammation** is referred to the scrotum via sensory nerve fibers that also supply the testicles.

V. Symptoms
A. Inflammatory lesions
    1. Patients with **acute epididymitis** present with unilateral scrotal pain and swelling. The pain is often intense. Dysuria, malaise, fever, and chills are often present.

    2. **Orchitis** is characterized by unilateral or bilateral testicular pain and swelling. In patients who develop orchitis from mumps, this pain typically occurs 4–10 days after onset of parotitis.

B. Torsion
    1. **Testicular torsion** causes a sudden onset of severe unilateral testicular pain, often accompanied by nausea and vomiting. Occasionally, the pain is intermittent, representing spontaneous detorsion and retorsion. Approximately 33–50% of patients will have experienced similar pain transiently in the past. Rarely will an episode of torsion be preceded by minor scrotal trauma. Torsion is not associated with dysuria, frequency, urgency, or hesitancy.

    2. **Torsion of the testicular appendages** causes unilateral scrotal pain with swelling, usually less pronounced than in testicular torsion. Urinary symptoms are absent.

C. Testicular rupture causes severe unilateral or bilateral testicular pain.

D. Testicular neoplasms are usually asymptomatic, but in 20% of cases, they cause a heaviness or a unilateral discomfort. Acute hemorrhage into the tumor, causing capsular distention, may also occur.

E. Extrascrotal causes
    1. The pain of an **inguinal hernia** is often reported as a dullness or heaviness in the scrotum. If incarceration with strangulation of the hernia has occurred, the patient presents with intense lower abdominal and scrotal pain.

    2. Patients with **ureteral colic** typically present with severe intermittent flank pain that can radiate to the suprapubic, scrotal, and inner thigh areas. Nausea, vomiting, fever, chills, and frequency of urination are often present.

    3. **Prostatitis** causes fever, chills, dysuria, urgency, frequency, myalgias, and intense perineal, scrotal, and back pain.

VI. Signs
A. Inflammatory lesions
    1. **Acute epididymitis** causes unilateral swelling and induration of the epididymis. If the testicle becomes involved (epididymo-orchitis), the testicle and epididymis eventually become a single mass that is swollen, firm, and tender. Fever is often present. The overlying scrotal skin often becomes erythematous, and later the spermatic cord may become tender, making it difficult to differentiate acute epididymitis from testicular torsion.

        a. The **cremasteric reflex** is present in patients with acute epididymitis but is absent in those with testicular torsion. This reflex is elicited by stroking the front and inner sides of the thigh, causing an ipsilateral retraction of the testicle toward the inguinal canal. This reflex is very useful in determining whether torsion is absent.

        b. **Prehn's sign** is somewhat useful in differentiating torsion and epididymitis. When the patient is supine and the scrotum is elevated, pain will be relieved in epididymitis but worsened in testicular torsion. This sign is not pathognomonic, however.

    2. **Orchitis** causes unilateral or bilateral swelling and tenderness in the testicle. The epididymis is not involved unless epididymo-orchitis is present.

B. Torsion
    1. In **testicular torsion,** the testicle is usually retracted on the involved side and is lying in a transverse position. It rapidly becomes firm and tender, and later the hemiscrotum becomes red and edematous. As the swelling continues, the testis and the epididymis become a single mass.

    2. **Torsion of the testicular appendages** produces a firm, tender nodule at the upper pole of the testis. This nodule is usually distinct from the epididymis. The testis itself will not be tender.

        a. The cyanotic appendix often can be seen through nonpigmented scrotal skin. This finding is termed the "blue dot" sign and is specific for a torsion of the testicular appendages.

    b. As edema progresses, the intrascrotal structures may become confluent and the skin of the scrotum becomes edematous, making diagnosis more difficult.

  C. Testicular rupture causes a tender, indurated scrotal mass with overlying ecchymosis. Distinguishing the testicle from the epididymis may be difficult or even impossible. The hemiscrotal mass caused by hematoma formation does not transilluminate.

  D. Testicular neoplasms are usually firm to hard, nontender masses on the testicle that do not transilluminate. Occasionally, a palpable left supraclavicular node or epigastric mass will be found. Some patients have associated gynecomastia from chronic gonadotropin or estrogen secretion. A hematoma that appears after minimal trauma should be considered a testicular tumor until proven otherwise.

  E. Extrascrotal causes

    1. Inguinal hernias cause a scrotal mass, and the examiner will not be able to palpate the spermatic cord above the mass. The mass will usually transilluminate, and bowel sounds occasionally may be heard.

    2. Ureteral colic may be characterized by flank tenderness. Scrotal examination is usually unremarkable. Hematuria may be present.

    3. Prostatitis usually causes a warm, tender, swollen prostate on rectal examination (see Chapter 64).

VII. Laboratory tests. Although most diagnoses of acute scrotum will be made or suspected on the basis of the history and the physical examination, laboratory analysis is often helpful.

  A. Urinalysis can detect pyuria, bacteriuria, and hematuria, which are common in infectious causes such as epididymitis and prostatitis. Microscopic or macroscopic hematuria will almost always be present in ureteral colic. Rarely is urinalysis helpful in detecting the other causes of acute scrotum.

  B. Urethral smear is helpful in the diagnosis of epididymitis in males under 35 and may demonstrate white blood cells (WBCs) and the presence of bacteria. In patients over age 35, this test is less useful because of a lower yield of WBCs and bacteria.

  C. An **elevated WBC count** and **erythrocyte sedimentation rate** may occur with inflammatory conditions and therefore may help in detecting these conditions. However, WBC elevation can also occur in testicular torsion.

  D. A **Doppler stethoscope** can often be used to distinguish between epididymitis and testicular torsion. The stethoscope head should be lubricated with a water-based gel and placed over the inferior pole of the involved testicle. The examiner must then compress the involved spermatic cord between his or her fingers and listen for the cessation of pulses. Findings include reduced or absent blood flow with testicular torsion and increased vascular perfusion with epididymitis. With epididymitis, arterial pulsation can be "turned on and off" by spermatic cord compression. The opposite testicle and spermatic cord can be used as a control to determine normal blood flow sounds. Diagnostic accuracy can be as high as 88%.

  E. A **radionuclide testicular scan** with technetium-99m can help the physician differentiate between testicular torsion and epididymitis. Visualization of the testis on scintigraphy almost always rules out testicular torsion. Diagnostic accuracy is in the range of 80–100% (sensitivity 85%, specificity 95%). The drawbacks of testicular scanning include cost, lack of immediate availability, and diagnostic uncertainty in a testis less than 2 cm in size. Testicular blood flow should not be compromised in testicular appendage torsion. Radionuclide scanning is extremely reliable and is the diagnostic test of choice.

  F. Scrotal ultrasonography is often helpful in eliminating the possibility of scrotal abscess formation from epididymitis, or scrotal trauma from hematoma or rupture. Scrotal ultrasonography is also useful in evaluating a testicular mass for potential neoplasm, which consists of a solid, irregular mass.

  G. Color Doppler ultrasonography is a combination of real-time ultrasonography and duplex sonography for noninvasive imaging of arterial and venous blood vessels. This study has become the most valuable diagnostic modality in the evaluation of the acute scrotum, with a sensitivity in testicular torsion of 82% and a specificity of 100%. In epididymitis, the sensitivity is 70% and the specificity, 88%. Color-coded ultrasonography readily demonstrates testicular perfusion.

H. Doppler sonography is another modality that can successfully measure blood flow to the testicle. Sensitivity is 80–89%, with a specificity of 97–100%.

I. Magnetic resonance imaging (MRI) can be used in cases of inconclusive clinical and ultrasound evaluation. MRI has been found to be highly accurate (91%) in such rare cases.

VIII. Treatment

A. Inflammatory lesions

1. **Acute epididymitis** generally can be managed in the ambulatory setting. Treatment varies according to age and severity. The two goals of treatment are to provide pain relief and to treat the underlying infection.

   a. **Pain relief.** Bed rest or sedentary activity with scrotal elevation and support is essential. Ice packs are beneficial in the first 24-48 hours, and nonsteroidal anti-inflammatory drugs (eg, **indomethacin,** 50 mg orally every 6–8 hours, or **ibuprofen,** 400–800 mg every 6–8 hours with a meal or snack) are helpful. **Acetaminophen with codeine** (eg, Tylenol 3), one to two tablets every 4–6 hours, or **acetaminophen with oxycodone** (eg, Tylox), one tablet every 4–6 hours, may be necessary to control scrotal pain. A cord block with 5–8 mL of a 50:50 mixture of 1% **lidocaine** and 0.5% **bupivacaine** can be given for immediate pain relief by physicians experienced with this block.

   b. **Antibiotics.** For sexually active males under the age of 35, the treatment of choice is **ceftriaxone** (Rocephin), 125 mg intramuscularly, plus **tetracycline,** 500 mg orally four times a day for 7 days, or **doxycycline,** 100 mg orally twice a day for 7 days. An alternative is **ofloxacin,** 300 mg orally twice a day for 7 days. For men over age 35, the drug of choice is **ciprofloxacin** (Cipro), 500 mg orally twice daily, **ofloxacin,** 200 mg orally twice a day, or **trovafloxacin,** 200 mg orally once a day, for 10–14 days. Alternative regimens include **ampicillin-sulbactam** (Unasyn), **piperacillin-tazobactam,** and **ticarcillin-clavulanate** (Timentin).

   c. **Hospitalization** is recommended for patients with fever and toxic appearance. Intravenous antibiotics and enforced bed rest are required for these patients.

   d. **Surgical drainage, orchiectomy,** or **both** is warranted when severe epididymo-orchitis results in abscess.

   e. **Urologic consultation** and **surgical exploration** are indicated in patients with complications, in diagnostic dilemmas, and for any case of suspected testicular torsion.

2. **Orchitis,** especially mumps orchitis, should be treated with bed rest and scrotal elevation. Anti-inflammatory therapy, described in section VIII,A,1,a, should be instituted. Corticosteroids, estrogens, and gamma globulin have been used in the past, but their usefulness is controversial and they are not generally recommended.

B. Torsion

1. Unless the possibility of **testicular torsion** can be eliminated via color Doppler ultrasonography or timely testicular scanning, emergency surgery is warranted, since the testicle will die from complete torsion within 3–48 hours. Testicular viability of 70–100% can be obtained if detorsion is obtained within 10 hours (Edelsberg and Surh, 1988). Viability after 10–12 hours of ischemia is approximately 20% and approaches 0% after 24–48 hours of ischemia. No testicle is typically salvageable after 48 hours. A less aggressive approach will lead to "castration by neglect." In patients with testicular torsion, bilateral orchidopexy is necessary because of the increased chance of contralateral testicular torsion in the future, since the bell-clapper deformity usually exists in both testicles.

2. **Testicular appendage torsion** is managed conservatively and nonsurgically with analgesics and ice. If the diagnosis is unclear, prompt scrotal exploration should be performed to rule out testicular torsion. If pain and swelling are severe, local nerve block or excision of the twisted appendage may be necessary.

C. Testicular rupture should be treated with prompt scrotal surgery, particularly if a hematoma is found on examination or ultrasonography.

D. Testicular neoplasia requires confirmation by biopsy through an inguinal approach and therapy as directed based on tissue identification.
E. Extrascrotal causes
  1. Inguinal hernia is treated surgically or nonsurgically as indicated.
  2. Ureteral colic (see Chapter 37).
  3. Prostatitis (see Chapter 64).

REFERENCES

Cilento BG, et al: Cryptorchidism and testicular torsion. Pediatr Clin North Am 1993;**40:**1133.

Edelsberg JS, Surh YS: The acute scrotum. Emerg Med Clin North Am 1988;**6:**521.

Gilbert DN, et al: *The Sanford Guide to Antimicrobial Therapy.* Antimicrobial Therapy, 1998:16, 19.

Kass EJ, Lundak B: The acute scrotum. Pediatr Clin North Am 1997;**44:**1251.

Lewis AG, et al: Evaluation of acute scrotum in the emergency department. J Pediatr Surg 1995;**30:**277.

Prater JM, Overdorf BS: Testicular torsion: A surgical emergency. Am Fam Physician 1991; **44:**834.

Serra AD, et al: Inconclusive clinical and ultrasound evaluation of the scrotum: Impact of magnetic resonance imaging on patient management and cost. Urology 1998;**51:**1018.

Wilbert DM, et al: Evaluation of the acute scrotum by color-coded Doppler ultrasonography. J Urol 1993;**149:**1475.

Yazbeck S, Patriquin H: Accuracy of Doppler sonography in the evaluation of acute conditions of the scrotum in children. J Pediatr Surg 1994;**29:**1270.

---

4   Alopecia

Frank S. Celestino, MD

I. Definition. Alopecia is the partial or complete loss of hair from areas where it normally grows. This loss may be localized, patchy, diffuse, or total.
II. Common diagnoses (Table 4–1). Traditionally, the alopecias have been classified as scarring (cicatricial) or nonscarring (noncicatricial). Scarring alopecias are those in which hair is unable to regrow because of follicle loss. The nonscarring forms, in contrast, are those in which the hair follicles are retained and the process of hair loss

---

TABLE 4–1. DIAGNOSES AND ETIOLOGIC CLASSIFICATIONS OF ALOPECIA

Cicatricial (scarring) alopecias
 1. **Neoplastic:** localized or metastatic
 2. **Nevoid:** nevus sebaceous, epidermal nevus
 3. **Physical or chemical:** burns, freezing, trauma, radiation, acids, alkalis
 4. **Infectious:** bacterial, fungal, protozoal, viral, mycobacterial
 5. **Congenital or developmental:** aplasia cutis, Darier's disease, recessive X-linked ichthyosis, keratosis pilaris atrophicans
 6. **Dermatosis-related:** lichen planus, necrobiosis lipoidica diabeticorum, cicatricial pemphigoid, folliculitis decalvans
 7. **Systemic disease:** lupus erythematosus, sarcoidosis, scleroderma, dermatomyositis, amyloidosis

Noncicatricial (nonscarring) alopecias
 1. **Drug-induced:** antimetabolites, anticoagulants, beta blockers, antidepressants, lithium, levodopa
 2. **Congenital:** ectodermal dysplasias, hair shaft disorders
 3. **Infectious:** secondary syphilis, tinea capitis, human immunodeficiency virus infection
 4. **Toxic:** arsenic, boric acid, thallium, vitamin A
 5. **Nutritional:** anorexia nervosa, marasmus, kwashiorkor, "crash" diets, iron or zinc deficiency
 6. **Traumatic:** trichotillomania, traction, friction, chemical, thermal
 7. **Endocrine:** hyper- or hypothyroidism, hypopituitarism, hyper- or hypoparathyroidism
 8. **Immunologic:** alopecia areata
 9. **Genetic or developmental:** male and female pattern baldness (androgenetic alopecia)
10. **Radiation-induced:** x-ray epilation
11. **Physiologic:** telogen effluvium (postpartum, postsurgical, febrile illness, severe psychological stress, puberty)

is potentially reversible. Nonscarring alopecias account for >95% of the hair loss seen by primary care physicians. The six causes listed below are the most common and important.

A. **Androgenetic alopecia,** including male and female pattern baldness.
B. **Traumatic alopecia.**
C. **Infectious alopecia,** related primarily to **tinea capitis.**
D. **Physiologic alopecia.**
E. **Alopecia areata.**
F. **Hair loss caused by systemic diseases,** especially endocrinopathies and malnutrition.

III. **Epidemiology.** Before the era of approved medical therapy for common male baldness, approximately 1 of every 2000 office visits to family physicians was for some form of hair loss. This figure is expected to increase three- to fivefold during the 1990s.

A. **Androgenetic alopecia** affects nearly three quarters of men to some degree, while less than one fifth of women suffer such hair loss. It is more common than all other causes of alopecia combined. One third of males show signs of this type of loss by age 30, and over half are affected by age 50. Certain racial groups (Japanese, Chinese, Native Americans, and some black Africans) have a much lower incidence of androgenetic alopecia.

B. **Traumatic alopecia** is relatively common in newborns (on the occiput) and in persons using certain hairstyling techniques, such as "cornrows," tight ponytails, and hair curlers. Compulsive, self-induced hair plucking (trichotillomania) is seen most often accompanying underlying psychological distress.

C. **Tinea capitis** most commonly affects children and young adults.

D. **Physiologic alopecia** may occur 2–3 months after major surgery, delivery, febrile states, severe psychological stress, and medication changes. This process, called **telogen effluvium,** is most often seen postpartum or after the discontinuation of oral contraceptives or corticosteroids.

E. **Alopecia areata** occurs in approximately 0.1% of the general population and exhibits no sex differential. Thirty-three percent of the cases start by age 20; only 25% of the cases occur after age 40. Familial occurrence is estimated to be 20–25%. Alopecia areata occurs more frequently in patients with other presumed autoimmune diseases, such as pernicious anemia, vitiligo, and Hashimoto's thyroiditis, and in patients with atopy or Down syndrome.

F. Of the **systemic processes causing hair loss,** thyroid disease is the most common.

IV. **Pathophysiology.** There are two types of human hair: **vellus hair,** which is fine, hypopigmented, and almost invisible; and **terminal hair,** which is coarse and usually pigmented. For both types of hair, growth involves alternating periods of growth (anagen) and rest (telogen), which are separated by a transition (catogen) phase. Normally, scalp hair has a 2- to 5-year anagen phase with a 3-month telogen phase. Eighty-five to 90% of scalp hairs are anagen, and 10–15% are telogen. Up to 1% of all telogen hairs may be shed diffusely each day.

The rate of new hair growth decreases with age, resulting in gradual thinning. Certain hormones, such as estrogen, progesterone, testosterone, and thyroid hormone, influence hair growth.

The primary pathogenic mechanisms of hair loss involve hair matrix or follicle destruction by physical or chemical agents, or both, and by infectious or immunologically mediated inflammation. Alopecia also may result from a slowing of hair growth from metabolic diseases, antimetabolites, or other drugs. Physiologic alterations can lead to hair loss by changing the relationship of the anagen and telogen phases of hair follicles.

A. **Androgenetic alopecia** results from the effect of androgenic hormones on scalp hair growth in genetically susceptible males and females. Follicles that produce terminal hair are gradually transformed into vellus-like follicles; in the late stages, the follicles actually become atrophic. Androgenetic alopecia is controlled by one dominant, sex-limited, autosomal gene that may be incompletely expressed because of polygenic modifying factors.

B. **Traumatic alopecia** is caused by constant friction, traction (eg, excessive combing or tight braiding), or recurrent hair plucking.

C. **Infectious alopecia** related to **tinea capitis** injures hair follicles by invoking an intense inflammatory response.

    D. In the **physiologic alopecia** process, **telogen effluvium,** an unusually large number of follicles (25–45%) abruptly end the anagen phase and move into transition (catogen), then into the rest (telogen) phase. Large numbers of telogen hairs then synchronously fall out.

    E. In **alopecia areata,** there is evidence to suggest cell-mediated immunologic injury.

    F. **Systemic processes** slow the rate of hair growth or alter the balance between the anagen and telogen phases of the hair follicles.

V. Symptoms. The vast majority of processes leading to alopecia are remarkably symptom-free locally. Systemic diseases have associated symptoms. Local disorders, especially physical trauma or infectious processes such as tinea capitis, may cause itching and pain. Many patients exhibit psychological distress over their hair loss.

VI. Signs. A careful review of the duration and location of the hair loss, major life changes, physical trauma, drug intake, and hair care habits, together with the signs below, will rapidly narrow the range of diagnostic possibilities. One initial clinical clue is the presence of follicular orifices on inspection, which implies a noncicatricial process.

    A. Androgenetic alopecia
        1. Male pattern baldness is most often characterized by frontotemporal hairline recession with variable hair loss at the scalp vertex.
        2. Female pattern baldness shows a predominance of diffuse or vertex hair loss.

    B. Traumatic alopecia usually shows patchy hair loss but may also be diffuse. Localized breakage with variously shortened hairs suggests mechanical damage.

    C. Infectious alopecia, which is related to tinea capitis, exhibits discrete patches of partial hair loss and breakage overlying scaly, inflamed skin. Less commonly, a **kerion** induced by the dermatophyte *Trichophyton tonsurans,* causes a deep, purulent folliculitis. With severe fungal infections or marked cellulitis, inflammation and suppuration can cause destruction and scarring. Secondary syphilis, in contrast, leads to a diffuse, moth-eaten appearance of the scalp.

    D. Physiologic alopecia is suggested by acute, diffuse, yet reversible hair thinning. When present, transverse nail lines (Beau's lines) imply a subacute physiologic injury.

    E. Alopecia areata is characterized by abrupt, patchy, but very well-demarcated hair loss. This process leaves discrete areas of smooth, hairless, noninflamed skin that is surrounded by easily plucked hairs. Another helpful (and some say pathognomonic) finding is that of "exclamation point" hairs, which are short, heavily pigmented shafts with wide, brushlike distal ends that taper at the skin surface. There can be complete loss of scalp hair (**alopecia totalis**) or of all body hair (**alopecia universalis**), although this is less common than other types of hair loss. Pitted nails are seen in up to one third of patients.

    F. Systemic diseases, such as thyroid disease, exhibit their specific associated signs in addition to diffuse hair loss and thinning.
        1. Signs of masculinization mandate an endocrinologic evaluation.
        2. Loss of the lateral one third of the eyebrows suggests hypothyroidism.

VII. Laboratory tests. Most cases of alopecia can be diagnosed by a thorough personal history and a careful physical examination. Ancillary tests may be helpful in certain situations.

    A. The **hair pull or pluck test** involves a moderately firm pull of 10–20 closely grouped hairs. Normally, less than 20% of the shafts will be removed, but in telogen effluvium and active androgenetic alopecia, over 40% of the shafts will be uprooted. This test is also helpful in advising patients on the prognosis of alopecia areata, since a positive result at the periphery of a patch implies advancing disease.

    B. **Wood's light examination, potassium hydroxide (KOH) preparation,** and, more rarely, **fungal cultures of hair shafts** aid in diagnosing fungal infection.

    C. A **trichogram** involves the microscopic analysis of at least 50 plucked hairs to determine hair structure and the proportion of telogen follicles. These hairs are removed from one area by a hemostat. Telogen hairs have small, unpigmented, ovoid bulbs and no internal root sheath. Anagen hairs have larger, elongated, pigmented bulbs shaped like the end of a broom, with a narrow internal root sheath. More than 20% of the patient's hair, and often up to 60%, will be telogen hairs if the patient has telogen effluvium. Anagen hairs that show atrophied bulbs are typical in patients with androgenetic alopecia.

D. A **hair count** is the actual count of all hairs lost over several days. Up to 100 hairs per day is considered normal. Elevated counts are typical of telogen effluvium.

E. **Scalp biopsy** is usually reserved for cases of uncertain origin but may be helpful in determining the prognosis of patients with alopecia areata and lupus erythematosus based on the degree of perifollicular lymphocytic infiltrate and antibody deposition, respectively.

F. **Assessment of endocrine dysfunction** may include thyroid tests and serum levels of dehydroepiandrosterone sulfate, testosterone, androstenedione, and sex hormone–binding globulin. All balding females should receive such an evaluation.

G. **Hematologic, serologic, rheumatologic,** and **blood chemistry tests** should be performed only when systemic disease is suspected, except for balding women, in whom a complete blood cell count, antinuclear antibody test, and ferritin are routinely indicated.

VIII. Treatment. Fortunately, most of the alopecia seen in primary care is noncicatricial, and thus may respond at least partially to specific therapy. Because of the often intense psychological impact of any degree of hair loss, emotional support of the patient remains paramount.

A. **Androgenetic alopecia.** Despite advertising claims of remarkable "cures" or treatments for androgenetic baldness, few truly effective agents exist. The long-term prognosis for such patients remains suboptimal, despite increasingly intense research efforts. The following therapies are recommended.

1. **Topical minoxidil (Rogaine),** now available without prescription, is recommended for both male and female pattern baldness. The drug's exact mechanism of action is uncertain. In large-scale, randomized, placebo-controlled trials, 2% and 5% minoxidil in an alcohol/propylene glycol vehicle improved hair growth and density by increasing the numbers of new vellus and terminal hairs. Positive prognostic factors for growth with minoxidil include a balding history of less than 5 years, vertex baldness smaller than 10 cm, and the presence of many indeterminate hairs (between vellus and terminal). Minoxidil is not effective in temple areas where hair is receding.

a. The **optimum therapeutic benefit** is achieved by the application of 1 mL of 2% or 5% minoxidil twice daily. Application once daily is ineffective. Treatment must be continued indefinitely, since discontinuation causes regression to pretreatment status within 2–3 months.

Responders notice a decrease in shedding by 2 months, with hair growth ensuing within 3–8 months of treatment. Approximately 40% of individuals experience moderate hair growth by 1 year, with stabilization of hair counts noted thereafter. Fewer than one half of these responders express satisfaction with the degree of regrowth. Efficacy (and side effects) are higher for the 5% solution, which is the preferred starting concentration in men.

b. **Side effects** are minimal. Only a minority of patients experience contact dermatitis, drying, or pruritus. No significant systemic adverse effects have been noted.

2. **Finasteride (Propecia),** an inhibitor of type 2 5α-reductase, is the only oral agent available and is to be used only in men. In studies of men ages 18–41 with mild to moderate hair loss in the vertex and anterior midscalp region, a 1-mg daily dose resulted in visible hair regrowth in 66% of subjects. Eight-eight percent of participants stabilized their hair counts. As with minoxidil, regrowth is usually not seen for 3–4 months. A 12-month trial is usually needed before declaring the drug ineffective. Side effects are mild, with less than 2% experiencing sexual dysfunction.

3. **Other medicinal treatments** that are under investigation but show some promise in early studies include minoxidil plus 0.05% tretinoin, spironolactone 100–200 mg daily, and minoxidil plus finasteride. Cyproterone acetate, cimetidine, topical progesterone, or oral estrogens (in the form of oral contraceptives) may be helpful for female pattern baldness. Hormone replacement therapy may benefit postmenopausal women.

4. **Surgical approaches** that may provide definitive therapy include hair transplantation, scalp reduction, transposition flaps, and soft tissue expansion. Because diffuse thinning is more common in women, these techniques are less suitable for them.

B. Traumatic alopecia responds to cessation of the underlying process. Psychotherapy may be, but rarely is, needed. Trichotillomania may be helped by the use of clomipramine, a drug that is useful in treating obsessive-compulsive disorder.

C. Infectious alopecia is corrected by direct treatment of the offending organism. For **tinea capitis,** systemic treatment is necessary. Adults respond to **griseofulvin,** ultramicrosize, 10–15 mg/kg/day for 6–8 weeks, in single or divided doses. Children should receive 10 mg/kg of the ultramicrosize agent. The drug is best absorbed when taken with food. **Oral ketoconazole** and **itraconazole** are used only in more resistant cases and are not approved for children less than 16 years of age. These two agents must not be coadministered with the antihistamines terfenadine or astemizole because of the risk of inducing malignant ventricular arrhythmias.

D. Telogen effluvium is managed by appropriate recognition of the inciting events. The patient should be assured that hair regrowth is expected within several months.

E. Alopecia areata

  1. Intradermal injection of corticosteroids remains the most common and effective treatment.

    a. Triamcinolone, 0.05 mL of the acetonide (10 mg/mL) or 0.1 mL of the hexacetonide (5 mg/mL), is systematically injected into the dermis of the involved area every 0.5–1 cm. Such therapy is best used for small patches of hair, since the total treatment dose should not exceed 15–20 mg/month. Injections are repeated monthly.

    b. Efficacy of treatments may be hard to judge because of the high rate (60–90%) of spontaneous remissions by 12–18 months, but in general, intralesional steroids hasten resolution by 6 months.

    c. For larger areas, topical high-potency steroid ointments (triamcinolone acetonide 0.5%, halcinonide 0.12%, fluocinonide 0.05%) with or without occlusion may be used with somewhat less success and more potential toxicity.

    d. Unfavorable prognostic signs for permanent regrowth include onset before puberty, alopecia totalis or universalis, recurrent attacks, or lack of response after 1 year. Fewer than 5% of the cases progress to alopecia totalis or beyond.

    e. Recurrences of areata are possible even after 20 years. Vigilance for the appearance of other autoimmune diseases is appropriate.

  2. Topical 5% minoxidil has shown moderate benefit in early studies. It can be combined with topical or intralesional corticosteroids for added benefit.

  3. Other therapies which have shown promise but which must be used at the dermatologist's discretion include the induction of allergic contact dermatitis with skin sensitizers, immunomodulation, topical anthralin (Dritho-Scalp), PUVA (psoralens plus ultraviolet light) therapy, and systemic corticosteroids.

F. Systemic disease–related hair loss usually responds to specific therapy of the underlying disease unless scarring is involved.

REFERENCES

Drake LA et al: Guidelines of care for androgenetic alopecia. Am Acad Dermatol 1996;**35:**465.
Habif TP: Hair diseases. In Habif TP (editor): *Clinical Dermatology.* 3rd ed. Mosby; 1996:739.
Sawaya ME: Clinical update on hair. Dermatol Clin 1997;**15:**37.
Shapiro J, Price VH: Hair regrowth—Therapeutic agents. Dermatol Clin 1998;**16:**341.
Sinclair R: Male pattern androgenetic alopecia. Br Med J 1998;**317:**865.

---

5   Amenorrhea

Laura B. Frankenstein, MD

I. Definition. Primary amenorrhea is the absence of menses by age 14 in girls without breast or pubic hair development or by age 16 in girls with normal breast and pubic hair development. Secondary amenorrhea is the absence of menses for ≥6 months in a female with previously normal menstrual cycles (21–35 days) or the absence of menses for ≥12 months in a female with previous menstrual cycles >35 days.

II. Common diagnoses
  A. Pregnancy and lactation.
  B. Hypothalamic dysfunction caused by emotional stress, strenuous exercise, anorexia nervosa, severe dieting, and chronic illness.
  C. Hyperprolactinemia resulting from idiopathic causes, medications (Table 5–1), nipple stimulation, chest wall trauma, prolactinoma, or hypothyroidism.
  D. Ovarian failure caused by premature menopause, anovulation, hypothyroidism, chemotherapy, radiation therapy, or hyperandrogenic chronic anovulation (polycystic ovaries and other causes).
  E. Uterovaginal abnormalities, including Asherman's syndrome, testicular feminization, and müllerian anomalies or agenesis (eg, Turner's syndrome).
III. Epidemiology. Secondary amenorrhea has a prevalence rate of 4% in the US population. This figure does not include pregnancy, which is the most common cause of amenorrhea. Primary amenorrhea is much less common.

In normal individuals, the mean age of menarche is 13.3 years (range, 11–17 years). By 16 years of age, 99% of healthy teens begin their menses. The mean age of menopause is 50 years (range, 35–55 years).

Risk factors for hypothalamic amenorrhea are weight loss, nulliparity, and a pre-existing tendency to menstrual irregularity. A single excessive fast may be associated with menstrual irregularities.

Ballet dancing and long-distance running are the activities most often associated with menstrual irregularities. The intensity of the training often correlates with the occurrence of menstrual disorders. The risk of amenorrhea approaches 20% when a woman runs more than 20 miles a week and increases to as much as 50% with further distance. Girls beginning rigorous training before menses begin may experience a delay in menarche for as long as 3 years.

Up to one third of secondary amenorrhea is the United States not due to pregnancy is due to prolactin-secreting adenomas.

Twenty percent to 40% of premature ovarian failure is associated with autoimmune disorders.

Seventy percent of hyperandrogenic chronic anovulation is due to polycystic ovaries. Excess androgen accounts for 37% of amenorrhea in women not pregnant or lactating. A 10–20% decrease in lumbar bone density is found in women with hypoestrogenic amenorrhea; their cardiovascular disease risk is increased.

Asherman's syndrome is most likely to occur after vigorous curettage or after endometritis associated with abortion or delivery.

"Postpill amenorrhea" does not exist. Ninety-nine percent of women resume menses within 6 months of discontinuing oral contraception. Women with no menses 6 months after stopping oral contraception or 1 year after their last dose of **medroxyprogesterone** (Depo-Provera) are amenorrheic for other reasons.
IV. Pathophysiology. Normal menses require a favorable environment, adequate hormonal stimulation of the endometrium, the ability of the endometrium to respond to hormones, and a patent outflow tract for endometrial shedding.
  A. Pregnancy and lactation interrupt menses fairly predictably. Postpartum mothers who do not breast-feed can expect to miss as many as two menses. Lactation causes amenorrhea because suckling stimulates prolactin release from the pituitary; this can last as long as 18 months while the mother is nursing.
  B. Hypothalamic dysfunction can be caused by reversible stresses that interfere with normal gonadotropin-releasing hormone (GnRH) and cyclic luteinizing hormone (LH) secretion and render estrogen production inadequate. Once the stress is resolved, GnRH and LH appear to normalize, and menses resume.

TABLE 5–1. MEDICATIONS THAT CAN INCREASE PROLACTIN

Phenothiazines	Meclizine
Butyrophenones	Tripelennamine
Thioxanthenes	Cimetidine
Methyldopa	Amitriptyline
Reserpine	Imipramine
Metoclopramide	

C. **Hyperprolactinemia.** Prolactin inhibits gonadotropin release.
   1. **Elevations in prolactin** are most often idiopathic but may be caused by drugs (Table 5–1) or mechanical factors.
   2. **Prolonged hypothyroidism** can elevate prolactin levels; the longer the level of thyroid-stimulating hormone (TSH) has been elevated, the greater the elevation of prolactin.
   3. **Prolactin-producing tumors** are less common than the above causes of hyperprolactinemia but are potentially more serious, as compromise of the optic chiasm can cause loss of vision and invasion of other structures. Prolactinomas are not related to oral contraceptive use, as was once thought. Microprolactinomas are <1 cm in diameter; macroprolactinomas are >1 cm in diameter.

D. **Ovarian failure**
   1. **Premature ovarian failure** occurs when a woman under 35 years of age is depleted of estrogen-producing follicles. Such ovarian failure is often idiopathic; there may be an accelerated loss of follicles because of genetics, autoimmune disease, infection, or iatrogenic trauma.
   2. **Anovulation** has many causes because any disorder or chronic illness affecting the hypothalamus, the pituitary, or the ovary can cause a woman to fail to ovulate. Often temporary, this condition is not accompanied by estrogen deficiency.
   3. **Hyperandrogenic chronic anovulation** is marked by excessive androgen production with increased levels of LH and decreased levels of follicle-stimulating hormone (FSH). Excess androgen can be produced by the ovaries or the adrenals.

E. **Uterovaginal abnormalities**
   1. **Asherman's syndrome** occurs when enough adhesions cover the endometrium that normal shedding is prevented.
   2. **Müllerian anomalies** or **agenesis** involves congenital discontinuity or absence of part of the outflow tract. An imperforate hymen is one anomaly that causes primary amenorrhea.

F. **Genetic disorders.** Turner's syndrome (XO karyotype) presents with primary amenorrhea due to failure of ovarian development; testicular feminization (46XY karyotype with androgen insensitivity) presents with amenorrhea due to absent outflow tract (uterus and vagina).

V. **Symptoms** other than missed menses may be few.
   A. **Nausea, fatigue, breast tenderness,** and **urinary frequency** may accompany pregnancy.
   B. **Previous menstrual history** is valuable.
   C. **Radical changes** in eating behavior, weight, or exercise habits may indicate hypothalamic dysfunction. This dysfunction may also be indicated when symptoms of a chronic disease are present.
   D. **Galactorrhea, headaches,** and **visual changes** may accompany hyperprolactinemia. If any of these three symptoms is present, there is an increased possibility of a prolactinoma.
   E. **Hot flashes, vaginal dryness,** and **dyspareunia** often indicate ovarian failure.
   F. **Hirsutism** is a complaint of 70% of the women with hyperandrogenic chronic anovulation. Many of these women also complain of **acne** and **oily skin.**

VI. **Signs.** The physical examination is usually normal.
   A. **Emotional stress,** such as sadness or emotional lability, and pronounced **weight loss** or other signs of anorexia may be present in patients with hypothalamic dysfunction.
   B. **Abnormal muscle stretch reflexes** and other stigmata of thyroid disease, which are signs of a chronic illness, may be found in patients with hypothalamic dysfunction.
   C. **Atrophic mucosa** (pale vaginal mucosa lacking normal rugal folds) accompanies ovarian failure.
   D. **Skin changes** suggestive of masculinization (eg, acne, increased facial and body hair, or loss of scalp hair) may be present in women with hyperandrogenic chronic anovulation. Sometimes it is discovered upon examination of these patients that

their ovaries are larger than normal. Hyperandrogenic chronic anovulation is more common in women who are obese.

E. If **breast and pubic hair development** has not begun by age 14, uterovaginal abnormalities should be suspected. Congenital abnormalities such as imperforate hymen are easily detected; other abnormalities may be more subtle and therefore more difficult to detect.

F. **Short stature (height <5 feet), sexual infantilism, and neck webbing** characterize Turner's syndrome.

G. **Large breasts with immature nipples, absent axillary or pubic hair, absent uterus or vagina, and possibly gonads palpable in the inguinal canal** characterize testicular feminization syndrome.

VII. **Laboratory tests.** Unless the diagnosis is obvious from the history and physical examination, testing will be necessary. An accurate diagnosis is the only way to determine proper management. The work-up can be performed in a stepwise fashion (Figure 5–1) to prevent unnecessary testing.

A. A **pregnancy test** is always indicated when periods are missed, even if the woman is convinced that she is not pregnant.

B. A test to determine the **level of TSH** is indicated because, although hypothyroidism is uncommon, the problem cannot always be detected based only on history and physical examination.

C. **Prolactin values** >30 ng/mL are significant. Prolactinoma is associated with prolactin levels >100 ng/mL.

D. The **progestin challenge** separates women with estrogen deficiency from those with normal or excess estrogen. It is therapeutic as well as diagnostic. **Medroxyprogesterone acetate** (Provera), 10 mg, is given orally once a day for 5 days. Any bleeding, even slight bleeding, during the week after the final dosage indicates that the patient has sufficient estrogen and that her amenorrhea is caused by anovulation. No bleeding during the week after the final dosage indicates that the patient has an estrogen deficiency or outflow tract problem that is preventing normal menses.

E. A **chemistry panel** may find unrecognized systemic disease such as diabetes mellitus, renal disease, lipid disorders, or liver disease.

F. **Gonadotropin levels**
   1. An **FSH level** >40 mIU/mL suggests premature or true menopause, depending on the patient's age. A high FSH level with a normal LH level indicates that the patient is premenopausal and may still be able to conceive.
   2. If a woman is of average menopausal age or has a family history of menopause at her age, an FSH level should be determined before following the procedures suggested in Figure 5–1. An LH level is useful if polycystic ovaries are suspected, because the LH-FSH ratio will be >2:1 when polycystic ovaries exist.

G. A **coned-down view of the sella turcica** is appropriate for women with a prolactin level that is elevated but is <100 ng/mL and for women with galactorrhea, even if the prolactin level is normal.

H. **X-ray evaluation of the sella turcica** by computerized tomographic (CT) scan with contrast is necessary only if the prolactin level is >100 ng/mL, if the coned-down view is abnormal, or if the patient has headaches or visual disturbances.

I. **Estrogen/progestin challenge** is performed if there is no bleeding after a progestin challenge and there is reason to suspect an outflow tract problem. To ensure endometrial proliferation, 2.5 mg of **conjugated estrogen** is taken daily for 21 days, and **medroxyprogesterone acetate** (Provera), 10 mg/day, is added to the last 5 days (days 17–21). Absence of bleeding during the week following the last dosage implies an outflow tract problem; bleeding during that week confirms that the patient has an estrogen deficiency. If an estrogen deficiency is strongly suspected, an FSH level should be obtained prior to this challenge.

J. Before withdrawal bleeding is induced, an **endometrial biopsy** is required in women with prolonged amenorrhea and signs of androgen or estrogen excess.

K. **Testosterone levels with dehydroepiandrosterone sulfate (DHEA-S)** need to be performed in women with excessive virilization to ensure that the excess androgenic state is not from a neoplastic source. Testosterone levels >200 ng/dL or

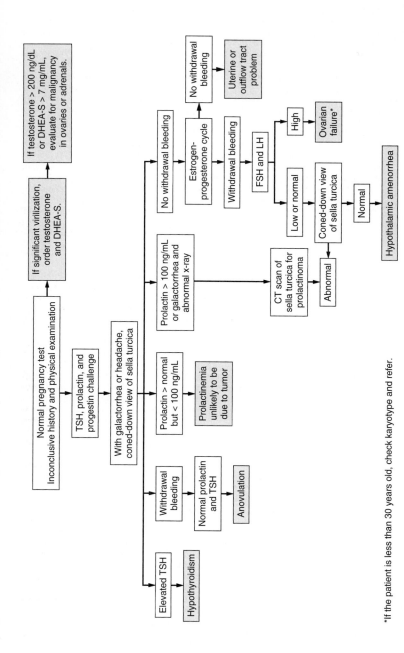

FIGURE 5-1. Laboratory evaluation of amenorrhea.

*If the patient is less than 30 years old, check karyotype and refer.

DHEA-S levels >7 mg/mL require a CT scan of the adrenals and ultrasound examination of the ovaries to look for tumors.
  L. Karyotyping is needed in women with premature ovarian failure at <30 years of age or with stigmata of testicular feminization or Turner's syndrome.
  M. Hysteroscopy is commonly used by specialists to diagnose and assess Asherman's syndrome and other uterine anomalies.
  N. Bone densitometry is indicated for women of any age with prolonged amenorrhea.
VIII. Treatment must be based on a firm diagnosis and must attempt to resolve underlying problems while restoring menses and treating problems associated with estrogen deficiency or androgen excess, such as osteoporosis and excess cardiovascular risk.
  A. Pregnancy and lactation. All mothers should be reminded that ovulation will occur before the first menses and is unpredictable; contraception is necessary if child spacing is desired. Breast-feeding is not an adequate contraceptive.
  B. Hypothalamic dysfunction is resolved when the stress causing the abnormal GnRH secretion lessens. In the meantime, other interventions are important.
    1. Relieving stress. For exercise-induced amenorrhea, a decrease in intensity of training or a weight gain of 2–3% usually results in normal menses within 1–2 months. Young athletes have more stress fractures when menses are absent; once training is decreased or weight is increased slightly, allowing menses to resume, the fracture rate returns to normal. A woman who is anorexic or who fasts excessively should be encouraged to change her eating habits enough to regain a small percentage of her weight or body fat; counseling or a support group may be necessary.
    2. Estrogen supplementation. A woman preferring to maintain her current lifestyle (eg, as a thin ballerina) may require years of counseling to cope with her emotional stress, or may have a chronic disease that has been corrected as much as possible. In such cases, estrogen should be provided until normal hormonal function resumes, in order to protect the patient from bone loss.
      a. Oral contraceptives are useful estrogen supplements because they provide contraception in case ovulation spontaneously resumes. They can be used safely until menopause if the woman does not smoke.
      b. Combination therapy is the best choice for smokers in their mid-30s or older and for women with contraindications to the pill. Any of the regimens used for menopausal replacement are appropriate (see Chapter 82).
    3. Smoking should be discouraged and adequate calcium intake should be encouraged to help the patient prevent bone loss (see section VIII,D,6 and Chapter 84).
  C. Hyperprolactinemia is resolved when the stimulus is found and corrected or when suppressive medication is used. Some women choose to live with elevated prolactin levels and require intervention to restore cyclic menses, to prevent excessive endometrial proliferation (this increases the risks of dysfunctional uterine bleeding and endometrial cancer), and to protect their breasts from unopposed estrogen (this increases the risk of breast cancer).
    1. Bromocriptine (Parlodel) is the drug most often used for hyperprolactinemia because it inhibits the secretion of prolactin and suppresses prolactin levels as long as the medication is taken. This drug shrinks prolactinomas, eliminates galactorrhea, and reestablishes fertility as well as normal menses.
      a. Starting with 2.5–5 mg at bedtime helps prevent the common side effects of orthostatic hypotension, nausea, and vomiting.
      b. For microprolactinomas and idiopathic causes, 2.5–5 mg twice a day is often enough to normalize prolactin levels.
      c. The dose of bromocriptine is raised by 2.5–5 mg a day every 3–4 weeks until prolactin levels are normalized.
      d. Menses usually return in 6–12 weeks once prolactin levels are normalized.
    2. Medroxyprogesterone acetate (Provera), 10 mg/day taken for 10 days each month, is useful to induce menses if a woman does not desire fertility, has no galactorrhea or does not mind the galactorrhea, or cannot tolerate bromocriptine. Provera will not shrink a tumor and does not normalize prolactin levels. The use of this drug on less than a monthly basis may protect

against endometrial cancer but may not be as effective in protecting against breast cancer.

   3. **Microadenomas** grow very slowly. In the absence of headaches or visual disturbances, prolactin levels should be followed yearly, with magnetic resonance imaging every 2–3 years.
   4. An **endocrinologist** or **neurosurgeon** should follow up on macroprolactinomas (>1 cm in diameter). Most smaller tumors can be followed on a yearly basis with prolactin level tests by a primary care physician.
   D. **Ovarian failure** may or may not be associated with lack of estrogen.
   1. **Weight loss** is helpful in women with polycystic ovaries in order to slow down estrogen production.
   2. **Clomiphene citrate** (Clomid) and other medications can be administered by physicians specializing in infertility to induce ovulation when fertility is desired. These drugs are not used merely for control of menses.
   3. Women with the polycystic ovary syndrome have three times the risk of hypertension and six times the risk of type II diabetes mellitus. They also have abnormal lipids. Based on these findings, women with **hyperandrogenic chronic anovulation** have a projected sevenfold risk of developing coronary heart disease and can be at increased risk for endometrial cancer. Weight loss, exercise, and dietary interventions are valuable for these women.
   4. **Surgical evaluation** is required with testicular feminization, for removal of testicular tissue to prevent malignancy.
   5. **Hormone treatment** options are the same as those for women who are estrogen deficient and for women with normal or excessive estrogen. Oral contraceptives are used to induce menses for any woman without contraindications to them and are particularly useful for women with polycystic ovary disease because the contraceptives suppress ovarian androgens, thus minimizing hirsutism. The usual dose of estrogen, 0.625 mg orally daily, used for menopausal women is only one fifth as potent as the usual dose of estrogen in oral contraceptives and may not be as effective at preventing bone loss in young women.
   6. **Calcium supplementation** (1500 mg/day) is helpful for women who are hypoestrogenic to prevent bone loss and allow for attainment of peak bone mass.
   E. **Uterovaginal abnormalities** require referral in most cases. Asherman's syndrome is usually treated by curettage or hysteroscopy and hormonal therapy. Congenital anomalies of the reproductive system may require exploratory and reconstructive surgery.

IX. **Patient follow-up**
   A. The patient should be reevaluated every few months to be sure further testing is not necessary. Hormonal replacement should be periodically discontinued in anovulatory and hypothalamic amenorrheic patients to see whether ovulation and menses will resume, whether pregnancy is desired, or whether alternative birth control is preferable.
   B. The incidence of spontaneous ovulation is higher in women predisposed to irregular menses. Thus, women should be reminded that amenorrhea does not necessarily protect them from becoming pregnant.
   C. The office visit for menstrual problems is a perfect time to review a woman's birth control needs and to ascertain whether her chosen method remains effective, safe, and acceptable for her and her partner(s) (see Chapter 100).

REFERENCES

Dahlgren E, et al: Polycystic ovary syndrome—Long-term metabolic consequences. Int J Gynecol Obstet 1994;**44:**3.

Kiningham RB, et al: Evaluation of amenorrhea. Am Fam Physician 1996;**53:**1185.

McIver MB, et al: Evaluation and management of amenorrhea. Mayo Clin Proc 1997;**72:**1161.

Putukian M: The female triad: Eating disorders, amenorrhea, and osteoporosis. Med Clin North Am 1994;**78:**345.

Serri O: Progress in the management of hyperprolactinemia. N Engl J Med 1994;**331:**942.

Speroff L, et al: *Clinical Gynecological Endocrinology and Infertility.* 5th ed. Williams & Wilkins; 1994.

6 Anemia

Mel P. Daly, MD

I. **Definition.** Anemia exists when the quantity or quality of circulating erythrocytes falls below normal. Under normal physiologic conditions, red blood cell production and turnover are carefully regulated. Anemia usually is the result of an acquired or hereditary disorder of red blood cells or may be a manifestation of an underlying non-hematologic disorder. Relying strictly on numerical definitions may be misleading, since normal values for hemoglobin depend on age, sex, race, altitude, smoking status, socioeconomic class, plasma volume, and presence of concomitant disease (Table 6–1).

II. **Common diagnoses** (Table 6–2)

III. **Epidemiology.** Using as a definition for *anemia* "hemoglobin values below the 95% reference range," the National Health and Nutrition Examination Survey (NHANES II) estimated anemia to be most prevalent in infants (5.7%), adolescent girls (5.9%), elderly females (5.8%), and elderly males (4.4%). Red blood cell parameters do not decline in healthy elderly individuals, yet the prevalence of anemia increases with age and institutionalization. Iron deficiency predominates as a cause of anemia in infants and young women, while inflammatory disease is the major cause of anemia in the elderly population.

   A. **Iron deficiency anemia** is the most common cause of nutritional anemia worldwide, with an increased prevalence in developing countries. Bleeding is the most common cause of iron deficiency anemia. It is uncommon for iron deficiency anemia to occur as a result of nutritional deficiencies in developed countries. Dietary restrictions of iron for 5 years or longer are required for the development of iron deficiency anemia in the presence of normal iron physiology. Most cases are caused by menstrual blood loss and increased iron requirements of pregnancy. Infants from impoverished families, adolescent children with lead poisoning, food faddists, patients with celiac disease, and those who have had gastrectomy are at greatest risk for developing iron deficiency anemia.

   B. **Anemia of chronic disease** is the most common form of anemia after the age of 60 because of the higher prevalence of concomitant infectious, inflammatory, and neoplastic diseases that may affect hematopoiesis (eg, chronic renal insufficiency, endocrine disorders, cancer, liver diseases, rheumatoid arthritis, and myelophthisis).

   C. **Vitamin B_{12} deficiency** is almost always due to pernicious anemia (PA). The peak age at onset is over 60 years. Less than 0.5% of the population over 80 years of age is affected by PA. The only source of cobalamin is animal products; thus, vegetarians who eat no meat, eggs, or cheese for a number of years may develop a nutritional deficiency state.

TABLE 6–1. NORMAL VALUES FOR HEMOGLOBIN (g/dL) BY AGE, SEX, AND RACE

Age (yr)	Males		Females	
	Median	Range	Median	Range
1–2	12.3	10.7–13.8	12.3	10.7–13.8
3–8	12.5	10.9–14.3	12.5	10.9–14.4
9–11	13.2	11.4–14.8	13.2	11–14.8
12–14	14	12–16	13.4	11.5–15.0
15–17	14.8	12.3–16.6	13.5	11.7–15.3
18–44	15.3	13.2–17.3	13.5	11.7–15.5
45–64	15.2	13.1–17.2	13.7	11.7–16
65–74	14.9	12.6–17.4	13.9	11.7–16

In black children between 3 and 5 years of age, hemoglobin levels are a median of 0.4 g/dL lower than in white children of the same age. In black men between 65 and 74 years of age, hemoglobin levels are a median of 1.1 g/dL lower than in white men of the same age.

TABLE 6–2. CLASSIFICATION OF ANEMIA BY MEAN RED BLOOD CELL VOLUME

Microcytic anemia or hypochromic microcytic anemia (MCHC, <30 g/dL; MCV, <85 fL)
  Iron deficiency
  Thalassemia
  Sideroblastic anemia
  Anemia of chronic disease (rare)

Normochromic macrocytic anemia (MCHC, 31–35 g/dL; MCV, >100 fL)
  Megaloblastic anemia
    Vitamin B_{12} deficiency
    Folate deficiency
  Nonmegaloblastic anemia
    Reticulocytosis
    Liver disease
    Myxedema
    Myelodysplasia, leukemia
    Aplastic anemia
    Lead poisoning
    Anemia associated with autonomic dysfunction

Normochromic or normocytic anemia (MCHC, 31–35 g/dL; MCV, 85–100 fL)
  Acute bleeding
  Marrow failure (aplasia, toxic, myelophthisic)
  Hemolysis
  Anemia of chronic disease

MCHC, mean corpuscular hemoglobin concentration; MCV, mean corpuscular volume.

D. Folic acid deficiency can occur in patients on diets deficient in fresh green vegetables, nuts, yeast, and liver. Folic acid stores in the body will deplete in 4 months. Elderly patients, pregnant women, and alcoholics are at risk for nutritional folate deficiency. There is an increased requirement for folic acid during growth spurts, during hemodialysis, in chronic hemolytic anemia, and in exfoliative skin disease.

E. Hemolytic anemia (Table 6–3)
  1. Sickle cell disease is inherited as an autosomal trait and occurs in the heterozygous state as sickle trait in 8–10% of blacks in the United States. Sickle trait rarely occurs in Eastern Mediterranean people or in people of Indian or Saudi Arabian ancestry. Disease develops in persons who are homozygous for the sickle gene (*HbSS*). About 2% of blacks in the United States have sickle cell anemia. Other sickle syndromes, such as sickle-β-thalassemia and sickle C disease, are uncommon in this country.

TABLE 6–3. CLASSIFICATION OF HEMOLYTIC ANEMIA

Intrinsic red blood cell membrane defects
  Hereditary spherocytosis, hereditary elliptocytosis, paroxysmal nocturnal hemoglobinuria

Red blood cell enzyme defects
  Glucose-6-phosphate dehydrogenase deficiency, pyruvate kinase deficiency

Hemoglobinopathies
  Sickle syndromes, thalassemias, unstable hemoglobins, methemoglobinemia

Immune hemolytic anemia
  Autoimmune or secondary to drugs and disease

Microangiopathic conditions
  Valve hemolysis, thrombotic thrombocytopenic purpura, hemolytic-uremic syndrome, disseminated intravascular coagulation, hemodialysis, cardiopulmonary bypass

Hypersplenism

Infections and toxins

2. The **thalassemias** are most common in Mediterranean and Asian populations. Sporadic cases of thalassemia are found among Africans and American blacks.

3. **Autoimmune hemolytic anemia** is rare and may occur on an idiopathic basis or secondary to other disorders, such as systemic lupus erythematosus, chronic lymphocytic leukemia, non-Hodgkin's lymphoma, Hodgkin's disease, and cancer. Drugs such as α-methyldopa, phenacetin, penicillin, rifampin, sulfonamides, quinidine, and chlorpropamide may induce an immune hemolysis, clinically indistinguishable from immune hemolytic anemia.

4. **Glucose-6-phosphate dehydrogenase (G6PD) deficiency** is one of the most common disorders causing hemolysis in the world, affecting 10% of black males in the United States. The gene for G6PD is carried on the X chromosome, and female carriers are rarely affected.

5. **Hereditary elliptocytosis** and **hereditary spherocytosis** are autosomal dominant disorders affecting about 200–300 million people worldwide, although these conditions are uncommon in the United States.

F. **Myelodysplastic syndromes** (MDSs) are disorders of stem cells that result in inadequate and abnormal maturation of bone marrow hematopoietic precursors. These disorders may progress to acute leukemia. MDSs are diagnosed in 1–10 per 100,000 people every year, and are more common in elderly males.

IV. **Pathophysiology.** The difference in hemoglobin levels between males and females, which becomes apparent in the second decade of life, is largely due to the hematopoietic effect of androgens. This sex difference in hemoglobin values diminishes with age, because of a reduced androgen effect.

A. **Iron deficiency anemia.** In the absence of physiologic drains on iron, such as pregnancy or menstruation, iron deficiency occurs as a result of bleeding. The usual source of blood loss is the gastrointestinal (GI) tract. The erosive effects of nonsteroidal anti-inflammatory drugs are often a precipitant. In elderly patients, colonic carcinomas, diverticular disease, and vascular malformations are other major causes of bleeding. Concomitant lesions of both the upper and lower GI tract are rare. Rare causes of blood loss include chronic hemolysis, hemoptysis, and bleeding disorders. Newborn infants who are breast-fed or who are taking non–iron-enriched formulas may become iron deficient in the first year of life. Malabsorption resulting from disease, from resection of the small bowel, or from partial gastric resection accounts for a small percentage of iron deficiency.

B. **Anemia of chronic disease** is due to a reduced utilization of storage iron and impaired incorporation of iron into hemoglobin, despite the presence of adequate iron stores in the reticuloendothelial system. The cause is unknown, but may result from immune activation and production of cytokines (eg, interleukin-1 or tumor necrosis factor) that directly inhibit the maturation of erythroid progenitors (burst-forming unit [BFU] and colony-forming unit [CFU]) and erythropoietin production. Other mechanisms related to the underlying primary disorder may also contribute to the anemia, such as blood loss, hemolysis, malabsorption, malnutrition, or bone marrow replacement or suppression by infection or drugs.

C. **Vitamin B_{12} deficiency.** Failure to absorb vitamin B_{12} because of reduced production or secretion of intrinsic factor occurs in pernicious anemia, a familial autoimmune disorder characterized by severe atrophic gastritis. Chronic treatment with histamine blockers and hydrogen ion pump inhibitors and *Helicobacter pylori* gastritis may also be implicated. Small bowel overgrowth, ileal malfunction, and certain drugs (*p*-aminosalicylic acid, neomycin, and potassium chloride) may account for malabsorption at the terminal ileum. Acidification of the small intestine and pancreatic disease may also cause cobalamin malabsorption by impairing the transfer of the vitamin from R-binder to intrinsic factor. Ineffective erythropoiesis that results in increased destruction of red blood cell precursors in the bone marrow may cause hyperbilirubinemia and elevated lactate dehydrogenase (LDH) levels. Vitamin B_{12} deficiency increases the likelihood of subsequent development of gastric cancer or polyps.

D. **Folic acid deficiency** occurs because the amount of folic acid in the average diet is not greatly in excess of nutritional requirements and because body folate reserves are relatively small. Decreased intake may occur in the elderly and in alcoholics. Other causes of folate deficiency include loss of food folate through excessive cooking and various forms of folate malabsorption (eg, jejunal atrophy caused by celiac disease). The increased nutritional demands of pregnancy and the increased requirements of chronic hemolytic anemia and exfoliative psoriasis may deplete folic acid reserves. Drugs such as phenytoin or sulfasalazine may interfere with folate absorption. Certain chemotherapeutic agents, antiviral drugs (eg, azidothymidine [AZT] and zidovudine), folate antagonists (eg, methotrexate), trimethoprim, nitrous oxide, primidone, and phenobarbital may cause megaloblastic anemia by antagonizing the effects of folate.

E. **Hemolytic anemia.** These disorders shorten red blood cell survival through immunologic mechanisms, intrinsic red blood cell defects, red blood cell enzyme deficits, and mechanical hemolysis (Table 6–3).

    1. **Sickle cell anemia** and other sickling disorders (HbS-β-thalassemia and HbSC) are associated with abnormal hemoglobin molecules that polymerize under reduced oxygen conditions. Sickle cell trait occurs in individuals who are heterozygous for HbS.

    2. **Hereditary red blood cell structural abnormalities** result in membrane defects that cause intravascular hemolysis (G6PD deficiency and pyruvate kinase deficiency).

    3. **Autoimmune hemolytic anemia** is caused by either warm (temperature >37 °C [98.6 °F]) **or cold antibodies directed at red blood cells.**

    4. **Drug-induced hemolytic anemia** results from immune complex, antibody, or hapten formation that directly or indirectly results in red blood cell destruction.

    5. **Microangiopathic hemolytic anemia** is a syndrome of traumatic intravascular hemolysis that may be associated with disseminated intravascular coagulation, vasculitis, hemolytic-uremic syndrome, thrombotic thrombocytopenic purpura, and eclampsia.

    6. **Paroxysmal nocturnal hemoglobinuria** is a rare disorder of bone marrow stem cells that results in abnormal complement activation and intravascular hemolysis.

F. **MDSs** are clonal disorders of stem cells causing inadequate and abnormal maturation of red blood cells. Previous treatment with radiation or mutagenic chemicals may result in MDSs.

G. **Sideroblastic anemia** may be hereditary or acquired and may result from an abnormality of porphyrin synthesis, which may occur idiopathically or secondarily to alcohol, drugs, or a number of chronic diseases, such as lymphoma or myeloma.

H. **Aplastic anemia** occurs because of a functional intrinsic marrow disturbance that results in quantitative or qualitative defects in red blood cell synthesis. This condition may be secondary to marrow infiltration by tumor or fibrosis; dose-related, idiosyncratic, or hypersensitivity effects of drugs (eg, antithyroid medications, gold, chemotherapeutic agents, AZT, phenytoin, and phenylbutazone); radiation; autoimmune suppression (eg, with systemic lupus erythematosus); and infections such as tuberculosis, atypical mycobacterial infections, brucellosis, hepatitis A and B, and, rarely, mumps, rubella, infectious mononucleosis, influenza, human immunodeficiency virus (HIV), parvovirus, and fungal and parasitic infections.

V. **Symptoms** of anemia are usually nonspecific and occur when hemoglobin levels fall to <8 g/dL. These symptoms include weakness and fatigue.

A. Elderly patients with impaired cardiopulmonary reserves may complain of chest pain, exertional dyspnea, and dizziness. Other symptoms seen in elderly patients with anemia are confusional states, reduced physical activity, memory loss, and even depression.

B. Many iron-deficient patients develop pica, an unusual craving for specific foods (eg, chewing ice). Advanced iron deficiency may cause dysphagia because of formation of esophageal webs (Plummer-Vinson syndrome).

C. Burning and soreness of the tongue is a symptom of vitamin B_{12} deficiency. In advanced cases of vitamin B_{12} deficiency, patients may be totally asymptomatic or may complain of numbness, paresthesia, unsteadiness, and weakness. Impaired memory, depression, and psychosis may also occur.

D. In severe cases of hemolytic anemia, such as that which occurs in sickle cell crises, fever and pain may be predominant symptoms. Common sites of acute painful episodes include the bones (back and long bones), chest, and abdomen.

Stroke, visual disturbances, hematuria, chronic skin ulcers, and painful priapism may also occur secondary to micro- or macroinfarcts.

VI. **Signs** of anemia are nonspecific; however, some signs characterize certain conditions.

A. **Iron deficiency anemia** results in pallor of the buccal and lingual mucosae and the nail beds. Other signs include atrophic glossitis, angular stomatitis, brittle nails, and cheilosis.

B. **Vitamin B_{12} deficiency** usually develops insidiously. The skin may look slightly yellow. Vitiligo may be seen, and the hair may become prematurely gray or white.

1. Glossitis is an important sign of vitamin B_{12} deficiency and may be intermittent, preceding the general symptoms of anemia by a long period. A smooth, shiny, atrophic tongue is common, and patchy areas of acute glossitis may be superimposed.

2. Hepatomegaly is common, especially if there is cardiac failure; splenomegaly occurs in 10% of cases or less and is usually mild.

3. Mental changes may predominate, with evidence of dementia. Signs of peripheral neuropathy together with posterior column lesions (paraplegia and sensory ataxia) may be found in cases of subacute combined degeneration of the cord secondary to longstanding vitamin B_{12} deficiency. These changes may occur in the absence of anemia.

C. **Folic acid deficiency.** Patients may appear malnourished and wasted. Diarrhea, cheilosis, and glossitis are common findings. Neurologic abnormalities do not occur. Other, nonspecific signs include mild confusion, depression, apathy, and intellectual loss.

D. **Hemolytic anemia**

1. **Autoimmune hemolytic anemia** may have a dramatic clinical presentation. The anemia may be of rapid onset and may be life-threatening. Patients may present with angina or congestive heart failure. Jaundice and hemoglobinuria may occur over a 1- to 3-day period. Hemolysis is usually less dramatic in onset. Signs of accelerated metabolism of hemoglobin, including jaundice, hemoglobinemia, hemoglobinuria, and hemosiderinuria, occur over a few days. Patients with thrombotic thrombocytopenic purpura may present with petechiae, fever, altered mental status, or focal neurologic findings.

2. Patients with **sickle cell anemia** often are chronically ill. Common signs include jaundice, hepatomegaly, cardiomegaly, a hyperdynamic precordium, and systolic murmurs. In patients with visual disturbances, retinal infarcts, vitreous hemorrhage, or retinal detachment may be found. Less common are splenomegaly, hemiplegia, and poorly healing ulcers of the lower tibia.

3. Children with **ß-thalassemia** are normal at birth, but bony deformities, growth failure, hepatosplenomegaly, and jaundice develop in childhood. In severe cases, hypogonadism, cardiomyopathy, progressive hepatomegaly, and endocrine dysfunction occur.

E. **Anemia of primary autonomic failure** is characterized by signs of autonomic dysfunction (orthostatic hypotension without an increase in heart rate, sinus arrhythmia, impaired blood pressure response to stressors, and absence of other causes) is associated with normocytic anemia.

VII. **Laboratory tests** (Table 6–4)

A. **Iron deficiency anemia.** The essential diagnostic features are absent marrow iron stores, serum ferritin <20 ng/mL, or transferrin saturation ≤0.08 in association with serum ferritin levels ≤50 ng/mL. The serum iron is low, and iron-binding capacity is high. Microcytic and hypochromic red blood cells on the peripheral smear are usual in the later stages of iron deficiency anemia. A normal red blood cell distribution width (RDW) effectively eliminates iron deficiency as a cause of microcytic anemia. Circulating transferrin receptor assays may, in the future, become a widely accepted measure of early iron deficiency. Upper and lower GI endoscopy is indicated if laboratory studies suggest iron deficiency, especially if stool testing for occult blood is positive.

B. **Megaloblastic anemia** is characterized by macrocytosis and hypersegmented granulocytes in the peripheral blood smear. The mean corpuscular volume is frequently >110 fL (but may be normal in patients with coexisting thalassemia), indirect hyperbilirubinemia and elevated LDH levels are usual, and the mean

TABLE 6–4. APPROACH TO EVALUATION OF ANEMIA

Routine database
Hematocrit, hemoglobin, MCV, MCHC, RDW, reticulocyte count, blood smear
What is the MCV?
Microcytic, normocytic, macrocytic
What is the underlying mechanism?
Decreased production, bleeding, increased destruction (hemolysis)
Does the patient have another problem associated with the anemia?
Race, genetic and family history, concomitant disease

MCV, mean corpuscular volume; MCHC, mean corpuscular hemoglobin concentration; RDW, red blood cell distribution width.

corpuscular hemoglobin concentration (MCHC) is normal (range, 31–35 g/dL). The reticulocyte count is low, and leukocyte and platelet counts may be decreased. An increase in the RDW precedes the macrocytosis of vitamin B_{12} and folate deficiencies. If macrocytosis is present, serum B_{12} and red blood cell folate levels should be obtained.

1. The normal range for serum vitamin B_{12} is 150–650 pg/mL. Some elderly patients have low B_{12} levels yet show no evidence of megaloblastic changes and have normal Schilling test results. This is thought to be due to an inability to mobilize B_{12} from foods. This group of patients may eventually go on to develop symptomatic B_{12} deficiency. Patients with low normal vitamin B_{12} levels are at risk for deficiency and should be followed up at regular intervals. The diagnosis of PA should be confirmed by a Schilling test.
2. In patients who are B_{12} deficient, serum folate is usually normal or elevated unless there is a coexisting folate deficiency.
3. The normal range for serum folic acid is 6–20 ng/mL. Red blood cell folate turns over more slowly than serum folate, and since folic acid remains in the red blood cells throughout their life span, current red blood cell folate levels indicate the folate status of the patient for the previous 4 months. Normal values of red blood cell folate are 150–600 ng/mL.
4. Serum levels of cobalamin metabolites, methylmalonic acid, and homocysteine are highly sensitive for diagnosing cobalamin deficiency. Normal levels rule out a deficiency with virtual certainty. Serum homocysteine levels are markedly increased in folate deficiency. Bone marrow biopsy may be necessary to rule out MDSs and malignancy, since these disorders may present with peripheral megaloblastosis.

C. **Anemia of chronic disease** is usually mild in degree and not progressive, with the hematocrit (hct) rarely falling below 25%, except in renal failure. The peripheral blood smear shows normochromic, normocytic red blood cells, low reticulocyte production, low or normal serum iron, and total iron-binding capacity usually <250 mg/dL. The RDW is usually normal. Reticuloendothelial iron stores are usually adequate, and serum ferritin levels are >50 ng/mL. Bone marrow iron is normal or increased. Serum erythropoietin levels are reduced in inflammatory disorders. The marrow is usually hypocellular, with decreased myeloid precursors. Serum protein electrophoresis should be ordered if the erythrocyte sedimentation rate is high or serum globulin levels are elevated.

D. **MDSs** are usually associated with cytopenias involving one or more cell lines. The anemia is usually normocytic, serum iron and transferrin levels are normal, and reticulocyte counts are low (reflecting decreased marrow production). A frequent finding in MDSs is an increase in numbers of monocytes, also found in patients with chronic myelomonocytic leukemia.

E. In **sideroblastic anemia,** there is moderate microcytic anemia (hct, 20–30%), increased serum iron and serum ferritin levels, with a significant number of ringed sideroblasts, and increased marrow iron stores. The peripheral blood smear shows a dimorphic population of red blood cells (normal and hypochromic).

F. **Hemolytic anemia.** The cardinal diagnostic feature of hemolytic anemia is the presence of significant reticulocytosis. This can be determined by calculating the reticulocyte production index (RPI), which corrects the reticulocyte count for the lower erythrocyte concentration and for the longer maturation time of these immature cells,

$$RPI = \frac{Reticulocytes}{Maturation\ time} + \frac{Observed\ hct}{45}$$

where 45% is used as a normal hct, and maturation time equals 1 day at hct of 45%, 1.5 days at hct of 35%, 2 days at hct of 25%, 2.5 days at hct of 15%, etc. If the RPI is >3, hemolytic anemia is likely; if it is <2.5, hemolytic anemia is unlikely.

1. In **extravascular hemolysis,** serum indirect bilirubin is elevated. In brisk hemolysis, conjugated bilirubin may also rise. Severe hemolysis elevates plasma hemoglobin concentrations, at times high enough to give the plasma a brown color. Plasma haptoglobin levels become diminished, and hemoglobinuria and hemosiderinuria ensue. In sustained and severe hemolytic anemia, nucleated red blood cells may enter the circulation.

2. **Immunohemolysis** is diagnosed based on the presence of autogenous antibodies or complement attached to the patient's red blood cells. Human antibody coating the red blood cell surface is detected with the direct Coombs' test. Circulating antibody to red blood cells is detectable with the indirect Coombs' test. Cold agglutinins will be found in patients with immune hemolysis due to cold-reactive antibodies.

3. **Sickle cell anemia** and the other hemoglobinopathies may be diagnosed by hemoglobin electrophoresis. Hemoglobin S will usually make up 85–95% of hemoglobin, and in homozygous S disease, no hemoglobin A will be present. Hemoglobin levels range between 5 and 10 g/dL, and neutrophil and platelet counts are frequently elevated. The blood smear in patients with sickle cell anemia shows sickle cells, Howell-Jolly bodies, reticulocytosis, and usually high white blood cell and platelet counts. Elevated levels of hemoglobin A_2 on hemoglobin electrophoresis and a positive family history of thalassemia are characteristic of sickle-β-thalassemia.

4. The **thalassemias** are characterized by a peripheral smear showing hypochromia and microcytosis with basophilic stippling. This condition may be confused with iron deficiency anemia; however, patients with iron deficiency anemia have a reduced red blood cell count, an elevated RDW, and reduced serum iron, whereas patients with β-thalassemia minor have normal or minimally reduced red blood cell counts, profound microcytosis, normal serum iron, and normal RDW. Patients with β-thalassemia will have increased levels of hemoglobin A_2 and hemoglobin F.

5. **Hereditary spherocytosis** is diagnosed by the finding of spherocytes and reticulocytes on the smear. The Coombs' test is negative, and the MCHC is elevated. Confirmation of the diagnosis is made by the 24-hour osmotic fragility test.

6. The **microhemangiopathic hemolytic anemias** are characterized by hemoglobinemia, hemoglobinuria, and fragmented red blood cells, helmet cells, and schistocytes on the peripheral smear.

VIII. **Treatment.** The only indication for red blood cell transfusion is to increase oxygen-carrying capacity in anemic patients. Among patients who have lost blood, transfusion may be indicated when hemoglobin levels are <8 g/dL or <10 g/dL if patients have symptomatic coronary or cerebrovascular disease. Transfusion should not be used to expand volume, enhance wound healing, or improve general well-being.

A. **Iron deficiency anemia** can usually be treated by correcting the cause of blood loss. **Iron preparations** such as **ferrous sulfate, ferrous gluconate, ferrous fumarate,** or polysaccharide-iron complexes (ferric polymaltose) can be used to replenish iron deficiency. The usual dose is 100–200 mg of elemental iron daily (ferrous sulfate, 325 mg, three times a day). Reticulocytosis should follow within a few days, and a rise in hemoglobin of 2 g/dL should occur within 3 weeks. Therapy should continue for a period of 6 months to replenish iron stores.

1. Approximately 10% of patients experience unpleasant GI side effects such as nausea, vomiting, epigastric pain, abdominal cramps, diarrhea, and constipation. To minimize these symptoms, the patient should begin taking one

tablet a day with meals, and the dose should be gradually increased. Ferrous gluconate, ferrous fumarate, and ferric polymaltose are less likely to cause GI side effects but are more expensive than ferrous sulfate.

2. Failure to respond to iron therapy is usually the result of noncompliance. Other reasons for failure to respond include incorrect diagnosis (eg, anemia of chronic disease or thalassemia), ongoing GI blood loss, or, rarely, poor absorption.

B. Anemia of chronic disease. There is no specific treatment other than that indicated for the underlying illness. Recombinant erythropoietin should be considered for all patients with anemia of renal failure, patients undergoing chemotherapy, or acquired immunodeficiency syndrome (AIDS) patients in whom AZT treatment may have to be discontinued because of anemia. Patients with multiple myeloma, malignancy, rheumatoid arthritis, and others with anemia of chronic disease have benefited from treatment with erythropoietin. An additive deficiency state will worsen the anemia; however, in the absence of a specific deficiency state, treatment with iron, vitamin B_{12}, and folic acid is useless.

C. Vitamin B_{12} or folate deficiency. Patients with confirmed vitamin B_{12} deficiency secondary to pernicious anemia must be given B_{12} therapy for the duration of their lives. The initial dosage should be 100 µg/day for the first week, then 100 µg twice weekly until hematologic values return to normal (or if neurologic complications exist for at least 6 months), then 100 µg monthly for life. Folic acid is given by mouth, usually in a dose of 1 mg/day for folate deficiency.

D. Hemolytic anemia. Consultation with a hematologist is usually indicated. Treatment should be directed toward removing the underlying cause if possible. If drugs are implicated, they should be discontinued. Patients with sickle cell anemia and the thalassemias should be referred for genetic counseling.

1. **Autoimmune hemolytic anemia (AIHA)** often responds to a regimen that includes steroids, immunosuppression, and sometimes splenectomy. Intravenous immunoglobulin is effective for severe life-threatening warm-antibody AIHA. Cold-antibody AIHA is managed by avoidance of cold temperatures and plasmaphoresis. Blood transfusions should be avoided in the presence of hemolysis.

2. Treatment of **sickle cell crises** consists of rest, hydration, and analgesia. Oral fluids (400 mL/h), oxygen, and 60 mg of oral morphine sulfate may avert admission to the hospital. If pain control cannot be achieved in 8 hours, hospital admission is indicated. Patients should be maintained chronically on folic acid supplements. Transfusions should be reserved for aplastic or hemolytic crises and for patients in the third trimester of pregnancy. Patients with sickle cell disease should be immunized with the pneumococcal vaccine and infections should be treated early and aggressively. Antibiotic prophylaxis with penicillin should be given to children between the ages of 2 months and 5 years because of the high risk of pneumococcal infection. Regular ophthalmologic examination should be done because of a high incidence of retinopathy. No treatment is required for patients with sickle trait.

3. Therapy for **ß-thalassemia** major involves aggressive transfusion aimed at keeping the hemoglobin level at about 12 g/dL, thus avoiding complications of cardiac failure, fluid overload, and skeletal abnormalities. Iron chelation may be required. Patients should take folic acid daily. Where feasible, bone marrow transplantation should be considered. ß-Thalassemia minor requires no specific therapy.

E. The treatment of **MDSs** involves transfusion and supportive care. Many patients benefit from combinations of erythropoietin, colony-stimulating factor, and immunosuppressant agents.

F. In patients with **sideroblastic anemia,** the offending drug or toxin should be eliminated. Most patients should be given a trial of **pyridoxine phosphate.** Occasionally, patients have been found to respond to combinations of pyridoxine (100–200 mg/day) and folate (1 mg/day). Elderly patients should be transfused with packed red blood cells when their hct falls below 25%, to prevent cardiorespiratory complications. Transfusions should be kept to a minimum, as they may exacerbate the already present iron-overloaded state.

REFERENCES

Ania BJ, Suman VJ, Fairbanks VF, et al: Prevalence of anemia in medical practice: Community vs. referral patients. Mayo Clin Proc 1994;**69**:730.

Biaggioni I, Robertson D, Krantz S, et al: The anemia of primary autonomic failure and its reversal with recombinant erythropoietin. Ann Intern Med 1994;**121**(3):181.

Carmel R: Pernicious anemia—The expected findings of very low serum cobalamin levels, anemia, and macrocytosis are often lacking. Arch Intern Med 1988;**148**:1712.

Francis RB Jr, Johnson CS: Vascular occlusion in sickle cell disease: Current concepts and unanswered questions. Blood 1991;**77**:1405.

Krantz SB: Pathogenesis and treatment of the anemia of chronic disease. Am J Med Sci 1994;**307**(5):353.

Means RT: Clinical application of recombinant erythropoietin in the anemia of chronic disease. Hematol/Oncol Clin North Am 1994;**8**:935.

Pruthi RK, Tefferi A: Subspecialty clinics: Hematology, pernicious anemia revisited. Mayo Clin Proc 1994;**69**:144.

Ridley DM, Dawkins F, Perlin E: Erythropoietin: A review. J Natl Med Assoc 1994;**86**:129.

San Miguel JF, Sanz GF, Vallespi T, et al: Myelodysplastic syndromes. Crit Rev Oncol Hematol 1996;**23**(1):57.

Savage DG, Lindenbaum J, Stabler SP, et al: Sensitivity of serum methylmalonic acid and total homocysteine determinations for diagnosing cobalamin and folate deficiencies. Am J Med 1994;**96**:239.

Timiras M-L, Brownstein H: Prevalence of anemia and correlation of hemoglobin with age in a geriatric screening clinic population. J Am Geriatr Soc 1987;**35**:639.

Welch HG, Meehan KR, Goodnough LT: Prudent strategies for elective red blood cell transfusion. Ann Intern Med 1992;**116**:393.

---

7   Ankle Injuries

Richard B. Birrer, MD

I. **Definition.** Ankle injuries involve trauma to the bony or soft tissue structures of the ankle.

II. **Common diagnoses**
   A. **Sprains** (85% of all ankle injuries).
   B. **Strains** (5% of all ankle injuries).
   C. **Tenosynovitis** (5% of all ankle injuries).
   D. **Contusions** (<5% of all ankle injuries).
   E. **Fractures** (<5% of all ankle injuries).

III. **Epidemiology.** Ankle injuries account for 0.5% of visits in the primary care ambulatory setting.
   A. **Sprains** are particularly common in individuals who play basketball, volleyball, football, or racquetball. Between 10% and 15% of all ankle sprains involve the medial compartment, and this is usually a more serious injury than a lateral sprain.
   B. **Strains** are common in persons who engage in explosive activities, such as track and field events. These injuries result from overuse of the muscle-tendon unit, particularly in endurance running, dancing, or gymnastics.
   C. **Tenosynovitis** most often occurs in individuals who are running, jumping, dancing, or cycling. This condition results from a direct blow or overuse with repetitive overloads and faulty technique.
   D. **Contusions** involving the ankle are significantly underreported and occur in persons who participate in contact sports. Such injuries also result from faulty footwear and poor field conditions.
   E. **Fractures** are more common than sprains in prepubertal children. They occur most frequently in persons who engage in high-velocity, high-impact sports (eg, football, soccer, skiing, hockey, or automobile racing).
      1. Stress fractures occur in running, gymnastics, or dancing.
      2. Salter type I and II fractures of the fibula are the most common ankle injuries in children.

IV. Pathophysiology

A. Sprains. Forceful inversion of the foot causes two types of sprains.

1. Lateral ligament sprain and sequential tearing of anterior talofibular, calcaneofibular, and posterior talofibular ligaments.
2. Medical compartment sprains and sequential tearing of the superficial deltoid ligament (tibionavicular), anteromedial capsule, anterior deep deltoid component, anterior tibiofibular ligaments, interosseus membrane, and remaining superficial and deep components.

B. Strains. Sudden and explosive or chronic stress causes partial or complete tearing of the muscle-tendon unit.

C. Tenosynovitis. Inflammation of the synovial sheath and peritendon occurs following a direct blow or overuse microtrauma.

D. Contusions. Capillary rupture, infiltrative bleeding, edema, and inflammation of the underlying tissue and bone occur.

E. Fracture. There are four basic injury mechanisms for fractures (Table 7–1). Lateral displacement of the talus (type A) is the most common, followed by medial displacement of the talus (type B), axial compression of the talus (type C), and repetitive microtrauma (type D).

V. Symptoms

A. Painful injuries that affect weight-bearing ability may be sprains.

1. Grade 1 sprains, which are microtears involving 20–30% of the ligament, cause minimal pain and disability. Weight bearing is not impaired.
2. Grade 2 sprains, which are microtears involving 25–75% of the ligament, cause moderate pain and disability. Weight bearing is difficult in such cases.
3. Grade 3 sprains, which are microtears involving >75% of the ligament, cause severe swelling, pain, and discoloration. Weight bearing is impossible.

B. The **location of pain** provides a clue to the diagnosis of **strains.**

TABLE 7–1. PATHOPHYSIOLOGY OF COMMON ANKLE INJURIES

Mechanism of Injury	Injury Examples
Lateral displacement	
Eversion with supinated ankle	Rupture of anterior inferior tibiofibular ligament, spiral oblique fracture of the fibula, posterior malleolar fracture, medial malleolar fracture, or deltoid ligament rupture
Eversion with pronated ankle	Rupture of deltoid ligament or fracture of medial malleolus, spiral fracture of fibula 2–3 inches above the top of the interosseus membrane, avulsion fracture of posterior malleolus, tear of interosseus membrane, in children (eg, type II or IV Salter fracture of tibia)
Adduction with pronated ankle	Fracture of medial malleolus or rupture of deltoid ligament, rupture of anterior inferior ligament, oblique fracture of distal fibula, posterior malleolar fracture
Adduction with dorsiflexed or plantar-flexed ankle	Medial malleolar fracture or tibiofibular diastases, medial or lateral osteochondral fractures
Medial displacement	
Inversion, plantar flexion, and adduction	Sequential tearing of the anchor talofibular, calcaneofibular, and posterior talofibular ligaments, avulsion fracture of the distal fibula, and transverse fracture of the medial malleolus
Adduction with supinated ankle	Avulsion of lateral malleolus or rupture of talofibular ligament, vertical fracture of the medial malleolus, in children (eg, type I or II Salter fracture of fibula, type III [Tilaux] or N of medial malleolus)
Axial compression of the talus	Impaction fracture, marginal fractures, tibiofibular diastases
Repetitive microtrauma	Medial osteochondral fractures or distal fibular stress fractures

1. Posterior pain on ambulation indicates a strain of the Achilles tendon.
2. Pain at the posterior interior medial malleolus suggests a strain of the tibialis posterior tendon.
3. A painful anterior tibia and ankle and medial foot indicate a strain of the tibialis anterior tendon.
4. Posterior inferior lateral malleolar pain suggests a strain of the peroneal tendons.

C. **Pain and swelling over the affected tendon indicate tenosynovitis.**
D. A **painful lump** may be caused by a **contusion.**
E. **Abrupt moderate to severe pain and swelling.** Immediate disability and discoloration and a patient report of an audible "pop" or crack indicate **acute fracture.** Patients with **chronic fracture** typically present with a history of a "sprained" ankle that resists all treatment, dull ache with slight swelling after excessive walking, increased pain with activity, and complete relief with rest.

VI. **Signs** (Table 7–2)
  A. **Tenderness, swelling, and associated findings**
  1. **Grade 1 sprains** of the lateral compartment result in slight tenderness and swelling over the ligaments and no laxity. Anterior drawer and talar tilt tests are negative. Medial compartment sprains cause tenderness and swelling over the deltoid ligament, no laxity, and slight pain with stress.
  2. **Grade 2 sprains** of the lateral compartment produce moderate tenderness and edema, hemarthrosis (40–50% of cases), and ecchymosis (30–40% of cases). Anterior drawer and talar tilt test results are positive. Medial compartment sprains cause tenderness and swelling over the ligament on eversion, as well as ecchymosis.
  3. **Grade 3 sprains** of the lateral compartment typically produce pronounced edema, loss of function, and severe pain, but may be painless. Hemarthrosis occurs in 80–90% of cases, and ecchymosis is present in 60–70% of cases. Anterior drawer and talar tilt test results are positive. Medial compartment grade 3 sprains cause diffuse swelling, tenderness, ecchymosis, and a positive talar tilt.
  4. **Sprains of syndesmosis** suggested by positive compression test (squeezing the midthird of the calf).
  B. **Crepitus ("packed snow" sensation)** over the involved tendon indicates a **strain.** Additional specific findings include the following signs.
  1. Positive Thomas-Doherty squeeze test (Table 7–2) in Achilles tendon strain.
  2. Loss of medial longitudinal arch height and forefoot abduction in tibialis posterior tendon strain.
  3. Weakness or loss of foot elevation with tibialis anterior tendon strain.
  4. Weakness of eversion and dorsiflexion in strain of the peroneal tendons.
  C. **Tenderness, thickening, erythema, crepitus, edema, weakness,** and **nodule formation** are signs of tenosynovitis.
  D. **Tenderness, ecchymosis,** and **edema,** particularly over the malleolus, are evidence of contusions.
  E. **Localized** or point **tenderness, edema,** and possible **crepitus and ecchymosis** are signs of an acute fracture. Abnormal osteophony (ie, loss of sound trans-

TABLE 7–2. MANEUVERS IMPORTANT IN EXAMINING THE INJURED ANKLE

Maneuver[1]	Findings
Anterior drawer test, which involves drawing the calcaneus and talus anteriorly while stabilizing the tibia	3–14 mm indicates grade 2 sprain; >15 mm indicates grade 3 sprain
Talar tilt test, which involves stressing the ankle laterally (inversion) and medially (eversion) while stabilizing the patient's leg	5- to 10-degree difference between ankles indicates grade 2 sprain; >10-degree difference indicates grade 3 sprain
Thomas-Doherty squeeze test, which involves squeezing the midthird of the calf with the knee flexed 90 degrees	Loss of plantar flexion with Achilles tendon rupture

[1]The anterior drawer, talar tilt, and stress tests can be facilitated by joint block. Lidocaine, 5–10 mL, is infiltrated into the joint opposite the side of injury and around the injured ligaments if necessary.

mission) may also occur. In chronic fractures, the physical examination is usually negative, except for point tenderness over the distal fibula (stress fracture) or on the talar dome with ankle plantar flexion (osteochondral fracture).

VII. Laboratory tests. Routine studies need not be performed if strains, tenosynovitis, and contusions are suspected.

  A. X-rays. X-rays are indicated if there is **pain near the malleoli** and any of the following findings.

    1. Bone tenderness at the tip of either malleolus or at the posterior edge of the malleoli.

    2. Inability to bear weight both immediately and in the emergency department (four steps).

    3. Stress films (ie, x-raying the ankle while applying varus or valgus stress) will be normal in grade 1 sprains. Such films will show a 5- to 10-degree tilt and 3- to 14-mm anterior displacement of the talus in grade 2 sprains and more than a 20-degree tilt with an anterior displacement of the talus of >15 mm in grade 3 sprains. Stress films should be performed to rule out associated ligamentous injury and joint instability if these findings are unclear from the physical examination.

    4. Comparing anteroposterior, lateral, oblique, and mortise views between affected and uninjured ankles demonstrates fracture fragments. **Mortise and oblique views** are useful for detecting **osteochondral fragments.** Routine films will not show stress fractures for the first 2–3 weeks following injury.

  B. Arthrography

    1. Arthrography is indicated in order to define the extent of damage. This technique is diagnostic for calcaneofibular tears (shown by extravasation of dye).

    2. Disadvantages of arthrography include expense, the need to schedule the procedure, allergic reactions to dye, and false-negative results several days after the injury. It should be used selectively in competitive athletes with significant disability.

  C. Computerized tomography (CT) and magnetic resonance imaging (MRI) are >80% sensitive and specific in detecting soft tissue damage. These tests are recommended for locating fragments and determining the percentage of joint surface involved in osteochondral fractures. Compared to arthrography, CT and MRI have a greater predictive value and better patient acceptance.

  D. Bone scans are helpful in detecting **stress fractures** in individuals with suggestive symptoms and normal plain films.

VIII. Treatment

  A. Sprains

    1. Management of **acute injuries**

      a. It is best to err on the conservative side when diagnosing the severity of a sprain and to be on the liberal side when treating and rehabilitating a sprain. Orthopedic consultation is recommended for grade 3 injuries and repeated sprains of any degree.

      b. Rest, ice, compression, and elevation (RICE) posterior splint or aircast; and non–weight-bearing activities may be useful in treating sprains. Non-steroidal anti-inflammatory drugs (NSAIDs) (eg, ibuprofen, 400–800 mg every 6–8 hours with food) and analgesics (eg, acetaminophen, 650 mg every 4–6 hours) should be given until edema and pain subside.

    2. Long-term management

      a. Grade 1 sprains should be immobilized in a weight-bearing brace or cast for 2–3 weeks, followed by strapping, bracing, or both for another 2–3 weeks.

      b. Grade 2 lateral ligament sprains should be immobilized for 2–4 weeks in a well-padded dorsiflexion walking cast, Unna boot, weight-bearing brace, or air cast. This should be followed by strapping at 90 degrees for 2–4 weeks. Severely swollen limbs should not be placed in a cast.

      c. Surgical repair is indicated for **grade 2 and 3 medial sprains.** Orthopedic consultation is also indicated for **grade 3 lateral sprains,** since the best approach (surgery versus immobilization) is unclear.

      d. Isometric **exercises** should be done for 15–20 minutes three times daily while the cast is in place. Range of motion (ROM), progressive resistance exercises (PRE) (ie, progressive muscle loading with weights), isometrics or isokinetics, proprioceptive exercises (with a balance or wobble board), and functional activity should be performed for 15–20 minutes three times daily following brace or cast removal.

3. **Prevention** of injury or reinjury involves the following measures.
   a. Using a **conditioning program** for the peroneal muscles that includes both isometric and isotonic exercises, emphasizing eversion and dorsiflexion.
   b. Teaching players to land with a relatively **wide-based stance.**
   c. **Taping, strapping, or bracing** previously injured ankles as well as uninjured ones.
   d. Using an **outer heel wedge** to avoid lateral sprains.
   e. Coordination training on a **balance board.**
   f. **Strengthening** of posteromedial muscles to prevent medial sprains.
   g. Using an **inner heel wedge** to avoid medial sprains.

B. **Strains** should be managed as described above for sprains (see section VIII,A).

C. **Tenosynovitis**
   1. **Initial treatment** includes **RICE, NSAIDs, and analgesics** as needed. **Injection of a corticosteroid** (eg, methylprednisolone acetate, 4 mg, with an equal volume of 1–2% lidocaine [Xylocaine]) may be helpful. This treatment is contraindicated in Achilles tendinitis, in the presence of infection, or if the patient has received a similar injection within the past 4 weeks or has a history of more than three such injections.
   2. **Long-term management** includes application of a **short leg, non–weight-bearing cast, or protective strapping for 1–3 weeks.** ROM and PRE should be used for 1–3 weeks after cast removal (see section VIII,A,2,d).
   3. **Surgical consultation** is indicated in cases of refractory pain and disability that are unresponsive to conservative therapy. Tenolysis and debridement may prove helpful in such cases.

D. **Contusions** should be treated with **RICE and PRE.** Large hematomas should be aspirated and protected from further injury with foam and felt padding.

E. **Fractures**
   1. **Initial management** of all fractures includes **RICE, NSAIDs, and analgesics** as needed. A **posterior splint** should be used, and no weight bearing should be permitted until pain and swelling subside. Consultation is advised for unstable, epiphyseal, and osteochondral fractures.
   2. **Long-term management** of stable fractures includes a neutral, positioned **walking cast for 4–6 weeks. Rehabilitation** includes 2–4 weeks of ROM, PRE, and proprioceptive and functional exercises, as already described for ankle sprains (see section VIII,A,2,d).

REFERENCES

Baldini C, et al: Management and rehabilitation of ligamentous injuries to the ankle. Sports Med 1987;**4**:364.

Birrer RB: Ankle injuries and the family physician. J Am Board Fam Pract 1988;**1**:274.

Keeno JS, Lange RH: Diagnosis dilemmas in foot and ankle injures. JAMA 1986;**256**:247.

Molnar ME: Rehabilitation of the injured ankle. Clin Sports Med 1988;**7**:193.

Nemeth VA, Thrasher E: Adhesive strapping techniques. Clin Sports Med 1983;**2**:217.

Rijke AM, Jones B, Vierhout PA: Injury to the lateral ankle ligaments of athletes. Am J Sports Med 1988;**16**:256.

Smith RW, Rerschl SF: Treatment of ankle sprains in young athletes. Am J Sports Med 1986; **14**:465.

Stiell IG, Greenberg GH, McKnight RD, et al: Decision rules for the use of radiography in acute ankle injuries: Refinement and prospective validation. JAMA 1993;**269**:1127.

---

8   Arm & Shoulder Pain

Richard Viken, MD

I. **Definition.** Arm and shoulder pain is localized or generalized discomfort in the upper extremity.

II. **Common diagnoses.** See the chapters indicated for the following causes of arm and shoulder pain: fibromyalgia (Chapter 48); rheumatoid arthritis, osteoarthritis, and gout

(Chapter 71); cervical disk disease (Chapter 50); and thoracic outlet syndrome and carpal tunnel syndrome (Chapter 53).
   A. **Impingement syndrome.**
   B. **Glenohumeral instability.**
   C. **Cubital tunnel syndrome.**
   D. **Lateral epicondylitis.**
   E. **Medial epicondylitis.**
   F. **Olecranon bursitis.**
III. **Epidemiology.** The exact prevalence of arm and shoulder pain is unknown, but the complaints of such pain are very common in primary care practice. The various types of this pain are described below.
   A. **Impingement syndrome** is the most common cause of shoulder pain in the over-40 age group, affecting men and women, as well as dominant and nondominant arms, with equal frequency. In the older population, intrinsic degenerative factors involving bone and tendon are the principal causes. In the younger, more active population, trauma, overuse, and poor training technique are primary sources of the problem.
   B. **Glenohumeral instability** occurs most commonly in the anterior direction, less so in the posterior and inferior directions. Some patients have multidirectional instability. Predisposing factors include active participation in throwing activities and inherent "double jointedness," or capsular laxity.
   C. **Cubital tunnel syndrome,** or entrapment of the ulnar nerve at the elbow, is the most common cause of ulnar nerve compression. It ranks just behind carpal tunnel syndrome as the most common peripheral compression neuropathy. The condition may result from a direct blow to the elbow or from activities that involve repetitive elbow flexion and extension (eg, those performed by carpenters, painters, or switchboard operators) or prolonged elbow flexion (eg, those by string musicians or jewelers). Patients with diabetes or alcoholism are at increased risk for this condition.
   D. **Lateral epicondylitis,** also called "tennis elbow," is a common cause of elbow pain in adults. It is associated with repeated extension of the wrist and pronation/supination of the forearm, particularly against resistance. Repeated actions such as turning screws, hammering nails, turning doorknobs, opening jars, and shaking hands may lead to this condition. It commonly develops in individuals between 40 and 60 years of age.
   E. **Medial epicondylitis** is much less common than the lateral form. It occurs in adults of all ages and is associated with activities that involve repetitive flexion of the wrist. This condition has been called "golfer's elbow," to indicate a common predisposing activity.
   F. **Olecranon bursitis** is less frequent than lateral epicondylitis as a cause of elbow pain. It is most common in middle-aged men and is usually secondary to repeated mild trauma that is often occupationally related. This condition may be secondary to involvement of the bursa by rheumatoid arthritis, crystal deposition disease (gout or pseudogout), or infection.
IV. **Pathophysiology**
   A. **Impingement syndrome** reflects degenerative changes in the components of the subacromial space: the acromioclavicular joint, the rotator cuff tendons, the subacromial bursa, and the biceps tendon. Recent studies further implicate malfunction of the pericapsular and glenohumeral muscular units. These changes are brought on by repetitive use of the arm in a position above the horizontal plane, which impinges the above structures between the humeral head and the acromion. A progressive syndrome of acute bursal swelling, chronic tendon thickening, and eventual tearing of avascular portions of the rotator cuff ensues. The untreated process results in glenohumeral joint effusion, instability, and arthropathy.
   B. **Glenohumeral instability** reflects the inherent instability of the shoulder joint, ranging from mild to extensive. With a subluxation, the humeral head slips partially out of the glenoid fossa. With a dislocation, the head slips completely off the glenoid, so that the articular surfaces are not touching. Two acronyms—TUBS and AMBRI—are used to characterize unstable shoulders, depending on whether an injury caused the instability. TUBS signifies an instability that is **t**raumatic, **u**nidirectional, associated with a **B**ankart lesion (detachment of the anterior capsule and labrum from the glenoid rim), and requires **s**urgical treatment. AMBRI

indicates an **a**traumatic condition that is **m**ultidirectional, and **b**ilateral and that usually responds to rehabilitation, but may need an inferior capsular surgical procedure.

C. The **cubital tunnel,** through which the ulnar nerve courses, is formed by the two heads of the flexor carpi ulnaris connected by a fibrous arch, the arcuate ligament. A decrease in tunnel size—as may occur with trauma-induced changes in musculoligamentous anatomy, the development of osteophytes, and the presence of ganglia or lipomas—is thought to be a cause of ulnar nerve compression. Another suggestion is that repetitive elbow motion may initiate a cycle of inflammation and edema, producing additional compressive forces on the nerve, amplified by its superficial location. Finally, 10–16% of the healthy population may be victims of idiopathic, recurrent ulnar nerve subluxation. Discussions of metabolic neuropathy are found in the chapters on diabetes mellitus (Chapter 78) and alcoholism (Chapter 92).

D. **Lateral epicondylitis.** In most cases, the exact pathophysiology of lateral epicondylitis is uncertain, but this condition is thought to involve inflammation of a tendon, periosteum, or ligament.

E. **Medial epicondylitis.** The pathophysiology of this condition is thought to involve inflammation of the tendons that insert into the medial epicondyle of the elbow.

F. **Olecranon bursitis** is an inflammation of the olecranon bursa, a synovium-lined space between the olecranon process and the skin. Under normal conditions, this bursa contains only a drop or two of synovial fluid. With inflammation, fluid volume increases and the bursa may become very swollen and painful.

V. Symptoms

A. **Impingement syndrome** produces pain with overhead motion in the presence of a full, or near-full, passive range of motion. Pain may radiate to the insertion of the deltoid muscle. Associated symptoms include nocturnal pain, pain on combing the hair or reaching up behind the back, and trapezius spasm. Arm weakness and clicking or popping as the arm is raised suggest a rotator cuff tear.

B. **Glenohumeral instability**

    1. **Traumatic instability** usually involves a single event that tears the anterior glenohumeral ligament complex, such as a fall on an outstretched arm or striking an arm as it is cocked to throw a football. Forced abduction, extension, and external rotation levers the humeral head out of the glenoid, depositing it anteroinferiorly beneath the coracoid. The patient holds the arm in abduction and external rotation, supported by the uninjured hand. Attempts to adduct or internally rotate the arm cause pain. The rarer posterior dislocation occurs with either a direct blow to the anterior shoulder or forced adduction, flexion, and internal rotation. The humeral head vacates the glenoid through a disrupted posterior capsule and reestablishes itself in a subacromial position. The patient holds the arm firmly across the chest, resisting painful attempts at abduction and external rotation.

    2. **Atraumatic instability,** a reflection of generalized ligamentous laxity, usually prompts patients to report that their shoulder "slips out of joint." Painless, often bilateral, subluxations among these patients are common, as are frank dislocations, with many of the latter voluntarily induced. Pain, when present, is most often a vague, persistent glenohumeral ache; or it may consist of intermittent flares similar to those of impingement syndrome. Episodes of activity-induced paralyzing pain followed by a sensation of numbness and a period of weakness, termed the "dead arm" syndrome, are highly suggestive of shoulder instability.

C. **Cubital tunnel syndrome** presents with tingling and numbness of the small and ring fingers, often at night, loss of hand coordination, decreased grip and pinch strength, and tenderness along the medial aspect of the elbow. Symptoms usually begin insidiously unless acute trauma is a factor.

D. **Lateral epicondylitis.** The most common complaint is pain in the elbow with radiation into the forearm that is produced or exacerbated by wrist extension, by gripping an object, or by forearm supination.

E. **Medial epicondylitis.** Pain is localized medially over the elbow with radiation into the forearm and exacerbation by flexion of the wrist.

F. **Olecranon bursitis.** Pain and swelling are localized to the posterior part of the elbow. The onset may be acute or gradual. A history of repeated mild trauma to the olecranon is frequently present. Occasionally, systemic symptoms such as fever, chills, or weakness are present.

VI. Signs

A. The most reliable finding in **impingement syndrome** is elicitation of pain by forcibly flexing and internally rotating the arm, while manually stabilizing the scapula (a positive "impingement sign"). A "painful arc" can be produced by having the patient slowly lower the arm in the scapular plane from 180 degrees of forward elevation. Pain occurs in the 60- to 120-degree range and is accentuated by resistance to abduction. The size of the painful arc correlates with the amount of impingement. Other positive signs include tenderness to palpation over the entire shoulder, the subdeltoid bursa, the acromioclavicular joint, and the biceps tendon.

B. Glenohumeral instability

    1. Traumatic instability results in palpable displacement of the humeral head into the axilla with relative prominence of the acromion (anterior dislocation) or into the subdeltoid area with relative prominence of the coracoid process (posterior dislocation). Compromise of the axillary and musculocutaneous nerves is suggested by anesthesia over the lateral shoulder and radial aspect of the forearm, respectively, as is a loss of static contraction of the deltoid and biceps muscles.

    2. Atraumatic instability followed by spontaneous reduction frequently yields a normal examination. The Apprehension Test is useful after the initial episode of subluxation. The patient's relaxed arm should be moved into abduction and external rotation, as in a throwing position. If this maneuver elicits pain and a feeling of apprehension that the shoulder will slip out of joint again, the test is positive and indicates anterior instability. Recurrent dislocators have a blunted Apprehension Test and demonstrate generalized ligamentous laxity in many joints. These patients may show the ability to hyperextend their elbow or to touch their thumb to the volar surface of the forearm.

C. Palpation or gentle tapping over the **cubital tunnel** elicits pain around the medial elbow and tingling in the ring and small fingers (positive Tinel's sign). Long-standing ulnar nerve compression may cause intrinsic hand muscle wasting and impaired two-point discrimination. Anhydrosis, suggested by dry, pale skin over the ring and small fingers, indicates chronic nerve irritation.

D. Lateral epicondylitis. Tenderness and occasionally swelling are present over the lateral epicondyle. Wrist extension against resistance reproduces the pain.

E. Medial epicondylitis. Tenderness and occasionally swelling are localized over the medial epicondyle, and pain is often exacerbated by flexion of the wrist.

F. Olecranon bursitis. A tender and frequently tense collection of fluid is noted over the olecranon, and the skin is often erythematous. Extension of the elbow is unimpaired and not painful; extreme flexion may be limited by pain produced by stretching of the inflamed bursa. When septic bursitis occurs, fever and generalized malaise may be present, although these signs are frequently absent with septic bursitis.

VII. Laboratory tests

A. Plain radiography of the shoulder can be helpful in locating a mechanical source for impingement syndrome. Sclerosis or spur formation, causing anatomic narrowing of the subacromial space, may be seen on the undersurface of the anterior acromion. Large tears of the rotator cuff may demonstrate a decrease in the acromiohumeral interval, a finding amplified by stress views, in which active deltoid contraction causes superior humeral migration, normally prevented by the head-depressing function on an intact cuff. **X-rays** may demonstrate soft tissue calcification just inferior to the acromion in patients with subacromial bursitis. Pre-reduction and postreduction (see section VIII,E,2) shoulder radiographs should be obtained in all patients with suspected traumatic dislocation. True anteroposterior, axillary, and scapular Y views will confirm the direction of the dislocation. More subtle lesions, such as a Bankart lesion or a humeral head impression fracture (Hill-Sachs lesion) may be evaluated by other radiographic views usually ordered preoperatively by an orthopedic surgeon. **X-ray of the elbow** is indicated when trauma has occurred prior to onset of cubital tunnel syndrome or olecranon bursitis, in order to identify fracture, malalignment, or osteomyelitis as possible contributing factors.

B. **Glenohumeraᵢ arthrography** has 95% diagnostic accuracy for rotator cuff tears, if contrast material enters the subacromial space. Patients older than 35 years with traumatic instability are candidates for arthrography to look for rotator cuff tears associated with dislocation.

C. Ulnar **nerve compression studies** showing a reduction in velocity of 30% or more suggest significant compression.

D. **Aspiration** of the bursa using sterile technique is indicated in patients suspected of having olecranon bursitis to assess the possibility of infection. The fluid should be gram-stained and cultured. Examination of aspirated fluid under the polarizing microscope may confirm a diagnosis of crystal deposition disease (see Chapter 71).

VIII. Treatment

A. **Conservative measures** are preferred initially in the management of most arm and shoulder disorders. Relative rest for a short period followed by supervised physical therapy is critical to effective rehabilitation. Patients should refrain from all activities that aggravate the pain. Ice packs should be applied for 20 minutes three or four times per day to painful or swollen areas. A sling may be used for comfort, but it should be removed three or four times during the day in order to perform gentle range-of-motion exercises such as **pendulum circles.** (While standing, the patient is instructed to lean over and face the floor, to let the sore arm dangle straight down, then draw circles in the air with the dangling arm, starting with small circles and working up to bigger ones for about 1 minute.) Because prolonge i immobilization is deleterious, **aggressive physical therapy** is most importan in treating these conditions. **Activity modification** to avoid repetitive trauma oɾ direct pressure to the olecranon is important in the resolution of olecranon bursitis. Patients with cubital tunnel syndrome should keep the elbow straight as much as is practical. Altering the work station or job description is often helpful.

B. **Strapping and splinting devices** may be used when persistent symptoms or inordinate pain accompany lateral and medial epicondylitis. Firm placement of a 2- to 3-inch Velcro band circumferentially around the proximal forearm effectively shortens the muscle length at the epicondylar level, resulting in less pull and strain with activity. Splinting the wrist in a position of function while awake accomplishes the same purpose. Patients with cubital tunnel syndrome may wear a nighttime elbow extension splint. A towel wrapped around the elbow is an inexpensive alternative. A sports elbow protector worn at work may prevent unexpected trauma.

C. **Systemic analgesics** are an effective adjunct to conservative measures. Preferred agents are the nonsteroidal anti-inflammatory drugs (NSAIDs): **aspirin,** 650 mg every 4–6 hours; **ibuprofen,** 400–600 mg every 6–8 hours; or **naproxen,** 250–375 mg every 8–12 hours. A one-week "burst" of corticosteroids is often effective for an acute, severe episode of cubital tunnel syndrome. A typical dose of **prednisone** is 40–60 mg/day. It is not necessary to taper this dose over a short period, but many physicians prefer to do so.

D. **Injections** of combined corticosteroid-lidocaine preparations (20–40 mg of **triamcinolone acetonide** added to 1–2 mL of 1% **lidocaine**) may be very helpful when selectively placed in the subacromial bursa or around the biceps tendon. The substantial reduction of pain is not only therapeutic, but it also helps to confirm the diagnostic impression of impingement syndrome. A similar confirmation of medial or lateral epicondylitis can be expected following injections into painful areas surrounding the medial and lateral epicondyles. Direct injection into tendon or bone should be avoided, and no more than three injections should be given in a 12-month period.

E. **Surgical intervention**

1. Failed conservative therapy of impingement syndrome (6 months in the over-40 age group, 12 months at younger ages) is the indication for a **subacromial decompression procedure.** Any or all of the following may be accomplished either through the arthroscope or through an open incision: anterior acromioplasty, coracoacromial ligament release, acromioclavicular arthroplasty, rotator cuff repair, and biceps tendon repair. Surgical decompression of the cubital tunnel and transposition of the ulnar nerve is indicated for patients with muscle atrophy, persistent sensory changes, or other disabling symptoms that defy nonoperative measures.

   2. Orthopedic manipulation under controlled conscious sedation will successfully reduce most acute shoulder dislocations. Following the first dislocation, the shoulder should be protected in a sling with a torso strap for 3 weeks. Recurrent dislocators should begin range-of-motion exercises as soon as tolerated.
   3. Open reduction may be necessary in first-time shoulder dislocation if closed reduction is not achieved after a couple of good efforts. Other surgical indications are large bony glenoid fragments, a fractured humerus, vascular damage, or the appearance of significant peripheral nerve injury immediately after closed reduction.
   4. Surgical stabilization of the glenohumeral capsular structures should be considered in the TUBS patient if 6 months of conservative therapy fails to show clinical improvement. Surgery is discouraged in the AMBRI patient, because the underlying ligamentous laxity tends to stretch out the repair.
   5. An infected olecranon bursa should be treated with prompt **aspiration,** followed by a pressure dressing and 3 weeks of antibiotics (**dicloxacillin,** 250 mg by mouth four times daily; or **ciprofloxacin,** 750 mg by mouth twice daily). **Surgical excision of the bursa** is indicated for recurrence of septic bursitis or for a chronically draining and infected bursa, particularly when olecranon osteomyelitis is present.

REFERENCES

Belzer JP, Durkin RC: Common disorders of the shoulder. Prim Care 1996;**23:**365.
Bozentka DJ: Cubital tunnel syndrome pathophysiology. Clin Orthop 1998;**351:**90.
Daigneault J, Cooney LM: Shoulder pain in older people. J Am Geriatr Soc 1998;**46:**1144.
Fongemie AE, Buss DB, Rolnick SJ: Management of shoulder impingement syndrome and rotator cuff tears. Am Fam Physician 1998;**57:**667.
Johnson TR: Elbow and forearm. In Snider RK (editor): *Essentials of Musculoskeletal Care.* American Academy of Orthopaedic Surgeons; 1997:124.
Sykes TF: What to do for the painful shoulder. Patient Care 1997;**31:**56.

---

9   Bites & Stings

Brenda Powell Crownover, MD, & Louise S. Acheson, MD, MS

   I. Definition
   A. A **mammalian bite** is a skin wound caused by the teeth of a human or other mammal.
   B. An **insect or arachnid bite or sting** involves penetration of the skin by some part of the animal with release of substances that cause local or systemic symptoms.
   II. Common diagnoses. The majority of bites and stings that afflict humans in the United States are caused by the following animals.
   A. Mammals, including humans and other mammals, both domestic and wild.
   B. Insects, including diptera (eg, mosquitoes, flies, and gnats); fleas and bedbugs; hymenoptera (eg, bees, wasps, hornets, yellow jackets, and ants); and pubic, head, and body lice.
   C. Arachnids, including mites that cause scabies, chiggers, hard and soft ticks, and brown recluse and black widow spiders.
   D. Less common bites and stings not discussed in this chapter include **marine envenomations** and **snake bites** (see references at the end of the chapter for further discussion of these envenomations).
   III. Epidemiology. Human, animal, and many insect bites occur most frequently during spring and summer evenings. About 1 million animal bites require medical attention each year in the United States. Eighty percent to 90% of these are dog bites. Human bites, which constituted 3.6% of bites reported to the New York City Health Department in 1 year (1977), are less commonly treated by physicians. Lice, scabies, and Lyme disease are increasing in prevalence. Hymenoptera stings cause more deaths than any other venomous animal (six deaths per 100,000 people per year).

A. Mammalian bites

1. **Humans.** Bite injuries from fights are common in teenagers and in alcohol-intoxicated males aged 30–35. Accidental bites are most common in children. Abused and sheltered children and residents and staff members of institutions for the mentally retarded are at especially high risk for human bites.

2. **Other mammals.** Seventy-five percent of animal bites are considered "unprovoked." Sixty percent of all dog bites involve neighborhood pets, and half of dog bite victims are children under the age of 15. In the United States, rabies is found almost exclusively in unvaccinated domestic mammals and in wild mammals such as skunks, raccoons, and bats.

B. Insect bites

1. **Mosquitoes** breed in stagnant water during the warm season.

2. **Fleas and bedbugs. Flea bites** usually result from contact with cats or dogs. Fleas can be found in grass, rugs, upholstery, floor cracks, and pet bedding, especially during warm, humid months. **Bedbugs,** which feed nocturnally on mammals and birds, may survive in clothing, furniture, and bedding for 6–8 weeks without a blood meal.

3. **Hymenoptera. Bee and wasp stings** are common in suburbs and rural areas. The bites of **fire ants** are a significant problem in the southeastern United States.

4. **Lice. Pubic lice** are usually transmitted by close body contact and are rarely spread by fomites. **Head lice,** which are commonly transmitted by the exchange of hats, combs, and brushes, may also be spread by close personal contact. Epidemics occur in schools. **Body lice,** associated with poor hygiene, are rare.

C. Arachnid bites

1. **Mites. Scabies** (adult mites or eggs) are readily transmitted by personal contact, especially within families or in crowded living situations. **Chiggers,** which are prevalent in brush in the southern and midwestern United States, bite gardeners, hikers, and campers.

2. **Ticks.** These arachnids can be acquired by contact with pets, vegetation, or the burrows of host animals such as mice. Several human diseases are transmitted by ticks. Rocky Mountain spotted fever and tick-borne relapsing fever are endemic to the western mountain states. Tularemia from tick bites occurs mainly in western states. Lyme disease, which is endemic to semiwooded areas in New England, New York, and Wisconsin, occurs sporadically in the Midwest and the West.

3. **Spiders.** The bites of two spiders described below cause serious morbidity and result in about 5% of all deaths from contact with venomous animals.

   a. **Brown recluse spiders** are endemic to the south central United States. These spiders, which are active nocturnally, hide both indoors and outdoors. They bite humans only when disturbed.

   b. **Black widow spiders** are found throughout the United States and Canada. They nest outdoors in crevices near the ground, especially where flies are present (eg, outhouses).

IV. Pathophysiology

A. Mammalian bites

cause morbidity both by mechanical disruption of tissue and by introduction of pathogens. Wound infections from both human and animal bites usually contain a mixture of aerobic and anaerobic mouth flora.

Clenched fist injuries are the most serious type of human bite and usually occur in the dominant hand when a fist strikes a tooth. In clenched fist injuries, the metacarpophalangeal joint is in flexion, making it easier for a tooth to penetrate the joint capsule.

Human bites can transmit such diseases as hepatitis B and even syphilis. Rabies, a fatal viral encephalitis, can be acquired if the saliva, urine, or other secretions of an infected animal or person come into contact with mucous membranes or broken skin. The incubation period is 10 days to several months.

B. Insect bites

1. **Mosquito "bites"** are local hypersensitivity reactions to substances in the saliva of the insect. Although mosquitoes do spread malaria and encephalitis, there is no evidence that insects transmit human immunodeficiency virus (HIV).

    2. **Fleas and bedbugs** feed on blood. Repeated flea bites cause sensitization. Fleas can transmit plague and typhus, and bedbugs can spread hepatitis B.

    3. **Hymenoptera** (eg, vespids, bees, and ants) **venoms,** which contain a mixture of enzymes, peptides, acetylcholine, and histamine, can cause local and systemic symptoms directly or through immune hypersensitivity.

    4. **Lice** bites cause a delayed hypersensitivity reaction.

C. Arachnid bites

    1. **Mites**

       a. **Scabies.** These parasitic mites burrow into the epidermis and lay eggs. A delayed hypersensitivity reaction to mites and their feces causes pruritus and skin eruptions.

       b. **Chiggers (harvest mites).** These bites also cause an allergic reaction.

    2. **Ticks** attached to the skin release neurotoxins. Mouth parts embedded in the skin may cause a granuloma. Local infection may complicate tick bites. See Chapter 41 for a discussion of **Lyme disease. Rocky Mountain spotted fever** is caused by the parasite *Rickettsia rickettsii,* and **tularemia** is caused by the gram-negative coccobacillus *Francisella tularensis.*

    3. **Spiders**

       a. **Brown recluse spider bites** inject venom that causes local thrombosis, arteriolar spasm, and hemorrhagic necrosis extending outward from the bite. Although severe envenomation may cause disseminated intravascular coagulopathy and hemolysis, it is rarely fatal.

       b. **Black widow spider venom** is a neurotoxin that releases and depletes acetylcholine from nerve terminals. Five percent to 10% of these spider bites are fatal.

V. Symptoms

A. Skin wounds are the result of **mammalian bites.** Symptoms of **wound infection** include increasing pain, impaired movement or sensation, purulent discharge from the wound, fever, or malaise. Rabies begins with pain and numbness in the area of the bite, followed by fever, dysphagia, pharyngeal spasms ("hydrophobia"), paralysis, convulsions, and death.

B. Itching is a symptom of **mosquito, flea, bedbug, lice, mite, and tick bites.** The itching from lice begins about 21 days after infestation.

C. Intense pain follows the bites or stings of some **hymenoptera and arachnids. Systemic symptoms** of envenomation (with multiple stings or bites of **hymenoptera**) include nausea, vomiting, faintness, headache, fever, numbness, and muscle spasms. **Allergic reactions** range from slowly developing pruritus and swelling around the sting, to generalized pruritus, cough, sneezing, itchy eyes, to rapidly developing generalized urticaria, dyspnea, and collapse from anaphylactic shock. A **delayed hypersensitivity reaction (serum sickness)** with fever, arthralgias, and malaise may occur 10–14 days after the sting.

    A **brown recluse spider bite** is often unnoticed until local pain and itching begin. These are followed by skin and subcutaneous tissue necrosis that spreads from the site for 3–4 days. Systemic symptoms include headache, fever, chills, malaise, weakness, nausea, vomiting, and joint pains.

    The **black widow spider bite** is a mild prick, followed in 1–3 hours by severe, cramping pain at the bite site, spreading to adjacent parts of the body. Pain, cramps, anxiety, weakness, sweating, salivation, lacrimation, bronchorrhea, nausea, vomiting, and fever may subside in hours, but may recur for up to 3 days.

D. Initially painless, tick bites most often go unnoticed. The neurotoxin from a tick attached for 4–6 days can cause malaise, weakness, difficulty in swallowing, and involuntary movements of the eyes, which abate within hours after the tick is completely removed. Patients may present early in the course of **Lyme disease** with a flulike illness (see Chapter 41). Symptoms of **Rocky Mountain spotted fever,** including severe headache, nausea, vomiting, and abdominal pain, begin 3–12 days after a tick bite, followed 2–6 days later by a rash. Patients with **tickborne relapsing fever** have recurrent bouts of myalgia, arthralgia, and fever, usually without a history of tick bite. **Tularemia** is characterized by chills, myalgia, headache, and fever. Some patients present with painful lymph nodes, conjunctivitis, or severe sore throat.

VI. Signs

A. Type of wounds. Human and animal bite wounds may be **superficial abrasions; puncture wounds that are sometimes arcinate; lacerations, often**

with crushed and macerated edges; or **wounds that may involve avulsion of tissue.** Seventy-five percent of human bites in children and 40% of dog bites are superficial abrasions. Over 50% of human bites are on the hands. The wound should be examined for visible evidence of damage to underlying structures, diminished circulation or excessive bleeding, decreased sensation, weakness, limited movement, or pain with movement. Since the extent of subcutaneous damage is notoriously difficult to determine, some clinicians advocate exploring all full-thickness **bites on the dorsum of the hand** under direct vision for tendon or joint involvement. A 2- to 3-cm incision is made after the application of local anesthesia and a tourniquet. There are no controlled studies comparing this method to wound care without routine exploration.

B. **Infection.** Signs of **infection—redness, warmth, swelling, tenderness, purulence, and limitation of movement**—may become evident within hours of a bite. More than one third of deeper human bite wounds and a smaller proportion of animal bites become infected; abrasions seldom reach that stage. Even apparently insignificant bites on the hand are prone to infection.

C. **Papules and vesicles.** The bites of mosquitoes, fleas, bedbugs, lice, chiggers, and ticks are **pruritic red papules or vesicles.** They often occur in clusters or in a linear pattern on exposed areas, especially the wrists, ankles, and legs for fleas, chiggers, and ticks and the hands, face, and neck for bedbugs. The bites of chiggers and flies have central puncta or vesicles, which may become hemorrhagic.

D. Sometimes the **appearance of the biting insect or arachnid** is the best clue to the diagnosis. Fleas (or their feces, which resemble tiny flakes of dried blood) may be found on pets. Pubic lice live in pubic and axillary hair and skin, but move all over the body and may be found in eyelashes, eyebrows, and the hairline, especially in children. Head lice live on the scalp. The seams of clothing and folds of bedding should be searched for body lice. Nits of pubic and head lice attach to hairs at the skin level; since hairs grow 1 mm every 3 days, one can determine how recently nits were deposited by their distance from the skin on the hair shaft. This information is particularly helpful in deciding whether nits represent a new infestation following a course of treatment.

Brown recluse spiders have a 3- to 5-cm leg span and a 1- to 2-cm brown, fuzzy body, with a violin-shaped dark band on the dorsum. Black widow spiders have 1- to 2-cm shiny, black bodies, with a red hourglass mark on the underside.

E. **Development of skin lesions**
   1. **Hymenoptera** (eg, bees and vespids). The normal **local reaction to venom is heat, redness, and tenderness.** A **local allergic reaction** consists of a red papule surrounded by a pale zone of edema, with varying amounts of local swelling. More severe **immediate hypersensitivity reactions** manifest the signs of generalized urticaria, redness, swelling, and anaphylaxis. Fire ants cause multiple papules, which become necrotic pustules within several hours.
   2. **Scabies.** The female mite's burrow typically takes the form of a short, serpiginous lesion on wrists, elbows, finger webs, or intertriginous areas. Myriad other skin lesions, including erythematous papules, nodules, scaly patches, excoriations, and secondary impetigo, can occur. Except in infants, scabies does not infest the scalp or the face.
   3. **Ticks.** After a hard tick has been attached for several days, its neurotoxin can cause an ascending progressive paralysis, similar to Guillain-Barré syndrome, with hyporeflexia. **Lyme disease** usually begins with a slowly spreading, annular skin lesion—erythema chronicum migrans—which resolves after about 3 weeks. The skin lesions of **Rocky Mountain spotted fever** are typically red macules on the peripheral extremities that may become purpuric and confluent. **Tularemia** is characterized by pain and ulceration at the bite site, with acutely inflamed, sometimes draining lymph nodes, or occasionally by severe pharyngeal inflammation with exudate, conjunctivitis, hepatosplenomegaly, or pneumonia.
   4. **Spiders**
      a. A **brown recluse spider bite** becomes a hemorrhagic bulla surrounded by induration and erythema after 6–12 hours. The area of skin and subcutaneous necrosis may progress over a few days, forming an ulcer, which heals slowly over 2–4 months. Signs of systemic intoxication, including morbilliform rash, tachycardia, hypotension, intravascular coagulopathy

(petechiae, purpura, and bleeding diathesis), and hemolysis, may appear 1–3 days after the bite.

    b. A **black widow spider bite** may result in local erythema and hyperhidrosis within 30 minutes. The skin lesion develops a pale center with a red-blue border. Muscle rigidity, with tremor and fibrillations, develops in body parts near the bite. Signs of **cholinergic excess,** such as fever, lacrimation, rhinorrhea, and bradycardia, and of **sympathetic activation,** such as hypertension and tachyarrhythmias, intensify over the next several hours.

VII. Laboratory tests
A. Mammalian bites
1. **Culture with sensitivity studies** is recommended for mammalian bite wounds with a high likelihood of infection (ie, deep puncture wounds, all bite wounds that are sutured, wounds that are clinically infected or require hospital treatment, and full-thickness bites on the hand).
2. A **radiograph** should be obtained when osteomyelitis is suspected. Forceful injuries, such as a hand bite from a blow to a tooth, require an x-ray to look for fractures and embedded tooth fragments.
3. An **animal suspected of being rabid** should be killed and its head should then be sent to a health department laboratory, where the brain will be examined for rabies antigens by fluorescent antibody staining.

B. Possible scabies infestation.
Scabies mites, eggs, or feces may be found by scraping open a pruritic lesion (especially the end of a burrow) with a No. 15 scalpel blade dipped in mineral oil, and then examining this material microscopically under a coverslip. The sensitivity of this procedure, which varies from 30% to 90%, may be increased by dropping fountain pen ink onto the skin and then wiping it away. The burrows retain the ink.

C. Suspected tick-borne diseases.
For laboratory evaluation of suspected Lyme disease, see Chapter 41. Spirochetes can be seen in the blood smear in 70% of cases of tick-borne relapsing fever. Rocky Mountain spotted fever and tularemia are diagnosed by antibody titers.

D.
If a **brown recluse spider bite with systemic involvement** is suspected, order blood type and screen, coagulation studies, complete blood cell count, electrolytes, blood urea nitrogen (BUN), creatinine, and urinalysis.

VIII. Treatment
A. Mammalian bites
1. **Wound care** is similar for human and other mammalian bites.
    a. **Thorough cleansing** is necessary. At home, this means repeatedly flushing the wound with soap and water, 3% hydrogen peroxide, or iodine solution. In the office, this involves pressure irrigation or scrubbing with gauze sponges (under local anesthesia if necessary) and 1% benzalkonium or povidone-iodine solution. The edges of a full-thickness wound should be debrided (see Chapter 43). Pressure irrigation should follow. A high-pressure stream of irrigant can be directed into the wound through a 20-gauge needle attached by intravenous tubing to a bag of sterile saline inside a transfusion cuff inflated to 300 mm Hg.

    b. **Primary closure** with sutures or wound tapes (Steri-Strips) may be considered for dog bites and for human and other animal bites on the face if treated within 3–6 hours after injury and apparently uninfected. Subcutaneous sutures should be avoided; a single layer of skin sutures may be replaced with Steri-Strips after 5–7 days. A pressure dressing should be applied for 24 hours, and the wound should be inspected for signs of infection after 48 hours.

        Bite wounds on the hands should never be closed primarily. A bitten hand should be immobilized, by splinting from the fingertips to the mid forearm, and elevated. Because of the risk of infection, the wound should be reexamined within 24 hours. After about 5 days, movement should be encouraged in order to avoid swelling and stiffness.

        Other bite wounds should be packed with gauze impregnated with an antibacterial agent and seen 2 and 4–7 days later. Revision and delayed primary closure may be considered at that time.

    c. The reporting of animal bites (and of human bites in some locales) to the local health department is mandatory.

2. Antibiotic therapy

a. **Indications.** Infected bite wounds require antibiotic therapy. Patients with such bites on the hand should be hospitalized for intravenous antibiotics. Use of antibiotics in the absence of signs of infection is controversial. A meta-analysis of eight randomized clinical trials suggests that prophylactic antibiotics reduce the incidence of infection in dog bites by about 40%.

Prophylactic antibiotics should be considered for cat and human bites and for dog bites that are >8 hours old. It is reasonable to treat with antibiotics bite wounds that have been sutured or followed up for possible delayed closure, all bites on the hand, bites causing deep puncture wounds, and all bites in diabetics or immunosuppressed persons.

b. **Agents of choice and treatment regimens.** Animal bites (especially cat bites) may become infected with *Pasteurella multocida,* and human bites with *Eikenella corrodens* and *Bacteroides* spp, which are sensitive to penicillin and ampicillin, but relatively resistant to clindamycin, first- and second-generation cephalosporins, and penicillinase-resistant penicillins. Staphylococci and other penicillinase-producing organisms are present in up to 41% of bite wound infections.

   (1) **Amoxicillin with clavulanic acid** (Augmentin) is the oral drug of choice for treatment (10-day course) or prevention (5-day course) of bite wound infection. The adult dose is 250 mg orally every 8 hours. Children should receive 30–50 mg/kg/day in three divided doses.

   (2) **Penicillin V,** 250 mg orally every 6 hours (30–50 mg/kg/day for children), may be adequate initial therapy for animal but not human bites. Infection developing within the first 24 hours suggests *Pasteurella* infection and constitutes an indication for penicillin.

   (3) Patients allergic to penicillin may receive the following antibiotics.

      (a) For adults and children aged 8 years or older: **erythromycin** (eg, **erythromycin ethylsuccinate,** 400 mg every 6–8 hours) *and* **tetracycline hydrochloride,** 250 mg orally every 6 hours, or **doxycycline,** 100 mg orally every 12 hours.

      (b) For children younger than 8 years old, for whom tetracycline is contraindicated: **erythromycin** *alone,* 30–50 mg/kg/day in three divided doses.

3. Hospitalization is indicated in the following situations.

a. Bites to the hand, except those that are very superficial and do not appear to be infected.

b. Bites involving tendon, joint capsule, bone, or facial cartilage.

c. Signs of infection despite antibiotics or when treatment has been delayed.

d. Severe disfigurement, or tissue loss that may require plastic surgery or grafting.

e. Potential poor compliance with outpatient therapy.

4. Rabies postexposure prophylaxis

a. **Indications** (Table 9–1). Contact the local health department or the Rabies Investigation Unit, Centers for Disease Control and Prevention, Atlanta, Georgia, at (404) 639-3534 or (800) 311-3435 for additional information.

b. **Regimen.** This involves passive immunization with human rabies immune globulin, 20 immunizing units/kg, half intramuscularly and half infiltrated around the wound, up to 8 days after exposure. Begin active immunization with human diploid cell rabies vaccine, 1 mL injected intramuscularly on days 0, 3, 7, 14, and 28. Pregnancy is not a contraindication. Immunosuppressive drugs such as corticosteroids should be avoided if possible.

5. Tetanus prophylaxis should be administered according to the indications outlined in Chapter 43.

B. **Insect bites. Symptomatic relief** is all that is needed for most bug bites, including those of mosquitoes, flies, fleas, and bedbugs. Topical lotions or creams such as **Calamine** or **0.5% hydrocortisone** or applications of ice may relieve itching. Occasionally, an oral antihistamine, such as **diphenhydramine** (Benadryl), 25 mg three times a day for adults, ameliorates the urticarial reaction. Other, more specific treatments are discussed below.

TABLE 9–1. RABIES POSTEXPOSURE PROPHYLAXIS

Animal	Animal Condition	Appropriate Treatment
Wild carnivores (eg, skunks, bats, or raccoons)	Available	Obtain fluorescent rabies antibody (FRA) test on animal. Begin HRIG[1] and HDCV.[2] Discontinue HDCV if FRA test is negative.
	Unknown	Assume rabid. Begin HRIG[1] and HDCV.[2]
Domestic dog or cat	Healthy/available	Observe animal for 10 days. If animal stays healthy, no treatment is necessary.
	Rabid/suspected rabid	Obtain FRA test on animal. Begin HRIG[1] and HDCV.[2] Discontinue HDCV if FRA test is negative.
	Unknown	Low risk of rabies in most areas. Consult local health department.
Rodents	Generally unknown	Prophylaxis rarely indicated. Consult local health department.

Adapted from the Centers for Disease Control and Prevention recommendations, 1991.

[1] Human rabies immune globulin, 20 U/kg intramuscularly on day 0. Before HRIG is given, serum should be drawn for measurement of rabies antibody titer.

[2] Human diploid cell vaccine, 1 mL intramuscularly on days 0, 3, 7, 14, and 28.

1. **For flea and mite infestations,** thorough **housecleaning,** including vacuuming, along with washing clothes and bedclothes, is indicated.
2. **Eradication of fleas and bedbugs** is best performed by a professional exterminator. After **fumigation,** pets, children, and pregnant women should stay away for at least 4 hours.
3. **Pets with fleas should be treated with insecticide** (eg, pyrethrum or malathion) after consultation with a veterinarian. This treatment should be repeated every 2 weeks in summer. The pet should wear a flea collar.
4. **Hymenoptera**
    a. The **stinger** (if present) **should be removed** by scraping sideways so as not to squeeze the attached venom sac.
    b. **Local pain and swelling** may be helped by applying ice and a protease (eg, a paste of meat tenderizer and water) to the site.
    c. **Local allergic reactions** should be treated with elevation to reduce swelling. **Antihistamines,** such as **diphenhydramine,** 25–50 mg (up to 1–2 mg/kg for children) orally every 6–8 hours, and **prednisone,** 1 mg/kg/day for 3 days, may also be effective.
    d. If **cellulitis** is present, an antibiotic, such as erythromycin, should be added to the above regimen (see Chapter 11).
    e. **Immediate hypersensitivity reactions** must be treated promptly with **epinephrine,** 1 : 1000, 0.01 mL/kg, up to 0.5 mL, injected subcutaneously, and repeated, if necessary, in 5–10 minutes. A large-bore intravenous line should be started and the patient should be observed for at least 6–8 hours, since the vast majority of rebound or biphasic anaphylactic reactions will occur during this period. Additional measures for treatment of anaphylaxis should be available if necessary. Intravenous diphenhydramine, 50 mg, is given to block H_1 receptor sites. Aerosolized bronchodilators such as albuterol, 2.5 mg (0.5 mL of 5 mg/mL solution) in 3 mL of normal saline, should be used for bronchospasm. Simultaneous use of H_2 blockers (eg, ranitidine, 50 mg intravenously every 8 hours, or cimetidine, 300 mg intravenously every 6 hours) provides additional benefit.
    f. For **serum sickness** that occurs 10–14 days after hymenoptera stings, give **prednisone,** 1–2 mg/kg/day orally in divided doses, tapering over 2 weeks.
    g. **Prophylaxis.** Any individual who has had *any* systemic allergic symptoms or progressively severe local reactions from hymenoptera stings should carry a kit with injectable epinephrine (eg, **Epi-Pen**), wear a medical identification bracelet, and avoid walking barefoot or wearing bright-colored clothing, flowers, or scent outdoors. Patients with allergic reac-

tions may be evaluated by an allergist for desensitization treatment with venom extracts.

5. Lice

    a. The patient should apply **1% lindane shampoo** (Kwell) to affected areas and allow it to remain in place for 4 minutes before rinsing. Clothing and bed linens should be laundered using the hot cycle. This treatment should be repeated after 1 week if new nits are visible close to the skin. Insecticides should be kept away from the eyes; on eyelashes, a thick coating of petroleum jelly should be applied twice a day for 8 days. Nits should be removed as much as possible by combing.

    b. Lindane is contraindicated for **infants** and **pregnant or lactating women.** These patients should apply **pyrethrin** (Rid) and leave it on for 10 minutes; treatment should be repeated in 1 week.

6. Scabies. Treat all household members simultaneously.

    a. Permethrin 5% (Elimite cream), 1 oz per person, is massaged into the skin from the neck to the toes (and also on the head in infants) and left on for 8–14 hours, then thoroughly washed off.

    b. A less expensive and equally effective treatment is **1% gamma-benzene hexachloride** (lindane [Kwell or Scabene]) **lotion,** applied to cool skin from the neck down for 8–12 hours, then washed off with soap and water. Since systemic absorption and neurotoxicity can occur, it should not be used on children under 2 years old, pregnant or lactating women, patients with seizures or other neurologic disease, or those with extensively inflamed skin.

    c. Despite elimination of live mites, pruritus and existing skin lesions may persist for several weeks. The itching may be treated with **hydrocortisone** or **0.1% triamcinolone cream.**

7. Ticks

    a. Hard ticks should be removed. After applying petroleum jelly or an organic solvent, grasp the tick very close to the skin with blunt forceps, and pull or twist. If the tick is not completely removed, it should be excised (eg, using a skin biopsy punch). Sometimes a diligent search is required to locate an attached tick.

    b. Skin infections should be treated with antibiotics (see Chapter 11).

    c. Early Lyme disease may be treated for 10–21 days with **doxycycline,** 100 mg twice a day, or **amoxicillin,** 250–500 mg three times a day (20–40 mg/kg/day for children) (see Chapter 41). It is probably not cost-effective to treat the patient prophylactically with antibiotics after a tick bite.

    d. For **Rocky Mountain spotted fever,** treatment should be started promptly with oral **tetracycline** (if the patient is older than 8 years), 25–30 mg/kg/day in four divided doses, or with one dose of **chloramphenicol,** 50 mg/kg, followed by 50 mg/kg/day in four divided doses. When the patient becomes afebrile, the dose should be halved, then discontinued after 2–3 days.

    e. Adults with **tularemia** can be treated with **streptomycin,** 0.5 g intramuscularly twice a day for 1 week.

    f. Tick-borne relapsing fever in adults is treated with **tetracycline,** 500 mg orally four times daily for 10 days.

8. Spider bites

    a. Hospitalization is indicated for patients with black widow spider bites who are symptomatic, elderly, or very young. Hospital treatment may also be necessary for patients with brown recluse spider bites if they have systemic symptoms or if laboratory evidence of intravascular coagulation and hemolysis exists.

    b. For **local lesions caused by brown recluse spider bites,** good wound care is important. A bitten extremity should be splinted and elevated. Soaks and sterile dressings, and possibly topical antibacterial agents such as silver sulfadiazine, are applied to the necrotic ulcer. Systemic antibiotics such as **erythromycin ethylsuccinate,** 400 mg orally four times a day, have been used but are not routinely indicated. **Excision** of the bite wound is ineffective and **contraindicated.** Local and systemic corticosteroids are of no benefit. The following treatments are **experimental:**

antivenom, hyperbaric oxygen, and dapsone, a polymorphonuclear cell inhibitor (dosage, 50–200 mg/day). The latter agent has potentially serious side effects.

   c. Tetanus prophylaxis should be given (see Chapter 43).

   d. Initial therapy for black widow spider bites consists of application of ice and extremity elevation. Calcium gluconate in a 10% solution (10 mL given by intravenous push over 5 minutes) may provide relief from muscle spasm. Narcotics and diazepam in standard doses can be initiated to relieve pain and muscle spasm.

   e. Before administering **black widow spider antivenom,** testing for sensitivity to horse serum should be done. The test packaged with the antivenom can be used. One 2.5-mL ampule of black widow spider antivenom intramuscularly or intravenously in 10–15 mL of normal saline over 10–15 minutes can then be administered.

C. Prevention

   1. Hepatitis B. Those at occupational risk of human bites, including health and dental workers and employees of institutions for the mentally retarded, should receive hepatitis B vaccine.

   2. Rabies. Veterinary workers occupationally exposed to animal bites and people traveling to areas where rabid dogs are common should be immunized with 1 mL of human diploid cell rabies vaccine intradermally on days 0, 7, and 21 or 28.

   3. Outdoor insect bites can be prevented by avoidance of their habitats, by covering the skin with clothing, and by use of effective insect repellents that contain diethyltoluamide (DEET). Repeated applications to the skin can cause allergic and toxic effects. **Permethrin** (Permenone Tick Repellent) sprayed on clothing protects against mosquitoes and ticks.

REFERENCES

Agre F, Schwartz R: The value of early treatment of deer tick bites for the prevention of Lyme disease. Am J Dis Child 1993;**147**:945.

Benenson AS (editor): Rabies. In: *Control of Communicable Diseases in Man.* 15th ed. American Public Health Association; 1990:353.

Bunzli W, Wright D, Hoang A, et al: Current management of human bites. Pharmacotherapy 1998;**18**:227.

Dire DJ: Emergency management of dog and cat bite wounds. Emerg Med Clin North Am 1992; **10**:719.

Hogan DJ, Schachner L, Tanglertsampan C: Diagnosis and treatment of childhood scabies and pediculosis. Pediatr Clin North Am 1991;**38**:941.

Insect repellents. Med Lett Drugs Ther 1989;**31**(792):45. (Editorial.)

Jerrard DED: Management of insect stings. Am J Emerg Med 1996;**14**:429.

Johnson CA: Management of snakebite. Am Fam Physician 1991;**44**:174.

Kelleher A, Gordon S: Management of bite wounds and infection in primary care. Cleveland Clin J Med 1997;**54**:137.

Kemp E: Bites and stings of the arthropod kind. Postgrad Med 1998;**103**:88.

Magid D, Schwartz B, Craft J, et al: Prevention of Lyme disease after tick bites: A cost-effectiveness analysis. N Engl J Med 1992;**327**:534.

Norris R: Managing arthropod bites and stings. Physician Sports Med 1998;**26**(7):47.

---

10   Breast Lumps & Other Breast Conditions

Diane J. Madlon-Kay, MD

  I. Definition. Breast lumps are any areas of the breast that feel different from surrounding breast tissue. The normal breast is lumpy due to its cystlike architecture.

  II. Common diagnoses

    A. Fibrocystic changes.

    B. Cancer.

    C. Fibroadenoma.

    D. Mastitis.

III. Epidemiology. Benign breast disease affects almost all women. Breast cancer will eventually develop in one of every nine women.

    A. Fibrocystic changes are the most common benign condition of the breast. The incidence of this disorder increases with age; approximately 25% of premenopausal women and up to 50% of postmenopausal women have this condition.

    B. Breast cancer is associated with the following risk factors.

        1. Age. As women age, they are more likely to develop breast cancer. Seventy-five percent of breast cancers occur in women over age 50, 23% occur in women aged 30 to 50, and only 2% occur in women under age 30.

        2. Genetic background. Women whose mothers or sisters had breast cancer are two to three times more likely to develop the disease. This risk increases further if these relatives had breast cancer before menopause or in both breasts.

        3. Hormonal factors. Early menarche, late menopause, nulliparity, first pregnancy after age 30, and early oophorectomy are associated with an increased incidence of breast cancer.

    C. Fibroadenomas, rarely seen postmenopausally, are most prevalent in women under age 25 and in black women.

    D. Mastitis is almost always associated with lactation.

IV. Pathophysiology

    A. Fibrocystic changes. Cysts may range in size from 1 mm to large macrocysts >1 cm. As women age, macrocysts are more common, probably because of changes in female sex hormones.

    B. Cancer. Viruses, chemicals, radiation, and diet have been implicated as causes of breast cancer. No specific causative factor has been found, however.

    C. Fibroadenomas. These neoplasms, which have both fibrous and epithelial components, probably arise from terminal ducts and lobules. Circulating estrogen levels may play a role in the growth of these lesions, since they tend to grow toward the end of the menstrual cycle and during pregnancy. They may calcify and regress after menopause.

    Fibroadenomas have been classified into juvenile and adult types. The adult type is usually a slow-growing, solitary lesion. The juvenile form is frequently multiple and rapidly enlarging.

    D. Mastitis. This condition results from the entrance of *Staphylococcus aureus* or streptococci into the breast tissue through abraded skin or a cracked nipple. Streptococcal infection usually leads to cellulitis, whereas staphylococcal infection may lead to abscess formation.

V. Symptoms

    A. Breast lumps. In approximately 70–80% of women who develop breast cancer, the first and only symptom is the incidental discovery of a mass by the patient.

    B. Breast pain is the most common symptom of fibrocystic changes. The pain is usually bilateral and often in the upper outer quadrants. Characteristically, the pain begins 1 week before menstruation and diminishes with the onset of menstrual flow. The pain is caused by breast swelling; breast volume may increase up to 15%.

    C. Nipple discharge of a yellow or greenish-brown color occurs in up to one third of patients with mastitis. The second most frequent symptom of breast cancer, nipple discharge in women over age 50 years, is of more concern than it is in younger women. If the discharge is associated with a mass, the mass is the primary concern. Spontaneous, recurrent, or persistent discharge requires surgical exploration. The character of the discharge cannot be used to distinguish benign from malignant causes. However, bloody, serous, serosanguineous, or watery discharges should be regarded with suspicion.

VI. Signs

    A. Breast lumps. Ideally, examination of the patient should take place 7–9 days after the onset of menstrual flow.

    In general, fibrocystic areas are slightly irregular, easily movable, bilateral, and in the upper outer quadrants. Compression often causes tenderness, especially premenstrually.

    On palpation, a cancerous lesion is usually solitary, irregular or stellate, hard, nontender, fixed, and not clearly delineated from surrounding tissues.

Fibroadenomas are usually rubbery, smooth, well-circumscribed, nontender, and freely mobile.

B. Breast inflammation. Mastitis is characterized by inflamed, edematous, erythematous, indurated tender areas of the breast.

C. Surface of the breast

   1. Retraction. Breast cancer frequently causes fibrosis. Contraction of this fibrotic tissue may produce dimpling of the skin, alteration of the breast contours, and flattening or deviation of the nipple.

   2. Edema of the skin. Lymphatic blockage produces thickened skin with enlarged pores characteristic of the so-called pigskin or "orange peel" (*peau d'orange*) appearance in breast cancer.

   3. Venous pattern may be prominent unilaterally in breast cancer.

VII. Laboratory tests. Diagnostic testing is unnecessary in women with multiple, bilateral, diffuse, symmetric breast lumps without dominant masses.

A. Mammography

   1. Indication. A woman over age 30 with a solitary or dominant mass or an area of asymmetric thickening in the breast should undergo mammography. A breast lump is described as a dominant mass when the breasts are diffusely nodular but one mass is clearly larger, firmer, or asymmetric in location.

   2. Contraindication. Since breast tissue is very dense in young women, mammograms are *not* recommended in women under age 30. In older women, some fatty displacement of breast tissue has occurred, and mammograms are more worthwhile.

   3. Efficacy. Although 85% of all breast cancers are documented by mammography, as many as 15% of women with breast cancers have a normal mammogram. Therefore, a palpable mass is of concern even if a mammographic report shows no evidence of malignancy. **A biopsy is the only test that definitively excludes cancer.**

   4. Interpretation. A mammogram is usually interpreted in one of three ways.

      a. Normal. No breast cancer is identified.

      b. Indeterminate. This usually means that an area of possible cancer or asymmetry is visible. It is not sufficiently suspicious to warrant immediate biopsy, however. A repeat mammogram in 3–6 months is often recommended.

      c. Suspected breast cancer. Mammogram findings suspicious for malignancy include a dominant or asymmetric mass, a typical microcalcification, a stellate pattern of denser tissue, an extension of streaks of denser tissue into the subcutaneous fat, retraction of the skin or nipple, and thickening of the skin.

B. Other imaging techniques. Although ultrasonography is not useful as a screening tool for breast cancer, it is useful for discriminating solid from cystic lesions. Other imaging techniques considered experimental or of no proven benefit for evaluation of breast conditions include thermography, diaphanography, computerized tomography, magnetic resonance imaging, and digital imaging.

C. Aspiration of a suspected breast cyst. Needle aspiration may be used to define the cystic nature of any breast mass.

A 20- or 22-gauge needle attached to a 10- or 20-mL syringe should be used. After the skin is cleaned with alcohol, the cyst is fixed between the fingers of one hand while the needle is directed into the cyst with the other. The aspirated fluid is usually amber to green in color. If the fluid is bloody or if the mass is still palpable or reappears within 1 month of observation, a biopsy is necessary. The fluid is usually discarded.

D. Breast biopsy. The cytologic or histologic characteristics of a clearly dominant breast mass should be confirmed by biopsy, regardless of other clinical or mammographic findings.

   1. Fine-needle aspiration biopsy is used to determine the cytology of suspected breast cancer. Accurate interpretation requires proper smearing and fixation of the slides as well as an experienced pathologist. In expert hands, the false-negative rate is 1.4% and the false-positive rate is near 0%.

   2. Excisional biopsy

      a. Excisional biopsy is indicated if the results of the physical examination or mammogram suggest cancer even when the cytologic findings of aspiration are benign, or if a breast mass may be cancerous and fine-needle aspiration biopsy and cytologic evaluation are not available.

    b. The biopsy is usually performed as an outpatient procedure using local anesthesia. Removal of the entire mass is the objective.

  3. Incisional biopsy may be performed in the following circumstances.

    a. To confirm the diagnosis of advanced cancer. If the mass is strongly suspected of being malignant, a cutting-edge core needle can be used.

    b. To evaluate a breast mass that is too large to be excised easily and completely.

VIII. Treatment

A. Fibrocystic changes

  1. General measures

    a. Supportive measures that may be helpful include the use of loose, light clothing and a comfortable, supporting, well-padded bra.

    b. Dietary changes

      (1) Caffeine intake. Although studies of dietary restriction of **caffeine** and other methylxanthines are conflicting, some reports suggest that eliminating consumption of such substances may be efficacious.

      (2) Vitamin E. This vitamin has not been found to be beneficial in placebo-controlled studies.

      (3) Evening primrose oil is often used by British physicians because of its significant response rate (60%), low incidence of side effects, and nonhormonal composition. The average dose is two 500-mg capsules three times a day for a minimum of 3–4 months. Evening primrose oil can be obtained without a prescription and costs about $1 a day.

  2. Pharmacologic therapy (Table 10–1). Before beginning treatment, carefully evaluate the woman's symptoms. Minimal symptoms for only a few days of the month do not require drug therapy. It may take 3–4 months for evidence of improvement with any treatment regimen.

    Although other drugs can be used for this purpose, **danazol** is the only pharmacologic agent approved by the US Food and Drug Administration for use in the treatment of fibrocystic changes. Since danazol therapy is associated with significant side effects, however, this agent should be administered only by a physician familiar with its use.

  3. Surgery. A subcutaneous mastectomy with implants or bilateral reduction mastectomies may be considered in the following patients.

    a. In women with an extremely high risk of breast cancer (eg, a history of breast cancer in a mother and a sister).

    b. In women with ductal or lobular atypical hyperplasia on biopsy. The risk of breast cancer is increased by a factor of approximately 5 in these women.

    c. In women with breast pain that is resistant to nonsurgical treatment.

TABLE 10–1. PHARMACOLOGIC THERAPY FOR FIBROCYSTIC CHANGES

Drug	Dosage	Effectiveness (%)	Significant Side Effects
Danazol[1]	100–400 mg by mouth daily for 4–6 months	60–90	Yes
Oral contraceptives (eg, Loestrin 1/20)	1 tablet by mouth daily for 1–2 years	70–90	Some
Medroxyprogesterone acetate	10 mg by mouth on days 15–25 of the menstrual cycle for 9–12 months	85	Some
Tamoxifen	10–20 mg by mouth daily for 4 months	70	Yes
Bromocriptine	1.25–5.0 mg by mouth daily for 2–4 months	50–80	Yes

[1] The only drug approved by the US Food and Drug Administration for the treatment of fibrocystic changes.

B. Breast cancer. The objective of treatment is to provide the greatest chance for cure or long-term survival. Whether this objective can be met while preserving the major portion of the breast is controversial. Radical mastectomy is now performed rarely, since modified radical mastectomy results in comparable survival. Lumpectomy is an option for some women.

   1. Surgery. The primary care physician is responsible for referring the patient to a surgeon, who should provide individualized counseling to the patient so that the appropriate option is selected. Breast cancers are staged at surgery, at which time tissue is obtained for estrogen and progesterone receptors.

   Most women can be fitted with a **prosthesis** within 3–6 weeks of surgery. The option of breast reconstruction should be discussed prior to surgery because it can often be performed at the same time.

   2. Chemotherapy, hormonal therapy, and radiation therapy should be directed by an oncologist.

   3. Careful and frequent follow-up is important. The history and the physical examination should be directed toward the breasts, bones, liver, chest wall, and nervous system. An annual mammogram of both breasts is recommended.

   4. Discussion of social and emotional issues is crucial. The American Cancer Society's Reach to Recovery program is a valuable resource for patients.

C. Fibroadenoma. Surgical excision, preserving as much normal breast tissue as possible, is the preferred treatment. After excision, the patient should be reassured that she is at no increased risk of cancer.

D. Mastitis. Lactating women should be encouraged to continue nursing.

   1. Ten days of an antibiotic effective against *S aureus* and streptococci should be sufficient.

   a. A penicillinase-resistant synthetic penicillin, such as dicloxacillin, 500 mg orally every 6 hours, should be used.

   b. For patients who are allergic to penicillin, erythromycin, 500 mg orally every 6 hours, is a reasonable alternative.

   2. Local heat is also of benefit.

   3. Failure of symptoms to respond to treatment in 48 hours or the development of a mass may indicate a breast abscess that requires incision and drainage. Inflammatory breast cancer must be considered in any mastitis that does not respond to treatment after 5 days or in nonnursing women with mastitis. A biopsy will establish the diagnosis.

REFERENCES

Drukker BH: Breast disease: A primer on diagnosis and management. Int J Fertil 1997;**42:**278.
Hansen N, Morrow M: Breast disease. Med Clin North Am 1998;**82:**203.
Marchant DJ: Controversies in benign breast disease. Surg Oncol Clin North Am 1998;**7:**285.
Sitruk-Ware R: Benign breast disease. Curr Ther Endocrinol Metab 1997;**6:**396.

---

11   Cellulitis & Other Bacterial Skin Infections

Donald B. Middleton, MD

I. Definition. Infections of the skin, such as cellulitis, follow bacterial invasion into the superficial or deep layers or specialized structures of the skin. The hallmarks of infection are pain, swelling, redness, and warmth. Infection may be a primary skin process or may reflect infection of some other organ system. At least 100 bacterial pathogens have been reported to produce skin infection.

II. Common diagnoses. Most bacterial skin infections have a pathognomonic appearance. Nonetheless, bacterial infection must be distinguished from allergic conditions (eg, eczema), contact dermatitis (eg, poison ivy), insect stings, trauma, and viral or fungal infections. The common bacterial skin infections are listed below.

A. Cellulitis, including erysipelas, erythrasma, and ecthyma.

B. Impetigo.

C. Folliculitis.

D. **Furuncle (boil).**

E. **Carbuncle.** Some less common but important infections include bacillary angiomatosis and chancriform lesions. Table 11–1 lists other possibilities.

III. **Epidemiology.** In the primary care setting, bacterial skin infections account for 2% of ambulatory visits.

A. **Cellulitis** follows traumatic disruption of the skin's protective barrier or occurs spontaneously in the young, elderly, diabetic, alcoholic, edematous, or immunocompromised. Cases develop throughout the year. Some specific forms of cellulitis are listed below.

1. **Erysipelas** is common in alcoholics, diabetics, or immunocompromised hosts, but occasionally arises spontaneously in preschool children or older adults.

2. **Erythrasma** affects young men. In tropical climates, 20% of men develop this infection.

3. **Ecthyma** occurs in children or the elderly, often after insect bites or excoriation.

4. **Necrotizing cellulitis** occurs most commonly in the elderly, a minority of whom have diabetes mellitus or myxedema. Intravenous drug abusers and those with malignancy, anal fissure, peripheral vascular disease, or penetrating trauma are also at risk for necrotizing cellulitis.

B. **Impetigo** is endemic in children, especially preschoolers. At least 20% of children have one or more bouts of this infection. The incidence of impetigo peaks in late summer and early fall, when minor trauma from insect bites or abrasions promotes infection. Close person-to-person contact or scratching from winter dryness or underlying chickenpox, scabies, or pediculosis can cause the infection and result in spread. Epidemics of impetigo occur occasionally, for example, infecting a whole wrestling team.

C. **Folliculitis** usually follows events such as shaving or immersion in a hot tub.

D. **Furuncles** and **carbuncles** arise in areas subject to friction and perspiration, usually in adults. Obesity, immunologic defects, and recurrent trauma (eg, from squeezing sebaceous cysts) are important factors.

E. **Bacillary angiomatosis** occurs in acquired immunodeficiency syndrome (AIDS) patients.

F. **Chancriform lesions** occur sporadically, especially in those with a sexually transmitted disease.

IV. **Pathophysiology.** A breach of the skin's surface barrier allows bacteria to penetrate and produce infection. Factors facilitating bacterial invasion are primary skin diseases (eg, eczema or psoriasis), trauma (eg, burns or bites), immunologic defects (eg, AIDS, alcoholism, multiple myeloma, or diabetes mellitus), contaminated wounds (eg, from soil or feces), viral or fungal infections (eg, varicella or athlete's foot), bacterial infection in structures contiguous to the skin (eg, osteomyelitis, tooth abscess, or sinusitis), circulatory dysfunction (eg, congestive heart failure or lymphedema), and bacteremia (eg, sexually transmitted diseases or subacute bacterial endocarditis). The inflammatory reaction mediated by cytokines and lymphokines probably worsens the warmth and erythema.

A. **Cellulitis** involves the epidermis and subcutaneous tissue. The major pathogens are *Streptococcus pyogenes,* usually group A, and *Staphylococcus aureus.* Numerous other bacteria are capable of producing cellulitis, including *Haemophilus*

TABLE 11–1. LESS COMMON BACTERIAL SKIN INFECTIONS

Tuberculosis
Necrotizing fasciitis: group A streptococcus or mixed flora
Paronychia: *Staphylococcus aureus* or group A streptococcus
Chronic ulcers: stasis ulcers
Intertrigo
Pilonidal cyst infection: coliforms, anaerobes
Sebaceous cyst infection
Gangrene: gas gangrene (*Clostridium perfringens*), Fournier's gangrene (mixed flora)
Decubitus ulcers
Erysipeloid: *Erysipelothrix rhusiopathiae*
Lyme disease: *Borrelia burgdorferi*

influenzae type b in the buccal cellulitis of young infants, pneumococcus in preseptal or postseptal orbital cellulitis, mouth anaerobes such as peptostreptococcus from human bites, soil bacteria such as *Clostridia* in necrotizing cellulitis, *Pasteurella multocida* from cat bites, and coliform organisms in decubitus ulcers. Specific conditions are described below.

1. **Erysipelas** involves the skin and the lymphatic tissues and is caused by group A, uncommonly C or G, or rarely B *S pyogenes.*
2. **Erythrasma** is a superficial infection produced by *Corynebacterium minutissimum.*
3. **Ecthyma** is a deep, ulcerating invasion of the skin caused by streptococcus or pseudomonas.
4. **Necrotizing ("flesh-eating") cellulitis** usually reflects group A streptococcus infection alone or mixed with other, usually anaerobic, bacteria.

B. **Impetigo** is a superficial infection traditionally produced by *S pyogenes.* Recent studies suggest that *S aureus,* usually phage group II, is a major pathogen. About 10% of all cases are bullous impetigo definitely resulting from staphylococcal invasion. Glomerulonephritis may complicate streptococcal impetigo. Scalded skin syndrome or, rarely, toxic shock may follow staphylococcal disease.

C. **Folliculitis** develops in hair follicles, may spread superficially, and is caused by staphylococcus or streptococcus or, when it occurs following hot tub use, by *Pseudomonas aeruginosa.*

D. **Furuncles** (single boils) and **carbuncles** (a conglomeration of boils) are deep infections that are usually caused by staphylococcus or streptococcus. These problems often follow sebaceous cyst manipulation.

E. **Bacillary angiomatosis** is the result of *Rochalimaea henselae* or *quintana* infection.

F. **Chancriform lesions** are seen in venereal diseases (eg, syphilis), anthrax, mycobacterial illness (eg, fish tank granuloma), and tularemia.

V. **Symptoms**

A. **Pain** at the site of infection occurs with most infections, except perhaps impetigo and erythrasma.

B. **Pruritus** is common in impetigo, cellulitis, folliculitis, and erythrasma. Scratching often causes further trauma and promotes spread of infection.

C. **Feverishness, chills,** and **malaise** can develop acutely. These symptoms often reflect invasion of deeper tissues or the bloodstream, especially when they occur with cellulitis, erysipelas, or carbuncles. Severely ill patients may become septic, slip into coma, or die.

VI. **Signs.** The physical appearance of these illnesses generally provides the clue to diagnosis.

A. **Cellulitis is acutely tender, red, and hot.** Allergic reactions are seldom as warm or tender. In cellulitis, the leading edge is not raised but may be well defined. Propagation, often from a central traumatic lesion, is centripetal and rapid, often resulting in lymphangitis or lymphadenopathy. Infection is occasionally indolent or can spread to regional lymph nodes, blood, fascia, or muscle, creating a life-threatening situation. Special situations are listed below.

1. **Cellulitis of the head. Preseptal orbital cellulitis,** involving only the eyelids, and **postseptal orbital cellulitis,** including orbital structures, both make the eyelids swollen and red. In postseptal cellulitis, gaze is dysconjugate, proptosis is present, and eye movement intensifies pain. Cheeks that are marked by a bluish discoloration and feel woody indicate **facial** or **buccal cellulitis.**
2. **Cellulitis of the extremity. Hand cellulitis** often follows puncture wounds, such as animal bites or foreign body insertion. **Cellulitis of the foot or the leg** often coexists with osteomyelitis in the immunocompromised or diabetic host.
3. **Erysipelas** is a fulminating cellulitis with a raised, demarcated edge and systemic fever. Seventy percent of cases are on the lower extremity. The forehead, face, and abdomen are other sites of infection. A *peau d'orange* ("orange peel") appearance is typical.
4. **Erythrasma,** a chronic, red-brown infection located in the genital area, is finely scaled.
5. **Ecthyma** is an acute, deep, penetrating, 0.5- to 3-cm-wide ulcer that initially resembles impetigo. Lesions can be multiple and surrounded by raised violaceous rims.

      6. Necrotizing cellulitis has an abrupt, painful onset. Despite apparent toxicity, initially the skin is only mildly abnormal, yet exquisitely tender. In 1–3 days, cyanosis and edema evolve into necrosis.

  B. Impetigo can be acute or chronic and may last for months.

      1. Streptococcal impetigo is characterized by small vesicles that gradually enlarge to 1–2 cm with a red halo and develop central honey crusts. "Kissing" lesions occur where two skin surfaces touch. Autoinoculation and multiple lesions are common. Underlying viral or fungal infections can be distinguished from impetigo by the appearance of the primary lesions, such as the smaller vesicles of chickenpox or the circinate raised edge and central clearing of tinea corporis.

      2. Staphylococcal impetigo may mimic streptococcal disease but classically is bullous with little surrounding erythema. A varnishlike finish coats ruptured bullae.

  C. Folliculitis produces small, red, dome-shaped pustules over the hair follicles. Hair may be broken or loose. Infection may be acute or chronic.

  D. A **furuncle** is a localized, deep-seated, pus-containing boil, often associated with a traumatized cyst or folliculitis. The nodule is hot and tender. Common sites are the neck, axillae, buttocks, and thighs.

  E. A **carbuncle** is a widely spread lesion with suppuration and many pus-draining ports. **Hidradenitis suppurativa** is a carbuncle of the axilla or the groin involving the apocrine sweat glands.

  F. Chancriform lesions are ulcerlike. Syphilitic ulcers are painless.

  G. Bacillary angiomatosis produces cherry hemangioma–like or nodular pyogenic granuloma–like lesions.

VII. Laboratory tests. In the usual case, attempts to identify a causative agent by cultures of the leading edge, central abrasions, or blood are of equivocal benefit. Paired antibody titers; counterimmunoelectrophoresis on urine, tears, and other fluids; and cultures of skin biopsies have marginal value. On the other hand, Gram's stain and culture of pus or deeply necrotic material have proven value. With an atypical presentation, all attempts to define the causative agent are justifiable.

  A. Cultures are warranted in the situations described below. **Blood cultures** and **cultures of pus** should be obtained from toxic patients, those with preseptal or postseptal cellulitis, those with necrotic cellulitis, and immunocompromised patients.

      1. Blood cultures are positive in 80% of patients with *H influenzae* cellulitis of the eye or the face.

      2. Needle aspiration of unruptured bullae or pus from incised abscesses provides reliable culture data.

      3. Conjunctival cultures may be useful in preseptal or postseptal cellulitis.

  B. Special procedures are sometimes helpful.

      1. Plain radiographs may detect tissue gas, as well as bone or sinus infection.

      2. Magnetic resonance imaging (MRI) or **computerized tomographic (CT) scans** can distinguish preseptal from postseptal cellulitis. MRI is useful with severe cellulitis in diabetes mellitus to detect underlying osteomyelitis. Either technique can be used to identify complicating subcutaneous abscesses common in diabetic or immunocompromised hosts. These abscesses may require surgical drainage.

      3. Bone scans are beneficial in selected cases of cellulitis to reveal concomitant osteomyelitis.

      4. Bone biopsy with culture is the definitive test to diagnose coexistent osteomyelitis.

      5. Wood's lamp lumination is useful in erythrasma because the infected skin fluoresces coral red.

VIII. Treatment. Antibiotic therapy is required for nearly all bacterial skin infections for a 7- to 10-day period. Ordinarily, complete resolution is achievable, but recurrences are common. (See Table 11–2 for details regarding medications.)

  A. Cellulitis

      1. Erythromycin, cephalosporins, fluoroquinolones, amoxicillin-clavulanate, azithromycin, clarithromycin, and **clindamycin** are all effective drugs. **Cephalexin, cefadroxil, cefaclor, cefuroxime,** and **cefixime** are the most often utilized cephalosporins. Cefixime is not effective for staphylococcus.

TABLE 11–2. ANTIBIOTICS FOR SKIN INFECTIONS

Drug (Trade Name)	Route of Administration[1]	Pediatric Dose (mg/kg/day)[2,3]	Adult Dose (g/day)[2]	Interval (dose/day)
Penicillins				
Penicillin V	PO	25–50	1–2	4
Penicillin G	IV, IM	100,000–250,000 U	1–24 million U	4–6
Amoxicillin	PO	20–40	0.75–1.5	3
Ampicillin	PO, IV, IM	25–200	1–12	4
Ampicillin-clavulanate (Augmentin)	PO	20–40	0.75–1.5	3
Ampicillin-sulbactam (Unasyn)	IV, IM	Dose based on ampicillin content 25–200; safety not established under age 12 years	6–12 (4–8 ampicillin)	4
Nafcillin	PO, IV, IM	50–200	1–12	4
Oxacillin	PO, IV, IM	50–200	1–12	4
Dicloxacillin	PO	12.5–25	1–2	4
Piperacillin	IV	Dose based on piperacillin content, 100–300; safety not established under age 12 years	6–24	4–6
Piperacillin-taxobactam (Zosyn)	IV	Dose based on piperacillin content, 150–400; safety not established under age 12 years	9–18	4
Ticarcillin	IV	Dose based on ticarcillin content, 100–300; safety not established under age 12 years	4–24	4–6
Ticarcillin/clavulanate (Timentin)	IV	Dose based on ticarcillin content, 150–300; safety not established under age 12 years	4.1–24.8 (4–24 ticarcillin)	4–6
Cephalosporins				
For use against gram-positive cocci and some gram-negative agents				
Cefadroxil (Duricef)	PO	30	1–2	1–2
Cefazolin (Kefzol)	IV, IM	25–100	1–12, 1–4	3
Cephalexin (Keflex)	PO	25–100	1–4	4
Cephalothin (Keflin)	IV	80–160	2–12	4–6
Cephradine (Velosef)	PO	25–50	1–4	2–4
For use against above plus *Haemophilus influenzae*				
Cefaclor (Ceclor)	PO	20–40	0.75–4	2–3
Cefonicid (Monocid)	IV, IM	Not used	0.5–2	1
Cefoperazone (Cefobid)	IV, IM	50–200	2–12	2
Cefoxitin (Mefoxin)	IV, IM	80–160	2–12	4–6
Cefprozil (Cefzil)	PO	15–30	0.5–2	1–2
Ceftibuten (Cedax)	PO	9	0.09–0.4	1
Cefuroxime axetil (Ceftin)	PO	20–30 or 125 or 250 mg/dose	0.5–1	2
Cefuroxime (Ceftin)	IV, IM	50–150	2–9	3–4
Loracarbef (Lorabid)	PO	15–30	0.4–0.8	2
For use against primarily gram-negative agents and most gram-positive cocci				
Cefepime (Maxipime)	IV, IM	Not used	1–2	2
Cefixime (Suprax)	PO	8	0.4	1
Cefotaxime (Claforan)	IV, IM	50–200	2–12	3–4
Cefpodoxime (Vantin)	PO	10	0.2–0.8	1–2
Ceftazidime	IV, IM	90–150	2–6	2–3

(*continued*)

TABLE 11–2. (*continued*)

Drug (Trade Name)	Route of Administration[1]	Pediatric Dose (mg/kg/day)[2,3]	Adult Dose (g/day)[2]	Interval (dose/day)
Ceftizoxime (Cefizox)	IV, IM	150–200	2–12	3–4
Ceftriaxone (Rocephin)	IV, IM	50–100	1–4	1–2
Other Antibiotics				
Erythromycin	PO, IV	30–50	1–2	3–4
Clarithromycin (Biaxin)	PO	15	0.5–1	2
Clindamycin	PO, IV	10–40	0.6–2.7	3–4
Metronidazole	PO, IV	15–30	0.75–2	3
Azithromycin (Zithromax)	PO	5–10	0.5 initial, then 0.25	1
Aztreonam (Azactam)	IV, IM	120–200	1.5–6	3–4
Imipenem-cilastatin (Primaxin)	IV	40–50	1–4	4
Gentamicin[4]	IV, IM	3–6	3 mg/kg/day	3
Tobramycin[4]	IV, IM	3–6	3 mg/kg/day	3
Vancomycin[4]	IV	10–50	1–2	4
Fluoroquinolones				
Ciprofloxacin (Cipro)	PO, IV	Not used	0.5–1.5	2
Grebafloxacin (Raxar)	PO	Not used	0.4–0.6	1
Levofloxacin (Levaquin)	PO, IV	Not used	0.25–0.5	1
Lomefloxacin (Maxaquin)	PO	Not used	0.4	1
Ofloxacin (Floxin)	PO, IV	Not used	0.4–0.8	2
Sparfloxacin (Zagam)	PO	Not used	0.2	1
Trovafloxacin (Trovan)	PO, IV	Not used	0.1–0.2	1

[1] PO, Oral; IV, intravenous; IM, intramuscular.
[2] Dosage may require adjustment in renal failure. U, Units.
[3] Not to exceed the adult dose.
[4] Serum levels indicated; gentamicin and tobramycin—peak, 4–12 µg/mL; trough, 1–2 µg/ml; vancomycin—peak, 35–45 µg/ml; trough, 5–10 µg/ml.

Cost and side effect profile should be considered. In streptococcal disease, penicillin is the drug of choice, while synthetic penicillins such as oxacillin are highly effective for both staphylococcus and streptococcus. Severely ill or immunocompromised patients should be initially broadly treated with an aminoglycoside and penicillin–β-lactam combination or a third-generation cephalosporin until cultures direct narrowing of the antibiotic given. The characteristic appearance of some infections points to specific treatment.

2. **Supportive care** includes limb elevation, moist warm soaks, and analgesics (eg, acetaminophen, aspirin, or ibuprofen in appropriate doses). Because of counter-inflammatory effects, nonsteroidal anti-inflammatory drugs (NSAIDs) may speed recovery. Patients with underlying congestive heart failure, stasis ulceration, or diabetes mellitus frequently develop recurrent cellulitis of the legs. Support stockings or Unna boot therapy may help. Hyperbaric oxygen is of limited value.

3. **Hospitalization** is recommended for toxic patients and for patients with mixed aerobic and anaerobic infections, postseptal cellulitis, necrotizing cellulitis, or gram-negative cellulitis, especially pseudomonas. Patients with preseptal cellulitis, cellulitis of the hand, or immunocompromised status have been successfully treated as outpatients, although some benefit from hospitalization. After a patient has an initial response to parenteral therapy, oral ciprofloxacin or ofloxacin offers a satisfactory alternative to prolonged hospitalization, except in children, in whom these drugs are currently contraindicated.

4. **Erysipelas** is treated with **penicillin** or **erythromycin,** usually with defervescence in 24–48 hours. Recurrences are common.

5. **Erythrasma** requires 14–21 days of **erythromycin.** Relapses can evolve into asymptomatic infection that can last for years.

      6. **Ecthyma** often necessitates weeks of an antipseudomonal drug (eg, **ciprofloxacin**) or an antistreptococcal agent (eg, penicillin).

      7. **Necrotizing cellulitis** requires surgical debridement.

B. Impetigo

    1. **Impetigo** may be treated with penicillin or **erythromycin.** Alternative antibiotics include any agent that eradicates streptococci and staphylococci, such as **clindamycin, cephalexin, azithromycin, clarithromycin,** or **amoxicillin-clavulanate.** Topical agents are effective for small areas, especially **mupirocin** applied three times a day. Agents such as **hexachlorophene** are not highly efficacious. With treatment, impetigo responds rapidly in over 98% of cases. The spontaneous resolution rate is 60% in 10 days.

    2. Although good hygiene is helpful, scrubbing tends to spread infection. Topical **isotretinoin** applied to areas of recurrent infection once a day has proven prophylactic value, especially for **hidradenitis suppurativa.**

    3. Eradication of nasal carriage of staphylococci or streptococci with topical mupirocin or oral **rifampin** may interrupt repetitive infections.

C. Folliculitis is treated with antistaphylococcal (eg, **erythromycin**) or antipseudomonal (eg, **ciprofloxacin**) antibiotics, normal saline compresses, and avoidance of hot tubs or cosmetics. In recurrent cases, topical antibiotics may be used for prophylaxis.

D. Furuncles require moist heat and, if fluctuant, incision and drainage. Squeezing can cause bacteremia.

E. Carbuncles demand systemic antibiotics directed against staphylococci (eg, **nafcillin, cefazolin,** or **clindamycin**) and often require incision and drainage with appropriate cultures.

F. Hidradenitis suppurativa is treated with antistreptococcal and antistaphylococcal antibiotics, warm compresses, surgical excision, avoidance of shaving and deodorants, topical daily isotretinoin, and occasionally **prednisone,** 40–60 mg/day for a limited course, to diminish scarring.

G. Bacillary angiomatosis may be treated with **erythromycin** or with **doxycycline,** 100 mg twice daily for 2 weeks.

H. Chancriform lesions are treated according to the identified cause.

REFERENCES

Bisno AL, Stevens DL: Streptococcal infections of skin and soft tissue. N Engl J Med 1996; **334:**240.

Demidovich CW, et al: Impetigo. Current etiology and comparison of penicillin, erythromycin, and cephalexin therapies. Am J Dis Child 1990;**144:**1313.

Hacker SM: Common infections of the skin. Characteristics, causes, and cures. Postgrad Med 1994;**96:**43.

Kremer M, Zuckerman R, Avraham Z, et al: Long-term antimicrobial therapy in the prevention of recurrent soft-tissue infections. J Infect Dis 1991;**22:**37.

Lindbeck G, Powers R: Cellulitis. Hosp Pract 1993;**28**(suppl 2):10.

Lowy FD: *Staphylococcus aureus* infections. N Engl J Med 1998;**339:**520.

Sachs MK: The optimum need of needle aspiration in the bacteriologic diagnosis for cellulitis in adults. Arch Intern Med 1990;**150:**1907.

Schwartzman WA: Infections due to *Rochalimaea:* The expanding clinical spectrum. Clin Infect Dis 1992;**15:**893.

Swartz MN: Cellulitis and subcutaneous tissue infections. In Mandell GL, et al (editors): *Principles and Practice of Infectious Diseases.* Churchill Livingstone; 1995:909.

Weinberg AN, Swartz MN: Bacterial diseases with cutaneous involvement. In Fitzpatrick TB, et al (editors): *Dermatology in General Medicine.* McGraw-Hill; 1993:2297.

---

12   Chest Pain

Joseph Hobbs, MD

I. Definition. Chest pain is the sensory response to noxious stimuli caused by trauma or dysfunction of the chest wall, thoracic organs, and contiguous structures. Psychological disorders can cause chest pain where no organic disease exists and can precipitate and exacerbate organic causes of chest pain.

II. Common diagnoses

  A. **Cardiac chest pain,** including myocardial ischemia, infarction, and pericarditis.

  B. **Aortic chest pain** caused by acute aortic aneurysmal distention and aortic dissection.

  C. **Tracheal and pleural chest pain** from tracheitis, pulmonary embolus or infarction, pneumonia, or pneumothorax.

  D. **Diaphragmatic chest pain** from adjacent pericarditis, pneumonia, acute pancreatitis, subdiaphragmatic abscess, and penetrating and perforated peptic ulcers.

  E. **Gastrointestinal (GI) chest pain** caused by esophagitis, esophageal spasm, esophageal obstruction, or esophageal rupture; peptic ulcer disease; pancreatitis; biliary tract disease; or acute liver distention.

  F. **Integumental, skeletal, and muscular chest pain** from herpes zoster, chest wall trauma, costochondritis, or rib, cervical, and upper thoracic spine disease.

  G. **Breast-related chest pain** from fibrocystic breast disease, mastitis, trauma, cellulitis, herpes zoster, or other dermatoses.

  H. **Psychogenic chest pain** as a result of somatization disorders or panic attacks.

III. Epidemiology. Chest pain is one of the most frequent causes of unscheduled office visits in family medicine and of admission to intensive care units in primary care practice. Patients with chest pain fear that the pain may represent a life-threatening situation, but most chest pain experienced by the general population usually is self-limited and physically harmless and poses no significant consequence.

  A. In pediatric or adolescent age groups, chest pain is most frequently musculoskeletal or psychogenic. Exercise of infrequently used muscle groups often precedes the development of chest pain of musculoskeletal origin.

  B. Cardiac chest pain caused by coronary artery disease is most likely in older patients, males, postmenopausal females, and those with risk factors for coronary heart disease, such as family history, hypercholesterolemia, smoking, diabetes mellitus, or preexisting coronary artery disease.

  C. Immunocompromised patients or those with chronic lung disease are at risk for pneumonia.

  D. Immobilization, estrogen use, pregnancy, congestive heart failure, long-bone fractures, disruption of venous endothelium, metastatic cancer, and other hypercoagulable states predispose individuals to pulmonary embolus with infarction.

IV. Pathophysiology

  A. **Cardiac chest pain** is caused by an imbalance between myocardial oxygen supply and demand that results in myocardial ischemia (see Chapter 81). In pericarditis, irritation of contiguous mediastinal structures such as the parietal pleura must occur to produce chest pain, since the pericardium is insensitive to pain.

  B. **Aortic chest pain.** In aortic dissection, acute stretching of the vascular wall of the aortic arch results in transmission of pain impulses through neural tracks similar to those carrying pain impulses from the heart.

  C. **Tracheal and pleural chest pain**

   1. **Tracheobronchial pain** is referred to sites in the neck and the anterior chest at about the same level as the point of irritation in the upper airways.

   2. A **pulmonary embolus** results in a zone of ventilated lung that is not perfused, leading to generalized bronchoconstriction, hypoxia, hypocapnia, lung tissue injury, and irritation of surrounding parietal pleura. Pulmonary fat embolism occurring after the fracture of a large bone can result in a similar process.

   3. **Pneumonia and pneumothorax** cause chest pain through parietal pleural irritation.

  D. In **diaphragmatic chest pain,** irritation of the peripheral portion of the diaphragmatic pleura may cause pain to radiate into the epigastrium, subchondral regions, lumbar spine, and lower chest. Diaphragmatic pleurisy caused by pneumonia or pericarditis irritating the central diaphragmatic peritoneum can cause pain along the trapezius or the costal margins.

  E. **GI chest pain** is caused by gastric mucosal irritation or disruption by ingestion of ulcerogenic substances, excess gastric acidity, and unknown factors that expose submucosal gastric structures to noxious stimuli. GI pain also can be caused by luminal obstruction and distention. Pancreatitis, acute distention of a hollow viscus such as the gallbladder, acute liver distention, and subdiaphragmatic abscess can result in referred chest pain. Esophageal chest pain is caused by irritation of the esophageal mucosa or by intense muscular contraction of esophageal smooth muscle.

F. **Integumental, skeletal, and muscular chest pain** may be caused by irritation, trauma, and compression of the nerves, muscles, bone, and cartilaginous structures of the chest wall.

G. **Breast-related chest pain** may result from trauma or from inflammatory and infectious processes of the breast.

V. **Symptoms.** Generally, somatic chest pain is referred to a specific level of the spinal cord and is localized, while visceral chest pain is transmitted to several levels and is likely to be diffuse. Chest pain arising from two separate sources can significantly modify the patient's perception of pain.

A. **Cardiac chest pain.** This pain is variable and is sometimes described as tightness, pressure, or burning of moderate to severe intensity that is located substernally and diffusely over the left chest. Less frequently, the pain may radiate to the right chest and the right upper extremity, and it may be described as tingling, numbness, or other nonspecific discomfort. Cardiac chest pain lasting 2–5 minutes that is precipitated by a predictable stress and relieved by cessation of the stress usually represents stable angina. When the discomfort of angina increases in frequency, duration, and severity and becomes increasingly resistant to rest, removal of other provoking causes, and antianginal medications, the possibility of impending myocardial infarction or unstable angina must be considered. The pain and associated symptoms of an acute myocardial infarction may not be preceded by predictable precipitating factors seen in stable angina, since myocardial ischemia and injury are precipitated by acute cessation of coronary blood flow secondary to thrombus formation. Myocardial pain caused by coronary spasm likewise may not have consistent precipitating events. Women and the elderly are more likely to have atypical presentations.

1. Symptoms associated with **ischemic cardiac disease** include palpitations, sweating, cool skin, shortness of breath, weakness, nausea, emesis, syncope (or near-syncope), and a sense of impending doom. Syncope or near-syncope associated with myocardial ischemia could represent left ventricular dysfunction, rhythm disturbances, or volume contraction.

2. The sharp paroxysmal pain of **pericarditis** is usually substernal or to the left of the sternum, and it can be exacerbated by swallowing, deep breathing, and torsion of the trunk. The pain may radiate to the left shoulder, upper back, and neck and may be associated with fever.

3. When cardiac pain is referred to the upper abdominal area, symptoms may simulate acute appendicitis, intestinal obstruction, and perforation of a peptic ulcer. Referral of cardiac pain to the back and the right upper quadrant may simulate cholecystitis and biliary colic.

4. Patients who are elderly and who have diabetes mellitus may have significant coronary artery disease with myocardial ischemia but have no chest pain.

B. **Aortic chest pain.** Acute aortic dissection causes pain that is severe and described by some patients as tearing. Aortic arch dissection usually causes diffuse substernal upper anterior chest pain with radiation into the shoulders. Progression of the dissection into the descending aorta causes pain at the base of the neck and along the back in the interscapular area. Dissection can impair blood supply to the carotid or vertebral arteries, causing syncope, coma, hemiplegia, and blindness. Renal artery involvement may cause acute oliguria, and mesenteric artery involvement may result in abdominal pain because of bowel ischemia. If the base of the aortic root is involved in the dissection, aortic pressures may be reduced, thus decreasing coronary artery blood flow.

C. **Tracheal and pleural chest pain**

1. The pain of **acute tracheitis** is perceived under the upper portion of the sternum and may be described as a burning sensation. Coughing and sneezing tend to exacerbate this discomfort. The pain is usually lateral to the sternum if its origin is in the major bronchi.

2. **Pulmonary embolism.** Although the most prominent symptom associated with pulmonary embolus is acute shortness of breath secondary to diffuse pulmonary bronchoconstriction, acute pleuritic chest pain can be present when the embolus is massive or associated with infarction or parietal pleural inflammation. Hemoptysis associated with the symptoms of a pulmonary em-

bolus suggests the presence of pulmonary infarction. If symptoms of a pulmonary embolus occur 1–5 days after the fracture of a large bone such as the hip, a fat embolus should be considered a source of lung injury.

   3. **Pneumonia** may cause pleuritic chest pain, chills, fever, shortness of breath, and fatigue (see Chapter 16).
   4. A **pneumothorax** is associated with an acute, sharp, unilateral, pleuritic chest pain and shortness of breath. Pneumomediastinum can be associated with a pneumothorax and can be caused by coughing, vomiting, bronchial asthma, or heavy lifting.

D. **Diaphragmatic chest pain** from pleurisy caused by pericarditis, pneumonia, or subphrenic abscess is sharp pain along the trapezius muscle or the costal margins that is made worse by coughing and deep breathing. A considerable amount of distortion of other mediastinal structures must occur in order to cause pain. Such distortion occurs with carcinoma of the esophagus and the apex of the lungs, large aortic aneurysms, spontaneous mediastinal emphysema, acute inflammatory disease, and traumatic rupture of the esophagus.

E. **GI chest pain**
   1. Irritation of the esophageal mucosa is accompanied by a burning sensation in the upper thoracic, cervical, and nasopharyngeal regions. Large meals and recumbent position may precipitate or exacerbate the chest discomfort from an incompetent lower esophageal sphincter. The pain of diffuse esophageal spasm is a nonlocalized heavy sensation, at times associated with dysphagia and located mostly to the left of the sternum. The association of substernal pain, vomiting, difficulty in swallowing, and weight loss suggests esophageal cancer. Forceful vomiting and retching may precede esophageal rupture.
   2. Burning chest pain occurring after meals suggests gastritis or peptic ulcer disease, especially if the pain is relieved by food and antacids. Chest pain following the ingestion of aspirin, nonsteroidal anti-inflammatory drugs (NSAIDs), slow-release potassium products, or alcohol may indicate not only the presence of gastritis or peptic ulcer disease but also the possible inciting agent.
   3. Sharp chest pain radiating to the back associated with the chronic use of alcohol may indicate acute or chronic pancreatitis.
   4. Colicky right-sided chest pain radiating to the back implies the possible presence of biliary colic caused by stone, stricture, or neoplasm. Colicky chest pain following a large meal containing fatty foods may indicate gallbladder disease and pylorospasm. The presence of an elevated temperature associated with right-sided chest pain suggests cholecystitis.
   5. Sharp chest pain preceded by retching, vomiting, or hematemesis suggests Mallory-Weiss syndrome.

F. **Integumental, skeletal, and muscular chest pain**
   1. Chest pain caused by herpes zoster is usually intense, often burning, or knife-like, and precedes and often persists after the vesicular rash has subsided.
   2. Bone pain is usually intense, well localized, and described as exquisitely tender over the affected area. Sharp, stabbing chest pain may be associated with costochondritis, chest wall contusion, rib fracture, and primary or secondary bone disease. Costochondral and chondrosternal pain, swelling, or both may simulate angina. The pain is usually well localized, but it may radiate across the chest and over the arms. Musculoskeletal chest pain tends to occur with movement of the inflamed muscle and involved body part and may be caused by trauma, incorrect posture, and nonspecific inflammatory processes of bone and muscles.
   3. Thoracic outlet syndromes may cause chest pain. Nerve compression is frequent and is usually associated with paresthesia. Vascular compression is less common and is associated with diffuse pain and coldness and weakness of the involved extremity.

G. **Breast-related chest pain.** Inflammatory processes of the breast produce sharp, cutting, and aching pain that may be referred to the medial aspect of the arm. Chest pain occurring premenstrually suggests fibrocystic breast disease.

H. **Psychogenic chest pain.** Chest pain that is absent during weekends or when the patient is away from stressful situations implies anxiety-tension syndromes. Such chest pain may be difficult to detect because the patient may be reluctant to discuss personal matters that are emotionally painful.

VI. Signs

    A. Cardiac chest pain. Fast, slow, or irregular pulses may be associated with myocardial ischemia. Pulse amplitude may be decreased if the force and volume of cardiac output are decreased. Cardiac chest pain may be associated with cool, sweaty skin and, in the presence of cardiac failure, with pulmonary edema and venous hypertension. An S_4 and a paradoxically split S_2 may accompany angina. A midsystolic click and a late systolic murmur suggest the presence of mitral valve prolapse. Pericarditis may cause a transient three-component friction rub and pulsus paradoxus. If the effusion associated with pericarditis is large, venous distention and other signs of cardiac tamponade may be present.

    B. Aortic chest pain from dissection may be associated with hypotension, discrepancies in blood pressure of the upper extremities, absence of peripheral pulses, and a murmur of aortic insufficiency. Patients may also present with congestive heart failure, stroke, and paraplegia.

    C. Tracheal and pleural chest pain

        1. In young children, **acute tracheitis** is characterized by a barking cough and may cause signs of respiratory distress.

        2. **Pulmonary embolus** may cause tachypnea and tachycardia. Chest auscultation may reveal rales, wheezes, and pleural friction rubs and increased S_2. Unilateral leg edema and pain may represent thrombophlebitis, which may be the origin of a pulmonary embolus.

        3. **Pneumonias** can be characterized by fever, tachycardia, pulmonary rales, and signs of pulmonary consolidation.

        4. If a **pneumothorax** is stable and small, there may be no associated signs. A large tension pneumothorax may cause tracheal deviation, hyperresonance, decreased breath sounds, decreased tactile and vocal fremitus, and respiratory distress.

    D. Chest pain from other mediastinal organs. Signs associated with disorders of other mediastinal organs occur late in the disease process and are associated with disruption of ventilation by tumor or expansion of vascular or other benign lesions. If a malignant neoplasm of a mediastinal structure is present, weight loss may occur. Obvious bleeding may indicate traumatic rupture of the esophagus. Fever is usually associated with inflammation of the mediastinum.

    E. GI chest pain

        1. **Peptic ulcer disease** is often associated with epigastric tenderness, signs of gastric outlet obstruction, and the peritoneal signs associated with peptic ulcer perforation and penetration.

        2. **Gallbladder inflammation or stones** may cause biliary tract distention and right upper quadrant tenderness, at times associated with abdominal rebound and jaundice.

        3. **Pancreatitis** causes signs of peritoneal inflammation (eg, rebound abdomen tenderness) and volume depletion (eg, hypotension or tachycardia).

        4. **Esophagitis** and **diffuse esophageal spasm** do not produce detectable signs. However, esophageal neoplasia may result in esophagitis and weight loss in late stages.

        5. **Spontaneous esophageal rupture** causes signs of mediastinitis (eg, fever).

    F. Integumental, skeletal, and muscular chest pain. Localized tenderness and pain with movement characterize disorders of skin, bone, and muscle that cause chest pain. Vesicular rash and tenderness in a dermatomal distribution suggest herpes zoster.

    G. Breast-related chest pain. Physical examination of the breast may reveal evidence of trauma, localized or diffuse tenderness, or skin disease (eg, herpes zoster or breast abscess).

    H. Psychogenic chest pain. Few physical signs are present with psychogenic chest pain other than signs of depression, such as weight loss or gain.

VII. Laboratory tests (see Chapters 10, 16, 22, 29, 45, and 86)

    A. Electrocardiography (ECG) and **serial cardiac isoenzyme tests** should be performed immediately for all patients with suspected cardiac chest pain.

        1. ST-segment elevation or depression, T-wave inversion, new Q waves of greater than 0.04 seconds, dysrhythmias, varying degrees of arteriovenous block, and reduction in aortic pressures may be associated with myocardial ischemia and infarction.

        2. ST-segment elevation, in most leads except aVR and V_1, is associated with pericarditis.

      3. Evidence of acute cor pulmonale, sinus tachycardia, and right axis deviation is associated with pulmonary embolus.

  B. Creatine phosphokinase (CPK) elevated with an MB fraction (CPK-MB) elevation suggests myocardial muscle infarction. Levels begin to rise within 4 hours of the acute event and peak within 18–24 hours.

  C. Cardiac troponins. Cardiac-specific troponin I and troponin T increase 3–12 hours after myocardial infarction and reach maximal levels at 12–24 hours. These cardiac-specific troponins are more specific and have greater sensitivity for myocardial injury than CPK-MB. Cardiac troponins remain elevated for 5–14 days, increasing the likelihood of diagnosing a recent myocardial infarction, when evaluation of chest pain is delayed because of atypical presentation or current clinical events suggest a recent "silent" myocardial infarction.

  D. Lactate dehydrogenase (LDH) levels are usually not specific for myocardial injury, although LDH-1 levels greater than LDH-2 levels suggest the possibility of myocardial infarction.

  E. Two-dimensional echocardiograms detect cardiomegaly, cardiac chamber size, valvular abnormalities, the presence of pericardial effusion, ejection fraction, and cardiac wall motion abnormalities.

  F. An elevated **erythrocyte sedimentation rate** and leukocytosis may be present with pericarditis.

  G. Blood cultures, viral serology, autoimmune studies (eg, antinuclear antibodies), **thyroid-stimulating hormone, blood urea nitrogen, creatinine, and cold agglutinin tests** may reveal the cause of pericarditis.

  H. Arterial blood gases may reveal hypoxia and acute respiratory alkalosis caused by pulmonary embolus and some pneumonias.

  I. Occult blood on stool examination may indicate the presence of esophageal and gastric lesions associated with GI bleeding.

  J. Chest x-rays may reveal evidence of left ventricular failure as a consequence of severe coronary artery disease, a widened mediastinum from aortic dissection, small pleural effusion and wedge-shaped zones of consolidation and hyperinflation from pulmonary embolus, consolidated areas of lung in pneumonia or a hyperlucent area between the chest wall, and the visceral pleura of the lung from pneumothorax. A large pneumothorax may cause mediastinal contents to shift toward the unaffected lung. Chest x-rays may also reveal fractures, spinal osteoarthritis, or malignant primary or metastatic processes.

  K. Exercise stress tests may reveal evidence of myocardial ischemia.

  L. Radionuclide scans using thallium with exercise tests may reveal hypoperfused portions of myocardium and abnormal ventricular wall movement suggestive of coronary artery disease.

  M. Coronary angiography and left ventriculography are used to determine the location and extent of coronary artery obstruction and the presence of left ventricular wall motion abnormalities.

  N. Venography and impedance plethysmography will reveal evidence identifying lower-extremity deep vein thrombosis in patients with pulmonary embolus originating from that source.

  O. Upper GI series and gastroscopy can detect duodenal and gastric ulcers and strictures, and esophagogastroscopy can detect mucosal lesions in addition to the above.

  P. Ventilation-perfusion lung scans may reveal ventilation-perfusion mismatches in patients with pulmonary embolus, but these mismatches can also be seen with chronic lung disease.

  Q. Pulmonary angiography is reserved for those patients in whom the diagnosis of pulmonary embolus is uncertain after less invasive tests although clinical suspicion remains high.

  R. Computerized tomography scans can identify the level and extent of aortic dissection and can identify cervical and thoracic spinal disk disease.

  S. Barium swallows can reveal esophageal motility disorders, benign and malignant esophageal neoplasms, and evidence of the reflux of gastric contents through an incompetent lower esophageal sphincter.

VIII. Treatment

  A. Cardiac chest pain

    1. Myocardial ischemia and/or infarction causing chest pain can be acutely, partially, or completely relieved by sublingual nitroglycerin, which also has the potential to relieve chest pain associated with esophageal spasm. Triage for reperfusion therapy must be made rapidly to enhance possible myocardial salvage. Patients should have intravenous access, morphine sulfate for pain, an aspirin to reduce platelet aggregation, heparin, beta blockers, oxygen supplementation, and thrombolytic therapy when indications warrant. Coronary angioplasty may be indicated when thrombolytic therapy is contraindicated. Acute, chronic, or recurrent chest pain caused by myocardial ischemia and myocardial infarction can also be relieved and prevented with the use of short- and long-acting nitrates and aspirin and by efforts to reduce cardiac work (eg, afterload reduction or cardiac rate control) and the improvement in myocardial oxygenation (coronary angioplasty and coronary artery bypass) (see Chapter 81).

   2. **Pericarditis** is usually treated with aspirin or other NSAIDs. Corticosteroids may be required if there is no response to more conservative therapy. Hospitalization is required if there are any signs of cardiac tamponade.

B. **Aortic dissection** is an acute medical emergency requiring hospitalization for aggressive antihypertensive therapy (see Chapter 80) and pain control. Pain relief is afforded only with potent narcotics. Acute proximal aortic dissection requires emergency surgical intervention.

C. **Tracheal and pleural chest pain** (see Chapter 16)

   1. **Pulmonary embolus and infarction** require hospitalization and acute intravenous anticoagulation to retard propagation and promote organization of deep vein thrombi. Long-term oral anticoagulation to prevent recurrence of thrombus formation is also necessary.

   2. A small, stable **pneumothorax** without evidence of respiratory compromise may require only observation, over several days, to ensure stabilization and resolution. A large, expanding tension pneumothorax may require hospitalization for chest tube insertion for lung reexpansion.

D. Treatment of **diaphragmatic pleurisy** caused by adjacent structures is directed to the specific diseased organ.

E. **GI chest pain** (see Chapters 22 and 86)

   1. **Cholelithiasis.** Symptomatic gallstones are treated with cholecystectomy, gallstone dissolution, or lithotripsy.

   2. **Pancreatitis** requires hospitalization for bowel rest, pain control, volume replacement, and removal of any offending agent or substance leading to this disorder.

F. **Musculoskeletal chest pain** is treated with rest and NSAIDs and other analgesics (eg, **ibuprofen,** 200–800 mg every 6 hours; **aspirin,** 1000–2000 mg every 4 hours; or **naproxen,** 250–500 mg twice a day).

G. **Breast-related chest pain** (see Chapter 10).

H. **Psychogenic chest pain.** Counseling and psychotherapy may be helpful (see Chapters 93, 96, and 100).

REFERENCES

Achem SR, Kolts BE, MacMath T, et al: Effects of omeprazole versus placebo in treatment of noncardiac chest pain and gastroesophageal reflux. Dig Dis Sci 1997;**42:**2138.

Eagle KA: Medical decision making in patients with chest pain. N Engl J Med 1991;**324:**1282.

Everts B, Karlson BW, Wahrborg P, et al: Localization of pain in suspected acute myocardial infarction in relation to final diagnosis, age and sex, and site and type of infarction. Heart Lung 1996;**25:**430.

Hackshaw BT: Excluding heart disease in the patient with chest pain. Am J Med 1992;**92**(5A):46S.

Hoffman RS, Hollander JE: Evaluation of patients with chest pain after cocaine use. Crit Care Clin 1997;**13:**809.

Mayou R: Chest pain, palpitations and panic. J Psychosomat Res 1998;**44:**53.

Nanbu R, Satou I, Nishijima H, et al: Differentiation of vasospastic angina from noncardiac chest pain by history and coronary risk factors in patients with chest pain at rest. Intern Med 1997;**36:**676.

Richter JE: Practical approach to the diagnosis of unexplained chest pain. Med Clin North Am 1991;**75:**1203.

Shima MA: Evaluation of chest pain. Back to the basics of history taking and physical examination. Postgrad Med 1992;**91:**155, 161.

13   Cold & Heat Injuries

Frank S. Celestino, MD

I. **Definitions.** The term *cold injuries* refers to a group of systemic or localized illnesses caused by excessive exposure to cold, sometimes wet, environments. The term *heat injuries* represents a heterogeneous group of disorders caused by excessive exercise in or prolonged exposure to warm environments.

II. **Common diagnoses**
   A. **Cold injuries**
      1. **Frostnip** is transient, localized, very superficial skin cooling without tissue destruction.
      2. **Chilblain** (pernio) is a form of nondestructive, cold-induced hypersensitivity reaction in the skin.
      3. **Immersion foot** (trench foot) is a nonfreezing pedal tissue injury caused by prolonged exposure to wet and cold.
      4. **Frostbite** represents tissue injury or death from acute freezing.
      5. **Accidental systemic hypothermia** involves an unintended decrease from the body's average 37 °C (98.6 °F) homeothermic core body temperature to <35 °C (95 °F) because of environmental exposure or immersion. Hypothermia may mimic drug or alcohol overdose, head trauma, stroke, overwhelming sepsis, myxedema coma, and central nervous system infections.
   B. **Heat injuries**
      1. *Heat edema* refers to swelling of the feet and ankles associated with prolonged sitting or standing in warm environments.
      2. **Heat syncope** involves sudden unconsciousness after prolonged standing or vigorous activity in the heat.
      3. **Heat cramps** are intense painful spasms of heavily exercised muscles, often the calves. They may occur during or after intense exertion.
      4. *Heat tetany* refers to acral and circumoral paresthesias, carpopedal spasm, and frank tetany.
      5. **Heat exhaustion** (prostration) is a clinical syndrome characterized by elevated core body temperature (<40 °C [104 °F]) with systemic symptoms and signs, excluding central nervous system dysfunction. **Heat stroke,** a true medical emergency, is characterized by marked elevations of core body temperature (>40.6 °C [105 °F]) combined with severe systemic symptoms, including serious central nervous system dysfunction. Early or mild heat stroke may be difficult to distinguish from heat exhaustion.
      6. **Thyroid storm** and **central nervous system infection** may, although rarely, mimic an environmentally induced heat injury.

III. **Epidemiology.** Cold injuries account for as many as 0.1% of ambulatory patient visits and 0.03% of civilian hospital admissions. Heat injuries are responsible for 0.2–0.3% of outpatient encounters and as many as 0.05% of civilian hospital admissions. Four percent to 9% of military recruits undergoing basic training in the southern United States during the summer suffer some form of heat-related illness.
   A. **Cold injuries**
      1. **Predisposing factors** for cold-related illnesses are listed in Table 13–1. In some studies, black race is listed as a risk factor, although the validity of such findings is clouded by the lack of control for socioeconomic variables. Environmental factors that modify the nature and extent of injury include wind speed, wind chill factor, temperature, duration of exposure, altitude, and degree of wetness.
      2. **Mortality rates** from cold injuries are rising. Increasing numbers of hypothermia-related deaths occur among the growing elderly population.
   B. **Heat injuries**
      1. **Predisposing factors** for heat-related illnesses are listed in Table 13–2. Men are affected two to three times more often than women. Blacks have a six- to 10-fold higher attack rate compared to whites, according to most surveys.

TABLE 13-1. PREDISPOSING FACTORS FOR COLD-RELATED ILLNESSES

Prolonged outdoor activities (eg, recreational or vocational)
Cold climate
Immobility
History of cold injuries
Inappropriate, wet, or tight-fitting clothing
Lack of acclimatization
Extensive skin damage
Psychiatric illness
Extremes of age
Preexisting central nervous system or cardiovascular disease
Malnutrition
Tobacco use
Sedative drugs, especially alcohol
Fatigue
Hypothyroidism
Blood loss

2. **Mortality rates** from heat-related illnesses are rising. Nearly 70% of all deaths occur among the poor, urban elderly population.

IV. Pathophysiology
A. Cold injuries
1. **Frostnip** is caused by the direct, reversible effects of cold on sensory nerves and dermal capillaries.
2. **Chilblain** involves edema of the papillary dermis and a mild lymphocytic vasculitis of both superficial and deep dermal vessels.
3. **Immersion foot** is caused by ischemic injury due to sustained severe vasoconstriction.
4. **Frostbite** is characterized by tissue destruction from (1) extracellular ice crystal formation, which increases the extracellular osmotic gradient and leads to intracellular dehydration, electrolyte imbalance, protein denaturation, and cell death; and (2) progressive vascular ischemic thrombosis and occlusion that is abetted by red blood cell sludging, platelet aggregation, and arterio-

TABLE 13-2. PREDISPOSING FACTORS FOR HEAT-RELATED ILLNESSES

Increased heat production

Exercise or exertion (eg, by athletes, military recruits, or manual laborers)
Infection (febrile state)
Labor (childbirth)
Hyperactivity (delirium, psychosis, alcohol withdrawal, status epilepticus, use of amphetamines, lysergic acid diethylamide [LSD], cocaine, or phencyclidine [PCP])
Hyperthyroidism
Malignant hyperthermia
Generalized tetanus

Impaired heat dissipation

Lack of acclimatization
High ambient temperature (including urban living, factories, and foundries)
High humidity
Obesity
Extremes of age
Heavy clothing
Dehydration
Cardiovascular disease
Autonomic dysfunction
Sweat gland dysfunction (cystic fibrosis, miliaria, or ectodermal dysplasia)
Skin disorders (scleroderma, ichthyosis, and burn sequelae)
Drugs (phenothiazines, anticholinergics, diuretics, antihistamines, beta blockers, and tricyclic antidepressants)
Previous episode of heat stroke
Alcoholism

venous shunting. Inflammatory mediators, prostaglandin F_2 and thromboxane A_4, play a key role in the ischemic vascular injury.

   5. **Accidental systemic hypothermia.** The primary form is characterized by normal thermoregulatory mechanisms but overwhelming cold exposure, as in cold water immersion or mountaineering accidents, while the secondary form, which usually affects elderly individuals, involves only mild to moderate cold stress but abnormal thermoregulation caused by drug- or disease-related alterations in heat production or loss (especially cardiovascular disease).

B. **Heat injuries**
   1. **Heat edema** involves muscular and cutaneous vasodilatation combined with venous stasis, leading to the accumulation of interstitial lower-extremity fluid.
   2. **Heat syncope** is characterized by cutaneous vasodilatation, peripheral pooling, and decreased venous return, causing cerebral hypoperfusion.
   3. **Heat cramps** are caused by profuse sweating, usually in acclimatized individuals or athletes who suffer disproportionate sodium loss despite adequate water repletion.
   4. **Heat tetany** is caused by marked respiratory alkalosis due to the hyperventilatory response to heat exposure.
   5. **Heat exhaustion** involves prolonged exposure or intense physical exertion in a warm environment that leads to profound water and salt depletion. There is no failure of thermoregulatory control. Although very often dehydration is isotonic, sometimes salt loss is in excess of water depletion (**hypotonic exhaustion**), while at other times water loss predominates (**hypertonic dehydration**). **Heat stroke** involves the failure of normal thermoregulatory mechanisms to compensate for the heat burden imposed by environmental temperature or exertional heat production. The body conserves central circulatory volume through peripheral vasoconstriction and sweat gland shutdown, at which point the core temperature precipitously rises to levels (>41.1 °C [106 °F]) that damage organs throughout the body by uncoupling oxidative phosphorylation and crippling cellular enzymes.

V. **Symptoms**
   A. **Cold injuries**
      1. **Localized numbness of affected areas** of exposed skin with tingling on rewarming is characteristic of **frostnip. Skin lesions that itch and burn significantly** are **chilblains.**
      2. **Coldness and anesthesia** followed by intense pain, burning, and tingling on rewarming is characteristic of **immersion foot.** Chronic cold hypersensitivity, pain and weakness on weight bearing, and hyperhidrosis may be sequelae.
      3. **Tingling or stinging sensations accompanied by painful dysesthesias,** and possibly prickly or itchy sensations, are the initial symptoms of **frostbite.** Eventually, paresthesias progress to numbness and anesthesia, possibly with stiffness and immobility. In 40–80% of cases, late symptoms include sensory deficits of touch, pain, and temperature as well as cold feet or hands, hyperhidrosis, numbness, pain, and joint discomfort. These symptoms can persist for years and can be quite debilitating. Thawing of frostbitten limbs causes tingling and burning sensations, and patients often experience throbbing pain and electric shock–like pain during the healing process as a result of ischemic neuritis and axonal degeneration.
      4. **Increasingly disturbing neuromuscular symptoms,** which correlate with the degree of temperature depression, are seen in **systemic hypothermia** (Table 13–3).
   B. **Heat injuries**
      1. A **vague sensation of fullness** in the affected part is usually the only symptom in otherwise asymptomatic patients with **heat edema.**
      2. **Pain from spastic abdominal or extremity muscles** with no systemic symptoms is indicative of **heat cramps.**
      3. **Acral and circumoral paresthesias** and often painful carpopedal spasm are involved in **heat tetany.**
      4. **Loss of consciousness** occurs when patients suffer from **heat syncope.**
      5. **Intense thirst, weakness, orthostatic dizziness,** faintness, anxiety, giddiness, impaired judgment, irritability, and muscular incoordination are common in patients with the **hypertonic dehydration form of heat exhaustion.**

TABLE 13–3. CLINICAL SYMPTOMS AND SIGNS AT DIFFERENT LEVELS OF SYSTEMIC HYPOTHERMIA

Temperature (°C)	Signs or Symptoms
34–36	Lethargy, moderate confusion, tachycardia, normal or raised blood pressure, hyperventilation, prominent shivering, stumbling and incoordination, exaggerated deep tendon reflexes (DTRs) and pupillary responses, peripheral vasoconstriction, normal electrocardiogram (ECG)
30–34	Delirium, bradycardia, hypotension, hypoventilation, minimal shivering, muscular rigidity (gelling), dilated pupils, normal to depressed DTRs, hypoxia, acidosis, cyanosis, depressed bowel sounds, cold diuresis, cardiac arrhythmias, Osborn (J) wave may be seen on ECG
<30	Unconsciousness (even appearing dead), profound bradycardia (even cardiac standstill), severe hypotension, shock, marked hypoventilation, extreme muscular rigidity simulating rigor mortis, absent DTRs and bowel sounds, fixed and unresponsive pupils, marked risk of spontaneous ventricular fibrillation

Nausea, vomiting, diarrhea, fatigue, malaise, headaches, anorexia, and muscle cramps are associated with **hypotonic exhaustion,** although overlap in these two groups of symptoms often exists (eg, isotonic exhaustion).

6. **Any constellation of neurologic symptoms** is possible with **heat stroke.** Headache, irritability, mild confusion, weakness, and dizziness are early symptoms; delirium, seizures, ataxia, and coma may occur as the body temperature rises. The severity of central nervous system involvement distinguishes heat stroke from heat exhaustion. Gastrointestinal symptoms such as nausea, vomiting, and diarrhea may predominate.

VI. **Signs**

A. **Cold injuries**

1. **Pale skin that retains some ability to blanch** with pressure is indicative of **frostnip.**

2. **Lesions on the face or extremities** consisting of discrete patches of warm, edematous, reddish-blue or violaceous skin are **chilblains.** Blisters may occur in rare cases.

3. **A cold, nearly anesthetic, mildly swollen, white or cyanotic limb** in which pulses are greatly diminished indicates **immersion foot.** During the first few days after rewarming, the extremity becomes hyperemic, hot, and edematous with bounding pulses. Blistering, ecchymosis, ulceration, and, in severe cases, gangrene may occur. Skin depigmentation, hyperhidrosis, and cold sensitivity usually develop during the next several weeks, and edema subsides.

4. **Skin and subcutaneous tissue that appear white, nonblanchable, waxy, and frozen,** accompanied by underlying structures that are soft and resilient when depressed before thawing indicate **superficial frostbite.** Erythema, mild edema, and bleb formation may subsequently occur, but no permanent tissue loss occurs. An icy, hard, or wooden appearance without deep tissue resilience represents **deep frostbite.** Hemorrhagic bullae, massive edema, cyanosis, gangrene, and even mummification often develop in these cases.

5. **Signs of severe neuromuscular, cardiovascular, and central nervous system dysfunction** emerge as the core body temperature descends in **systemic hypothermia** (Table 13–3).

B. **Heat injuries**

1. **Swelling of the feet and ankles** is common in patients with **heat edema.** Carpopedal spasm and even frank tetany are characteristic of **heat tetany.**

2. **Cool, moist skin, a weak and rapid pulse, and transient hypotension with accompanying orthostasis** may occur with **heat syncope.** The patient's mental status is normal upon regaining consciousness, and the core temperature is normal.

3. **Tense, tender muscles with associated fasciculations** are usually present with **heat cramps.**

4. **Orthostasis, hypotension, tachycardia, tachypnea, oliguria, weight loss, and pallor** are common to various degrees in patients with **heat exhaustion.** Ashen, cold, clammy, or intensely diaphoretic skin and a modestly elevated

core temperature (even as high as 40 °C [104 °F]) may be apparent. Mucous membranes and skin show signs of dehydration. Cognitive functioning remains intact, except for mild giddiness and slight impairment of judgment.

5. **Core temperature elevation to 40.6 °C (105 °F) or higher, sinus tachycardia, hyperventilation, anhidrosis (usually) with dry, hot, even cyanotic skin, orthostatic hypotension or shock, focal neurologic signs of almost any type, and signs of coagulopathy (ecchymoses, petechiae, hematuria, hematemesis)** are characteristic of **heat stroke.**

VII. Laboratory tests

A. Cold injuries. Laboratory tests can help detect any of the multisystem complications of hypothermia, such as bronchopneumonia, pulmonary edema, congestive heart failure, myocardial infarction, arrhythmias, acute renal failure, disseminated intravascular coagulation (DIC), pancreatitis, myoglobinuria, and hypoglycemia.

1. **Routine laboratory studies** are not indicated in cases of frostnip, chilblain, and immersion foot. A **complete blood cell count** is the only necessary routine study for patients with frostbite.

2. **Wound and blood cultures** are recommended if complications of immersion injury (eg, cellulitis, thrombophlebitis, or wet gangrene) occur. Such cultures may also be desirable in more serious cases of frostbite.

3. **Ongoing clinical surveillance** for infectious complications is required for all patients with frostbite.

4. **Arteriography** or, preferably, a **noninvasive vascular investigation** (eg, Doppler ultrasonography, digital plethysmography, or triple-phase radioactive isotope scanning) should be performed on all patients with frostbite except those with clearly very superficial injury. Unfortunately, none of these imaging modalities can reliably predict the extent of future tissue damage at the time of initial examination. Rather, they are most useful 1–3 weeks after injury to assess the boundaries of tissue viability and help plan for surgical therapy of devitalized tissues. Recently, magnetic resonance scanning was shown to be superior to traditional triple-phase isotope scanning in assessing tissue viability.

5. **Liver enzyme, glucose, amylase, electrolytes, blood urea nitrogen (BUN), creatinine, complete blood cell count, platelet count, fibrinogen, fibrin degradation products, prothrombin time (PT), partial thromboplastin time (PTT), urine myoglobin determination, chest x-ray, electrocardiography (ECG), and blood culture tests** must be performed as initial studies for all patients with accidental systemic hypothermia.

B. Heat injuries. Laboratory tests often show severe heat stroke complications such as dehydration, leukocytosis, hemoconcentration, hyperuricemia, lactic acidosis, hypokalemia, thrombocytopenia, hypocalcemia, hypophosphatemia, abnormal clotting, DIC, respiratory alkalosis, metabolic acidosis, and evidence of myocardial, hepatic, or renal damage. Hepatic and myocardial enzymes often reach into the tens of thousands in heat stroke victims, and arrhythmias may occur.

1. **Routine laboratory studies** are not required for patients with heat edema, heat syncope, heat cramps, and heat tetany.

2. **Serum electrolytes** may be useful in severe cases of heat cramps to detect sodium alterations or hypokalemia.

3. **Urinalysis, serum electrolytes, BUN, and creatinine tests** should be performed in all patients with heat exhaustion to detect any serious disturbances in sodium, potassium, fluid status, and renal function.

4. **Complete blood cell and platelet counts, coagulation studies, arterial blood gases, liver function tests, and a urine myoglobin evaluation** should be performed to distinguish heat stroke from heat exhaustion. Occult mild rhabdomyolysis and modest elevation in liver enzymes may occur with heat exhaustion, but high levels (tens of thousands) of liver enzymes occur only with heat stroke.

5. **Complete blood cell count, platelets, PT, PTT, fibrinogen, fibrin degradation products, electrolytes, BUN, creatinine, blood sugar, urinalysis, calcium, phosphorus, liver function tests, ECG, creatine kinase, urine myoglobin, amylase, blood lactate, uric acid, and arterial blood gas determinations** should be included as initial laboratory tests for all patients with heat stroke.

VIII. Treatment

A. Cold injuries

1. **Frostnip** requires no special treatment other than gradual spontaneous rewarming. There are no sequelae.

2. **Chilblain.** Mild cases need only spontaneous rewarming with protection from the environment. In more symptomatic patients, warm (<41.1 °C [106 °F]) water immersion is used. Analgesics and antipruritics are adjuncts. The area should not be rubbed or massaged. Because the lesions may recur yearly on exposure to cold, windy conditions, protective covering is advised. **Nifedipine,** 20–60 mg/day orally, has been shown to provide rapid clearing of acute lesions and symptoms and to prevent development of new lesions.

3. **Immersion foot.** Initial treatment consists of removing constrictive wet footgear and protecting the limb from trauma and continued cold exposure. Gentle gradual rewarming and drying are accomplished by exposure to room air without massaging. Hospitalization is preferable in all but the mildest cases.

4. **Frostbite.** Thawing in the field should be avoided if there is any risk of refreezing, and the cold-injured part should never be rubbed or massaged and should never bear weight. Hospitalization is required except in clear-cut cases of minor superficial injury since the extent of tissue damage is often difficult to predict at the time of initial evaluation. If there is associated systemic hypothermia, raising of the core body temperature should take precedence over treatment of the frostbitten appendage.

   a. Rewarming in a rapid yet controlled manner is the critical element of therapy. The affected part should be immersed for 20–30 minutes in a circulating warm water bath that is precisely controlled at 40–42 °C (104–108 °F).

   b. Narcotics may be administered for pain (especially during rewarming). Supportive measures include protection of the limb from infection and trauma, twice-daily hydrotherapy in a warm (40 °C [104 °F]) water/hexachlorophene bath, tetanus prophylaxis, nicotine avoidance, limb splinting and elevation to minimize edema, at least twice-daily application of aloe vera cream (at least 70% concentration and alcohol-free), which is a potent antiprostaglandin, and use of sterile dressings. Blisters containing clear or milky fluid, which is rich in inflammatory mediators, should be debrided prior to aloe vera application. Hemorrhagic blisters can be aspirated or left intact.

   c. Anecdotal and experimental evidence suggests improved outcomes from the use of ibuprofen (800 mg orally three times daily or 12 mg/kg/day) and prophylactic intravenous penicillin (500,000 units every 6 hours for 72 hours). Further antibiotics are given only if infection arises. Vasodilators (reserpine, 0.5 mg intra-arterially once, or phenoxybenzamine, 10–60 mg/day orally) have been advocated by some, but remain an optional therapy. Reserpine accomplishes a medical sympathectomy by depleting arterial wall norepinephrine for up to 4 weeks, thus improving distal blood flow. Other promising agents not yet adequately studied in humans include superoxide dismutase, a free radical scavenger, pentoxifylline (platelet antiaggregation), and hyperbaric oxygen.

   d. Unproven or controversial therapies include heparin, low-molecular-weight dextran, steroids, calcium channel blockers, dipyridamole, vitamin C, streptokinase, dimethyl sulfoxide, and surgical sympathectomy.

   e. Escharotomy or fasciotomy is performed if circulation is impaired or a compartment syndrome develops. Definitive amputation should be delayed until 3–5 weeks after injury when tissue demarcation becomes clear.

   f. Preventive measures are necessary, since the patient will have heightened susceptibility to subsequent cold stress.

5. **Accidental systemic hypothermia** is a medical emergency. All patients should be hospitalized for definitive rewarming therapy in an intensive care unit. Initial management should include provision of supplemental oxygen, gentle manipulation to prevent ventricular fibrillation, establishment of intravenous access, removal of wet clothing, and transfer to a warm room. Recurrent hypothermia is a significant risk for recovered hypothermia victims because of residual subclinical impairment of thermoregulatory reflexes. Education concerning risk factors and preexposure planning are necessary.

B. Heat injuries

1. **Heat edema** is self-limited. Treatment involves the use of support hose and simple periodic evaluation of the lower limbs. Diuretics are not indicated.

2. **Heat syncope** responds to rest in a recumbent position, cooling, and oral rehydration.

3. Patients with **heat cramps and heat tetany** respond to cessation of physical exertion, rest in a cool place, gentle stretching of the involved muscle groups, and oral rehydration with salt water or commercially available electrolyte/glucose solutions (eg, Gatorade). In more severe cases, intravenous normal saline, 1 L over 1–2 hours, can be effective. Salt tablets should not be used.

4. **Heat exhaustion.** Hospitalization may be necessary. All patients need rest from exercise, a cool environment, and recumbency. Mild to moderate illness may be treated with oral electrolyte solutions unless nausea or vomiting supervenes. More severe cases will require intravenous fluids (1–2 L over 2–4 hours), electrolyte repletion, and cooling measures such as ice packs to the groin and axillae and/or tepid water spraying with electric fanning.

5. **Heat stroke.** All patients should be hospitalized for definitive treatment. Initial therapy includes supplemental oxygen, transfer to a cool place, removal of clothing, and intravenous access for fluid repletion. The goal of treatment is to reduce the core temperature to 39 °C (102 °F) within 60 minutes while limiting iatrogenic effects and minimizing illness sequelae. Evaporative cooling using whole-body sprays of lukewarm water with fan-blown air is the easiest and most efficient method of reducing the core body temperature. This can be combined with strategic ice packing in the groin, axillae, and neck. Other, less optimal techniques include cold water submersion, cold gastric or peritoneal lavage, and cool intravenous fluids. Intravenous diazepam (5–10 mg) or chlorpromazine (5–10 mg) is helpful in abolishing shivering that will occur with cooling.

   Education is important, since heat stroke survivors suffer from persistent thermolability and an increased risk of recurrent heat injury.

REFERENCES

Cold Injuries

Braun R, Krishel S: Environmental emergencies. Emerg Med Clin North Am 1997;**15**:451.

Danzl DF: Frostbite. In Rosen P, Barkin R (editors): *Emergency Medicine: Concepts and Clinical Practice.* 4th ed. Mosby; 1998:953.

Danzl DF: Accidental hypothermia. In Rosen P, Barkin R (editors): *Emergency Medicine: Concepts and Clinical Practice.* 4th ed. Mosby; 1998:963.

Leikin JB, Aks SE, Andrews S, et al: Environmental injuries. Disease-a-Month 1997;**43**:821.

Reamy BV: Frostbite: Review and current concepts. J Am Board Fam Pract 1998;**11**:34.

Heat Injuries

Armstrong LE, Epstein Y, Greenleaf JE, et al: American College of Sports Medicine position stand: Heat and cold illness during distance running. Med Sci Sports Exerc 1996;**28**:1.

Barrow MW, Clark KA: Heat-related illnesses. Am Fam Physician 1998;**58**:749.

Hales JR: Hyperthermia and heat illness: Pathophysiologic implications for avoidance and treatment. Ann NY Acad Sci 1997;**813**:534.

Hett HA, Brechtelsbauer DA: Heat-related illness. Postgrad Med 1998;**103**:107.

Yarbrough B: Heat illness. In Rosen P, Barkin R (editors): *Emergency Medicine: Concepts and Clinical Practice.* 4th ed. Mosby; 1998:986.

---

14   Confusion

Bruce M. LeClair, MD, MPH

I. **Definition.** *Confusion* is a general term frequently used to describe some aspect of global cognitive impairment, usually disorientation or inappropriate reaction to environmental stimuli. For the purposes of this chapter, the disturbance should be clinically significant and a change from a previous level of functioning (as opposed to confusion due to mental retardation or transient disorientation due to unfamiliarity with surroundings).

II. **Common diagnoses.** Common causes of clinically significant confusion include **delirium, dementia,** and **depressive pseudodementia.** In addition to the common causes of confusion described here, **age-associated memory disorder, amnestic disorder, malingering,** and **factitious disorder** must be entertained.

   A. **Delirium** is also termed acute confusional state (ACS), metabolic encephalopathy, toxic psychosis, acute brain syndrome, and psychosis associated with organic brain syndrome. *ACS* and *delirium* are the preferred terms. The fourth edition of the American Psychiatric Association's *Diagnostic and Statistical Manual of Mental Disorders* subdivides the causes into general medical conditions, substances, or a combination of these factors. Diagnostic features of delirium are given in Table 14–1.

      1. Due to a **general medical condition**

         a. **Metabolic disorders,** such as electrolyte and fluid imbalances; hepatic, renal, or pulmonary failure; diabetes; hyperthyroidism or hypothyroidism and other endocrinopathies; nutritional deficiencies; and hypothermia and heat stroke.

         b. **Infections,** including pneumonia, urinary tract infection, bacteremia and septicemia, meningitis or encephalitis, septic emboli, neurosyphilis, human immunodeficiency virus (HIV) dementia, and brain abscess.

         c. **Cardiovascular disorders,** such as congestive heart failure, arrhythmia, myocardial infarction, hypovolemia, aortic stenosis, transient ischemic episodes and stroke, chronic subdural hematoma, vasculitis, arteriosclerosis, subarachnoid hemorrhage, and hypertensive encephalopathy.

         d. **Neoplastic disease,** including systemic primary intracranial or metastatic disease to the brain. Cancer is the most common cause of death among delirious patients; the 6-month mortality rate is 25%.

         e. **Postoperative state.**

         f. **Seizure disorders** (ie, ictal and postictal states).

         g. **Acute psychoses.**

         h. **Other disorders,** especially in the elderly, including fecal impaction and urinary retention.

      2. Due to **substances** (Table 14–2). Drug intoxication is the most common cause of acute confusion in late adolescents and young adults.

   B. **Environmental factors,** such as the transfer of an elderly individual to unfamiliar surroundings, may cause confusion.

   C. **Dementias,** such as Alzheimer's disease, multi-infarct dementia, and Parkinson's disease as well as reversible or partially reversible causes such as thyroid disease, vitamin deficiencies (eg, B_{12} or folate), infections, metabolic abnormalities, and normal pressure hydrocephalus.

   D. **Depressive pseudodementia.** Depression may coexist with dementia in over one third of outpatients with dementia and in an even larger portion of patients with dementia in nursing homes.

TABLE 14–1. DIAGNOSTIC CRITERIA FOR DELIRIUM

A. The ability to focus, sustain, or shift attention is impaired.

B. There is an accompanying change in cognition (which may include memory impairment, disorientation, or language disturbance).

C. The disturbance develops over a short period and tends to fluctuate over the course of the day. Associated features and disorders:

    1. Disturbance of the sleep-wake cycle

    2. Disturbed psychomotor behavior

    3. Emotional disturbances such as anxiety, fear, or depression

Because of a general medical condition, A through C plus . . .

D. There is evidence from the history, physical examination, or laboratory findings that the disturbance is caused by the direct physiologic consequences of a general medical condition.

Due to substance intoxication, A through C plus . . .

E. There is evidence from the history, physical examination, or laboratory findings of either of the following:

    1. The symptoms in A and B developed during substance intoxication.

    2. Medication use is causally related to the disturbance.

III. Epidemiology. The reported prevalence and incidence of confusion vary, depending on the definition, the patient's perceptions, and the setting. Patients who perceive confusion as memory loss or a temporary lapse are more likely to report episodes than those who perceive it as a permanent, progressive process.

Age alone is not a predictor of confusion. Poorer health, change in health status, and education level (often a proxy for socioeconomic status) have been shown to be better predictors of self-referred, ambulatory episodes of confusion.

In a study of 1365 persons aged 55 and older living in the community, 3.3% reported being "frequently," 14.4% "sometimes," 16.3% "rarely," and 66% "never" confused during the previous year. Of the 34% reporting confusion, only 17.2% reported episodes occurring more frequently than in the prior year.

A. The elderly are the population subgroup most vulnerable to acute confusion. Factors placing the elderly at risk include polypharmacy, physiologic changes occurring with aging, and prevalence of underlying chronic diseases. Dementia is a known risk factor for delirium. As many as 22% of community-dwelling elderly persons with dementia have coexisting delirium. Patients with two diagnoses have a 49% incidence of delirium, and patients with three or more diagnoses have a 65% incidence. Relocation, bereavement, sensory deprivation or overload, and disruption in pattern or meaning of life experiences place the elderly at risk.

TABLE 14–2. DRUGS COMMONLY IMPLICATED IN ACUTE CONFUSIONAL STATES

Therapeutic drugs
Analgesics
Anesthetics (eg, ketamine)
Anticholinergics
Anticonvulsants
Antidepressants
Antihistamines
Antihypertensives
Antiparkinsonian agents
Antipsychotics
Antispasmodics
Cimetidine and ranitidine
Corticosteroids
Digitalis
Disulfiram
Insulin
Lithium
Oral hypoglycemics
Sedatives
Stimulants (eg, amphetamines)

Addictive drugs being withdrawn from use
Alcohol
Amphetamines
Benzodiazepines
Bromides
Carbon monoxide
Industrial poisons
Poisoning agents
Poisonous plants (eg, mushrooms)
Sedatives and hypnotics
Snake bite

Intoxicating agents
Cannabis
Cocaine
Ethyl alcohol
Hallucinogens
Inhalants (eg, glue, ether, nitrites, or nitrous oxide)
Methyl alcohol
Opioids
Phencyclidine (PCP)

B. **Patients who abuse drugs** such as ethanol and cocaine are at increased risk for development of delirium.
C. **Patients with structural brain disease,** such as dementia and Parkinson's disease, have an increased risk of developing delirium.
D. **Patients with underlying depressive illness** are at increased risk for delirium.
E. **The terminally ill** or hospice patient may become confused as a result of depression, anxiety, discomfort, or pain as well as from progression of the disease. Although psychological adjustment reactions occur after diagnosis or relapse, about 10–20% of patients develop formal psychiatric disorders that require specific care. As more terminal patients are cared for in the home or hospice setting, it is important not to mistake confusion due to depression, anxiety, or pain as a natural reaction to or course of the underlying disease.

IV. **Pathophysiology**
A. **Disturbance of cerebral metabolism, systemic illness, or toxic conditions** may reduce the production or effect of neurotransmitters in the brain, particularly acetylcholine and epinephrine. Acetylcholine is essential for attention, learning, memory, and information processing. The frontal and temporal lobes are most commonly affected.
B. Certain **physiologic changes that occur with aging** account for the sensitivity of the elderly to metabolic insults or other disorders. These changes include alterations in pharmacodynamics, pharmacokinetics, and sleep physiology; sensory impairment; central nervous system fallout; and decreased synthesis of neurotransmitters, especially in the cholinergic system.
C. The **pathophysiology of delirium in drug abusers** varies with each drug and is beyond the scope of this text. Many of the biochemical disturbances that most commonly cause confusional states are at the level of the reticular activating system.

The pathophysiology of dementia is discussed in Chapter 77. The pathophysiology of depression is discussed in Chapter 96.

V. **Symptoms** (Tables 14–1 and 14–3 and Chapters 77 and 96)
VI. **Signs** (Tables 14–1 and 14–3 and Chapters 77 and 96)
A. **Administration of a mental status test** may be helpful when delirium is suspected. The Mini-Mental State Examination (MMSE) has high sensitivity and specificity in this situation (Table 14–4). In validation studies, using a cutoff score of 23 or below, the MMSE has a sensitivity of 87%, a specificity of 82%, a false-positive rate of 39.4%, and a false-negative rate of 4.7%. These rates refer to the capacity of the MMSE to accurately distinguish patients with clinically diagnosed dementia or delirium from patients without these syndromes. Only after delirium and depression have been ruled out can dementia be diagnosed in a patient with cognitive impairment. If dementia is suspected in an otherwise asymptomatic person, assessment of risk factors and the clinician's knowledge of the patient's condition, history, and social situation may help guide the decision to initiate an assessment for dementia. The use of a functional activities questionnaire may be useful for early detection. Clinicians should take into consideration factors such as hearing or visual problems and physical disabilities in the selection of tests, as well as confounding factors such as age, educational level, and cultural influences in the interpretation of these tests.
B. A **physical examination** may provide helpful clues to the cause of delirium. These findings are listed below.
1. If **diastolic blood pressure** is >120 mm Hg, hypertensive encephalopathy should be considered.
2. If **systolic blood pressure** is <90 mm Hg, confusion may be from impaired cerebral perfusion secondary to shock. Drug overdose, adrenal insufficiency, and hyponatremia should also be considered.
3. **Tachycardia** suggests sepsis, delirium tremens, hyperthyroidism, hypoglycemia, or an agitated, anxious patient.
4. **Fever** may indicate infection, delirium tremens, cerebral vasculitis, or fat embolism syndrome. *Hypothermia* is defined as a core temperature (rectal or esophageal) below 35 °C (95 °F) and may cause confusion.
5. **Tachypnea** suggests hypoxia. A patient with chronic obstructive lung disease receiving fractional inspiratory oxygen of >0.28 may be confused from hypercarbia.

TABLE 14–3. CLINICAL FEATURES OF DELIRIUM, DEMENTIA, AND DEPRESSIVE PSEUDODEMENTIA

Feature	Delirium	Dementia	Pseudodementia
Onset	Sudden, often at night	Insidious	Sudden
Duration prior to presentation to physician	Hours to weeks	Months to years	Days to weeks
Course over 24-hour period	Fluctuating, with nocturnal exacerbation	Stable over day	Stable
Consciousness, awareness, alertness	Reduced	Clear	Clear
Attention	Globally disordered, hypoalert, or hyperalert; distractible; fluctuates over the course of the day	Normal, except in severe cases	May be disordered
Cognition	Globally disordered	Globally impaired	May be selectively impaired
Hallucinations	Usually visual or visual and auditory	Often absent	Usually absent
Delusions	Fleeting, poorly systematized	Often absent	Usually absent
Orientation	Usually impaired, at least for a time	Often impaired	May be impaired
Psychomotor activity	Increased, reduced, or shifting unpredictably	Often normal	Varies from psychomotor retardation to near normal
Memory	Immediate and recent impairment	Recent and remote impairment	May be normal, poor effort
Speech	Often incoherent, slow, or rapid	Patient has difficulty finding words, perseveration	Normal or slow
Sleep-wake cycle	Always disturbed	Often fragmented	May be unchanged
Involuntary movements	Often asterixis or coarse tremor	Often absent	Usually absent
Appearance	Appears ill	Appears well	Appears well
Physical illness or drug toxicity	One or both are present	Often absent, especially in senile dementia of the Alzheimer's type	Usually absent
Focal neurologic signs	Absent	Favors multi-infarct dementia	Absent
Electroencephalogram	Usually diffuse slowing of background activity; with withdrawal, excessive low-amplitude fast activity	Usually diffuse slowing; seizure activity and focal abnormalities can be detected	Normal

6. **Hyperalert confusion** may result from alcohol withdrawal. A person who is excited, hyperalert, and hallucinating may be experiencing toxicity from amphetamines, lysergic acid diethylamide (LSD), cocaine, or phencyclidine (PCP).
7. **Papilledema** suggests hypertensive encephalopathy or an intracranial mass.
8. **Dilated pupils** suggest sympathetic outflow, which is common with delirium tremens. Pinpoint pupils suggest narcotic excess or constricting eyedrops. An agitated, confusional state without focal signs may occur with head trauma.
9. **Bibasilar crackles** indicate congestive heart failure with hypoxia. Asymmetric crackles suggest pneumonia with hypoxia.
10. **Acute confusion, ataxia, bilateral sixth-nerve palsies, and nystagmus** suggest Wernicke-Korsakoff encephalitis.
11. **Confusion, irritability, insomnia, and a photosensitive rash with diarrhea** suggest pellagra.
C. See Tables 14–1 and 14–3 and Chapters 77 and 96 for further information.

TABLE 14–4. MINI-MENTAL STATE EXAMINATION (MMSE)

		Score	Points
ORIENTATION			
1. What is the:	Year	_____	1
	Season	_____	1
	Date	_____	1
	Day	_____	1
	Month	_____	1
2. Where are we?	State	_____	1
	County	_____	1
	Town or city	_____	1
	Hospital	_____	1
	Floor	_____	1
REGISTRATION			
3. Name three objects, taking 1 second to say each. Then ask the patient to repeat all three after you have said them. Give 1 point for each correct answer. Repeat the answers until the patient learns all three.		_____	3
ATTENTION AND CALCULATION			
4. Serial sevens. Give 1 point for each correct answer. Stop after five answers. Alternate: spell the word *world* backwards.		_____	5
RECALL			
5. Ask for names of three objects learned in question 3. Give 1 point for each correct answer.		_____	3
LANGUAGE			
6. Point to a pencil and a watch. Have the patient name them as you point.		_____	2
7. Have the patient repeat, "No ifs, ands, or buts."		_____	1
8. Have the patient follow a three-stage command: "Take a paper in your right hand. Fold the paper in half. Put the paper on the floor."		_____	3
9. Have the patient read and obey the following: "Close your eyes." (Write it in large letters.)		_____	1
10. Have the patient write a sentence of his or her choice. (The sentence should contain a subject and an object and should make sense. Ignore spelling errors when scoring.)		_____	1
11. Have the patient copy a line drawing of intersecting pentagons. (Give one point if all sides and angles are preserved and if the intersecting sides form a quadrangle.)		_____	1
Add points for each correct response	**TOTAL**	_____	30

Adapted with permission from Folstein MF, Folstein SE, McHugh PR: "Mini Mental State: A Practical Method for Grading the Cognitive State of Patients for the Clinician." *Journal of Psychiatric Research,* 12(3):189–198, 1975. © 1998, MMLLC.

VII. Laboratory tests. Unless the cause of the confusional state is obvious from the history and the physical examination, the following tests should be considered.
   A. Basic screening studies include complete blood cell count with differential count and sedimentation rate; serum chemistry profile, including levels of electrolytes, blood urea nitrogen, magnesium, and calcium; toxicologic screen of urine, blood, or both; urinalysis; chest x-ray; electrocardiogram; and serum drug levels of prescribed medications as indicated.
   B. A **lumbar puncture** should be performed on every patient with delirium to evaluate the possibility of bacterial, fungal, or tumor meningitis, unless there is a reason not to proceed with this test. Relative contraindications include rapid improvement in the patient's clinical status and concerns about increased intracranial pressure because of a mass lesion.
   C. An **electroencephalogram** may identify partial complex seizure disorder, metabolic encephalopathy, or sedative use and should be considered in patients suspected of having these disorders.
   D. Computerized tomography (CT) of the head is the method of choice for the initial evaluation of confused, obtunded patients in order to rule out subdural hematoma, epidural hematoma, stroke, cerebral abscess, or neoplasm. Repeat CT after

24–48 hours should be done if acute infarct is considered. Magnetic resonance imaging with magnetic resonance arteriography may be useful to rule out chronic subdural hematoma, regional blood flow abnormalities, or an aneurysm.

E. Additional tests that may be considered when the foregoing tests fail to reveal a likely cause of the patient's confusion are arterial blood gas analysis, blood cultures, serum ammonia levels, liver function studies, thyroid function tests, cortisone levels, antinuclear antibodies, serum protein electrophoresis, serum B_{12} and folate levels, syphilis test (VDRL), serum and urine osmolality, HIV titer, and urine tests for heavy metals, porpholilinogen, and metanephrines.

VIII. Treatment

A. Patients with delirium require hospitalization for close monitoring and identification and correction of the underlying cause. The mortality rate for delirium has been reported to be as high as 30%. When a specific cause cannot be found, certain principles of behavior management should be used. A quiet, private room with familiar objects and a family member present, when possible, can be beneficial. Maintenance of a normal sleep-wake pattern should be established early.

The terminally ill hospice patient may be managed at home or in an in-patient hospice setting, depending on the desires and needs of the patient and family. Often, control of pain and anxiety is all that is needed. Treatment for psychosis or depression may also be indicated.

Medical management is controversial and varied. **Haloperidol** (0.25–2 mg) given intramuscularly may be helpful in the urgent setting. Occasionally, maintenance doses of haloperidol (2–5 mg orally two or three times daily) may be used until the underlying cause of delirium can be determined. If a benzodiazepine is used, **lorazepam (Ativan)** is usually the drug of choice because of its relatively short half-life. **Chloral hydrate** (500 mg orally at bedtime) or **trazedone hydrochloride (Desyrel,** 50–150 mg orally at bedtime) can be useful. **Resperidone** (0.5 mg orally twice daily up to 4–6 mg daily) has been shown to be effective in aggressive, angry, or violent patients with dementia. Paradoxic reactions can occur with all of these medications. Care should be taken not to overly sedate patients, especially the elderly.

B. The management of dementia and depression is discussed in Chapters 77 and 96, respectively.

C. The incidence of delirium may be decreased by limiting polypharmacy in the elderly, by closely monitoring drug usage by the elderly, and by recognizing the prodromal symptoms of insomnia, nightmares, fleeting hallucinations, and anxiety.

D. Finally, open communication with family members about the suspected causes and prognosis of the delirium is essential.

REFERENCES

Agency for Health Care Policy and Research: Guideline 19: Early identification of Alzheimer's disease and related dementias, available at www.ahcpr.gov/clinic or through the Office of the Superintendent of Documents at (202) 512-1800.

American Psychiatric Association: *Diagnostic and Statistical Manual of Mental Disorders (DSM-IV).* 4th ed. American Psychiatric Association; 1994.

Barraclough J: ABC of palliative care: Depression, anxiety and confusion. Br Med J 1997;**315:** 1365.

Espino DV, Jules-Bradley AC, Johnston CC, et al: Diagnostic approach to the confused elderly patient. Am Fam Physician 1998;**57:**1358.

Feske SK: Coma and confusional states: Emergency diagnosis and management. Neurol Clin 1998;**16:**237.

---

15   Constipation

Russell L. Anderson, MD

I. Definition. Constipation occurs when a patient has fewer than three bowel movements per week. Many patients also consider hard stools, straining, and abdominal discomfort to be symptoms of constipation.

II. **Common diagnoses.** Constipation may result from a number of organic or functional sources.
  A. **Functional causes** are the most common and include the following problems.
    1. Suppression of normal gastrocolic reflex because of time constraints or impaired mobility.
    2. Inadequate dietary fiber and bulk, often combined with inadequate fluid intake.
    3. Increased intestinal transit time and colonic motility disorders such as irritable bowel syndrome.
  B. **Drugs,** particularly those with anticholinergic activity and those with smooth muscle depressant action, are frequent causes of constipation. Iron supplements, aluminum- and calcium-based antacids, and bismuth preparations are common contributors to constipation.
  C. **Anal and rectal lesions,** such as hemorrhoids and anal fissures, can cause pain and stricture.
  D. **Neurologic diseases and spinal cord lesions** that disrupt colon parasympathetic and abdominal motor nerves.
  E. **Megacolon,** either from Hirschsprung's disease or from secondary causes such as chronic laxative abuse.
  F. **Intermittent or partially obstructing lesions** of the bowel, such as the following.
    1. Intrinsic lesions of the bowel.
    2. Intra-abdominal lesions causing pressure on the bowel and partial obstruction.
    3. Adhesions from earlier surgery or injury to the bowel.
  G. **Metabolic disorders** such as diabetes mellitus, hypothyroidism, hypokalemia, hypercalcemia, and uremia.
III. **Epidemiology.** Approximately 4 million people in the United States have constipation on a frequent basis. This figure corresponds to a prevalence of 2%, making constipation the most frequent gastrointestinal problem seen in ambulatory medicine.
  A. Constipation is reported more frequently by patients over the age of 65. The problem may be more a result of physical inactivity among this group rather than intrinsic bowel changes caused by the aging process.
  B. Constipation is three times more common in women than in men.
  C. Nonwhite patients report constipation about 1.3 times more frequently than do white patients.
  D. The prevalence of constipation is highest in the southern region of the United States.
  E. Patients from low-income families report constipation more frequently than patients from high-income families.
IV. **Pathophysiology.** The basic pathophysiologic mechanism of constipation involves increased transit time through the colon with inspissation of bowel contents.
V. **Symptoms.** The primary symptom of constipation is the occurrence of fewer than three bowel movements per week. Associated symptoms that may indicate contributing factors include the following.
  A. **Straining at stool,** which may indicate the presence of a rectal stricture.
  B. **Pain**
    1. **Sharp anal pain** is common with external hemorrhoids.
    2. **Crampy abdominal pain** in the lower abdomen is usually caused by bowel distention, which can result from irritable bowel syndrome, intermittent obstruction, or adhesions.
    3. **Noncrampy dull pain in the left abdomen** is often associated with diverticulosis.
  C. **Bleeding**
    1. **Bright red blood in the stool** indicates hemorrhoids, fissures, or a possible mass in the rectum.
    2. **Brisk bleeding** is rarely caused by hemorrhoids and must be thoroughly investigated immediately.
    3. **Melena** results from bleeding proximal to the anal canal, and the cause must be diagnosed to rule out carcinoma or other serious conditions.
  D. **Alternating episodes of constipation and diarrhea** are characteristic of irritable bowel syndrome.
  E. The **duration** of the problem can be important in determining the cause of the constipation.

1. **Recent onset** usually relates to changes in lifestyle or health status, such as the following.
   a. **Use of drugs** with the potential for constipation, including drugs prescribed by the physician, over-the-counter drugs, and herbal supplements.
   b. **Dietary changes** such as restrictive weight loss diets or dietary changes because of the aging process or poor dentition.
   c. **Partially obstructing lesions** caused by masses or adhesions of the bowel.
2. **Long duration** indicates a functional cause or chronic organic disease.
   a. **Inadequate amounts of fiber or fluids** in the diet are the most common cause of chronic constipation. The diet should contain a daily intake of at least 25 g of fiber and 2000 mL of fluids.
   b. **Concurrent illnesses** may present as constipation. Disorders that may present this way include hypothyroidism, diabetes mellitus, hypokalemia, and hypercalcemia.

VI. **Signs** of the causes of constipation that may be found during the examination of the patient include the following.
   A. **Findings in the abdominal examination** that indicate possible organic causes of constipation, such as:
      1. **Palpable abdominal masses or organomegaly.**
      2. **Silent or abnormal bowel sounds.**
      3. **Areas of tenderness.**
   B. A **rectal examination** can reveal painful areas indicating external hemorrhoids, strictures, anal tears, or abrasions.
   C. The **presence of a mass** in the rectum indicates an impaction or obstructing lesion.
   D. The **amount and consistency of the contents** of the rectum, both of which are increased by most causes of constipation but may be decreased in obstructions proximal to the rectum.
   E. **Anal sphincter tone** is increased in functional problems and strictures but is decreased in neurologic diseases.
   F. The **diameter of the rectal ampulla** is markedly increased in megacolon.

VII. **Laboratory tests** are usually not required in acute constipation; however, cases resistant to treatment may require some of the following tests in order to establish the cause of the problem.
   A. **Fecal occult blood testing**
      1. This test may indicate ulcerative or cancerous lesions. Although sensitivity for detecting colorectal cancers and adenomas ranges from 50% to 90%, this procedure is an inexpensive and noninvasive method of screening for bleeding lesions of the bowel.
      2. This test is not indicated when the patient has hemorrhoids or fissures that may cause misleading positive results. If there is reason to suspect a bleeding lesion of the anal canal, the test should be delayed briefly until the local condition is resolved, or other methods of discovering a more proximal lesion should be used.
   B. **Blood or serum studies**
      1. **Serum electrolytes** can detect hypokalemia, which may present as constipation.
      2. **Blood or serum glucose** will eliminate diabetes mellitus as a cause of the constipation.
      3. **Thyroid-stimulating hormone** level can detect hypothyroidism.
      4. **Serum calcium level** determinations can eliminate hypercalcemia as a cause of the constipation.
   C. **Proctoscopy** is recommended if digital examination indicates hemorrhoids, fissures, strictures, or masses in the anus or the rectum.
   D. **Sigmoidoscopy or colonoscopy** is indicated in cases that are resistant to conservative treatment or in cases in which a lesion of the bowel is suspected. This test can detect masses, cicatrizing obstructions, bleeding points, and inflammatory lesions in the colon. If megacolon exists, colonoscopy is necessary to obtain biopsies.
   E. **Barium enemas** can be valuable in demonstrating the extent of dilated bowel in megacolon and in revealing diverticula and most masses.

VIII. Treatment

A. Correction of any existing underlying conditions that may be causing the condition is the first step in treatment.

    1. The physician should treat the patient for any concurrent problems that may present as constipation.

    2. Any drugs that may produce or aggravate constipation should be eliminated or reduced to the minimum effective dose if possible (Table 15–1).

B. Patient education is a critical step in the management of constipation. The patient should be informed of the wide variability of normal bowel function and encouraged to establish a regular pattern of bowel movements. The recommended time for attempting bowel movement is after meals, which allows the patient to take advantage of the normal gastrocolic reflex.

C. Nonpharmacologic treatment should be instituted as the next step in the treatment of constipation.

    1. Adequate fluid intake is necessary in the treatment of constipation. The patient should be instructed to maintain a **daily fluid intake of at least 2000 mL,** which is equivalent to eight 8-oz glasses, or 2 quarts, of fluid. This amount may be **contraindicated** in conditions such as congestive heart failure, renal insufficiency, and diabetes insipidus. Water is preferable, but other acceptable fluids include clear soups, nonalcoholic beverages, and gelatin (eg, Jell-O). Caffeinated beverages should be carefully controlled because of the weak diuretic effect of caffeine and possible adverse effects on the heart, blood pressure, and central nervous system.

    2. Dietary changes are a keystone in the treatment program. Dietary fiber should be increased to a total of 25–50 g/day through the addition of whole-grain or rye bread, bran muffins, rye crisp, bran-based cereals, and other high-fiber cereals, such as oatmeal. Cream cereals (rice, wheat, grits, and farina) and puffed cereals are low in fiber. High-fiber fruits include dried dates, raisins, pears, and apples (including applesauce). Bananas are a poor source of fiber. Vegetables such as broccoli, Brussels sprouts, dry beans, greens, carrots, beets, peas, and other legumes are good sources of fiber. Lettuce, potatoes, cabbage, celery, and onions are poor sources of fiber. High-fiber foods should

TABLE 15–1. DRUGS THAT CAN CAUSE CONSTIPATION

Antihypertensives
Clonidine
α-Methyldopa
β-Adrenergic blockers
Calcium channel blockers

Gastrointestinal
Atropine
Belladonna alkaloids and combinations
Antispasmodics
Aluminum hydroxide antacids
Calcium carbonate antacids
Cimetidine
Ranitidine
Sucralfate

Psychiatric drugs
Tricyclic antidepressants
Trazodone

Analgesics
Opiates and derivatives
Propoxyphene

Decongestants and bronchodilators
Phenylpropanolamine
Pseudoephedrine
Phenylephrine
Terbutaline

be added to the diet slowly in order to minimize symptoms of flatulence, cramping, and borborygmus.

   3. **Addition of extra fiber** in the form of bran and bran products is necessary if the patient is unable to achieve the required amount in the regular diet. One-quarter to one-half cup (0.5–1 oz) of bran is usually an adequate supplement to the patient's diet. Bran may be added in the form of muffins (average of 6–7 g of bran per muffin) or may be mixed with other cereals or sprinkled over fruit.

D. **Pharmacologic agents** should be used in cases resistant to simple measures.

   1. **Bulk laxatives** are the first agents that should be added. These agents are the safest and are effective.

      a. **Psyllium seed** preparations (**Metamucil, Perdiem, Effer-Syllium, Hydrocil,** and others). The usual dose of psyllium mucilloid is approximately 3.5 g suspended in 4–6 oz of water or juice one to three times daily.

      b. **Methylcellulose-based** products (eg, **Citrucel**). The average dose of methylcellulose is 2 g in 8 oz of water one to three times a day.

      c. **Polycarbophil** (eg, **Fibercon**). The recommended dose is 500–1000 mg (two to four tablets) with 6 oz of fluid one to three times a day.

   2. **Other laxatives**

      a. The laxatives listed below may be used episodically to relieve constipation, but regular use should be avoided because of possible adverse effects.

         (1) **Milk of Magnesia,** 30–60 mL at bedtime, is usually effective and relatively safe.

         (2) **Bisacodyl** (eg, **Dulcolax**), a 5-mg oral tablet or 10-mg rectal suppository, acts rapidly but may cause severe cramping.

         (3) **Citrate of Magnesia,** 240 mL or less taken at bedtime. Large doses can cause diarrhea, resulting in severe fluid and electrolyte losses. Patients with decreased renal function can develop toxic magnesium levels.

         (4) **Saline enemas** (eg, **Fleet**) may be used for relief of episodic constipation or as preparation for bowel studies.

         (5) **Hyperosmolar agents.** Lactulose, 15–30 mL/day orally, and sorbitol, 70% solution, 15 mL/day, are effective laxatives. Lactulose is more expensive and offers no clear advantage over sorbitol. Common side effects are belching, flatulence, and abdominal cramping.

      b. Other laxatives may be effective but offer no advantages. Their adverse effects often outweigh their value.

         (1) **Irritant agents** containing **casanthranol, cascara, danthron, phenolphthalein,** and combinations of these drugs can result in degeneration of myenteric neurons, loss of colon activity, secondary megacolon, cramping, abdominal discomfort, and melanosis coli, a harmless darkening of the colonic mucosa.

         (2) **Lubricating laxatives,** such as mineral oil, when taken orally, cause aspiration lipoid pneumonia in patients with impaired swallowing. These agents may also block absorption of calcium, phosphate, and vitamins A and D with chronic use.

   3. **Stool softeners** can be used alone or can be used to augment bulk laxatives. **Docusate calcium** (eg, **Surfak**), starting with a dose of 240 mg, or **docusate sodium** (eg, **Colace**), beginning at a dose of 100 mg, can be given daily at bedtime. The dose should be reduced over a period of weeks until the minimum effective dose is reached.

   4. **Herbal or "natural" laxatives** are widely available and may contain multiple herbal ingredients; however, the active ingredients in the vast majority are cascara sagrada or senna, both of which are irritant laxatives unsuitable for treating chronic constipation.

E. **Combination therapy** may be necessary for certain patients.

   1. Patients who have a **history of chronic laxative use** may require a progressive program to eliminate dependence.

      a. **The patient must be educated about normal bowel physiology and the procedures to reinforce it, and the dietary changes described above should be instituted.**

    b. The current regimen of laxatives should be replaced with a program of combined stool softeners and bulk laxatives. If necessary, doses can be increased to establish a normal pattern, then slowly reduced until the minimum dose necessary to maintain a normal pattern is reached.

    c. Glycerine or bisacodyl suppositories can be used by the patient on an episodic basis if necessary.

2. Patients who are **bedridden, demented,** or suffering from **neurologic diseases** or **spinal cord injury** frequently require a program of multiple laxative agents. The goal of treatment is to avoid impaction without inducing diarrhea.

    a. Dietary fiber and supplemental fiber are given at levels as near to optimal as possible.

    b. Fluid intake of 2000 mL/day is instituted if not contraindicated by other medical conditions.

    c. A daily schedule must be established that is conducive to regular bowel movements. The patient can take advantage of the gastrocolic reflex by attempting bowel movement after the first meal of the day. The patient should be given as much privacy and time as the situation and the patient's condition allow. The patient should be placed in a sitting position or as upright a position as possible. A bedside commode is superior to a bedpan. The use of a footstool with the commode produces a more physiologic posture that is conducive to bowel movements.

    d. Maximum doses of bulk laxatives and stool softeners can be instituted. Once bowel action is established, the doses of the agents are slowly reduced, over a period of weeks, until the minimum dose necessary to maintain normal bowel function is reached.

    e. Bisacodyl oral tablets can be given if the previous steps have not been successful. The bisacodyl should be started at half the usual adult dose and increased at intervals of 3 or 4 days until a maximum dose of 15 mg (three tablets) is reached. Oral doses work best when given at bedtime. A 10-mg suppository of bisacodyl 30 minutes after breakfast may be added to the regimen if necessary.

    f. A **hypertonic phosphate solution enema** (eg, **Fleet**) may be given to the patient on an episodic basis as needed.

F. Prevention is the best treatment for impaction. Decreasing frequency and increasing stool consistency are indications that a rectal examination is necessary. If an impaction is discovered:

    1. Manual fragmentation will usually reduce most impactions to passable dimensions.

    2. Hypertonic phosphate solution enemas are usually effective in managing impactions that are not totally cleared by manual fragmentation. If necessary, these enemas can be followed by softening agent enemas, such as **mineral** or **cottonseed oil (Fleet Oil Retention)** enemas, 150 mL, or **docusate sodium, 1% solution (Colace),** 30 mL diluted to 100 mL with water, given as an enema.

    3. An impaction that is not cleared by the previous methods may require mechanical reduction with a sigmoidoscope. In rare cases, surgery may be necessary to remove an impaction.

REFERENCES

Devrode G: Constipation. In Sleisenger M, Fordtran J (editors): *Gastrointestinal Disease.* 5th ed. Saunders; 1993;837.

Floch S, Arnold W: Clinical evaluation and treatment of constipation. Gastroenterologist 1994; **2:**50.

McEvoy G (editor): *American Hospital Formulary Service Drug Information 93.* American Society of Hospital Pharmacists; 1993.

Nelson J, Moxness K, Jensen M, et al (editors): *Mayo Clinic Diet Manual.* 7th ed. Mosby; 1994.

Prather C, Oritz-Camacho CP: Evaluation and treatment of constipation and fecal impaction in adults. Mayo Clin Proc 1998;**73:**881.

Read N, Celik A, Katsinelos P: Constipation and incontinence in the elderly. J Clin Gastroenterol 1995;**20:**61.

16   Cough

Richard D. Clover, MD

I. **Definition.** A cough is the sudden noisy expulsion of air from the lungs, usually initiated when the lining of the airways in the respiratory tract is irritated.

II. **Common diagnoses**
   A. **Viral infections.**
   B. **Bacterial and other infections.**
   C. **Respiratory irritants.**
   D. **Allergic rhinitis or asthma.**
   E. **Chronic obstructive pulmonary disease (COPD) or chronic bronchitis.**
   F. **Cancer.**
   G. **Aspiration** of a foreign body or from gastroesophageal reflux.
   H. **Psychogenic cough.**

III. **Epidemiology.** Although essentially everyone experiences an acute episode of
coughing at some time, most studies report a prevalence of chronic cough in only
8–14% of the population.
   A. **Viral infections** are especially prominent during the winter months and occur
   more frequently in children than in adults.
   B. **Bacterial and other infections.** Factors that interfere with defense mechanisms
   and predispose patients to bacterial infections include cigarette smoke, alcohol,
   hypoxia, viral infections, mechanical obstructions, immunosuppressive agents,
   and alterations in the level of consciousness.
      1. Acute sinusitis is usually a complication of a viral infection of the upper res-
      piratory tract. It occurs in persons with allergic rhinitis or anatomic abnor-
      malities of the nose.
      2. Bacterial pneumonia usually results from a failure of normal pulmonary de-
      fense mechanisms.
      3. Tuberculosis (TB) cases have increased partly because of human immuno-
      deficiency virus (HIV)–associated TB, immigration from countries with high
      TB prevalence, substance abuse, homelessness, and poverty.
   C. **Respiratory irritants**
      1. Cigarette smoke is a common cause of cough. Nonsmokers who are ex-
      posed to a smoke-filled room frequently cough. Cough rates in smokers in-
      crease with the number of cigarettes smoked; about 25% of persons who
      smoke one-half pack per day, 50% of persons who smoke one pack per day,
      and most who smoke two packs or more per day report a daily cough.
      2. Other common air pollutants that cause coughs are sulfur dioxide, nitrogen
      oxide, ammonia, ozone, and dust.
   D. **Allergic rhinitis or asthma**
      1. Cough associated with allergic rhinitis varies with the seasonal or environ-
      mental occurrence of the allergens producing the rhinitis.
      2. Cough is a common manifestation of asthma and may be the initial and pre-
      dominant manifestation of asthma.
   E. **COPD or chronic bronchitis.** Cough is seen in all patients with COPD.
   F. **Cancer.** In patients with lung cancer, cough occurs in 70–90% at some time in
   their clinical illness, although it is an early sign in <20% of patients. Risk factors
   for lung cancer include exposure to cigarette smoke, asbestos, radioactivity, and
   certain chemicals, including chloromethyl ethers and metals.
   G. **Aspiration** from gastroesophageal reflux is most commonly encountered in elderly patients, although it may occur in patients with neuromuscular disorders that
   interfere with normal swallowing or in patients with primary esophageal disease.
   Cough occurs in >90% of children who aspirate a foreign body.
   H. **Psychogenic cough** is uncommon and usually occurs in older children and adolescents. This cough does not occur at night. School phobia is frequently an associated finding.

IV. **Pathophysiology.** In general, mechanical, inflammatory, or chemical factors stimulate afferent fibers in the vagus, trigeminal, glossopharyngeal, or phrenic nerves.

These nerves convey this information to the brain's "cough center" in the medulla. Returning fibers from the cough center carry motor impulses to the larynx and muscles of the diaphragm, chest wall, and abdomen.

  A. **Viral infections,** including influenza, parainfluenza, adenovirus, respiratory syncytial virus, rhinovirus, and coronavirus, are the most common causes of cough. The inflammation from these infections directly simulates cough receptors. In patients with excessive sputum production, increased secretions stimulate coughing.
  B. **Bacterial and other infections** generally result in inflammatory stimulation of the cough receptors. Common causes of bacterial pneumonia include *Streptococcus pneumoniae, Mycoplasma pneumoniae, Staphylococcus aureus, Haemophilus influenzae,* and mixed anaerobic bacteria. As with viral infections, bacterial infections cause an increase in sputum production, which may also elicit the cough reflex. Primary TB in childhood may produce a cough similar to that caused by any infection, but it also produces cough by exuberant hilar or mediastinal lymphadenitis compressing central bronchi. In chronic pulmonary TB, cough is produced both by inflammatory stimulation of cough receptors and by caseous areas liquefying and draining into the bronchial tree.
  C. **Respiratory irritants.** Most environmental irritants, including smoke, have a direct stimulatory effect on the cough reflex.
  D. **Allergies or asthma.** In allergic rhinitis and asthma, the cough reflex is stimulated either by inflammatory changes that result from the allergens or by thick mucous secretions. Patients with these illnesses complain of nocturnal cough from the drainage; allergic rhinitis, in particular, may cause postnasal drainage. Furthermore, bronchoconstriction may cause mechanical stimulation of the cough receptors.
  E. **COPD or chronic bronchitis.** Cough in COPD is usually elicited in one of three ways: (1) a direct irritant effect from cigarette smoking, (2) decreased mucociliary clearances of secretions, or (3) increased secretions overwhelming the mucociliary apparatus and predisposing the patient to secondary infections from *S pneumoniae, H influenzae,* and other respiratory organisms.
  F. **Cancers** produce cough by mechanical compression of the airways.
  G. **Aspiration.** Foreign bodies produce direct mechanical stimulation of the cough receptors.

V. **Symptoms**
  A. Symptoms of **viral infections** generally include coryza, sore throat, postnasal drip, and fever. The cough is usually paroxysmal and occurs both day and night.
  B. **Bacterial infections**
    1. Cough, postnasal drip, headache, facial pain, swelling, and low-grade fever are common symptoms of **acute sinusitis.**
    2. In **pneumonia,** the cough is usually productive of mucopurulent secretions and is associated with fever, chills, sweats, and other constitutional symptoms, such as weakness, fatigue, and general malaise.
    3. In chronic lower respiratory tract infections, such as **TB, fungal infections,** and **lung abscesses,** a chronic cough associated with vague constitutional symptoms, including weakness, fatigue, and malaise, may be the presenting complaint.
    4. A cough with minimal to no sputum production is the predominant complaint of patients with *Mycoplasma* infections.
  C. **Respiratory irritants.** Cough is usually the only symptom of this problem. Shortness of breath may be associated with the cough if significant bronchoconstriction occurs as a result of the irritant.
  D. **Allergic rhinitis or asthma.** Patients with allergic rhinitis present with sneezing, rhinorrhea, nasal congestion, postnasal drip, and cough. The three cardinal symptoms of asthma are wheezing, dyspnea, and cough. The cough is nonproductive and paroxysmal.
  E. **COPD or chronic bronchitis.** Persons with COPD may also complain of dyspnea on exertion, shortness of breath, wheezing, and significant sputum production, depending on the severity of the underlying disease.
  F. **Cancer.** Cough as the result of pulmonary cancer is frequently associated with hemoptysis. Patients may also complain of anorexia, weight loss, malaise, and fever.
  G. **Aspiration.** A cough or choking sensation may be the only complaint of a person who has aspirated a foreign body. A patient with recurrent aspiration of oral or

gastric secretions may have a history of difficulty swallowing either liquids or solids. Symptoms of gastroesophageal reflux may not be present in elderly persons with recurrent aspiration.

   H. Psychogenic cough is generally diagnosed by exclusion. The cough is usually nonproductive, and symptoms of anxiety, especially school phobia, may be present.

VI. Signs

   A. Viral infections produce a boggy nasal mucosa and an erythematous swollen posterior nasopharynx. The patient may have rales, rhonchi, or wheezes, depending on the degree of lower airway inflammation. Infants with bronchiolitis may experience tachypnea, nasal flaring, and intercostal muscle retractions, depending on the severity of the infection.

   B. Bacterial and other infections

      1. In **sinusitis,** the sinuses may be tender to percussion, the nasal mucosa may be boggy, and purulent rhinorrhea may be noted. Oral examination may reveal a granular or cobblestone-appearing posterior oropharynx that is caused by posterior nasal drainage.

      2. In **bronchitis,** rhonchi and wheezes are the predominant physical findings on pulmonary examination.

      3. In **bacterial pneumonias,** localized rhonchi, rales, and tubular breath sounds with signs of consolidation may be noted.

   C. Respiratory irritants. The physical examination is generally normal unless wheezing from bronchial constriction is present.

   D. Allergic rhinitis or asthma

      1. In **allergic rhinitis,** the nasal mucosa is moist, edematous, and generally pale blue. Examination of the eyes reveals injected conjunctivae.

      2. In **asthma,** wheezing is the most prominent physical finding. An acute exacerbation, if severe, may be associated with nasal flaring and intercostal muscle retraction. However, physical findings are not sensitive; frequently, the patient with asthma has no significant findings.

   E. COPD or bronchitis

      1. In **chronic bronchitis,** the patient has essentially normal chest diameter and resonance and may have coarse breath sounds with rhonchi and wheezes. Peripheral cyanosis may also be present.

      2. In **emphysema,** the patient is usually thin and has a "barrel-shaped" chest with a greater diameter and increased resonance, decreased breath sounds, and no peripheral cyanosis.

   F. Cancer. Physical findings of an individual with cancer frequently relate to the underlying or associated lung disease (eg, COPD).

   G. Aspiration of a foreign body. The physical examination is often normal. Localized findings of wheezing, rales, or rhonchi may be found in the segments associated with the aspiration.

VII. Laboratory tests. The patient's history and physical examination are the two most important aspects of the evaluation of a patient with cough. In one study (Irwin, 1981), 72% of patients were correctly diagnosed on the basis of history and examination alone. The following laboratory tests may be helpful in confirming or evaluating the severity of the cause of the cough.

   A. X-rays. X-rays should be considered when the diagnosis and management of the patient's illness cannot be adequately determined from the history and physical examination. Sinus x-rays, x-rays of the soft tissues of the neck, and chest x-rays, although nondiagnostic, may be helpful. For example, diffuse alveolar infiltrate in the setting of acute pneumonia suggests a viral or mycoplasmal infection, whereas a consolidated segment of the lung indicates bacterial infection. Cavitary lesions suggest staphylococcal, anaerobic, or mycobacterial infections. Alveolar infiltrates associated with cardiomegaly suggest congestive heart failure with associated pulmonary edema. Diffuse interstitial infiltrates in a patient with a progressive cough and dyspnea may signify interstitial fibrosis. X-rays do have limitations in evaluating patients with coughs (see Chapter 59).

   B. Sputum smears. Gram stains of sputum are of disputed value, although the presence of many white blood cells without significant organisms and epithelial cells should raise the suspicion of causes such as virus, chlamydia, legionella, and mycobacterium. Other stains and assays are useful in diagnosing a variety of infections. **Acid-fast bacilli (AFB) stains** are useful in diagnosing TB. Giemsa or silver stains are used to detect *Pneumocystis*. **Monoclonal antibodies** for immunofluorescence assays and **enzyme-linked immunosorbent assay (ELISA)** are used to rapidly detect legionella and viral infections.

   C. **Cultures.** Cultures of sputum are helpful if the possibility of a resistant or unusual organism exists, that is, gram-negative organisms, penicillin-resistant *S pneumoniae, Mycobacterium* species, and fungi.

   D. **Pulmonary function tests.** Pulmonary function tests are helpful in evaluating persons with asthma and COPD, for confirming the diagnosis, for determining the response to beta-agonists, and for establishing the severity of the disease (see Chapters 72 and 74).

   E. **Fiber-optic bronchoscopy.** If the exact cause of the patient's cough cannot be confirmed or if other studies have revealed abnormalities for which biopsies are needed to make the diagnosis, fiber-optic bronchoscopy should be performed.

   F. **Arterial blood gases.** In persons with significant respiratory distress, arterial blood gas values are helpful in evaluating the degree of hypoxemia and carbon dioxide retention as well as the response to oxygen therapy. Abnormal blood gas values indicate other possible causes of the cough, including pulmonary embolism or cardiovascular abnormalities producing significant arteriovenous shunting.

   G. **Intradermal antigen testing.** For diagnosing TB, purified protein derivative (PPD) testing is important. Guidelines for interpretation of PPD results are summarized in Table 16–1.

VIII. Treatment

   A. **General measures.** Treatment should be directed toward a specific underlying cause. However, two classes of agents are commonly prescribed for the symptomatic treatment of cough, usually as adjuncts to specific treatment.

      1. **Antitussive drugs.** In general, antitussive agents act centrally or peripherally.

         a. The most commonly prescribed **centrally acting** agent is **codeine phosphate,** 15–30 mg every 4–6 hours in adults. The most commonly used nonnarcotic antitussive is **dextromethorphan,** the highly advertised active ingredient in a number of proprietary cough suppressants.

         b. **Peripherally acting** antitussive drugs anesthetize cough receptors. **Benzonatate** (Tessalon Perles), 100 mg orally three times a day, has theoretical value, although it frequently cannot be delivered at the site of irritation (ie, the lower respiratory tract). **Topical agents** (eg, lidocaine) are used effectively to reduce cough during fiber-optic procedures.

      2. **Mucolytic agents.** These agents affect bronchial secretions by increasing their volume, decreasing their viscosity, and promoting their motility and removal from the airways. In well-controlled studies, **guaifenesin** has been ineffective in chronic bronchitis at the most commonly prescribed doses when

TABLE 16–1. CRITERIA FOR DETERMINING NEED FOR PREVENTIVE THERAPY IN PERSONS WITH POSITIVE TUBERCULIN REACTIONS

Category	Age Group	
	<35 Years	≥35 Years
With risk factor[1]	Treat at all ages if reaction to 5TU purified protein derivative (PPD) ≥10 mm (or ≥5 mm and patient has had recent contact, is HIV-infected, or has radiographic evidence of old TB).	
No risk factor	Treat if PPD ≥10 mm.	Do not treat.
High-incidence group[2]	Treat if PPD ≥15 mm.[3]	Do not treat.

[1] Risk factors include HIV infection, recent contact with infectious person, recent skin-test conversion, abnormal chest radiograph, intravenous drug abuse, and certain medical risk factors.

[2] Foreign-born persons, medically underserved low-income populations, and residents of long-term-care facilities.

[3] Lower or higher cut points may be used for identifying positive reactions, depending on the relative prevalence of *Mycobacterium* tuberculosis infection and nonspecific cross-reactivity in the population.

Adapted from the Centers for Disease Control and Prevention: Screening for tuberculosis and tuberculous infection in high-risk populations and the use of preventive therapy for tuberculous infection in the United States. MMWR 1990;**39:**RR-8.

compared with placebo; at higher doses (1200–2400 mg/day), however, this drug may be effective. The clinical usefulness of **iodides** (potassium iodide, saturated solution of potassium iodide) is significantly limited by the high incidence of side effects. **Water** may reduce cough by soothing the irritated receptors and moistening the mucous membranes.

B. **Viral respiratory infections.** Most of these infections require no specific therapy, although in certain instances antiviral agents are beneficial.

1. In infants with severe bronchiolitis, **ribavirin** administered as a continuous aerosol is effective in diminishing the rate of excretion of the virus and in promoting symptomatic improvement. The use of this drug should be limited to only the most severe cases and preferably delivered in a closed system because of its potential toxicity, especially to pregnant health care workers.

2. **Amantadine** may be used in the treatment and prophylaxis of influenza infections, especially in person at high risk for developing complications. The dosage is 100 mg orally two times a day for adults and 5 mg/kg in divided doses for children.

3. **Rimantadine,** a structural analog of amantadine, which generally has fewer side effects, also may be used in influenza therapy. Adults may be given 100 mg orally two times a day, and children younger than 9 years should receive 5 mg/kg/day up to 150 mg/day.

C. **Bacterial infections**

1. In patients with **pneumonias,** therapy should be directed toward the underlying etiologic agent.

   a. Infants less than 2 months of age should be admitted to a hospital for intravenous antibiotic therapy because of the high rate of associated sepsis.

   b. Older infants and children with mild to moderate disease may be treated as outpatients, although initiation of therapy with **ceftriaxone** (Rocephin), 50 mg/kg/day (intramuscularly or intravenously), should be considered pending culture results. Two equally effective oral medications include **amoxicillin/clavulanic acid** (Augmentin), 40 mg/kg/day three times a day, and **cefuroxime** (Ceftin), 125–250 mg twice a day. Neither of these drugs is adequate for penicillin-resistant *S pneumoniae,* which requires treatment directed by sensitivity results.

   c. **Erythromycin,** 500 mg orally four times a day, is the drug of choice for adolescents and young adults with community-acquired pneumonia. Alternatives include **azithromycin** (Zithromax), 0.5 g on the first day, then 0.25 g every day for the next 4 days, or **clarithromycin** (Biaxin), 0.5 g twice a day for 7–10 days. In addition, the newer fluoroquinolones (levofloxacin, 500 mg daily, or trovafloxacin, 200 mg daily for 7–14 days) may be used in adults because of their enhanced activity against *S pneumoniae.*

   d. Hospitalization should be considered for the elderly and for people with underlying lung disease.

2. **TB**

   a. The usual **preventive therapy** for TB is isoniazid (10 mg/kg daily for children up to a maximum adult dosage of 300 mg daily), taken continually for 6–12 months.

      (1) Twelve months of therapy is recommended for persons with HIV infection and persons with stable abnormal chest radiographs consistent with past TB.

      (2) Other groups should receive a minimum of 6 continuous months of therapy (Table 16–1).

   b. Because administration of a single drug often leads to the development of bacteria resistant to that drug, effective regimens for the treatment of active TB must contain multiple drugs to which the organisms are susceptible (Tables 16–2 and 16–3). These drugs have significant side effects, depending on the patient's age and underlying conditions. Protocols to monitor these side effects and for compliance with treatment are frequently beneficial when treating TB.

D. **Respiratory irritants.** Smoking cessation promotes a remarkable reduction in coughing. Coughs from environmental pollutants can be reduced by decreasing the exposure to the pollutants.

TABLE 16–2. DOSAGE RECOMMENDATIONS FOR THE INITIAL TREATMENT OF TUBERCULOSIS AMONG CHILDREN[1] AND ADULTS

Drugs	Daily (mg/kg)		2 times/week (mg/kg)		3 times/week (mg/kg)	
	Children	Adults	Children	Adults	Children	Adults
Isoniazid	10–20 (max 300 mg)	5 (max 300 mg)	20–40 (max 900 mg)	15 (max 900 mg)	20–40 (max 900 mg)	15 (max 900 mg)
Rifampin	10–20 (max 600 mg)	10 (max 600 mg)	10–20 (max 600 mg)	10 (max 600 mg)	10–20 (max 600 mg)	10 (max 600 mg)
Pyrazinamide	15–30 (max 2 g)	15–30 (max 2 g)	50–70 (max 4 g)	50–70 (max 4 g)	50–70 (max 3 g)	50–70 (max 3 g)
Ethambutol[2]	15–25 (max 2.5 g)	5–25 (max 2.5 g)	50 (max 2.5 g)	50 (max 2.5 g)	25–30 (max 2.5 g)	25–30 (max 2.5 g)
Streptomycin	20–30 (max 1 g)	15 (max 1 g)	25–30 (max 1.5 g)	25–30 (max 1.5 g)	25–30 (max 1 g)	25–30 (max 1 g)

[1] Children ≤12 years of age.
[2] Generally not recommended for children whose visual acuity cannot be monitored (<6 years of age). However, ethambutol should be considered for all children who have organisms resistant to other drugs, whose susceptibility to ethambutol has been demonstrated, or when susceptibility is likely.
Adapted from the Centers for Disease Control and Prevention: Initial therapy for tuberculosis in the era of multidrug resistance. MMWR 1993;**41**:RR-7.

TABLE 16–3. REGIMENS FOR THE INITIAL TREATMENT OF TUBERCULOSIS AMONG CHILDREN AND ADULTS

	Without HIV Infection		With HIV Infection
Option 1	Option 2	Option 3	
Isoniazid, rifampin, and pyrazinamide daily for 8 weeks followed by 16 weeks of isoniazid and rifampin daily or 2–3 times/week[1] in areas where the isoniazid resistance rate is not documented to be <4%. Add ethambutol or streptomycin to the initial regimen until susceptibility to isoniazid and rifampin is demonstrated. Continue treatment for at least 6 months and 3 months beyond culture conversion. Consult a TB medical expert if patient is symptomatic or smear- or culture-positive after 3 months.	Administer daily isoniazid, rifampin, and pyrazinamide and streptomycin or ethambutol for 2 weeks, then the same drugs 2 times/week[1] for 6 weeks (by directly observed therapy [DOT]), and subsequently, with 2 times/week administration of isoniazid and rifampin for 16 weeks (by DOT). Consult a TB medical expert if the patient is symptomatic or smear- or culture-positive after 3 months.	DOT 3 times/week[1] with isoniazid, rifampin, pyrazinamide, and ethambutol, or streptomycin for 6 months.[2] Consult a TB medical expert if the patient is symptomatic or smear- or culture-positive after 3 months.	Option 1, 2, or 3 can be used, but continue treatment regimens for a total of 9 months and at least 6 months beyond culture conversion.

[1] All regimens administered 2 times/week or 3 times/week should be monitored by DOT for the duration of therapy.
[2] The strongest evidence from clinical trials is the effectiveness of all four drugs administered for the full 6 months. There is weaker evidence that streptomycin can be discontinued after 4 months if the isolate is susceptible to all drugs. The evidence for stopping pyrazinamide before the end of 6 months is equivocal for the 3 times/week regimen, and there is no evidence of the effectiveness of this regimen with ethambutol for less than the full 6 months.
Adapted from the Centers for Disease Control and Prevention: Initial therapy for tuberculosis in the era of multidrug resistance. MMWR 1993;**41**:RR-7.

    E. Allergic rhinitis or asthma. See Chapters 59 and 72.

    F. COPD or chronic bronchitis. See Chapter 74.

    G. Cancer. The primary care physician should coordinate the referral of patients with lung cancer to specialists for tissue diagnosis and consideration of chemotherapy, radiation therapy, or both.

    H. Aspiration of a foreign body or from gastroesophageal reflux. Patients who have aspirated a foreign body should be immediately referred to a pulmonologist for removal of a foreign body (see Chapters 22 and 86 for management of gastroesophageal reflux).

    I. Psychogenic cough. Persons with psychogenic coughs can be referred for counseling. No data are available to determine a preferred type of psychotherapy.

REFERENCES

American Thoracic Society: Control of tuberculosis in the United States. Am Rev Respir Dis 1992;**146:**1623.

Bartlett JG, Breiman RF, Mandell LA, et al: Community-acquired pneumonia in adults. Clin Infect Dis 1998;**26:**811.

Bloch AB, Cauthen GM, Onorato IM, et al: Nationwide survey of drug-resistant tuberculosis in the United States. JAMA 1994;**271:**665.

Braman SS, Corrao WM: Cough: Differential diagnosis and treatment. Clin Chest Med 1987; **8:**177.

Centers for Disease Control and Prevention: Initial therapy for tuberculosis in the era of multidrug resistance. MMWR 1993;**41:**RR-7.

Centers for Disease Control and Prevention: Screening for tuberculosis and tuberculous infection in high-risk populations and the use of preventive therapy for tuberculous infection in the United States. MMWR 1990;**39:**RR-8.

Chaulk CP, Moore-Rice K, Rizzo R, et al: Eleven years of community-based directly observed therapy for tuberculosis. JAMA 1995;**274:**945.

Irwin RS, Corrao WM, Pratter MR: Chronic persistent cough in the adult: The spectrum and frequency of causes and successful outcome of specific therapy. Am Rev Respir Dis 1981; **123:**413.

Pickwell SM: Positive PPD and chemoprophylaxis for tuberculosis infection. Am Fam Physician 1995;**51:**1929.

Reismann JJ, Canny GJ, Levison H: The approach to chronic cough in childhood. Ann Allergy 1988;**61:**163.

Telzak EE, Sepkowitz K, Alpert P, et al: Multidrug-resistant tuberculosis in patients without HIV infection. N Engl J Med 1995;**333:**907.

US Department of Health and Human Services (DHHS): *Executive Summary: Guidelines for the Diagnosis and Management of Asthma.* DHHS; 1994.

Utell MJ: Cough. In Poe PH, Israel RH (editors): *Problems in Pulmonary Medicine for the Primary Physician.* Lea & Febiger; 1982.

---

17   Dermatitis & Other Pruritic Dermatoses

William G. Phillips, MD, Marjorie Shaw Phillips, MS, RPh, FASHP
& Christopher L. Krogh, MD, MPH[†]

   I. Definition. Pruritus is a sensation that causes one to itch, which is a peculiar irritating sensation in the skin that arouses the desire to scratch. **Dermatitis** is inflammation of the skin, whereas **dermatosis** is defined as any disease of the skin in which inflammation is not necessarily a feature.

  II. Common diagnoses

    A. Pityriasis rosea.

    B. Nummular eczema.

    C. Lichen simplex chronicus.

    D. Psoriasis.

    E. Xerosis.

[†] Died on February 24, 1994, in a plane crash in Minot, North Dakota, during one of his regular flights to an Indian reservation as part of his work as Maternal and Child Health Consultant for the Indian Health Service.

     F. **Scabies.**
     G. **Tinea infections.**
     H. **Seborrhea.**
     I. **Contact dermatitis** (irritant and allergic).
     J. **Atopic eczema.**
     K. **Dyshidrosis.** Other pruritic dermatoses discussed elsewhere in this book include insect bites and stings (Chapter 9) and folliculitis (Chapter 11).

III. **Epidemiology.** Approximately 15% of all patients presenting to generalist physicians do so for care of a skin disease or lesion.

     A. **Pityriasis rosea** is most commonly seen in children and young adults in the spring and fall. Outbreaks in institutions suggest an infective origin, possibly viral; however, no causative agent has been identified.

     B. **Nummular eczema** typically occurs in young adults and, less commonly, in children. The cause is unknown, although the history is usually positive for asthma and hay fever. In the elderly, a history of a low-protein diet is often found.

     C. **Lichen simplex chronicus** is most common in middle-aged women, atopic individuals, and persons suffering from extreme stress.

     D. **Psoriasis** affects more than 2% of people of European ancestry. It has a presumed autoimmune pathogenesis. Sunlight, relaxation, and the summer season are usually beneficial, while upper respiratory infections, trauma to the skin, lithium, and beta blockers can exacerbate psoriasis. About 15% of patients with psoriasis develop a seronegative inflammatory arthritis that has many clinical features of rheumatoid arthritis.

     E. **Xerosis,** or dry skin, most commonly results from the aging process. In younger patients, often there is a history of frequent bathing with hot water and use of harsh soaps combined with the effects of cold air, low humidity, and/or central heating.

     F. Distribution of **scabies** is worldwide, and it occurs in all social classes. Major outbreaks of scabies occur roughly every 30 years and last about 15 years. Scabies is much more likely to be acquired from direct personal contact than from touching contaminated bedding or clothing.

     G. The estimated lifetime risk of acquiring a **dermatophyte** infection is between 10% and 20%. **Tinea capitis** is most common in 3- to 8-year-olds, particularly males. It may occur in epidemics. Farmers and children with pets are classically at risk for **tinea corporis.** Obesity, heat, humidity, perspiration, and chafing predispose individuals to **tinea cruris,** which is four times more common in young adults and males than in other population groups. Acquisition of **tinea pedis** appears to depend on a susceptibility factor. More males than females are affected with this condition, which is rare in children.

     H. **Seborrhea** is often familial and is most common in adult males. It shows an association with diabetes mellitus, sprue, Parkinson's disease, and epilepsy. Seborrhea typically worsens in cooler seasons.

     I. **Irritant contact dermatitis** affects 1 of every 1000 workers each year. Sixty-five percent of all industrial illnesses are dermatoses, and approximately three sevenths of occupational dermatosis is believed to be **allergic contact dermatitis.**

     J. **Atopic eczema** is a common disease affecting 7–24 individuals per 1000. It is more common in infancy and childhood than in adulthood; however, some individuals are affected throughout life. Heredity is thought to be the single most important predisposing factor.

     K. **Dyshidrosis** is most common in adolescent or young adult males. A personal or family history of atopy is often present.

IV. **Pathophysiology.** In acute dermatitis, the histologic examination reveals intercellular edema (spongiosis) that eventually separates the epidermal cells and forms vesicles and bullae. Rupture of numerous tiny blisters can lead to crusting. The final stage, lichenification, is characterized by parakeratosis (imperfect keratinization) or hyperkeratosis (stratum corneum produced faster than it can be shed), either of which results in scaling.

     A. In **pityriasis rosea,** there is a moderately dense, mainly lymphocytic dermal infiltrate with papillary edema and a few extravasated red blood cells.

     B. In **nummular eczema,** parakeratosis and hyperkeratosis, with scaling and crusting, are prominent.

C. **Lichen simplex chronicus** is characterized by excoriation and lichenification without other specific findings.

D. **Psoriasis** is characterized by inflammation, hyperproliferation of the epidermis, altered maturation of the epidermis (resulting in scaling), and vascular alterations. In both the dermis and the epidermis, there may be a leukocytic infiltrate and pustule formation. More than 90% of patients who present with psoriasis have symmetrical discrete plaques.

E. In **xerosis,** the horny cell layer gives up water to the atmosphere.

F. **Scabies** is caused by the mite *Sarcoptes scabiei,* which is 0.3–0.4 mm long and, when on human skin, burrows through the horny layer of the stratum granulosum. Symptoms are believed to arise in part from a host reaction to mites and their eggs and feces. Initial infestations may take several weeks before an eruption manifests due to the time delay of sensitization, whereas subsequent reactions in a previously treated individual can occur in less than a day.

G. In **tinea infections,** pruritus may be caused by fungal keratolytic enzymes and exotoxins. Occasionally, dermatophytid, a sensitivity reaction to the fungus, also occurs. People with atopic tendencies and those who have zoophilic fungi infections tend to have more inflammation.

H. **Seborrhea** presents no diagnostic microscopic changes and may be described as a skin condition rather than a disease. Neutrophils are sometimes seen in the stratum corneum with focal spongiosis.

I. In **contact dermatitis,** mononuclear cells often aggregate around minute blood vessels, and edema may separate deep epidermal from adjacent dermal cells.

J. **Atopic eczema** appears to be associated with a deficiency in cell-mediated immunity, although some researchers postulate that an immunoglobulin A deficiency early in life allows ingested allergens to enter the bloodstream, producing immune responses that would not otherwise occur. Established lesions show edema and variable infiltration with mononuclear cells and eosinophils.

K. **Dyshidrosis** is distinguished by deep (1- to 2-mm) vesicles between, but not involving, sweat glands. These vesicles usually resorb without rupturing.

V. **Symptoms.** The above conditions are characterized by varying degrees of pruritus. Scabies can be especially pruritic, while the itching of pityriasis, nummular eczema, and seborrhea may be minimal.

VI. **Signs** (see Table 17–1). With some exceptions, primary changes (eg, erythema, edema, vesicles, and weeping) become overlaid with secondary changes (eg, excoriation, crusting, erosions, scales, and scars) that are produced by conscious or unconscious scratching.

VII. **Laboratory tests.** The history and the physical examination are generally all that are necessary to diagnose the conditions discussed in this chapter. Laboratory tests are occasionally indicated to differentiate common dermatoses from rarer conditions. The tests listed below are also sometimes useful to confirm a particular diagnosis.

A. **Microscopic examination** of burrow scrapings in mineral oil may reveal scabies mites, eggs, or feces.

B. **Potassium hydroxide (KOH)** preparations are the classic tests for tinea. Skin scrapings are placed on a glass slide, one or two drops of 10–20% KOH are added, and the slide is heated gently to dissolve cellular material and reveal the hyphae and spores characteristic of tinea.

C. **Wood's light examination** is useful in the differential diagnosis of tinea of the scalp, which fluoresces bright yellow-green, or of the skin (*Corynebacterium minutissimum*), which resembles tinea but fluoresces red.

D. **Patch testing** is the classic test for allergic contact dermatitis. Allergen is applied to the skin for 48 hours and then removed. The skin is observed 20 minutes later. Reactions may take place in one area of tissue but not in others.

E. **Biopsy**
1. If lesions of atopic eczema involve the nipple and do not subside with simple treatment, Paget's disease must be excluded by biopsy. Unilateral eczema of the breast may be the only indication of a ductal adenocarcinoma.
2. In cases of pityriasis, the physician should strongly consider a serologic test or a biopsy to rule out syphilis.
3. In any case in which the diagnosis is in doubt, a biopsy should be considered.

VIII. **Treatment.** Overall goals of treatment include (1) relief of itching and scratching; (2) identification and treatment of underlying causes, where possible; and (3) cosmetic improvement.

TABLE 17–1. LOCATIONS AND SIGNS OF COMMON PRURITIC DERMATOSES

Condition	Usual Sites	Acute Changes	Chronic Changes
Pityriasis rosea	Chest and trunk	Herald patch, salmon-pink, 3–4 cm on trunk	Macular papular lesions with a Christmas tree distribution
Nummular eczema	Extensor surfaces, shoulders, breasts, buttocks	Erythema, mild edema with occasional vesiculation	Crusting with excoriation
Lichen simplex chronicus	Areas within easy reach of fingers	Excoriation	Lichenification, exaggerated skin markings
Psoriasis	Knees, elbows, scalp	Erythematous papulosquamous lesions; pustules may occur	
Xerosis	Extremities, neck	Platelike scaling, eczematous changes	
Scabies	Groin, hands, lower abdomen, back	Scaly, grayish burrows	Obscured by excoriations
Tinea capitis	Scalp	Grayish scaling, round areas with broken hairs	
Seborrhea	Scalp	Moist, greasy scales; crusted pinkish or orangish scalp patches	
Contact dermatitis	Exposed area or previously sensitized area	Darkening, edema	Weeping, vesicles, bullae
Atopic eczema	Dorsa of hands, feet, ears, skin creases	Dryness	Thickening, excoriation, scaling
Dyshidrosis	Palms, soles, sides of fingers	Weeping patches, deep vesicles	Desquamation, vesicles dry up

A. General measures

1. Relief of itching and scratching

a. First-generation sedating **antihistamines** can be useful in combating the urge to scratch. Agents include **hydroxyzine** (Vistaril or Atarax), 25–100 mg for adults, 12.5–25 mg for children aged 6 and older, or 0.5 mg/kg up to 12.5 mg for children younger than 6 years, up to three or four times a day; **trimeprazine** (Temaril), 5 mg twice a day for adults, 1.25 mg up to three times a day as needed for children aged 2–3 years, or 2.5 mg up to three times a day as needed for children over 3 years old; or **diphenhydramine** (Benadryl), 50 mg at bedtime for adults and 12.5 mg every 4–6 hours for children aged 6–12 years.

b. **Topical therapy**

(1) **Acute and subacute conditions** are best treated with nonocclusive creams, gels, or soaks. Soaks offer the potential advantages of low cost, immediate soothing effect, low risk of sensitization, and safety even with chronic use. **Burow's solution,** rather than water, is recommended to minimize bacterial overgrowth and is easily prepared using one commercial Burow's tablet in 1 pint of cool water. This can be applied to the skin by pouring over a dressing appropriate to the lesion size and then allowing the dressing to dry for 15–20 minutes. Alternatively, the patient can immerse him- or herself in a cool bath to which baking soda or oatmeal has been added.

(2) **Chronic conditions** are often most easily treated with occlusive ointments than with soaks. Hydrophobic (greasy) ointments such as **white petrolatum** (USP) or **zinc oxide ointment** (USP), applied two or three times a day, infrequently produce reaction or sensitization.

(3) **Topical steroids** (see Table 17–2) fall into three groups: low, moderate, and high potency. As a general rule, only low-potency topical steroids (eg, **hydrocortisone** 2.5% or less, **fluocinolone** 0.01%, or **triamcinolone** 0.025%) are recommended for the conditions

TABLE 17–2. TOPICAL STEROIDS FOR DERMATOSES

Generic Name of Product	Dosing[1]	Trade Name(s)	Cost[2]
Lowest potency			
Hydrocortisone (cream, ointment, lotion) 0.5–2.5% 2.5% cream 0.5–1% available without prescription	qd–qid	Generic Hytone, Synacort, etc	$–$$ $$–$$$
Dexamethasone (topical aerosol) 0.01%	bid–qid	Aeroseb-Dex[3]	$$$$
Low potency			
Betamethasone valerate (cream) 0.01%	qd–tid	Valisone Reduced Strength	$$$$
Fluocinolone acetonide (cream, ointment) 0.01%	bid–qid	Generic, Flurosyn Synalar	$–$$ $$
Flurandrenolide (cream,[3] ointment,[3] lotion) 0.025%	bid–tid	Cordran, Cordran SP	$$$$
Triamcinolone acetonide (cream, ointment, lotion, aerosol) 0.025%	tid–qid	Generic	$
		Aristocort, Aristocort A, Kenalog	$$$
High potency (for acute, self-limited dermatosis; avoid on face)			
Fluocinolone acetonide (cream) 0.2%	bid–qid	Synalar-HP	$$$$
Fluocinonide (cream, gel, ointment, solution) 0.05%	bid–qid	Generic Lidex, Lidex-E	$$$ $$$$
Halcinonide (cream, ointment, solution) 0.1%	qd, bid–tid	Halog, Halog-E	$$$$
Triamcinolone acetonide (cream, ointment) 0.5%	bid–qid	Generic Aristocort, Aristocort A, Kenalog	$ $$$$$

[1] Usual adult doses. Patients should be instructed to apply sparingly to skin in a light film and rub in gently.
[2] Average wholesale cost to the pharmacist for 15 g of ointment or cream: $, <$2; $$, $2–5; $$$, $5–10; $$$$, $10–20; $$$$$, >$20.
[3] Available as a 58-g spray.

described in this chapter. Sensitivity to steroids may develop, especially in atopic individuals.

   c. Systemic steroids are reserved for conditions not responding to the treatments above. Using the smallest possible dosage for the shortest period is advisable. Specific goals of treatment should be established prior to the use of oral steroids to help ascertain their effectiveness.

      Prednisone can be administered as "bursts" of 40–60 mg each morning for 4–7 days, then stopped. Side effects and dangers appear to be minimized with this regimen.

2. Elimination of aggravating factors

   a. Rapid temperature changes, low humidity, alcohol, caffeine, and excessive cleansing or washing may aggravate each condition. Other irritants include synthetic or rubber shoes, dyed socks, cosmetics, hair spray, jewelry, and tight or very soft clothing or furs.

   b. Previous treatment history should be obtained. Part of the present clinical picture may be the result of prior treatment. Topical anesthetics, topical antihistamine-containing products such as Caladryl, and even hydrocortisone cream may themselves produce sensitization.

B. Condition-specific treatments

   1. Pityriasis rosea is a self-limited disease that usually resolves in 6–8 weeks. Oral antihistamines (see section VIII,A,1,a) are helpful with the pruritus. Steroids are not indicated.

   2. Nummular eczema is treated with topical steroids, oral antihistamines, and oral antibiotics when a secondary infection occurs. **Coal tar solutions** (eg, Zetar, 30% emulsion, 1–2 tbsp mixed in a lukewarm bath, with immersion for 15–20 minutes repeated three to seven times weekly) help in resistant cases. Foods with excessive iodides and bromides should be avoided; these include chocolate, salted nuts, cheeses, seafood, iodized salts, tomatoes, melons, and dark greens. In older patients, increasing the intake of protein-rich foods such as beef and gelatin may be helpful.

3. **Lichen simplex chronicus** can be treated with oral antihistamines and soaks in ice-cold **Burow's solution** for 15 minutes. Should moderate-potency corticosteroid ointments or creams not control the lesions, then **coal tar solution** (3–10%) may be added to the regimen as a soak, combined with the Burow's solution.

4. **Psoriasis** treatment is related to reducing epidermal cell turnover.
   a. **Mild lesions** can be treated with emollients (eg, **Desitin ointment,** applied three times a day to affected areas, or **A and D ointment,** applied three times a day) chronically to affected areas. Keratolytic agents, such as **salicylic acid** (eg, salicyclic acid soap), applied daily, can bring limited improvement but can irritate inflamed skin. Mild to moderate corticosteroid ointments (see Table 17–2) are one of the mainstays of treatment but can cause localized skin atrophy.
   b. **Moderate lesions** may respond to **ultraviolet (UV) light** or **tar preparations** (eg, Estar applied at bedtime to affected areas, allowing the gel to remain for 5 minutes and then removing any excess by patting with tissues) or a combination of UV light and tar preparation. **Calcipotriene** (Dovonex), a new topical treatment for psoriasis of mild to moderate severity, is a vitamin D derivative that inhibits epidermal cell proliferation in vitro. Calcipotriene should be applied twice daily to psoriatic plaques on the trunk and/or the extremities, avoiding application to the face and the groin, where it may cause irritant dermatitis. Topical calcipotriene is about as effective as moderate- to high-potency topical steroids. Absorption of calcipotriene is a problem only if large quantities (>100 g/week) are applied. It should not be used by patients with demonstrated hypercalcemia or evidence of vitamin D toxicity. It has a pregnancy category of C.

5. **Xerosis** is best managed by decreasing skin dryness. Patients should bathe less frequently and use an emollient soap such as Dove, Aveeno bar, Neutrogena, Basis, or Oilatum. Emollients such as Nivea skin oil or cream, Keri lotion or cream, and Eucerin lotion or ointment may be placed liberally on moist skin after bathing.

6. **Scabies** can be treated with a variety of agents.
   a. The drug of choice is **5% permethrin** (Elimite). Permethrin should be massaged into the skin from the neck down. The cream should be removed by washing after 8 hours. Infants should be treated on the scalp, temples, and forehead. One application is curative. Elimite has a pregnancy category of B. It is not known whether it is excreted in human milk. Because of the evidence for tumorigenic potential of permethrin in animal studies, consideration should be given to discontinuing nursing temporarily or withholding the drug while the mother is nursing. Elimite is reported to be safe and effective in children 2 months of age and older. Compared with **lindane** (Kwell), permethrin is considered much less toxic.
   b. **Crotamiton** (Eurax) lotion or cream has proved much less reliable than permethrin in the treatment of scabies. It should be massaged into the skin from the chin to the toes after the patient has showered. A second application is advisable 24 hours later. A cleansing bath should be taken 48 hours after the last application. Crotamiton has a category C for use in pregnancy. Crotamiton should therefore be given to a pregnant woman only if clearly needed. Safety and effectiveness in children have not been established.

7. **Tinea infections**
   a. Care should be given to treatment in women who are or might soon become pregnant. Griseofulvin has a pregnancy category of X, fluconazole and itraconazole are category C, and terbinafine is category B.
   b. **Tinea capitis** (mycosis of the hair) is best treated with oral therapy. **Griseofulvin** is the only oral antifungal agent approved by the US Food and Drug Administration for first-line treatment of tinea capitis. In adults with tinea capitis, **ultramicrosize griseofulvin** (Fulvicin P/G, Gris-PEG, or Grisactin Ultra) is given in dosages of 330–375 mg/day for 4–6 weeks. **Itraconazole** (Sporanox, 100 mg/day with food for 6 weeks in adults) and **terbinafine** (Lamisil, 250 mg/day for 4–6 weeks in adults) are alternatives.

    c. Tinea barbae is treated with the same agents as used for tinea capitis.

    d. Tinea corporis should be treated orally unless only one or two small, isolated lesions are present. **Terbinafine** (Lamisil, 250 mg/day for 2–4 weeks) and **itraconazole** (Sporanox, 100–200 mg/day with a meal for 2 weeks) are equally effective in treating tinea corporis in adults.

    e. Tinea cruris involves the medial aspect of the inner thighs. It does not usually involve the scrotum or penis, as yeast infections do. **Topical therapy** often works, but if the infection spreads to the lower thighs or buttocks, oral therapy with **itraconazole** (Sporanox, 100–200 mg/day with meals for 2 weeks in adults) or **terbinafine** (Lamisil, 250 mg/day for 2–4 weeks in adults) may be needed.

    f. Tinea pedis is often treated with topical therapy. **Miconazole lotion** (Monistat-Derm) may be applied twice daily for 2–4 weeks. **Tolnaftate powder** (Tinactin) is also effective when applied locally twice daily. Hyperkeratotic tinea pedis often requires oral therapy. Good choices for oral therapy in adults are **itraconazole** (Sporanox, 100 mg/day with a meal for 30 days), **terbinafine** (Lamisil, 250 mg/day for 2–4 weeks), or **ultramicrosize griseofulvin** (250–375 mg every 12 hours for 4–8 weeks).

    g. Tinea manuum, a fungal infection of the hands, is treated similarly to tinea pedis.

8. Seborrheic dermatitis

    a. In **adults,** conventional therapy for **seborrheic dermatitis** of the scalp is a shampoo containing one of the following compounds: **salicylic acid** (eg, X-Seb T or Sebulex), **selenium sulfide** (eg, Selsun or Exsel), **coal tar** (eg, DHS Tar, Neutrogena T-Gel, or Polytar), or **pyrithione zinc** (eg, DHS Zinc, Danex, or Sebulon). Each of these shampoos can be used two or three times a week. After application, shampoos should be left on the hair and scalp for at least 5 minutes to ensure that the medication reaches the scalp skin. In more severe cases, adults may massage topical steroid lotions such as **2.5% hydrocortisone** (eg, Hytone) into the scalp once or twice daily.

    b. For **infantile seborrheic dermatitis,** the usual approach is conservative, with the use of a mild, nonmedicated shampoo (eg, baby shampoo used twice a week) first, followed by the use of a shampoo containing coal tar in resistant cases. Topical steroids should be avoided in infants if possible, because of significant percutaneous absorption.

9. Contact dermatitis is best treated by identifying and removing the offending agent. For the active phase, topical steroids are helpful. For acute, weepy vesicular lesions, wet dressings in the form of soaks or lotions may be needed.

10. Atopic eczema can be treated in the acute stage with wet compresses using **Burow's solution.** Judicious use of low-potency topical steroids and oral antihistamines such as **cyproheptadine** (eg, Periactin, 4 mg three times a day for adults and 0.25 mg/kg/day for children over 2 years of age) or **trimeprazine** (Temaril, 2.5 mg four times a day for adults, 1.25 mg at bedtime for children aged 6 months to 3 years, and 2.5 mg at bedtime or up to three times a day as needed for children over 3 years) are helpful. **Coal tar solutions** may also provide relief. Affected individuals should avoid contact with herpes simplex and live virus vaccine.

11. Dyshidrosis often responds well to mild steroid creams, which may be alternated with Burow's soaks. Plain leather shoes and frequent changes of clean, undyed, cotton socks may also be helpful.

REFERENCES

Greco PJ, Ende J: An office-based approach to the patient with pruritus. Hosp Pract (Off Ed) 1992;**27**(5A):121.

Janniger CK, Schwartz RA: Seborrheic dermatitis. Am Fam Physician 1995;**52:**149.

Kirsner RS, Federman D: Treatment of psoriasis: Role of calcipotriene. Am Fam Physician 1995;**52:**237.

Noble S, Forbes R, Stamm P: Diagnosis and management of common tinea infections. Am Fam Physician 1998;**58:**163.

Peterson CM, Eichenfield LF: Scabies. Pediatr Ann 1996;**25:**97.

Stern RS: Psoriasis. Lancet 1997;**350:**349.

18   Dermatologic Neoplasms

George A. Nixon, MD

I. **Definition.** A dermatologic neoplasm is a lesion produced by the abnormal proliferation of cells normally found in skin.

II. **Common diagnoses**

   A. **Benign dermatologic neoplasms,** such as seborrheic keratoses and nevi (moles), verrucae (warts), lentigines, lipomas, and keratoacanthomas.

   B. **Premalignant dermatologic neoplasms,** such as actinic keratoses, atypical mole syndrome, and giant congenital nevus.

   C. **Malignant dermatologic neoplasms,** such as basal cell carcinoma, squamous cell carcinoma, and malignant melanoma.

III. **Epidemiology.** Of the patients who consult primary care physicians for skin problems, 20% are diagnosed as having a skin neoplasm or tumor.

   A. **Benign neoplasms**

   1. All individuals develop **nevi** (eg, moles, birthmarks, or beauty marks). Approximately 1% of infants have one or more nevi at birth. These increase during adolescence to an average of 20–40 lesions by the third decade, and few remain by age 90. These lesions are more prevalent in whites, and their number increases as a result of sun exposure.

   2. **Seborrheic keratoses** (seborrheic or senile warts) are very common skin growths in middle-aged adults and the elderly. Although the cause of these lesions is unclear, they demonstrate an autosomal dominant mode of inheritance and are associated with oily-seborrheic skin.

   3. **Verrucae** (warts) can occur at any age, but are more common during the teenage years. Their appearance and clinical course are unpredictable, but their incidence, severity, and prevalence are greater in the immunocompromised patient.

   4. **Lentigines** are hyperpigmented macular lesions found most commonly in children or young adults with light complexions. In elderly individuals, these lesions become more prevalent in sun-exposed areas, where they are recognized as "age" or "liver" spots.

   5. **Keratoacanthomas** occur on sun-exposed areas in the elderly as rapidly growing solitary lesions.

   B. **Premalignant neoplasms**

   1. **Actinic keratoses** are the most common premalignant skin lesions. They are found most often on sun-exposed areas (eg, the face, head, and dorsal surface of the hands) of middle-aged to elderly persons with light complexions who have a history of prolonged or repeated intense sun exposure. Lifetime risk of an individual with actinic keratosis developing a cutaneous squamous cell carcinoma is estimated at 20%.

   2. **Giant congenital nevus** (bathing trunk nevus) is a large but rare nevus apparent at birth on the lower torso or buttocks. It is brown to black and often contains hair. Four percent to 6% will give rise to malignant melanoma; this transformation occurs in 50% prior to puberty.

   3. **Atypical mole syndrome** (formerly dysplastic nevus syndrome) is a familial autosomal dominant syndrome in which an individual's risk for the development of cutaneous melanoma is 10–100 times that of the general population.

   C. **Malignant neoplasms.** The skin is the most common cancer site, with over 1 million new cases of skin cancer diagnosed each year. Risk factors for skin cancer development are listed in Table 18–1.

   1. **Basal cell carcinoma.** This is the most common skin cancer. Two thirds of these neoplasms develop in sun-damaged areas, and the remainder occur in covered areas where genetic disposition plays a role.

   2. **Squamous cell carcinoma.** A higher proportion of skin cancers arising from squamous cells develop in sun-exposed areas. The incidence of squamous cell cancer is higher in individuals with fair skin, immune disorders, outdoor occupations, and exposure to hydrocarbon fractions such as soot, coal tar, and lubricating oils.

TABLE 18–1. RISK FACTORS FOR DEVELOPMENT OF SKIN CANCER

Racial and ethnic factors
White race, especially individuals of northern European descent whose features include fair complexion, freckled skin, blond or red hair, and blue eyes. The incidence of skin cancer is 15 times higher in whites than in blacks.

Sun exposure
More skin cancers occur in persons whose occupations or hobbies involve increased sun exposure (eg, farmers, construction workers, sailors, or sunbathers). The prevalence of these lesions increases as one surveys populations living closer to the equator, in sunny regions, and at high altitudes.

Chronic skin damage or irritation
Immunosuppression, radiation, burns, scars, and chronic ulcers

Chemical carcinogens
Ongoing exposure to reagents such as radium, creosote, pitch tar, coal tar products, or arsenic ingestion

---

3. **Malignant melanomas.** Melanoma accounts for 2–3% of all skin cancers, but two thirds of skin cancer mortality. The incidence of malignant melanoma has increased by 500% over the past four decades. Melanoma rates are highest in developed countries and, worldwide, the closer one moves to the equator. Increased ultraviolet light exposure through depletion of the ozone layer may be a contributing factor; however, correlation with sun exposure is less frequent for melanoma than for basal and squamous cell cancers. Rather than duration, *intensity* of sun exposure (ie, a history of blistering sunburn before age 20) doubles the risk of melanoma. A positive family history and a history of a previous primary lesion are also risk factors.

Most individuals are diagnosed between the ages of 40 and 55. The occurrence of melanoma exhibits no sexual preference. In males, lesions tend to occur in the interscapular area, and in females, on the back and the lower legs.

IV. **Pathophysiology**
   A. **Benign neoplasms**
      1. **Nevi** are aberrant collections of melanocytes in the epidermis, in the dermis, or at the epidermal junction. The appearance of a nevus depends on the location of the melanocytes. In **juvenile (flat) nevi,** the melanocytes are in the dermoepidermal junction. Juvenile nevi often evolve into **compound (domed) nevi,** with epidermal and dermal components.
      2. **Seborrheic keratoses** consist of hyperplastic epithelium with increased melanin and numbers of immature epidermal cells in relation to maturing keratinocytes.
      3. **Verrucae** (warts) are caused by a papillomavirus.
      4. **Lentigines** are 0.2- to 2-cm collections of melanocytes and hyperpigmented basilar cells with prolonged rete pegs.
      5. **Keratoacanthomas** represent an aberrant growth of epithelial cells, resembling squamous cell cancer histologically. Researchers believe that these tumors are induced by viruses, ultraviolet light, or chemical irritants.
   B. **Premalignant neoplasms**
      1. **Actinic keratoses** represent epidermal dysplasia produced by chronic sun exposure. This results in loss of orientation, atypia, and hyperkeratosis of epidermal cells.
      2. In **giant congenital nevi,** the melanocytes are situated deep within the dermis and within the sweat glands, hair follicles, and sebaceous glands.
      3. **Atypical moles** are nevi that demonstrate persistent lentiginous melanocytic hyperplasia and atypia, as well as patchy lymphocytic infiltration.
   C. **Malignant neoplasms**
      1. **Basal cell carcinomas** originate from basal cells that have lost the ability to differentiate into normal keratinizing cells, often because of solar damage. Untreated basal cell carcinoma grows slowly, invading contiguous soft tissue, bone, and cartilage; metastasis rarely occurs distant from the primary lesion.
      2. **Squamous cell carcinomas** result from damage to the DNA of keratinocytes by one or more of the agents listed in Table 18–1, most commonly ultraviolet light.

Sixty percent of squamous cell carcinomas arise from actinic keratosis. Spread is most commonly by local extension and, less commonly, by metastasis. Locations prone to metastasis include mucocutaneous squamous cell cancer (11% of cases) and squamous cell carcinoma arising at sites of inflammatory or degenerative change, such as chronic ulcers, burns, or scars (up to 30% of cases).

3. **Malignant melanomas** originate from melanocytes normally found along the basal layer of the epidermis. They are very aggressive cancers with a tendency for rapid spread and early metastasis. Evidence of thickness >1.70 mm or distal spread at the time of diagnosis forecasts a poor prognosis for survival.

   a. Recognized precursor lesions include atypical and congenital nevi. The majority of melanomas arise from apparently normal skin. Occasionally, melanomas occur in the eye or the vagina, or on the palms and soles of patients of dark-skinned races.

   b. Each of the histologic types of melanoma occurs, grows, and metastasizes at a different rate. The four types and their frequencies of occurrence relative to other melanomas are:

      (1) **Superficial spreading melanoma** (70%).
      (2) **Lentigo maligna melanoma** (12%).
      (3) **Nodular melanoma** (10%).
      (4) **Acral lentiginous melanoma** (8%).

V. Symptoms. Symptoms are not useful in the classification of skin neoplasms as benign or malignant. Lesions of either type may be asymptomatic. Most persons seek no medical evaluation of skin neoplasms. Medical advice, when sought, is frequently motivated by displeasure with cosmetic appearance or location. Patients are annoyed when these lesions become entangled in necklaces, are irritated by skin folds or clothing (eg, collars, bras, or belts), interfere with shaving, or are judged to produce disfigurement. Consultation, when prompted by anxiety over changes in appearance, size, number of lesions, local discomfort, bleeding, discharge, or ulceration, should heighten suspicion for malignancy.

VI. Signs of particular neoplasms

   A. Benign neoplasms

      1. **Nevi** may be found on any skin surface, but are more common above the waist.

         a. The common types of nevi are described below.

            (1) **Junctional nevi** are usually flat, oval, well-circumscribed, darkly pigmented lesions 0.1–0.6 cm in diameter.
            (2) **Compound nevi** are slightly elevated, with a domed or warty appearance, and may contain hairs. These symmetrically round or oval lesions are flesh-colored or darker.
            (3) **Intradermal (dermal) nevi** are extremely pleomorphic and may be sessile or pedunculated, warty or polypoid, and either dark to flesh-colored or translucent. They occur most frequently about the face and neck. As an individual ages, the structural tissue of these lesions is replaced by fat and fibrous tissue.

         b. Pigmented lesions resembling nevi include the following.

            (1) **Mongolian spots,** which are large, irregular, gray to bluish-black congenital macular lesions, are frequently present in the sacrum-buttock region in infants of dark-skinned race. These lesions fade after the first few months or years of life.
            (2) **Lentigines** (age or liver spots) are large (1- to 3-mm), macular lesions of tan to dark brown color with a scaly surface. They appear most commonly in sun-exposed regions of older persons, but unlike freckles, their pigmentation is not affected by sunlight.
            (3) **Ephelides** (freckles) are pigmented macules <0.5 cm in diameter, seen most often on sun-exposed areas of fair-skinned persons. Their number and pigmentation increase with sun exposure.

      2. **Seborrheic keratosis.** The appearance of these lesions can be quite varied and can be smooth, warty, domed, or plaque-like. Typically, they have a "stuck-on" or "dropped candle wax" appearance. They are found on sun-exposed as well as covered skin areas, especially the face, neck, and trunk, but are never present on the soles or palms.

3. **Verrucae** (warts). The common types of warts are described below.
   a. **Flat warts** (verruca plana), slightly elevated macular lesions of 1–3 mm with smooth, flesh-colored surfaces, are generally found on the face, neck, hands, and lower legs in a linear distribution.
   b. **Periungual warts** are hypopigmented nodular lesions with rough surfaces found adjacent to and sometimes extending beneath the nails.
   c. **Plantar warts** appear as thick, superficial, coalescing lesions extending deep into the dermis that reveal pinpoint-sized bleeding points when pared. These lesions occur on the feet, typically at points of maximal pressure, and are thus often painful with walking or standing.
   d. **Genital warts** (condylomata acuminata or venereal warts) are velvety, moist, slightly raised, cauliflower-like lesions that occur singularly or in clusters on the genitalia or in perianal areas.
4. **Keratoacanthomas** appear over 1–2 weeks in sun-exposed areas as rapidly growing solitary nodules or papules with a central keratin plug. Early, rapid growth is classically followed by slow, spontaneous regression with scarring.

B. Premalignant neoplasms
1. **Actinic keratosis** (solar or senile keratosis). These precursors of squamous cell cancers appear as rough, scaly skin in irregular, erythematous, or tan plaques on the scalp, face, neck, forearms, and dorsa of the hands. Removal of the adherent yellow crust frequently induces bleeding.
2. **Congenital nevi** vary in diameter from a few millimeters to several centimeters. Flat at birth, they may later become thickened, slightly elevated, and covered with many coarse hairs. Most of the lesions are small and remain benign, but occasionally they are extensive and cover a large area of the chest, back, shoulders, sacrum, and buttocks with a significant potential for malignant change.
   a. Bathing trunk nevus is so called because it often occurs in a truncal distribution and can involve an entire hand or leg or the scalp. Scalp involvement may be associated with epilepsy or mental retardation.
   b. Congenital nevi should be differentiated from mongolian spots, which are more common in black infants and fade after the first few months or years of life.
3. **Atypical mole syndrome** is heralded by the sudden appearance in an adolescent of multiple nevi with wide variation in size, shape, and color. Usually, these nevi are located on the back, but they are also common on the scalp, upper and lower limbs, buttocks, groin, and female breasts. They differ from common nevi in size (5–10 mm in diameter compared to <6 mm for common nevi), shape and contour (irregular borders with poor margination compared to symmetric, uniform borders for common nevi), and color (intra- and interlesional variations of brown, black, or red compared to more homogenous variations of tan, brown, or black for common nevi).

C. Malignant neoplasms
1. **Basal cell carcinomas** appear as papular or nodular lesions with raised, pearly borders and numerous superficial telangiectases. There is often a central area of ulceration (rodent ulcer) with an irregular, rolled border.
2. **Squamous cell carcinomas** initially appear as thickened skin with scaling and hyperkeratosis in sun-exposed areas. Induration is the first clinical sign of malignancy. Over time, these lesions become larger, deeply nodular, and ulcerated. Dilated superficial blood vessels are present within the lesion and the surrounding tissue.
3. **Melanomas** are classically described by the *ABCD* mnemonic: **a**symmetry, **b**order irregularity, **c**olor variation, and **d**iameter ≥5 mm. The diagnosis should be considered in any nevus exhibiting an increase in size, erratic growth, or a change in color.

VII. Laboratory tests
A. The lesions listed below should be biopsied.
1. Newly discovered moles in a patient over 40.
2. Any mole >0.5 cm that is accompanied by any tenderness, itching, bleeding, or ulceration.
3. Lesions with a history of recent growth, ulceration, or clinical characteristics suggestive of melanoma.

B. Several techniques may be used to remove skin neoplasms.

    1. Shave excision is useful for elevated lesions or those in which depth of excision is unimportant. Anesthetic is injected beneath the lesion so as to elevate its base on the wheal created. The surrounding skin is then held taut while the blade of a No. 15 scalpel lying nearly horizontal to the skin surface is passed through the base using long, smooth, cutting strokes. Bleeding is easily controlled with simple pressure, Monsel's solution, silver nitrate sticks, or electrocautery.

    2. Skin biopsy is performed with either a scalpel or a skin punch biopsy instrument. Both techniques provide full-thickness diagnostic specimens, but punch biopsy is not practical when complete excision is required of irregular, large, or cystic lesions.

        a. Punch biopsy. The skin is prepared with an aseptic solution, and the lesion is injected with anesthetic (lidocaine [Xylocaine], 1% or 2%) to produce a wheal around the base of the biopsy site. Care should be taken to avoid direct injection into the lesion, since this may distort the structural anatomy. With the skin stretched perpendicular to wrinkle (Langer's) lines, the dermal punch is then pressed onto the biopsy site using a firm, twisting motion. Resistance decreases when subcutaneous tissue is reached. The punch is then withdrawn and the lesion is cut away with a scalpel or iris scissors and immediately placed in preservative. After hemostasis is achieved, the wound may be closed with suture or left to heal secondarily.

        b. Excisional biopsy. The skin is washed and prepared with an aseptic solution. Local anesthetic (lidocaine [Xylocaine], 1% or 2%) is injected along the planned lines of excision, producing a wheal along the skin. The tip of the needle can be used to mark the lines of intended excision. These should parallel skin wrinkle lines. Using the tip of a No. 15 scalpel, the lesion is then excised and placed in preservative. The excision site is then closed with suture.

VIII. Treatment

A. Benign neoplasms

    1. Nevi usually require no treatment except for cosmetic or diagnostic purposes. Most are easily removed by shave or excisional biopsy as described above.

    2. Seborrheic keratoses. Removal may be achieved by cryosurgery or by shave or curette excision after anesthetizing the skin with a local anesthetic. Monsel's solution, silver nitrate stick, or electrodesiccation can then be used to achieve hemostasis.

    3. Warts

        a. Flat warts may be treated with **cryosurgery** or **topical keratolytics.** Alternatively, **tretinoin (retinoic acid)** cream or lotion (0.025%, 0.05%, or 0.1%) can be applied once or twice daily to produce mild inflammation and subsequent regression. Successful treatment may require several weeks. **Fluorouracil** (Efudex) cream, 5%, applied once or twice a day for 3–5 weeks, is also effective.

        b. Periungual warts. The proximity of these warts to, and occasionally involvement of, the nail bed dictate cautious treatment. **Cryosurgery** can be used, taking care to avoid injury to the nail matrix and superficial nerves. Alternatively, **cantharidin** (Cantharone), **bichloroacetic acid,** or **salicylic acid** may be applied weekly until the wart regresses. Occasionally, these treatments fail; eradication in these instances can be achieved only through the performance of a digital block followed by blunt dissection.

        c. Plantar warts. Foot pain at the site of these warts leads patients to seek treatment. Successful treatment methods include the application of **40% salicylic acid** under occlusion to a wart that has been pared to its core, or the application of a 40% salicylic acid pad. After 24–48 hours, the plaster is removed, whitened skin is scraped away, and a new plaster is applied. Treatment may require several weeks. Topical treatment with **bichloroacetic acid** or other similar keratolytic agents may be used. Intralesional injection of a 1 U/mL solution of **bleomycin sulfate** is reported to have a cure rate of 48%. Cryosurgery or excision of these warts is discouraged, as both methods tend to cause considerable pain and temporary loss of mobility.

    d. Anogenital warts (condylomata acuminata or venereal warts). Treatment options include patient- and physician-applied topicals, intralesional interferon injections, cryotherapy, laser, and conventional surgery. Treatment choice should be guided by the preference of the patient. **Imiquimod cream 5%** (Aldara) induces the production of interferon alfa, which acts directly against human papillomavirus. The cream is applied by the patient at bedtime 3 nights a week for up to 16 weeks. Effective cure is reported in 54% with initial treatment. **Podofilox gel 0.5%** (Condylox) is self-applied every 12 hours for 3 days, then discontinued for 4 days for a maximum of four treatment cycles. The reported response is 45–88%. Burning and irritation are common local side effects. Physician-applied topicals of 10–25% **podophyllin solution** and **trichloroacetic** and **bichloroacetic acid** 25% or 50% solutions at weekly intervals have reported cure rates of 32–80%, but with disadvantages of inconvenience and cost to the patient. With the surrounding skin protected by petrolatum, podophyllin or trichloroacetic acid solution is applied to external warts with a cotton swab. Podophyllin is allowed to dry and washed off in 1–2 hours; the trichloroacetic acid solution, after a few moments. Patients should be followed up in 1 week, at which time a second application may be performed. *Note:* Caution should be exercised when treating unusually large lesions or lesions of the mouth, vagina, or anorectal region. Systemic toxicity can occur from absorption of podophyllin through mucous membranes. Intralesional injection of **interferon** achieves wart eradication in 36–62%, but is expensive and requires multiple office visits.

        Cryosurgery and **electrosurgery** may be used for treatment of limited lesions on the vulva or the shaft of the penis. Management of large or anorectal lesions with these modalities should be left to those experienced in their treatment, as scarring and pain may occur.

  4. Lentigines. These lesions pose no health threat. Attempts at removal by topical or surgical techniques are unsatisfactory because of the tendency toward recurrence. They can be masked or made less noticeable by the routine use of sunscreens or creams containing hydroquinone.

  5. Keratoacanthoma. Simple excision of these lesions provides a high cure rate and excellent cosmetic results. Nonexcisional therapies producing acceptable results include intralesional 5-fluorouracil, cryosurgery, electrodesiccation, and oral isotretinoin.

B. Premalignant lesions are treated mainly to prevent malignant degeneration and for cosmetic reasons. Patients with these lesions should specifically be educated regarding **sun protection** (ie, covering exposed areas), **use of sunscreens** with a sun protection factor of 15 or more, **avoidance of sun exposure** between 10 AM and 4 PM, regular **skin self-examination,** and avoidance of tanning salons.

  1. Actinic keratoses. Electrodesiccation with curettage or excision or **cryosurgery** is practical if lesions are few in number. For patients with more extensive lesions, **topical 5-fluorouracil** (Efudex) is an effective alternative method of treatment available to primary care physicians. For lesions on the face or lips, a 1–2% solution or cream is applied twice daily in an amount sufficient to cover the lesions. Over a period of 2–4 weeks, lesions undergo a process of inflammation, necrosis, and ulceration. When ulceration occurs, treatment is discontinued and healing should begin to occur. Actinic lesions on the scalp, neck, thorax, and extremities are treated with a 5% concentration of 5-fluorouracil cream.

        Tretinoin (0.05% or 0.1%) **cream,** applied once a day, may be used in patients with mild actinic damage. **Dermabrasion** and **chemical peel** are also effective treatments, but these procedures should be performed only by physicians trained and experienced in these techniques.

  2. Giant congenital nevi. Patients with congenital nevi >20 cm in diameter should be referred to a plastic surgeon within the first decade of life for evaluation for removal.

  3. Atypical mole syndrome should be followed up by a dermatologist. Frequent examinations, serial photographs, and early excision of any suspicious lesions are necessary.

C. Malignant lesions should be excised and submitted for pathologic examination.
   1. **Basal cell cancers.** The method of removal depends on lesion size, location, and physician preference. Treatment techniques include **excision, electrodesiccation and curettage, cryosurgery, Mohs' micrographic surgery,** and **radiation.** Basal cell cancers >2 cm and those located on the nose, eye, or ear should be referred for expert surgical removal.
   2. **Squamous cell carcinomas.** The management of these cancers is similar to that of basal cell neoplasms, except that topical fluorouracil may be used for lesions arising within actinic keratoses. Squamous cell lesions arising within scar tissue or in mucous membranes have a high metastatic potential, and patients with such lesions should be referred to a specialist.
   3. **Malignant melanomas.** Patients with suspected melanoma should be referred to an experienced surgeon for excision and follow-up of recurrent disease.

REFERENCES

Edwards L, Ferenczy A, Eron L, et al: Self-administered topical 5% imiquimod cream for external anogenital warts. Arch Dermatol 1998;**134**:25.
Habif TP: *Clinical Dermatology: A Color Guide to Diagnosis and Therapy.* 3rd ed. Mosby; 1995.
MacKie RM: Epidermal skin tumours. In Champion RH, Burton JL, Burns DA, et al (editors): *Textbook of Dermatology.* 6th ed., vol 2. Blackwell; 1998:1651.
MacKie RM: Melanocytic naevi and malignant melanoma. In Champion RH, Burton JL, Burns DA, et al (editors): *Textbook of Dermatology.* 6th ed., vol 2. Blackwell; 1998:1717.
Sams WM Jr, Lynch PJ: *Principles and Practice of Dermatology.* Churchill Livingstone; 1990.
Tyring S, Edwards L, Cherry LK, et al: Safety and efficacy of 0.5% podofilox gel in the treatment of anogenital warts. Arch Dermatol 1998;**134**:33.

---

19   Diarrhea

David P. Losh, MD

I. Definition. Acute diarrhea is a change in bowel movements characterized by increased frequency or looseness of less than 3 weeks' duration.

II. Common diagnoses
   A. Viral diarrhea. Rotaviruses, enteric adenoviruses, and the Norwalk virus are the agents that most often cause diarrhea. Viruses may be responsible for up to 58% of all cases of diarrhea in children. Rotavirus, the most frequently occurring agent, accounts for 16–35% of cases of diarrhea in children and up to 10% of cases in adults. Enteric adenoviruses, which are the second most common viral pathogen, are responsible for up to 13% of cases. The Norwalk virus is a common cause of outbreaks of diarrhea in older children and adults. It accounts for fewer cases in children than do rotaviruses and enteric adenoviruses. Less common viruses associated with diarrheal outbreaks in children include astroviruses and calciviruses.
   B. Bacterial diarrhea. Bacteria account for at least 10% of all cases of diarrhea. The bacterial agents that cause diarrhea are divided into toxigenic, invasive, cytotoxic, and adherent bacteria. Toxigenic strains of *Escherichia coli* are the most common cause of traveler's diarrhea. Other toxigenic bacteria include sources of food poisoning such as *Staphylococcus aureus, Bacillus cereus,* and *Clostridium perfringens.* Enterohemorrhagic *E coli* is a toxin-producing bacterium that is both adherent and cytotoxic. It is considered a major pathogen because of the severity of the primary illness and its sequelae. Of the invasive bacteria, *Campylobacter* spp are the most frequently occurring bacterial agents, followed by *Salmonella* spp, *E coli,* and *Shigella* spp. *Campylobacter jejuni* accounts for 90% of the cases of diarrhea that are caused by *Campylobacter* spp. Of the 2000 serotypes of *Salmonella,* only 10 are responsible for 75% of the *Salmonella*-caused diarrheas. *Shigella sonnei* and *Shigella flexneri* are the most common species of *Shigella* that cause diarrhea. Other bacterial agents, such as *Yersinia enterocolitica* and *Vibrio parahaemolyticus,* are less frequent but may be the predominant organism during some diarrheal outbreaks.

C. **Protozoal diarrhea.** Protozoa are an uncommon cause of diarrhea in the general population but may have a higher prevalence among children in day-care centers, immunocompromised persons, or persons exposed to untreated water. *Giardia lamblia,* the most common cause of parasitic gastroenteritis, is found in 5–10% of the total US population and can be found in 20–30% of children in day-care centers. In the United States, *Entamoeba histolytica* is much less common than *Giardia lamblia. Cryptosporidium* is becoming a more frequently recognized cause of diarrhea, occurring in immunocompromised persons, among children in day-care centers, and in large outbreaks resulting from contaminated water.

D. **Diarrhea related to medication use.** Some drugs, especially laxatives, antibiotics, and excess caffeine or alcohol, can cause diarrhea. In addition, any new medication or recent dosage change may result in diarrhea.

E. **Diarrhea associated with eating nondigestible carbohydrates.** Substances such as lactose may cause diarrhea.

F. **Chronic or recurrent diarrhea.** Patients with conditions such as irritable bowel syndrome, inflammatory bowel diseases, malabsorption syndromes, diabetic enteropathy, dumping syndrome, or villous adenoma may present with diarrhea.

G. **Traveler's diarrhea** is transmitted by organisms that are food- and water-borne (eg, from raw vegetables and unpeeled fruits, meats, seafood, milk, and ice). Such diarrhea is particularly common in visitors to Mexico, Latin America, Africa, the Middle East, and Asia.

H. **Diarrhea associated with acquired immunodeficiency syndrome (AIDS).** Patients with AIDS are at high risk for venereally transmitted enteric infections. Multiple organisms (*Cryptosporidium* spp, *Microsporida, Cyclospora, Neisseria gonorrhoeae, Campylobacter jejuni, Chlamydia trachomatis, Shigella* spp, *Salmonella* spp, *Mycobacterium avium* complex, *Giardia lamblia, Entamoeba histolytica, Blastocystis,* and viruses such as cytomegalovirus, adenovirus, and herpesvirus), in combination with oral-anal sexual practices and the immunocompromised condition, result in diarrhea. An organism is unable to be found in about 15–20% of AIDS patients with diarrhea and the condition is attributed to AIDS enteropathy.

III. **Epidemiology.** Acute diarrhea accounts for up to 5% of visits to physicians' offices and emergency rooms and is particularly prevalent in children.

A. **Viral diarrhea.** Diarrhea caused by viruses is most common during the winter months. Rotaviruses are spread by the fecal-oral route and are prevalent in day-care centers. Most cases occur between the ages of 3 months and 2 years. The Norwalk virus, which is also transmitted by the fecal-oral route, can be found in contaminated water and shellfish. It occurs most often in outbreaks among children over the age of 5 years and in adults. All viruses, including adenoviruses, may be spread by the fecal-oral route, but may also be contracted from contaminated fingers, inanimate surfaces, and possibly even from inhaling contaminated aerosols.

B. **Bacterial diarrhea**

1. **Toxigenic bacteria.** *Staphylococcus aureus* toxins are most frequently found in cooked foods that are later refrigerated, such as custard, pastries, and processed meats. *Clostridium perfringens* most often occurs in improperly refrigerated foods that are heated on steam tables. *Clostridium difficile* is found in low numbers in the stool of about 4% of the population. Antibiotic use may allow for overgrowth of this organism, with the elaboration of toxins that cause diarrhea and pseudomembranous colitis. *Bacillus cereus* usually occurs in unrefrigerated fried rice. Toxin-producing strains of *E coli* are responsible for the majority of cases of traveler's diarrhea and are found in feces, contaminated water, or food.

2. **Cytotoxic and adherent bacteria.** *E coli* O157:H7 is the most common serotype associated with bloody diarrhea caused by enterohemorrhagic *E coli.* It has been associated with contaminated meat such as undercooked ground beef, contaminated water, and unpasteurized milk or fruit juice.

3. **Invasive bacteria.** *Campylobacter jejuni* is often associated with animal sources and is common among travelers and backpackers. *Salmonella* spp most often are found in children or in patients with lack of gastric acidity. Eggs and poultry are common sources, and outbreaks occur in late summer or fall. *Shigella* spp, which most commonly affect young children, are spread by fecal-oral transmission. Diarrhea caused by *Shigella* spp, most frequent in the summer or the fall, is common in day-care settings and low socioeconomic

living situations. *Yersinia enterocolitica* is associated with contaminated meat or dairy products and may cause illness that mimics appendicitis or Crohn's disease. *Vibrio parahaemolyticus* is associated with raw seafood, such as oysters and fish (eg, sushi).

C. **Protozoal diarrhea.** *Giardia lamblia* is endemic to parts of the Rocky Mountains in the United States and frequently affects travelers and backpackers who drink untreated water. It is also found among children in day-care centers and in sexually active homosexual males. *Entamoeba histolytica,* another cause of traveler's diarrhea, is also transmitted by sexual contact and is found in up to 30% of homosexual males. *Cryptosporidium* spp causes diarrhea in individuals who work with animals, among children in day-care centers, and in immunocompromised patients, such as persons with AIDS. In 1993, it affected over 400,000 persons in Milwaukee, Wisconsin, from a contaminated public water source.

D. **Diarrhea related to medication use.** The young and the elderly are at particular risk.

E. **Diarrhea associated with eating nondigestible carbohydrates.** Lactase deficiency is found in the majority of the world's population but is less prevalent in those of northern European descent.

IV. **Pathophysiology**

A. **Viral diarrhea.** Viruses cause diarrhea by increasing fluid secretion by the small bowel. Such diarrhea, called **secretory diarrhea,** is characterized by normal electrolyte concentrations, low stool osmolality, and large stool volume that remains despite fasting. Secretory diarrhea is usually free of blood, pus, and large amounts of mucus.

B. **Bacterial diarrhea**

1. **Toxigenic bacteria** (eg, *Staphylococcus aureus, Clostridium perfringens, Clostridium difficile, Bacillus cereus,* and *E coli*.) cause diarrhea by elaborating either preformed toxins or toxins that have been released after bacterial growth in the intestines. These poisonous substances generally result in secretory diarrhea. *Clostridium perfringens* releases a toxin after producing spores in the intestines.

2. **Cytotoxic and adherent bacteria** (eg, enterohemorrhagic *E coli* O157:H7) adhere to the bowel surface and release a potent cytotoxin in the large bowel that can cause bloody diarrhea and hemolytic-uremic syndrome.

3. **Invasive bacteria** (eg, *Campylobacter* spp, *Salmonella* spp, *Shigella* spp, *Yersinia enterocolitica,* and *Vibrio parahaemolyticus*) invade the cell walls and are more likely to produce **exudative diarrhea.** This type of diarrhea is characterized by the outpouring of plasma, blood, serum proteins, or mucus from inflammatory or ulcerative lesions.

C. **Protozoal diarrhea.** Direct cell damage or interference with absorption by coating of the intestinal wall results in protozoal diarrhea.

D. **Diarrhea related to medication use.** Medications may cause diarrhea by several mechanisms. Saline laxatives, certain antacids, and substances containing magnesium, phosphate, or sulfate cause **osmotic diarrhea** by limiting reabsorption of fluid. Alcohol and caffeine increase bowel motility. Antibiotics cause diarrhea by both direct bowel irritation and alteration of normal flora. Antibiotics such as lincomycin, clindamycin, neomycin, tetracycline, and ampicillin may cause diarrhea in 10–50% of patients. These antibiotics may alter normal bowel flora, possibly resulting in pseudomembranous colitis. However, the most common cause of diarrhea by antibiotics such as erythromycin, ampicillin, and tetracycline is a direct irritant effect with mucosal damage. Neomycin sometimes produces fat malabsorption during the first week of therapy.

E. **Diarrhea associated with eating nondigestible carbohydrates.** Lactase is the enzyme necessary to digest lactose, the sugar found in dairy products. Without enough lactase, the undigested lactose may cause an osmotic diarrhea.

V. **Symptoms**

A. A **self-limited diarrhea** without fever, dehydration, or hematochezia is usually the result of a virus. Symptoms usually last from 1–2 days to 1 week. The diarrhea may be accompanied by nausea, vomiting, headache, low-grade fever, cramping, and malaise. Vomiting is especially common with the Norwalk virus.

B. Diarrhea of **sudden onset** that lasts a short time (ie, 2–12 hours) is generally caused by toxigenic bacteria. The toxins cause a variety of symptoms. Nausea and vomiting are variable findings. Some abdominal cramping frequently occurs with the diarrhea. Fever, severe abdominal pain, headache, prolonged nausea and vomiting, malaise, and myalgia are usually absent. Toxins produced from enterohemorrhagic *E coli* produce frequent loose stools that are often bloody as well as abdominal cramping, vomiting, and low-grade fever. Severe cases may lead to hemolytic-uremic syndrome (bloody diarrhea, thrombocytopenia, hemolytic anemia, and renal failure).

C. Diarrhea of a more **gradual onset** that lasts 1–7 days may result from invasive bacteria. Generalized symptoms of fever, cramping, headache, nausea, malaise, and myalgia are common. Dehydration may be a significant threat. *Yersinia enterocolitica* may produce fever and right lower quadrant pain that are suggestive of acute appendicitis.

D. **Protozoal diarrhea.** Diarrhea with periumbilical or epigastric pain of variable intensity may be caused by *Giardia lamblia. Entamoeba histolytica,* another protozoan, produces acute bloody diarrhea that ranges from mild to severe. *Cryptosporidium* results in a watery diarrhea that may last as long as 1–2 months in healthy patients but may be severe and long-lasting (ie, months to years) in immunocompromised individuals.

E. Hematochezia, tenesmus, or rectal pain as well as watery, large-volume diarrhea or abdominal bloating should suggest the possibility of multiple causative agents in homosexual males or patients with AIDS.

VI. **Signs.** Determination of the cause of diarrhea from physical signs alone is often difficult. In cases of mild toxigenic diarrhea, the physical signs may be normal or limited to mild hyperactivity of the bowel. However, diarrhea caused by invasive bacteria, enterohemorrhagic bacteria, or parasites may yield bloody or mucus-laden stools. In contrast, viral diarrhea and toxigenic bacterial diarrheas are much less likely to contain blood or mucus.

A. Watery, greasy, or mucus-laden stools may indicate the presence of *Giardia lamblia*. In contrast, the stools of patients with diarrhea caused by *Entamoeba histolytica* are more likely to be bloody.

B. In more severe cases of diarrhea, such as enteropathic diarrhea, fever may be present and signs of dehydration are more likely.

   1. **Mild dehydration** (3–5% of body weight or <50 mL/kg fluid deficit). Signs include mild dryness of the mucosal membranes and restlessness. Blood pressure is normal.

   2. **Moderate dehydration** (6–9% of body weight or 50–100 mL/kg fluid deficit). The patient's pulse may be rapid and weak, respirations may be deep and rapid, blood pressure may be low or demonstrate a postural drop only, the eyes may appear sunken, the voice may be hoarse, the skin may retract slowly, and restlessness or irritability may be present.

   3. **Severe dehydration** (10% or more of body weight or >100 mL/kg fluid deficit). The patient's pulse is very rapid and feeble, respirations are deep and rapid, blood pressure is low, the skin retracts very slowly (>2 seconds), the eyes are quite sunken, the voice may be inaudible, and the patient may be drowsy, with cold or sweaty extremities.

   4. In infants, the fontanelles may be sunken in cases of moderate dehydration. This condition is even more pronounced in severe dehydration.

VII. **Laboratory tests.** No testing is necessary if the patient appears to have viral or mild toxigenic bacterial diarrhea, since the disease is mild and self-limited. In patients who are ill or who have had diarrhea for more than several days, the following testing sequence should be performed.

A. **Stool sample**

   1. Obtain stool to check for **fecal leukocytes.** A fleck of stool is placed on a slide and mixed with two drops of methylene blue solution, and a coverslip is applied. Large numbers of white blood cells suggest an inflammatory or invasive diarrhea. Bloody diarrhea without large numbers of leukocytes is suggestive of amebiasis.

   2. In addition, the same stool specimen should be examined for occult blood. The test is also simple and inexpensive, and it is more likely to be positive in cases of diarrhea from invasive bacteria, enterohemorrhagic bacteria, or protozoa than in other forms of diarrhea.

   3. Stool cultures and examination for ova and parasites should be reserved for relatively ill-appearing patients with signs of invasive or persistent diarrhea.

Signs of invasive diarrhea are severe diarrhea, a temperature >38.5 °C (101.3 °F) orally, stools with fecal leukocytes, or stools containing blood. If a child has bloody diarrhea, a search for *E coli* O157:H7 is indicated. Routine stool cultures cannot be justified from a cost-benefit standpoint in all cases of mild diarrhea. (The laboratory should be notified when looking for *Vibrio, Cryptosporidium*, or *E coli* O157:H7. These agents require special testing.)

    a. The best specimen for laboratory analysis is fresh stool. The sample may be refrigerated overnight, if necessary, however. When obtaining a specimen for ameba, three stool specimens should be obtained and a glass collecting rod, not a cotton swab, should be used.

    b. Highly sensitive serologic tests are available for amebic disease. Seroconversion takes 2–4 weeks, however.

  4. Immunologic assays on the stool to detect virus-associated antigens should be ordered when viral diarrhea is a possible diagnosis. Determining the causative agent of a diarrhea epidemic in a day-care center or diagnosing severe diarrhea in an infant are examples of when immunologic tests may be helpful.

B. Complete blood cell count (CBC), electrolytes, blood urea nitrogen (BUN), and creatinine. In most cases, these tests are necessary only if the patient is severely ill or dehydrated.

C. Sigmoidoscopy (without preparatory enemas). This procedure is reserved for cases that persist beyond 1 week with initial negative diagnostic studies. Biopsies and direct rectal smears of the bowel wall mucus are the most sensitive tests for amebiasis. Sigmoidoscopy may yield generalized inflammation with invasive bacteria, discrete yellow plaques in *Clostridium difficile* pseudomembranous colitis, or melanosis coli in chronic laxative abusers.

D. When the above evaluation fails to reveal a cause and more extensive testing is indicated, other tests, including determination of fecal fat content, alkalinization of the stool to detect phenolphthalein laxatives, lactose tolerance tests, D-xylose tests, immunoglobulin A (IgA) antibodies for celiac sprue, and tests for pancreatic insufficiency, are available. They should be ordered on an individual basis, based on the patient's history and physical findings.

VIII. Treatment

A. Rotavirus vaccination. Rotavirus vaccination was removed from the market on October 15, 1999. The removal was based on scientific data that indicated an association between the rotavirus vaccination and intussusception among some infants during the first 2 weeks following vaccination. The data did not indicate an ongoing risk to children who were given the vaccination in the past. The Advisory Committee on Immunization Practices of the Centers for Disease Control and Prevention (CDC) no longer recommends the vaccination as a part of the childhood immunization schedule in the United States. Educational materials for parents about childhood diarrhea is available on the CDC Web site (see references).

B. Maintenance of hydration and rehydration

  1. Oral hydration. Mild diarrhea requires only maintenance of hydration through oral solutions containing glucose. Glucose aids in the transport of water and sodium. Commercially available oral electrolyte solutions are preferable to clear fluids such as nondiet soft drinks, apple juice, lemonade, Kool-Aid, etc. While these clear liquids may be diluted and used in adults with mild diarrhea, they should be avoided in infants and young children with acute diarrhea because these drinks may have a very high carbohydrate content, a high osmolality, and a very low electrolyte content. The ideal level of glucose in an oral rehydration solution (ORS) is approximately 2%. There is some evidence that solutions containing rice-syrup solids may decrease stool output in infants and promote more absorption and retention of fluid and electrolytes than solutions containing glucose alone. ORSs recommended by the United Nations Children's Fund and the World Health Organization may also be used. This solution is available in packets containing 20 g of glucose and 90 meq of sodium per liter along with potassium and bicarbonate or trisodium citrate. Commercially available ORSs have between 45 and 75 meq of sodium per liter. In a child with mild to moderate dehydration, 60–80 mL/kg of an ORS should be given over 4–6 hours. The additional fluid required to meet all replacement needs should be administered over the next 18–20 hours. If vomiting is present, 5 mL of an ORS should be given every 2–5 minutes. Breast-feeding may be continued during oral rehydration therapy.

2. **Parenteral rehydration.** If a child or elderly adult is severely dehydrated, parenteral rehydration will be required in the hospital. Initial rehydration is usually accomplished within 3–4 hours of admission. Once the patient is able to take fluids, further rehydration is accomplished with oral fluids. In the moderately ill adult patient who does not require hospitalization, intravenous fluids may be given in the ambulatory setting. Adults may be given 1–2 L over a period of 1–2 hours. Solutions of 5% dextrose and Ringer's lactate, 5% dextrose and 0.9 N saline, and 5% dextrose and 0.45 N saline are all acceptable.

C. **Symptomatic treatment.** Preparations that reduce diarrhea and enhance patient comfort may be considered in selected patients with mild viral or toxigenic diarrhea. Antimotility drugs should not be used in patients with fever or bloody stools.

1. **Solutions containing kaolin and pectin** (eg, Kaopectate or Donnagel). These agents may add some bulk to the stool, but great care must be used with formulations containing additional ingredients such as atropine. Such formulations are best avoided in young children.

2. **Bismuth subsalicylate** (eg, Pepto-Bismol). This product may be used in doses of 2–3 tbsp every 3 hours. It may reduce the duration of diarrhea in some cases and is the preferred agent when vomiting is present. In children, the dose is 20 mg (1.14 mL)/kg, five times a day for up to 5 days. Bismuth subsalicylate is not recommended in immunocompromised patients.

3. **Opiates.** These drugs may afford some temporary relief in cases of mild, crampy diarrhea in the mildly ill, afebrile adult patient. They inhibit intestinal motility and allow for increased invasion of the organisms or absorption of toxin. Opiates should *not* be used in cases of invasive, infectious diarrhea, and they should be avoided in children. Typical doses are diphenoxylate (eg, Lomotil), 2.5–5 mg orally usually four times daily, up to 20 mg/day; or loperamide (eg, Imodium), 4 mg orally initially, followed by 2 mg after each loose stool, up to 16 mg/day. Loperamide is the preferred agent due to its safety and efficacy.

4. **Patient bed rest** will also help slow cramping and excess bowel motility.

D. **Dietary therapy.** Children should be fed continuously during a diarrheal illness with their usual diet. "Bowel rest" and clear fluids may actually prolong the course of diarrhea. A mixed diet, such as one with wheat noodles or other complex carbohydrate food, may reduce the severity and duration of diarrhea. Breast-feeding may be continued during diarrheal illness.

E. **Antibiotic therapy.** Patients with infectious bacterial diarrheas who either have relatively mild symptoms or have become asymptomatic usually *do not* require antibiotic therapy.

Antibiotics should be prescribed when the patient exhibits toxicity or has persistent diarrhea. It is best to first attempt to identify the specific diarrhea-causing organism; however, empiric antibiotic therapy may be considered when the patient has fever along with leukocytes or blood in the stool or has a moderate to severe case of traveler's diarrhea. Empiric treatment consists of a quinolone, either norfloxacin (400 mg), ciprofloxacin (500 mg), or ofloxacin (300 mg), orally twice a day for 3–5 days. Empiric treatment of presumed giardiasis may also be considered, since at least half of the stools of patients with *Giardia* test negative for the parasite. Recommended antibiotic regimens used to combat specific organisms are listed below.

1. ***Campylobacter.*** Erythromycin, 500 mg orally four times a day for 5–7 days.

2. ***Salmonella* spp.** Antibiotics may result in a high incidence of carrier states. If severe, these cases usually require hospitalization and treatment with ampicillin, trimethoprim-sulfamethoxazole, or chloramphenicol. If outpatient therapy is used, the dose of trimethoprim-sulfamethoxazole, double strength, is one tablet orally twice a day for 2 weeks.

3. ***Shigella* spp.** Trimethoprim-sulfamethoxazole, double strength (160 and 800 mg, respectively), one tablet orally twice a day for 3–5 days. If the infection is acquired during travel, a quinolone is indicated due to high rates of resistance to trimethoprim-sulfamethoxazole.

4. ***Yersinia enterocolitica.*** Diarrhea caused by this organism is usually self-limited and does not require antibiotics. If the patient shows signs of septicemia,

however, he or she will require hospitalization and intravenous amino-glycosides, intravenous trimethoprim-sulfamethoxazole, or a third-generation cephalosporin.

5. **Clostridium difficile** (pseudomembranous colitis). Metronidazole, 1–2 g/day orally in three or four divided doses for 7–14 days. A more expensive alternative is oral vancomycin, 125–500 mg orally every 6 hours for 7–14 days.

6. **Enterohemorrhagic E coli.** The use of antibiotics is controversial and may predispose the patient to hemolytic-uremic syndrome. Antibiotic therapy is not currently recommended for patients with E coli O157:H7. Supportive care is the mainstay of therapy.

7. **Giardia.** Metronidazole, 250 mg orally three times a day for 7–10 days (pediatric dose: 15 mg/kg/day, divided into three doses for 7–10 days). An alternative is quinacrine hydrochloride; however, it is no longer available in the United States. The only effective liquid oral medication is furazolidone, in a dose of 100 mg orally four times a day (pediatric dose: 2 mg/kg orally three times daily), for 7–10 days.

8. **Entamoeba.** Metronidazole, 750 mg orally three times a day for 10 days for the trophozoites, and iodoquinol, 650 mg orally three times a day for 20 days, or paromomycin, 500 mg orally three times a day for 7 days, for cysts (pediatric dose: metronidazole, 35–50 mg/kg/day divided into three doses for 20 days).

9. **Cryptosporidium.** Currently, there is no effective antibiotic for cryptosporidiosis.

F. **Treatment of particular kinds of diarrhea**

1. **Traveler's diarrhea** should first be treated with solutions of fluids that contain sugars. **Diphenoxylate** or **loperamide** may provide some symptomatic relief in mild cases without fever or in those with stools without blood or mucus. (**Bismuth subsalicylate,** two tablets orally four times a day, may be helpful in treating the diarrhea.) For most travelers, treatment at the onset of diarrhea is preferable to prophylaxis. Since E coli is the most common cause of traveler's diarrhea, **trimethoprim-sulfamethoxazole,** one double-strength tablet orally twice daily for 3–5 days, or **doxycycline,** 100 mg orally twice daily for 3–5 days, may be used. Alternatives are norfloxacin, 400 mg orally every 12 hours for 5 days, or **ciprofloxacin,** 500 mg orally every 12 hours for 5 days. Antibiotics should especially be considered if the diarrhea is accompanied by fever, vomiting, or bloody stools. If diarrhea persists, treatment should be guided either by stool cultures and examination for ova and parasites or by sigmoidoscopy for mucus examination and biopsies.

2. **Diarrhea caused by lactose intolerance** may be treated by avoiding excess dairy products. Commercially prepared low-lactose milk, cheese, ice cream, and yogurt are available. One or two 250-mg **lactase** capsules may be taken orally with dairy products. Lactase (eg, Lactaid) may also be added to milk, five to 15 drops per quart.

3. **Diarrhea in the immunocompromised patient.** Immunocompromised patients with diarrhea should have a limited evaluation followed by specific or symptomatic treatment. Recommended testing includes examination for routine cultures, parasitology, Clostridium difficile toxin, and blood cultures for bacteria and mycobacteria. If a specific pathogen is identified, it may be treated; otherwise, empiric quinolone therapy for 10 days may be considered. Persistent symptoms or evidence of colitis may prompt endoscopy with biopsy and cultures for additional organisms.

REFERENCES

Dick L: Travel medicine: Helping patients prepare for trips abroad. Am Fam Physician 1998; **58**:383.

DuPont HL, Practice Parameters Committee of the American College of Gastroenterology: Am J Gastroenterol 1997;**92**:1962.

Farthing MJ: Giardiasis. Gastroenterol Clin North Am 1996;**25**:493.

Hogan DE: The emergency department approach to diarrhea. Emerg Med Clin North Am 1996; **14**:673.

Koutkia P, Mylonakis E: Enterohemorrhagic Escherichia coli O157:H7—An emerging pathogen. Am Fam Physician 1997;**56**:853.

Kroser JA, Metz DC: Evaluation of the adult patient with diarrhea. Prim Care 1996;**23**:629.

Lew EA, Poles MA, Dieterich DT: Diarrheal diseases associated with HIV infection. Gastroenterol Clin North Am 1997;**26**:259.

Lifschitz CH: Treatment of acute diarrhea in children. Curr Opin Pediatr 1997;**9**:498.

National Immunization Program, Centers for Disease Control and Prevention: Rotavirus. http://www.cdc.gov/nip/news/rota-news.htm

Provisional Committee on Quality Improvement, Subcommittee on Acute Gastroenteritis: Practice parameter: The management of acute gastroenteritis in young children. Pediatrics 1996;**97**:424.

20   Dizziness

Diane J. Madlon-Kay, MD

I. **Definition.** *Dizziness* is an imprecise term commonly used by patients to describe symptoms such as faintness, giddiness, lightheadedness, or unsteadiness.

II. **Common diagnoses.** The various diagnoses of dizziness can be divided into three main categories.

   A. **Peripheral vestibular disorders,** which account for up to 36% of cases in university dizziness clinics, include vestibular neuronitis, benign positional vertigo, Meniere's disease, acoustic neuroma, and otitis media.

   B. **Systemic diseases,** such as cardiac problems, drugs, metabolic abnormalities, anemia, infection, and psychogenic causes, may result in dizziness. Twenty percent to 30% of all cases of dizziness are believed to be psychogenic.

   C. **Central nervous system diseases,** such as stroke, transient ischemic attack, or multiple sclerosis, are responsible for dizziness in 5% of patients.

III. **Epidemiology.** Approximately 1% of patient visits per year in primary care are for dizziness. Dizziness rarely results in hospitalization or referral.

   A. The frequency of dizziness as a presenting complaint rises steadily with age. Although children rarely have symptoms of dizziness, this condition is the most common presenting complaint of ambulatory patients aged 75 years and older.

   B. Dizziness is more common in women than in men in all age categories.

IV. **Pathophysiology.** In up to 19% of cases, a definitive cause of dizziness cannot be found. The pathophysiology of dizziness is described below.

   A. **Peripheral vestibular disorders.** Some patients who experience dizziness have a disorder at some point along the course of the vestibular nerve other than at its origin in the brain stem. Most often, the problem is at the termination of the nerve in the inner ear, known as the labyrinth.

   B. **Systemic diseases.** Disorders in almost any organ system can cause dizziness. Spatial orientation depends on the complex interaction of adequate sensation, central integration, and the proper motor response.

   C. **Central nervous system diseases.** Any disease that disrupts the pathway between the vestibular apparatus and the brain may result in dizziness. Normally, impulses from this apparatus proceed through the eighth cranial nerve to the vestibular nuclei of the brain stem. From the brain stem, they are transmitted to the cerebellum and the cerebral cortex.

V. **Symptoms**

   A. Complaints of **vertigo** (ie, a sensation of turning or spinning) accompanied by **nausea, vomiting, diaphoresis,** and **difficulty with balance** suggest peripheral vestibular disorders. Patients may also have **auditory symptoms** such as decreased hearing, tinnitus, or ear pain. Symptoms of particular disorders are described below.

      1. **Vestibular neuronitis or acute labyrinthitis.** After an acute onset of severe vertigo lasting several days, gradual improvement follows for several weeks. Symptoms frequently follow a viral illness.

      2. **Benign positional vertigo.** Instances of vertigo related to position are extremely brief, can be associated with nausea, and often will wake the patient from sleep when turning over in bed. Although the disorder is generally self-limited, its course is variable.

      3. **Meniere's disease.** Patients with this disease have discrete attacks of vertigo of abrupt onset. The attacks last for several hours, not days, and are often accompanied by nausea and vomiting. The interval between attacks may be

weeks to months. Between attacks, the patient is asymptomatic. Fluctuating hearing loss, typically accompanied by tinnitus and a feeling of pressure in the ear, is usually present during attacks. Irreversible hearing loss and chronic tinnitus develop in the affected ear over time.

    4. Acoustic neuroma. Few patients have vertigo initially. Typically, the earliest symptoms are unilateral tinnitus and hearing loss. Symptoms are slowly progressive, and continued growth of the tumor is associated with facial weakness and ataxia.

  B. Patients with central nervous system diseases also have **vertigo.** The vertigo is almost always accompanied by other central nervous symptoms, such as facial numbness, hemiparesis, or diplopia.

  C. Patients with systemic diseases may describe **lightheadedness, feeling "about to pass out,"** or various vague feelings in the head. The physician should ask questions to elicit symptoms of specific causes such as heart disease, anemia, hyperventilation, medications, and psychiatric problems.

VI. Signs

  A. Dysarthia, facial numbness, hemiparesis, or diplopia may be found in central nervous system diseases.

  B. The Dix-Hallpike (Nylen-Barany) maneuver can be helpful in distinguishing peripheral from central vestibulopathy. Have the patient sit on the edge of the examining table and lie down suddenly, with the head hanging 45 degrees backward and turned 45 degrees to one side. Then repeat the test twice, once with the head turned to the other side and once with the head in the middle position. The patient's eyes should be kept open to observe (1) the development of vertigo and (2) the time of onset, duration, and direction of nystagmus. This maneuver will reveal a central or peripheral pattern of vertigo, as shown in Table 20–1.

  C. Inspection of the eardrum may reveal otitis media or serous otitis.

  D. Orthostatic blood pressure determinations are helpful when the history suggests dizziness due to hypovolemia from blood loss or dehydration. A drop in systolic blood pressure of as much as 20 mm Hg, a decline in diastolic pressure of up to 10 mm Hg, and a rise in pulse rate of up to 20 beats per minute can be normal findings with standing. If standing causes a greater blood pressure drop or pulse rise and reproduces the patient's symptoms, some form of hypovolemia is the most likely cause.

  E. If the history suggests a psychological cause, have the patient hyperventilate. Ask the patient to blow vigorously for 3 minutes on a paper towel held 6 inches from the mouth. This action may cause some circumoral and digital numbness, as well as reproduce the patient's dizziness.

VII. Laboratory tests

  A. Few patients with suspected peripheral vestibular disorders require laboratory testing. Patients whose symptoms are progressive or recurrent should have an **audiologic evaluation** that includes a pure tone audiogram, speech discrimination testing, and tympanometry. Such patients should also undergo vestibular examination by **electronystagmography.**

    Laboratory testing of patients whose dizziness may be caused by systemic diseases must be guided by history and physical examination. Most "screening" laboratory tests, such as complete blood cell counts and electrolyte determinations, are rarely helpful.

  B. **Brain stem evoked response (BSER)** testing is a useful screening in patients with suspected central causes of dizziness. A normal BSER safely excludes an acoustic neuroma. If the BSER is abnormal, an imaging procedure, such as magnetic resonance imaging, the most informative radiographic study, is indicated.

TABLE 20–1. DISTINGUISHING PERIPHERAL FROM CENTRAL VERTIGO WITH POSITION TESTING

	Peripheral	Central
Latency (time to onset of vertigo or nystagmus)	3–10 s	None; begins immediately
Fatigability (lessening signs and symptoms with repetition)	Yes	No
Nystagmus direction	Fixed	Changing
Intensity of signs and symptoms	Severe	Mild

VIII. Treatment

  A. Peripheral vestibular disorders. The symptoms of vertigo are frightening to patients. The physician must be supportive and reassuring, since most causes of vertigo are not a serious health threat.

   1. Initial treatment of acutely vertiginous patients usually involves having them lie still in a darkened room and avoid head movement. It is important to have patients mobilized as soon as the most severe nausea and vertigo subside, to avoid protracted disability.

   2. Drug therapy may provide symptomatic relief.

    a. Antihistamines, the most commonly prescribed drugs for vertigo, suppress the vestibular end organ receptors and inhibit activation of vagal responses. Patients should take the medication for a few weeks and then try discontinuing the drug. The major side effects are dry mouth and sedation. Commonly recommended drugs are meclizine, 25 mg orally every 4–6 hours, and diphenhydramine, 50 mg orally every 4–6 hours.

    b. Antiemetics can be tried when nausea and vomiting are pronounced. These agents suppress central vestibular pathways, which activate a vagal response. Their major side effect is sedation. Commonly recommended antiemetic drugs are prochlorperazine, 5–10 mg orally every 6 hours *or* 25-mg suppository by rectum twice daily, and trimethobenzamide, 250 mg orally every 6 hours *or* 200-mg suppository by rectum every 6 hours. Acute dystonic reactions may occur occasionally with prochlorperazine.

   3. Vestibular exercises may be helpful, especially in cases of prolonged benign positional vertigo.

    a. Instruct the patient to reproduce the vertigo by assuming the appropriate ear down, supine position and hold that position until the vertigo subsides. The vertigo usually returns upon resumption of sitting. Have the patient repeat these maneuvers, usually five times, until the vertigo no longer recurs.

    b. Performing this exercise at least four times a day leads to longer symptom-free intervals and a reduction in the duration of symptoms.

   4. The **canalith repositioning maneuver** eliminates symptoms of benign positional vertigo in up to 80% of patients after one treatment.

   5. Surgery may be indicated if other medical therapies fail to adequately relieve severe vertigo. Surgical procedures include sectioning of the vestibular nerve, repair of an inner ear fistula, labyrinthectomy, or placement of a lymphatic shunt. Unilateral deafness may result.

  B. Systemic diseases causing dizziness require treatment that is specific to the particular cause.

  C. Central nervous system diseases. Symptomatic treatment of vertigo as described above may be helpful. Treatment of the underlying central nervous system condition is crucial.

REFERENCES

Hotson JR, Baloh RW: Acute vestibular syndrome. N Engl J Med 1998;**339:**680.
Kroenke K: Dizziness: A focused 5-minute workup. Consultant 1996;**36:**1715.
Lambert PR: Evaluation of the dizzy patient. Comp Ther 1997;**23:**719.
Vernick DM: Benign paroxysmal positional vertigo: Diagnostic and therapeutic maneuvers. Hosp Med 1996;**32:**37.

21   Dysmenorrhea

Rhonda Agnes Sparks, MD, & Denise LeBlanc-Ziegler, MD

  I. Definition. Dysmenorrhea is pain with menstruation, usually cramping in nature, involving the lower abdomen and, in some women, the lower back and inner thighs. The distinction must be made between **primary dysmenorrhea,** in which no identifiable pelvic pathology is present, and **secondary dysmenorrhea** (pain secondary to organic pelvic pathology).

II. Common diagnoses
A. Primary dysmenorrhea
B. Secondary dysmenorrhea. Underlying causes include:
1. **Endometriosis.**
2. **Leiomyomas (fibroids).**
3. **Adenomyosis.**
4. **Ovarian cysts** (see Chapter 55).
5. **Pelvic inflammatory disease (PID)** (see Chapter 55).
6. **Intrauterine devices (IUDs).**
7. **Miscellaneous causes.** Congenital abnormalities (bicornuate or septate uterus), cervical stenosis, imperforate hymen, uterine polyps, or uterine adhesions may cause secondary dysmenorrhea.

III. Epidemiology
A. Primary dysmenorrhea is the most commonly reported gynecologic symptom in the United States, affecting 40–70% of women of childbearing age. Ten percent to 15% of women report symptoms severe enough to limit daily activities (usually days 1–3 of menses). The reported incidence of dysmenorrhea in parous women is one third that in nulliparous women and is much more likely in adolescents. Cigarette smoking has been associated with an increased duration of dysmenorrhea with each cycle. Other risk factors for dysmenorrhea include obesity and frequent alcohol consumption. Studies have shown decreased prevalence and improvement of dysmenorrhea symptoms with exercise.
B. The prevalence of **secondary dysmenorrhea** varies depending on the prevalence of the underlying pelvic pathology, and increases with age.
1. **Endometriosis** occurs in 3–10% of women of reproductive age. Twenty-five percent to 35% of women with infertility have endometriosis.
2. **Leiomyomas (fibroids)** develop in 20% of women by age 40, the majority being asymptomatic. Black women have an increased incidence of uterine fibroids.
3. **Adenomyosis** is observed most frequently in women in the fifth and sixth decades. Fifteen percent of women with adenomyosis have associated endometriosis.
4. **Ovarian cysts** (see Chapter 55).
5. **PID** (see Chapter 55).

IV. Pathophysiology
A. Primary dysmenorrhea
1. **Prostaglandin production** is two to seven times greater in women with dysmenorrhea than in women who do not report menstrual pain. The increased production of prostaglandin $F_{2\alpha}$ ($PGF_{2\alpha}$) and prostaglandin E_2 (PGE_2) or an inadequate $PGF_{2\alpha}$:PGE_2 ratio increases uterine resting tone, myometrial contractile pressure, frequency of uterine contractions, and dysrhythmic uterine contractions. These abnormalities lead to vasoconstriction, ischemia, and hypoxia of the uterus, all of which result in pain. In addition, prostaglandins hypersensitize pain fibers to bradykinin and other physical stimuli.

   Endometrial concentrations of PGE_2 and $PGF_{2\alpha}$ are relatively low in the proliferative phase but rise throughout the secretory phase, reaching their highest levels during menstruation. This suggests that sex steroids, especially progesterone, play a role in producing the concentration of prostaglandins required for dysmenorrhea to occur. This is also consistent with the occurrence of dysmenorrhea almost exclusively in ovulatory cycles.
2. **Other possible factors** contributing to primary dysmenorrhea have been implicated in the literature. These include leukotrienes, platelet activating factor, and vasopressin.
3. **Psychosocial factors** involving the patient and/or her family may modulate the pain of primary dysmenorrhea. These factors are no more unique to the pain from dysmenorrhea than to pain from any other source.

B. Secondary dysmenorrhea
1. **Endometriosis.** Endometrial implants that produce prostaglandins can be found on the ovaries, uterosacral ligaments, cul-de-sac, or elsewhere in the peritoneum.
2. **Leiomyomas** (fibroids) are benign uterine tumors composed mainly of smooth muscle with some connective tissue component. Fibroids are often associated with menometrorrhagia and thus excess prostaglandin production.

      3. Adenomyosis is the extension of endometrial glands and stroma into the myometrium. The endometrial tissue does not appear to be hormonally responsive, and the exact mechanism of this type of dysmenorrhea is unknown.

      4. IUDs can cause or contribute to dysmenorrhea, by unknown mechanisms.

V. Symptoms

  A. Primary dysmenorrhea is associated with ovulation and therefore usually presents 6–12 months after menarche when ovulation is established. Pain usually begins just prior to or 1–2 hours after menses and usually lasts <72 hours. Associated symptoms may include nausea and vomiting, fatigue, diarrhea, low back pain, inner or anterior thigh pain, and headache. Sixty percent of women with migraines have an increased incidence of headaches during menses.

  B. The pain of **secondary dysmenorrhea** may be atypical or chronic and may vary in description and temporal relation to menses.

    1. Endometriosis is usually a deep aching pain that begins several days prior to menses, may last throughout the cycle, and may be associated with dyspareunia, infertility, or menorrhagia.

    2. Leiomyomas. The majority of fibroids are asymptomatic. Women may experience pelvic pressure, bloating, heaviness of the lower abdomen, menorrhagia, or metrorrhagia, depending on the location and size of the tumor.

    3. Adenomyosis is usually associated with severe dysmenorrhea and menorrhagia. Thirty percent to 40% of patients are asymptomatic.

    4. IUDs. Pain associated with an IUD occurs after IUD placement.

VI. Signs

  A. Primary dysmenorrhea. Most commonly, the physical examination will be normal. Tenderness on uterine palpation may be present.

  B. Secondary dysmenorrhea

    1. Endometriosis is classically associated with palpable nodules in the posterior cul-de-sac and a tender fixed uterus on bimanual examination, but may be present in a patient with a normal exam.

    2. Leiomyomata are suspected if the uterus is irregularly enlarged or nodular.

    3. Adenomyosis is associated with a symmetrically enlarged uterus.

    4. Ovarian cysts (see Chapter 55).

    5. PID (see Chapter 55).

VII. Laboratory tests

  A. Primary dysmenorrhea. With a suggestive history and a normal physical examination, no laboratory evaluation is indicated.

  B. Secondary dysmenorrhea workup may include:

    1. Gonococcal and chlamydia cultures if signs or symptoms suggest PID or the patient is at risk for sexually transmitted diseases.

    2. Pelvic ultrasound to diagnose fibroids, ovarian cysts, or mass lesions found on examination.

    3. Hysterosalpingography if a uterine anomaly is suspected.

    4. Laparoscopy for diagnosing endometriosis (visualize endometrial implants) and if other tests do not reveal the cause of secondary dysmenorrhea.

VIII. Treatment (Figure 21–1)

  A. Prostaglandin synthetase inhibitors (ie, NSAIDs) (Table 21–1). Most nonsteroidal anti-inflammatory drugs (NSAIDs) are effective in relieving primary dysmenorrhea in 70–90% of cases. NSAIDs inhibit prostaglandin production without affecting endometrial development, can be started with the onset of pain associated with menses, and are rarely needed for >72 hours.

    If a patient is unresponsive to NSAIDs after 3 months and no new history or physical findings suggest secondary dysmenorrhea, another NSAID should be tried. If the patient remains unresponsive to NSAIDs, a workup for underlying gynecologic pathology is warranted (Figure 21–1).

    Contraindications to NSAIDs include gastrointestinal ulcers and hypersensitivity. Side effects are mild and well tolerated and occur in <5% of patients (Table 21–2).

  B. Oral contraceptives (OCPs) suppress both menstrual fluid volume and prostaglandin release, but not synthesis. This is achieved by causing endometrial hypoplasia. OCPs are effective in 60–80% of patients and are an alternative to NSAIDs or an additional therapeutic option in patients desiring contraception. If OCPs and NSAIDs in combination do not provide relief after 3–6 months, reevaluation and workup for underlying gynecologic pathology should be done (Figure 21–1).

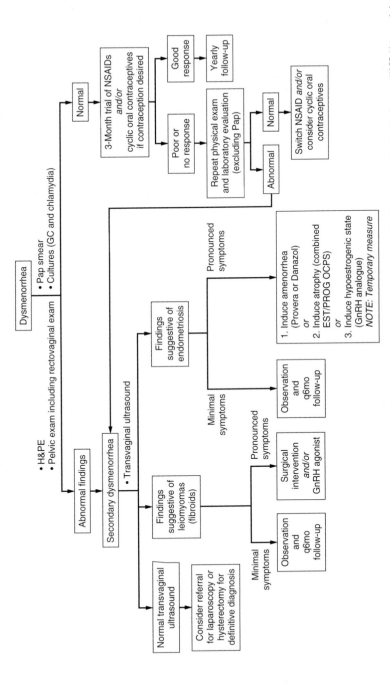

FIGURE 21-1. Evaluation and treatment of dysmenorrhea. EST/PROG OCPs, Estrogen/progestin oral contraceptives; GC, gonococcal culture; GnRH, gonadotropin-releasing hormone; H&PE, history and physical examination; NSAIDs, nonsteroidal anti-inflammatory drugs.

TABLE 21–1. NONSTEROIDAL ANTI-INFLAMMATORY DRUGS MOST COMMONLY USED IN THE TREATMENT OF PRIMARY DYSMENORRHEA

Drug[1] (mg)	Initial Dose (mg)	Subsequent Dosage (mg)
Propionic acids		
Ibuprofen (Motrin, Advil)	400	400–600 qid
Ketoprofen (Orudis)	50	50 tid
Naproxen sodium (Anaprox)	550	275 q6h
Naproxen (Naprosyn)	500	250–375 bid
Acetic acids		
Sulindac (Clinoril)	200	200 bid
Diclofenac (Cataflam)	50	50 tid
Etodolac (Lodine)	400	300–400 bid

[1] Consult full prescribing information before administering any of these drugs.

TABLE 21–2. SIDE EFFECTS OF PROSTAGLANDIN SYNTHETASE INHIBITORS

Gastrointestinal symptoms	Indigestion, heartburn, nausea, abdominal pain, constipation, vomiting, diarrhea, melena
Central nervous system symptoms	Headache, dizziness, vertigo, visual disturbances, hearing disturbances, irritability, depression, drowsiness, sleepiness
Other symptoms	Allergic reaction, skin rash, edema, bronchospasm, hematologic abnormalities, eye effects, fluid retention, liver and kidney effects

    C. Calcium antagonists are being investigated as possible therapeutic agents for dysmenorrhea because of their potent uterine-relaxing effects; however, their use is still experimental.

    D. Transdermal nitroglycerin is also under investigation as a possible treatment modality for primary dysmenorrhea.

    E. Secondary dysmenorrhea treatment options

        1. Endometriosis can be treated with OCPs, which induce endometrial atrophy and decrease symptoms. Danazol and progestin-only contraceptives can improve symptoms by inducing amenorrhea. Gonadotropin-reducing hormone (GnRH) agonists are sometimes used as a temporary measure or preoperatively to reduce endometrial implant size.

REFERENCES

Hacker NF, Moore JG: *Essentials of Obstetrics and Gynecology.* 3rd ed. Saunders; 1998.
Harlow SD, Park M: A longitudinal study of risk factors for the occurrence, duration and severity of menstrual cramps in a cohort of college women. Br J Obstet Gynecol 1996;**103:**1134.
Osathanondh R: Dysmenorrhea. In: Bardin WC, ed. *Current Therapy in Endocrinology and Metabolism.* 5th ed. Saunders; 1997.
Rakel RE: *Saunders Manual of Medical Practice.* Saunders; 1996.
Speroff L, Glass RH, Kase NG: *Clinical Gynecologic Endocrinology and Infertility.* 5th ed. Williams & Wilkins; 1994.

---

22   Dyspepsia

Alan M. Adelman, MD, MS

  I. Definition. Dyspepsia is characterized by epigastric discomfort or pain and can be associated with epigastric heaviness or fullness, belching or regurgitation, bloating, early satiety, heartburn, food intolerance, nausea, or vomiting. Lower bowel function is usually not affected.

II. Common diagnoses
  A. Nonulcer dyspepsia (NUD). This disorder represents 30–50% of patients with dyspepsia.
  B. Peptic ulcer disease (PUD), which includes gastric and duodenal ulcers, gastritis, and duodenitis (20–30% of patients with dyspepsia). Together, NUD and PUD probably account for 50–80% of all cases of dyspepsia.
  C. Gastroesophageal reflux disease (GERD), accounting for 5–10% of patients with dyspepsia.
  D. Gastric or pancreatic cancer, afflicting fewer than 1% of patients with dyspepsia.
  E. Cholecystitis or **cholelithiasis** (see Chapter 1) and **irritable bowel syndrome** (see Chapter 1).
  F. Other causes of dyspepsia, such as Zollinger-Ellison syndrome, chronic pancreatitis, abdominal angina, and coronary artery disease, are uncommon.
III. Epidemiology. Dyspepsia is a common complaint, occurring in 20–30% of the general population. It accounts for approximately 5–10% of all visits to general practitioners in England. The prevalence is greatest in patients 18–45 years of age and then declines with increasing age. Males and females are equally likely to complain of dyspepsia. Medications may be a risk factor. Examples of drugs that can cause upper abdominal discomfort include aspirin, nonsteroidal anti-inflammatory drugs (NSAIDs), erythromycin, tetracycline, alcohol, and potassium supplements.
  The epidemiology of some of the common diagnoses associated with dyspepsia is described below.
  A. NUD. The incidence of NUD is age dependent; approximately 70% of patients under age 40 have NUD, as opposed to only 40% of those over age 60.
  B. PUD. PUD of the duodenum affects males twice as frequently as females. Peak incidence is between ages 45 and 64 in males and at age 55 in females. Gastric ulcer occurs much less frequently than duodenal ulcer and increases in incidence with advancing age.
  C. Gastric or pancreatic cancer. The incidence of gastric cancer and pancreatic cancer increases with advancing age.
  D. Impaired gastric emptying is most often associated with other medical problems, such as GERD, postoperative paralytic ileus, vagotomy, antrectomy, pregnancy, postoperative opiate analgesia, and medical conditions including uremia, diabetes mellitus, and scleroderma. The cause may also be idiopathic.
IV. Pathophysiology
  A. NUD. The exact cause of NUD is unknown. Excess gastric acid, disordered motility of the upper gastrointestinal (GI) tract, functional disturbances of GI peptide hormones, stress and psychosocial factors, environmental factors, diet, and genetic factors have all been implicated. No link between NUD and *Helicobacter pylori* has been established.
  B. PUD. There is a clear link between *H pylori* and PUD. Normally, there is a balance between acid/peptic activity and mucosal defense. When acid is overproduced in the presence of pepsin and pepsinogen or when mucosal defense is impaired, PUD occurs. Impaired mucosal defense is the most common factor in the occurrence of PUD. NSAIDs and *H pylori* can impair mucosal defense.
  C. GERD. Incompetence of the lower esophageal sphincter (LES) is the single most important factor. Acid and bile reflux may result in GERD, and impaired gastric emptying may also play a role.
  D. Gastric or pancreatic cancer. Toxins (eg, nitrosamines or polycyclic hydrocarbons), genetic factors, pernicious anemia, and atrophic gastritis have been associated with gastric cancer. The cause of pancreatic cancer is unknown, although chemical carcinogens and cigarette smoke are suspected.
  E. Gastroparesis. There are three main mechanisms for delayed gastric emptying: (1) mechanical obstruction, such as PUD or tumor; (2) disorders of gastric motility, such as scleroderma; and (3) autonomic neuropathy, as in diabetes. GI hormones may also play a role.
V. Symptoms. In general, symptoms seem to be of little help in making a specific diagnosis in a patient with dyspepsia.
  A. In addition to age greater than 45 years, **historical features** more often associated with a **specific lesion** include constant, daily pain; significant weight loss (>10–15 lb); persistent vomiting; past history of PUD; previous gastric surgery;

male gender; cigarette smoking, which is associated with both gastric and duodenal ulcers; and heartburn and regurgitation, which are reliable symptoms of reflux, with positive predictive values of 59% and 66%, respectively.

B. Symptoms poorly discriminating between specific disease and NUD are
listed below.

1. **Relief with antacids or food.** Relief of pain with food or antacids is more
   common in patients with NUD than in those with duodenal ulcer.
2. **Nocturnal pain.** There is no difference between patients with organic disease and those with functional disease in the occurrence of nocturnal pain
   severe enough to awaken the patient.
3. **Food intolerance.** Intolerance to specific types of food cannot distinguish
   PUD from other causes of dyspepsia.
4. **Duration of pain.** In patients under age 50, pain of more than 1 year's duration predicts some abnormality on upper GI series.
5. **Pain** that occurs within 1 hour of eating.
6. **Anorexia.**

C. Depending on the predominant symptoms, **NUD** may be divided into the following **clinical syndromes.** Unfortunately, these syndromes do not predict response
to therapy.

1. **Ulcerlike dyspepsia,** in which burning and other classic symptoms of PUD
   predominate.
2. **Refluxlike dyspepsia,** characterized primarily by heartburn and regurgitation.
3. **Dysmotility-like dyspepsia,** in which symptoms of bloating, early satiety,
   distention, nausea, and retching predominate.
4. **Aerophagia,** abdominal bloating after abnormal air swallowing, often relieved
   with belching.
5. **Idiopathic NUD,** characterized primarily by epigastric discomfort.

D. Symptoms that may identify patients with **complications of PUD or other specific causes of dyspepsia** are listed below.

1. **Hematemesis, melena,** or both indicate GI bleeding.
2. **Dizziness,** especially upon sitting or standing, or **syncope** may indicate significant blood loss.
3. **Persistent vomiting** is a symptom of gastric outlet obstruction.
4. **Pain that radiates straight through to the back** may indicate a perforated
   ulcer, leaking abdominal aneurysm, pancreatitis, or pancreatic cancer.
5. **Pain radiating to the shoulder** may result from diaphragmatic irritation due
   to pus, blood, or free air.

VI. Signs. In general, the **physical examination** is not helpful in determining the cause
of dyspepsia. In uncomplicated cases, the examination usually reveals only mild to
moderate epigastric tenderness.

The following signs may be helpful in identifying patients with **complications of
PUD or serious systemic illness.**

A. Unexplained tachycardia (pulse >120) or **postural hypotension** (orthostatic
change in blood pressure >20 mm Hg) may indicate significant blood loss from
GI bleeding.

B. Abdominal rebound or rigidity suggests peritoneal irritation. A perforated viscus, blood, or infection can cause peritoneal irritation.

C. Blood in the stool may indicate upper GI bleeding.

D. Jaundice may indicate biliary tract obstruction from pancreatic cancer or cholelithiasis.

VII. Laboratory tests. The laboratory approach to dyspepsia is evolving. Many experts
recommend testing for *H pylori* in individuals less than 45 years of age and without
signs of serious disease (see Figure 22–1).

A. Indications for further testing. A diagnostic investigation should be started
promptly in patients with clinically obvious conditions, such as severe systemic
illness, bleeding, perforation, symptoms of upper GI obstruction, or evidence of
cancer.

1. Dyspeptic patients over age 45 should have their diagnosis confirmed because of the decreasing incidence of NUD as age increases.
2. Persistence of symptoms after empiric treatment in patients previously not
   evaluated with endoscopy or upper GI series requires further evaluation.

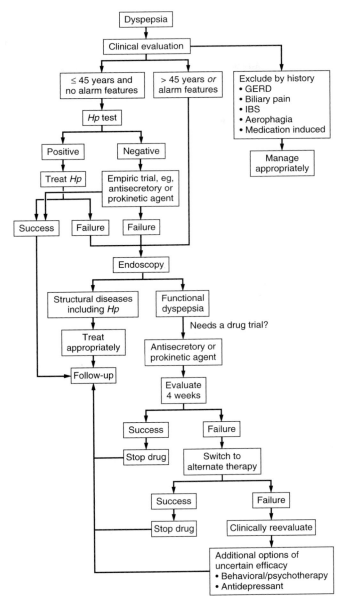

FIGURE 22–1. Management algorithm for patients presenting with dyspepsia who have not been previously investigated. GERD, Gastroesophageal reflux disease; *Hp, Helicobacter pylori;* IBS, irritable bowel syndrome. (Adapted with permission from Clinical Practice and Practice Economics Committee, American Gastroenterological Association: American Gastroenterological Association medical position statement: Evaluation of dyspepsia. Gastroenterology 1998;**114:**579.)

   3. In patients who experience a recurrence of dyspepsia and who have previously been treated empirically for the condition, a specific diagnosis should be made.
   B. **Tests that may be useful** include those listed below.
   1. **Upper GI series.** The upper GI series is noninvasive and relatively inexpensive. The false-negative rate of this technique exceeds 18%, while the false-positive rate is between 13% and 35%. Even with double-contrast studies, the false-negative rate is still between 9% and 17%, and the false-positive rate is approximately 10%. In a patient with GERD, only severe esophagitis may be detected, although reflux and motility disorders of the esophagus can be seen. The presence of a hiatal hernia does not correlate with GERD.
   2. **Upper GI endoscopy.** Upper GI endoscopy is a relatively safe procedure with a complication rate of 1.32 or less per 1000 cases. Over half of the complications in one study were the result of the medication used for sedation (eg, hives and thrombophlebitis), with cardiopulmonary complications, perforation, bleeding, and infection representing the remainder. Some argue that, despite its cost, upper GI endoscopy is preferable because lesions can be directly visualized and biopsy can be performed. One study has shown that prompt endoscopy followed by appropriate treatment was more cost-effective than empiric treatment.
   3. **Intraesophageal pH monitoring.** Most physicians consider this procedure to be the single best test for diagnosis of GERD. Coupled with a symptom diary, 24-hour monitoring has a sensitivity between 87% and 93% and a specificity of 92–97% for GERD.
   4. **Scintigraphy** is best used to detect delayed gastric emptying. GERD and delayed gastric emptying can be detected using [99mTc]sulfur colloid, although intraesophageal pH monitoring is a better test for reflux.
   5. **Esophageal manometry** is useful to document esophageal pressures, especially lower esophageal incompetence in GERD. There is an inverse relationship between LES resting pressure and the incidence of GERD. Measurement of LES pressure alone will misclassify more than 30% of patients, however.
   6. **Tests for *H pylori*** can be either noninvasive (serology or urea breath test) or invasive (rapid urease test, obtained at the time of upper endoscopy). Serology is the easiest and least costly, but urea breath test is more accurate.
VIII. **Treatment.** Figure 22–1 presents an approach to dyspeptic patients. A practical approach for dyspeptic patients less than 45 years of age without complications of PUD or serious systemic illness is to test for *H pylori,* and if positive, treat (see Chapter 86). Another approach is empiric treatment with an antiulcer or antireflux regimen. Patients should also be encouraged to discontinue ulcerogenic medications (eg, alcohol or NSAIDs) and cigarette smoking. For those individuals with dyspepsia who are over 45 years of age, empiric treatment should be followed by the establishment of a definitive diagnosis. If symptoms worsen or persist despite therapy, the patient should undergo further evaluation (see section VII,A and B). When the cause of the patient's dyspepsia is known, the following therapeutic measures may be helpful.
   A. **NUD.** At present, the best therapy for NUD is unclear. Fortunately, in most individuals, abdominal discomfort resolves within several weeks. The physician can use the descriptions of the clinical NUD syndromes (see section V,C) to guide therapy. Treatment for *H pylori* is not appropriate.
   1. Ulcerlike dyspepsia should be treated as PUD (see Chapter 86).
   2. Conditions similar to GERD should be treated as such (see section VIII,C).
   3. Dysmotility-like dyspepsia should be treated as impaired gastric emptying (see section VIII,E).
   4. **Aerophagia.** The patient should be advised to eat slowly, keep the chin tucked in, and avoid the following: gum chewing, carbonated beverages, artificial sweeteners (eg, sorbitol), legumes, and the cabbage food family. Exercise, discontinuation of or decrease in smoking, and a heating pad to the abdomen have been reported as helpful to some individuals. Medications such as simethicone or sedatives are usually not helpful.
   5. **Idiopathic NUD.** Research has shown that the use of antacids or cimetidine, as compared with placebo, does not have a beneficial effect. Age, gender, and gastric acid production are not predictive of pain resolution. Only reduc-

tion in cigarette smoking has been shown to be predictive of a reduction in pain and ultimate pain resolution.
- **B. PUD** (see Chapter 86).
- **C. GERD.** Initial treatment of GERD includes antireflux measures and antiulcer agents (see Chapter 86 for a discussion of antiulcer agents). Antireflux measures include weight reduction; avoiding lying down or bending over after meals; consuming few large meals and bedtime snacks; elevating the head of the bed on 4- to 8-inch blocks; dietary modifications such as avoidance of caffeine, chocolate, peppermint, and fatty foods; and discontinuation of alcohol consumption and cigarette smoking.
  - **1.** If symptoms persist or worsen, a prokinetic agent (see Chapter 49) may be helpful.
  - **2.** Antireflux surgery should be considered if documented reflux persists despite full medical therapy.
- **D. Gastric or pancreatic cancer.** The primary treatment of gastric or pancreatic cancer is surgery. At present, surgery offers the only chance for cure; chemotherapy and radiation therapy are experimental.
- **E. Gastroparesis.** Once mechanical obstruction has been ruled out, a prokinetic agent is indicated (see Chapter 49).

REFERENCES

Bytzer P, Hansen JM, de Muckadell OBS: Empirical H_2-blocker therapy or prompt endoscopy in management of dyspepsia. Lancet 1994;**343**:811.

Clinical Practice and Practice Economics Committee, American Gastroenterological Association: American Gastroenterological Association medical position statement: Evaluation of dyspepsia. Gastroenterology 1998;**114**:579.

National Institutes of Health Consensus Statement: *Helicobacter pylori in Peptic Ulcer Disease.* February 7–9, 1994;**12**(1):1.

Talley NJ, Silverstein MD, Agreus L, et al: AGA technical review: Evaluation of dyspepsia. Gastroenterology 1998;**114**:582.

---

23   Dyspnea

Scott A. Fields, MD, & William L. Toffler, MD

- **I. Definition.** Dyspnea is an unpleasant subjective sensation of difficult breathing (breathlessness).
- **II. Common diagnoses.** Diagnoses of dyspnea, listed in descending order of likelihood, include the following conditions.
  - **A. Pulmonary disorders**
    - **1. Obstructive lung disease** (asthma, acute bronchitis, chronic bronchitis, and emphysema).
    - **2. Restrictive lung disease** (pneumothorax, pleural effusions, neoplasms, interstitial lung disease, diaphragmatic paralysis, and scoliosis).
    - **3. Pneumonia.**
  - **B. Cardiac diseases** (acute myocardial infarction, left ventricular heart failure, pericarditis, and arrhythmias).
  - **C. Vascular diseases** (pulmonary embolism, drug-induced vascular shunting, and hypotension).
  - **D. Neurologic diseases** (Parkinson's disease and amyotrophic lateral sclerosis).
  - **E. Upper airway obstruction** (epiglottitis and foreign body aspiration) and **other diseases** (anemia, thyrotoxicosis, and carbon monoxide poisoning).
- **III. Epidemiology.** Dyspnea is an extremely common complaint of patients presenting for acute medical care; 16–25% of nonsurgical admissions from the emergency room involve patients who present with a chief complaint of shortness of breath.
  - **A.** The younger the patient, the more intense the sensation of dyspnea. Recent studies indicate that males and females are equally likely to perceive dyspnea.
  - **B.** Those patients with a history of frequent airway symptoms report greater levels of dyspnea. In general, few data show a clear relationship between the intensity

of the sensation of shortness of breath and changes in the caliber of the airway; however, evidence indicates that these patients have been sensitized so that they respond to small changes in the airway.

   C. Patients who smoke cigarettes complain of dyspnea less often than nonsmokers. The number of pack-years of smoking is unrelated to the intensity of complaints of dyspnea.

   D. Occupational exposure to asbestos, coal, silica, uranium, or beryllium places patients at risk for lung disease that may result in dyspnea.

IV. Pathophysiology. Many mechanisms have been postulated for the sensation of dyspnea. No single mechanism is specific for any of the diseases listed in section II; however, any or all mechanisms may be involved in any given case.

   A. Vascular stimuli. Pressure receptors located in the heart are important in sensing such conditions as congestive heart failure, pulmonary stenosis, and mitral heart disease.

   B. Mechanical stimuli. Muscle receptors located in the intercostal muscles, as well as receptors located within the lung interstitium, are important sensors for such conditions as pleural effusions and pneumothorax.

   C. Humoral stimuli. The carotid body serves as a receptor for hypoxemia, hypercapnia, and acidosis. Anemia leads to decreased oxygen-carrying capacity, and therefore reduced oxygen delivery. Thyrotoxicosis results in increased oxygen demand. Carbon monoxide binds to hemoglobin with 200 times the affinity of oxygen, severely compromising oxygen delivery to tissue.

   D. Psychogenic factors. Neurologic receptors located in the cerebral cortex may be important for psychoneurosis.

V. Symptoms

   A. Orthopnea, dyspnea on exertion, chest pain, previous angina, myocardial infarction, or evidence of cardiac dysfunction, such as arrhythmia, may signify a cardiac condition (eg, congestive heart failure [see Chapter 76]). Anginal chest pain and pressure (see Chapter 81) may be associated with dyspnea.

   B. Coughing has been shown to increase the sensation of shortness of breath, possibly through bronchoconstriction. Coughing or production of phlegm on a daily basis is commonly associated with lung disease. Exercise-induced cough, wheezing, or nighttime cough may suggest reactive airway disease.

   C. Bronchitis without bronchospasm usually will not cause dyspnea.

   D. Sore throat, pain and difficulty with swallowing, respiratory distress, and muffled voice are associated with epiglottitis.

VI. Signs. Special attention should be given to the patient's general appearance, such as qualitative evaluation of breathing difficulty. Dyspnea at rest is a nonspecific finding.

   A. Vital signs. The patient's respiratory rate, temperature, pulse, and blood pressure should be determined. An increased respiratory rate (>20 respirations per minute) helps quantitate dyspnea, but it is a nonspecific sign. Fever (>38.5 °C [101 °F]) is associated with respiratory infection. An increased pulse rate (>100 beats per minute) or elevated blood pressure above the patient's baseline may indicate the level of respiratory distress.

   B. Respiratory conditions

      1. The presence of rhonchi and wheezing are associated with lung disease. An increased thoracic anterior-posterior diameter, clubbing, and localized fine rales are indicative of chronic lung disease.

      2. Intrapulmonary processes, such as pleural effusions and the absence of breath sounds, may indicate lung cancer. Dullness to percussion can help establish the presence of effusions or pneumonia.

   C. Cardiovascular findings. The examination should entail an evaluation of abnormal heart sounds (S_3 and S_4) and rub. Signs of heart failure include increased regular venous distention, peripheral edema, and pulmonary rales in the lower lung fields.

   D. Neurologic findings. The nature of dyspnea caused by neurologic disease varies, depending on the location of the lesion.

      1. Involvement of the midbrain may lead to central hyperventilation. Hyperventilation is the response to the sensation of dyspnea.

      2. A lesion in the spinal cord may result in peripheral and respiratory muscle paralyses associated with inability to take a deep breath.

3. Involvement of the pontine nucleus may be associated with respiratory ataxia (ie, loss of coordination of respiratory function).
4. A medullary lesion will cause loss of autonomic control of breathing, but not breathlessness. The patient will not feel short of breath, yet cannot regulate his or her respiratory rate.

VII. **Laboratory tests.** The need for laboratory tests should be based on the patient's history and physical examination. In situations in which the diagnosis is obvious, laboratory testing will not be helpful. In other cases, in which the cause of dyspnea will be unclear even after a thorough history and physical examination, a stepwise approach to laboratory testing may decrease both diagnostic cost and patient discomfort.

A. A **peak expiratory flow rate** of <200 L/min (normal value, 400–600 L/min) indicates significant obstructive airway disease that may require hospitalization. This rate, which is easily measured with a hand-held flowmeter, can be compared to the patient's subjective assessment of shortness of breath and can be especially useful in the presence of wheezing.

B. **Arterial blood gas analysis** provides levels of oxygenation, carbon dioxide, and pH (normal values: pH, 7.40; P_{CO_2}, 40 mm Hg; P_{O_2}, 90–100 mm Hg). An arterial blood gas profile should be considered in cases of severe dyspnea as well as to help define dyspnea of unclear origin.

C. A **chest x-ray** demonstrates infiltrates, a pneumothorax, or signs of congestive heart failure.

D. A **complete blood cell count** can establish a possible underlying infection or the presence of anemia.

E. An **electrocardiogram** is imperative for evaluation of cardiac arrhythmia or ischemic changes. **Other useful cardiac studies** may include right cardiac catheterization, echocardiography, measurement of ejection fraction, left heart catheterization, and exercise treadmill testing.

F. A determination of the **carbon monoxide level** (normal value, <2%) may document a toxic exposure. Levels are elevated in active smokers (<10%), thereby decreasing oxygen-carrying capacity. Lethal levels (>50%) can occur despite relatively normal arterial blood gas.

G. **Formal spirometry** (see Chapter 74) is useful in the interpretation of spirometry in patients with dyspnea. In restrictive disease, forced vital capacity (FVC) is low, and forced expiratory volume in 1 second (FEV_1) and the maximal midexpiratory flow ($FEV_{25-75\%}$) may be low. The FEV-FVC ratio may be normal or even high. In obstructive disease, FVC, FEV, FEV_1-FVC ratio, or $FEV_{25-75\%}$, or all four, may be low. In mixed disease, all of these values are low.

H. **Exercise testing** is helpful in the evaluation of cardiac abnormalities as well as in the diagnosis of exercise-induced asthma.

I. The use of a **ventilation/perfusion** (V/Q) **scan** in the evaluation of a suspected pulmonary embolism requires that a thorough clinical evaluation be integrated with the results of the nuclear medicine laboratory evaluation.
   Patients with suspected deep venous thrombosis should undergo evaluation by noninvasive vascular evaluation, including **Doppler flow studies** and **plethysmography. Venography** is not without risk and should be reserved for cases that cannot be managed by noninvasive testing alone (see Chapter 44).

VIII. **Treatment.** Once the underlying diagnosis has been made, treatment strategies should involve increasing oxygen delivery and correction of the underlying disease process. See the appropriate chapter for treatment of asthma (Chapter 72), chronic obstructive pulmonary disease (Chapter 74), congestive heart failure (Chapter 76), cough (Chapter 16), ischemic heart disease (Chapter 81), peripheral vascular disease (Chapter 87), stroke (Chapter 90), thyroid disease (Chapter 91), and wheezing (Chapter 68). Management of other important causes of dyspnea is discussed here.

A. **Pulmonary embolism**
   1. If testing is positive for the presence of deep venous thrombosis or pulmonary embolism, the patient should be hospitalized for anticoagulation therapy. If the patient has no previous history of pulmonary embolism or known risk factor, treatment should last for only 6 months.
   2. Otherwise, the patient will require permanent anticoagulation. Prior to deciding on this treatment, the patient should be evaluated for contraindications, such as history of falls, to determine whether the benefits outweigh the risks.

If anticoagulation is contraindicated in a patient with recurrent pulmonary embolism, filters placed in the inferior vena cava may be used.

B. Pneumothorax
   1. A stable pneumothorax (<10%) should be treated with rest, observation, and daily clinical follow-up until the patient is asymptomatic. If the patient is symptomatic, oxygen should be administered to decrease dyspnea, and pain control should be obtained without decreasing respiratory drive. The patient with a larger or symptomatic pneumothorax may need to be treated in the hospital, and a thoracostomy tube may be indicated.
   2. Recurrent pneumothorax may require attempting to sclerose the pleural linings, using an agent such as tetracycline. If this fails, open thoracotomy may be necessary to obtain closure of the air leak.

C. Epiglottitis. Acute management of epiglottitis involves preservation of the airway. If the patient is seen in the outpatient setting and acute epiglottitis is suspected, examination with a tongue blade should be avoided because of the possibility of complete airway obstruction, and the patient should be taken to the hospital. The patient should be sent by ambulance to an emergency care center for possible intubation. Intubation in the outpatient setting should be avoided.

Oxygen administration should be initiated, and a humidifier should be used. Anterior-posterior and lateral neck x-rays should be obtained. Patients with x-ray findings suggestive of epiglottitis (thickening of the epiglottis or "thumb sign") should be admitted to the hospital for intense monitoring and parenteral antibiotics (eg, ampicillin or chloramphenicol). A first-generation cephalosporin may be used as an alternative therapy.

D. Foreign body aspiration
   1. Bronchoscopy is the treatment of choice to remove the foreign body. Cultures should be obtained during the procedure if postobstructive pneumonia is suspected. Treatment with appropriate antibiotics would be started based on these cultures. Empiric-use antibiotics effective against common respiratory pathogens, such as ampicillin or a first-generation cephalosporin, may be indicated.
   2. Mechanical efforts to dislodge the object, such as the Heimlich maneuver, should be used only if complete airway obstruction is apparent.
   3. If the patient is in significant respiratory distress, he or she should be transferred to the hospital setting for acute treatment and observation.

REFERENCES

Date H, Goto K, Souda R, et al: Bilateral lung volume reduction surgery via median sternotomy for severe pulmonary emphysema. Ann Thorac Surg 1998;**65**:939.

Gift AG, Narsavage G: Validity of the numeric rating scale as a measure of dyspnea. Am J Crit Care 1998;**7**:200.

Murata GH, Kapsner CO, Lium DJ, et al: Patient compliance with peak flow monitoring in chronic obstructive pulmonary disease. Am J Med Sci 1998;**315**:296.

Rietveld S: Symptom perception in asthma: A multidisciplinary review. J Asthma 1998;**35**:137.

Seemungal TA, Donaldson GC, Paul EA, et al: Effect of exacerbation on quality of life in patients with chronic obstructive pulmonary disease. Am J Respir Crit Care Med 1998;**157**:1418.

---

24   Dysuria in Women

L. Peter Schwiebert, MD

   I. Definition. Dysuria is a burning sensation associated with urination.
   II. Common diagnoses
   A. **Acute bacterial cystitis** (25–35% of cases).
   B. **Vulvovaginitis** (see Chapter 67) (21–38% of cases).
   C. **Pyelonephritis** (up to 30% of cases).
   D. **Dysuria without pyuria,** including interstitial cystitis (15–30% of cases).
   E. **Urethritis** (3–10% of cases).
   III. Epidemiology. Clinical syndromes associated with dysuria account for 5–15% of visits to family physicians. Urinary tract infection (UTI) accounts for over 7 million visits

by women to US physicians annually; by age 30, half of all women have had at least one UTI per year. Twenty percent of these women suffer recurrent UTIs.

A. Acute bacterial cystitis. Factors that contribute to development of acute and recurrent bacterial cystitis include sexual intercourse, use of a diaphragm and spermicidal gel for contraception, postponement of micturition, and douching.

Factors that increase the likelihood of "complicated" UTI (ie, a UTI caused by resistant organisms, an infection that is difficult to eradicate, or a recurrent infection) include pregnancy, indwelling urinary catheter, recent urinary tract instrumentation, known urinary tract abnormality or stone, recent systemic antibiotic use, diabetes mellitus, or other immunosuppressed condition.

B. Vulvovaginitis. In college-aged women, vaginal infections are a more frequent cause of dysuria than UTIs.

C. Pyelonephritis. Factors associated with acute or subclinical pyelonephritis include the presence of symptoms for 7 or more days before seeking medical consultation, lower socioeconomic status, dysuria occurring in an inner-city emergency room setting, pregnancy, known urinary tract abnormalities or stone, recurrent UTIs (more than three UTIs in the past year), history of first UTI occurring before age 12, diabetes mellitus or other immunosuppressed disorders, or occurrence of another UTI within 7 days after completion of an appropriate course of antimicrobial therapy. Approximately one third of patients with lower UTI symptoms will have unrecognized or subclinical pyelonephritis.

D. Dysuria without pyuria. Risk factors include urethral trauma and exposure to physical or chemical irritants (eg, citrus, ethanol, chocolate, coffee, carbonated beverages, sugar, or spicy foods). Ninety percent of patients with interstitial cystitis are women, with a median age of 40 and a likely past history of childhood or adult UTIs.

E. Urethritis. Factors that increase the likelihood of urethritis in a patient with dysuria include a history of a recent new sexual partner, a partner with urethritis, or multiple sexual partners.

IV. Pathophysiology

A. Acute bacterial cystitis. Organisms normally inhabiting the lower bowel gain access through the short female urethra and multiply in the bladder. Eighty-five percent to 90% of "uncomplicated" UTIs are caused by *Escherichia coli,* 5–10% result from *Staphylococcus saprophyticus,* and a few are caused by *Klebsiella pneumoniae* or *Proteus mirabilis.*

Organisms implicated in complicated infections include *Serratia, Pseudomonas, Klebsiella, Enterococcus,* and Enterobacteriaceae species.

B. Pyelonephritis results when bacteria invade renal tissue, causing a severe inflammatory response.

C. In dysuria without pyuria, inflammation of the urethra, sometimes caused by irritants, occurs and produces pain. In interstitial cystitis, it is hypothesized that alterations in the bladder epithelium's protective glycosaminoglycan mucus layer occur, enhancing the irritant effect of urinary solutes. Also, fluid restriction concentrates urine and increases its irritant effect on bladder mucosa.

D. Urethritis. Urethritis results when organisms, often sexually transmitted, are present in large numbers in the urethra and the periurethral glands. This causes a local inflammatory response.

Chlamydia trachomatis is the most common pathogen, although *Neisseria gonorrhoeae, Trichomonas vaginalis,* and herpes simplex virus may also cause urethritis. (For the pathophysiology of these conditions, see Chapter 67.)

V. Symptoms.
The onset of symptoms is usually abrupt, and the patient may describe "internal" dysuria (ie, suprapubic pain) as opposed to stinging of the skin without vaginal discharge.

A. Dysuria

1. Dysuria is the cardinal symptom of acute bacterial cystitis. Other symptoms of this condition include urinary frequency, mild anorexia or nausea, nocturia, urgency, voiding small amounts, urinary incontinence, and suprapubic pain.
2. The dysuria accompanying urethritis often has a stuttering, gradual onset and is "internal." Increased frequency and urgency of urination may indicate dysuria without pyuria.
3. Patients who complain of external dysuria, or a burning sensation as the urine passes the inflamed labia, may have vulvovaginitis.

B. Vaginal discharge
1. Dysuria and an associated increase in vaginal discharge from concomitant cervicitis may indicate urethritis.
2. Patients with vulvovaginitis complain of vaginal discharge, odor, or itching.

C. Pain. Localized pain in the flank, low back, or abdomen and systemic symptoms, such as fever, rigors, sweats, headaches, nausea, vomiting, malaise, and prostration, can occur with UTI, particularly pyelonephritis.

VI. Signs

A. Acute bacterial cystitis
1. Fever almost never develops when a UTI is localized to the bladder.
2. Suprapubic tenderness is present in only about 10% of patients with cystitis. If this sign is present, however, it has a high predictive value for cystitis.

B. Vulvovaginitis. For signs of this condition, see Chapter 67.

C. Pyelonephritis. The patient often has a fever of 38–39 °C (101–102 °F) costovertebral angle tenderness, and tachycardia.

D. Dysuria without pyuria. In this case, the physical findings just described are absent. The pelvic examination may show some periurethral or vulvar irritation, however.

E. Urethritis is frequently associated with mucopurulent cervicitis.

VII. Laboratory tests

A. Urinalysis. A clean-catch midstream urinalysis (UA) is the most important test in the evaluation of dysuria.
1. Pyuria (>5 white blood cells [WBCs] per high-powered field in a centrifuged specimen) is a highly sensitive indicator for the presence of UTI (*UTI* is defined as 100 or more uropathogenic bacteria per milliliter of urine). Using this definition, pyuria is found in up to 95% of patients with acute bacterial cystitis and more than 10^5 bacteria per milliliter, in more than 70% of patients with acute cystitis and 10^2 to 10^5 bacteria per milliliter, but in only 1% of asymptomatic, nonbacteriuric patients.

   The leukocyte esterase "dipstick" method is 75–95% sensitive in detecting pyuria and is an acceptable alternative if microscopy is unavailable.
2. Microscopic hematuria is found in up to 60% of cases of acute bacterial cystitis. Microscopic bacteriuria (one bacterium per high-power field) occurs in 90% of cases of acute cystitis with more than 10^5 uropathogenic bacteria per milliliter. Microscopic hematuria and bacteriuria are therefore fairly sensitive for UTI, but their absence does not rule out acute cystitis.
3. In interstitial cystitis, UA is negative for both white blood cells and bacteria; approximately 20% of these patients have gross hematuria.

B. Colony count
1. Traditionally, *significant bacteriuria* is defined as more than 10^5 uropathogenic bacteria per milliliter of urine.
2. Recent studies have documented that one third of women with acute bacterial cystitis have colony counts of 10^2 to 10^4 bacteria per milliliter. Acute pyelonephritis has also been associated with these lower counts. Therefore, *significant bacteriuria* has been redefined as 10^2 colonies or more of a known uropathogen.

C. Culture
1. Culture is indicated in the following situations.
   a. If acute bacterial cystitis is suspected, but clinical findings and UA leave the diagnosis in question.
   b. If the patient has symptoms and signs of upper or complicated UTI (see section III,C).
   c. Two to four days after a patient completes treatment for a complicated UTI.
   d. After a patient self-administers antibiotics (see below).
2. Rapid culture tests using a dipslide are up to 98% sensitive, as compared to conventional culture, in detecting more than 10^5 colonies of the uropathogen per milliliter. These tests cannot detect bacteriuria at 10^2 to 10^4 colonies per milliliter.
3. **Cultures for gonorrhea** (urethral and endocervical) and **rapid assay for chlamydia** should be performed if clinically warranted, that is, in the pres-

ence of suggestive symptoms and signs with pyuria, but without bacteriuria or hematuria.
   D. Pelvic examination is indicated if clinical data suggest urethritis or vaginitis.
   E. Urodynamic studies (demonstrating a bladder capacity <350 mL and urge to void at 150 mL) and possibly **cystoscopy** (to rule out other causes, such as carcinoma in situ) are indicated if interstitial cystitis is suspected.
VIII. Treatment. Complicated UTI (see section III,C) requires at least 7–10 days' antibiotic treatment. In the absence of complicated UTI or pyelonephritis, symptoms and signs of acute bacterial cystitis, along with pyuria, hematuria, or bacteriuria or a combination of these, make a diagnosis of UTI likely enough to warrant treatment without culture.
   A. Acute, uncomplicated bacterial cystitis
   1. A **3-day regimen** using amoxicillin, trimethoprim (TMP), trimethoprim-sulfamethoxazole (TMP-SMX), or norfloxacin (Table 24–1) is associated with less frequent side effects and cure rates comparable to a 7- to 14-day course of treatment. A recent study found 3 days' treatment with TMP-SMX to be more effective and less expensive than 3 days of nitrofurantoin, cefadroxil, or amoxicillin.
   2. **Treatment of recurrent UTIs.** Occurrence of at least three symptomatic UTIs over 12 months, or more than two over 6 months, warrants prophylaxis. Certain measures that have been shown to decrease the number of recurrences of UTIs include frequent bladder emptying, especially following sexual intercourse; discontinuation of diaphragm use; and urine acidification using cranberry juice (>300 mL/day) or oral ascorbic acid. This last method is often impractical, since dyspepsia often occurs with the large dose of ascorbic acid necessary to reduce urinary pH.
      a. Since 85% of patients with recurring infections develop symptoms within 24 hours following sexual intercourse, postcoital antibiotics (one dose orally after sexual intercourse) may be helpful. Acceptable regimens include TMP-SMX, one single-strength tablet; nitrofurantoin, 50–100 mg; or sulfisoxazole, 500 mg.
      b. If a postcoital regimen is not effective, long-term prophylaxis is indicated. Recommended regimens include one of the following: TMP-SMX, one single-strength tablet taken at bedtime or three times weekly; TMP, 100 mg once daily at bedtime; norfloxacin, 200 mg once daily at bedtime; or nitrofurantoin, 50–100 mg once daily at bedtime. Antibiotics should be discontinued 3–6 months after initiating treatment to identify patients who

TABLE 24–1. ANTIBIOTICS RECOMMENDED FOR URINARY TRACT INFECTIONS IN WOMEN

Drug	Dosage (mg)
Trimethoprim (TMP)[1,2]	100 bid or 200 daily
Trimethoprim-sulfamethoxazole (TMP-SMX)[1,2]	160/800 bid
Nitrofurantoin[3]	100 qid
Amoxicillin[4]	250 tid
Amoxicillin-clavulanate[2,5]	500 tid
Cefpodoxime proxetil[5]	100 bid
Ciprofloxacin[5]	250 bid
Exoxacin[5]	200 bid
Norfloxacin[2,5]	400 bid
Loracarbef[5]	200 daily
Lomafloxacin[5]	400 daily
Ofloxacin[5]	200 bid
Sulfisoxazole[4]	500 qid

[1] Preferred agents for acute cystitis, 3-day or 10- to 14-day regimen.
[2] Preferred agents for oral therapy of mild acute pyelonephritis.
[3] One hundred milligrams twice daily for the monohydrate/crystal form.
[4] Twenty-five percent to 35% of *Escherichia coli* are resistant to this agent.
[5] Expensive relative to other agents.

will remain disease-free; women experiencing recurrences should receive extended (1- to 2-year) prophylaxis.

   c. Patients with one or two bouts of uncomplicated UTIs per year can be given an antibiotic prescription for a 3-day treatment course when symptoms occur.

B. Vulvovaginitis (see Chapter 67).

C. Pyelonephritis. Patients with pyelonephritis generally should be hospitalized for parenteral treatment. Patients with mild symptoms in whom close follow-up can be assured can be managed in the ambulatory setting with a 2-week course of treatment. Patients with complicated UTI are at risk for subclinical pyelonephritis and should be treated with a standard 10- to 14-day regimen (see Table 24–1).

D. Dysuria without pyuria. Offending agents such as local irritants, caffeine, and ethanol should be eliminated. Warm baths, increasing fluid intake (to dilute urine), a heating pad applied suprapubically, or drinking a cup of water mixed with 1 tsp of baking soda may help relieve symptoms. If urinary frequency is a prominent feature, antispasmodics, eg, **phenazopyridine** (Pyridium), 100–200 mg orally three times a day, or **hyoscyamine sulfate** (Levsin), 0.125–0.250 mg orally every 4 hours, may be helpful. A variety of oral agents have been used for interstitial cystitis without convincing evidence of efficacy in large, placebo-controlled trials. These agents include amitriptyline, 25–150 mg at bedtime; hydroxyzine, 25–50 mg at bedtime; cimetidine, 200 mg three times daily; and nifedipine, sustained release, 30–60 mg/day. The only agent approved for interstitial cystitis by the US Food and Drug Administration is pentosan polysulfate (Elmiron), 300 mg daily, which may act by augmenting the bladder's glycosaminoglycan mucus layer. Patients responding poorly to oral therapies and patients with severe symptoms may benefit from urologic referral for further management, such as intravesical dimethyl sulfoxide (DMSO).

E. Urethritis (see Chapter 64).

REFERENCES

Barry HC, Ebell MH, Hickner J: Evaluation of suspected urinary tract infection in ambulatory women: A cost-utility analysis of office-based strategies. J Fam Pract 1997;**44**:49.

Hooten TM, Winter C: Randomized comparative trial and cost analysis of 3-day antimicrobial regimens for treatment of acute cystitis in women. JAMA 1995;**273**:41.

Kurowski K: The woman with dysuria. Am Fam Physician 1998;**57**:2155.

Pinson AG, Philbrick JT, Lindbeck GH, et al: Oral antibiotic therapy for acute pyelonephritis: A methodologic review of the literature. J Gen Intern Med 1992;**7**:544.

Stamm WE, Hooten TM: Management of urinary tract infections in adults. N Engl J Med 1993;**329**:1328.

---

25   Earache

David W. Euans, MD

I. **Definition.** Earache (otalgia) is pain or discomfort perceived in the area of the ear.

II. **Common diagnoses**

   A. Acute otitis media.

   B. Otitis externa.

   C. Barotrauma.

   D. Direct trauma, including cold injury.

   E. Referred otalgia or ear pain from a source other than the ear (see Table 25–1).

III. **Epidemiology**

   A. Otitis media occurs most frequently during the winter months, thus coinciding with the peak incidence of viral upper respiratory tract infections. The peak age incidence is 6 months to 7 years. Native Americans and Eskimos experience otitis media more frequently than do people of other races. Otitis media is also more prevalent in children with Down syndrome or cleft palate and in children whose parents smoke cigarettes.

TABLE 25–1. CAUSES OF REFERRED OTALGIA

Cause	Mechanism	Symptoms	Laboratory Signs	Tests	Treatment	Comments
TMJ dysfunction	Internal derangement of joint, malocclusion, poorly fitting dental prostheses, bruxism	Deep pain that becomes worse with eating	Pain on palpation, crepitus, asymmetry of motion	None	Ibuprofen, 200–400 mg tid–qid; moist heat; mechanical soft diet. Refer to dentist if not relieved in 3–4 weeks	
Dental disease	Inflammation or pressure on nerves by abscessed teeth, impacted third molars	Dull to lancinating pain that becomes worse with eating, tooth very sensitive to cold	Carious teeth, tender teeth, red or necrotic gingiva	None	Dental referral; codeine, 30–60 mg, and/or aspirin or acetaminophen, 325 mg q4h; penicillin V, 250–500 mg qid	
Head and neck tumors	Traction on or inflammation of nerves	Hoarseness, lump, dysphagia, slowly increasing pain or pressure	Tumor in nasopharynx or larynx	None	Refer for excision or biopsy and possible radiation or chemotherapy	
Infection of sinuses, pharynx	Nerve irritation from infection	Retro-orbital or frontal pain, sore throat	Sinus tenderness, poor transillumination, exudative pharyngitis	Sinus x-rays, strep screen	See Chapters 59 and 61	
Carotodynia	Pain referred along same nerve pathways as the ear	Throat pain, dysphagia	Tender bifurcation of carotid artery	None	Aspirin, 650 mg qid, moist heat to affected side of neck	
Temporal arteritis	Collagen vascular disease with inflammation	Pain near affected arteries, weight loss, fever, jaw claudication	Tender, indurated temporal artery	Elevated ESR	Prednisone, 60 mg/day; taper by 10% weekly to 10 mg/day after 4–6 weeks; then taper 1 mg/week	Treat to prevent blindness. Use ESR to monitor therapy
Trigeminal, glossopharyngeal, or sphenopalatine neuralgia	Compression of nerves	Lancinating pain triggered by chewing or swallowing cold liquids	Trigger points in nasopharynx	None	Carbamazepine, 200 mg/day, up to 1600 mg/day; phenytoin, 300–400 mg/day; or baclofen, up to 20 mg tid. Surgical decompression, ablation for nonresponders	Aplastic anemia can occur with carbamazepine

ESR, Erythrocyte sedimentation rate; TMJ, temporomandibular joint.

131

    B. Otitis externa is 10–20 times more common in the summer than in cooler months. This condition is more likely to affect individuals with diabetes than those people who do not have this disease.

    C. Barotrauma most commonly occurs either after flying in an unpressurized aircraft or after scuba diving. Acute upper respiratory infections and allergies increase susceptibility to this condition.

    D. Direct trauma is seen more frequently in young males, in whom it may result from fights or automobile accidents; in military personnel or miners, who may work near explosions; or in hikers, mountain climbers, or outdoor workers in cold climates, who may suffer frostbite.

    E. Referred otalgia

        1. Temporomandibular joint (TMJ) dysfunction tends to occur in patients with the following conditions: (1) dental malocclusion or poorly fitting dental prostheses, (2) bruxism (nocturnal tooth grinding), (3) trauma to the mandible, or (4) degenerative TMJ disease—especially in women in the third or fourth decade of life.

        2. Individuals with poor oral hygiene are likely to develop dental diseases, such as abscesses.

        3. Patients with a history of heavy tobacco or alcohol use or serous otitis (in adults), those of Chinese ancestry, and those with dysphagia or hemoptysis are at increased risk for cancers of the ear, nose, and throat region.

IV. Pathophysiology

    A. Otitis media causes ear pain through pressure and inflammation of the middle ear cavity. The factors described below affect the development of this disorder.

        1. Eustachian tube dysfunction is the fundamental prerequisite for otitis media. Experts believe that viral upper respiratory infections cause a loss of tubal ciliated epithelium and increase bacterial adherence to the epithelium. These infections may even have an immunosuppressive effect on the host.

        2. Viruses associated with acute otitis media include influenza type A, respiratory syncytial virus, and adenovirus.

        3. Bacteria in acute otitis media originate in the patient's nasopharyngeal flora. *Streptococcus pneumoniae, Haemophilus influenzae,* and *Moraxella catarrhalis* are the bacteria most commonly isolated from middle ear effusions. *Streptococcus pneumoniae* accounts in up to 50% of episodes of otitis media. *Haemophilus influenzae* is responsible for up to 30% of cases of acute otitis media in children under 5 years of age. *Moraxella catarrhalis* may cause up to 25% of otitis media. Coagulase-positive staphylococci, group A streptococci, and Enterobacteriaceae account for very small numbers of culture-proven bacterial infections. Bacterial products, especially endotoxins and pneumococcal cell walls, are partially responsible for middle ear inflammation and effusion.

    B. Otitis externa results when water—particularly if the water is bacteria-laden, as is found in swimming holes—remains in the external auditory canal and macerates the skin of the canal. Abrasions of the canal from attempts to clean it or irritation from foreign bodies make it vulnerable to bacterial infection. Bacteria commonly cultured in external otitis include *Pseudomonas aeruginosa, Proteus vulgaris,* staphylococci, and Enterobacteriaceae. Fungi, such as *Aspergillus, Candida,* and *Penicillium,* also play a role, especially in tropical climates. Severe infections with *Pseudomonas,* especially in patients with diabetes, cause a necrotizing vasculitis with bacterial invasion and destruction of the surrounding cartilage. Osteomyelitis often accompanies these infections.

    C. Barotrauma occurs when a diver or flier descends and is unable to equalize the pressure between the middle ear and the nasopharynx. The resulting pressure differential causes pain. Barotrauma is commonly associated with conditions such as allergies or upper respiratory infections that may decrease eustachian tube patency.

    D. Direct trauma to the external ear causes injury and pain due to hematomas, lacerations, abrasions, or rupture of the tympanic membrane (TM). Fractures involving the auditory canal or the middle ear and frostbite may also cause otalgia.

    E. Referred otalgia is due to the complex innervation of the ear. The ear is supplied by sensory branches of the trigeminal, facial, vagus, and glossopharyngeal cranial nerves and by the lesser occipital and great auricular cervical nerves.

V. Symptoms
A. Pain
1. **Severe deep pain** in the ear is a sign of otitis media. The pain increases over hours or days unless treatment is given or the TM ruptures from increasing middle ear pressure. Fever, dizziness, nausea, and vomiting may also be present. Hearing loss in the affected ear is common.
2. Patients with **barotrauma** present with feelings of pressure in the ear that progress to **moderate or, frequently, severe pain** in a few hours. Patients may also complain of hearing loss, tinnitus, and vertigo.
3. **Direct trauma** causes **pain** in the injured part of the ear. Injuries to the middle ear are less well localized than those of the auricle or the canal. Patients with frostbite of the auricle usually present with a burning pain that lasts for several hours.
4. The nature of the pain in **referred otalgia** depends on the cause (see Table 25–1).
B. Itching. Patients with **otitis externa** present with itching that progresses to mild to moderate pain. External ear or jaw movement aggravates the pain. A low-grade fever may also be present. Complaints of impaired hearing are rare unless the canal is so edematous as to be partially to totally blocked.

VI. Signs of particular conditions
A. Otitis media. The usual findings are a normal canal and a reddened TM, which may be either bulging with middle ear fluid under pressure or retracted, because of negative pressure in the middle ear. A purulent discharge will be seen if the membrane has ruptured. Pneumatic otoscopy shows the TM to be immobile or, at most, only poorly mobile. The presence of a reddened TM alone, without evidence of immobility, is not sufficient to diagnose acute otitis media. Bullae present on the TM are pathognomonic of *Mycoplasma* or viral infections (bullous myringitis).
B. Otitis externa. This condition results in redness or crusting of the auricle if this portion of the ear is involved. Movement of the auricle or pressure on the tragus elicits pain. Otoscopic examination shows a red, edematous canal, usually with a purulent drainage. Surrounding inflammation may cause the TM to be erythematous. Tympanic otoscopy is usually normal, but may show a slight decrease in mobility.
C. Barotrauma. In this condition, abnormal findings are generally limited to the TM. Otoscopy at an early stage will show a red TM. Later in the course of this condition, the membrane becomes blue or yellow. If the eustachian tube remains blocked, bubbles or air-fluid levels may be seen.
D. Direct trauma. Injury to the auricle is usually easy to diagnose by inspection. Patients with frostbite may present initially with an area of pallor on the auricle. Erythema, and sometimes bullae, may appear at a later stage. Canal injuries will be evident as lacerations, abrasions, or hematomas. TM perforations will be noted upon otoscopic examination.
E. Referred pain (see Table 25–1 for details).

VII. Laboratory tests. The cause of otalgia is usually evident from the history and examination. Laboratory tests may be helpful in the following situations.
A. While no specific testing is usually necessary if otitis media is suspected, tympanometry may be useful in equivocal cases. It may also be helpful for follow-up examination of patients treated for acute otitis media, especially those who are very young. The presence of significantly reduced pressure and poor TM movement helps diagnose a middle ear effusion.
B. The **white blood cell count** in cases of acute otitis media is frequently elevated and shifted to the left, particularly in children.
C. Radiography and computerized tomography are useful to determine the presence of other associated injury when occult fractures of the skull or intracerebral injury is suspected. These techniques are usually not needed to diagnose ear injuries, however.
D. Referred pain (see Table 25–1 for details).

VIII. Treatment
A. Otitis media
1. **Acute otitis media** (see Table 25–2).
   a. Infants under the age of 2 months should be hospitalized and treated with parenteral antibiotics. Children over the age of 2 years may be treated

TABLE 25–2. ORAL DRUG THERAPY FOR ACUTE OTITIS MEDIA

Drug	Dosage		Comments
	Pediatric	Adult	
Amoxicillin[1]	50 mg/kg/day tid	500 mg tid	Least costly, but treatment failures associated with resistant organisms
Amoxicillin plus clavulanate[2]	40 mg/kg/day tid	250–500 mg tid	Diarrhea common
Azithromycin[2]	10 mg/kg/day, day 1; 5 mg/kg/day, days 2–5	500 mg, day 1; 250 mg, days 2–5	Long half-life allows short course of treatment
Cefaclor[2]	40 mg/kg/day tid	500 mg tid	
Cefixime[2]	8 mg/kg/day daily or bid	400–800 mg daily	Gastrointestinal side effects common
Cefpodoxime proxetil[2]	10 mg/kg/day	200 mg bid	
Cefprozil[2]	30 mg/kg/day	250–500 mg bid	Excellent antimicrobial spectrum
Ceftibuten[2]	9 mg/kg/day	400 mg daily	Not indicated for *Streptococcus pneumoniae* infections
Cefuroxime axetil[2]	30 mg/kg/day bid	250–500 mg bid	Diarrhea common; suspension may have unpleasant aftertaste
Clarithromycin[2]	15 mg/kg/day bid	250–500 mg bid	No specific indication for otitis media
Erythromycin[3]	40 mg/kg/day qid	250–500 mg qid	For penicillin-allergic patients over age 4 years
Erythromycin (E) plus sulfamethoxazole (S)[3]	50 mg/kg/day qid (E) plus 150 mg/kg/day qid (S)		For penicillin-allergic patients between 2 months and 4 years of age
Loracarbel[2]	30 mg/kg/day q12h	200 mg q12h	
Trimethoprim-sulfamethoxazole[3]	1 tsp/10 kg bid	1 double-strength tablet bid	Not effective against group A streptococci

[1] Drug of choice for initial treatment of non–penicillin-allergic patients.
[2] Second-line antibiotics, used if less-expensive first-line antibiotics fail.
[3] Alternative drugs for penicillin-allergic patients.

with a 5- to 7-day course of antibiotics if there is no TM perforation, craniofacial abnormality, recurrent or chronic infection, or immunocompromise. A follow-up examination should take place in 14 days.

b. No studies have documented the efficacy of decongestants or antihistamines in the treatment of otitis media. These drugs are not indicated, except as symptomatic treatment (see Chapter 59 for dosage).

c. The patient should be re-evaluated in 48–72 hours if fever or pain exists at pretreatment levels. If fever or pain persists, a 10-day course of a different antibiotic should be instituted. The patient should be re-evaluated at 2-week intervals if the effusion has not resolved. An effusion may require up to 3 months to clear. Antibiotics are not indicated for persistent middle ear effusion in the absence of acute otitis media. Effusions persisting beyond 3 months should be evaluated by an otolaryngologist.

d. The parents of young patients with acute otitis media should be educated concerning the importance of having the child take all the medication as well as keeping follow-up appointments. They should also be made aware of signs of possible meningitis (ie, extreme irritability or somnolence).

2. Recurrent otitis media

    a. Underlying conditions predisposing to recurrent disease (defined as three episodes of acute otitis media in a 6-month period or four or more episodes in a 12-month period) should be treated. Such disorders include enlarged adenoids, allergies, immunodeficiencies, nasal septal deviation, and sinusitis.

    b. The insertion of **tympanostomy tubes,** which results in immediate improvement in hearing, has been advocated for the prevention of recurrent otitis media. However, surgical management has not been proven superior to antibiotic prophylaxis or interval treatment of recurrences.

    c. Antibiotics used for prophylaxis of recurrent otitis media include **amoxicillin,** 25 mg/kg/day at bedtime; **sulfisoxazole,** 75 mg/kg/day at bedtime; and **trimethoprim-sulfamethoxazole,** 25 mg/kg/day at bedtime, based on the sulfamethoxazole component.

B. Otitis externa

  1. First, the canal is gently and thoroughly cleansed of debris using a cotton-tipped applicator. Then a mixture of polymyxin B, Neosporin, and hydrocortisone (eg, Cortisporin otic solution) should be instilled into the ear canal four times daily. Adults should use four drops, and children, three drops, each time. If TM perforation has possibly occurred, a suspension should be used instead of the solution, to minimize patient discomfort. An effective alternative is 2% acetic acid in propylene glycol (**V̄oSol** or **V̄oSol HC**) used in the same manner. Likewise, ofloxacin otic solution has been shown to be effective when used twice daily.

  2. If the auditory canal is very edematous, the placement of a small absorptive wick in the canal will help to distribute the medication to the deeper parts of the canal. The wick may be removed once the edema has resolved.

  3. External otitis with cellulitis of the auricle should be treated with systemic antibiotics effective against *Staphylococcus aureus* and β-hemolytic streptococci (see Chapter 11).

  4. Patients with malignant otitis externa, a severe infection involving the deeper periauricular tissue, should be hospitalized and treated with parenteral antibiotics.

C. Barotrauma

  1. The acute episode may be treated with decongestants (eg, **pseudoephedrine,** 30–60 mg every 4–6 hours) and analgesics (**acetaminophen,** 325–650 mg every 4–6 hours, or **codeine,** 30–60 mg every 4–6 hours).

  2. Patients with multiple episodes of barotrauma should use a long-acting oral decongestant, such as timed-release **pseudoephedrine,** 120 mg once or twice daily, or a topical nasal decongestant such as **phenylephrine,** two sprays 5 minutes apart in each nostril 30 minutes prior to flying or diving. Individuals who use topical decongestants should be cautioned to apply them only intermittently to avoid rhinitis medicamentosa. To prevent future recurrences, the diver or flier should be instructed in the proper methods of equalizing middle ear and ambient pressure, such as swallowing hard or exhaling against closed nostrils.

D. Direct trauma

  1. Abrasions and small lacerations of the auricle should be treated as are other minor skin injuries (see Chapter 43).

  2. Hematomas of the auricle should be aspirated, and a pressure dressing should be applied to prevent formation of a cauliflower ear.

  3. Traumatic perforations of the TM are treated by keeping the canal dry. If the perforations do not heal within several weeks, the patient should be referred to an otolaryngologist.

E. Referred otalgia (see Table 25–1).

REFERENCES

Culpepper L, Froom J: Routine antimicrobial treatment of acute otitis media. JAMA 1997;**278:** 1643.

Dowell S, Schwartz B, Phillips W: Appropriate use of antibiotics for URIs in children: Part I. Otitis media and acute sinusitis. Am Fam Physician 1998;**58:**1113.

Gilbert D, Moellering R, Sande M (editors): *The Sanford Guide to Antimicrobial Therapy.* Antimicrobial Therapy; 1998.

Jones R, Milazzo J, Seidlin M: Ofloxacin otic solution for treatment of otitis externa in children and adults. Arch Otolaryngol Head Neck Surg 1997;**123:**1193.

Yanagisawa K, Kveton JF: Referred otalgia. Am J Otolaryngol 1992;**13:**323.

---

26   Edema

P. Richard Olson, MD*

I. **Definition.** Edema is puffiness or swelling, usually in the most dependent parts of the body resulting from positive sodium balance.

II. **Common diagnoses**

  A. Edema caused by **perceived underfilling of the arterial system** (eg, congestive heart failure [CHF], tricuspid valve disease, pericardial effusion, or orthostatic [idiopathic] edema).

  B. Edema caused by **overfilling of the vascular system** (eg, glomerulonephritis syndromes, nephrotic syndrome, cirrhosis, or adrenal hyperplasia or tumor).

  C. **Capillary edema** (eg, allergic reactions, vasculitis, or toxic reactions).

  D. **Regional venous disease** (eg, venous thrombosis, lower extremity venous insufficiency, or extravenous compression).

  E. **Lymphedema**

    1. **Primary lymphedema** due to congenital disorders of regional lymphatics.

    2. **Secondary lymphedema** (eg, surgical removal of the lymphatics, fibrosis of the lymph nodes secondary to radiation therapy, or infiltration by cancer or lymphoma).

  F. **Drug-induced edema** (eg, nonsteroidal anti-inflammatory drugs [NSAIDs], vasodilators, or beta blockers). See Table 26–1.

  G. **Hypoalbuminemia** due to impaired synthesis or excessive loss.

III. **Epidemiology.** Edema is a very common physical finding in primary care.

  A. Edema caused by **underfilling of the arterial system**

    1. **CHF** (see Chapter 76) is the result of several insults to the heart muscle, most commonly hypertension but also ischemic disease, valvular disease, and cardiomyopathies.

    2. **Tricuspid valve disease** is usually associated with other more obvious valvular disease and dilated ventricles.

TABLE 26–1. MEDICATIONS CAUSING EDEMA

Drug	Incidence (% of Patients)
Nonsteroidal anti-inflammatory drugs	
Flurbiprofen (Ansaid)	3–9
Naproxen (Naprosyn or Anaprox)	3–9
Tolmetin (Tolectin)	3–9
Ketoprofen (Orudis)	>3
Antihypertensives	
Nifedipine (Procardia)	10–30
Diltiazem (Cardizem)	5–9
Pindolol (Visken)	6
Labetalol (Normodyne)	3
Other agents	
Estramustine (Emcyt)	20
Tamoxifen (Nolvadex)	4–11
Etretinate (Tegison)	1–10
Interferon (Roferon-A)	9

Phenothiazines, estrogens, androgens, and corticosteroids may also cause edema.

---

* Retired.

    3. Pericardial effusion is an uncommon cause of edema. The effusion is often infectious in origin (viral or tuberculosis), autoimmune (systemic lupus erythematosus [SLE] or rheumatoid arthritis), and occasionally neoplastic.

    4. Orthostatic (idiopathic) edema is primarily a problem in women and has only recently been recognized as an underfilling problem.

B. Edema caused by **overfilling of the vascular system**

    1. Glomerulonephritis syndromes. Poststreptococcal glomerulonephritis, immune globulin A nephropathy, Goodpasture's syndrome, and idiopathic rapidly progressive glomerulonephritis are seen primarily in male patients.

    2. Nephrotic syndrome results from systemic diseases (diabetes or hypertension) or primarily renal diseases (minimal change disease).

    3. Cirrhosis is most commonly associated with alcohol. Up to 25% of end-stage cirrhosis is secondary to hepatitis C.

    4. Adrenal hyperplasia and tumor are rare causes of edema.

C. Capillary edema

    1. Atopic individuals are prone to localized histamine-induced allergic reactions.

    2. Vasculitis is seen in autoimmune diseases such as SLE and periarteritis nodosa.

    3. Toxic reactions to venoms (arthropod or reptilian) can lead to massive local edema.

D. Regional venous disease

    1. One third of patients over age 40 hospitalized for major surgery or myocardial infarction develop deep vein thrombosis. The incidence increases with age and after stroke, hip surgery, and prostatectomy (see Chapter 44). Chronic venous insufficiency is a complication of varicose veins and a sequela of deep vein thrombosis.

    2. Extravenous compression results from casts, tumors, or restrictive appliances.

E. Lymphedema

    1. Primary lymphedema is an uncommon genetic disease (Milroy's disease).

    2. Patients who have undergone cancer surgery or radiation therapy are at risk for **secondary lymphedema.** Parasitic infection (filariasis) is rare in the United States.

F. Drug-induced edema is particularly common in patients taking NSAIDs, beta blockers, calcium channel blockers, and other vasodilators. It is more common in elderly individuals, since they are likely to be taking multiple medications.

G. Hypoalbuminemia

    1. Impaired synthesis is seen in severe malnutrition and malabsorption syndromes.

    2. Excessive albumin loss contributes to the edema in severe burns, enteropathy, and severe desquamating skin disease.

IV. Pathophysiology. The pathophysiology of the edematous states is complex. Edema can be precipitated by arterial underfilling, altered Starling forces, primary renal sodium retention, and altered volume/capacitance ratios which lead to a positive sodium balance, increased total blood volume, and increased venous pressure.

A. Edema caused by **perceived underfilling of the arterial system.** Baroreceptors in the aortic arch and the carotid bodies sense "underfilling" of the arterial system from diminished cardiac output or decreased peripheral vascular resistance. The resultant increased sympathetic activity, activation of the renin-angiotensin aldosterone system, and nonosmotic release of vasopressin combine to decrease glomerular filtration and increase proximal tubular reabsorption of sodium, resulting in renal sodium and water retention. To restore perfusion, a reflex hormonal cascade involving catecholamines, antidiuretic hormone (ADH), angiotensin II, endothelins, prostaglandin H_2, thromboxane A_2, and aldosterone results in renal retention of salt and water as well as increased vascular resistance. Unfortunately, the effect on the failing heart is increased afterload and preload, resulting in a vicious cycle of perceived underfilling at the arterial receptor level.

B. Edema caused by **overfilling of the vascular system.** Primary renal retention of sodium and water mediated at the tubule level is currently thought to be the initiating event in glomerulonephritis, nephrotic syndrome, cirrhosis, and the edema of pregnancy. The retention of sodium and water overwhelms the defenses against edema (increased lymphatic flow, parallel decline in capillary and interstitial oncotic pressure, and increased interstitial hydrostatic pressure).

C. **Capillary edema** results from increased capillary permeability, which can be caused locally by histamine from allergic reactions or toxins such as snake venom and systemically by anoxia. The decreased venous return leads to secondary hyperaldosteronism.

D. **Regional venous disease** such as thrombosis or venous insufficiency causes locally increased hydrostatic pressure, resulting in more filtered interstitial fluid than the lymph vascular system can transport.

E. **Lymphedema.** Reduction of lymphatic transport capacity below normal values results in a protein-rich edema fluid. Consequences of the increased oncotic pressure of the interstitial fluid are decreased capillary reabsorption and secondary hyperaldosteronism.

F. **Drug-induced edema**
1. NSAIDs cause hyperreninemia and stimulation of the aldosterone system via their effect on renal prostaglandins, resulting in renal retention of sodium and water.
2. Vasodilators cause decreased peripheral vascular resistance, with accompanying increased blood volume and systemic venous pressure.
3. Beta blockers have a negative inotropic effect on the heart, leading to reduced cardiac output, with its attendant increased systemic venous pressure.

G. **Hypoalbuminemia.** Low serum albumin results in decreased oncotic pressure at the capillary level and decreased reabsorption of interstitial fluid. When the interstitial fluid exceeds the lymph vascular system's ability to transport, edema occurs. Venous return is also decreased, resulting in secondary hyperaldosteronism, a vicious cycle of renal sodium and water retention, and further dilution of the serum albumin.

V. **Symptoms** vary with the underlying disease process and the extent of the edematous state. Patients with CHF may have edema of several organ systems (see Chapter 76). Patients with venous thrombosis may have minimal or no symptoms, making the diagnosis extremely difficult.

A. **Pressure, fullness, pain, and limitation of ambulation** may be experienced in varying degrees with edema of the lower extremities, depending on the severity of the condition.

B. **Mild exertional dyspnea** or the **distress of acute pulmonary edema** may occur with edema of the lungs.

C. **Abdominal bloating** and distention from ascites is common in patients with cirrhosis.

D. Significant **weight variation** between morning and evening, **increased thirst, headaches,** and a **sense of generalized swelling** may result from idiopathic edema.

VI. **Signs**

A. **Weight gain and accumulation of edema fluid in dependent body parts** are the earliest signs of CHF. Edema is first seen in the submalleolar spaces in the ambulatory patient and overlying the sacrum, flanks, and lateral thighs in the bedridden patient.

B. A **positive Homan's sign** (calf pain with passive dorsiflexion of the foot) and **tenderness along the veins** are suggestive of thrombotic disease, but a high index of suspicion in the appropriate clinical settings is important to make the diagnosis.

C. **Increased pigmentation of the skin** may accompany swelling in patients with chronic venous insufficiency. Change in skin creases and tautness of the skin are present in significant idiopathic edema. Edema of periorbital tissues, where tissue elasticity is high, may be present in patients with hypoalbuminemia. Significant hypoalbuminemia may result in edema of the arms and hands, as well as the legs and feet.

D. **Local swelling** that is firm and nonpitting is the major sign of capillary edema. Such swelling in a severe form is common in patients with lymphedema.

E. **Diurnal variations in weight** of 4–5 lb are highly suggestive of idiopathic cyclic edema in women.

VII. **Laboratory tests**

A. **Urinalysis** provides important information about the renal status and may be indicative of renal disease. It may differentiate between renal losses with significant proteinuria and underproduction in patients who may have hypoalbuminemia. An abnormal result with proteinuria may occur when the patient's edema is drug-induced.

B. A **chemistry panel** assesses renal function and electrolyte status and indicates the severity of hepatic or renal involvement. Impaired renal function may be a sign of drug-induced edema.

C. A **chest x-ray** can reveal the presence of pleural effusions, increased vascular congestion, cardiomegaly, and specific patterns suggestive of pericardial disease.

D. **Echocardiography** can be helpful in assessing overall cardiac function and valvular heart disease.

E. **Thyroid-stimulating hormone (TSH)** results may indicate hyper- or hypothyroidism.

F. **Ultrasonography** can often determine the absence of flow in the deep venous system, which indicates venous thrombosis.

G. The **venogram,** though attended by significant morbidity, is the "gold standard" and provides an anatomic diagnosis of occlusive venous disease.

H. Assessment of **prothrombin time and partial thromboplastin time and proteins C and S** is useful when looking for hypercoagulable states and in preparation for anticoagulation in patients with regional venous disease.

I. **Complete blood cell count.** Hemoglobin and hematocrit indicating severe anemia may signify high-output heart failure.

VIII. Treatment. Nowhere in medicine is the axiom "treat the underlying disease" more appropriate than in the treatment of edematous states. General measures to facilitate mobilization of edema fluid include bed rest and moderate sodium restriction (ie, 1–2 g of sodium chloride per day). The use of diuretics is adjunctive to specific therapy.

Patients on diuretic therapy should be monitored with regard to (1) daily weight, aiming for diuresis of 1–2 lb/day; (2) orthostatic blood pressure, to monitor adequacy of intravascular volume; (3) serial serum creatinine and blood urea nitrogen (BUN) levels, to assess prerenal azotemia; and (4) electrolytes, looking for alterations in sodium and potassium concentrations necessitating concomitant fluid restriction and possibly potassium supplementation.

A. Edema caused by **perceived underfilling of the arterial system**

   1. **CHF** can be treated with angiotensin-converting enzyme (ACE) inhibitors such as **captopril** (Capoten), 6.25–25 mg twice a day. In mild to moderate heart failure, a **thiazide diuretic** (HydroDIURIL), 25–100 mg/day, or **metolazone** (Zaroxolyn), 2.5–20 mg/day, is effective. In patients with more severe disease, the more potent diuretics acting on the loop of Henle are utilized (eg, **furosemide** [Lasix], 20–200 mg/day, or **bumetanide** [Bumex], 0.5–2 mg/day). Occasionally, patients will require combination therapy (see Chapter 76).

   2. **Orthostatic (idiopathic) edema** is often resistant to usual diuretic management and is best managed by (1) patient education, (2) sodium restriction, and (3) use of an aldosterone antagonist such as spironolactone (Aldactone), 50–100 mg three or four times a day. Vasoconstrictor therapy with ephedrine, 25 mg three times a day, or amphetamine, starting at 5 mg twice a day, has been shown to be quite effective for many patients.

B. Edema caused by **overfilling of the vascular system**

   1. **Glomerulonephritis syndromes** are best referred to a nephrologist.

   2. **Nephrotic syndrome** is primarily treated with immunosuppressive agents, such as prednisone. Initial treatment with an ACE inhibitor and a low-protein diet will reduce proteinuria. This condition is best managed in consultation with a nephrologist.

   3. Edema secondary to **cirrhosis** can be difficult to manage. Avoidance of hepatotoxins is essential, as is an adequate diet. Diuretics can be useful, but must be monitored very carefully to avoid precipitating hepatic coma and hepatorenal syndrome (see Chapter 75).

   4. **Adrenal hyperplasia** can be treated medially or surgically. Tumor should be treated by resection.

C. **Capillary edema**

   1. Allergic reactions are treated according to etiology and severity with antihistamines, steroids, or epinephrine. Envenomations are treated with specific antivenom (see Chapter 9).

D. Deep venous thrombosis is treated with anticoagulation for 4–6 months. Chronic venous insufficiency is managed by elevating the extremities, wearing support hosiery, and using diuretics as an adjunct (see Chapter 44).

E. Lymphedema. This condition can be particularly disabling because of the magnitude of the swelling. The therapy of lymphedema is difficult and controversial. Diuretics are not indicated, since they can cause further concentration of the high-protein edema fluid, aggravating fibrotic changes. Sequential pneumatic pressure devices can reduce the amount of swelling, and elastic stockings (TED or Jobst) or compression dressings are necessary to maintain an edema-free state. These devices are usually ordered in conjunction with a knowledgeable physical therapist. Meticulous hygiene should be maintained to reduce the incidence of infection. Controversial and experimental approaches include lymphatic microsurgery and complex decongestant therapy (Földi, 1989).

F. Drug-induced edema is treated by removing the offending agent.

G. Edema caused by hypoalbuminemia. Malnutrition is treated by gradually refeeding the patient.

REFERENCES

Andreoli TE: Edematous states: An overview. Kidney Int 1997;**51**(suppl 59):S2.

Földi E, Földi M, Clodius L: The lymphedema chaos. Ann Plast Surg 1989;**22**:505.

Martin P, Schrier RW: Renal sodium excretion and edematous disorders. Endocrinol Metab Clin North Am 1995;**24**:459.

Palmer BF, Alpern RJ: Pathogenesis of edema formation in the nephrotic syndrome. Kidney Int 1997;**51**(suppl 59):S21.

Sapira JD: *The Art and Science of Bedside Diagnosis.* Urban & Schwarzenberg; 1990.

Schrier RW, Niederbengen M: Paradoxes of body fluid volume regulation in health and disease. A unifying hypotheses. West J Med 1994;**161**:393.

Streeten DH: Idiopathic edema: Pathogenesis, clinical features and treatment. Endocrinol Metab Clin North Am 1995;**24**:S31.

Wyngaarden JB, Smith LH, Bennett JC (editors): *Cecil's Textbook of Medicine.* 19th ed. Saunders; 1992.

---

27   Failure to Thrive

Jack A. Yanovski, MD, PhD, & Susan Zelitch Yanovski, MD

I. Definition. *Failure to thrive* (FTT) is the term used to characterize infants and young children who are not growing adequately. The possibility of FTT should be investigated in any child whose weight or height is less than the fifth percentile for age, whose weight or height has slowed enough to cross two percentile lines on the standard growth charts, or whose weight for height is less than the fifth percentile.

II. Common diagnoses. Traditionally, FTT has been considered to be either organic (related to physical illness) or nonorganic (also called psychosocial) in origin, depending on whether a specific cause can be discovered. However, the differential diagnosis (see Table 27–1) is more useful when categorized in the following manner.

  A. Nutrition-dependent FTT (>80% of all cases).

    1. Inadequate intake of nutrients (>80% of nutrition-dependent FTT).

    2. Inadequate absorption of nutrients (<5%).

    3. Increased utilization of nutrients (<10%).

    4. Increased loss of nutrients (<5%).

  B. Nutrition-independent FTT (<20% of all cases).

    1. Familial short stature (>30% of nutrition-independent FTT).

    2. Constitutional delay of growth (>30%).

    3. Endocrine abnormalities (<10%).

    4. Genetic syndromes (<10%).

    5. Intrauterine growth retardation (IUGR) (<20%).

III. Epidemiology. Five percent of the population falls below the fifth percentile for weight or height; thus, 5% of all children in the primary care setting may have FTT. The exact

TABLE 27-1. DIFFERENTIAL DIAGNOSIS, PRESENTATION, AND LABORATORY EVALUATION OF FAILURE TO THRIVE

Cause	Symptoms	Signs	Laboratory Tests
Nutrition-dependent FTT			
Inadequate intake			
Psychosocial factors	See text	See text	See text
Cleft palate	Nasal regurgitation	Cleft on examination	None
Thrush	Refuses bottle	White plaque on oral mucosa	None
Neurodevelopmental disorders	History of developmental delay	Spasticity, microcephaly	Head CT or MRI
Inadequate uptake			
Severe lactose intolerance	Watery diarrhea, abdominal pain	Abdominal distention, dehydration	Lactose tolerance test, stool pH
Cystic fibrosis	Frequent infections, foul stools	Tachypnea, wheezing, fatty stools	Electrolytes, sweat test
Intestinal malabsorption	Diarrhea	Abdominal distention	Stool pH, fecal fat, jejunal biopsy
Infectious diarrhea	Diarrhea, melena	Abdominal distention, pain	Stool Wright's stain, culture
Inflammatory bowel disease	Abdominal pain, diarrhea, melena	Heme-positive stool, fever	Stool hematest, ESR, BE
Increased utilization			
Infections (UTI, HIV, Tb)	Depends on infection	Fever, lymphadenopathy	CBC, U/A & culture, HIV, PPD
Cardiac dysfunction (congestive heart failure)	Shortness of breath, swelling, blue lips	Cyanosis, rales, edema	Chest x-ray, ECG, echocardiogram
Chronic renal failure	Lassitude, pruritis	Pallor, edema	Serum BUN and creatinine
Inflammatory bowel disease	Abdominal pain, diarrhea, melena	Heme-positive stool, fever	Stool hematest, ESR, BE
Connective tissue diseases	Fever, arthralgia, myalgia	Arthritis, rash, myositis	ESR, CBC, ANA
Renal tubular acidosis	Polyuria, vomiting in infancy	Tachypnea, muscular weakness	U/A, electrolytes, blood gas
Increased loss			
Gastroesophageal reflux	Very frequent "wet burps"	Emesis, cough, wheezing	Esophageal pH probe, milk scan
Pyloric stenosis	Projectile vomiting after meals	Palpable olive, dehydration	Electrolytes, abdominal ultrasound
Diabetes mellitus	Polydipsia, polyphagia, polyuria	Lethargy, Kussmaul respirations	U/A, serum glucose, pH

(continued)

141

TABLE 27–1. (*continued*)

Cause	Symptoms	Signs	Laboratory Tests
Nutrition-independent FTT			
Familial short stature	Short members of family	Normal exam	Bone age x-rays
Constitutional delay of growth	Family history of late puberty	Normal exam, delayed puberty	Bone age x-rays
Genetic syndromes			
Turner's syndrome	Hand puffiness, loose neck skin	Short/webbed neck, cubitus valgus	Chromosomes
Down syndrome	Advanced maternal age	Epicanthal folds, simian crease	Chromosomes
Skeletal dysplasias	Positive family history	Short extremities, trident hands	Pelvic, lumbar, extremity x-rays
Endocrine abnormalities			
Growth hormone deficiency	May have none	Prominent forehead, large abdomen	"Provocative" growth hormone test
Thyroid hormone deficiency	Dry skin, cold intolerance	Slow movements, cold skin	Serum thyroxine, TSH
Cushing's syndrome	Obesity, poor sleeping	Hypertension, diabetes mellitus	Urine free cortisol, plasma ACTH
Intrauterine growth retardation	Infant small for gestational age	Hepatosplenomegaly, chorioretinitis	Viral antibody titers, urine for CMV

ACTH, Adrenocorticotropic hormone; ANA, antinuclear antibodies; BE, barium enema; BUN, blood urea nitrogen; CBC, complete blood cell count; CMV, cytomegalovirus; CT, computerized tomography; ECG, electrocardiogram; ESR, erythrocyte sedimentation rate; FTT, failure to thrive; HIV, human immunodeficiency virus; MRI, magnetic resonance imaging; PPD, purified protein derivative; Tb, tuberculosis; TSH, thyroid-stimulating hormone; U/A, urinalysis; UTI, urinary tract infection.

prevalence of FTT has not been determined in the outpatient setting. FTT accounts for 3–5% of hospitalizations in pediatric referral centers.

Nutrition-dependent FTT accounts for at least 80% of all FTT in the outpatient setting. **Inadequate intake of nutrients** is causative in >80% of patients with nutrition-dependent FTT, and is the result of psychosocial factors >95% of the time.

A. Nearly 10% of all children from low-income families present in the primary care setting with psychosocial FTT.

B. Up to 10% of children with FTT show evidence of nonaccidental injury.

C. Premature infants are at particular risk. Twenty percent to 30% of premature infants have psychosocial FTT even when their growth points are plotted with a correction for gestational age.

IV. Pathophysiology

A. Nutrition-dependent FTT. The common characteristic is insufficient nutrition to meet the growth requirements of the child.

    1. Inadequate intake may be caused by the following factors.

        a. Parental and familial factors. An insufficient food supply may result from an inability to pay for appropriate foods, lack of knowledge of formula preparation, difficulties with breast-feeding (eg, sore nipples or inadequate milk supply), or parental impairment (eg, mental or physical illness, addiction, or lack of parenting skills). Divorce, spouse abuse, lack of support for a new parent, child abuse or neglect, or a "chaotic family style" with multiple caretakers may also cause the infant to have insufficient nutrition.

        b. Child factors. Emotional problems, personality variables (eg, the undemanding infant who is breast-fed), and physical illnesses (eg, cleft palate, choanal atresia, or thrush) may make feeding difficult. Once malnutrition is established, the child tends to become irritable and to have feeding difficulties, and a vicious cycle is thus established.

    2. *Inadequate absorption* refers to children who have adequate or even increased food intake, but who cannot absorb enough nutrients to sustain normal growth.

    3. Increased utilization of nutrients leads to FTT despite normal intake and absorption because of an increase in energy expenditure.

    4. Increased loss of nutrients through vomiting, diarrhea, or urinary excretion means that the nutrients cannot be used by the body for growth.

B. Nutrition-independent poor growth can result from any of the following.

    1. Familial short stature. In general, short parents are likely to have short children. Expected height based on parents' heights can be predicted by the midparental height formula.

        a. For a male child:

$$0.5 \times (\text{mother's height [in cm]} + \text{father's height [in cm]} + 13 \text{ cm})$$

        b. For a female child:

$$0.5 \times (\text{mother's height [in cm]} + \text{father's height [in cm]} - 13 \text{ cm})$$

        c. Midparental height predictions have a standard deviation of 5 cm.

    2. Constitutional delay. Children may start out short but attain a fairly normal height because they enter puberty at a later age than the average individual. Therefore, these children grow for a greater number of years. Their parents or other relatives often have a history consistent with relatively late onset of puberty.

    3. Endocrine diseases. Growth hormone and thyroid hormone deficiencies cause short stature via lack of hormonal factors that support bone and tissue growth; glucocorticoid excess (Cushing's syndrome) also diminishes linear growth.

    4. Genetic abnormalities. Children with chromosomal abnormalities may have altered cellular processes that prevent normal growth.

    5. IUGR. The growth of fetal cells is affected; examples of causes of IUGR include insufficient delivery of nutrients (including oxygen) to the fetus as well as infectious damage.

V. Symptoms. The majority of children with FTT are discovered upon routine medical examination. Presenting complaints include gastrointestinal symptoms such as anorexia, vomiting and diarrhea, respiratory symptoms, and behavioral difficulties.

Symptoms of gastrointestinal problems, frequent infections, cardiac problems, respiratory difficulties, or endocrine dysfunction may suggest organic disease (Table 27–1).

A. A **detailed medical history** should include information regarding maternal health, events of the pregnancy and of the early neonatal period, and the use of alcohol, cigarettes, or other drugs during pregnancy. Medical history should also include information regarding previous hospitalizations, accidents, medications, and infections.

B. A **feeding history** will include both information on dietary intake and the psychosocial events surrounding feeding time. Both the quantity and quality of food should be evaluated. The nursing pattern of breast-fed babies should be assessed. The possibility of maternal ingestion of milk suppressants (eg, alcohol or diuretics), inadequate milk supply or let-down reflex, and poor sucking should be investigated. Juice consumption should also be evaluated, as excessive fruit juice intake may displace more calorie- and nutrient-dense foods.

C. The **parents' or guardians' knowledge and beliefs** about child nutrition (eg, food restriction for religious or health reasons or understanding proper dilution of formula) must be examined.

D. Information about **stress in the family** may be revealing. The current family situation, including who lives in the home, the existence of parental supports, and the possibility of financial difficulties or substance abuse, should be considered.

VI. **Signs**

A. **Growth rate** (also called growth velocity) is extremely valuable in determining the cause of FTT (see Table 27–2).

1. Normal infants grow approximately 25 cm and 7 kg in the first year, then decrease growth velocity to a steady 5–6 cm/year and 2–3 kg/year by age 3. Children continue to grow at this rate until they approach puberty. However, 50% of children, especially those with constitutional delay, cross percentiles during years 1 and 2 before settling into a growth channel and demonstrating a normal growth rate parallel to a percentile line. Detailed weight and height velocity charts in 3-month increments are now available (Guo et al, 1991), and may be useful for determining the adequacy of the child's height and weight velocity.

2. Accurate measurements of height, weight, and head circumference are essential and should be **plotted on standard growth charts** so that the child's growth percentile and growth rate can be determined. These percentiles can be used to help categorize FTT (see Table 27–3).

    a. Asymmetric FTT, also called "head sparing," in which the child's weight is most affected and the head circumference is either normal or at least the closest of the three measurements to the fifth percentile, is seen in children with nutrition-dependent FTT.

TABLE 27–2. DETERMINING THE ETIOLOGY OF FAILURE TO THRIVE BY COMPARISON OF THE LINEAR GROWTH RATE, BONE AGE, CHRONOLOGIC AGE, AND HEIGHT AGE

Linear Growth Rate	Bone Age Versus Chronologic Age	Bone Age Versus Height Age	Possible Cause
Decreased	BA ≤ CA	BA ≥ HA	Nutrition-dependent FTT
Normal or slightly decreased	BA = CA	BA > HA	Familial short stature
Decreased or normal	BA < CA	BA = HA	Constitutional delay
Decreased	BA = CA	BA > HA	Genetic syndromes
Decreased	BA < CA	BA ≥ HA	Growth hormone deficiency
Decreased	BA < CA	BA ≤ HA	Hypothyroidism
Normal or slightly decreased	BA ≤ CA	BA > HA	IUGR

The linear growth rate and bone age may be used to determine the cause of FTT. The growth rate is decreased when the child's height increases by <5 cm/year after the age of 2.5 years, or if the infant's length crosses percentiles on standard anthropometric growth charts before that age. *Height age* is defined as the age on the growth chart for which a child's actual height would be at the 50th percentile. BA, Bone age; CA, chronologic age; FTT, failure to thrive; HA, height age; IUGR, intrauterine growth retardation.

TABLE 27-3. DETERMINING THE ETIOLOGY OF FAILURE TO THRIVE BY COMPARISON OF WEIGHT, HEIGHT, AND HEAD CIRCUMFERENCE PERCENTILES

Weight	Height	Head Circumference	Possible Cause
<3%	~3%	>3%	Mild nutrition-dependent FTT; may be psychosocial or organic
<<3%	<3%	~3%	Severe nutrition-dependent FTT; may be psychosocial or organic
<3%	<3%	<3%	Organic disease in 70%; may reflect IUGR
~3%	~3%	~3%	Familial short stature or constitutional delay
>3%	<3%	>3%	"Short stature"; rule out endocrine or genetic disorder
≤3%	≤3%	<<3%	Primary central nervous system dysfunction

The percentiles of a child's weight, height, and head circumference as determined on standard anthropometric growth charts can be compared to help determine the etiology of failure to thrive (FTT). The third percentile is listed for illustrative purposes. IUGR, Intrauterine growth retardation.

    b. Symmetric FTT, in which weight, height, and head circumference are all equally and severely affected, is usually seen in children with organic disease. Symmetric FTT is an indication for a detailed search for occult medical disease.

  B. Signs of psychosocial FTT. Children with this condition may exhibit the following characteristics.

    1. Stereotypical **behavioral disturbances** include apathetic and withdrawn behavior, minimal smiling, decreased vocalizations, lack of "cuddliness," "hypervigilance," and self-stimulatory behavior. Children 3 years or older with **psychosocial short stature** may show depression, pain agnosia, and bizarre food habits (eg, polydipsia, drinking from rain puddles, eating from garbage cans, stealing food, or unusual food preferences).

    2. Poor muscle tone may exist even though deep tendon reflexes are normal. There may be a persistence of infantile postures, such as flexed and abducted arms and legs, beyond the normal 4–5 months of age.

    3. Developmental delay may be seen in these children, especially in areas that require social stimulation, such as speech and language.

    4. Evidence of **child abuse or neglect** (eg, poor hygiene, bruises in different stages of healing, and characteristic patterns of injury) may be present.

  C. Signs of malnutrition (eg, prominent skin folds, stomatitis, or pallor) may appear in children with nutrition-dependent FTT, regardless of the cause.

  D. A **normal physical examination** is most common in children with FTT. However, the physical examination must be thorough in order to exclude organic causes of FTT (Table 27–1).

VII. Laboratory evaluation. Routine medical examination allows identification of FTT in the majority of children with this problem. A thorough history, combined with the physical examination, has a positive predictive value of approximately 80% for the presence of an underlying organic disease. Conversely, in the absence of suggestive historical or physical findings, organic disease will be found in <1% of patients.

  A. If the history and physical examination suggest no organic basis for the child's poor growth, and the growth chart shows asymmetric FTT, the FTT is probably nutrition-dependent, and psychosocial FTT is overwhelmingly the most likely diagnosis.

    1. A **24-hour diet recall** and a **7-day food diary** may help the physician confirm or disprove suspicions of inadequate intake.

    2. Extensive **laboratory evaluation** will have a low yield in finding occult disease as a cause of the patient's FTT. However, the "screening" tests described below, which are inexpensive and involve minimal risk, should be obtained for all children with a low growth rate, nonsuggestive history, and physical examination.

      a. Complete blood cell count to look for anemia, chronic infection, or neutropenia.

   b. Erythrocyte sedimentation rate to screen for collagen-vascular disease, inflammatory bowel disease, and chronic infection.
   c. Urinalysis and culture to look for signs of renal tubular acidosis, chronic renal insufficiency, urinary tract infection, or diabetes mellitus.
   d. Chemistry panel to look for chronic renal disease or renal tubular acidosis, salt-losing adrenogenital syndromes, rickets or other skeletal disorders, or hypercalcemia. An isolated decreased bicarbonate (between 16 and 20 meq/dL; normal, 22–30 meq/dL) may be seen in undernutrition.
   e. Purified protein derivative (PPD) intradermal test to rule out tuberculosis.
   f. "Bone age" x-rays of the left hand and wrist to help differentiate causes of poor growth and to determine a child's future growth potential.
   g. Thyroid function tests to screen for occult hypothyroidism.
   h. Stool for fecal fat as a malabsorption screen.
   B. If the growth records, history, and physical examination are consistent with **IUGR, constitutional delay,** or **familial short stature,** laboratory testing usually will not be useful.
   1. Bone age x-rays can confirm the diagnosis (Table 27–2). If the bone age is significantly less than the chronologic age (ie, >2.5 years delayed), consultation with a pediatric endocrinologist is recommended.
   2. Follow-up for patients with these diagnoses should be scheduled for no later than 6 months from the time of initial evaluation. If the growth rate over 6 months is normal and there have been no further losses in height or weight percentiles, the patient does not need additional laboratory evaluation, but careful follow-up of height and weight should be continued at 6-month intervals. If the growth rate decreases, the initial laboratory tests suggested in the previous section are indicated.
   C. Other laboratory studies are likely to be productive only when the history or physical examination or screening laboratory tests are suggestive (see Table 27–1).
   D. Any patient with a **low growth rate** which has been present for more than 1 year (determined by growth points that fall progressively further below the fifth percentile line on the growth chart) and which has no known cause should be referred for further evaluation.
VIII. Treatment
   A. Nutrition-dependent FTT
   1. Outpatient treatment may be attempted for those patients whose weight for age is >75% of the median or >80% of the median for height.
   2. Hospitalization is indicated in children whose weights are <60% of the median for age, whose weights are <70% of the median for height, or who fail to gain adequate weight after a trial of outpatient therapy. For children with intermediate values, the decision to hospitalize should depend on factors such as underlying medical conditions and the family's ability to participate in the patient's treatment. Sometimes a patient does not require hospitalization in the acute care setting, but may benefit from an extended stay in a pediatric rehabilitation facility, where nutritional rehabilitation can be combined with medical and psychological therapies. For those managed in the outpatient setting, structured home health visits, even by relatively unskilled staff, can significantly improve growth.
   3. Any **underlying organic disease** that is discovered should be addressed with the goal of optimizing the child's ability to incorporate and retain nutrients.
   4. Adequate nutrition is the primary therapy for children with nutrition-dependent FTT, regardless of origin. To facilitate catch-up growth, an intake of one and a half to two times the average caloric intake for age should be the goal. Nutritional rehabilitation should be started while diagnostic evaluation is in progress.
   a. Micronutrient deficiencies are common in children with FTT. A **multivitamin supplement** with iron and zinc should be prescribed during nutritional rehabilitation. Additional vitamin D is indicated if rickets is present.
   b. Refeeding must be gradual in children with severe malnutrition, because of the possibility of gastrointestinal or circulatory decompensation. Small, frequent feedings should be offered. Weight gain will usually commence

within 14–21 days from the start of refeeding. Accelerated weight gain must continue for 4–9 months before a child can attain a normal weight for height.

5. A **multidisciplinary approach** involving primary care physicians, nurses, nutritionists, and social workers, with consultation as needed from specialists such as mental health professionals or occupational/physical therapists, should be developed. Multidisciplinary team treatment may be used in either the inpatient or outpatient setting.

6. **Enrollment in an early intervention or infant stimulation program** is recommended.

7. **Prognosis.** Through long-term follow-up of children hospitalized for nutrition-dependent FTT, the following points have been observed.
   a. Sixty percent to 80% of children with FTT will attain a weight and height greater than the third percentile.
   b. Gross motor function normalizes in >80% of these children.
   c. Intellectual development has been reported to be statistically impaired in 40–60% of children with nutrition-dependent FTT, but the average loss of IQ is <10 points.

B. **Nutrition-independent FTT**
   1. **Familial short stature** currently has no treatment, although several studies using growth hormone to augment growth are under way. Children with this condition will be short adults.
   2. **Constitutional delay** usually requires no treatment beyond reassurance, since most of the children in this category will attain a fairly normal adult height.
   3. Children with **hypothyroidism** require thyroid hormone replacement, and will grow well once this is appropriately replaced (see Chapter 91). Children with suspected growth hormone deficiency should be referred to a pediatric endocrinologist for evaluation and treatment. If therapy is initiated early, good adult height may be attained.
   4. Children with suspected **genetic syndromes** such as Turner's syndrome or skeletal dysplasias should be referred to a pediatric endocrinologist, since some of these children may benefit from growth hormone or other hormone therapy.
   5. **IUGR** has no specific therapy. Approximately one third of such children remain small. The remainder experience catch-up growth during the first year of life. Children with IUGR frequently have superimposed nutrition-dependent FTT of both medical and psychosocial origin that must be addressed to maximize growth potential.

REFERENCES

Black MM, Dubowitz H, Hutcheson S, et al: A randomized clinical trial of home intervention for children with failure to thrive. Pediatrics 1995;**95:**807.

Boddy JM, Skuse DH: The process of parenting in failure to thrive. J Child Psychol Psychiatr 1994;**35:**401.

Gahagan S, Holmes R, Hutcheson JJ, et al: A stepwise approach to evaluation of undernutrition and failure to thrive. Risk status and home intervention among children with failure-to-thrive: Follow-up at age 4. Pediatr Clin North Am 1998;**45:**169.

Guo SM, Roche AF, Fomòn SS, et al: Reference data on gains in weight and length during the first two years of life. J Pediatr 1991;**119:**355.

Hobbs C, Hanks HG: A multidisciplinary approach for the treatment of children with failure to thrive. Child Care Health Dev 1996;**22:**273.

Leung AK, Robson WM, Fagan JE: Assessment of the child with failure to thrive. Am Fam Physician 1993;**48:**1432.

Maggioni A, Lifshitz F: Nutritional management of failure to thrive. Pediatr Clin North Am 1995;**42:**791.

Sills RH: Failure to thrive: The role of clinical and laboratory evaluation. Am J Dis Child 1978; **132:**967.

Skuse DH, Gill D, Reilly S, et al: Failure to thrive and the risk of child abuse: A prospective population survey. J Med Screen 1996;**2:**145.

Wright CM, Callum J, Birks E, et al: Effect of community based management in failure to thrive: Randomised controlled trial. Br Med J 1998;**317:**571.

28   Fatigue

Anthony F. Valdini, MD, MS

I. **Definition.** Fatigue is a subjective complaint of tiredness, weariness, or lack of energy.
II. **Common diagnoses.** Fatigue may result from virtually every physical and psychological illness. Four major classes of fatigue that are useful in evaluating the tired patient are listed below.
  A. **Physiologic fatigue** is that caused by overwork, lack of sleep, or a defined physical stress, such as pregnancy. This is "appropriate" fatigue for the condition that caused it.
  B. **Physical fatigue** may result from infections, endocrine imbalances, cardiovascular disease, anemia, and medication side effects, or, less commonly, from cancer, connective tissue diseases, and other ailments.
  C. **Psychological illness,** including depression, anxiety, stress, and adjustment reaction, can cause fatigue.
  D. **"Mixed" fatigue,** which is often overlooked, involves any of the above categories occurring in combination.
III. **Epidemiology.** Fatigue is the seventh most common symptom in primary care and accounts for more than 10 million office visits every year (Kroenke et al, 1988). Various studies have found the prevalence of fatigue in primary care to be between 10% and 20%. One group of investigators found that 6.7% of patients presenting to a family medicine clinic had a primary complaint of fatigue.
  A. **Gender.** Women visit physicians for fatigue more often than men, even when the greater frequency of female visits is taken into account. This may be cultural or may be a result of the open-ended nature of the work many females perform. Females, as a group, work more hours in a day and more years in their lives than males. Other possible reasons for the more frequent complaints of fatigue by females include hormonal changes, reducing diets, and relative lack of physical fitness.
  B. **Age** is not a reason for fatigue. In other words, old age is not a cause of fatigue.
  C. **Race** is not a risk factor for fatigue. One study, however, reported that fatigued nonwhites were less likely to improve over the course of a year (Valdini et al, 1988).
  D. **Family constellation** represents a cause of fatigue in at least two cases: (1) parents of children who are less than 6 years old and (2) children of alcoholics. Neither cause is well defined. In the first group, sleep disturbance and other environmental stresses associated with this life-cycle stage may be responsible. Fatigue and depression are known to be more common in the second group.
  E. **Duration.** Fatigue lasting 1 month or less is commonly a result of physical causes; fatigue lasting 3 months or more is likely to be caused by psychological factors.
  F. **Medications.** A thorough drug history, including the use of over-the-counter medications, alcohol, and drugs of abuse, can reveal that fatigue is a side effect.
  G. **Lifestyle and environment.** Information gathered about life habits (eg, irregular or inadequate sleep patterns, reducing diets, too much or too little exercise, and long hours spent commuting and working) helps the physician assess the presence of physiologic fatigue. Exposure to pollution, including noise and tobacco smoke, also might be significant. Travel history should be obtained.
  H. **Utilization of health care resources.** Patients identified as fatigued visit the physician and are admitted to the hospital more often, incur greater charges for prescription medications, develop more new diagnoses, and have a greater proportion of their diagnoses containing a psychological component than do their nonfatigued counterparts.
IV. **Pathophysiology.** The pathophysiology of fatigue stems from its underlying cause.
  A. A **review of systems,** with an emphasis on the endocrine and cardiovascular systems, can often identify common physical causes.
  B. A detailed **psychological history** will often yield clues of a mixed or primary psychological cause.
V. **Associated symptoms**
  A. **Fever, chills, sweats,** and **significant weight loss** are associated with infection and carcinoma.

TABLE 28–1. CHARACTERISTICS PROPOSED TO DISTINGUISH PSYCHOLOGICAL FATIGUE FROM PHYSICAL FATIGUE

Characteristic	Psychological	Physical
Duration	Chronic	Acute
Primary deficit	Desire	Ability
Onset	Stress related	Unrelated to stress
Diurnal pattern	Worse in morning	Worse in evening
Course	Fluctuates	Progressive
Effect of activity	Relieves	Worsens
Associated symptoms	Multiple and nonspecific	Few and specific
Previous problems	Functional	Organic
Family	Stressful	Supportive
Appearance	Anxious/depressed	Ill
Family history	Psychological/alcoholism	None
Placebo effect	Present	Absent
Effect of sleep	Unaffected/worsened	Relieved
Decreased activity to cope	No	Yes

Adapted with permission from Katerndahl DA: Differentiation of physical and psychological fatigue. Fam Pract Res J 1993;**13**:82.

B. **Specific historical features** (see Table 28–1) may indicate psychological or physical origins of fatigue (Katerndahl, 1993). The feature most solidly linked with physical versus psychological causes is the chronicity of fatigue; that is, acute fatigue is likely to be caused by physical or physiologic events, while chronic fatigue is associated with psychological and mixed causes. Fatigue should be distinguished from weakness and hypersomnolence, which indicate a different origin.

C. **Chronic fatigue syndrome (CFS)** is a distinct diagnostic category. The International Chronic Fatigue Syndrome Study Group has recently revised the case definition (Fukada et al, 1994). It includes a duration of 6 months or longer, absence of an identified cause, and the presence of at least four specific symptoms (see Figure 28–1). Among the symptoms and signs associated with CFS, Komaroff and Buchwald (1991) found the following frequencies: low-grade fever (60–95%), myalgias (20–95%), sleep disorder (15–90%), impaired cognition (50–85%), depression (70–85%), headaches (35–85%), pharyngitis (50–75%), anxiety (50–70%), weakness (40–70%), postexertional malaise (50–60%), arthralgias (40–50%), and painful lymph nodes (30–40%). Despite the findings of "subtle and diffuse" immunologic abnormalities and associated viruses—Epstein-Barr virus, enteroviruses, herpesvirus type 6, retroviruses, and others—the syndrome remains enigmatic; its cause remains to be determined.

   1. **Chronic idiopathic fatigue.** Not all patients with chronic fatigue symptoms meet the criteria for CFS. Persons tired for 6 months or longer for no apparent cause who do not meet CFS criteria for severity or specific symptoms are classified as having "chronic idiopathic fatigue" (Fukada et al, 1994).

   2. Most patients who are tired for more than 1 year have significant psychological problems.

VI. **Signs**

A. The **physical causes** of acute fatigue (eg, rales, edema, and gallops of congestive heart failure) may be obvious.

B. **Subtle signs** of infections (eg, lymphadenopathy or temperature elevation), connective tissue disease (eg, extra-articular manifestations), and cancer should not be overlooked.

VII. **Laboratory tests.** Laboratory investigation based on signs will be more productive than screening based on the complaint of fatigue alone. The patient often needs the reassurance of a laboratory investigation. The clinician should bear in mind, however, that laboratory investigations of persons fatigued for more than 1 year have been remarkably unproductive (Kroenke et al, 1988).

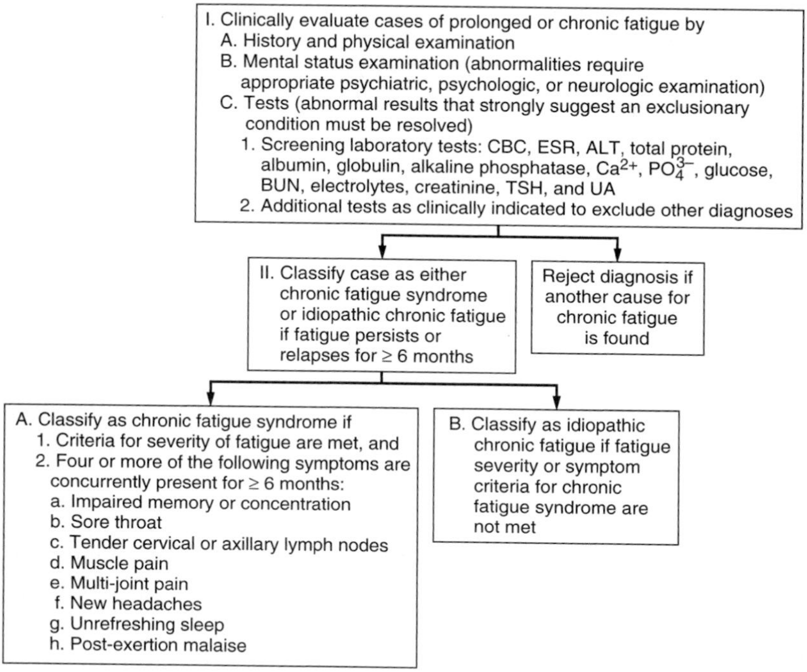

I. Clinically evaluate cases of prolonged or chronic fatigue by
   A. History and physical examination
   B. Mental status examination (abnormalities require
      appropriate psychiatric, psychologic, or neurologic examination)
   C. Tests (abnormal results that strongly suggest an exclusionary
      condition must be resolved)
      1. Screening laboratory tests: CBC, ESR, ALT, total protein,
         albumin, globulin, alkaline phosphatase, Ca^{2+}, PO_4^{3-}, glucose,
         BUN, electrolytes, creatinine, TSH, and UA
      2. Additional tests as clinically indicated to exclude other diagnoses

II. Classify case as either chronic fatigue syndrome or idiopathic chronic fatigue if fatigue persists or relapses for ≥ 6 months

Reject diagnosis if another cause for chronic fatigue is found

A. Classify as chronic fatigue syndrome if
   1. Criteria for severity of fatigue are met, and
   2. Four or more of the following symptoms are
      concurrently present for ≥ 6 months:
      a. Impaired memory or concentration
      b. Sore throat
      c. Tender cervical or axillary lymph nodes
      d. Muscle pain
      e. Multi-joint pain
      f. New headaches
      g. Unrefreshing sleep
      h. Post-exertion malaise

B. Classify as idiopathic chronic fatigue if fatigue severity or symptom criteria for chronic fatigue syndrome are not met

FIGURE 28–1. International Chronic Fatigue Syndrome Study Group recommendations for evaluation and classification of unexplained chronic fatigue. ALT, Alanine aminotransferase; BUN, blood urea nitrogen; CBC, complete blood cell count; ESR, erythrocyte sedimentation rate; PO_4, phosphorus; TSH, thyroid-stimulating hormone; UA, urinalysis. (Adapted with permission from Fukada K, et al, and the International Chronic Fatigue Syndrome Study Group: The chronic fatigue syndrome: A comprehensive approach to its definition and study. Ann Intern Med 1994;**121**:955.)

A. Since the most common physical causes of fatigue are infectious (viral infections are the most common), endocrine (thyroid disease and diabetes mellitus predominate), and cardiovascular, a level 1 laboratory evaluation would consist of the following tests.
   1. Complete blood cell count with differential, **sedimentation rate, urinalysis, and chemistry panel** (SMA-23).
   2. Thyroid panel.
   3. Pregnancy testing in females of childbearing age.
B. A second-level investigation is rarely useful, but such an evaluation would include the following tests.
   1. Chest x-ray to look for adenopathy, signs of congestive heart failure, pulmonary infections, and tumors.
   2. Electrocardiogram to look for silent infarction or ischemia.
   3. Serologies (ANA, anti-RO, and anti-LA) to test for connective tissue diseases presenting with fatigue.
   4. A **drug screen** for unreported drug (including alcohol) use can occasionally be productive.
   5. In appropriate patients and geographic areas, **human immunodeficiency virus (HIV) tests, skin tests for tuberculosis** with controls, **Lyme titers,** and **VDRL tests** should be performed.
C. Third-level tests for Addison's disease, multiple sclerosis, myasthenia gravis, and poisoning are best considered last, since these problems represent uncom-

mon causes of fatigue. Third-level testing should be prompted by a specific suspicion or sign.

D. **Abnormal laboratory findings.** Treatment of the abnormality until it resolves is necessary to determine whether the abnormality represents the cause of the fatigue. One should be prepared to resume the search for a cause if a particular laboratory value returns to normal but the patient's condition does not.

VIII. Treatment

A. **Etiology identified.** Specific treatments for defined physical and psychological causes should be administered when possible.

B. **Etiology undetermined**
  1. **Behavioral treatment.** Despite intensive investigation and follow-up, the cause of the fatigue often remains undetermined. In such a case, behavioral methods to amend self-imposed limits on activity and to decrease vocalization of the complaint, an aerobic exercise program, and group therapy may provide the patient with some relief. These modalities should be offered to all fatigued patients whose problems do not resolve with more specific treatment.
  2. **Drug therapy.** A host of medications have been used with limited success to provide relief from fatigue of unknown origin. The list includes vitamins, thyroid supplementation (for subclinical hypothyroidism), amphetamines, and pemoline. The use of any medication for treatment of a symptom without a specific, identified cause is problematic. However, the likelihood of depression or fibromyalgia causing fatigue in persons with no obvious cause probably warrants a 2-month therapeutic trial of antidepressants.
  3. **Diet therapy.** Several unproven diets have been proposed (Morris and Stare, 1993). Although fatigue has been associated with a body mass index of 45 or greater, it is not certain that weight loss will alleviate fatigue in greatly obese persons. Nevertheless, achieving and maintaining ideal body weight through balanced nutrition is recommended for general health and may be helpful in fatigued patients.

IX. Patient follow-up

A. **Frequency of visits.** It is not known exactly how often the fatigued patient should return to the physician. A few bimonthly visits early in the investigation of the complaint will serve to cement the patient-doctor relationship and establish good faith. If no identifiable cause of fatigue is determined, the physician should avoid the inclination to stop seeing the patient for the problem. Regularly scheduled visits, even as seldom as twice a year, remind the patient that he or she is not adrift and that the reported changes in the patient's condition will receive serious consideration.

At each visit, a review of physical, environmental, and psychological symptoms and signs should be conducted. Physician support, reassurance, and follow-up are important for the patient whose fatigue appears to have no clear cause.

X. **Natural history.** In one series, in which 73 fatigued and 72 nonfatigued subjects were reevaluated after 1 year, 41% of the fatigued patients were no longer fatigued, based on Rand Index of Vitality scores. Fifteen of the 72 nonfatigued subjects became fatigued after 1 year (Valdini et al, 1988). The difference in improvement between fatigued patients with physical diagnoses and those with psychological diagnoses was not significant.

REFERENCES

Fukada K, et al, and the International Chronic Fatigue Syndrome Study Group: The chronic fatigue syndrome: A comprehensive approach to its definition and study. Ann Intern Med 1994; **121**:953.

Katerndahl DA: Differentiation of physical and psychological fatigue. Fam Pract Res J 1993; **13**:81.

Komaroff AL, Buchwald D: Symptoms and signs of chronic fatigue syndrome. Rev Infect Dis 1991;**13**(suppl 1):S8.

Kroenke K, et al: Chronic fatigue in primary care. Prevalence, patient characteristics and outcome. JAMA 1988;**260**:929.

Morris DH, Stare FJ: Unproven diet therapies in the treatment of the chronic fatigue syndrome. Arch Fam Med 1993;**2**:181.

Valdini AF, et al: A one year follow-up of fatigued patients. J Fam Pract 1988;**26**:33.

29   Fluid, Electrolyte, & Acid-Base Disturbances

Joseph Hobbs, MD

I. **Definition.** Fluid, electrolyte, and acid-base disturbances occur when there is excessive loss, retention, or distribution of fluids and electrolytes or failure to replace obligate or excessive losses.

II. **Common diagnoses**

   A. **Volume depletion.** Hypovolemia and decreased effective circulating volume resulting from actual volume losses are frequently seen as complications of diarrhea, vomiting, excessive sweating, and increased renal diuresis. Decreased effective circulating volume without actual volume losses caused by redistribution of fluids is seen in septic, anaphylactic, vasodilating drug-induced, and cardiogenic shock.

   B. **Volume excess.** Hypervolemia caused by decreased effective circulating volume with renal sodium and water retention occurs in congestive heart failure, hepatic cirrhosis, and nephrosis, and with the chronic use of drugs such as vasodilators. Hypervolemia and increased effective circulating volume result from the ingestion or administration of increased sodium chloride and increased intrinsic or extrinsic mineralocorticoid activity.

   C. **Hyponatremia,** or hypo-osmolality, occurs with renal, gastrointestinal (GI), and skin volume loss; congestive heart failure; hepatic cirrhosis; nephrotic syndrome, in which water ingestion exceeds renal water clearance because of hypovolemic-induced antidiuretic hormone (ADH) secretion; and syndromes of inappropriate antidiuretic hormone secretion (SIADH) and primary polydipsia.

   D. **Hypernatremia,** or hyperosmolality, occurs with increased insensible, renal, and GI water loss; decreased water ingestion secondary to age, debility, or hypothalamic disorders; and excess sodium administration.

   E. **Hypokalemia** can be caused by the use of diuretics, diarrhea, vomiting, hyperglycemia-induced osmotic diuresis, metabolic and respiratory alkalosis, posttreatment of severe megaloblastic anemias, decreased potassium intake, increased insensible loss, mineralocorticoid excess, and delirium tremens.

   F. **Hyperkalemia** occurs in excess potassium intake, acute and chronic renal failure, hypoaldosteronism, type I renal tubular acidosis (RTA), metabolic acidosis, excessive tissue destruction (eg, acute hemolysis), and digitalis intoxication.

   G. **Metabolic acidosis** occurs in chronic renal failure; types I, II, and IV RTA; diarrhea; diabetic ketoacidosis; lactic acidosis; salicylate intoxication; and with the ingestion of methanol, paraldehyde, ethylene glycol, and ammonium chloride.

   H. **Metabolic alkalosis** frequently occurs in diuretic overuse, vomiting, mineralocorticoid excess, postchronic hypercapnia, chloride-losing diarrhea, and excessive oral ingestion of absorbable alkali.

   I. **Respiratory acidosis** can occur in chronic and acute obstructive lung disease, with the use of central nervous system (CNS) depressants, and in severe pulmonary edema, diffuse pneumonia, large pneumothorax, upper airway obstruction, oxygen administration in chronic hypercapnia, and cardiac arrest.

   J. **Respiratory alkalosis** is frequently seen in hyperventilation syndromes, anxiety, fever, salicylate intoxication, cerebrovascular accidents, pulmonary emboli, pulmonary edema, and hepatic failure.

III. **Epidemiology.** In primary care settings, fluid, electrolyte, and acid-base disturbances represent one of the 12 most frequently encountered clinical problems. These disorders often appear as a complication of other diagnoses, such as chronic renal disease and congestive heart failure.

   A. In primary care settings, absolute volume loss (eg, vomiting, diarrhea, and febrile states) and reduction in effective circulating volume (eg, congestive heart failure, hepatic cirrhosis, and nephrosis) frequently predispose individuals to fluid, electrolyte, and acid-base disorders.

   B. Frequently used pharmacologic agents such as diuretics, CNS depressants, nonsteroidal anti-inflammatory drugs, angiotensin-converting enzyme inhibitors, oral hypoglycemic agents, β-adrenergic blockers, and vasodilators, in appropriate and inappropriate dosages, can cause fluid, electrolyte, and acid-base disorders.

C. The most frequent fluid disorder in infants and children, isotonic and hypotonic volume contraction, is caused by febrile states such as viral gastroenteritis.

D. The incidence of acid-base fluid and electrolyte disorders increases with age as a result of declining renal function, decreased thirst response, CNS disease, chronic debility, and increased sensitivity of organs to hypoperfusion.

IV. Pathophysiology

A. **Volume depletion** caused by GI, renal, dermal, and insensible losses can result in renal, cerebral, and cardiac hypoperfusion and compensatory increased cardiac output; tachycardia; and systemic vasoconstriction in skeletal muscle and GI tract, thus shunting perfusion to more vital organs.

   1. Volume depletion causes catecholamine, ADH, and angiotensin II–enhanced proximal and distal renal reabsorption of sodium chloride, suppression of atrial natriuretic peptide, and aldosterone-induced distal reabsorption of sodium bicarbonate which is associated with excessive loss of potassium and hydrogen, especially in hypochloremia.

   2. Volume depletion–stimulated ADH secretion causes hyponatremia if isotonic volume losses are replaced with hypotonic fluids.

B. **Volume excess** is usually caused by decreased effective circulating volume, which results in renal sodium and water conservation and edema formation. Volume excess can also occur in states such as chronic renal failure and hyperaldosteronism, in which the effective circulating volume is increased. Excess sodium intake causes renal sodium wasting and water conservation.

C. **Hyponatremia** is most frequently caused by volume depletion and the resulting renal conservation of ingested water in place of isotonic volume losses. SIADH causes hyponatremia in the absence of the volume and osmolality stimulus to ADH secretion.

   1. Hyponatremia can occur in primary polydipsia when renal water excretion is normal but the volume of ingested water overwhelms normal renal excretory mechanisms.

   2. Hyponatremia with normal water content (ie, pseudohyponatremia) occurs with severe hyperlipidemia and hyperproteinemia. Hyponatremia with hyperosmolality is found in hyperglycemia and mannitol infusions.

D. **Hypernatremia** results when water is lost at rates that exceed water replacement or when hypertonic salt substances are ingested.

E. **Hypokalemia** with decreased total body potassium occurs frequently as a result of urinary potassium losses caused by diuretics, although hypokalemia resulting from GI and skin losses is not uncommon. Hypokalemia can also occur in osmotic diuresis (eg, hyperglycemia), sodium-losing nephropathies, primary mineralocorticoid excess, hypercalcemia, and hypomagnesemia. Hypokalemia with normal total body potassium is found in association with intracellular potassium shifts induced by alkalosis, acute increases in erythropoiesis, increased insulin activity, delirium tremens, and hypothermia.

F. **Hyperkalemia** results from increased potassium intake; cellular extrusion of potassium induced by metabolic acidosis, hyperglycemia, tissue catabolism, and severe exercise; digitalis overdose; and decreased urinary excretion induced by renal failure, volume depletion, hypoaldosteronism, and RTA.

G. **Metabolic acidosis** occurs when the concentration of bicarbonate decreases as a result of GI or renal bicarbonate loss or bicarbonate titration with fixed acids (eg, diabetic ketoacidosis or lactic acidosis) at rates exceeding bicarbonate generation. The physiologic compensation for bicarbonate loss is increased excretion of CO_2 by hyperventilation (ie, decreased P_{CO_2}).

H. **Metabolic alkalosis** is caused by the excess bicarbonate retention coupled with excess hydrogen loss or the intake of bicarbonate at rates exceeding renal excretory capacity. The physiologic compensation for the increased bicarbonate concentration is hypoventilation, which results in an increased P_{CO_2}.

I. **Respiratory acidosis** is caused by a primary increase in P_{CO_2} as a result of inhibition of respiratory centers, respiratory muscle and chest wall dysfunction, and pulmonary ventilation and perfusion dysfunctions. The physiologic compensation for the increased P_{CO_2} is cellular and renal generation of increased amounts of bicarbonate, resulting in increased bicarbonate ion concentration.

J. **Respiratory alkalosis** occurs when there is a primary decrease in P_{CO_2} as a result of hyperventilation. The physiologic compensation for the decreased P_{CO_2} is increased cellular sequestration and renal loss of bicarbonate, resulting in decreased bicarbonate concentration.

V. Symptoms

A. Volume depletion. If the volume loss is acute, postural dizziness and syncope may occur. Chronic volume losses of great magnitude may exist without postural symptoms, with progressive fatigue being a more prominent complaint.

B. Volume excess. In congestive heart failure, associated symptoms include exercise-induced fatigue, orthopnea, paroxysmal nocturnal dyspnea, and swelling in the lower extremities. Symptoms of hepatic cirrhosis include increased abdominal girth, easy bruisability, abdominal pain, and early satiety. In nephrosis, an antecedent history of streptococcal skin infection and coffee-colored urine may be present. In mineralocorticoid excess, edema and other signs of glucocorticoid excess may be present as well as a history of the ingestion of drugs with mineralocorticoid activity.

C. Hyponatremia. The severity of the symptoms associated with hyponatremia is directly related to the rate and degree of sodium concentration lowering. The symptoms include headache, lethargy, obtundation, seizures, and coma.

D. Hypernatremia. Early findings of hypernatremia include weakness, irritability, seizures, and coma. Severity is determined by the rate and amount of water loss. Symptoms of hypernatremia include weakness and irritability. Seizures, coma, and symptoms of volume depletion may develop later.

E. Hypokalemia. Generalized weakness is the most common symptom; anorexia, nausea, vomiting, constipation, and muscle cramps may also occur. Hypokalemia increases the sensitivity of cardiac muscle to the toxic effects of digitalis, which may include anorexia, nausea, vomiting, changes in color perception, and palpitations.

F. Hyperkalemia. Significant elevation in serum potassium levels (ie, >8 meq/L) can cause muscle weakness, initially involving the lower extremities and progressively moving to the trunk and the upper extremities, as well as palpitations.

G. Metabolic acidosis. Patients may report symptoms associated with hypokalemia, hyperkalemia, and volume depletion, as well as hyperventilation. Depending on the origin of metabolic acidosis, alteration in the level of consciousness caused by the toxic effect of ingestions may be present.

H. Metabolic alkalosis. The symptoms associated with metabolic alkalosis are those caused by volume depletion and hypokalemia or volume retention if metabolic alkalosis is caused by mineralocorticoid excess. There also may be a history of excessive absorbable alkali ingestion.

I. Respiratory acidosis. The symptoms associated with respiratory acidosis include shortness of breath, headache, irritability, delirium, obtundation, and coma. Patients with chronic respiratory acidosis usually tolerate greater amounts of CO_2 retention with fewer symptoms than patients with acute respiratory acidosis. There may be apneic episodes at night with snoring and daytime fatigue and sleepiness in patients with sleep apnea.

J. Respiratory alkalosis. The symptoms associated with respiratory alkalosis include circumoral and digital paresthesias, lightheadedness, and irritability. Carpopedal spasm, tetany, and syncope may occur if the P_{CO_2} reduction is acutely severe and sustained. Patients may report palpitations that are manifestations of ventricular or supraventricular dysrhythmias caused by hypocapnia.

VI. Signs

A. Volume depletion. If the volume loss is acute, findings such as hypotension, tachycardia, and abnormal postural blood pressure and pulse changes (a systolic blood pressure drop of >15 mm Hg and pulse rise of >20 mm Hg from supine to sitting) are readily apparent. If there is an absolute volume loss, there is usually weight loss, and depending on the severity and the chronicity of the loss, flat neck veins and reduction in skin turgor, tearing, and urinary output may be present.

B. Volume excess may result in hypotension, tachycardia, abnormal postural blood pressure and pulse changes, weight gain, and lower extremity or presacral edema. In congestive heart failure, venous hypertension, pulmonary edema, and a left ventricular gallop rhythm may be present. Volume excess in renal failure or mineralocorticoid excess may cause hypertension in an edematous patient.

C. Hyponatremia. Signs of volume depletion are frequently present when there is absolute volume loss. Relative volume loss caused by decreased effective circulating volume results in edema formation (see section VI,B). Patients with SIADH and primary polydipsia may have slight weight gain without evidence of edema.

D. Hypernatremia is most frequently associated with signs of volume depletion (see section VI,A). Hypernatremia caused by ingestion of hypertonic solution may cause edema, weight gain, hypertension, and pulmonary edema.

E. Hypokalemia. Severe hypokalemia may be associated with objective evidence of proximal muscle weakness and cardiac rate and pulse irregularities.

F. Hyperkalemia. Muscle weakness and cardiac and pulse irregularities may be the only manifestations of severe hyperkalemia.

G. Metabolic acidosis. Metabolic acidosis is associated with signs of volume depletion and hypokalemia (see above). Depending on the severity of the acidosis, varying degrees of altered mental status and increased rate and depth of pulmonary ventilation may be present.

H. Metabolic alkalosis. Volume depletion in metabolic alkalosis leads to neurologic and cardiovascular compromise because of hypoperfusion. The associated hypokalemia causes cardiac rhythm disturbances and decreased muscle strength. In saline-resistant metabolic alkalosis, there may be evidence of volume excess, glucocorticoid excess, hypertension, and hypokalemic-induced muscle weakness.

I. Respiratory acidosis. Respiratory acidosis may be associated with increased respiratory rate and effort progressing to decreasing respiratory rate and effort as fatigue ensues and CO_2 retention increases. Severe respiratory acidosis can cause hypotension, cardiac dysrhythmias, and respiratory arrest.

J. Respiratory alkalosis causes increased rate and volume of ventilation. In acute respiratory alkalosis, tachypnea is obvious, but in chronic hyperventilation, increased depth of ventilation may replace tachypnea.

VII. Laboratory tests

A. Volume depletion causes the urine specific gravity and osmolality to be high. The urine sodium concentration is <10 meq/L, and the fractional excretion of sodium (FENa) is <1% unless diuretic use or intrinsic renal disease disrupts the renal salt- and water-conserving mechanisms. Blood urea nitrogen (BUN) urinary excretion is also impaired, resulting in a BUN–serum creatinine ratio of >20 : 1 (prerenal azotemia). The urine sediment is acellular in prerenal azotemia, but it may show renal tubular epithelial cells and casts in acute tubular necrosis.

B. In **volume excess** or retention caused by decreased effective circulating volume depletion (eg, congestive heart failure), the chest x-ray may show cardiomegaly and pulmonary edema, and the electrocardiogram (ECG) may reveal evidence of left ventricular enlargement.

C. Hyponatremia with a low calculated serum osmolality (ie, 2[sodium] + glucose/18), in the absence of severe hyperlipidemia, hyperproteinemia, or hyperglycemia, is indicative of true water excess relative to sodium or hypo-osmolality. If water excess has been caused by renal water retention secondary to volume depletion or SIADH, the urine specific gravity will be high (>1.020) and the urine osmolality will be higher than the serum osmolality. Urine sodium concentration will be <10 meq/L in hyponatremia induced by volume depletion, assuming no underlying renal sodium wasting disorder or diuretic use, but mild urinary sodium wasting occurs in hyponatremia secondary to SIADH caused by water-induced volume expansion. If hyponatremia has been caused by polydipsia, the urine specific gravity and osmolality will be low and sodium will be present in the urine.

D. Hypernatremia is identified by the presence of elevated serum osmolality, urine specific gravity, and urine osmolality (>600 mosm/kg). The urine sodium concentration is <10 meq/L. Hypernatremia occurs without maximally concentrated urine in diabetes insipidus, in osmotic diuresis, and with loop diuretic use.

E. Hypokalemia associated with urine potassium <10 meq/L implies a nonrenal route of potassium loss. Hypokalemia with urine potassium >10 meq/L suggests renal potassium loss. Changes on ECG associated with hypokalemia include decreased amplitude of T waves, U-wave formation, ST-segment depression, and cardiac arrhythmias.

F. Hyperkalemia. Advancing hyperkalemia (ie, serum potassium >5.5 meq/L) may be associated with peaked T waves, arteriovenous block, QRS widening, ST-segment depression, complete heart block, and ventricular fibrillation.

G. Metabolic acidosis. Electrolyte changes include decreased serum pH, decreased plasma bicarbonate concentration, decreased P_{CO_2} (ie, 1.2 mm Hg decrease in

Pco_2 for every 1.0 meq/L reduction in bicarbonate concentration), hyperchloremia in normal anion gap metabolic acidosis, normochloremia in increased anion gap metabolic acidosis, and a maximally acidic urine. Metabolic acidosis and suboptimal urinary acidification suggest RTA. Hyperkalemia, normokalemia, and hypokalemia may all be associated with total body potassium depletion. Findings of volume depletion and renal disease may be present. Toxicology may reveal the metabolic by-products of an acid toxin ingestion (ie, salicylates).

H. Metabolic alkalosis results in an elevated serum pH, increased bicarbonate concentration, increased Pco_2 (ie, 0.7 mm Hg reduction in Pco_2 for every 1.0 meq/L rise in bicarbonate concentration), hypokalemia, acidic urine, and hypochloremia. Metabolic alkalosis caused by alkali ingestion is associated with an alkaline urinary pH.

I. Respiratory acidosis. In acute and chronic respiratory acidosis, there are compensatory increases in the plasma bicarbonate concentration of 1.0 and 4.0 meq/L, respectively, for every 10 mm Hg rise in Pco_2 resulting in a decreased pH.

J. Respiratory alkalosis. In acute and chronic respiratory alkalosis, there are compensatory decreases in the bicarbonate concentration of 2.0 and 5.0 meq/L, respectively, for every 10 mm Hg decrease in Pco_2 resulting in an elevated pH.

VIII. Treatment

A. Volume depletion. The primary aim of therapy is the restoration of effective circulating volume by the termination of the volume loss and the ingestion of fluids and electrolytes or infusion of isotonic and hypotonic fluids at rates and volumes titrated to blood pressure, pulse, urinary output, and weight normalization. Acute small-volume losses can be managed in the office (eg, as in viral gastroenteritis), but large acute or chronic volume losses or relative losses in patients with severe congestive heart failure may require hospitalization. Initial volume repletion in hemodynamically unstable patients requires rapid isotonic fluid replacement to restore vital organ perfusion.

B. Volume excess

1. In patients with edema caused by decreased effective circulating volume, treatment is aimed at increasing cardiac output and restoring intravascular oncotic forces. Diuretics may be required, especially if the retained fluid compromises ventilation (eg, pulmonary edema and tense ascites). Potentiation of the diuretic effect can be obtained by using two or more diuretics which act on different segments of the renal tubule. Overdiuresis can further compromise cardiac output.

2. In states of **aldosterone excess** (hepatic cirrhosis with ascites), an aldosterone antagonist (eg, spironolactone) is used to decrease sodium reabsorption and excess edema formation.

3. Angiotensin-converting enzyme inhibitors, when used for afterload reduction in patients with congestive heart failure, may decrease the need for diuretics.

C. Hyponatremia caused by true volume depletion is treated by isotonic volume repletion. Once effective circulating volume has been restored, a water diuresis will ensue and plasma sodium will normalize. In edematous states, SIADH, primary polydipsia, and renal failure, water restriction is used in order to restore normal osmolality. In symptomatic SIADH with significant hyponatremia, the acute treatment is water restriction plus the utilization of hypertonic saline in the hospital setting.

D. Hypernatremia. The repletion of the patient's circulating volume (see above) with isotonic fluids is the initial aim of therapy, usually in the hospital setting, followed by the administration of hypotonic solution to decrease the patient's hyperosmolality at rates that will avoid cerebral edema.

E. Hypokalemia. Treatment includes increased dietary intake of potassium-rich foods (eg, fruits and vegetables), administration of potassium chloride (KCl), and halting renal, GI, and skin losses of potassium. KCl can be given as an elixir or as a slow-released preparation. In diuretic-induced hypokalemia that is resistant to replacement therapy, a magnesium deficiency may be present that must be corrected in order to maximize the effectiveness of potassium repletion.

F. Hyperkalemia. Treatment of severe hyperkalemia may require hospitalization to antagonize the cellular effect of hyperkalemia, enhance potassium cellular entry, and remove excess potassium from the body.

G. Metabolic acidosis. The aims of treatment are the cessation of acid production and retention, the halting of pure bicarbonate loss, and the restoration of normal effective circulating volume. Use of alkali is reserved for severe and continuous acidosis (ie, pH <7.2 or <7.0 for diabetic ketoacidosis). Alkali is also used to promote tissue removal of salicylates and renal salicylate excretion.

H. **Metabolic alkalosis,** if saline responsive, requires volume and chloride repletion with normal saline (NaCl) and appropriate amounts of potassium in the form of KCl. In patients with saline-resistant metabolic alkalosis, efforts should be made to remove or inhibit the source of mineralocorticoid excess (eg, by administering spironolactone) and to restore potassium and chloride hemostasis.

I. **Respiratory acidosis.** Treatment is aimed at increasing the effectiveness of the patient's pulmonary ventilation (eg, through bronchodilation) and reversing or stabilizing the primary disease process, which impedes CO_2 removal (eg, upper airway obstruction).

J. **Respiratory alkalosis.** Treatment is aimed at the primary disorder responsible for the enhanced pulmonary ventilation. An example is the use of rebreathing for patients with anxiety-induced hyperventilation.

REFERENCES

Bidani A: Electrolyte and acid-base disorders. Med Clin North Am 1986;**70**:1013.
Haber RJ: A practical approach to acid-base disorders. West J Med 1991;**155**:146. (See comments.)
Haber RJ: Acid-base disorders: Classification and management. Am Fam Physician 1995;**52**:584.
Hobbs J: Fluid, electrolyte and acid-base disorders. In Taylor RB (editor): *Family Medicine: Principles and Practice*. 5th ed. Springer-Verlag; 1998:825.
Hojer J: Management of symptomatic hyponatremia: Dependence on the duration of development. J Intern Med 1994;**235**:497.
Kaehny WD: Respiratory acid-base disorders. Med Clin North Am 1983;**67**:915.
Kovacs L, Robertson GL: Syndrome of inappropriate antidiuresis. Endocrinol Metab Clin North Am 1992;**21**:859.
Oster JR, Singer I: Hyponatremia: Focus on therapy. South Med J 1994;**87**:1195.
Paulson WD: Diagnosis of mixed acid-base disorders in diabetic ketoacidosis. Am J Med Sci 1993;**306**:295.
Phillips PA, Rolls BJ, Ledingham JG, et al: Reduced thirst after water deprivation in healthy elderly men. N Engl J Med 1984;**311**:753.
Phillips PA, Johnston CI, Gray L: Disturbed fluid and electrolyte homeostasis following dehydration in elderly people. Age Ageing 1993;**22**:S26.
Sterns RH: The management of hyponatremic emergencies. Crit Care Clin 1991;**7**:127.
Vieweg WV: Treatment strategies in the polydipsia-hyponatremia syndrome. J Clin Psychiatry 1994;**55**:154.

---

30   Foot Pain

Kent W. Davidson, MD

I. **Definition.** The foot, which has 26 bones and 33 joints, acts as a platform and shock absorber to support the weight of the body as well as a powerful lever to propel the body. Foot pain is usually related to an inflammatory process resulting from trauma, a deformity, or a foot-shoe incompatibility.

II. **Common diagnoses.** Diagnosis can be facilitated by considering three distinct regions of the foot: the forefoot, the midfoot, and the hindfoot.

A. **Forefoot.** Conditions of the forefoot include calluses, corns, and plantar warts; bunions (hallux valgus); interdigital (Morton's) neuromas; and stress (fatigue or march) fractures. Problems related to the toes include ingrown toenail and fracture of the phalanges.

B. **Midfoot.** Problems in the midfoot region are generally a result of flatfoot (pes planus).

C. **Hindfoot.** Conditions include plantar fasciitis, infracalcaneal bursitis, and posterior heel problems such as Achilles tendinitis and posterior calcaneal bursitis.

III. **Epidemiology.** Although 40% of the US population has foot problems annually, only a relatively small number of these individuals visit their physicians. The most commonly reported foot problems are corns and calluses, flatfoot, and bunions.

Foot problems generally develop in response to the following predisposing factors.

A. **Structural abnormalities,** which may result in the development of bunions and symptomatic flatfoot.
B. **Overuse or trauma,** which may lead to the development of fracture, plantar fasciitis, Achilles tendinitis, or posterior calcaneal bursitis.
C. **Inappropriate footwear,** which may make patients susceptible to interdigital neuroma, ingrown toenail, calluses, or posterior calcaneal bursitis.

IV. **Pathophysiology**

A. **Calluses, corns, and plantar warts.** Calluses, which are accumulations of hyperkeratotic epithelium, occur primarily at weight-bearing sites such as beneath the metatarsal heads or on the heel. Corns, generally smaller and with more well-defined margins than calluses, usually develop between the toes from friction or bony prominences. Both are more likely to develop from inappropriate footwear or from abnormal foot mechanics. Plantar warts are caused by a papillomavirus and usually occur on weight-bearing surfaces.

B. **Bunions.** Congenital or acquired medial deviation of the first metatarsal shaft, with lateral deviation of the great toe, can lead to chronic irritation of the medial aspect of the first metatarsophalangeal joint. This process results in callus formation and a tender bursa (bunion).

C. **Interdigital neuroma,** also known as Morton's neuroma or intermetatarsal neuritis, is caused by compression and irritation of an interdigital nerve between the metatarsal heads.

D. **Stress fractures** commonly involve the distal aspect of the metatarsals. They may also occur in other regions of the foot, including the heel (os calcis stress fracture), the sesamoid bones around the first metatarsophalangeal joint, and the midfoot (tarsal navicular stress fracture). Stress fractures are usually related to excessive or repetitive activity as opposed to acute trauma.

E. **Ingrown toenail** results when the nail becomes embedded in the lateral nail fold. Its development is related to incorrect nail trimming, incurving of the nail plate, and wearing shoes that constrict the toes.

F. **Fractured phalanges** most commonly result from direct trauma, as with dropping a heavy object on the toe or striking an object with the toe while walking.

G. **Flatfoot (pes planus)** is characterized by flattening of the medial longitudinal arch of the foot. In the geriatric population, flatfoot is frequently associated with degenerative arthritis and rupture of the posterior tibial tendon.

H. **Plantar fasciitis.** The plantar fascia a rises from the plantar aspect of the calcaneus and extends to the proximal phalanges. Plantar fasciitis results from small tears near the origin of the plantar fascia, causing localized inflammation and pain.

I. **Infracalcaneal and posterior calcaneal bursitis.** Inflammation of the bursae located beneath or behind the calcaneus is responsible for these conditions. A posterior calcaneal exostosis, variously referred to as a heel spur, "pump bump," or "runner's bump," develops from traction of the heel cord on the os calcis, usually in association with tight heel cords.

J. **Achilles tendinitis** results from inflammation or small tears of the Achilles tendon occurring near its attachment onto the calcaneus.

V. **Symptoms**

A. **Pressure-related discomfort** is characteristic of corns, calluses, or warts.

B. Patients who present to the physician with a **painful swelling or deformity** at the medial aspect of the first metatarsophalangeal joint usually have bunions.

C. Reports of **intermetatarsal pain** with radiation into the third and fourth toes in association with a tender nodule between the same metatarsal heads are characteristic of an interdigital neuroma. Symptoms may also occur between other metatarsal heads.

D. **Pain of insidious onset,** usually involving the metatarsals, which resolves with rest but recurs with weight bearing, indicates a stress fracture.

E. **Pain involving the lateral aspect of the nail,** usually associated with edema and drainage, characterizes ingrown toenail.

F. **Fractures of the phalanges** present with acute pain in the involved digit and pain with ambulating.

G. **Pain and stiffness** in the midfoot, associated with degenerative arthritis or laxity of the posterior tibial tendon, are common symptoms of pes planus (flatfoot). This condition, particularly the flexible variety, in which the deformity occurs only with weight bearing, is usually asymptomatic.

   H. Patients report **subcalcaneal pain,** which sometimes radiates to the arch of the foot with running or walking, in plantar fasciitis. Typically, the pain is present in the morning and improves after taking a few steps.

   I. An **aching sensation** in the midplantar aspect of the calcaneus is typical of infracalcaneal bursitis. In contrast to plantar fasciitis, symptoms usually increase with the duration of weight bearing.

   J. Patients with Achilles tendinitis present with **pain at or proximal to the insertion of the Achilles tendon onto the calcaneus. Heel pain** from posterior calcaneal bursitis occurs in a similar location.

VI. Signs

   A. Tenderness, pain, and swelling

   1. Point tenderness and swelling over the involved bone occur with stress fractures.

   2. A tender prominence at the first metatarsal head with valgus deviation of the first toe is a sign of bunions.

   3. A nodule between the metatarsal heads is occasionally present with an interdigital neuroma. Symptoms may be reproduced by compression of the metatarsal heads.

   4. Ingrown toenail typically presents with swelling and erythema of the involved lateral nail groove. More severe forms will be associated with the development of granulation tissue and purulent drainage.

   5. Phalangeal fractures are associated with swelling and ecchymosis of the involved digit. Often there is an associated subungual hematoma. Any movement of the digit will produce pain. Angulation may occur, particularly with proximal phalangeal fractures.

   6. Tenderness to palpation usually occurs along the medial plantar border of the sole with flatfoot. Flattening of the medial longitudinal arch of the foot and often a valgus deflection of the heel are indicative of this condition.

   7. Tenderness is present along the medial plantar aspect of the calcaneus in plantar fasciitis. Pain is increased by forced dorsiflexion of the digits.

   8. Tenderness to palpation in the midplantar aspect of the calcaneus is characteristic of infracalcaneal bursitis.

   9. Swelling and erythema near the attachment of the Achilles tendon onto the calcaneus are usually associated with Achilles tendinitis. Dorsiflexion of the ankle elicits pain and may produce crepitus. Heel pain in a similar location is also a sign of posterior calcaneal bursitis.

   B. Hyperkeratotic lesions. Calluses and corns, which both appear as hyperkeratotic lesions, may be indistinguishable from each other. Calluses are more common beneath the metatarsal heads or on the heel, while corns usually develop between the toes. Other hyperkeratotic painful lesions, plantar warts, can be differentiated from calluses if trimming the lesion reveals punctate bleeding associated with the virus-induced wart.

VII. Laboratory tests. Since most of the problems affecting the feet are structural or traumatic in nature, laboratory tests are usually not diagnostic. If an inflammatory arthropathy is suspected, however, a complete blood cell count, erythrocyte sedimentation rate, rheumatoid titer, and uric acid determination should be performed. Arthritis is particularly likely with inflammatory conditions involving the heel or first metatarsophalangeal joint or in association with a bony deformity. X-rays may prove useful in establishing the origin of foot pain, however (see also Chapter 71).

   A. Indications. X-rays should be performed on initial presentation in three instances: (1) when bony deformity is present, (2) when fracture is suspected, or (3) when the diagnosis is in question. Typically, the anterior-posterior (AP), oblique, and lateral views are obtained. If x-rays are not taken initially, failure to respond to empiric treatment may prompt x-ray evaluation on subsequent visits.

   Interdigital neuroma, ingrown toenail, superficial lesions of the foot, bursitis, and tendinitis that affect the heel are generally *not* associated with x-ray findings.

   B. Findings

   1. X-rays show an increased angle between the first and second metatarsals in bunions (normal, 10–12 degrees).

2. Although x-rays may be negative initially in stress fractures, after 2–3 weeks they may reveal the fracture or the presence of callus. A bone scan is more sensitive in the early phases, and this test may be necessary if x-rays fail to reveal the abnormality. Computerized tomography and magnetic resonance imaging (MRI) may be helpful to visualize the fracture or to distinguish a stress fracture from a neoplastic process.

3. Crush injuries usually result in fractures of the distal or middle phalanx. Fractures of the proximal phalanx typically occur through the mid-shaft. AP and oblique views are best for diagnosis, since overlapping toes may obscure fracture identification on the lateral view.

4. X-rays performed while bearing weight will demonstrate loss of integrity of the longitudinal arch and may demonstrate degenerative changes in cases of flatfoot.

5. In plantar fasciitis, x-rays are usually unremarkable unless a bone spur, which usually extends distally from the anterior calcaneus, has developed. When posterior calcaneal exostosis is present, a bone spur extending upward from the calcaneus into the Achilles tendon can be seen on x-ray.

6. Although, in most instances, the diagnosis of an interdigital neuroma is made clinically, the use of ultrasonography or MRI scanning for confirmation has been suggested when the clinical findings are atypical or when initial treatment is unsuccessful.

VIII. Treatment
A. General principles

1. **Appropriate footwear** can prevent and, in some cases, resolve many problems related to the foot. Characteristics of good footwear include roomy toe boxes, supportive arches, and low heels. Primary care physicians should familiarize themselves with basic podiatric appliances such as heel lifts, cushioned inner soles, and arch supports and use them, when appropriate, in the management of foot problems.

2. **Acute treatment of inflammation** involves the use of rest, ice, and nonsteroidal anti-inflammatory drugs (NSAIDs) (eg, ibuprofen, 400–600 mg every 6–8 hours).

3. **Invasive procedures** should be undertaken with caution and topical keratolytics should be avoided when treating patients with diabetes or vascular insufficiency to avoid development of infection or chronic ulceration.

4. **Orthopedic or podiatric referral** may be necessary for more specialized needs such as molding orthotics, placing metatarsal bars, or performing surgery.

B. Treatment of specific problems

1. **Calluses, corns, and plantar warts**

   a. Simple trimming of calluses or corns may provide temporary relief of pressure-related discomfort, but does not permanently resolve the causative structural or footwear-related problem. Use of cushioning materials or orthotic devices or switching to more appropriate footwear addresses many of these underlying causes.

      Softening calluses with lotion and keeping the callus thin by filing or using a pumice stone will minimize the discomfort related to the thickened epithelium.

   b. Trimming the hyperkeratotic surface and applying **salicylic acid** solution or plasters (eg, **Occlusal-HP** or **Duofilm**) daily is usually successful in treating plantar warts. Other therapies for plantar warts include cryotherapy, curettage, and photocoagulation with a flashlamp-pulsed tunable dye laser.

2. **Acute management of bunions** includes a combination of foot rest, avoidance of pressure on the tender bunion, and administration of NSAIDs. The use of appropriate footwear, protective shields, or orthotic devices constitutes conservative treatment. Surgery should be considered in cases involving marked deformity or chronic pain.

3. Conservative therapy for **interdigital neuromas** may be provided via shoe modification (eg, wide toe box, metatarsal bar, and soft inner soles) or through measures to reduce inflammation, such as NSAID treatment or local steroid

injection (eg, prednisolone tebutate, 10–20 mg). Surgical excision or neurolysis may be required if conservative efforts fail.

4. Treatment of **stress fractures** involves rest and efforts to disperse weight away from the fracture to promote healing. This can be accomplished with a stiff-soled shoe, metatarsal bar, or walking cast. Healing usually takes 4–6 weeks.

5. Treatment of **ingrown toenail** depends on the severity of the condition. With mild involvement, use of warm-water soaks, topical or oral antibiotics (cephalexin [Keflex], 250–500 mg four times daily, or amoxicillin/clavulinic acid [Augmentin], 250–500 three times daily), and elevation of the corner of the nail are usually successful. When associated with drainage and infection or when recurrent, a partial nail avulsion, lateral matricectomy, and destruction of the lateral wall granulation tissue are usually curative. A description of this procedure follows.

   a. Following a surgical prep with povidone-iodine (Betadine), a digital block is performed. One to 2 mL of lidocaine without epinephrine is injected on either side of the base of the toe plus a small quantity across the dorsum to anesthetize any small branches of the digital nerves. For hemostasis, a tourniquet made from a Penrose drain may be placed at the base of the toe.

   b. Following adequate anesthesia, a strip of nail (usually no more than 25% of the width) on the involved side is elevated using a blunt spatula and cut from the distal edge to the proximal nail fold using heavy scissors or a nail splitter. The cut is then extended beneath the nail fold to the germinal epithelium, taking care not to disrupt the nail fold.

   c. Once the nail has been cut to the level of the germinal epithelium, the lateral nail is grasped with a straight artery clamp and removed using a twisting action. Redundant pieces of nail or granulation tissue are then removed using a sharp spoon curette.

   d. When ablation of the involved nail is desired, application of 89% phenol is used to destroy the nail matrix. Phenol is applied to the nail matrix via a soaked swab or wooden applicator for 1 minute for two applications, taking care to avoid normal tissue. Flushing the area with 70% isopropyl alcohol will "neutralize" the phenol.

   e. Following removal of the tourniquet, the wound is dressed with an antibiotic ointment, a nonstick dressing, and tube gauze, which should remain in place for the next 24 hours. Daily dressing changes and application of an antibiotic ointment should be done until healing is complete.

6. **Nondisplaced fractures of the phalanges** are usually treated by splinting ("buddy taping") to the adjacent toe for 2–3 weeks. The use of cotton wadding between the toes helps prevent maceration. Wearing a stiff-soled shoe is usually adequate to allow painless ambulation, but on occasion a walking cast or removable boot may be required. Open fractures, severe comminution, dislocation of the joint, or gross displacement will require orthopedic consultation. If a **subungual hematoma,** usually involving the great toe, is present, drilling or burning a hole through the toenail using the end of a heated paper clip can relieve it.

7. No treatment is necessary for **asymptomatic flatfoot,** although arch support is recommended. Should patients with flatfoot become symptomatic, use of flexible arch supports, heel cord stretching, and exercises to strengthen the arch (eg, spreading, flexing and extending toes, and picking up objects with the toes) will usually prove beneficial.

8. **Plantar fasciitis and infracalcaneal bursitis**

   a. Heel lifts, padded heel cups, or orthotic devices may be beneficial, particularly in the presence of foot deformities or abnormal footstrike.

   b. Rest, ice, NSAIDs, and local injections of steroids are used in the acute treatment of plantar fasciitis and infracalcaneal bursitis.

   c. Heel cord stretching is an important preventive measure for plantar fasciitis.

   d. A **dorsal night splint,** designed to maintain ankle dorsiflexion and toe extension, may be beneficial, especially in individuals refractory to the conventional treatments just described.

      e. Release of the plantar fascial bands via an open or endoscopic proce-
      dure is a measure of last resort in refractory cases.
   9. Initial treatment of posterior heel problems involves rest, ice, and use of
   NSAIDs. With **Achilles tendinitis,** immobilization may be required. Steroid
   injections are contraindicated, since such injections may lead to tendon rupture. Surgical referral even for **posterior calcaneal exostoses** is usually not
   required unless the condition becomes chronic. Use of heel lifts or orthotics,
   regular heel cord stretching, avoidance of rigid heel counters, and prophylactic application of ice are usually sufficient to prevent recurrence.

      Should Achilles tendinitis develop while a patient is taking fluoroquinolone
   antibiotics, discontinuation may be necessary, as they have been implicated
   in the development of tendinitis and subsequent tendon rupture.

REFERENCES

Clanton TO, Porter DA: Primary care of foot and ankle injuries in the athlete. Clin Sports Med 1997;**16:**435.

Powell M: Effective treatment of chronic plantar fasciitis with dorsiflexion night splints: A crossover prospective randomized outcome study. Foot Ankle Int 1998;**19:**10.

Wyngarden TM: The painful foot. Part I: Common forefoot deformities. Am Fam Physician 1997; **55:**1866.

Wyngarden TM: The painful foot. Part II: Common rearfoot deformities. Am Fam Physician 1997; **55:**2207.

Zuber TJ, Pfenninger JL: Management of ingrown toenails. Am Fam Physician 1995;**52:**181.

---

31   Fractures

Ted C. Schaffer, MD

  I. Definition. A fracture is a complete or incomplete break in the continuity of a bone.
  II. Common diagnoses
    A. The following conditions should be differentiated from fractures.
      1. A **sprain** is a joint injury to the ligaments that attach to a bone.
      2. A **strain** is an injury to the musculotendinous unit that attaches to a bone.
      3. A **contusion** is an injury to the soft tissue surrounding the bone.
      4. A **dislocation** is the complete loss of continuity between two articular surfaces.
      5. A **subluxation** is a partial loss of continuity between opposing articular
      surfaces.
    B. The **Salter-Harris classification** of pediatric fractures should be understood (see
    Figure 31–1).
      1. Salter I fractures through the epiphyseal plate are clinical diagnoses. The
      prognosis is excellent.
      2. Salter II fractures through the metaphysis are also stable injuries.
      3. Salter III and IV fractures, which involve the epiphysis, and Salter V fractures,
      which are crush injuries to the growth plates, are more serious problems, es-
      pecially when involving the long bones of the body.
  III. Epidemiology. Fractures can occur at any time of the year and can involve anyone,
  regardless of age, gender, race, size, or occupation. One percent of family physician
  office visits each year are for the treatment of fractures. Evaluation of musculoskeletal injuries that are potential fractures (eg, sprains or strains) account for 3–5%
  of all office visits.
    A. Infants. As many as 1% of newborns may sustain a fractured clavicle at the time
    of delivery.
    B. Children. The incidence of fractures and other trauma increases during the sum-
    mer months because of the increase in outdoor activity.
    C. Elderly individuals. The incidence of fractures increases during cold or icy
    weather conditions because of the increased risk of falls that may result in fracture.
    Elderly persons with physical ailments such as visual impairment or vertebro-
    basilar insufficiency are particularly vulnerable to falls that may result in fractures.

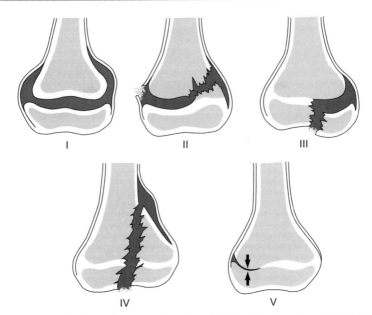

FIGURE 31–1. Salter-Harris classification of epiphyseal injuries in children. (Reproduced, with permission, from Way LW [editor]: *Current Surgical Diagnosis & Treatment.* 9th ed. Originally published by Appleton & Lange; 1991. Copyright © 1991 by the McGraw-Hill Companies, Inc.)

IV. Pathophysiology

A. Impact force. Direct impact to the bone or indirect forces generated around the bone cause most fractures. The greater the forces involved in the injury, the greater is the extent of bone and soft tissue damage.

B. Bone diseases. Abnormalities in bone may lead to pathologic fractures with only minimal trauma.

1. **Bone architecture** may be abnormal. The most common example is osteoporosis (see Chapter 84), a disease in which loss of calcium from bone results in weakening of the bone structure.

2. **Tumors,** either malignant (primary or metastatic) or benign, can cause bone weakness by replacing or destroying bone tissue.

C. Repetitive forces to the bone can lead to cumulative microtrauma, eventually causing a stress fracture.

V. Symptoms

A. Pain is the hallmark of new fracture occurrence. Often, however, the amount of pain experienced by the patient correlates poorly with the amount of bone damage. In children, pain at an epiphyseal plate is usually a Salter I fracture, not a joint sprain, since the growth plate is often the weakest area when a joint is stressed.

B. Loss of motion can occur with fractures, especially when the fracture is located near a joint surface.

C. Loss of function may be noted by the patient, either because of the pain involved or because of soft tissue swelling.

VI. Signs

A. Tenderness to palpation should be present over a new fracture site. If there appears to be radiographic evidence of a fracture but the area is not tender on examination, the diagnosis of a fracture is suspect.

B. Swelling of the area is usually caused by soft tissue injury around the fracture.

C. Deformity may be apparent when the area of injury is inspected. The deformity may appear either as an obvious angulation at the bone or simply as an abnormal manner in which the extremity is being held.

D. Crepitus can sometimes be noted with a displaced fracture.

E. Abnormal mobility may be observed. Motion of the joint above and the joint below the injured area should always be tested to ensure that these adjacent regions are not also affected by the injury.

VII. Laboratory tests

A. An **x-ray** of any suspected fracture must be performed, since this is the method by which most fractures are confirmed. At least two views directed 90 degrees apart are required, since a nondisplaced fracture may not be visible if only a single view is obtained.

Comparison x-rays of the opposite limb should be obtained in children in order to aid the physician in distinguishing a fracture line from a normal epiphyseal growth plate.

B. A **bone scan** is indicated when x-rays are not definitive (eg, in the case of certain wrist fractures) or are negative in the face of clinical evidence for fracture (eg, in the case of a stress fracture of the metatarsal).

VIII. Treatment

A. General principles for the management of a potential fracture are as follows.

1. The physician should assume a fracture has occurred until an x-ray examination has proven otherwise.

2. A **splint** should be applied to the fractured area in order to decrease bone motion and hold the bone in place. This procedure will alleviate pain and prevent further tissue damage.

3. Ice applied immediately for 20–30 minutes will curtail swelling and provide pain relief. The ice should not directly touch the skin. Ice therapy may be repeated at 90-minute intervals.

4. Dislocations or fractures should not be reduced until x-rays have been obtained. The medicolegal assumption will be that unsuspected postreduction fractures have been caused by the reduction unless the fractures were previously documented by x-ray. Reduction before x-ray is advisable when there is evidence of vascular compromise to an extremity that may be relieved by immediate reduction of the dislocation or fracture. Immediate posttraumatic reduction of a dislocation may also be permissible when the patient is having substantial pain and the reduction is easily accomplished, such as an anterior shoulder or a finger dislocation.

B. The following **specific fractures** can be managed in an ambulatory setting.

1. Finger fractures (see Chapter 34).

2. Hand fractures (see Chapter 34).

3. Arm fractures

a. Buckle (torus) fractures of the radius usually occur in children after a fall onto the wrist or hand. X-ray findings may be subtle, showing only a small disruption in the cortex of the distal radius. The patient should wear a short arm cast for 3–4 weeks.

b. Colles' fractures usually occur in elderly patients after falling on an outstretched hand. These fractures involve dorsal displacement of the distal radius and are often accompanied by a fracture of the ulnar styloid. Care must be taken in treating these fractures, since they are sometimes complicated.

(1) First, the fracture must be reduced, which may be difficult and painful for the patient. The physician should have knowledge of acceptable angles of relocation before attempting any reduction.

(2) Careful neurovascular examination should be performed before and after the reduction, since median nerve injury is common.

(3) A long arm cast is applied after the reduction, usually with the wrist placed in mild flexion, pronation, and ulnar deviation.

(4) Patient dissatisfaction with treatment of this fracture is high, and the physician should strongly consider orthopedic referral.

c. Humeral head fractures are common in elderly individuals after falling on an outstretched arm or sustaining a blow to the lateral arm. Eighty percent of proximal humerus fractures are minimally displaced. The shaft of the humerus is often impacted into the humeral head.

(1) Treatment, even if the shaft is impacted, consists of providing the patient with a shoulder sling for 1–2 weeks and, after the sling is removed, providing the patient with range-of-motion exercises. The major risk involved in humeral head fractures is loss of shoulder motion after immobilization.

   (2) Orthopedic referral is needed if the fracture involves displacement >1 cm.

4. Clavicle fractures

   a. Middle third (midclavicular) fractures account for 80% of clavicular fractures and are easily managed. A "figure-of-8" or clavicular strap is worn for 3–6 weeks by children and for 6 weeks by adults. A residual callous is often left, but the fracture usually heals well.

   b. Distal end fractures, which are present in 15% of these cases, can be more complicated than midclavicular fractures. The initial management is the same, but painful acromioclavicular joint arthritis may develop, necessitating resection of the distal clavicle.

   c. Proximal fractures occur in 5% of these cases and should be evaluated carefully. The physician should look for signs of vascular injury due to the close proximity of the great vessels of the neck. Orthopedic consultation should be strongly considered.

5. Simple torso fractures

   a. Rib fractures are common in the elderly with only minor trauma. In young adults and children, they are usually the result of greater traumatic force. A chest x-ray should be obtained to exclude pneumothorax or pulmonary contusion. Rib fractures are easily managed if the bones are not displaced.

   (1) Pain relief is the main focus of treatment. Systemic analgesics such as codeine or nonsteroidal agents are usually adequate, but intercostal nerve blocks can be considered if a patient is in severe pain. Rib belts should be avoided, since they cause substantial atelectasis and increase the incidence of pneumonia.

   (2) Hospitalization should be considered for multiple rib fractures (three or more) because of the increased risk to the patient of pulmonary contusion and atelectasis. In the elderly, even a single rib fracture can occasionally lead to pulmonary compromise.

   b. Lumbar compression fractures are common in elderly patients with osteoporosis and can occur with minimal trauma. They can be seen from the T-4 through L-5 vertebrae, and neurologic compromise is extremely rare. Treatment is aimed at pain relief, with immobilization for a few days followed by ambulation with support.

   c. Undisplaced pelvic fractures are another problem in the elderly, occasionally complicated by blood loss, even where the fractures are minor. Treatment is aimed at pain relief and ambulatory support.

6. Ankle fractures

   a. Fibular fractures **below the tibial dome** are avulsion fractures caused by ligamentous pulling during sudden inversion of the foot. Treatment is a posterior leg splint for 5–7 days until the swelling has subsided, followed by a short leg walking cast for 3–6 weeks. A pneumatic ankle support device may be considered as an alternative to casting. In children, tenderness over the epiphyseal plate of the distal fibula should be regarded as a Salter I fracture, not an ankle sprain. Treatment consists of a short leg walking cast for 3–4 weeks.

   b. When fibular fractures are **at or above the tibial dome,** greater ligamentous instability occurs, because the syndesmotic ligaments and interosseous membrane are involved. Referral is indicated in these cases, since surgery may be required.

7. Foot and toe fractures (see Chapter 30).

C. Special features of **pediatric fractures** are described below.

   1. The time needed for **cast or splint immobilization** for fractures in children is generally one half to one third the time needed for immobilization of an adult fracture, since bone healing occurs much faster in children than in adults.

   2. Growth plate injuries should be managed carefully.

   a. Salter I or II fractures are treated like any other fracture. The fracture is usually immobilized by a cast or splint for several weeks. Long bones usually require a cast, while phalangeal fractures may need only a splint.

    b. Parents of children with growth plate injuries should be advised of the possibility of bone abnormalities with further growth. These abnormalities are quite rare with Salter I and II fractures, except when the fractures are in the distal femur or the proximal tibia.

D. Fractures requiring referral. In an ambulatory setting, the physician must know which bone injuries should be managed by an orthopedist because of the increased risk of complication. The following list serves as a guideline for situations in which consultation is advisable.

    1. Open fractures increase the risk of infection, especially osteomyelitis, and of nonunion of the fracture fragments.

    2. Neurovascular compromise is an orthopedic emergency necessitating immediate care by a qualified surgeon.

    3. Unstable fractures, where bone alignment cannot be maintained without external forces, usually require open reduction and internal fixation.

    4. Intra-articular fractures create a high risk for the development of long-term traumatic arthritis in the patient. Open surgical reduction is often required in order to achieve the best possible bone alignment.

    5. Growth plate injuries of long bones that involve the epiphysis (Salter III, IV, or V fractures) create a high risk of complications, and therefore the patient may require long-term orthopedic management.

REFERENCES

Greenspan A: *Orthopedic Radiology: A Practical Approach.* 2nd ed. Lippincott; 1992.

Letts RM: *Management of Pediatric Fractures.* Churchill Livingstone; 1994.

Rockwood C, Green D, Bucholz R, et al (editors): *Fractures in Adults.* 4th ed. Lippincott-Raven; 1996.

Rockwood C, Wilkins K, Beaty J (editors): *Fractures in Children.* 4th ed. Lippincott-Raven; 1996.

Safran MR, McKeag DB, Van Camp SP (editors): *Manual of Sports Medicine.* Lippincott-Raven; 1998.

---

32   Gastrointestinal Bleeding

Jim L. Wilson, MD, & Mark A. Landis, MD

I. Definition. Blood loss from any part of the gastrointestinal (GI) tract constitutes GI bleeding.

II. Common diagnoses. The most common diagnoses of GI bleeding in the ambulatory care setting are described below.

    A. Upper GI bleeding makes up about 25% of GI bleeds.

        1. Peptic ulcers account for 51–62% of upper GI hemorrhages. Duodenal ulcers account for about 31–36% of bleeds, and gastric ulcers account for 20–24%.

        2. Mucosal erosions and gastritis account for about 14% of upper GI bleeding.

        3. Esophageal varices compose 6–11% of upper GI bleeding and result in the highest rate of mortality.

        4. Acute lacerations of gastroesophageal mucosa (Mallory-Weiss tears) occur in 3.5–7.2% of upper GI bleeding.

    B. Lower GI bleeding accounts for 75% of GI bleeds.

        1. Diverticulosis causes about 30–40% of lower GI bleeds.

        2. Inflammatory bowel disease accounts for 21% of lower GI bleeds.

        3. Neoplasms (eg, carcinoma of the colon or polyps) usually produce mild, occult blood loss with intermittent episodes of acute bleeding. They account for about 14% of lower GI bleeds.

        4. Arteriovenous malformations (angiodysplasia) cause about 2% of lower GI bleeding.

        5. Benign disease such as hemorrhoids, fissures, and fistulas makes up 11% of lower GI bleeding.

III. Epidemiology. Two recent studies estimate that 250,000–350,000 cases of upper GI bleeding require hospitalization yearly in the United States. Mass screening of asymptomatic populations has detected occult bleeding in 2–8% of those persons tested.

A. A worldwide geographic variation in the occurrence of **peptic ulcer disease** has been shown. Possible explanations include genetic differences, environmental factors, and diet. Risk factors include cigarette smoking and emotional stress.

B. Aspirin and other nonsteroidal anti-inflammatory drugs (NSAIDs) have been implicated as risk factors for **acute hemorrhagic gastritis** as well as **peptic ulcer disease.** Recent studies suggest that the overall increased risk of upper GI bleeding from NSAIDs is small. Elderly patients have a higher risk than other age groups for NSAID-induced upper GI bleeding.

C. Chronic, excessive alcohol ingestion may cause cirrhosis of the liver, which leads to **esophageal varices** up to 90% of the time. This is caused by portal hypertension.

D. Acute alcohol ingestion has been noted in a majority of patients with **Mallory-Weiss tears.**

E. A low-fiber diet is thought to be the single most important risk factor for the development of **diverticular disease** of the colon, which increases in frequency after age 50.

F. **Angiodysplasia** is estimated to occur in up to 30% of individuals over the age of 50. The incidence is equally common in both sexes. Most of the lesions are found in the right colon, especially in the cecum.

G. The incidence of **colorectal carcinomas** increases after age 50 and declines after age 75, peaking in the sixth and seventh decades. Recent statistics indicate that 140,000 new cases are diagnosed (70% in the colon and 30% in the rectum) and 60,000 deaths occur yearly. Significant risk factors for colorectal carcinoma include high-fat, low-fiber diets; hereditary polyps; and inflammatory bowel disease.

IV. **Pathophysiology** of GI bleeding depends on the type and location of the bleeding lesion.

A. Bleeding in **peptic ulcer disease** occurs from a break in the mucosa that extends through the muscularis layer. Acute and chronic inflammatory cells surround the ulcer crater. When the ulcer erodes into a blood vessel, bleeding occurs.

B. Diffuse, superficial mucosal lesions are the source of bleeding in **gastritis.** It is caused by local irritants, *Helicobacter pylori,* NSAIDs, and alcohol ingestion. NSAIDs work by inhibiting cyclooxygenase and therefore stop production of prostaglandins, which are protective.

C. In **esophageal varices,** bleeding occurs when the vessel ruptures because of increased pressure and increased size of the vessel.

D. Mucosal lacerations such as **Mallory-Weiss tears** are caused by mechanical forces, often brought about by severe retching.

E. **Diverticular bleeding** occurs when vasae rectae are displaced as the diverticulum enlarges. These are vessels that penetrate the muscularis layer to supply the mucosa.

F. The vascular lesions found in **angiodysplasia** are arteriovenous malformations considered to be caused by degenerative aging processes.

V. **Symptoms.** In a significant percentage of cases, GI bleeding produces no symptoms and is detected only during routine examination for fecal occult blood.

A. **Symptoms of significant GI blood loss** include weakness, lightheadedness, faintness, syncope, palpitations, sweating, clammy skin, nausea, vomiting, thirst, anxiety, and acute cardiovascular collapse (shock). GI bleeding may be accompanied by any of the following symptoms: indigestion, dysphagia, retching, abdominal pain, weight loss, and a change in bowel habits.

B. **Hematemesis** (vomiting of blood that may be either bright red or dark like coffee grounds) and **melena** (tarry black, foul-smelling, sticky stools characteristic of digested blood) usually are caused by upper GI bleeding (ie, bleeding above the ligament of Treitz). Note that bleeding from the nose and oropharynx should initially be included in the differential.

C. **Hematochezia** refers to the passage of bright red blood from the rectum and is usually associated with lower GI bleeding (ie, bleeding below the level of the ligament of Treitz). It can, however, come from brisk, upper GI bleeding in up to 10% of cases.

VI. **Signs**

A. **Vital signs.** Loss of 1 L or more of blood over 15–30 minutes will produce a pulse rate of 100 beats per minute or more and a systolic blood pressure of 100 mm Hg or less. A decrease in systolic blood pressure of 10 mm Hg or more and a heart rate increase of 20 beats per minute or more when the patient changes from a supine to a sitting position are also signs of significant blood loss.

B. When acute blood loss (ie, >2000 mL) occurs, signs of hypovolemic shock develop, including a systolic blood pressure of 80 mm Hg or less, pallor, cyanosis, and cool, clammy skin.

C. Physical examination. In addition to changes in vital signs, pertinent findings include the following.

   1. Skin. Telangiectasias and jaundice suggest cirrhosis of the liver, which may cause esophageal varices.

   2. Cardiovascular. Evidence of congestive heart failure (eg, rales or gallop) and systolic flow murmurs (as in anemia) may be a result of acute or chronic blood loss.

   3. Abdomen

   a. Epigastric pain on palpation suggests peptic ulcer disease.

   b. Hyperactive bowel sounds may indicate blood in the intestinal tract.

   c. Rigidity suggests peritoneal irritation from intra-abdominal blood resulting from a perforated ulcer.

   d. Hypoactive bowel sounds and distention may be caused by intestinal obstruction from a problem such as carcinoma of the colon. Masses may indicate colonic neoplasm or diverticular disease.

   4. Rectal examination

   a. Rectal carcinoma may be detected as a mass upon digital examination of the rectum.

   b. Melena usually signifies upper GI bleeding of any type.

   c. Bright red blood suggests lower GI bleeding and may be a result of hemorrhoids, fissures, diverticular disease, carcinoma, or angiodysplasia.

VII. Laboratory tests. The objectives of laboratory tests are to estimate the volume of blood loss and to determine the site(s) and cause(s) of bleeding.

A. Patients suspected of having GI bleeding should have a test for **fecal occult blood** to confirm the diagnosis. All persons over age 50 should be tested for fecal occult blood to screen for colorectal neoplasm. Multiple (at least three) samples should be obtained when intermittent bleeding is suspected. (For further discussion of screening tests, see Chapter 108.)

B. The following **blood tests** should be performed initially and monitored as necessary.

   1. Hemoglobin, hematocrit, or both.

   2. Prothrombin time, partial thromboplastin time, bilirubin, and ammonia level are useful when liver disease (eg, cirrhosis secondary to chronic ethanol ingestion) is suspected.

   3. Blood urea nitrogen (BUN) may be elevated in upper GI bleeding because of digested blood in the intestinal tract. A BUN/creatinine ratio >36 suggests an upper tract source.

C. If upper GI bleeding is suspected, a **nasogastric tube** should be passed initially for diagnostic purposes. A grossly bloody aspirate confirms the source of bleeding in the upper GI tract, but a grossly negative aspirate does not rule out the possibility of bleeding from that source.

D. In acute upper GI bleeding, **esophagogastroduodenoscopy (EGD)** is the most sensitive way of making a diagnosis. Best results are obtained if the procedure is performed in the first 12–24 hours of an episode of severe upper GI bleeding. Endoscopy can also be used in successful therapy of an acute upper GI bleed.

E. Flexible rectosigmoidoscopy. This procedure is most useful for screening or case finding in colorectal cancer or other causes of lower GI bleeding. Sixty-centimeter sigmoidoscopes offer greater sensitivity in detection of neoplasms than do 35-cm sigmoidoscopes.

F. Colonoscopy allows visualization of the lower GI mucosa and localization of the bleeding site. Forty percent of cases of rectal bleeding with previously normal sigmoidoscopy and barium enema results show an undetected lesion with colonoscopy. Profuse bleeding may preclude identification of the lesion. In some cases, it allows for treatment by coagulation.

G. Barium enemas are rarely useful in GI bleeding, as they are imprecise for this problem. They have no therapeutic benefit and may compromise other tests such as endoscopy or angiography. They are not generally recommended.

H. Arteriography should be considered when endoscopy cannot be performed because of massive bleeding. Total blood loss must be 0.5–1.5 mL/min in order to be detected. The use of this technique as a route of embolization of a bleeding lesion is an added advantage.

I. Nuclear medicine scans. Although these scans (technetium 99m [^{99m}Tc]) may not detect the precise location of bleeding, they are capable of demonstrating intermittent or low rates of bleeding and are useful screening tests prior to arteriography.

VIII. Treatment. In 70% of the cases, GI bleeding stops spontaneously, and the patient can be managed with general supportive measures and medication. Surgical intervention is not necessary.

A. Patients with **severe bleeding** (ie, tachycardia, hypotension, postural changes, or shock) require hospitalization for stabilization, diagnostic evaluation, parenteral volume replacement, and surgical consultation.

B. Patients with **mild bleeding** and stable vital signs can be managed as outpatients. Exceptions to this might include the elderly, those with a low initial hematocrit, and those with a coagulopathy. In some cases, early endoscopy may help with risk stratification and lead to fewer or shorter hospital admissions.

C. For discussion of the management of dyspepsia and peptic ulcer disease, see Chapters 22 and 86, respectively.

D. Oral iron therapy (ferrous sulfate), 325 mg three times daily, is useful to compensate for iron deficiency after the cause of bleeding has been detected.

E. Preventing the recurrence of GI bleeding should be a major treatment goal. Reduction of risk factors (eg, avoiding alcohol and cigarettes, modifying the diet, and reducing stress) is important in the overall management of patients. Patients with large varices should be placed on β-adrenergic blockers or long-acting nitrates long term.

REFERENCES

Billingham RP: The conundrum of lower gastrointestinal bleeding. Surg Clin North Am 1997;**77:** 241.

Grace ND: Diagnosis and treatment of gastrointestinal bleeding secondary to portal hypertension. Am J Gastroenterol 1997:**92:**1081.

McGuirk TD, Coyle WJ: Upper gastrointestinal tract bleeding. Emerg Med Clin North Am 1996; **14:**523.

Terdiman JP: Update on upper gastrointestinal bleeding. Basing treatment decisions on patients' risk level. Postgrad Med 1998;**103**(6):43.

Vernava AM III, Moore BA, Longo WE, et al: Lower gastrointestinal bleeding. Dis Colon Rectum 1997;**40**(7):846.

---

33   Genital Lesions

Tomás P. Owens Jr., MD

I. Definition. Genital lesions are any acquired abnormality of the external genitalia.

II. Common diagnoses
   A. Ulcerative lesions
   1. **Herpes simplex virus types 1 and 2** (HSV-1 and -2).
   2. **Primary syphilis** (chancre).
   3. **Chancroid.**
   B. Verrucoid/papillomatous lesions
   1. **Condylomata acuminata.**
   2. **Secondary syphilis** (condyloma latum).
   3. **Molluscum contagiosum.**
   4. **Pearly penile papules.**
   C. Pruritic lesions
   1. **Balanitis.**
   2. **Erythrasma.**

   3. *Phthirus pubis* (pubic lice).
   4. **Vulvar dystrophy.**
   D. **Cystic lesions**
      1. **Bartholin's gland cysts or inflammation.**
      2. **Spermatocele/epididymal cyst/varicocele.**
         Other causes of genital lesions discussed elsewhere include psoriasis, seborrheic dermatitis, scabies, tinea cruris, allergic/contact dermatitis (see Chapter 17); testicular torsion, epididymo-orchitis (see Chapter 3); folliculitis (see Chapter 11); urethritis (see Chapter 64), vaginitis, cervicitis, and chlamydia (see Chapters 24, 55, and 67). Causes of genital lesions not discussed here because of their relative rarity include penile cancer, bowenoid papulosis of the penis/vulvar epithelial neoplasia, testicular cancer, lymphogranuloma venereum, granuloma inguinale, lichen planus, fixed drug eruption, erythroplasia of Queyrat, Peyronie's disease, penile/vulvar trauma, penile prostheses, and priapism.
III. **Epidemiology.** The 1995 National Ambulatory Medical Care Survey describes diseases of the skin and subcutaneous tissue as being the principal diagnosis in 4.7% of all office visits and diseases of the genitourinary system as 5.5% of all office visits.
   A. **Ulcerative lesions**
      1. The presence of antibodies to **HSV-2** varies from 3% in nuns to 70–80% in prostitutes and seems to be directly proportional to sexual activity. **HSV-1,** which is present in 90% of the population, can cause genital herpes although much less frequently than **HSV-2.** Herpes is generally self-limited, with recurrences decreasing over the years.
      2. The United States has shown a steady decline in the number of cases reported since 1991. The incidence of primary and secondary syphilis dipped to a total of 11,387 cases (4.3 per 100,000) in 1996, but the incidence remains high among non-Hispanic blacks and in the South.
      3. **Chancroid** has declined steadily since 1987 to a total of 386 cases in 1996, 88% of which occurred in five states (Illinois, Louisiana, New York, North Carolina, and Texas). Occasional discrete outbreaks occur, commonly associated with the influx of Central American, Caribbean, and Southeast Asian immigrants. Underreporting is common because of the diagnostic difficulty. As many as 10% of patients with chancroid may be coinfected with *Treponema pallidum* or HSV. The disease has an important role in the transmission of the human immunodeficiency virus (HIV), primarily among heterosexuals.
   B. **Verrucoid/papillomatous lesions**
      1. **Condylomata** constitute only one of the expressions of human papillomavirus (HPV), which is now the most common sexually transmitted entity. Condylomata can also cause cervical and vulvar dysplasia. Condylomata are most common during the reproductive years and are commonly associated with other sexually transmitted diseases (STDs). Condylomata may grow dramatically with pregnancy, HIV, or corticosteroid use.
      2. **Secondary syphilis** occurs 6–24 weeks after untreated primary syphilis and is extremely contagious.
      3. **Molluscum contagiosum** is common in children. Genital lesions are associated with sexual transmission. HIV infection is associated with an increased number and size of lesions.
      4. **Pearly penile papules** first appear around puberty and are present in up to 30% of men. There are no known predisposing risk factors.
   C. **Pruritic lesions**
      1. **Balanitis** tends to occur in the uncircumcised, diabetics, those with poor hygiene, and those with phimosis. Chronic balanitis is a potential precursor of premalignant penile glanular changes and is a major indication for adult circumcision.
      2. **Erythrasma** occurs more often in obese dark-skinned men.
      3. *Phthirus pubis* (pubic lice) occurs most commonly in young adults, is very contagious, and is transmitted sexually or by sharing clothing, towels, or bed linens.
      4. **Vulvar atrophy/lichen sclerosus et atrophicus** is a common process in postmenopausal women but is seen in all age groups. In men, it is called bal-

anitis xerotica obliterans. Hyperplastic dystrophy and leukoplakia are less common and considered premalignant; vulvar carcinoma is uncommon.

D. Cystic lesions

1. **Bartholin's duct cysts** and abscesses account for 2% of all new patients in a gynecologic practice. These lesions are more common after menarche and before menopause; they are unrelated to STDs.

2. **Varicoceles, spermatoceles,** and **epididymal cysts** are relatively common benign processes. Varicoceles are more common in young men.

IV. Pathophysiology

A. Ulcerative lesions

1. Primary infection with either HSV-1 or HSV-2 can be associated with viremia. Direct local inflammatory changes and cytolysis account for most of the syndrome in recurrences. Transmission occurs by direct contact with secretions or lesions. The incubation period is 2–14 days. Maximal viral shedding occurs within 24 hours of the appearance of lesions and diminishes by the fifth day; nevertheless, viral shedding occurs intermittently in the absence of any signs in many persons.

2. Primary infection with *T pallidum* produces a **chancre** at the site of inoculation 10–90 days after direct contact with secretions of an infected person.

3. **Chancroid** is a highly contagious disease caused by *Haemophilus ducreyi,* a gram-negative coccobacillary organism. Transmission occurs from 10 days before the onset of symptoms through the convalescent period.

B. Verrucoid/papillomatous lesions

1. **Condylomata acuminata** is caused by HPV, with an incubation period from weeks to years. Warts are commonly associated with serotypes 6 and 11 and can disappear spontaneously in 6–12 months, but may persist with immunosuppression or corticosteroid intake. Recurrences are common during the first few years after infection or after immunologic strain (eg, viral illness, malignancy, or HIV). It can be transmitted sexually or not sexually.

2. **Secondary syphilis** appears 2–10 weeks after the chancre or, rarely, synchronously with the primary syphilitic lesion.

3. **Molluscum contagiosum** is caused by a poxvirus and is transmitted by close physical contact (commonly in children at day care or school). Lesions develop slowly over a 2- to 3-month period; when genital lesions are present, sexual transmission is likely.

4. **Pearly penile papules** histologically are angiofibromas.

C. Pruritic lesions

1. **Balanitis** is usually caused by irritation due to smegma or superimposed infection with *Candida* species. It can be precipitated by contact irritants. When it includes the foreskin, it is known as **balanoposthitis.** In uncircumcised males, a complication of balanitis is phimosis, a contraction of the distal foreskin over the glans. Paraphimosis can occur if the foreskin has been retracted, constricting the glans and causing ischemia.

2. **Erythrasma** is a chronic bacterial infection caused by *Corynebacterium minutissimum.*

3. Pubic lice ("crabs") is caused by *Phthirus pubis* and occurs only in humans. This louse prefers moist environments, seldom goes into neighboring skin, and has been described rarely on facial hair.

4. **Vulvar dystrophy** has been postulated to be an autoimmune, metabolic, and, more recently, infectious process (ie, *Borrelia burgdorferi*). Inflammation is definitely a feature.

D. Cystic lesions

1. Cystic lesions develop when **Bartholin's glands** located on either side of the lower vaginal vestibule become obstructed with detritus. When the lesions are infected, organisms include staphylococci, streptococci, coliforms, and anaerobes.

2. A **spermatocele** is a cyst containing sperm. **Epididymal cysts** arise from either the globus major or the globus minor of the epididymis and also contain sperm. A **varicocele** is a dilated plexus of the scrotal veins (pampiniform plexus).

V. Symptoms
A. Ulcerative lesions
1. **HSV-1 or -2.**
   a. Primary infection may manifest as fever, generalized myalgia, malaise, headaches, and weakness, peaking 3–4 days after the onset of lesions. Painful inguinal or deep pelvic lymphadenopathy arises 2–3 weeks later. Burning pain and pruritus along with vaginal or urethral discharge and dysuria are common.
   b. Recurrent infection rarely causes systemic symptoms. There is a prodrome of burning, lancinating pain 1–2 days before eruption.
2. **Chancres** are painless, unless secondarily infected. Patients present for evaluation of the lesion or for accompanying lymphadenopathy.
3. Patients with **chancroid** present with pain at the lesion and in surrounding tissue and with inguinal lymphadenitis.

B. Verrucoid/papillomatous lesions
1. **Condylomata acuminata** are painless. Rarely, a patient may complain of hematuria from a urethral condyloma.
2. **Condyloma lata** are painless lesions, although generalized myalgia, fever, chills, and arthralgia may occur in the early phase of eruption.
3. Patients with **molluscum contagiosum** rarely present with pruritus.
4. **Pearly penile papules** are asymptomatic but worrisome to some patients.

C. Pruritic lesions
1. **Balanitis** is associated with pruritus and burning pain on or after sexual intercourse or with excessive smegma production. Dysuria and more severe pain occur with more severe disease.
2. Pruritus and longstanding rash persisting after fungicidal therapy are common presentations for **erythrasma.**
3. ***Phthirus pubis*** infestation manifests as pruritus, rarely severe. Some patients describe nits on their pubic hair.
4. Patients with **vulvar dystrophy** present with varying degrees of pruritus and concerns about the lesion's appearance.

D. Cystic lesions
1. Small **Bartholin's gland cysts** are usually asymptomatic. Larger lesions cause discomfort, pruritus, and sometimes dyspareunia. As the lesions become infected, there is pain, at times very severe, external dysuria, and vulvar discharge. Systemic symptoms are rare.
2. **Spermatoceles** and **epididymal cysts** are usually painless scrotal masses. **Varicoceles** are almost always asymptomatic, but they may cause infertility, which may be the presenting complaint. Rarely, fullness or mild discomfort is present, commonly with abstinence. Sexual activity with a partner or masturbation may improve symptoms.

VI. Signs
A. Ulcerative lesions
1. **HSV-1 or -2** initially is an erythematous papule, which is followed hours to a few days later by small, grouped vesicles on the glans, on the distal and sometimes proximal shaft of the penis, or on the scrotum in males. The entire vulva can be involved. Pustules, erosions, or ulceration occur, which heal by crusting in 2–4 weeks, leaving some hypomelanosis or hypermelanosis. Scarring occurs only with manipulation or secondary infection. **Primary infection** produces larger numbers of lesions than **recurrent infection.**
2. The **chancre** is a papule that erodes into a single, round, beefy-red ulcer with hard, raised borders and yellow-green exudative material on its base. Chancres occur in the inside penile foreskin, coronal sulcus, shaft, or base, or on the cervix and vagina (where patients seldom detect it), vulva, or clitoris. Extragenital sites for chancres are the mouth, lips, breast, fingers, and thighs. Multiple chancres can be seen in HIV infection.
3. **Chancroid** is a tender papule that erodes into single or multiple round, oval, or serpiginous ulcers with sharp, flat, nonindurated borders. Ulcers can become confluent and large. Distribution of lesions is similar to that of chancre.

B. Verrucoid/papillomatous lesions
1. **Condylomata acuminata** are skin-colored or pink-red tumors, which are localized, fleshy, soft, moist, elongated, and dome-shaped with filiform or con-

ical vegetating projections in grape- to cauliflower-like clusters on moist surfaces. They can be keratotic and smooth papular warts in dry surfaces or subclinical "flat" warts. Large lesions occur perianally in immunosuppressed persons.

2. **Condylomata lata** are soft, flat-topped, moist, skin-colored or pale pink papules, warts, nodules, or plaques, which may become confluent. These lesions occur in any body surface, but have a preference for the anogenital area and intertriginous sites.

3. **Molluscum contagiosum** presents as pearly white papules or nodules 2–8 mm in diameter, which are mostly round or oval with a classic umbilicated top. The papules are localized in clusters, with preference for the genital area, neck, and trunk and may evolve to pustules and small crusts or plaques. Large size or large number of lesions, particularly in the face, suggests HIV.

4. **Pearly penile papules** are thin, conical, white, or pale pink uniformly sized groups of papules, forming multiple parallel lines mostly on the corona, but also in the balanoprepucial sulcus.

C. Pruritic lesions

1. Erythema, excess amounts of smegma, and flat white-gray "empty" or erythematous papules suggest **balanitis;** erosions and fine scaling sometimes associated with marked edema of the prepuce suggest **balanoposthitis.** **Phimosis** may be present, revealing only edema of the foreskin and obstructing the view of the glans.

2. An erythematous to brownish-red plaque with sharp borders and minimal scaling located on the inner thigh extending into the scrotum or vulva suggests **erythrasma.**

3. Minuscule white-gray nits are seen attached to hair shafts, and brownish-gray lice of similar size (1–2 mm) are seen on the perifollicular skin in *Phthirus pubis* infestation. Papules, lichenification, and excoriations from scratching can be seen.

4. **Vulvar dystrophy** varies from nonspecific thinned skin, to multiple flat, irregular pearly/ivory white or pink/reddish (less common) papules or macules in multiple sites. They may eventually coalesce into white plaques involving the entire perineum. Kraurosis vulvae (atrophy and shriveling of the skin or mucous membranes) with hypomelanosis, telangiectasias, and a "keyhole" vaginal opening is an old, now abandoned gynecologic term for the final outcome of this process.

D. Cystic lesions

1. A rubbery, soft, renitent bulge in the inner aspect of the lower vaginal vestibule (outside of the introitus) suggests **Bartholin's gland cyst;** if infected, the cyst is red and extremely tender.

2. **Spermatocele/cystocele** is a painless, cystic, or, rarely, firm mass that transilluminates just above and posterior to the testicle; it is commonly not noticed by the patient and found incidentally during examination. A **varicocele** is a "bag of worms" in the scrotal sac formed by hundreds of dilated tortuous vessels in the pampiniform plexus posterior and superior to the testis; it is mildly tender. The size of a varicocele increases with the Valsalva's maneuver and decreases with the supine position. Testicular atrophy may be present. Unilateral dilatation in an older man, which has occurred rapidly or doesn't abate with recumbency, suggests a malignancy obstructing the renal vein.

VII. Laboratory tests

A. Ulcerative lesions.
Testing for chlamydia, gonorrhea, and HIV (with adequate counseling) should be considered in persons with primary HSV-1 or -2, syphilis, or chancroid. In addition, testing for syphilis is recommended in those with primary HSV-1 or -2.

1. Laboratory studies are rarely necessary in HSV-1 or -2; they are reserved for situations in which the diagnosis is not clear and certainty is imperative, such as a primary infection soon before parturition or when strict confirmation is necessary for medicolegal cases.

   a. In the **Tzanck test,** a vesicle is unroofed and its fluid is smeared on a slide, dried, and stained with Giemsa or Wright's stain. Presence of giant multinucleated acanthocytes is considered a positive test result for **herpesviridae** (simplex or zoster).

      b. Viral culture is expensive and must incubate 7 days before being read. Positive cultures can occur in persons with nonherpetic lesions who shed the herpesvirus regularly.

      c. Microscopic pathology and **electron microscopy** can be used, although this is rarely necessary.

2. Primary syphilis

      a. Dark-field microscopic examination of the lesion's secretions is diagnostic but rarely available to the clinician. It reveals treponemes contracting and kinking, but these may not be seen if the chancre has been treated with topical antibiotics.

      b. Rapid plasma reagin (RPR) and VDRL tests, the nontreponemal tests, turn positive 1 week after the appearance of the chancre. These tests become negative up to 1 year after treatment, but may remain positive for life at a low titer in a small percentage of patients.

      c. Confirmatory treponemal tests such as the **fluorescent treponemal antibody-absorption** (FTA-ABS) or *T pallidum* **hemagglutination assay** (TPHA) may take 2 weeks to become positive. Treponemal tests remain weakly positive for life.

3. The diagnosis of **chancroid** is clinical and based on excluding other ulcerative processes such as syphilis. A repeat RPR performed 1 week after identification of the lesion is more reliable in ruling out syphilis. **Gram's stain** for coccobacillary clusters is unreliable, and **culture** is difficult and expensive.

B. Verrucoid/papillomatous lesions. Testing for chlamydia, gonorrhea, and HIV (with adequate counseling, including safe-sex information) should be considered in persons with condylomata acuminata, condyloma lata, or molluscum contagiosum. In addition, testing for syphilis is recommended in those with condylomata acuminata.

    1. The diagnosis of **condylomata acuminata** is clinical.

      a. Occasionally, a **biopsy** confirms the diagnosis.

      b. Subclinical lesions can be soaked with **5% acetic acid** (white vinegar) for 5 minutes, resulting in white epithelium that can be observed with a colposcope or magnifying glass of 4–10× magnification. White papules may be noted, although other changes such as mosaicism and punctation are possible.

    2. RPR and VDRL are always positive when **condyloma lata** are present. FTA confirmation is warranted.

    3. Sticking a needle through a lesion releases the semisolid core of **molluscum contagiosum,** which is considered diagnostic. Microscopic observation reveals inclusion "molluscum" bodies or Lipschütz cells.

    4. No laboratory is necessary to diagnose **pearly penile papules.** A biopsy reveals an angiofibroma.

C. Pruritic lesions

    1. Balanitis is a clinical diagnosis; however, biopsy of any associated glanular mass is needed.

    2. Wood's lamp examination shows a classic coral-red fluorescence in **erythrasma.** Scraping of the lesions may show gram-positive rods and do not show hyphae.

    3. Lice and nits can be observed microscopically in *Phthirus pubis* infestation. Testing for chlamydia, gonorrhea, syphilis, and HIV (with adequate counseling) should be considered in those who were infested by direct sexual contact.

    4. Biopsy is necessary in **vulvar dystrophy** to distinguish lichen sclerosus from leukoplakia, vitiligo, lichen planus, or carcinoma.

D. Cystic lesions

    1. Diagnosis of **Bartholin's gland cyst** is clinical. Cultures should be considered only when cellulitis is present.

    2. Diagnosis of **spermatocele/varicocele/epididymal cysts** is clinical.

      a. Transillumination or aspiration to confirm the presence of fluid differentiates epididymal cysts/spermatoceles from rare solid malignant tumors.

      b. Surgical exploration is sometimes warranted if a spermatocele has been growing rapidly or is located in such a position that a testicular mass cannot be ruled out.

      c. Ultrasonography is rarely used.

VIII. Treatment
  A. Ulcerative lesions
   1. Therapy does not eradicate **HSV-1 or -2** nor does it affect the severity or rate of recurrences after discontinuation. Significant clinical improvement is seen when therapy is started promptly after onset of symptoms.
     a. **For primary infection:** acyclovir 400 mg or famciclovir 250 mg po three times per day *or* valacyclovir 1 g po twice a day for 7–10 days; it is unclear whether higher doses (eg, acyclovir 400 mg five times per day) are warranted for stomatitis, pharyngitis, or proctitis.
     b. **Recurrent infection**
        (1) At onset: acyclovir 200 mg five times per day or 400 mg tid or 800 mg po bid for 5 days *or* famciclovir 125 mg or valacyclovir 500 mg po bid for 5 days.
        (2) Suppressive therapy: acyclovir 400 mg or famciclovir 250 mg bid for 1 year *or* valacyclovir 500 mg or 1 g po once a day, with consideration of a drug-free period at that point to assess the need for continued therapy.
     c. Counseling regarding potential for recurrence, amelioration of symptoms over the years, transmission in the absence of lesions, and the need for condom use is important.
   2. **Primary syphilis** is treated with benzathine penicillin G, 2.4 million U intramuscularly in a single dose. Persons who are allergic to penicillin should receive doxycycline 100 mg orally bid for 2 weeks.
   3. Persons with **chancroid** should be treated with azithromycin 1 g orally in a single dose *or* ceftriaxone 250 mg intramuscularly in a single dose *or* erythromycin base 500 mg orally qid for 7 days *or* ciprofloxacin 500 mg po bid for 3 days. Ciprofloxacin should not be given to children or pregnant patients. There has been intermediate resistance to ciprofloxacin and erythromycin worldwide.
  B. Verrucoid/papillomatous lesions
   1. **Condylomata acuminata** resolve spontaneously in 6–15 months, except in immunocompromised persons. Most clinicians treat to avoid persistent growth. Treatment removes only the wart and does not eliminate the virus, which could remain for months to years. Recurrences are common during the first year, even after adequate removal. An additional Papanicolaou smear is recommended in women at the time of diagnosis with warts.
     a. Most effective therapies include the following.
        (1) **Cryotherapy** with liquid nitrogen. The cryotherapy probe, spray "gun," or cotton-tipped applicator is applied until blanching occurs no more than 1 mm around the perimeter of the lesions, which fall off in 24–72 hours, leaving a shallow ulcer.
        (2) **Trichloroacetic acid** or **bichloroacetic acid** 80–90% can be applied, only to warts, and turns them white in seconds. Lesions should be powdered with talc or sodium bicarbonate immediately to remove unreacted acid. Treatment can be repeated weekly as necessary.
        (3) **Imiquimod** (Aldara) 5% cream is applied by the patient's finger on each lesion at bedtime and washed off in the morning, three times a week for as long as 16 weeks.
        (4) **Podophyllin,** 10–25%, in compound tincture of benzoin applied to warts. The total amount applied per session should be limited to 0.5 mL or less than 10 cm^2 to avoid systemic toxicity; medication should be washed off in 4 hours. Treatment may be repeated weekly and is contraindicated in pregnancy.
        (5) **Podofilox** (Condilox), 0.5% solution, for self-treatment is applied twice daily for 3 days followed by 4 days of no therapy. Treatment can be repeated up to four cycles and is contraindicated in pregnancy. The health care provider should teach the patient which lesions to treat and how to apply the drug.
        (6) **Electrodesiccation** or **electrocautery** is contraindicated in patients with anal lesions or with a pacemaker.
        (7) **Surgical tangential shave/scissor excision** or **curettage.**

      b. Alternative therapies include the following.

          (1) Carbon dioxide laser is necessary only with warts that are very extensive or very resistant to other therapies.

          (2) Interferon alpha-2b (Intron-A) can be injected on the base of lesions three times per week for 3 weeks and repeated as needed. This drug is extremely expensive, and its use should be restricted to extremely recalcitrant cases.

    2. Treatment of **secondary syphilis** is similar to that of primary syphilis.

    3. Spontaneous remission of **molluscum contagiosum** occurs in weeks to several months. **Cryotherapy, curettage,** or **electrocautery** can be done.

    4. Reassurance is all that is necessary with **pearly penile papules.**

C. Pruritic lesions

    1. Balanitis

      a. The foreskin should be kept retracted as much as possible.

      b. The glans should be dried thoroughly after showering and micturition.

      c. Candidiasis should be treated with an **imidazole** cream (ketoconazole, butoconazole, clotrimazole, econazole, miconazole, isoconazole, tioconazole, or terconazole), ciclopirox, or **nystatin** cream, topically twice daily, *or* fluconazole 150 mg po in a single dose. Ketoconazole and itraconazole might be as effective but have a higher potential for toxicity. Terbinafine should not be used as a primary agent for *Candida*.

      d. The glans and prepuce should be washed with soap and water and dried thoroughly after sexual intercourse.

      e. Circumcision may be needed in resistant cases or if phimosis develops.

    2. Povidone-iodine soap cleansing can be sufficient for **erythrasma. Econazole** cream twice daily for 7–10 days or **erythromycin base** 250 mg orally qid for 14 days is also effective.

    3. Lindane 1% shampoo applied for 4 minutes *or* **permethrin** 1% creme rinse or **pyrethrins with piperonyl butoxide** applied for 10 minutes and then thoroughly washed off are effective treatments for **pubic lice.** Lindane should be avoided in children and during gestation and lactation. **Permethrin** has less potential for toxicity than lindane.

    4. Vulvar dystrophy

      a. When biopsy reveals intraepithelial neoplasia, either **laser therapy** or conventional **surgical excision** is indicated.

      b. In lichen sclerosus **topical testosterone** is no longer recommended. Highly potent **topical steroids** (eg, clobetasol 0.05% should be carefully rubbed on the lesion bid for 1 month and then once daily for 2–3 weeks) followed by lower-potency steroids (triamcinolone acetonide 0.1% or betamethasone valerate 0.1%) bid for a few weeks. Leukoplakia requires close follow-up; 5-fluorouracil topically is often used instead.

D. Cystic lesions

    1. Bartholin's gland cysts/inflammation

      a. Hot, wet dressings or sitz baths may promote spontaneous drainage of cysts.

      b. Incision and drainage are effective in most abscesses.

      c. Marsupialization is recommended for recurrences.

      d. Antibiotic therapy is not necessary unless there is associated cellulitis.

    2. Spermatoceles/varicoceles/epididymal cysts

      a. No treatment is necessary for **epididymal cysts** or **spermatoceles** unless large and uncomfortable, in which case surgical resection is recommended.

      b. Asymptomatic **varicoceles** require no treatment. If associated with discomfort, scrotal support may help; if support is not helpful or if infertility is present, ligation of the internal spermatic veins at the inguinal ring either with an open procedure or transcutaneously via sclerotherapy results in pain control and could improve fertility.

REFERENCES

Clark JL, Tatum NO, Noble SL: Management of genital herpes. Am Fam Physician 1995;**51**:175.

Division of STD Prevention: *Sexually Transmitted Disease Surveillance, 1996.* US Department of Health and Human Services, Public Health Service/Centers for Disease Control and Prevention; September 1997.

Fitzpatrick TB, Johnson RA, Wolff K, et al: *Color Atlas and Synopsis of Clinical Dermatology.* 3rd ed. McGraw-Hill, 1997.

Gilbert DN, Moellering RC, Sande MA: *The Sanford Guide to Antimicrobial Therapy.* 28th ed. Antimicrobial Therapy; 1998.

Handsfield HH: Clinical presentation and natural course of anogenital warts. Am J Med 1997; **102**(5A):16.

Mayeaux EJ, Harper MB, Barksdale W: Noncervical human papillomavirus genital infections. Am Fam Physician 1995;**52**:1137.

MMWR 1998 Guidelines for Treatment of Sexually Transmitted Diseases MMWR 1998;**47**:RR-1.

National Ambulatory Health Care Survey: *1995 Advance Data From Vital and Health Statistics.* No. 286. National Center for Health Statistics; 1998.

Peter G (editor): *1997 Red Book: Report of the Committee on Infectious Diseases.* 24th ed. American Academy of Pediatrics; 1997.

34   Hand & Wrist Injuries

James L. Greenwald, MD

I. **Definition.** Hand and wrist injuries include a number of different conditions involving acute disruption of the normal structure and function of the soft and bony tissues of the hand and wrist through the action of external forces.

   II. **Common diagnoses** (see also Chapters 13, 31, 43, and 60). Referred pain from a process originating in the elbow, shoulder, cervical spine, or central nervous system must always be considered in the diagnosis of acute hand or wrist complaints (see Chapters 8 and 50).

   A. **Fractures:** phalanges, metacarpals, carpals, and distal ulna and radius.

   B. **Dislocations:** interphalangeal (IP), metacarpophalangeal (MP), lunate, and perilunate.

   C. **Ligamentous sprains:** IP and MP collateral ligaments, volar capsular plate of the fingers, and carpal ligaments.

   D. **Tendon injuries and deformities:** finger extensor distal avulsion (mallet finger), central slip avulsion (boutonniere finger), flexor profundus, flexor superficialis, de Quervain's disease, and inflammatory tenosynovitis.

   E. **Amputations.**

   F. **Other soft tissue conditions:** contusions, lacerations, infections, burns, and hand-arm vibration syndrome.

   III. **Epidemiology.** Injuries to the hand and wrist are very common. Sixty-two percent of emergency department visits are for injuries, and 28.6% of the injuries seen are hand and wrist injuries. Thirty percent of all injuries in children involve the hand and wrist, with boys having twice the injury rate of girls. Hand trauma is disproportionately common in the industrial setting, representing 30–40% of industrial accidents. Work-related hand pain has an overall prevalence of 10%. Alcohol ingestion is frequently associated with hand and wrist injuries, and the nonprofessional use of fireworks causes about 3000 hand injuries annually.

   A. **Fractures.** The phalanges are the most commonly fractured bones in the body. Carpal fractures are rare in children younger than 10 years of age. The fifth metacarpal (boxer's fracture) is a common fracture often resulting from altercation.

   B. **Dislocations** often occur in individuals who participate in sports. Dislocations of the proximal interphalangeal (PIP) and MP joints are most common.

   C. **Sprains** of the IP and MP ligaments occur frequently in individuals engaged in sports, especially basketball, football, skiing, and racket sports. Ligamentous injuries in the distal interphalangeal (DIP) and wrist joints are less common.

   D. **Tendon injuries** may occur in a penetrating wound through industrial accidents, altercation, or forced movement of a fixed joint, as in playing basketball, baseball, or football. Extensor tendon injuries are more common than flexor tendon injuries in nonpenetrating trauma.

   E. **Amputations** are common in operators of heavy machinery, especially farmers, and in homeowners through operation of snow blowers, lawn mowers, chain saws, and electric saws.

F. Repetitive motion, vibration, or sports participation without proper preparation can cause a variety of **overuse syndromes,** most commonly **tenosynovitis.**

IV. **Pathophysiology**

   A. Fractures may result from a crushing injury (distal phalanx), downward transmission of shear forces (proximal phalanx), a fall on an outstretched hand (carpal scaphoid), or a direct blow to the hand (hamate). Oblique or spiral fractures tend to be unstable and heal with shortening or angulation.

   Angulation in fractures of the middle or proximal phalanx is caused by traction from the surrounding structures. **Anteroposterior angulation of a middle phalangeal fracture** is determined by the location of the fracture with respect to the insertion of the flexor sublimis tendon. Volar angulation commonly results from a fracture of the distal third; dorsal angulation, from a fracture of the proximal to middle third. Proximal phalangeal fractures often result in volar angulation due to the flexor sublimis tendon.

   The tenuous blood supply of some of the carpal bones may lead to nonunion or avascular necrosis following nondisplaced fractures of the lunate (Kienböck's disease) or scaphoid.

   B. Only certain joints are subject to simple **dislocation** without fracture. Forced hyperextension rarely dislocates the DIP joint. Downward transmission of force is more likely to result in dorsal PIP or MP joint dislocations. The rare perilunate dislocation involves disruption of the capitolunate joint with posterior dislocation of the hand and distal carpals. Dislocation of the carpal lunate anteriorly into the carpal tunnel may occur with a fall on the palm through disruption of wrist ligaments and simultaneous transmission of forces from the surrounding bones. Lunate subluxation may injure the median nerve that supplies some motor function and sensory innervation.

   C. Ligamentous sprains may be classified as grade I (injury to a few fibers), grade II (partial disruption of ligament integrity with significant impairment of function), and grade III (complete disruption).

   Traumatic rupture from a hyperextension injury is most likely to occur at the PIP joint, which can lead to a hyperextending joint (swan-neck deformity [Figure 34–1]). The volar capsular plate is intimately associated with the collateral ligaments, and both may be injured in dislocations. Lateral (radialward) dislocation of the thumb MP joint may result in a tear of the ulnar collateral ligament (game-

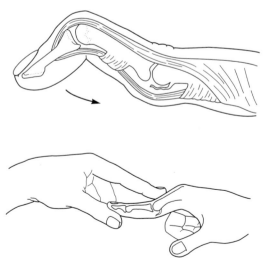

FIGURE 34–1. Volar plate rupture causes swan-neck deformity. A stress test shows an abnormal increase in extension.

keeper's thumb). The same injury mechanism in children generally causes an epiphyseal fracture, or bony gamekeeper's thumb. A number of injuries to the carpals may result in chronic pain and weakness as a result of ligamentous instability.

D. Tendon injuries. Overuse or misuse may lead to swelling of a tendon and its sheath, causing tendinitis. In chronic tenosynovitis, the swelling of the tendon sheath causes pinching, and a nodular deformity of the underlying tendon leads to triggering upon use (trigger finger or clutched thumb) or even loss of mobility. This commonly occurs from synovial swelling at the fibrous pulley, which restrains the flexor tendon as it crosses the metacarpal head (Figure 34–2).

    The **extensor tendon** is commonly injured when the extended finger is forced into flexion. Avulsion injuries can occur either at its insertion into the distal phalanx (mallet finger [Figure 34–3]) or the insertion of the central slip into the middle phalanx, which can lead to a boutonniere deformity (Figure 34–4). Flexor tendon injuries can occur with forceful hyperextension of the DIP joint or with a penetrating wound. With complete disruption, retraction of the proximal portion of the tendon always occurs.

E. The microvascular lesion underlying **hand-arm vibration syndrome** is characterized by vascular muscle hypertrophy, endothelial cell injury, and α_1-receptor dysfunction.

V. Symptoms

A. Pain is caused by fractures, dislocations, ligamentous sprains, and tendon injuries. **Swelling** is common with fractures and ligamentous sprains.

    1. Pain and **swelling** may result from an acute PIP volar plate injury from gamekeeper's thumb. **Persistent or severe pain** accompanied by swelling is an indication that nondisplaced fractures, as opposed to soft tissue injuries, of the hand and wrist may be present.

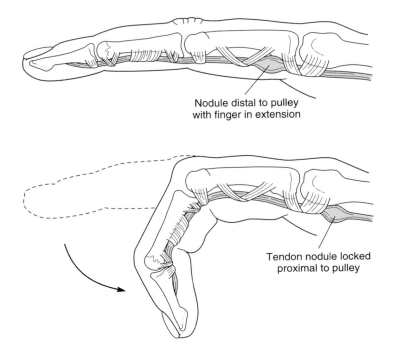

Nodule distal to pulley
with finger in extension

Tendon nodule locked
proximal to pulley

FIGURE 34–2. Trigger finger results from nodular constriction of the flexor tendon by inflammation of the fibrous sheath at the metacarpophalangeal joint. (Reprinted with permission from Snider RK [editor]: *Essentials of Musculoskeletal Care.* American Academy of Orthopedics; 1997:249.)

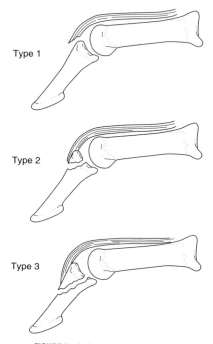

Type 1

Type 2

Type 3

FIGURE 34–3. The three types of mallet finger.

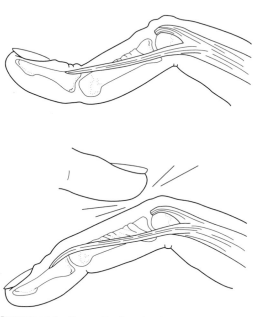

FIGURE 34–4. Boutonniere deformity caused by disruption of the central slip and volar displacement of the lateral bands. The point tenderness test elicits tenderness over the base of the middle phalanx.

2. **Chronic wrist pain** may be caused by a neglected carpal scaphoid or lunate fracture or by a neglected sprain. **Wrist pain with median nerve paresthesia** suggests the relatively rare lunate or perilunate dislocation. **Pain,** especially on wrist extension, and **loss of power in the wrist** are common with injuries to the scapholunate ligaments.

3. A **painful grasp with a weakened, unstable MP joint** occurs if gamekeeper's thumb is not properly treated in the acute phase.

4. **Pain on use** that is greater than would be expected from the findings on inspection is a clue to a more significant injury, such as a flexor tendon disruption or fracture. Pain with use and edema may also accompany tenosynovitis.

B. **Noise.** A **snapping** noise commonly occurs with tendon rupture and fractures. A palpable **click** on wrist extension may occur with a scapholunate sprain. **Clicking and popping** may be found in tenosynovitis.

C. Hand-arm vibration syndrome results in **Raynaud's phenomenon** (ie, cold-induced blanching of the fingertips) with paresthesias in a median and/or ulnar nerve distribution.

VI. **Signs.** Examination under local or regional anesthesia may be necessary to assess the full extent of an injury but must be deferred until thorough motor and sensory examinations have been performed.

A. **Rotational malalignment** is an indication of finger fractures.

B. **Angulation** of fractures may be determined by examination, but may not be apparent without x-ray.

C. **Tenderness**
1. **Tenderness over the anatomic snuff-box** suggests a carpal scaphoid fracture. This type of fracture is as common as a scapholunate sprain, which also causes tenderness over the snuff-box or dorsum of the wrist just distal to the radius. The two injuries may be difficult to distinguish on clinical and laboratory examinations.

2. **Anterior tenderness over the DIP joint** indicates injury of the volar plate in that joint.

3. **Tenderness over the ulnar side of the MP joint of the thumb** suggests a gamekeeper's thumb injury.

4. **Localized tenderness** may occur with tenosynovitis.

D. **Motor function and sensory examinations** can help detect muscle, tendon, ligament, and nerve injuries.

1. **Sensory examination** with a tuning fork and calipers is necessary if the median or ulnar nerve may have been injured in a dorsal lunate dislocation or hand-arm vibration syndrome. Discrimination of two points just under 5 mm apart is normal.

2. **Loss of extension** is a primary sign of extensor tendon injury, but the absence of loss of function may be misleading in certain instances (eg, the boutonniere deformity may develop gradually after the initial insult, and laceration of the thumb extensor tendon may be masked by action of the extensor pollicis brevis muscle).

3. **Flexor tendon function** should be carefully examined whenever there is a penetrating wound or acutely painful grip. Flexor profundus function can be tested by holding the PIP and MP joints in full extension and asking the patient to actively flex the finger. When the other fingers are held in full extension, the flexor sublimis can be examined. This test may not accurately reflect sublimis injury in the index and little fingers, however. **Blocked flexion** can be caused by a variety of ligamentous injuries, including entrapment of a ruptured volar plate, a buttonholing of a dislocated phalanx through a ruptured volar plate, and fracture-dislocations of the proximal end of the middle phalanx. **Triggering,** a sudden, often painful unblocking associated with a palpable or audible click, may occur with flexor tenosynovitis.

E. **Pain**
1. **Pain or hypermobility on lateral stress of a joint** may indicate collateral ligament disruption.

2. Complete disruption of the volar plate in the DIP joint can be confirmed by the presence of hyperextension on anesthetized examination. **Pain over the dorsal DIP joint on extension or lack of full extension** of the distal phalanx

indicates a mallet finger injury. **Pain over the DIP joint** on attempted flexion usually indicates a flexor profundus injury.

3. **Severe pain and edema of the PIP joint** should alert the physician to the possibility of injury to the central slip, as the boutonniere deformity may not occur until weeks later, when tightening and volar displacement of the lateral bands of the extensor tendon occur.

4. **Dorsal pain or weakness on opposed extension** may indicate an occult extensor tendon injury in a penetrating wound.

5. **Finkelstein's test** can detect tenosynovitis of the common sheath of the abductor pollicis longus and extensor pollicis brevis. When present, pain occurs when the wrist is deviated ulnarward with the thumb fully flexed and nested in the palm.

F. **Deformity**

1. An **unreducible deformity** may rarely occur after DIP subluxation. This results from entrapment of the proximal end of the middle phalanx in the complex web of tendons and ligaments surrounding this joint.

2. Athletes or trainers commonly reduce **finger dislocations** on the field and, if deformity is not immediately apparent, may not seek follow-up treatment. While most finger dislocations heal without difficulty in the absence of fractures, patients who neglect treatment after PIP dislocation may note the gradual onset of a boutonniere or swan-neck deformity.

3. In the **Watson test** for chronic scapholunate laxity, pressure is applied to the distal scaphoid while the hand is passively moved from ulnar to radial deviation. A painful deformity may be produced as the scaphoid subluxes dorsally, followed by a click upon release of the maneuver. One should compare the findings with the uninvolved side to avoid false-positives.

VII. **Laboratory tests.** X-rays are useful for detection of fractures, ligament or tendon avulsions, the presence of foreign bodies, and bony involvement in lacerations or amputations. An x-ray must be taken whenever a phalangeal dislocation occurs, to help determine the presence of a bony, ligamentous, or tendon disruption. X-rays are often unnecessary with ligamentous injuries when the diagnosis is obvious and treatment plans would not be altered by finding a concomitant fracture.

A. A carpal scaphoid fracture should always be suspected when there is pain in the wrist and tenderness around the anatomic snuff-box. **Special scaphoid views** must be ordered in addition to anteroposterior (AP), lateral, and oblique x-rays of the wrist, specifically AP views under full ulnar and radial deviation. A fracture of the hook of the hamate may require a special "carpal tunnel view."

B. Small or stress fractures may not be visible on x-ray at the time of injury. Bone resorption at the fracture site may widen the fracture line and enhance visibility on another x-ray in 2 weeks. **Radionuclide bone scanning** may also be helpful.

C. X-ray detection of **lunate dislocation** requires careful inspection of carpal alignment. The upward concavities of the radius, lunate, and capitate bones are axially arranged on the normal lateral carpal x-ray. Repeat x-ray in patients with persistent pain may demonstrate Keinböck's disease.

D. Small radiopaque chips on x-ray alert one to the presence of ligamentous avulsions in the volar plate, gamekeeper's thumb, and phalangeal collateral ligament injuries. **Stress x-rays** under anesthesia may be used by a specialist to diagnose significant gamekeeper's thumb or volar plate injuries.

E. A special posteroanterior x-ray with the fist clenched and in supination must be ordered when chronic laxity of the scapholunate ligaments is suspected. Widening of the joint space beyond 2 mm is abnormal. Injuries to the wrist ligaments are best confirmed by **arthroscopy. Arthrography** and **magnetic resonance imaging (MRI)** may also be used to delineate wrist ligament injuries, although only in scapholunate dissociation has MRI been shown to be equal to the other techniques.

F. The avulsed fragment may migrate with the retracted profundus or sublimis tendon in patients with tendon injuries.

G. X-rays in patients with finger fractures should be carefully assessed for angulation. Significant joint involvement may not be readily apparent in volar plate avulsion fractures of the base of the middle phalanx. The presence of a V at the dorsal joint line is associated with posterior dislocation in this unstable fracture (Figure 34–5).

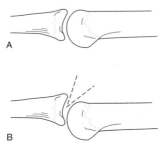

FIGURE 34–5. A lateral x-ray in the posterior fracture dislocation associated with volar plate avulsion may show the V sign (**B**) as well as loss of continuity of the posterior cortices. (Reprinted with permission from Eiff MP, Hatch RL, Calmbach WL: *Fracture Management for Primary Care.* Saunders; 1998:39.)

VIII. Treatment

A. Fractures. Preventive counseling should include discouragement of the use of fireworks and encouragement of the use of protective gloves for woodcutting. If a fracture is suspected on examination, it should be treated as if it indeed is one and x-rayed again in 1–3 weeks. Patients with the following should be referred for treatment by a specialist: displaced, unstable (eg, spiral or oblique phalangeal), articular, or open fractures; comminuted scaphoid fractures; fractures of the other carpals; metacarpal fractures with >30-degree angulation; or fractures involving neurovascular compromise. The injured limb may require a splint.

   1. **Fractures of the distal phalanx** that spare the articular surface are often comminuted. Good function is restored by using a splint that has a protective hood to prevent bumping of the fingertip.

   2. A **stable, nonangulated transverse proximal phalangeal or metacarpal fracture** may be supported in the position of function with a gauntlet cast with incorporated anterior aluminum/foam finger splints as needed for more distal fractures. Inclusion of an adjacent finger improves stability. In a finger fracture, protection with buddy taping or with a removable finger splint may be used for the following 2 weeks while range-of-motion exercises are begun. With metacarpal fractures, dorsal angulation of as much as 30 degrees is acceptable. The cast should extend to place the MP joint in 70- to 90-degree flexion. These fractures are quite unstable, and closed reduction with cast fixation is often ineffective in relieving angular deformity. While a boxer's fracture with volar angulation of 30–70 degrees will leave a mild deformity without reduction and internal fixation, this deformity should have little effect on function in patients who do not perform fine manipulations at work and may be acceptable to many.

   A primary care physician may choose to reduce transverse fractures with volar angulation involving the proximal phalanx of the lower to middle third of the middle phalanx using digital anesthesia before these fractures are immobilized. Transverse fractures of the distal third of the middle phalanx (distal to the insertion of the flexor sublimis) should be reduced and immobilized with both IP joints in extension. Stability should be evaluated by close follow-up and repeat x-ray in 1 week. Fractures including the articular surface or resulting in periarticular dislocation should be referred to a provider with specialty hand skills.

   3. **Fractures of the scaphoid or thumb proximal phalanx** must be fixed with the thumb in an opposed position using a spica short-arm cast. With carpal fractures, a long-arm extension may be necessary to prevent pronation and supination. In scaphoid fractures, delayed union is common, and nonunion or avascular necrosis, which occurs in 10% of cases, may require surgery and result in decreased function.

   4. **Patient instructions** following casting should include a warning to notify the physician immediately for burning pain, which could indicate ischemia or

impending pressure sores from cast compression. **Rehabilitation** after cast removal should include passive and active range-of-motion exercises. **Occupational therapy** should be considered for those patients who work with their hands and for those over 35 who would be more prone to develop arthritis.

B. Dislocations. Dorsal finger dislocations may be reduced with or without finger anesthesia, although anesthesia is desirable to evaluate stability after reduction. Reducible phalangeal dislocations should be examined for bone, volar plate, collateral ligament, and tendon injuries and then treated appropriately. Close follow-up will help detect volar plate or extensor hood instability or volar plate entrapment that may not be initially apparent. Any injury to the PIP joint will result in prolonged edema. Lunate dislocations require specialist referral; they are reduced by extension, manual traction, and manipulation of the dislocated portion.

C. Ligamentous sprains

    1. Finger collateral ligament sprains generally respond well to splinting in the position of function for 3 weeks. Tongue blade or Popsicle stick splints have no place in the treatment of jammed fingers.

    2. The collateral stability of a nondislocated or reducible **volar plate injury** can be confirmed by an anesthetized examination prior to closed treatment when excessive edema or lateral tenderness is present. Suspected volar plate injury with edema and anterior tenderness should be treated in the same fashion as an obvious injury with documented hyperextensibility.

    3. Gamekeeper's thumb can be treated with immobilization for 4–6 weeks in the absence of complete disruption, as shown by instability upon examination. Complete disruption, often accompanied by a fracture at the base of the proximal phalanx, requires surgical intervention.

    4. A **scapholunate sprain** and a **suspected scaphoid fracture** may both be treated by immobilization with a spica cast for 3 weeks. If tenderness persists, another x-ray may be taken with appropriate views to determine which condition is present. Persistent pain in sprains may indicate carpal instability and require referral. Mild wrist sprains can be adequately treated with a splint.

D. Tendon injuries

    1. Mallet finger. Treatment depends on the grade of the injury (Figure 34–2). Type I or II mallet finger can generally be treated by continuous splinting in mild hyperextension (approximately 110 degrees for 6 weeks). The splint should be periodically examined for its integrity. An unstable (type III) mallet finger requires referral for open reduction and internal fixation.

    2. Boutonniere finger. A suspected central slip injury must be treated by splinting the PIP joint in extension for 2 weeks. If posterior joint tenderness persists at 2 weeks, the diagnosis of central slip injury is assured and splinting should continue for at least another 2 weeks.

    3. Wrist tendinitis is treated by rest, nonsteroidal anti-inflammatory medications (eg, **ibuprofen,** 600 mg three times a day for 10 days), injection of the tendon sheath with a soluble steroid (eg, 0.5 mL of **triamcinolone,** 40 mg/mL) in multiple sites, or immobilization. Persistent triggering or clutching may require surgical division of the tendon sheath.

    4. Flexor tendon laceration or avulsion should generally be treated by a hand specialist. Some primary care physicians with extra training may elect to repair lacerated extensor tendons on their own.

E. Amputations that involve a small portion of the distal phalanx may be treated by careful debridement and then dressing changes. Referral should be considered when the amputation is below the midshaft of the distal phalanx, when the injury extensively reduces the fingertip pad, when extensive trauma to the nail bed will result in a deformed nail without anatomic repair, or when the occupation of the injured person demands rapid anatomic restoration.

    Microsurgical replacement of amputated digits will prolong recovery and may not always be successful. Severed digits should be placed in a sterile saline-soaked gauze dressing in a clean, preferably sterile, plastic bag and should be kept on ice, not dry ice.

F. Hand-arm vibration syndrome is treated by avoiding the injurious activity. Calcium channel blockers (eg, **nifedipine,** 30 mg/day) may be helpful.

REFERENCES

Anderson BP: *Office Orthopedics in Primary Care: Diagnosis and Treatment.* Saunders; 1995.

Behrens V, et al: The prevalence of back pain, hand discomfort and dermatitis in the US working population. Am J Public Health 1994;**84:**1780.

Bhende MS, Dandrea LA, Davis HW: Hand injuries in children presenting to a pediatric emergency department. Ann Emerg Med 1993;**22:**1519.

Eiff MP, Hatch RL, Calmbach WL: *Fracture Management for Primary Care.* Saunders; 1998.

Morgan RL, Linder MM: Common wrist injuries. Am Fam Physician 1997;**55:**857.

Schaffer TG: Common hand fractures in family practice. Arch Fam Med 1994;**3:**982.

Snider RK (editor): *Essentials of Musculoskeletal Care.* American Academy of Orthopedics; 1997.

---

35   Headaches

John P. Fogarty, MD

I. **Definition.** Headaches represent a subjective feeling of pain referable to a variety of intracranial and extracranial structures.

II. **Common diagnoses.** The Ad Hoc Committee's Classification of Headache, developed in 1962, is the most widely known classification used today. Daroff modified this system in 1988. The various types of headaches seen in the primary care setting are described below in terms of the original classification scheme (the more recent terminology is given in parentheses).

A. **Muscle contraction headaches** (tension headaches), either primary (without underlying disease) or secondary to head or neck injury, arthritis, trauma, or inflammation. The most common form of primary headaches, muscle contraction headaches occur in 20–25% of new cases. More than 50% of all headaches seen in primary care are of this type.

B. **Vascular headaches** (migraine headaches, including cluster headaches), either primary or secondary to systemic or local infection, hypoxia, alcohol ingestion, drugs and chemicals (eg, nitroglycerin or food preservatives), withdrawal (eg, caffeine or ergot preparations), or altitude or after seizures. These constitute 10–15% of new headaches and <10% of all headaches seen in primary care. Migraine headaches are further subdivided into common (migraine without aura), classic (migraine with aura), and complicated types.

C. **Mixed headaches,** which display features of both migraine and tension headaches. These constitute 10–15% of new headaches and 20–30% of chronic headaches.

D. **Traction or inflammatory headaches,** commonly known as "acute" headaches. Such headaches may result from either (1) intracranial causes, such as neoplasms (primary or metastatic), infections (meningitis, encephalitis, or abscess), hemorrhage (cerebrovascular accident, ruptured aneurysm, or trauma), or post-lumbar puncture; or (2) extracranial causes, such as eye, ear, nose, and throat diseases (eg, trauma, infections, neoplasms, and temporal arteritis). In ambulatory primary care, <0.4% of new headaches are due to serious intracranial disease, and patients with these headaches do not usually present with typical vascular or muscular headache symptoms.

III. **Epidemiology.** Seventy-five percent to 80% of adults in the United States every year have headaches, and about 50% of Americans have had severe or disabling headaches at some time in their lives. More than half of the patients who seek medical help for headaches visit family physicians, and most of these patients see the primary care physician only once for this symptom. The actual prevalence of headache is probably much higher than office data suggest, since the majority of headache sufferers do not seek medical attention at all.

A. **Muscle contraction headaches.** These headaches, which can occur at any age, are most common in young adulthood. Chronic muscle contraction headaches requiring medical attention usually occur in females, often with an underlying anxiety or depressive disorder. Forty percent of these patients have a positive family history of headaches.

B. **Vascular headaches.** Migraine headaches usually begin in adolescence or young adulthood. Seventy-five percent of these headaches occur in females, and 90% of these patients have a family history of migraine headaches. Cluster headaches, on the other hand, which usually affect males, occur at a later age (30–50 years) in individuals with no family history of migraines.

C. **Mixed headaches.** These headaches, which have the clinical features of both vascular and muscle contraction headaches, occur in individuals of either sex and have a variable age at onset. Mixed headaches are particularly common in patients with chronic headaches. Patients with mixed headaches typically also have associated depression, sleep disturbances, and a predilection toward substance abuse.

D. **Traction or inflammatory headaches.** These headaches are associated with particular physical conditions. Their occurrence depends on the underlying diagnosis, pre-existing medical conditions of the patient, and recent history (eg, trauma or infection).

IV. **Pathophysiology.** The classification referred to above implies a vascular mechanism for migraine headaches and a muscular mechanism for tension headaches. However, recent data suggest that migraine and tension headaches are physiologically similar entities with varied symptomatic expression. These conditions reflect either a primary central or a combined central and peripheral disturbance of neuroreceptor and neurovascular function. Although anxiety, worry, stress, and depression commonly trigger headaches, recent research challenges the assumption that the primary causal event is psychological. The "neuroreceptor/neurovascular" hypothesis more effectively explains the symptom overlap between migraine and tension headaches. Recent research on the neuropharmacology of serotonin suggests a significant role of this vasoconstrictor in headaches and explains the mechanism of action of several of the serotonin analogs or agonist medications now available for headache therapy. It is suggested that they have their effect by a receptor-mediated neural pathway in both the central nervous system and the trigeminal nerve, where they block neurogenic inflammation.

V. **Symptoms of particular types of headaches.** Differentiation among types of headaches is usually based on the history. Emphasis should be placed on the history of onset, quality and intensity of pain, frequency, provoking influences, and associated symptoms.

A. **Muscle contraction headaches** have the following characteristics: (1) they are usually bilateral, although they can be unilateral; (2) they last from hours to as long as months; (3) usually they are nonthrobbing; and (4) infrequently, they are associated with nausea or vomiting. The clinical picture can vary greatly in frequency, severity, location, and duration. Classically, muscle contraction headaches are headaches in the occipital and vertex regions that produce a bandlike ache around the head. Patients with these headaches may experience a variety of associated symptoms and signs, including depression, sleep and appetite disturbances, and difficulty with relationships, all of which may be precipitated by stress, recent or remote loss, and family dysfunction. Repeated careful history taking over a period of visits is frequently helpful in eliciting underlying stressors. Such tools as the family genogram may be helpful in evaluating family relationships, dysfunctions, and positive headache histories in other family members and prove therapeutic in helping the patient understand relationships and family history.

B. **Vascular headaches** are typically characterized by unilateral, pulsating pain and moderate to severe nausea or vomiting. Reversible visual or hemisensory symptoms (aura) may occur before, during, or after the attack (Table 35–1).

C. **Mixed headaches** are migraine-type headaches in individuals with a history of frequent tension headaches or vice versa. Mixed headaches should be considered in patients with a change in either (1) the pattern or character of their typical headache or (2) response to previously effective therapy.

D. **Traction or inflammatory headaches** may herald serious disease. A good history, including age, occupation, medications, and other medical conditions or recent infections, will, in most cases, determine the cause. Symptoms of a "worrisome" headache that should elicit a search for an underlying cause include the following.

1. Headache, new in onset, that is constant, prevents sleep, and progressively worsens over several weeks (indicative of possible intracranial mass lesion

TABLE 35-1. COMMON CHARACTERISTICS OF VASCULAR HEADACHE

	Classic Migraine	Complicated Migraine	Common Migraine	Cluster Headache
Prodrome	Stereotypical, usually visual scotomata; lasts 10–30 minutes; resolves with onset of headache	Significant neurologic signs and symptoms overshadow headache	Often absent, may be vague; irritability, fluid retention, insomnia, etc	None
Headache	Episodic, unilateral, throbbing; nausea and vomiting; lasts 1–6 hours; several attacks per year	Mild or inapparent; duration unpredictable	Unilateral or bilateral throbbing, usually with nausea; may last 1–3 days; frequency variable	Excruciating, periorbital, unilateral, nonpulsatile; occurs in "clusters" of 1–3 months; last approximately 1 hour; often occurs at night and is associated with alcohol
Examination	Nausea and vomiting, hibernation, photophobia	Neurologic deficit; aphasia, hemiplegia, confusion; ophthalmoplegia	Nausea and vomiting, no neurologic findings, hibernation, photophobia	Photophobia, tearing, nasal stuffiness, possible Horner's syndrome; possibly agitated or violent

or infection). The "first," or "new," headache, especially over the age of 35, is less likely to be migraine or tension.

2. Headache that is abrupt, explosive, and extremely severe (eg, "the worst headache of my life"), suggestive of intracranial hemorrhage.
3. Headache beginning with exertion (consider leaking aneurysm, increased intracranial pressure, or arterial dissection).
4. Headache in a drowsy or confused patient (consider sepsis, trauma, etc).
5. Headache in the elderly patient (possibly indicative of temporal arteritis, cerebrovascular accident, etc).

VI. **Signs of particular types of headaches.** A complete physical examination with emphasis on neurologic, otologic, and general physical conditions is necessary in the evaluation of the patient who presents with headache.

A. **Muscle contraction headaches.** A physical examination may reveal muscle tightness, or "trigger points," over the posterior cervical and occipital regions. The range of motion of the neck may provide clues to the secondary causes of muscle contraction headache, such as cervical arthritis (eg, stiffness, decreased range of motion, or crepitus with movement), inflammatory processes (eg, trigger points or nodules), or infectious causes (eg, lymphadenopathy).

B. **Vascular headaches.** Signs of migraine headaches may be mild or severe and dramatic, from a patient in obvious pain to actual neurologic dysfunction in complicated migraine. Photophobia, tearing, nasal stuffiness, or Horner's syndrome may occur in cluster headaches (Table 35–1).

C. **Mixed headaches.** Signs will depend on the predominant characteristics manifested by the headache, whether of the vascular or muscle contraction type.

D. **Traction or inflammatory headaches.** Signs of a "worrisome" headache are listed below.

1. Headache accompanied by fever may indicate meningitis, purulent sinusitis, otitis, dental abscess, etc.
2. Headache with a stiff neck may indicate pus or blood in the meninges.
3. Headache with abnormal physical signs (eg, focal neurologic deficits or high blood pressure [>200 mm Hg systolic or >120 mm Hg diastolic]) may indicate increased intracranial pressure from mass effect or accelerated hypertension.

VII. **Laboratory tests.** Diagnostic testing is unnecessary for most patients with chronic, recurring headaches and for low-risk patients (ie, young patients who [1] have prior or family history of headache, [2] are improving during their evaluation, [3] have none of the above-mentioned "worrisome" symptoms or signs, [4] are perfectly alert and oriented, and [5] have no focal neurologic signs). For these individuals, repeated history taking and physical examinations over time, in addition to observations of response to treatment, are the best diagnostic tools.

Further diagnostic tests are indicated in high-risk patients (ie, those individuals with severe headaches who do not meet the low-risk criteria). The following tests should be considered.

A. **Radiologic evaluation.** Plain skull films are rarely useful in the evaluation of headache. Specific studies (eg, sinus or temporomandibular joint series) should be ordered when clinical suspicion dictates.

1. **Computerized tomography (CT).** In the patient who presents with a severe and acute headache, this procedure is most helpful in diagnosing hemorrhage, whether subarachnoid or intraparenchymal. The acutely ill patient who requires monitoring will be most easily evaluated by CT.
2. **Magnetic resonance imaging (MRI).** This procedure is generally more informative in patients with chronic headaches. Characteristic findings have been described using MRI in patients with migraine, trigeminal neuralgia, and temporomandibular joint dysfunction. This procedure is also superior in showing a subacute subdural hematoma in patients with a history of trauma, and it is useful to further characterize and clarify lesions found on CT. MRI has excellent resolution in the posterior fossa.

B. **Lumbar puncture (LP).** The purposes of LP are (1) to establish the presence or absence of blood or inflammatory cells in the cerebrospinal fluid, (2) to differentiate between hemorrhage or meningitis in the patient with a stiff neck, and (3) to determine the cause of meningitis, if present. Although LP is easy to perform and readily available, it is an invasive, uncomfortable procedure that has no role in the routine headache evaluation. LP should *not* be performed when increased intracranial pressure is suspected.

C. Blood analysis. A complete blood cell count is rarely useful or definitive in the evaluation of headache and has no place except in the febrile patient. The erythrocyte sedimentation rate is indicated in the older patient with a new headache to rule out temporal arteritis. Significant elevations should be confirmed by arterial biopsy. Prompt steroid therapy should be initiated to avoid the complication of retinal artery occlusion.

D. Other studies. Radionucleotide imaging and angiography, which are usually less helpful than CT scans for identifying or ruling out significant intracranial disease, should be reserved for the few patients with normal CT scans and cerebrospinal fluid findings whose evaluations strongly suggest an intracranial lesion. MRI has largely replaced these studies. Electroencephalography is not routinely helpful for the patient with a new headache, although it may be useful in the patient with chronic headaches who does not respond to therapy to ensure that no seizure disorder is present.

VIII. Treatment

A. Muscle contraction headaches. A supportive cooperative relationship with the patient is essential. Education, insight into family and life events, consideration of environmental and emotional triggers, and counseling may help both decrease headache frequency and increase coping skills. Biofeedback, stress management, and muscle relaxation techniques as well as exercise programs and dietary changes may also help. For the patient with chronic tension headaches, a multidisciplinary approach using both drug and nondrug treatments with individual and family therapy is often necessary.

1. **Acute therapy** (see Table 35–2). Drug therapy should begin with mild analgesics (eg, aspirin or acetaminophen, 650–1000 mg at onset and every 4–6 hours as needed), nonsteroidal anti-inflammatory drugs (NSAIDs) (eg, ibuprofen, 600–800 mg at onset and repeated every 6–8 hours; naproxen, 250–500 mg at onset and repeated every 8–12 hours; or others in equivalent doses), or muscle relaxants (eg, cyclobenzaprine, 10 mg three times daily for up to 21 days; chlorzoxazone, 500–750 mg three times daily; methocarbamol, 1000–1500 mg four times daily; or diazepam, 5 mg two to four times daily), or a combination of the above may be used. Narcotic analgesics, which may lead to habituation and dependency, should be avoided at an early stage, since these headaches become chronic.

2. **Preventive therapy.** Medications used for migraine prophylaxis have also proven useful in the patient with frequent, recurrent tension headaches. Specifically, beta blockers and tricyclic antidepressants, alone or in combination, are very beneficial (see below). Physical therapy may be a useful adjunct in the management of chronic tension headaches.

3. **Patient follow-up.** The majority of acute headache patients will see their primary physician only once for this complaint. Early follow-up is recommended in the patient with new headaches to gauge response to therapy and reconfirm findings of the history and the physical examination. Review of headache diaries, precipitating factors, and life events may help avoid the chronic headache.

B. Vascular headaches

1. **Migraine headaches**

   a. **General measures** include education of the patient and avoidance of precipitating factors, such as alcohol, certain foods (eg, foods containing tyramine or monosodium glutamate), fatigue, and particular life stressors. Alternative therapies are frequently prescribed for migraine sufferers and include aerobic exercise, biofeedback, progressive self-relaxation, meditation, massage therapy, or acupuncture. The most widely researched botanical for migraine headache is a wildflower called feverfew (*Tenacetum parthenium*) in dosages of 125 mg of a standardized extract twice per day. It can be used for either acute treatment or prophylaxis of migraine.

   b. **Acute therapy** is most appropriate when migraine attacks are no more frequent than two to four times a month. Effective medications include the following agents (see also Table 35–2).

TABLE 35–2. TREATMENT APPROACHES TO HEADACHE

Mild to Moderate Migraine	Severe Migraine	Acute Cluster Therapy	Acute Tension Therapy
Simple analgesic PO	NSAIDs as in mild, ketorolac IM	Inhaled 100% O_2	ASA
ASA	5-HT agonist	DHE/antiemetic	NSAIDs
Acetaminophen	Sumatriptan SQ, PO, IN	Ergotamine	Acetaminophen
NSAIDs	Zolmitriptan PO	Parenteral narcotics	Combination analgesics
Naproxen	Naratriptan PO		Physical modalities
Ibuprofen	Rizatriptan PO		
Indomethacin	Ergot derivatives		
Ketorolac	Ergotamine/caffeine PO,		
Combination analgesics	PR, SL		
Midrin	DHE IV, IM, or IN with or		
Fiorinal/Fioricet	without metoclopramide		
Antiemetics PO, PR	IM, IV		
Metoclopramide	Opioid analgesics		
Promethazine	Butorphanol nasal spray		
	Meperidine IM, IV with or		
	without promethazine		
	Neuroleptics		
	Prochlorperazine IM, IV		
	Chlorpromazine IM, IV		
	Corticosteroids IM, IV		

ASA, Aspirin; DHE, dihydroergotamine; 5-HT, 5-hydroxytryptamine; IM, intramuscularly; IN, intranasally; IV, intravenously; NSAIDs, nonsteroidal anti-inflammatory drugs; PO, by mouth; PR, rectally; SL, sublingually; SQ, subcutaneously.

(1) **Ergot alkaloids.** These drugs are estimated to be effective within 2 hours in >90% of the cases when administered parenterally, 80% when given rectally, and up to 50% when given orally. They are also available in sublingual forms. Since ergotamine preparations may result in dependency and rebound headaches, they should not be used more often than 2 days/week.

(2) A **combination of acetaminophen, dichloralphenazone, and isometheptene mucate** (Midrin, a sedative and vasoconstrictor) is helpful taken in a dose of two capsules at onset, followed by one every 30 minutes as needed, to a maximum of five capsules per day.

(3) **NSAIDs** or **nonnarcotic analgesics** can be very effective if given early. The doses mentioned in section VIII,A,1 are appropriate.

(4) **Antiemetics** administered either by mouth, intramuscularly, or by rectal suppository may be necessary to offset the nausea and gastric stasis associated with migraine and may be helpful for their additive effect to narcotics. Chlorpromazine, 10–25 mg orally, 25–50 mg intramuscularly, or 50–100 mg rectally; promethazine, 12.5–25 mg intramuscularly, orally, or rectally; or prochlorperazine, 5–10 mg orally or intramuscularly or 25 mg rectally, may be tried.

(5) **Triptans,** the newest class of medications for migraine developed in the last several years, are selective serotonin receptor agonists. They have proven to be very effective in the treatment of migraines. **Sumatriptan** (Imitrex), the first medication of this class, is now available in an injectable form (6 mg subcutaneously), intranasal form (20–40 mg intranasally), and oral form (50–100 mg by mouth). Several oral formulations have been recently developed, including **zolmitriptan** (Zomig), 2.5–5 mg orally, **naratriptan** (Amerge), 1–2.5 mg orally, and **rizatriptan** (Maxalt), 5–10 mg orally, and all show good results in clinical studies. These agents have higher bioavailability than oral sumatriptan, and naratriptan has a longer half-life, which may have an advantage in preventing recurrence. These agents should be used with care in patients with suspected coronary artery, cerebrovascular, or peripheral vascular disease, since they have been associated with vascular vasospasm.

(6) Narcotic analgesics such as **codeine,** 30 mg, or **oxycodone,** 5 mg (both with or without acetaminophen), may benefit some patients during an acute attack, but their use must be carefully balanced with the risks of habituation and rebound headache. The potential for abuse is less with agonist-antagonist opioids than with receptor agonists. Transnasal **butorphanol tartrate** (Stadol NS), 1 mg followed by another 1 mg 1 hour later, has been shown to be effective for the acute treatment of migraine headache. Sedative hypnotics such as **secobarbital** (Seconal, 100 mg orally or intramuscularly) or **triazolam** (Halcion, 0.125–0.25 mg orally) may be helpful in allowing the patient to "sleep off" the headache.

c. **Preventive therapy** is indicated if either the number of attacks exceeds three or four per month or headaches occur on a predictable schedule (eg, with menses). Effective medications include the following drugs.

  (1) **Beta blockers.** These agents are the most important drugs for the prevention of migraine. Nadolol, starting at 20 mg/day, up to 80–160 mg/day, and propranolol, 20–40 mg three or four times daily, are equally effective. Once- or twice-daily dosing improves compliance.

  (2) **Cyproheptadine** (Periactin) in doses of 2–4 mg three times daily, has proven useful in children.

  (3) **Tricyclic antidepressants.** Amitriptyline, doxepin, or imipramine, 25–150 mg at bedtime, and nortriptyline, 25–75 mg at bedtime, have also proven useful, probably because of serotonin dynamics. The full dosages normally used for depression are not necessary to achieve benefit.

  (4) **Calcium channel blockers.** These drugs are not as effective as beta blockers for prophylaxis, but are the agents of choice for those patients who are unable to take beta blockers (eg, patients with asthma, congestive heart failure, and diabetes, who take insulin). Verapamil, 40–160 mg two to four times daily, and diltiazem, 30–90 mg two or three times per day, are the most effective agents to date. Nifedipine may actually increase headaches.

  (5) **Methysergide** (Sansert) is very effective in a dose of 2 mg three or four times daily. This drug should not be used for longer than 6 months without a 1-month "drug holiday" because of reported adverse effects, including retroperitoneal and cardiopulmonary fibrosis.

  (6) **Other agents.** Clonidine, 0.1–0.2 mg two or three times per day, or carbamazepine, 100–200 mg twice daily, may also be effective.

d. **Patient follow-up.** Patient education during an acute headache is not very effective. Subsequent visits to assess response to therapy, patient understanding, and frequency of attacks can be therapeutic. The mutually cooperative, understanding relationship critical to long-term success can be established only with frequent visits at the onset of the headaches, followed by gradual decreasing of visits as the patient assumes more responsibility.

2. **Cluster headaches**

  a. **Acute therapy** (see Table 35–2) includes (1) **inhalation of 100% oxygen** by mask at a rate of 7–10 L/min; (2) **inhaled ergotamine,** one puff every 5 minutes for a maximum of five puffs per day; and (3) **sublingual nifedipine,** 10–20 mg, repeated every 6–8 hours (not to be used with ergotamine).

  b. **Prevention** is preferable. Effective medications include (1) **methysergide,** 2–8 mg/day; (2) **lithium,** 300 mg three times per day (monitoring blood levels weekly to avoid toxicity); (3) **prednisone,** 40–60 mg/day for 5 days, followed by tapering over 10–14 days; and (4) **calcium channel blockers,** such as nifedipine, 10–20 mg three times daily, alone or in combination.

C. **Mixed headaches.** Patients with constant tension headaches, migraine headaches, or both have often seen many physicians without relief. They present a major challenge, especially because there is frequent habituation to narcotic and ergotamine medications. A combined approach consisting of counseling, migraine prophylactic medication (usually including antidepressants), education, and coping techniques is the best therapy. Continuity of care with a single knowledgeable physician is essential for these patients.

D. Traction or inflammatory headaches. Treatment of the underlying disease, whether medical or neurosurgical, is the best approach.

REFERENCES

Daroff RB: New headache classification. Neurology 1988;**38**:1138.
Maizels M: The clinician's approach to the management of headache. West J Med 1998;**168**:203.
Matthew NT: Serotonin 1D (5HT1D) agonists and other agents in migraine. Neurol Clin 1997; **15**:61.
Saper JR: Diagnosis and treatment of migraine. Headache 1997;**37**(suppl 1):S1.
Silberstein SD, Lipton RB: Overview of diagnosis and treatment of migraine. Neurology 1994; **44**(suppl 7):S6.

---

36   Hearing Loss

David Paul, MD, MPH, & Paula Root, MD, MPH

I. **Definition. Hearing loss** is a reduction of an individual's ability to perceive sound. **Sensorineural loss** results from deterioration of the cochlea, or lesions of the eighth cranial nerve. **Conductive loss** occurs when lesions of the external or middle ear impede the passage of sound waves to the inner ear. Combined sensorineural and conductive loss in the same ear is referred to as **mixed hearing loss. Central hearing disorders** result from lesions in the central auditory pathways.

II. **Common diagnoses** (Table 36–1)

   A. **Sensorineural loss**

      1. **Presbycusis.**

      2. **Acoustic damage.**

      3. **Ototoxicity.**

      4. **Meniere's disease.**

      5. **Other causes** of sensorineural loss not discussed in this chapter include neoplastic, metabolic, vascular, and viral disorders.

   B. **Conductive loss**

      1. **Obstruction of the external auditory canal.**

      2. **Otosclerosis.**

      3. **Otitis media.**

   C. Causes of **central hearing loss** not discussed in this chapter include demyelinating disease, ischemia, neoplasm, and hematoma.

III. **Epidemiology.** Approximately 15 million people in the United States are hearing impaired, and approximately 2 million Americans are functionally deaf. Approximately 90% of Americans over 65 years of age have some degree of hearing impairment, and approximately 15% of school-aged children have a 16-dB hearing loss. One of every 2000 individuals is deaf or severely hearing impaired. At least 90% of these hearing problems are secondary to middle ear disorders that are potentially treatable.

   A. **Sensorineural loss**

      1. **Presbycusis.** Eighty-three percent of those aged 57–89 in the Framingham Heart Study cohort had hearing loss because of the aging process, although many of these people had coexistent losses from cerumen impaction (30%) or ear canal collapse. Blacks had significantly less age-related hearing loss than did whites.

      2. **Acoustic damage,** or noise-induced hearing loss, may be caused by chronic exposure to excessive noise levels or from acoustic trauma, which occurs when a person is exposed to a specific noise event, such as a shotgun blast or a firecracker explosion.

         a. Over 9 million American workers are exposed to excessive noise levels, and as many as 17% of these workers have hearing loss.

         b. Noise exposure is not limited to the workplace. Noise-induced hearing loss has been demonstrated in children and adolescents.

TABLE 36–1. ETIOLOGY OF HEARING LOSS

Infectious
  Otitis media
  Mumps
  Rubella
  Herpes zoster
  Syphilis
  Tuberculosis
  Cytomegalovirus

Trauma
  Perforated tympanic membrane
  Temporal bone fracture

Environmental
  Acoustic trauma

Neoplastic
  Acoustic neuroma
  Meningioma
  Glomus tumor
  Cerebellopontine angle tumor

Systemic
  Sarcoidosis
  Giant cell granuloma
  Histiocytosis
  Collagen vascular disease
  Paget's disease
  Behçet's syndrome
  Hurler's syndrome

Local
  Obstructed ear canal from cerumen or foreign body
  Meniere's disease
  Otosclerosis
  Congenital cochlear deformity

Vascular
  Migraine
  Vascular compromise

Idiopathic

Ototoxic Agents
  Primarily reversible:
    Antimicrobials: Erythromycin, quinine,
      chloroquine
    Carbon monoxide diuretics: Furosemide,
      bumetanide, ethacrynic acid, acetazolamide,
      mannitol
    NSAIDs: Ibuprofen, indomethacin, piroxicam,
      naproxen, sulindac, ketoprofen, mefenamic
      acid
    Salicylates

  Primarily irreversible:
    Antimicrobials: Aminoglycosides (kanamycin,
      neomycin, gentamicin, tobramycin, strepto-
      mycin, netilmicin, amikacin), vancomycin
    Antineoplastics: Cisplatin, vincristine,
      vinblastine, nitrogen mustard, bleomycin
    Bromates heavy metals: Arsenic, mercury, lead
    Hydrocarbons: Toluene, xylene, styrene

3. **Ototoxicity** is caused primarily by exposure to drugs. The risk of ototoxicity increases for patients who are given parenteral drugs, who have decreased creatinine clearance, whose treatment is extended beyond 14 days, who are of an advanced age, or who are using other potentially ototoxic drugs. This condition is the most common cause of deafness in children. Environmental exposure and workplace exposure are less common causal agents. Cigarette smokers are 1.69 times as likely to have a hearing loss as nonsmokers.
4. **Meniere's disease** is most common between the fourth and sixth decades but may occur at any age.
   B. **Conductive loss**
1. Approximately 12% of the Framingham cohort had conductive hearing loss because of **impacted cerumen** or an **obstruction of the external canal** by a foreign body. This type of loss is more common in older males than in women or young males.
2. **Otosclerosis** results in adult deafness approximately 50% of the time. This condition is transmitted through autosomal dominant inheritance with variable expression and is common in young to middle-aged women. Otosclerosis typically occurs in patients during the second or third decade of life, and the disorder is 10 times more common among whites than blacks.
IV. **Pathophysiology**
   A. **Sensorineural loss**
1. **Presbycusis.** This condition results from atrophy of the organ of Corti at the basal end of the cochlea. It is a slow and progressive deterioration of hearing associated with aging and may begin in middle age.

2. **Acoustic damage.** Excessive noise exposure generally affects hair cells of the cochlea, causing noise-induced hearing loss. Once these cells are damaged, they cannot be replaced. Impulse noise or acoustic trauma can cause areas of the basilar membrane to become detached, which results in free-floating fragments in the cochlear duct.

3. **Ototoxicity.** Exposure to ototoxic agents may result in cochleotoxicity, vestibulotoxicity, or both. Hearing impairment may be either permanent (eg, when caused by drugs such as mercury, arsenic, lead, or aminoglycosides) or temporary (eg, when caused by drugs such as aspirin, quinine, or certain diuretics). Actual recovery may be delayed and is often incomplete. The correlation between ototoxicity and plasma levels of drugs is poor.

4. **Meniere's disease.** This disorder is typically unilateral and associated with fluctuating hearing loss, vertigo, and tinnitus. Recurrent episodes of endolymphatic hypertension (hydrops) are thought to cause dilation of the endolymphatic sac and atrophy of the hair cells.

B. **Conductive hearing loss**

1. **Obstruction.** Hearing loss often results from obstruction of the external ear canal by cerumen or foreign bodies, such as crayons, food, or toys. Cerumen sometimes accumulates in the auditory canal of individuals with either excessive production of cerumen or ineffective self-cleaning mechanisms. In the third and fourth decades of life, the hairs found in ear canals become coarser and longer, which secondarily reduces natural clearance of cerumen. Otitis externa may also obstruct the canal.

2. **Otosclerosis.** This is a progressive sclerotic fixation of the stapes in the round window, which results in a dampening of sound conduction to the cochlea.

3. **Otitis media** (suppurative or serous). The collection of fluid behind the tympanic membrane may cause hearing loss. Hearing should return to normal after the infection is treated, unless significant scarring or rupture of the tympanic membrane is present.

V. **Symptoms**

A. The **time at which symptoms occur** may indicate particular problems.

1. **Noise-induced hearing loss** may be most pronounced shortly after the patient leaves the workplace, and the patient's hearing may improve while away from work.

2. A temporal relationship between the use of a toxic agent and the symptomatology is generally present in patients with **ototoxicity.**

3. Symptoms of hearing loss from **impacted cerumen** frequently begin suddenly following bathing or swimming when a drop of water closes the passageway.

B. **Vertigo, imbalance,** and **disequilibrium** may occur in patients with ototoxicity. Nausea sometimes occurs in patients with this condition.

C. High-pitched **tinnitus** may occur in individuals with **presbycusis, noise-induced hearing loss,** and **otosclerosis.**

D. **Reduced hearing acuity**

1. Patients with **presbycusis** may not report reduced hearing acuity until late in the disease process. However, they often cannot understand what people are saying when ambient noise levels may be relatively loud, as in crowded or large areas or on the telephone. Some patients complain that people mumble.

2. Patients with **noise-induced hearing loss** first notice some muffling of sound, but they usually consult a physician only when they begin to experience difficulties hearing speech, which is a late finding.

3. Patients with **conductive hearing loss** tend to hear conversation better in noisy rooms than in quiet rooms. Reduced hearing acuity is common in patients with **impacted cerumen.**

E. **Intolerance of loud noises** sometimes occurs in individuals with **presbycusis.**

F. **Pain, discomfort, or itching** can occur in patients with hearing loss from **impacted cerumen, otitis media,** or **otitis externa.**

G. **Chronic cough** may be present in patients with impacted cerumen if the impaction abuts the tympanic membrane. The cough should disappear with removal of the impaction.

H. **Behavioral changes** resulting from isolation and depression caused by hearing loss may include fear, anger, depression, frustration, embarrassment, or anxiety.

(Elderly people with hearing loss suffer depression twice as often as the general population.)

VI. Signs. Physical findings may be limited.

A. Otoscopic examination

1. Impacted cerumen or a foreign body may be evident.
2. Findings consistent with otitis externa or otitis media (see Chapter 25) may be seen.
3. The medial wall of the middle ear or the promontory seen through the tympanic membrane may appear reddish in patients with **otosclerosis.**

B. Tuning fork tests

1. **Lateralization of the Weber's test to one side** means either a conductive loss on that side or a sensorineural loss on the opposite side. The Weber's test is performed by placing the handle of a vibrating tuning fork (512 cycles/s) against the midline of the patient's forehead. A patient with normal sensorineural function and no conductive loss hears the sound equally in both ears.
2. A **Rinne test** can assess both **air and bone conduction. Air conduction** persists longer than **bone conduction** in a patient with no hearing loss. To determine bone conduction, one places the tuning fork against the mastoid process until the patient can no longer hear the fork. To test air conduction, one places the fork near the ear, without touching it. Equal hearing levels at both positions are consistent with hearing loss of mixed cause. If air conduction is louder, either normal hearing or **sensorineural loss** may exist. If bone conduction is louder, **conductive loss** exists.

VII. Laboratory tests. An **audiogram** is the primary study generally indicated in patients with hearing loss. Tympanometry is a useful test to assess middle ear function. Referral to an otolaryngologist is appropriate if more sophisticated testing is required.

A. Indications

1. Audiometry is indicated in all patients with hearing loss, except those patients with a foreign body or acute infection whose hearing normalizes following treatment. Audiometry measures threshold levels (ie, the intensity at which the patient is able to perceive sound correctly 50% of the time). This level is usually measured by presenting pure tones to the individual at preset frequencies through air conduction and occasionally through bone conduction.
2. It is recommended that baseline audiometry be performed within 3 days of institution of therapy with ototoxic agents for patients who are alert enough to cooperate with the examination. Serial audiometry on an individual basis should be considered during the course of treatment and should be performed annually after treatment, if indicated by the patient's condition.

B. Findings

1. **Sensorineural loss** causes lower thresholds in low frequencies than in high frequencies.
   a. Individuals with **presbycusis** display a pattern with a greater high-frequency loss at 8000 than at 4000 cycles, often described as a smooth, ski slope–shaped curve. The loss is generally equal bilaterally. It is not always possible to distinguish, from an audiogram alone, whether the hearing loss is the effect of presbycusis, noise exposure, or ototoxic agents.
   b. The classic **noise-induced pattern** on the audiogram shows high-frequency loss, greatest at 4000 cycles, with improvement at 8000 cycles. The audiogram should be measured at least 14 hours after the last significant noise exposure in order to minimize the confusion of temporary versus permanent threshold shifts.
2. **Conductive loss** causes low-frequency (ie, 125–500 cycles) loss rather than high-frequency loss. Bone conduction testing in patients with conductive hearing loss reveals normal hearing thresholds.
3. **Mixed loss** causes audiometric patterns with features of both sensorineural and conductive hearing loss.

VIII. Treatment

A. Preventive measures. Effective measures to prevent or minimize hearing loss are described below.

1. Physicians should **minimize the use of ototoxic drugs** and **carefully monitor** patients taking these drugs.

    2. Individuals with exposure to noise at home or work (Table 36–2) should re-
ceive education concerning the use of **ear protection during noise exposure** and should be fitted for proper **ear protective devices.**

B. Sensorineural loss

    1. Presbycusis. Patients with a presumptive diagnosis of presbycusis should
be referred to an audiologist for further testing to confirm the diagnosis and
for rehabilitation. Patients may increase the effectiveness of communication
by using the following techniques: cupping the hand behind the ear, finding
a quiet environment in order to reduce distractions and background noise
levels, using good lighting in order to see the speaker and to understand gestures, and learning various lipreading techniques. Hearing aids or other assis-
tive devices may be beneficial. Psychological support, particularly for elderly
patients, is very helpful.

    2. Noise-induced loss. Patients with this type of loss should be referred to an
otolaryngologist if the following indications are present: asymmetric hearing
loss, rapid and progressive hearing loss, permanent threshold shift, or an occasional finding of low-frequency loss. All patients with losses presenting at
threshold levels of >25 dB are candidates for hearing aids.

    3. Ototoxicity. For patients with ototoxicity, time is of the essence. Early removal
of the offending agent will reduce the likelihood of permanent hearing loss.

C. Conductive loss

    1. Foreign bodies or **cerumen** in the external auditory canal can almost always
be removed by irrigation, forceps, or earloops. If the object is wedged in place,
the patient should be referred to an otolaryngologist because of the risk of
damage to the tympanic membrane or bony structures presented by attempts
at removal.

        a. Hard cerumen can be softened fairly quickly prior to irrigation with a few
drops of dishwashing detergent. The ear can be irrigated with water approximately 20 minutes after the detergent is applied. The use of water
at a temperature of 35–37.8 °C (95–100 °F) will prevent the patient from
experiencing vertigo.

        b. Water irrigation, which can cause foreign bodies consisting of vegetable
matter to swell, is contraindicated in the presence of such foreign bodies.
Alcohol solutions should be used in such cases. A perforation in the tympanic membrane is an absolute contraindication to irrigation.

    2. Otitis externa or **otitis media** should be treated with appropriate medica-
tions (see Chapter 25).

TABLE 36–2. TYPICAL NOISE LEVELS

Type of Noise	Decibels (dB)
Industrial	
Riveting machine	110
Textile loom	106
Farm tractor	98
Newspaper press	97
Lathe	81
Community	
Jet flyover at 1000 ft	103
Power mower	96
Motorcycle at 25 ft	90
Diesel truck 40 mph at 50 ft	84
Near freeway, auto traffic	64
Air conditioning unit at 20 ft	60
Home	
Rock band	<108–114>
Food blender	88
Garbage disposal	80
Dishwasher	75
Conversation	60

3. Otosclerosis can be successfully treated with stapedectomy. Patients with this condition should be referred to an otolaryngologist.

REFERENCES

Bahadori R: Adverse effects of noise on hearing. Am Fam Physician 1993;**47:**1219.

Brookhouser P, Northington D, Kelly W: Noise-induced hearing loss in children. Laryngoscope 1992;**102:**634.

Cruickshanks KJ, Klein R, Klein B, et al: Cigarette smoking and hearing loss. JAMA 1998; **279:**1715.

Morata T, Dunn D, Sieber W: Occupational exposure to noise and ototoxic organic solvents. Arch Environ Health 1994;**49:**359.

Moscicki EK, Elkins EF, Baum HM, et al: Hearing loss in the elderly: An epidemiologic study of the Framingham Heart Study cohort. Ear Hear 1985;**6**(4):184.

Niskar A, Kieszak S, Holmes A, et al: Prevalence of hearing loss among children 6 to 19 years of age. JAMA 1998;**279:**1071.

Pedersen K, Rosenhall U, Moller M: Changes in pure-tone thresholds in individuals ages 70–81: Results from a longitudinal study. Audiology 1989;**28:**194.

37   Hematuria

Leonard W. Morgan, MD, PhD

I. **Definition.** Hematuria is the presence of red blood cells (RBCs) in urine. It can be classified as gross or microscopic, depending on whether blood is visible or invisible to the unaided eye. Significant hematuria is three or more RBCs per high-power field in a centrifuged specimen.

II. **Common diagnoses**

   A. **Urinary tract infections,** such as cystitis and pyelonephritis (34% of all cases of gross hematuria, 28% of all cases of microscopic hematuria).

   B. **Prostatic diseases,** such as benign prostatic hypertrophy (BPH) and prostatitis (18% of all cases of gross hematuria, 13.2% of all cases of microscopic hematuria).

   C. **Neoplasms** resulting from renal, bladder, and prostatic cancer (22.5% of all cases of gross hematuria, 3–10% of all cases of microscopic hematuria).

   D. **Urinary stones** (5.3% of all cases of gross hematuria, 0.4% of all cases of microscopic hematuria).

   E. **Trauma** (2% of all cases of gross hematuria).

   F. **Renal diseases,** such as glomerulonephritis. Rare in adults, this condition is responsible for 50% of the cases of hematuria in children.

   G. **Drugs.** See Table 37–1.

III. **Epidemiology.** Gross hematuria is common, and microscopic hematuria occurs in 3–4% of the adult population.

   A. **Urinary tract infections.** Cystitis is more common in females than in males.

   B. **Prostatic diseases**

TABLE 37–1. DRUGS THAT MAY CAUSE HEMATURIA

Drug	Induced Condition
Aspirin-phenacetin combination	Papillary necrosis, analgesic nephropathy, uroepithelial tumors
Penicillins	Allergic interstitial nephritis
Cephalosporins	
Sulfonamides	
Phenytoin (Dilantin)	
Cyclophosphamide (Cytoxan)	Chemical hemorrhagic cystitis, uroepithelial tumors
Mitotane (Lysodren)	
Anticoagulants	Spontaneous urinary tract bleeding, bleeding from occult urinary tract neoplasm
Primaquine	Hemoglobinuria resulting from hemolysis in individuals with glucose-6-phosphate dehydrogenase deficiency
Nitrofurantoin (Furadantin, Macrodantin)	

        1. BPH. Clinically significant BPH affects an average of 23% of males by age 45 and 88% of males by age 90.

        2. Prostatitis. This disease occurs with equal frequency in postpubertal males of all ages.

   C. Neoplasms. The incidence of neoplasms increases after age 40.

        1. Carcinoma of the bladder, which accounts for two thirds of these neoplasms, occurs mainly after the sixth decade. The peak incidence occurs at an earlier age in patients who work in the printing, leather, and dye industries, however. The condition is also associated with cigarette smoking. Carcinoma of the bladder is three times more common in males than in females.

        2. Renal cell carcinoma accounts for up to 90% of all renal tumors. This type of carcinoma has a peak incidence after age 50 and affects males more often than females. Renal cell carcinoma has also been associated with cigarette smoking.

        3. Carcinoma of the prostate is a disease of old age that rarely occurs before age 50. It increases in incidence from 10% of all men in the fifth decade to 50% of all men over age 80.

        4. Wilms' tumor, the most common malignancy in children, occurs most often in children under 6 years old.

   D. Urinary stones. People who live in the southeastern United States have an increased incidence of such stones. Individuals with gout or leukemia (receiving chemotherapy), as well as those persons with a positive family history of nephrolithiasis, are at increased risk for developing stones.

   E. Trauma. Direct trauma to the abdomen or the pelvis is most often the cause of hematuria. Indirect trauma such as physical exertion (as by marathon runners) is also associated with hematuria, however.

   F. Renal diseases. Nephrogenic streptococcal pharyngitis is the most common cause of glomerulonephritis in children.

IV. Pathophysiology

   A. Urinary tract infections. See Chapter 24.

   B. Prostatic diseases. In BPH, the persistent contraction of the detrusor muscle produces enlargement and dilatation of the mucosal vessels. Bleeding then occurs by leakage of RBCs or vessel rupture.

   C. Neoplasms. Inflammation or obstruction causes vasodilatation and RBC leakage through the epithelial junction. Enlarging tumors cause bleeding by necrosis or erosion into adjacent blood vessels.

   D. Urinary stones. In passing down the ureters, the lodging and dislodging of stones causes mucosal and small vessel disruption. Inflammation from stones lodged for a significant amount of time can also contribute to the bleeding.

   E. Trauma. Blunt trauma can cause fracture of the kidney, rupture of subcortical vessels, and/or rupture of major vessels to the kidney, as well as ureteral, bladder, or urethral injury. Hematuria resulting from blunt trauma to the abdomen without obvious renal damage probably represents a contusion of the kidney and may be a predictor of other intra-abdominal injuries. Solid organs, such as the spleen and the liver, are most often involved.

   F. Renal diseases. Seventy-five percent of the glomerulopathies have an immunologic origin. The final common path is damage to the glomerulus with widening of the epithelial junction and subsequent loss of RBCs.

V. Symptoms

   A. Hematuria associated with **suprapubic pain, dysuria, urgency, frequency,** and **nocturia,** especially in women, makes cystitis a likely diagnosis (see Chapter 24).

   B. Dysuria, fever, suprapubic or back pain, and **urinary frequency and urgency,** occasionally associated with hematuria, are symptoms of acute prostatitis. Patients with chronic prostatitis usually present with isolated back pain, dysuria, or posterior urethral discomfort upon ejaculation. Prostatism is commonly associated with obstructive symptoms, such as dribbling, incomplete voiding, urgency, and hesitancy. Nocturia is also common and is probably related to incomplete voiding.

   C. The presence of **blood in the urine,** usually **unaccompanied by other symptoms,** is the most common presenting symptom of carcinoma of the bladder. Hematuria occurs in 85% of such patients. Urgency, frequency, and stranguria may also reflect the presence of cancer.

Hematuria is also present in 90% of cases of renal cell carcinoma. Sometimes the tumor is manifested primarily as constitutional symptoms, such as fever, malaise, weakness, and weight loss. These symptoms, however, are generally associated with metastatic disease. The classic association of pain, hematuria, and abdominal mass is rare.

D. Flank pain associated with gross or microscopic hematuria indicates the presence of urinary stones. Patients with stones present with silent (painless) hematuria or flank pain with hematuria.

E. Patients with **primary renal diseases** (conditions that originate in the kidney, such as glomerulonephritis) may present with gross or microscopic hematuria with or without flank pain. In contrast, secondary conditions (eg, systemic lupus erythematosus or endocarditis) are more likely to be silent or present with systemic symptoms.

F. In general, **gross hematuria** may be induced by exercise. Blunt trauma may result in pain at the site of injury.

VI. Signs

A. Pyelonephritis can usually be differentiated from cystitis by the presence of fever, costovertebral angle tenderness, and a "toxic" appearance (see Chapter 24).

B. In BPH, **digital rectal examination** may reveal enlarged but firm lateral lobes. The degree of obstruction generally correlates with median lobe hypertrophy, which cannot be evaluated by rectal examination.

In acute prostatitis, digital rectal examination reveals an enlarged, boggy prostate gland, occasionally with increased warmth to the touch. No specific physical finding of chronic prostatitis is evident.

C. Physical examination is of limited value in the evaluation of urologic malignancies. No specific findings of bladder cancer are apparent on physical examination. An abdominal mass is a late finding in renal carcinoma. Weight loss and muscle weakness are generally associated with metastatic disease. Digital rectal examination commonly reveals a stony-hard or nodular prostate in prostatic carcinoma. An abdominal mass is the most frequent and consistent physical finding of Wilms' tumor.

D. Patients with hematuria due to vigorous exercise usually have no clinical signs. However, those with blunt trauma may have tenderness, ecchymoses, or abrasions at the point of impact.

E. Patients with glomerulonephritis commonly present with hypertension and edema, but they may also show no signs of the disease. Secondary glomerulonephritis may be characterized by fever, rash, joint tenderness, heart murmur, or splinter hemorrhages of the nail beds.

VII. Laboratory tests. Figure 37–1 outlines the approach to patients with microscopic hematuria.

A. Urinalysis (UA). Dipstick and microscopic evaluation of a centrifuged urine specimen should be the initial step in the diagnostic work-up of patients with hematuria. This test is inexpensive and confirms the presence or absence of blood in the urine. Certain results point to the cause of the hematuria.

    1. Sample collection. A midstream specimen improves the chances of a good sample for analysis and culture. Catheterization may be necessary, especially in females of childbearing age. Iatrogenic hematuria may result from urethral trauma.

    2. Initial hematuria (hematuria with initiation of micturition) suggests a lesion in the urethra, whereas **terminal hematuria** (hematuria at the end of micturition) suggests a bladder neck or a prostatic urethral lesion. **Total hematuria** (hematuria occurring throughout micturition) occurs with bladder, ureteral, or renal lesions.

    3. Documentation of hematuria. True hematuria should be differentiated from **pseudohematuria.** Pseudohematuria can be derived from at least two sources: chemical agents (Table 37–2) or, in females, cervical or vaginal bleeding.

    4. Associated findings that can narrow the differential diagnosis include crystals in nephrolithiasis, bacteria in infections, and >2+ (100 mg of protein per deciliter) proteinuria or RBC casts in glomerular disease. Dysmorphic RBCs with a wide range of alterations in the urinary sediment also suggest glomerular disease. White blood cell casts may be seen in pyelonephritis. Pyuria with hematuria may be due to infection, stones, tumors, or glomerulonephritis.

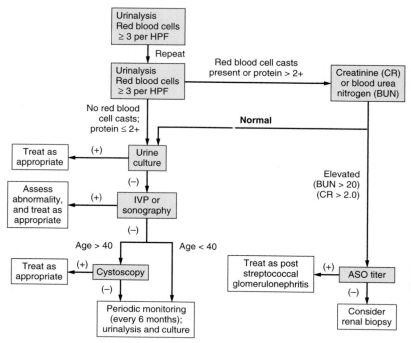

FIGURE 37–1. Algorithm for laboratory and radiologic work-up of hematuria. ASO, Antistreptolysin O.; HPF, high-power field; IVP, intravenous pyelography.

TABLE 37–2. CAUSES OF "RED URINE" (PSEUDOHEMATURIA)

Endogenous substances
  Red blood cells (hematuria)
  Free hemoglobin
  Myoglobin
  Bilirubin
  Urobilinogen
  Porphyrins

Exogenous substances
Dyes
  Beets
  Blackberries
  Rhubarb
Drugs
  Anthraquinone-containing laxatives
  Chloroquine (Aralen)
  Deferoxamine (Desferal)
  Doxorubicin (Adriamycin)
  Metronidazole (Flagyl)
  Phenothiazines
  Phenytoin (Dilantin)
  Rifampin (Rifadin, Rimactane)
  Sulfasalazine (Azulfidine)

5. Some urine dipsticks can test for the presence of nitrates, which are suggestive of a urinary tract infection. The dipstick can give a false-positive result. Therefore, it is important to corroborate dipstick findings with microscopic examination.

B. **Urine culture.** Regardless of the results of the UA, urine culture is a reasonable next step in the evaluation of hematuria. The patient's history and physical examination and the results of a urine culture can establish the diagnosis of pyelonephritis, cystitis, or prostatitis. A positive culture in patients over 40 years of age does not rule out malignancy, and further diagnostic work-up is therefore indicated.

C. **Phase contrast microscopy.** Evaluation of RBC morphology in urine to determine the site of bleeding in hematuria has been used extensively over the last few years. Phase contrast microscopy is the technique most often used to evaluate hematuria. It has a sensitivity of 90–95% and a specificity of 95–100% in differentiating glomerular from lower tract bleeding. This test is promising and should be used early in the evaluation of hematuria (after a urinary tract infection has been excluded).

D. **Multichemistry profile.** In patients with suspected glomerular disease, blood urea nitrogen (BUN), creatinine (Cr), serum protein, and serum lipid determinations can be helpful. For example, elevated BUN and Cr, a decreased albumin level, and hyperlipidemia may be seen in some cases of glomerulonephritis.

E. **Complete blood cell count (CBC).** A nonspecific test in the evaluation of hematuria, this test can document the degree of blood loss and indicate the presence of systemic involvement (eg, pyelonephritis or cystitis). Target cells or sickle cells suggest hemoglobinopathy as a possible cause of hematuria.

F. **Erythrocyte sedimentation rate (ESR).** This test, which is also nonspecific, should be considered only if a secondary glomerular disease is suspected. In cases of endocarditis and systemic lupus erythematosus, the ESR would likely be elevated.

G. **Intravenous pyelography (IVP).** This technique is the most effective method for evaluating the anatomy of the upper urinary tract. With the addition of a cysto-urethrogram, the lower urinary tract can also be viewed.

   1. An IVP is indicated if UA confirms hematuria on two separate specimens and urine cultures are negative. IVP has demonstrated utility in the evaluation of urolithiasis, renal tumors, renal trauma, carcinoma of the bladder, and BPH.
      Further studies may be necessary to completely rule out bladder or renal carcinoma. Bladder tumors 1 cm or larger can be visualized only 75% of the time. Therefore, the absence of a radiolucent bladder lesion does not exclude the presence of a bladder tumor. If bladder carcinoma is suspected, a cystoscopic evaluation is indicated even with a negative IVP. All patients with a history of renal trauma and hematuria should undergo an IVP or radiographic evaluation.
   2. Conditions that may preclude the use of IVP are allergy to the dye and diminished renal function.

H. **Nephrotomography.** This radiographic test, combined with an IVP, improves the capability of detecting small renal carcinomas.

I. **Ultrasonography.** This technique can be used to evaluate the same lesions as with IVP, with some limitations. It is not as effective as IVP in evaluating urolithiasis and carcinoma of the bladder. Ultrasonography can be quite helpful if the patient either is allergic to the dye used in IVP or has compromised renal function, or if a cystic lesion of the kidney is suspected.

J. **Cystoscopy.** This procedure should be used in the evaluation of all patients over 40 years of age who present with gross hematuria. It should also be used in patients over 40 with microscopic hematuria who have a negative urine culture, IVP, or sonogram. With cystoscopy, lesions can be visualized directly and biopsies can be taken. Even if cystoscopy is normal, a higher-yield sample for cytology may be obtained. Cystoscopy is the procedure of choice for evaluating patients suspected of having carcinoma of the bladder.

K. **Computerized tomography (CT).** This technique is used to evaluate small lesions of the kidney and for staging bladder carcinoma. Although it is an excellent diagnostic tool, it is not cost-effective in most instances.

L. **Angiography.** This procedure is rarely needed in the evaluation of hematuria because CT scans, ultrasonography, and other diagnostic tools can provide the same information more safely and cost-effectively.

M. Renal biopsy. This procedure is indicated in two instances: (1) when other diagnostic tests have yielded little information and hematuria persists, and (2) if the patient's history and laboratory data suggest that glomerulonephritis is the cause of hematuria.

VIII. Treatment
    A. Urinary tract infections. See Chapter 24.
    B. Prostatic diseases. See Chapter 64.
    C. Neoplasms. Surgery, chemotherapy, and radiation are possible modalities. Details of therapeutic interventions are beyond the scope of this chapter.
    D. Urinary stones
        1. Once ureteral obstruction is ruled out and the acute episode has passed, calyceal stones can be managed expectantly with hydration and analgesia. However, patients with ureteral stones too large to pass should be referred to a urologist.
        2. Patients with renal calculi can be considered for lithotripsy.
        3. Prophylactic therapy should be instituted after the acute episode has passed. Reasonable prophylaxis against recurrent stones is achieved by maintaining a urine flow rate of 3–4 L/day. Recurrence of uric acid stones may be prevented by a low-purine diet and uricosuric agents.
    E. Trauma. Exercise-induced hematuria is self-limited. Urologic trauma is best managed with the assistance of a urologist.
    F. Renal diseases. Therapy for poststreptococcal glomerulonephritis, a condition that can be managed by family physicians, is generally limited to treating the associated hypertension. Rapid or continued deterioration of renal indices (increasing BUN and Cr) requires consultation.

REFERENCES

Brendler CB: *History, Physical Examination, and Urinalysis. Campbell's Urology,* vol I. 7th ed. Saunders; 1998;146.

Copley JB, Hasbargen JA: "Idiopathic" hematuria: A prospective evaluation. Arch Intern Med 1987;**147:**434.

Crompton CH, Ward PB, Hewitt IK: The use of urinary red cell morphology to determine the source of hematuria in children. Clin Nephrol 1993;**39:**44.

Fuselier HA Jr, Rous SN, Sullivan JW: A practical workup for hematuria. Patient Care 1990; **24:**159.

Knudson MM, McAninch JW, Gomez R, et al: Hematuria as a predictor of abdominal injury after blunt trauma. Am J Surg 1992;**164:**482.

Mohammad KS, Bdesha AS, Snell ME, et al: Phase contrast microscopic examination of urinary erythrocytes to localize source of bleeding: An overlooked technique? Clin Pathol 1993; **46:**642.

Mohr DN, Offord KP, Melton LJ III: Isolated asymptomatic microhematuria: A cross-sectional analysis of test-positive and test-negative patients. J Gen Intern Med 1987;**2:**318.

Restrepo NC, Carey PO: Evaluating hematuria in adults. Am Fam Physician 1989;**40:**149.

---

38   Hip Pain

Richard Viken, MD

  I. Definition. Hip pain is pain in or about the hip that may be caused by processes in the hip joint or surrounding muscles, soft tissues, or neurovascular elements.
  II. Common diagnoses. Causes of hip pain may be diagnosed partially on the basis of the patient's age.
    A. Causes of hip pain in **children and adolescents,** in order of decreasing frequency, include transient (toxic) synovitis, bacterial infection, Perthes disease, and slipped femoral capital epiphysis.
    B. Hip pain in **adults** may result from several conditions, listed in order of decreasing frequency: osteoarthritis and rheumatoid arthritis (representing 90% of adult hip pain), fractures, referred pain, bursitis, meralgia paresthetica, avascular necrosis, and malignancy (see Figure 38–1).

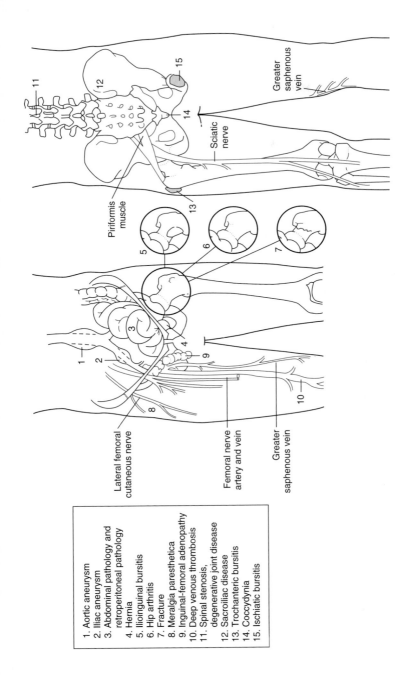

FIGURE 38–1. Hip pain can represent different musculoskeletal and nonmusculoskeletal problems.

1. Aortic aneurysm
2. Iliac aneurysm
3. Abdominal pathology and retroperitoneal pathology
4. Hernia
5. Ilioinguinal bursitis
6. Hip arthritis
7. Fracture
8. Meralgia paresthetica
9. Inguinal-femoral adenopathy
10. Deep venous thrombosis
11. Spinal stenosis, degenerative joint disease
12. Sacroiliac disease
13. Trochanteric bursitis
14. Coccydynia
15. Ischiatic bursitis

For epidemiology and further discussion of low back pain, rheumatoid arthritis, and osteoarthritis, see Chapters 46 and 71. To obtain more information about pelvic soft tissue disorders causing hip pain, see Chapter 55.

III. Epidemiology

A. **Transient synovitis** usually occurs in boys (male-female ratio, 3:2) aged 2–12 (average age, 6) years. It is considered the most common nontraumatic cause of hip pain in childhood.

B. **Infection** of the hip joint can occur at any age but is most common in infants and toddlers.

C. **Perthes disease** most often occurs in boys (male-female ratio, 5:1) aged 3–10 years. It is bilateral 12% of the time. The families of children with the disorder exhibit an increased incidence varying from 2% to 20%, although no consistent hereditary pattern exists. Within the general population, the incidence is 1 per 20,000. Low birth weight is a risk factor.

D. **Slipped femoral capital epiphysis** occurs in adolescence (male-female ratio, 2:1). The incidence varies from 2 to 10 per 100,000. About one third of the cases are bilateral. Two thirds of the children are obese.

E. **Bursitis** can be associated with a history of trauma or overuse. Trochanteric bursitis occurs predominantly in women during the fourth to sixth decades. Its onset is insidious, preceded by apparent trauma in only one quarter of the cases. Ischial bursitis is associated with prolonged sitting on hard surfaces, thus the name "weaver's bottom."

F. **Meralgia paresthetica** is most commonly seen in overweight, middle-aged men. Pregnancy and constrictive clothing also may cause this condition.

G. Nontraumatic **avascular necrosis** of the femoral head begins between the ages of 25 and 45. In 75% of the cases, predisposing factors include corticosteroid therapy, alcoholism, sickle cell disease, and dysbaric occupational exposure (eg, underground and undersea workers). This condition accounts for 10% of the total hip joint replacements in the United States.

H. In one series of 176 cases of **cancer,** 18% of metastases were to the pelvis or the femur, most commonly from cancer of the breast, prostate, lung, kidney, and thyroid (in that order). Additionally, multiple myeloma may cause hip pain in older adults.

IV. Pathophysiology

A. **Transient synovitis** may be related to antecedent viral or bacterial upper respiratory infection, recurrent microtrauma, or allergic hypersensitivity, although a cause-effect relationship has not been proven. Biopsies reveal nonspecific inflammatory congestion and synovial membrane hypertrophy.

B. **Infection** of the hip joint is usually caused by *Staphylococcus aureus* or *Haemophilus influenzae* via the skin, upper or lower respiratory tract, or umbilical structures. Femoral vein or artery puncture also can cause direct joint contamination. The relatively small hip joint space allows rapid pressure-induced destruction of vessels and cartilage by accumulating pus and proteolytic enzymes.

C. **Perthes disease** is an avascular necrosis of the femoral head. The cause is uncertain.

D. In **slipped femoral capital epiphysis,** the upper femoral epiphysis slips posteromedially off the metaphysis. This can occur either acutely with severe trauma (a worse prognosis) or gradually, as in 80% of patients, in response to chronic heavy loading.

E. In hip **bursitis,** excessive friction and direct trauma cause inflammation of the bursal wall with fluid exudate and occasional calcium deposition. In 15% of iliopsoas (iliopectineal) bursitis cases, the bursa communicates directly with the hip joint.

F. **Meralgia paresthetica** is compression of the lateral femoral cutaneous nerve, a sensory branch of L2–L3 innervating the anterolateral aspect of the thigh. The nerve is usually affected as it exits from the lateral aspect of the inguinal ligament.

G. Nontraumatic **avascular necrosis** is due to vascular insufficiency to the femoral head.

H. **Cancers** produce hip pain through osteoclast-induced bone resorption, which results in osteoporosis, microfractures, and possible pathologic fracture of the proximal femur or pelvis.

V. Symptoms

A. **Transient synovitis** most commonly causes a painful limp, acute in one half of the patients, insidious in the other half. Pain occasionally will awaken children at night.

B. In **bacterial infection,** patients appear apprehensive and toxic with constant hip pain that is worsened by movement. Neonates have poorly localized symptoms, are often septic, and present with failure to thrive, difficult feeding, lethargy, irritability, or abdominal distention.

C. **Perthes disease** first appears as pain and stiffness in the groin, lateral hip, or medial knee. A limp then develops. Knee pain alone may occur in 15% of the cases. The patient usually tolerates symptoms for 1–12 months before seeing a physician.

D. **Slipped femoral capital epiphysis** is characterized by simultaneous pain and limp in 50% of the patients, with pain preceding limp in the others. Pain is localized to the groin, buttock, or lateral hip. Knee pain alone may occur. About 20% of the patients present acutely with a history of a sudden twisting or falling injury.

E. The hip pain of **osteoarthritis** and **rheumatoid arthritis** is insidious in onset and is often referred to the groin, thigh, knee, and lateral side of the leg. It is frequently accompanied by subtle stiffening experienced as difficulty crossing the legs or engaging in sexual intercourse. Upper-extremity symptoms are commonly present (see Chapter 71).

F. **Bursitis**

   1. **Trochanteric bursitis** causes pain in the thigh and along the posterolateral hip margin. Running worsens the pain.

   2. **Ischial bursitis** results in pain or tenderness over the ischial tuberosities that is worsened by sitting.

   3. **Iliopsoas bursitis** causes pain over the superior anterior aspect of the joint and under the psoas muscle. The patient frequently limps with the hip in flexion and external rotation. The position of hip extension intensifies the pain, which is commonly noted on arising from a chair or assuming a supine position in bed.

G. **Meralgia paresthetica** causes pain or paresthesias over the anterior superior iliac spine and the anterior lateral thigh. Prolonged standing and walking may worsen the pain, while sitting may relieve it.

H. **Avascular necrosis** appears as abrupt hip pain followed by progressive, intermittent episodes in 85% of the patients. Motion and activity invariably worsen the pain. Pain at rest is present in two thirds of the patients, and night pain occurs in about 40% of those afflicted.

I. **Cancers** can cause acute pain and disability if a pathologic fracture occurs. More commonly, the condition is gradual in onset and exacerbated by movement.

VI. Signs

A. **Transient synovitis** produces voluntary limited hip motion. Thigh circumference may be diminished. Muscle spasm may occur. Patients are not ill or febrile.

B. In **bacterial infection,** the hip is in 20 degrees of flexion, abduction, and lateral rotation—a position that maximizes the joint's capacity for accumulating fluid. The proximal thigh is swollen. Fever is present.

C. **Perthes disease** produces an antalgic gait (an acute, one-sided limp in which the patient takes quick, soft steps to shorten the period of weight bearing on the involved extremity), limited hip motion, and occasionally a flexion contracture. Thigh and calf circumferences are diminished, and late in the process, the leg length may decrease.

D. **Slipped femoral capital epiphysis** causes a limp characterized by short steps with external rotation of the foot. Passive hip flexion elicits external rotation and abduction of the femur. One half of these patients will have thigh atrophy, and one half will have shortening of the extremity up to 1 in.

E. A limp is present in **osteoarthritis** and **rheumatoid arthritis.** Hip range of motion is limited in all directions, especially internal rotation and adduction. Flexion deformities may be present (see Chapter 71).

F. **Bursitis**

   1. Palpation over the greater trochanter reproduces the pain of **trochanteric bursitis.** External rotation and abduction against resistance worsen the pain.

2. Palpation of the ischial tuberosity elicits the pain of **ischial bursitis.** Straight leg raising is limited and painful.

3. Palpable tenderness over the involved bursa is found in **iliopsoas bursitis.** Hip extension may be limited. A cystic mass is present in about 30% of the patients. Quadriceps atrophy may be present in patients with profound bursal enlargement that encroaches on the femoral nerve.

G. The pain of **meralgia paresthetica** can be mimicked by palpating the lateral femoral cutaneous nerve against the medial aspect of the anterior superior iliac spine. Touch and pinprick sensation over the anteriolateral thigh is diminished. Muscle wasting or weakness is not present.

H. **Avascular necrosis** causes a limp and limited abduction and internal rotation.

I. In early **malignant** involvement of the hip, there are no significant signs. Later, swelling that is palpable and tender may develop over superficial bony prominences. Pathologic fracture of the femur will often result in immediate disability and lack of ambulation. However, an occult fracture may show normal range of motion except for exacerbation of pain at extremes of internal or external rotation.

VII. Laboratory tests

A. **Plain radiography** of the involved hip in adults and both hips in children is the single most cost-effective adjunctive test. When combined with age-adjusted history and thoughtful interpretation of physical signs, the routine x-ray approaches 90% sensitivity and 90% specificity for diagnosis.

1. Transient synovitis, bursitis, and meralgia paresthetica show no significant change.

2. Bacterial infection causes lateral displacement of the femoral head away from the acetabulum (see Figure 38–2).

3. Perthes disease shows the following sequence: lateral displacement of the femoral head (see Figure 38–2), widening and increased density of the femoral epiphysis, flattening of the femoral head and widening of the femoral neck, demineralization and fragmentation of the femoral head, and finally, reossification of the femoral head.

4. The slipped femoral capital epiphysis appears widened with irregular margins. The femoral head is displaced posteriorly and medially (see Figure 38–3).

5. Avascular necrosis is difficult to diagnose early because of a 19% false-negative rate. Later stages show bone collapse and degenerative arthritis.

6. Cancer produces punched-out circular areas of osteolysis with no reactive bone in the case of myeloma, and irregular lytic lesions with increased bone density in the case of metastases.

B. A **radioisotope bone scan** will demonstrate avascularity of the femoral head in Perthes disease before radiographic features are evident. This test is 97% sensitive in differentiating Perthes disease from nonspecific synovitis. Bone scans are more sensitive than radiographs for detecting bony metastases, plus they provide a survey of the entire skeleton. However, increased uptake on a bone scan is not specific for malignancy, and some neoplasms, including myeloma, are poorly detected.

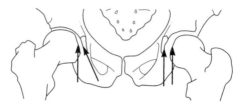

FIGURE 38–2. The interval between the ossified part of the femoral head or neck and the acetabulum, marked by arrows, is the teardrop distance. This distance is a useful criterion for early diagnosis of Perthes disease, and is also a good indication of the presence of excess joint fluid caused by bacterial infection. In 96% of normal patients, the teardrop distance in each hip is the same or differs by only 1 mm or less.

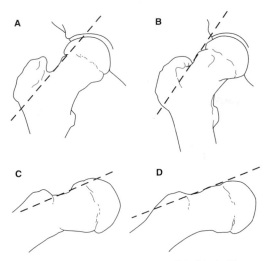

FIGURE 38-3. Anteroposterior view of slipped femoral capital epiphysis. A line superimposed on the superior femoral neck normally intersects part of the head (**A** and **C**). If the epiphysis is slipped, the line will not intersect the head (**B** and **D**). In some cases, only a frog view (**C** and **D**) will show a slip.

    C. Ultrasonography is very sensitive in detecting a hip effusion, as might be seen in suspected transient synovitis or septic arthritis. Ultrasound may also detect an enlarged iliopsoas bursa.

    D. Computerized tomography (CT) will confirm enlargement of the iliopsoas bursa.

    E. Subsequent ultrasound-guided **aspiration** of the hip joint will identify those with septic arthritis: turbid or purulent synovial fluid, a fluid white blood cell (WBC) count >20,000/μL^3 with a predominance of polymorphonuclear cells.

    F. An elevated **WBC count** and **erythrocyte sedimentation rate (ESR)** are very sensitive and specific for diagnosing a bacterial infection of the hip.

    G. Although costly, **magnetic resonance imaging (MRI)** is the most sensitive, specific, and low-risk noninvasive test for the early diagnosis of avascular necrosis. It has a positive predictive value of 96%, compared to 71% for nuclear scanning and 54% for CT. It is considered the procedure of choice for confirming the diagnosis of osteonecrosis.

    H. Evidence of abnormal **plasma** or **urine protein** patterns is a very sensitive, yet not very specific, indicator of myeloma. Elevated **serum calcium, alkaline phosphatase,** and **prostate specific antigen (PSA)** are sensitive indicators of bony metastases but, again, are not very specific.

VIII. Treatment

    A. Bed rest at home for 7–10 days, **local heat** and **massage,** and **aspirin** as needed will help relieve the pain of transient synovitis. Have patients use crutches to slowly resume weight bearing. Most children suffer only a single attack of transient synovitis, but it may recur. Approximately 6–15% of the patients with transient synovitis eventually develop Perthes disease.

    B. Minimization of risk factors such as obesity and constrictive garments is the crux of treating meralgia paresthetica. Abdominal muscle strengthening exercises are also helpful. Patients should be reassured that this condition is benign and self-limited.

    C. Systemic and local analgesics are effective for bursitis. Suggested oral therapy for adults is **indomethacin,** 25–50 mg three times a day, or **naproxen,** 375–500 mg twice a day. If pain persists or function is limited, the affected bursa should be injected with 20–40 mg of **prednisolone** (Hydeltra-T.B.A.) or **methylprednisolone** (Depo-Medrol) added to 1–2 mL of 1% lidocaine. No more than three injections should be given each year. Management of moderate to severe metastatic bone pain should begin with oral opioids in combination with a non-steroidal anti-inflammatory drug (NSAID) or acetaminophen. A usual starting dose is **codeine** 30 mg plus **acetaminophen** 300 mg (Tylenol No. 3), two tablets every 3–4 hours, or **hydrocodone** 7.5 mg plus **ibuprofen** 200 mg (Vicoprofen), one or two tablets every 3–4 hours. **Salmon calcitonin** (Miacalcin), a potent inhibitor of osteoclast-induced bone resorption, given subcutaneously at 100 IU/day, may also be helpful.

D. Surgical intervention

1. A patient with bacterial infection of the hip must be hospitalized for **arthrotomy** to drain all purulent material and for intravenous antibiotics. Poor prognosis is correlated with delayed action. Results of ultrasound-guided aspiration may allow selection of a smaller high-risk group for operative drainage and may also shorten operative time.

2. Perthes disease requires the orthopedic use of **braces, casts,** or **surgery** in order to retain the normal spherical shape of the femoral head during the natural repair process. Under the best of circumstances (eg, younger age or earlier diagnosis), minimal deformity and normal function will result. In other cases, degenerative arthritis will hinder adult life.

3. Slipped femoral capital epiphysis is best treated with immediate cessation of weight bearing and **surgical stabilization.** Follow-up studies reveal a high incidence of osteoarthritis, even in uncomplicated well-treated slips. Cancer patients with increasing pain not responsive to analgesics, in whom radiographs show destruction of more than 50% of the cortex or lesions larger than 3 cm in diameter, may have an impending pathologic fracture and should be considered for prophylactic internal fixation.

4. Under CT guidance, diagnostic and therapeutic **aspiration and drainage** of a massively enlarged iliopsoas bursa can be accomplished. Prophylactic intravenous antibiotics will lessen the need for repeat aspiration.

5. Avascular necrosis may be treated by **core decompression** if the diagnosis is made early. End-stage disease usually requires **replacement arthroplasty,** a less than durable solution for an active young adult.

E. Radiotherapy, while only palliative, remains an effective method of pain control for myelomatous and metastatic bone lesions in the area of the hip.

REFERENCES

Biundo JJ: Regional rheumatic pain syndromes. In Klippel JH (editor): *Primer on the Rheumatic Diseases.* 11th ed. Arthritis Foundation; 1997:136.

Buckwalter JA, Brandser EA: Metastatic disease of the skeleton. Am Fam Physician 1997;**55:**1761.

Hart JJ: Transient synovitis of the hip in children. Am Fam Physician 1996;**54:**1587.

Hedger S, Darby T, Smith MD: Unexplained hip pain: Look beyond the obvious abnormality. Ann Rheum Dis 1998;**57:**131.

Lieberman JR: Hip and thigh. In Snider RK (editor): *Essentials of Musculoskeletal Care.* American Academy of Orthopaedic Surgeons; 1997:264.

Menelaus MB: Perthes disease. In Broughton NS (editor): *A Textbook of Paediatric Orthopaedics.* Saunders; 1997:219.

Nattrass GR: Slipped upper femoral epiphysis. In Broughton NS (editor): *A Textbook of Paediatric Orthopaedics.* Saunders; 1997:229.

---

39   Insomnia

Jeffrey L. Susman, MD

I. **Definition.** Insomnia is the inability to initiate or maintain sleep when sleep should normally occur.

II. **Common diagnoses.** The major causes of insomnia are listed below.

A. **Transient conditions.**

B. **Psychiatric diseases.**

C. **Drug and alcohol use.**

D. Physiologic, age-, or gender-related insomnia.

E. Medical disorders. Common examples include symptomatic prostatic hypertrophy, congestive heart failure, and gastroesophageal reflux.

F. Primary sleep disorders
   1. Disturbances of the sleep-wake cycle.
   2. Sleep-related movement disorders.
   3. Disorders of excessive somnolence (eg, sleep apnea and narcolepsy).

III. Epidemiology. A Gallup survey of 2000 Americans showed that 36% had difficulty sleeping in the last year. Of these, 9% said that this was a chronic problem. Only 5% had visited a physician specifically for a sleep problem.

   A. Predisposing factors to **transient insomnia** include situational stress or conflict; environmental factors, such as excessive noise, bright light, and improper temperature; travel problems, including jet lag and adjustment to new sleeping environments; hospitalization or institutionalization; and shift work.

   B. Sleep disturbance is common in many **psychiatric illnesses,** including depression (Chapter 96), bipolar disease, mania, dementia (Chapter 77), and delirium, and in patients with excessive neurotic symptoms or the inability to deal effectively with anger and emotions (Chapter 96).

   C. People who use certain **drugs and alcohol** are at great risk for insomnia (see Table 39–1).

   D. Physiologic, age-, and gender-related insomnia
   1. **Age.** Complaints of insomnia increase with age. More than 50% of elderly people will admit to sleep problems, if asked.
   2. **Gender.** Females are more likely to complain of insomnia than males.

   E. Sleep problems are often secondary to concomitant **medical disorders.**

   F. Primary sleep disorders
   1. **Disturbances of the sleep-wake cycle** are common in people who are hospitalized, are institutionalized, or have jet lag.
   2. **Sleep-related movement disorders** include restless legs syndrome and nocturnal myoclonus. One third of patients with **restless legs syndrome** have a family history of this disorder. This problem is sometimes associated

---

TABLE 39–1. MEDICATIONS ASSOCIATED WITH SLEEP DISTURBANCE

Excessive wakefulness
  Theophylline
  Amphetamines
  Caffeine
  Anticonvulsants
  Alcohol
  Nicotine
  Triazolam (rebound phenomena)
  Thyroid hormone
  Methylphenidate
  Sympathomimetics

Nightmares
  Beta blockers (especially lipophilic agents such as propranolol)
  Tricyclics
  Antiparkinsonian agents
  Quinidine

Excessive somnolence
  Benzodiazepines
  Antihistamines
  Anticonvulsants
  Tricyclics (especially amitriptyline, doxepin, and trazodone)
  Monoamine oxidase inhibitors
  Antihypertensives (especially clonidine)

Other symptoms
  Diuretics (nocturia)
  Levodopa and tricyclics (sleep-related myoclonus)
  Caffeine (nonrepetitive muscle contractions at sleep onset or hypnic jerks)

with motor neuron disease, renal disease, or circulatory problems. **Nocturnal myoclonus** is more common in older individuals.

   3. **Disorders of excessive somnolence**
      a. **Sleep apnea syndrome.** Central sleep apnea usually has a readily apparent cause such as stroke, brain stem infarction, or neoplasia. Obstructive sleep apnea is associated with an upper airway abnormality and with medical conditions such as thyroid dysfunction, hypertension, cor pulmonale, obesity, and severe pulmonary dysfunction. Obstructive sleep apnea is most common in men and in older individuals.
      b. **Narcolepsy** is most likely to occur in young to middle-aged males.

IV. **Pathophysiology.** Normal sleep helps control tissue growth and repair, regulates immune function, and aids memory integration.
   A. Normal sleep may be divided into five stages. **Non–rapid eye movement (non-REM) sleep** includes the transition period from wakefulness to sleep or light sleep (stages 1 and 2) and deep sleep (stages 3 and 4). Deep sleep is characterized by decreased muscle tone, blood pressure, and respiratory rate. **REM sleep,** or "dream sleep" (stage 5), is associated with skeletal muscle atonia, variability of vital signs, and dreaming.
   B. A person normally goes from wakefulness through stages 1–4 during the early part of the night. After approximately 90 minutes of sleep, the first REM period begins. As the night progresses, cycles of REM and non-REM sleep occur at 1- to 3-hour intervals, and the amount of deep sleep in each cycle decreases.
   C. Approximately 2% of the population requires less than 5 hours of sleep, and another 2% requires more than 9 hours of sleep, each day. Most adults require 6–8 hours of sleep each day.

V. **Symptoms.** Patients with insomnia may present with unusual or nonspecific symptoms, such as headache and irritability, in addition to complaints of difficulty in initiating or maintaining sleep. A sleep diary (see Table 39–2), a tape recording of the patient's sounds while sleeping, and a history of the patient's sleep patterns provided by the patient's bed partner are useful tools in diagnosing the causes of insomnia.
   A. **Snoring** is common in the general population and becomes more common as the patient increases in age. Over 60% of men and 45% of women over the age of 60 snore. Unusual snoring, however, may be a symptom of a more serious problem such as sleep apnea syndrome.
   B. **Pain, paresthesias, cramps, cough,** and **breathlessness** may indicate that the insomnia is caused by illness or disease.
   C. **Sleep phase disorders**
      1. **Delayed sleep phase.** Patients with this problem have difficulty falling asleep, have no problems once asleep, and awaken later than usual.
      2. **Advanced sleep phase.** Patients cannot stay awake in the evening, have no difficulty once asleep, and awaken early in the morning.
      3. **Irregular sleep phase.** Patients complain of frequent drowsiness and naps and excessive time in bed.
   D. **Difficulty maintaining sleep, periodic hypersomnolence, headache, impotence, enuresis, personality changes, unusual movements,** and **loud sounds or snoring** during sleep may indicate sleep apnea syndrome.

TABLE 39–2. SLEEP DIARY

Date and day of the week
Habits prior to sleep, including food, drink (especially alcohol and caffeine), and medication
Activities prior to bedtime, including reading, television, telephone, sex, work, exercise, and socializing
Bedtime
Time it takes to fall asleep
Quality of sleep, including awakenings and nightmares
Dreams, snoring, or unusual movements
Time awake
Total sleep time
Symptoms and alertness upon awakening
Daytime sleepiness and naps
Other unusual or important factors

E. **Excessive daytime sleepiness** and **"sleep attacks,"** hypnagogic or bizarre **hallucinations,** and **cataplexy** (sudden muscle weakness) are common symptoms of narcolepsy. The symptoms usually begin when the patient is between 20 and 30 years of age.
   1. **Cataplexy** is pathognomonic; however, episodes of cataplexy may be very short, infrequent, and easily overlooked.
   2. **Periodic amnesia** or **accidents** may be the presenting symptoms because of the patient's "sleep attacks" and cataplexy.
VI. **Signs** of the psychiatric disorders and medical diseases mentioned previously should be sought, as discussed in detail elsewhere (see Chapters 77 and 96).
VII. **Laboratory tests.** In most cases, a careful history and physical examination will obviate the need for laboratory evaluation and will point to underlying medical conditions. A **sleep study** is indicated in the following situations.
   A. The diagnosis remains obscure or the problem persists or worsens.
   B. There is suspicion of sleep apnea, especially in patients with signs of cardiopulmonary difficulties and respiratory symptoms or daytime somnolence.
   C. Periodic hypersomnia is present. A sleep study is particularly important when this is associated with functional impairment.
   D. Serious disorders of the sleep-wake cycle occur that are not associated with transient changes in work or travel.
   E. The patient feels that the problem is becoming more severe.
VIII. **Treatment**
   A. **Transient insomnia**
      1. **Environmental factors** such as proper light, noise levels, and temperature should be optimized.
      2. **Psychiatric and medical disorders** associated with sleep disturbance should be treated. **Drug and alcohol use** should be carefully assessed.
      3. **Good sleep hygiene** (see Table 39–3) should be instituted.
      4. **Adjustments to new sleeping environments, shift work,** and **jet lag** should be addressed. Small delays in the sleep-wake cycle (ie, staying up longer and going to bed later before west-bound travel) are more easily accommodated prior to travel than in the opposite situation (ie, going to bed earlier before east-bound travel). Adjustment to shift work is difficult if the schedule rotates irregularly. If possible, a routine of sleep-wake periods should be established.
      5. **Pharmacologic agents** may be used in very select cases of transient sleep disorders unassociated with more serious problems (see Table 39–4). Some guidelines for hypnotic therapy are presented below.
      a. Make a presumptive diagnosis and rule out primary sleep disorders or underlying medical problems that pharmacologic therapy might aggravate.
      b. Determine the goals of therapy.
      c. Educate the patient on the use of medication.

TABLE 39–3. SLEEP HYGIENE

Awaken at a regular hour
Exercise daily on a regular basis (not close to bedtime)
Control the sleep environment (proper temperature, decreased noise and light)
Eat a light snack before bedtime (if not contraindicated)
Limit or eliminate alcohol, caffeine, and nicotine
Use hypnotics on a short-term basis only
Wind down prior to bedtime
Have a "worry time" early in the evening
Go to bed when sleepy
Avoid excessive sleep on weekends or extremes of sleep
Use relaxation and behavioral modification techniques
Use bed for sleeping only
Eliminate naps unless part of the schedule
Get up if you cannot get to sleep in 15–30 minutes
Sleep where you sleep best
Recognize the adaptation effect in new environments

TABLE 39–4. PHARMACOLOGIC THERAPY FOR TRANSIENT INSOMNIA

Class and Selected Agents	Initial Dose (mg)	Comments
Nonprescription		
Aspirin or acetaminophen (Tylenol)	325–650	May relieve troublesome aches or pains, thereby easing sleep
Antihistamines		
Diphenhydramine citrate (Excedrin PM)		May be effective transiently. Can have carryover anticholinergic side effects and induce paradoxic wakefulness
Diphenhydramine hydrochloride (Benadryl, Nytol)		
Doxylamine succinate (Unisom)		
Prescription		
Chloral hydrate	500–1000	May cause nausea. Can displace warfarin and phenytoin from albumin
Benzodiazepines		Effective for about 1 month with less potential for withdrawal and dependence. Will decrease sleep latency and nocturnal awakenings
Triazolam (Halcion)	0.125–0.25	Intermediate onset and rapid elimination. May cause rebound insomnia
Alprazolam (Xanax)	0.25	Have intermediate onset of action and elimination. Should be given at least 1 hour prior to bedtime
Lorazepam (Ativan)	1	
Temazepam (Restoril)	15	
Oxazepam (Serax)	15	Has slow onset of action and must be given several hours prior to bedtime
Estazolam (ProSom)	0.5–2	Intermediate half-life
Flurazepam (Dalmane)	15	Should be used cautiously because of their long half-lives and potential for accumulation when used habitually
Chlordiazepoxide (Librium)	5–10	
Diazepam (Valium)	1–5	
Quazepam (Doral)	7.5–15	
Zolpidem (Ambien)	5–10	Nonbenzodiazepine hypnotic that may have less potential for withdrawal and be more specific for sedative properties alone

    d. Begin with a low dose of medication and increase as needed based on improved sleep and daytime functioning.
    e. Follow up in 1 week to reassess the patient's condition. Telephone contact is reasonable for reliable patients.
    f. Medication use should be limited to no more than 3–4 weeks. Longer therapy is unlikely to be effective.
    g. Educate the patient about the possibility of withdrawal symptoms.
B. Physiologic or age-related insomnia
    1. The patient should be given **reassurance.**
    2. Good sleep hygiene should be recommended.
    3. Use of **medications** should be avoided.
    4. In the absence of underlying disease, patients who **snore** should be given the following advice.
        a. Exercise during the day or early evening.
        b. Avoid sedatives and alcohol.
        c. Sleep on the side, not on the back. Sewing a tennis ball in the back of the pajamas may make this position easier to maintain.
        d. Raise the head of the bed 6 inches.
        e. Use a soft collar.
        f. Drink a cup of coffee before going to bed.
C. Underlying **medical disorders** should be treated whenever possible. Certain problems may be associated with underlying primary sleep disorders (eg, hypertension and obesity with sleep apnea syndrome). In the absence of contraindications, short-term pharmacologic therapy is often useful for hospitalized patients.

D. Primary sleep disorders
 1. **Disturbances of the sleep-wake cycle.** Slow advancement or delay of the patient's bedtime, usually in conjunction with a sleep laboratory, is the therapy for this disorder. The irregular sleep phase disturbance will respond to strict structuring of a patient's waking and sleeping hours.
 2. **Sleep-related movement disorders.** These disorders may respond to the treatment of underlying medical conditions, the avoidance of stimulants, including caffeine, and the judicious use of **benzodiazepines. Clonazepam,** 1–4 mg, and carbidopa-levodopa, 25/100 mg at bedtime, are useful for restless legs syndrome.
 3. **Disorders of excessive somnolence**
    a. **Sleep apnea syndrome. Central sleep apnea** requires treatment by a pulmonary or neurologic specialist. For patients with **obstructive sleep apnea,** consultation with pulmonary and otorhinolaryngology specialists is indicated. Upper airway abnormalities may be amenable to ear, nose, and throat surgery. Obesity and underlying medical conditions should be treated aggressively. Patients should sleep on the side and should avoid depressants that affect the central nervous system. Nasal continuous positive airway pressure is the treatment of choice for most patients. Occasionally, tracheostomy is necessary if more conservative measures fail.
    b. **Narcolepsy** should be managed by a specialist skilled in the evaluation and control of this disorder.
IX. Follow-up of sleep disorders and insomnia should be dictated by the severity of the problem. For serious sleep disorders, close supervision and careful follow-up are necessary. On the other hand, when more serious problems have been ruled out, a 2- to 4-week trial of good sleep hygiene is indicated. The identification of hidden medical or psychophysiologic causes of sleep disturbance should be pursued.

REFERENCES

Allen R: Restless legs syndrome, part I. Psychiatric Times 1998;**April:**36.
Allen R: Restless legs syndrome, part II. Psychiatric Times 1998;**July:**16.
Coren S: *Sleep Thieves.* Free Press; 1996.
Cupp M: Melatonin. Am Fam Physician 1997;**56:**1421.
Dement W: The perils of drowsy driving. N Engl J Med 1997;**337:**783.
Kryger M, Roth T, Dement W: *Principles and Practice of Sleep Medicine.* 2nd ed. Saunders; 1994.
Nowell P, Mazumdar S, Buysse D, et al: Benzodiazepines and zolpidem for chronic insomnia. JAMA 1997;**278:**2170.
Susman JL: Sleep. In Ham JR, Sloane PD (editors): *Primary Care Geriatrics.* 3rd ed. Mosby–Year Book; 1997:397.

---

40   Jaundice

L. Peter Schwiebert, MD, & Gerry A. Steiner, MD

I. Definition. Jaundice is the yellow discoloration of the skin and mucous membranes caused by an elevated serum bilirubin. In adults, jaundice is visible at bilirubin levels of 2–3 mg/dL. In newborns, the threshold for visible jaundice is 5–6 mg/dL. Clinical jaundice may be divided into two groups.
 A. Unconjugated hyperbilirubinemia. The indirect fraction of bilirubin exceeds 80% of the total bilirubin.
 B. Conjugated hyperbilirubinemia. The direct fraction of bilirubin ranges from 20% to 60% of the total bilirubin.
II. Common diagnoses. The causes of jaundice are grouped below by the age at onset and the pathophysiologic mechanisms involved. It is important to realize that this scheme is an oversimplification and that more than one pathophysiologic process may be present in a single disorder. For example, cirrhotic patients may have both hepatocellular dysfunction and hemolysis.
 A. Adult onset
    1. **Unconjugated hyperbilirubinemia** may occur with overproduction of bilirubin (eg, hemolytic anemias), ineffective erythropoiesis (eg, thalassemias,

sideroblastic anemias, and pernicious anemia), and impaired uptake and conjugation of bilirubin (eg, Gilbert syndrome, which occurs in 3–7% of the US population, and Crigler-Najjar syndrome type II, an uncommon disorder).

  2. Conjugated hyperbilirubinemia occurs with impaired intrahepatic excretion or extrahepatic obstruction.

  a. Impaired intrahepatic excretion.

    (1) Viral hepatitis accounts for 75% of jaundice in patients less than 30 years of age but only 5% in patients over 60.

    (2) Cirrhosis causes about one third of jaundice in 30- to 60-year-old patients.

    (3) Congestive heart failure accounts for 10% of jaundice after age 60.

    (4) Metastatic disease causes 13% of jaundice after age 60.

    (5) Other causes include drug use, pregnancy, primary biliary cirrhosis, primary hepatocellular carcinoma, and Dubin-Johnson and Rotor's syndromes (both rare).

  b. Extrahepatic obstruction (eg, gallstones, strictures, and tumors, especially pancreatic cancer) accounts for 60% of jaundice in patients over 60 years of age.

B. Childhood jaundice

  1. Unconjugated hyperbilirubinemia

    a. Neonatal onset.

      (1) Physiologic jaundice is present in as many as 50% of newborns.

      (2) Hemolytic anemia is the most common pathologic cause of jaundice, usually resulting from ABO incompatibility or, less commonly, Rh incompatibility, spherocytosis, enzyme deficiency, or a hemoglobinopathy.

      (3) Other causes of unconjugated neonatal jaundice include breastfeeding, polycythemia, hematoma reabsorption, pyloric stenosis, and congenital hypothyroidism.

    b. Infancy and childhood onset. Jaundice may result from hemolytic diseases (eg, glucose-6-phosphate dehydrogenase [G6PD] deficiency and spherocytosis), Gilbert syndrome, and Crigler-Najjar syndrome.

  2. Conjugated hyperbilirubinemia

    a. Neonatal onset. Sepsis, neonatal hepatitis, TORCHS infections (**t**oxoplasmosis, **r**ubella, **c**ytomegalovirus [CMV], **h**erpes, and **s**yphilis), extrahepatic obstruction in biliary atresia or choledocholithiasis, and metabolic diseases, such as galactosemia, α_1-antitrypsin deficiency, or tyrosinemia may result in jaundice.

    b. Infancy and childhood onset. Viral hepatitis is the most common cause of jaundice in a previously healthy child. Less common causes include Wilson's disease and milder forms of galactosemia.

III. Epidemiology. Jaundice is very common in newborns; after the neonatal period, jaundice remains a common symptom, accounting for as many as 4% of admissions to acute care hospitals.

  A. Hepatitis. Risk factors for hepatitis A include ingestion of raw shellfish, travel to countries with unsanitary water supplies, household contact with infected persons, and exposure to diapered infants in a day care center. Risk factors for hepatitis B include origin in a country where the virus is endemic (eg, sub-Saharan Africa or Asia), birth canal exposure of the infant to an infected mother, and sexual contact with an infected patient. History of blood transfusions (especially before 1992), intravenous drug abuse, multiple sexual partners, hemodialysis, and health care occupations are risk factors for both hepatitis B and hepatitis C.

  B. Hemolytic anemias. African-Americans are prone to certain types of hemolytic anemias (eg, sickle cell disease and G6PD deficiency). Patients of Mediterranean descent and Asians are at increased risk for the thalassemias.

  C. Gender. Primary biliary cirrhosis, gallstones, and lupoid hepatitis are more common in females. Pancreatic carcinoma, alcoholic liver disease, and G6PD deficiency are more common in males.

  D. Family history of alcoholism, hemolytic anemias, Wilson's disease, or inherited disorders of bilirubin metabolism (eg, Gilbert syndrome) increase risk for the same disorder in a given patient.

E. Drugs such as erythromycin, nonsteroidal anti-inflammatory drugs, anabolic and contraceptive steroids, phenothiazines, and sulfonylureas place patients at risk for drug-induced jaundice (see also Chapter 45).

IV. Pathophysiology. There are three important pathophysiologic mechanisms.

   A. Overproduction. The major source of bilirubin is degradation of hemoglobin from senescent red blood cells. Excessive hemoglobin degradation and bilirubin over-production occur in immune hemolysis (eg, ABO incompatibility or Rh isoimmu-nization), nonimmune hemolysis (eg, G6PD deficiency or spherocytosis), extra-vascular hemolysis (eg, cephalhematomas in newborns), or intramarrow hemolysis (eg, "ineffective erythropoiesis" in thalassemia or pernicious anemia).

   B. Defective hepatic uptake and conjugation. Bilirubin from the periphery is tightly bound to albumin during transportation in the blood to the hepatocyte. Inside the hepatocyte, the nonpolar bilirubin is enzymatically conjugated by the action of uri-dine diphosphoglucuronyl transferase (UDPGT) to form water-soluble bilirubin glucuronides. UDPGT activity is physiologically decreased in neonates, increasing unconjugated bilirubin levels. Hereditary defects in bilirubin uptake and conjuga-tion occur in Gilbert syndrome and Crigler-Najjar syndrome. Diseases affecting the hepatocyte (eg, hepatitis) also impair bilirubin conjugation.

   C. Impaired excretion. After conjugation, bilirubin is excreted in the bile and trans-ported in the biliary system to the gastrointestinal tract. Obstruction at the cellu-lar level (eg, hepatocellular disease), at the ductule (eg, phenothiazine exposure), at the septal ducts (eg, primary biliary cirrhosis), or from mechanical blockage of the bile ducts (eg, pancreatic tumor) can result in conjugated hyperbilirubinemia. Since conjugated bilirubin is water soluble, but the unconjugated form is not, the level of bilirubin in the urine generally parallels the rise of conjugated bilirubin in the serum. Unconjugated (but not conjugated) bilirubin is reabsorbed from the in-testine via the enterohepatic circulation; neonates' unconjugated bilirubinemia, along with their decreased enteral intake and decreased levels of intestinal flora, contributes to hyperbilirubinemia in this group (eg, physiologic and breast milk jaundice).

V. Symptoms

   A. Onset of jaundice

      1. A rapid onset suggests infection, drug reaction, hemolytic anemia, or acute choledocholithiasis.

      2. Intermittent or fluctuating jaundice occurs in Gilbert syndrome (typically with fasting or intercurrent illness), Crigler-Najjar syndrome, Dubin-Johnson or Rotor's syndrome, recurrent common bile duct stones, and congestive heart failure.

      3. A gradual onset occurs in cirrhosis, intrahepatic metastases, pregnancy, or primary biliary cirrhosis.

   B. Pruritus. Severe pruritus and excoriations suggest extrahepatic obstruction.

   C. Abdominal pain occurs more often with obstructive jaundice than with hepato-cellular disease. Colicky, right upper quadrant pain prior to the onset of jaundice suggests choledocholithiasis, especially in middle-aged to older patients.

   D. Fever with chills suggests biliary obstruction and cholangitis. **Flulike symptoms** suggest viral or drug-induced hepatitis.

   E. Additional clues to **obstructive jaundice** include a >2-week history of acholic stools or severe jaundice without systemic symptoms.

   F. Sixty percent to 70% of patients with acute hepatitis C are asymptomatic, 20–30% have jaundice, and 10–20% complain only of fatigue, anorexia, or abdominal pain.

   G. In neonates, historical clues include history of premature rupture of membranes (sepsis), delay in clamping the cord (polycythemia), and previous history of a jaundiced baby (metabolic disorders or anemias).

VI. Signs

   A. Urticaria suggests hepatitis B infection.

   B. Cutaneous xanthomas suggest hypercholesterolemia seen in patients with chronic cholestasis (eg, primary biliary cirrhosis).

   C. Spider angiomata, palmar erythema, white nails, gynecomastia, testicular atro-phy, ascites, and signs of portal hypertension are signs of chronic hepatocellular disease or cirrhosis.

   D. Kayser-Fleischer ring of the cornea is pathognomonic of Wilson's disease.

   E. A **palpable (Courvoisier's) gallbladder** suggests malignant common duct obstruction (eg, cancer of the head of the pancreas) or, more commonly, an obstructing stone in the cystic duct.
   F. **Large nodules** in the liver suggest a metastatic cancer.
   G. **Splenomegaly** is found in many patients with cirrhosis, chronic active hepatitis, and acute alcoholic liver disease. However, splenomegaly is present in less than 5% of patients with acute viral hepatitis, gallstones, or malignant biliary obstruction. Hepatomegaly, especially if the liver span is ≥15 cm and tender, suggests alcoholic hepatitis or malignancy.
   H. In newborns, jaundice can be detected by examining the child in a well-lighted room and blanching the skin with digital pressure, revealing skin and subcutaneous tissue color. Icterus is first seen in the face and progresses to the trunk and the extremities; the degree of cephalocaudad progression correlates roughly with the bilirubin level (ie, the face, approximately 5 mg/dL; midabdomen, approximately 15 mg/dL; and the soles of the feet, approximately 20 mg/dL).
   I. Infants should be examined for signs of infection, increased hemoglobin load, a metabolic disorder, or biliary obstruction (see Table 40–1).
VII. **Laboratory tests.** Most causes of jaundice can be determined with a history, physical examination, and simple laboratory evaluation. Jaundice may be classified into two broad groups, based on preponderance of unconjugated bilirubin (overproduction or abnormal uptake or conjugation) or of conjugated bilirubin (abnormal secretion, biliary flow, or, rarely, intestinal transit or catabolism of bilirubin) (see Figure 40–1).
   A. **Jaundice in adults** (Figure 40–1)
      1. **Routine tests**
         a. A **complete blood cell count (CBC)** is required in all patients.
         b. A **peripheral smear and reticulocyte count** are required for all patients with unconjugated jaundice or anemia.
         c. A **liver battery** is required in all patients and should include the following tests.
            (1) **Total and direct bilirubin.**
            (2) **Alkaline phosphatase,** the level of which parallels the degree of cholestasis or obstruction. In classic hepatocellular disease, the

TABLE 40–1. RISK FACTORS AND EVALUATION OF JAUNDICED TERM NEONATES

Historical or Examination Risk Factors	Evaluation
Factors suggesting hemolysis, including family history of significant hemolytic disease *or* onset of jaundice at <24 hours of age *or* rise in bilirubin >0.5 mg/dL/hr *or* pallor/hepatomegaly *or* maternal Rh negative and infant Rh positive or maternal blood type O and infant blood type A or B *or* poor response to phototherapy	G6PD and pyruvate kinase testing (if RBC enzyme abnormality is suspected) RBC osmotic fragility testing (if spherocytosis is suspected) Hemoglobin electrophoresis (if hemoglobinopathy is suspected)
Factors suggesting sepsis or congenital viral infection, including vomiting, lethargy/irritability, abdominal distention, poor feeding, excessive weight loss, temperature instability, apnea/tachypnea, microcephaly, petechiae, cataracts, tachycardia/bradycardia, cyanosis, *or* maternal ruptured membranes >12–18 hours	TORCHS testing, septic work-up, blood/cerebrospinal fluid/urine cultures, with or without bacterial antigen testing
Factors suggesting cholestasis, including dark urine and light stools, jaundice persisting >3 weeks, *or* hepatomegaly	Right upper quadrant ultrasound, hepatobiliary scintigraphy if ultrasound is normal, TSH, LFTs, liver biopsy, urine/serum amino acids, urine reducing substances, sweat chlorides
Factors suggesting nonhemolytic causes of RBC destruction, including cephalhematoma, plethora, bruising, ileus, or gastrointestinal obstruction	Abdominal radiography if obstructive picture

G6PD, Glucose-6-phosphate dehydrogenase; LFTs, liver function tests; RBC, red blood cell; TORCHS, toxoplasmosis, rubella, cytomegalovirus, herpes, and syphilis; TSH, thyroid-stimulating hormone.

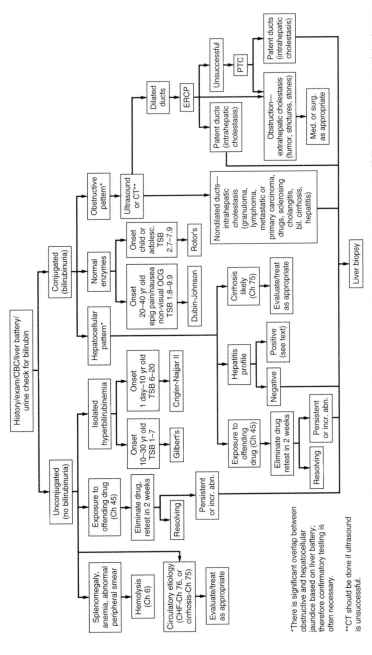

FIGURE 40-1. Evaluation of jaundice in adults. CBC, Complete blood cell count; CHF, congestive heart failure; CT, computerized tomography; ERCP, endoscopic retrograde cholangiopancreatography; OCG, oral cholecystogram; PTC, percutaneous transhepatic cholangiography; TSB, total serum bilirubin.

*There is significant overlap between obstructive and hepatocellular jaundice based on liver battery; therefore confirmatory testing is often necessary.

**CT should be done if ultrasound is unsuccessful.

217

alkaline phosphatase level is less than three times above normal, while in obstructive disease, it is greater than three times the normal value (see Chapter 45).

(3) Transaminases (ALT and AST) generally rise in proportion to the degree of active hepatocellular disease (see Chapter 45). In patients with typical obstructive jaundice, the transaminases are only mildly to moderately elevated (eg, two to three times normal), while they are usually at least five times normal in patients with hepatocellular disease.

d. A **prothrombin time** should be ordered if there is any suspicion of severe liver dysfunction or obstruction. In obstructive disease, a prolonged prothrombin time may respond dramatically to parenteral vitamin K, 10 mg subcutaneously. Minimal improvement in the prothrombin time after administration of vitamin K implies hepatocellular disease.

e. Urinalysis for bilirubin and urobilinogen can be helpful, in that it is inexpensive and only conjugated bilirubin is detectable.

2. Special tests

a. Viral hepatitis studies

(1) Immunoglobulin M (IgM) hepatitis A antibody appears at the onset of symptoms of hepatitis A infection and clears within 6 months during convalescence.

(2) Hepatitis B surface antigen (HBsAg) is the first serologic marker to appear in hepatitis B infection, starting 2–6 weeks before symptoms. The antigen generally clears within 6 months, but it persists in patients with chronic active or persistent infection.

(3) Hepatitis B core antibody (anti-HBc) is present in virtually all patients with an active hepatitis B infection. Since anti-HBc appears later than HBsAg but often before patients develop clinical symptoms, it thus serves to confirm hepatitis B infection when HBsAg is present. Anti-HBc persists for life.

(4) Hepatitis C antibody becomes detectable by enzyme immunoassay (EIA) in 90% of patients by 12 weeks after infection. Although EIA is >97% sensitive in detecting hepatitis C, it cannot differentiate acute, chronic, or resolved infection and should be confirmed by recombinant immunoblot assay (RIBA) testing. Negative EIA test or positive EIA coupled with negative RIBA rules out hepatitis C; an indeterminate RIBA should be followed with reverse transcriptase–polymerase chain reaction (RT-PCR) for hepatitis C RNA. Indeterminate RIBA coupled with negative RT-PCR and normal ALT rules out hepatitis C. Because of possible acquired maternal antibody, EIA testing in neonates at risk is not considered reliable until 12 weeks of age.

(5) IgM antibody to Epstein-Barr virus and CMV should also be considered in the appropriate clinical setting, although screening for hepatitis A and B should usually be done first.

b. Antimitochondrial antibody to screen for primary biliary cirrhosis should be considered in patients 30–60 years of age (especially females) with evidence of chronic cholestasis. Antibodies are positive in 85–90% of patients with primary biliary cirrhosis.

c. Serum iron, transferrin saturation, and ferritin to screen for hemochromatosis should be considered in patients with chronic liver disease without a defined cause. In hemochromatosis, the plasma iron exceeds 200 U/dL and transferrin saturation exceeds 70%.

d. Serum ceruloplasmin and urine copper levels to screen for Wilson's disease should be considered in patients under 30 years of age or in patients with hepatitis and neurologic dysfunction.

e. Antinuclear and smooth muscle antibodies are positive in about two thirds of patients with lupoid hepatitis (autoimmune hepatitis) and should be considered in patients (especially females) with evidence of chronic liver disease without a clear cause.

f. Serum protein electrophoresis is useful to screen for α_1-antitrypsin deficiency.

    g. One study indicated that **serum secretory component (SC)** is more reliable than alkaline phosphatase in differentiating mechanical from hepatocellular cholestasis.

3. Other diagnostic studies

    a. Ultrasonography to look for dilated biliary ducts is indicated in patients in whom extrahepatic obstruction is suspected. The presence of dilated biliary ducts indicates the presence of obstruction. Ultrasound is over 90% specific, and if jaundice has been present 1 week or more, it is close to 90% sensitive in detecting obstruction.

    A computerized tomographic (CT) scan is similar in sensitivity and specificity to an ultrasound scan, but it is more expensive. It should be used in cases in which ultrasonography is unsatisfactory because of equivocal findings or technical limitations (eg, overlying bowel gas).

    b. Endoscopic retrograde cholangiopancreatography (ERCP) or percutaneous transhepatic cholangiography (PTC) is indicated if extrahepatic obstruction is strongly suspected on clinical grounds (even if ultrasound results are negative) or if additional anatomic information is required for diagnosis.

    The choice of ERCP versus PTC depends mainly on local expertise and availability. ERCP is often preferred if the ducts are not dilated on ultrasonography or if planned therapy includes papillotomy, stenting, pancreatic stone removal, or biopsy.

    c. Liver biopsy may be useful in the following situations: (1) to differentiate chronic active from chronic persistent hepatitis, (2) to diagnose malignant involvement of the liver, and (3) to document or diagnose hepatocellular disease when the diagnosis is not otherwise possible on clinical grounds.

B. Jaundice in infants (Figure 40–2). Several factors influence evaluation and management decisions in the icteric term newborn. The first is **gestational age**—the lower the gestational age, the greater the risk of significant hyperbilirubinemia. This is partly because healthy term infants at 37–38 weeks may not nurse as well as infants born at 40 weeks. A second important factor is **age** at which jaundice first appeared—clinical jaundice at ≤24 hours of age is always abnormal and requires evaluation. The third factor determining evaluation and management is maternal or infant symptoms or signs increasing the likelihood of significant underlying abnormalities (see Table 40–1).

    1. Physiologic jaundice begins between the second and fourth days of life. Total serum bilirubin (TSB) levels are <15 mg/dL. The direct bilirubin is no more than 1.5 mg/dL, the bilirubin rises <5 mg/dL in 24 hours, and it resolves by 1 week (in term infants) or 2 weeks (in preterm infants).

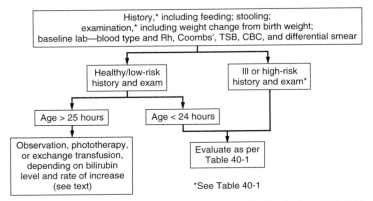

FIGURE 40–2. Evaluation of jaundice in term neonates. CBC, Complete blood cell count; TSB, total serum bilirubin.

2. **Breast milk jaundice** is characterized by progressive unconjugated hyperbilirubinemia in the first or second week of life, generally starting on or after the fourth day, peaking by 10–15 days of age, and is a diagnosis of exclusion. Breast milk jaundice resolves by 3–12 weeks of age, and approximately one third of breast-fed infants continue to have jaundice after 2 weeks. If the history (absence of dark urine or light stools) and physical examination are normal, continued observation without testing is appropriate. Jaundice in term breast-fed infants beyond 3 weeks should prompt urine bilirubin and total/direct serum bilirubin testing.

3. Jaundice persisting beyond 3 weeks in any term infant should prompt investigation for biliary atresia or other causes of cholestasis.

VIII. Treatment

A. **Pruritus.** Since pruritus may be disabling for some patients, leading to depression and even suicide, early treatment is advisable. Agents used to treat pruritus include **cholestyramine,** one packet or scoop in juice or applesauce three times a day, and antihistamines (eg, **diphenhydramine,** 25–50 mg three or four times a day).

B. **Viral hepatitis.** Most patients can be treated symptomatically on an outpatient basis. Hospital admission is indicated for inability to maintain hydration or for evidence of severe hepatocellular failure or ascites.

1. If the liver enzymes fail to return to normal within 6 months, liver biopsy is indicated.

2. Alfa-interferon can induce sustained remissions in some patients with chronic hepatitis B, C, and D. Consultation should be sought with a gastroenterologist familiar with its use.

C. **Extrahepatic obstruction**

1. If fever and chills develop, suggestive of cholangitis, prompt hospitalization for intravenous antibiotics and surgical consultation is necessary. Nonoperative biliary drainage can be performed in selected patients via ERCP on transhepatically placed stents.

2. Surgical therapy is generally required for extrahepatic biliary obstruction.

D. **Unconjugated hyperbilirubinemia** (eg, Gilbert, Dubin-Johnson, or Rotor's syndrome) beyond the neonatal period rarely requires treatment directed at lowering the bilirubin level. However, treatment for the primary disease process may be indicated (eg, corticosteroids for hemolytic anemias).

E. **Neonatal jaundice.** Therapy for neonatal jaundice is directed at both treatment of the underlying cause and prevention of kernicterus, a form of neurotoxic damage to the basal ganglia and the hippocampus of newborns from high levels of unconjugated bilirubin. In healthy term infants, the risk is low, even with TSB levels as high as 23 mg/dL, although the tolerable level is lower in premature infants.

1. **Phototherapy** exposes infants to blue-range lights or broad-spectrum white lights shone through a Plexiglas shield to screen out harmful ultraviolet radiation. This produces photoisomers of unconjugated bilirubin that are water soluble and may be excreted in bile or urine without conjugation.

   The eyes of the newborn must be covered during phototherapy to prevent retinal damage. Adequate fluid intake promotes the elimination of bilirubin and counteracts the dehydration associated with phototherapy. Phototherapy should be considered at TSB >15 mg/dL at 25–48 hours of age, >18 mg/dL at 49–72 hours of age, or >20 mg/dL past 72 hours of age. A favorable response to phototherapy is a decrease of 1–2 mg/dL within 4–6 hours, with subsequent continued decreases. Discontinuation of phototherapy should be considered once the TSB is 2 mg/dL below the threshold for initiation of therapy.

2. **Exchange transfusion** is traditionally performed when the TSB exceeds the threshold for phototherapy by 5 mg/dL or if phototherapy fails. The threshold for exchange transfusion should be lowered by 1–2 mg/dL when additional risk factors for kernicterus are present, such as perinatal asphyxia, respiratory distress, hypoglycemia, metabolic acidosis (pH ≤7.25), hypothermia (temperature, <35 °C [95 °F]), hypoproteinemia (protein, ≤5 g/dL), and signs of clinical or central nervous system deterioration.

3. **Breast milk jaundice** requires no treatment if the TSB is <20 mg/dL. One should consider close observation and increasing the frequency of breast-feeding to eight to 10 times every 24 hours. Depending on maternal preference and physician judgment, options beyond observation and increasing the frequency of breast-feeding include initiating phototherapy, supplement-

ing breast-feeding with formula with or without phototherapy, substituting formula, or temporarily substituting formula and initiating phototherapy. (Cow's milk formula inhibits intestinal reabsorption of unconjugated bilirubin; substituting formula for 2–3 days in a healthy jaundiced breast-fed infant may allow subsequent resumption of breast-feeding without further bilirubin increase.) If breast-feeding is interrupted, the mother should be reassured that the breast milk has caused the baby no harm and should be encouraged to resume breast-feeding.

4. **Physiologic jaundice** requires no treatment in term infants or in premature infants whose bilirubin is <10 mg/dL.
5. **Neonates with hemolytic jaundice** often become profoundly anemic at 2–4 weeks of age and may require transfusion of packed cells. Hemoglobin and hematocrit must be monitored serially in all infants with hemolytic jaundice.

F. **Cholestatic jaundice**
  1. **Ursodeoxycholate** (usual dose, 10–12 mg/kg/day) improves both biochemical abnormalities and symptoms in primary biliary cirrhosis and other forms of chronic cholestasis.
  2. Pruritus is treated as discussed above.

G. **Other hepatocellular disease.** Periodic monitoring of patients is necessary with clinical examination and liver function tests (see Chapter 75). When the disease is progressive, liver biopsy may be indicated for definitive diagnosis.

REFERENCES

Alter MJ, Mast EE: The epidemiology of viral hepatitis in the United States. Gastoenterol Clin North Am 1994;**23:**437.

American Academy of Pediatrics: Practice parameter: Management of hyperbilirubinemia in the healthy term newborn. Pediatrics 1994;**94:**558.

Barloon TJ, Bergus GR, Weissman AM: Diagnostic imaging to identify the cause of jaundice. Am Fam Physician 1996;**54:**556.

Buckley SE, DiPalma JA: Recognizing primary biliary cirrhosis and primary sclerosing cholangitis. Am Fam Physician 1996;**53:**195.

McKnight JY, Jones JE: Jaundice. Am Fam Physician 1992;**45:**1139.

Moyer LA, Mast EE, Alter MJ: Hepatitis C: Part I. Routine serologic testing and diagnosis. Am Fam Physician 1999;**59:**79.

Ostrow JR, Elfrink RPJO, Bos PJ: Jaundice and disorders of bilirubin metabolism. In Stein JH (editor): *Internal Medicine.* Mosby; 1998.

Pasha TM, Lindor KD: Diagnosis and therapy of cholestatic liver disease. Med Clin North Am 1996;**80:**995.

Rosenberg AA, Thilo EH: The newborn infant. In Hay WW Jr, Groothuis JR, Hayward AR, et al (editors): *Current Pediatric Diagnosis & Treatment.* 13th ed. Appleton & Lange; 1997:48.

Versland MR, Wu GY, Gorelick FS, et al: Serologic assay for secretory component distinguishes mechanical from hepatocellular cholestasis in humans. Dig Dis Sci 1997;**42:**2246.

---

41   Joint Pain

Pamela Sue Horst, MD

I. **Definition.** Joint pain is discomfort or tenderness in one or multiple joints regardless of whether a physical examination shows objective findings such as swelling, joint effusion, warmth, or tenderness.

II. **Common diagnoses**
  A. **Arthralgia** is joint pain without objective findings such as swelling, warmth, and tenderness. Examples of conditions with arthralgia complaints are viremia, the primary stage of Lyme disease, hypermobility syndromes, growing pains, fibromyalgia, and psychogenic rheumatism, which includes depression and school phobia.
  B. **Arthritis** is joint pain with objective findings. Examples of conditions with arthritis include osteoarthritis and rheumatoid arthritis (see Chapter 71), septic arthritis, tertiary Lyme disease, toxic synovitis, gout, and rheumatic fever.
  C. **Trauma,** the most common cause of joint pain, is not described here, since it is described in detail in other chapters (see Chapters 7, 8, 34, 38, and 42).

III. **Epidemiology.** Eleven percent of patients visiting general and family physicians in the United States had complaints related to the back and the upper or lower extremities. Unspecified arthritis is the 14th most common principal diagnosis seen by these physicians.

    A. Arthralgias

        1. **Viremia** can occur at any age. The influenza virus is usually seen in the early winter months. Rubella infection is more likely to cause arthralgias in young adult females than in children.

        2. **Lyme disease,** which is seen mostly in the northeastern states, south to Maryland and Virginia, as well as in portions of Wisconsin, Minnesota, and California, affects individuals of all ages. Most cases occur in the summer months.

        3. **Hypermobility syndromes** are found most commonly in children between 10 and 15 years of age. These conditions may be associated with other rheumatic diseases and collagen disorders such as Marfan syndrome.

        4. **Growing pains,** which occur in up to 18% of school-aged children, are more common in girls than in boys. Parents of a child with growing pains often had similar pains during childhood. Symptoms usually peak at age 11 and continue throughout adolescence.

        5. **Fibromyalgia** occurs most commonly in young females.

        6. **Psychogenic rheumatism.** Many depressed patients have multiple somatic complaints. School phobia is seen in children with persistent separation anxiety who are part of overly dependent parent-child interactions.

    B. Arthritis

        1. **Septic arthritis**

            a. Risk factors for nongonococcal septic arthritis in adults include bacteremia, immunosuppressive therapy or immunodeficiency, and underlying chronic disease (especially diabetes mellitus, malignancy, and liver disease).

            b. Ninety-six percent of pediatric septic arthritis occurs prior to age 6. Children with sickle cell anemia are more prone to salmonella arthritis.

        2. **Toxic synovitis** is seen in children under the age of 10 and occurs within 1 week of an upper respiratory infection.

        3. **Gout** is a common cause of acute monoarticular arthritis in men over age 40 and in women who are postmenopausal. A positive family history increases the likelihood of gout development.

        4. **Rheumatic fever** incidence has progressively declined in developed countries so that the rate of rheumatic heart disease is now 0.2–0.5 per 100,000. Local epidemics occurred in the mid-1980s in the United States (eg, 99 cases in Utah). In the 1990s, outbreaks of rheumatic fever have declined again.

IV. **Pathophysiology**

    A. Arthralgias

        1. **Viral infections** such as hepatitis B and rubella may cause circulating immune complexes that trigger joint inflammation. Influenza and coxsackieviruses can cause a painful myositis. Any febrile illness can cause arthralgias and myalgias, including acute human immunodeficiency virus (HIV) infection.

        2. **Lyme disease** occurs following the bite of a deer tick that hosts the spirochete *Borrelia burgdorferi.*

            In early disease, the spirochete causes local infection in the skin and joint responding to antibiotics. In late disease unresponsive to antibiotics, an autoimmune response may play a role in the symmetric oligoarthritis seen often in the knees.

        3. **Hypermobility syndromes.** A causative agent for this disorder has not been found. Hypermobility is not consistently associated with any other condition.

        4. **Growing pains.** The origin is unknown, but frequently an emotional component and a genetic component (pain-prone families) are involved.

        5. **Fibromyalgia.** No definite structural abnormality has been found. The associated sleep disturbance may actually be a causal factor by exaggerating the pain.

    B. Arthritis

        1. **Septic arthritis**

            a. *Neisseria gonorrhoeae,* which is responsible for over half of the cases of adult septic arthritis, causes pain through synovial inflammation.

    b. *Staphylococcus aureus,* various streptococcal bacteria, and gram-negative bacilli are the most common causes of nongonococcal bacterial arthritis in adults. Like *N gonorrhoeae,* these organisms usually enter the synovium via the bloodstream but occasionally directly penetrate the synovium at infected sites (eg, overlying cellulitis, infected bursitis, or skin ulcer).

    c. *Haemophilus influenzae* is the most common cause of septic arthritis in children.

  2. Toxic synovitis is probably a viral infection of the synovium. The joint most commonly affected is the hip.

  3. In **gout,** the deposition of uric acid crystals in the joint cavity induces articular inflammation. Prolonged hyperuricemia caused by overproduction of uric acid resulting from enzyme deficiencies or decreased renal excretion initially leads to supersaturation and then to precipitation of sodium urate in articular tissues.

  4. In **rheumatic fever,** infection with group A β-hemolytic streptococci stimulates an immune response to the M-associated surface protein molecules of the bacteria. Rheumatogenic strain M proteins include epitopes that are cross-reactive with epitopes found in the joints, brain, and cardiac tissue, thus permitting an autoimmune response in the host.

V. Symptoms. Certain symptoms help to distinguish the different types of joint pain.

  A. Number of joints involved

    1. Monoarticular complaints make infection, gout, toxic synovitis (of the hip), or trauma more likely.

    2. Polyarticular involvement suggests diffuse connective tissue disease, viremia, or rheumatic fever (Table 41–1). In the latter, migratory pains are common. **Symmetric joint involvement** indicates rheumatoid arthritis and is also seen in growing pains.

  B. Duration of pain

    1. Acute onset of pain suggests trauma, infection, or gout.

    2. Chronic recurrent pain makes a chronic disease (eg, growing pains, fibromyalgia, hypermobility syndromes, osteoarthritis, and rheumatic disease) more likely.

  C. Timing of pain

    1. Nocturnal pain indicates a malignant tumor, especially in adolescents or young adults. Growing pains also occur most often at night; they are gone by morning, however. Such pains can be severe enough to awaken a child. Gout often begins at night.

    2. Pain that increases with use suggests osteoarthritis, trauma, or overuse syndromes such as tennis elbow or other tendinitis. Growing pains can also be exacerbated by exercise.

    3. Limb pains that occur only on school days and disappear soon after the school bus leaves may indicate school phobia.

TABLE 41–1. SYMPTOMS OF RHEUMATIC FEVER

Major Manifestations	Minor Manifestations	Supporting Evidence of Antecedent Group A Streptococcal Infection
Carditis	Clinical findings	Positive throat culture of rapid streptococcal antigen test
Polyarthritis	Arthralgia	Elevated or rising streptococcal antibody titer
Chorea	Fever	
Erythema marginatum	Laboratory findings	
Subcutaneous nodules	Elevated acute phase reactants	
	Erythrocyte sedimentation rate	
	C-reactive protein	
	Prolonged PR interval	

If supported by evidence of preceding group A streptococcal infection, the presence of two major manifestations or one major and two minor manifestations indicates a high probability of acute rheumatic fever. (From Adnans D: Guidelines for the diagnosis of rheumatic fever: Jones criteria, updated 1992. Circulation 1993;**87**:302.)

D. History of preceding illness
   1. An upper respiratory infection in the past week suggests toxic synovitis.
   2. A recent sore throat makes rheumatic fever more likely.
   3. A deer tick bite in the last month makes Lyme disease a possibility. Only 50% of patients recall the tick bite, however.
   4. A recent rubella immunization could cause arthralgias.

E. Associated systemic symptoms
   1. **Diarrhea** suggests inflammatory bowel disease.
   2. **Anorexia** and **weight loss** make hepatitis B, acquired immunodeficiency virus (AIDS), or malignant tumors more likely.

VI. Signs

A. Appearance of skin
   1. A rash known as **erythema migrans** occurs in about 90% of patients with Lyme disease. This rash, which begins as a red macule or papule at the site of the tick bite, enlarges within several days to 1 month. Partial clearing follows, and the center of the rash may become dusky, indurated, or vesicular.
   2. **Erythema** over a joint indicates arthritis.
   3. A **generalized, evanescent, pinkish maculopapular rash** makes viremia a likely cause of arthralgias.

B. Joint swelling
   1. **Soft, symmetric, often fusiform joints** are signs of rheumatoid arthritis.
   2. **Exquisitely tender joints** indicate gout. Tophi may be seen nearby.

C. Range of motion (ROM) and stability
   1. Individuals who are able to **extend the wrist and the metacarpophalangeal joint** so that the fingers are parallel to the dorsum of the forearm, **passively appose the thumb to the flexor forearm, hyperextend the elbows and the knees** 10 degrees or more, and **flex the trunk** with the knees extended so that the palms rest on the floor have hypermobility syndrome.
   2. **Limitation of motion** due to pain, swelling, deformity, or muscle spasm may be a sign of trauma or arthritis.
   3. **Crepitation** suggests irregular joint surfaces, as in osteoarthritis.

D. Joint deformity
   1. **Irregular bony enlargements** on the proximal and distal interphalangeal joints of the fingers (respectively known as Bouchard's and Heberden's nodes) may indicate osteoarthritis.
   2. **Joint deformities** may be a sign of chronic inflammatory arthritis (eg, rheumatoid arthritis).
   3. A **tender bony mass near a joint** suggests a tumor.

E. Systemic signs of joint disease
   1. A **heart murmur** suggests rheumatic fever (Table 41–1).
   2. **Urethral or cervical discharge** makes gonococcal arthritis more likely.
   3. **Fever** suggests septic arthritis, rheumatic fever, or viremia.

VII. Laboratory tests (Figure 41–1). No diagnostic tests are indicated if hypermobility syndrome is suspected or if there is no inflammation and the patient's history is consistent with growing pains.
   A. If a joint effusion is present and the diagnosis is in doubt, or if septic arthritis is suspected, **arthrocentesis** is indicated (Table 41–2).
   B. Other tests, such as complete blood cell count, erythrocyte sedimentation rate, antinuclear antibodies, and uric acid, to evaluate for systemic disease and diffuse connective disease can be ordered, as indicated by the patient's history and physical examination (see Chapter 71).

VIII. Treatment

A. Arthralgias
   1. **Viremia** patients should be reassured as to the benign course of the disease. **Symptomatic treatment** includes **analgesics, such as nonsteroidal anti-inflammatory drugs (NSAIDs):** ibuprofen, 400–800 mg orally three times a day; naproxen, 250–500 mg orally two times a day; fenoprofen, 300–600 mg orally every 6–8 hours; acetaminophen, 5–10 mg/kg orally every 4–6 hours in children, and 325–650 mg orally every 4 hours for adults; or aspirin, 60–100 mg/kg/day in divided doses in children and 4 g/day in divided doses in adults.

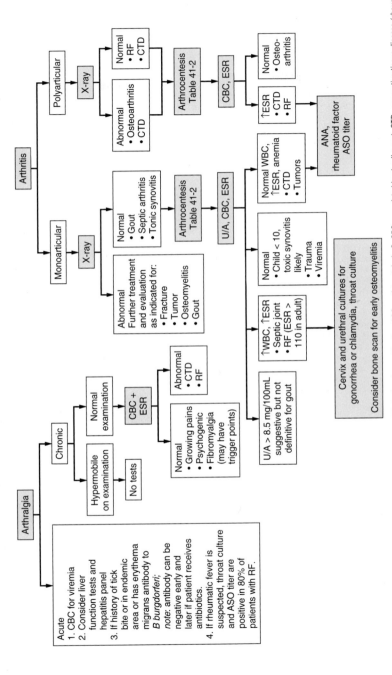

FIGURE 41–1. Approach to laboratory evaluation of patients with joint pain. ANN, Antinuclear antibodies; ASO, antistreptolysin 0; CBC, complete blood cell count; CTD, connective tissue disease (rheumatic diseases); ESR, erythrocyte sedimentation rate; RF, rheumatic fever; U/A, uric acid.

TABLE 41–2. JOINT FLUID FINDINGS

	Normal	Trauma	Infection	Crystalline Disease	Inflammatory
Color	Clear to yellow	Bloody to xanthro-chromic	Yellow to cloudy	Yellow to cloudy	Yellow to cloudy
Cell count (cells/μL) WBC/RBC	<200/0	<1000/many	1000–200,000/few	1000–2000/few	1000–20,000/few
Crystals	Negative	Negative	Negative	Yes; pseudo-gout and gout	Negative
Culture	Negative	Negative	Positive	Negative	Negative

RBC, Red blood cell count; WBC, white blood cell count.

2. **Lyme disease**
   a. Stage 1 disease (ie, erythema migrans, musculoskeletal pains, fatigue, headache, and stiff neck) can be treated by the primary care physician.
      (1) **Oral antibiotics** can shorten the duration of rash and prevent sequelae. Doxycycline, 100 mg twice daily, should be given for 21 days. Amoxicillin may be given to pregnant or lactating women; the dosage is 500 mg three times a day for 21 days. For children, the dosage is 20–40 mg/kg/day divided into three doses for 21 days. Children with penicillin allergy should receive erythromycin, 30 mg/kg/day for 21 days.
      (2) Patients should be told to report **complications** such as Bell's palsy or other neuropathies, arthritis, and any symptoms of congestive heart failure. Encourage patients to wear clothes that cover the wrists and the ankles when in an epidemic area in order to prevent tick bites. Use of insect repellents may discourage attachment of deer ticks.
         Treatment of patients with more severe neurologic conditions (eg, cranial neuropathies, meningitis, or encephalitis), cardiac problems (PR interval >0.3 seconds), or arthritic involvement requires consultation with a specialist in infectious diseases and hospitalization for parenteral administration of ceftriaxone or penicillin G.
3. **Hypermobility syndromes** should be treated with rest for acute symptoms, abstinence from activities causing pain, exercise to strengthen muscle groups around symptomatic joints, and analgesics (see section VIII,A,1 for dosage information). Assure the patient and the family that this condition is benign.
4. **Growing pains** can be effectively managed with heat and massage for pain and avoidance of excessive exercise if it exacerbates pain. If necessary, aspirin in a dose of 60–100 mg/kg/day in four divided doses can be given. Assure the family that this condition is not serious.
5. **Fibromyalgia**
   a. **NSAIDs** should be administered (see section VIII,A,1 for dosage information).
   b. The patient should obtain **adequate sleep and exercise** and should understand that the disease is neither crippling nor life-threatening. Oral medications at bedtime (eg, 10–25 mg of amitriptyline, 10 mg of cyclobenzaprine or zolpidem) can be used to promote sleep.
   c. **Injection** of tender soft tissue (trigger points) using 1% lidocaine (Xylocaine), 2–3 mL, with or without corticosteroid (eg, 0.5 mL of triamcinolone, 40 mg/mL), may be helpful for more severe pain.
   d. **Antidepressants** (eg, fluoxetine, 20–40 mg in the morning) are helpful for those patients with signs of depression such as decreased appetite, lack of interest in life, and malaise.

    e. Physical therapy that involves biofeedback treatment, massage, strengthening exercises, or transcutaneous nerve stimulation may be useful in patients with localized pain or significant muscle spasm.

    f. Psychotherapy is indicated for the management of persistent symptoms that do not respond to treatment or for patients with severe depression.

6. Psychogenic rheumatism. Depressed patients should be managed as described in Chapter 96.

    School phobia should be managed in the following ways.

    a. Quickly excluding organic causes and focusing on emotional issues.

    b. Mobilizing the affected extremity gradually (physical therapy is helpful).

    c. Encouraging normal daily activities, including early return to school.

    d. Referring the patient for psychotherapy, particularly if the patient is an adolescent, because more severe psychiatric disease is likely to occur in patients in this age group. The primary care physician can usually manage the prepubertal child.

B. Arthritis

1. For information concerning the treatment of osteoarthritis and rheumatoid arthritis, see Chapter 71.

2. Septic arthritis. For patients with this condition, hospitalization is indicated, with administration of parenteral antibiotics. Orthopedic consultation should be sought for consideration of joint drainage.

3. Toxic synovitis

    a. Bed rest (for a few days) is indicated until pain resolves.

    b. Aspirin, 60–100 mg/kg/day in four to six divided doses, should be given for pain.

    c. If the pain persists or recurs, frequent x-rays of the hip are required to rule out Legg-Calvé-Perthes disease (aseptic necrosis of the femoral head), which occurs in up to 20% of patients (see Chapter 38).

4. Gout. For a discussion of treatment, see Chapter 71.

5. Rheumatic fever

    a. Acute inflammation should be suppressed with **aspirin,** 80–100 mg/kg/day in children and 4–8 g/day in adults. After a serum salicylate level between 20 and 30 mg/dL has been maintained for 6–8 weeks, the aspirin dosage should be gradually decreased. If symptoms recur, the dosage should be increased again. Other NSAIDS may be effective, but this has not been documented.

    b. Streptococcal pharyngitis should be treated with **penicillin V potassium,** 250 mg four times daily for 10 days. For further information, see Chapter 61.

    c. If severe carditis (eg, congestive heart failure, pericarditis, or cardiomegaly) is present, consultation with a cardiologist is necessary. Bed rest or decreased activity is indicated. **Prednisone,** 2 mg/kg/day, is recommended for 2 weeks; the dosage should then be tapered at the rate of 5 mg every 2–3 days. **Aspirin** should be added when the prednisone dosage is decreased and should be continued for 1 month.

    d. Prevention of recurrence of rheumatic fever is important. Secondary prophylaxis with **penicillin V potassium,** 250 mg orally twice a day in adults and once a day in children, should be administered in the following situations.

        (1) To individuals age 18 and older, for 5 years after the last attack.

        (2) To individuals under age 18 who have had the disease.

        (3) To all patients who currently have rheumatic heart disease.

REFERENCES

Adnans D: Guidelines for the diagnosis of rheumatic fever: Jones criteria, updated 1992. Circulation 1993;**87**:302.

Biro F, Gervanter H, Baum J: The hypermobility syndrome. Pediatrics 1983;**72**:701.

Preslar AJ, Heckman JD: Emergency department evaluation of the swollen joint. Emerg Med Clin North Am 1984;**2**:425.

Sigal LH: Musculoskeletal manifestations of Lyme arthritis. Rheum Dis Clin North Am 1998;**24**:323.

Stollerman GH: Rheumatic fever. Lancet 1997;**349**:935.

Wallace DJ: The fibromyalgia syndrome. Ann Med 1997;**29**:9.

42   Knee Pain

Mitchell A. Kaminski, MD

I. **Definition.** Knee pain is discomfort localized to the knee joint. Knee pain can be acute, most often reflecting an injury, or chronic, reflecting a recurrent disorder with persistent inflammation.

II. **Common diagnoses**
   A. **Ligamentous injuries** (collateral, cruciate, or iliotibial band).
   B. **Meniscal injuries.**
   C. **Patellofemoral dysfunction.**
   D. **Bursitis** (prepatellar, infrapatellar, or anserine; Baker's cyst).
   E. **Fractures.**
   F. **Osgood-Schlatter disease, Sinding-Larsen-Johansson syndrome,** and **osteochondritis dissecans.**
   G. **Arthritis** (rheumatoid, osteo-, gout, or pseudogout).
   H. **Pain referred from the hip.**

III. **Epidemiology.** Knee pain is a frequent presenting symptom in primary care practice. Each year, 1 of every 10 persons in the United States suffers an injury to the leg warranting medical care or activity restriction. The knee and the leg, after the back, ankle, and foot, are the most common sites for arthritis. Acute knee pain is more likely in young and active patients, in whom it is often the result of injury.
   A. Collateral and cruciate ligament injuries are most common in sports involving contact or torsion of the lower extremities. Patellofemoral injuries occur most often in jumping sports. These are more frequent in tall, adolescent females. Iliotibial band syndrome occurs most frequently in runners.
   B. Chronic pain or increasing patient age makes inflammatory arthritis more likely. Arthritis of the knee has been associated with obesity and repetitive trauma, both occupational and recreational. Illnesses such as diabetes mellitus, sickle cell anemia, and recurrent infections often underlie septic arthritis.
   C. Osgood-Schlatter disease (traumatic apophysitis of the tibial tubercle) and osteochondritis dissecans occur in adolescents. Osgood-Schlatter disease is more common in males than in females.
   D. Referred pain from the hip should be considered especially in pediatric patients (see Chapter 38) and in older patients at risk for metastatic disease and fracture of the hip.

IV. **Pathophysiology.** Because the knee is a complex, weight-bearing hinge joint (Figure 42–1), it is susceptible to forces that can disrupt the ligaments and muscles providing its support. The mechanism of injury often describes these forces. Disruption of the articular surfaces between the femoral condyles and their tibial and patellar articulations leads to inflammation and pain.
   A. **Ligamentous injuries**
      1. **Collateral ligament injuries** are caused by medial or lateral external force or excessive sideways fulcrum action of the femoral condyles on the tibia. The medial collateral ligament is most often injured.
      2. Anterior or posterior **cruciate ligament injuries** result from excessive anterior or posterior impact with torsion on the knee. This usually severe trauma is often accompanied by other injuries.
      3. **Iliotibial band syndrome** is an overuse syndrome resulting from excessive friction between the iliotibial band and the lateral femoral condyle. It is precipitated by a change in footwear, increase in a running schedule, or prolonged downhill running.
   B. **Cartilaginous injuries. Meniscal tears** occur while bearing weight with excessive rotation of the femur on a fixed tibia. The medial meniscus is injured more often than the lateral one.
   C. **Patellofemoral dysfunction** encompasses a continuum of disorders from patellofemoral arthralgia to chondromalacia patellae and patellar subluxation. These disorders are often associated with an abnormal "Q" angle and abnormal tracking of the extensor mechanism (Figure 42–2). Strong isometric forces applied to the extensor muscles with slight knee flexion lead to acute and recurrent patellar sub-

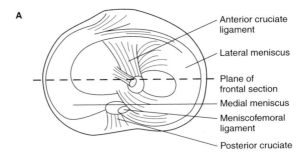

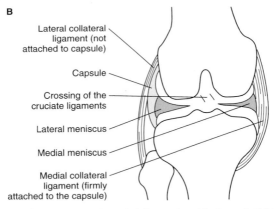

FIGURE 42–1. Relationship between the menisci, the capsule, and the ligaments of the knee. **(A)** A superior view of the menisci and cruciate ligaments. **(B)** A posterior view of a frontal section of the knee through the middle third. (Modified with permission from Steinberg GG, Akins CM, Baran DT, et al [editors]: *Ramamurti's Orthopaedics in Primary Care.* 2nd ed. Williams & Wilkins; 1992.)

    luxation. Direct trauma to the knee cap, recurrent dislocation, and chronic stresses lead to degeneration of the patellar cartilage (chondromalacia patellae). Chronic inflammatory change may lead to patellar or quadriceps tendon rupture.

  D. Bursitis may be caused by contusion over the bursa (prepatellar or superficial infrapatellar bursitis), overuse (deep infrapatellar or anserine bursitis), or acute or chronic intra-articular inflammation (Baker's cyst) (Figure 42–3).

  E. Direct trauma most commonly underlies **fractures** of the patella or the femoral condyles, while fractures of the tibial plateau result from compressive rotational or lateral stresses. Bone that is pathologically weaker than ligaments will fracture before the ligaments will tear. Distal femoral Salter type I fractures in adolescents may initially mask as a "ligament tear."

  F. Osgood-Schlatter disease is believed to be secondary to traction trauma to the calcifying apophysis in adolescents. **Sinding-Larsen-Johansson syndrome** is a traction tendinitis of the distal pole of the patella. The cause of **osteochondritis dissecans** is still uncertain.

  G. The pathophysiology of the various forms of inflammatory arthritis is discussed in Chapter 71.

  H. Hip disease leading to pain referred to the knee is discussed in Chapter 38.

V. Symptoms. Determining the onset, location, character, precipitant, and relieving factors of knee pain helps with diagnosis. Immediate pain and swelling suggest hemarthrosis and more serious injury. Symptoms of rheumatoid arthritis and osteoarthritis

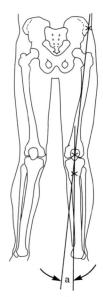

FIGURE 42–2. "Q" angle. A normal "Q" angle is <14–15 degrees.

are chronic, unlike the arthritis of gout or pseudogout, which flares acutely. The site of pain and swelling often helps to localize the abnormality. Some symptoms are suggestive of specific disorders.

A. Pain

1. **Mild pain** over the lateral side of the knee suggests iliotibial band syndrome. **Moderate to severe pain** usually occurs with fractures.
2. **Localized pain** and **effusion** occur with incomplete disruption of ligaments. **Diffuse pain,** especially with climbing stairs or getting up from a squatting position, is a hallmark of chondromalacia patellae.
3. **Pain with weight bearing** often occurs with meniscal tears and with osteochondritis dissecans. Inability to bear weight is common with fractures.

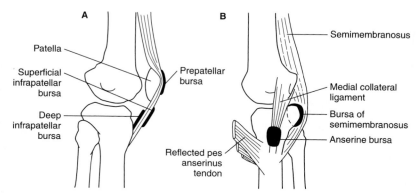

FIGURE 42–3. Bursae about the knee. **(A)** The lateral view; **(B)** the medial view. (Modified with permission from Steinberg GG, Akins CM, Baran DT, et al [editors]: *Ramamurti's Orthopaedics in Primary Care.* 2nd ed. Williams & Wilkins; 1992.)

      4. Pain with resisted knee extension (eg, from running, climbing, jumping, or kicking) occurs with Osgood-Schlatter disease, Sinding-Larsen-Johansson syndrome, and chondromalacia patellae.

      5. Aching pain in the knee, even at rest, may indicate osteochondritis dissecans. Knee pain from rheumatoid arthritis is worse after inactivity, while activity tends to precipitate pain in osteoarthritis.

      6. Pain limited to the knee is common with septic arthritis. **Knee pain referred from the hip** may be the only symptom of hip disease.

  B. Instability

      1. A "pop" followed by knee instability may occur with complete ligament disruption, particularly of the cruciate ligaments, and with patellar or quadriceps tendon rupture.

      2. "Locking" or "giveway" suggests a bucket handle meniscal tear.

      3. A loose joint body may cause locking or restricted range of motion in advanced cases of osteochondritis dissecans.

  C. Swelling

      1. Rapid swelling is usual with hemarthrosis.

      2. Swelling behind the knee with variable to no pain is seen with Baker's cyst.

      3. Swelling with pain over the tibial tubercle is seen with Osgood-Schlatter disease. **Swelling and pain over the respective bursa** is seen in prepatellar, infrapatellar, and anserine bursitis (Figure 42–3).

      4. Joint swelling is more common with rheumatoid arthritis than with osteoarthritis (see Chapter 71).

  D. Stiffness

      1. A patient may feel "something out of place" and be unable to flex or extend the knee with patellar dislocation.

      2. Stiffness that is worse after inactivity is common with rheumatoid arthritis.

  E. A **limp** may be noticed in patients suffering from knee pain referred from the hip.

  F. Systemic symptoms

      1. Rheumatoid arthritis is accompanied by systemic symptoms more often than is osteoarthritis.

      2. Fever and chills are common with septic arthritis.

VI. Signs. Examination after an acute injury is often limited by pain and swelling. Localization of tenderness to palpation provides valuable clues to the diagnosis (Figure 42–4). Special maneuvers (Table 42–1) may reveal signs of ligamentous or meniscal injury or patellar instability.

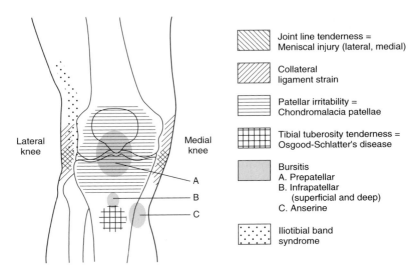

FIGURE 42–4. Sites of knee tenderness and suggested diagnoses.

TABLE 42–1. SPECIAL MANEUVERS IN THE KNEE EXAMINATION

Test	Method	Significance
McMurray's	Extend axially compressed knee with internal tibial rotation and then with external tibial rotation	Locking or popping suggests meniscal injury
Drawer sign	Pull/push tibia anteriorly and posteriorly with 90-degree flexion and foot planted	Laxity found with cruciate ligament tear
Lachman's maneuver	With knee flexed 20 degrees and femur supported, pull tibia anteriorly	Step-up from lower patella to tibial tuberosity indicates anterior cruciate ligament instability
Collateral ligament stressing	Valgus varus stress of knee in full knee extension then 30-degree flexion	Laxity with full extension suggests collateral and cruciate ligament injury. Laxity only at 30-degree flexion suggests collateral ligament tear
Apprehension sign	Valgus varus stress on patella with quadriceps relaxed, knee extended	Extreme guarding suggests patellar subluxation
Patellar irritability	Compress patella against femoral condyles	Tenderness indicates chondromalacia patellae
Thigh circumference measurement	Measure thigh circumference at an equal distance above both mid-patellae	Decreased circumference of thigh above affected knee suggests subacute or chronic disorder with quadriceps atrophy

A. **Localized swelling and tenderness** over the affected bursa will be found in bursitis. Tenderness is also common with femoral condylar fractures. Hip or groin tenderness and pain with rocking of the hip are the primary clues to knee pain referred from the hip.

B. **Erythema** may appear in patients with femoral condylar fractures, and it is present to varying degrees in patients with rheumatoid arthritis, osteoarthritis, and the arthritis of gout and pseudogout.

C. **Tense effusion** is seen in patellar fracture, and a tense, hot effusion is common with septic arthritis. Varying amounts of joint effusion are seen with rheumatoid arthritis, osteoarthritis, and the arthritis of gout and pseudogout.

D. **Limitation in range of motion** is common with septic arthritis, effusion, and muscle spasm. Irritation with range-of-motion testing, and possibly a restriction of range of motion caused by a loose body, are seen with osteochondritis dissecans and meniscal tear.

E. **Crepitance** is palpable with patellar fracture.

F. **Shortening** and **deformity** may occur with femoral condylar fractures and to varying degrees with rheumatoid arthritis, osteoarthritis, and the arthritis of gout and pseudogout.

G. **Hemarthrosis** may occur with femoral condylar fractures.

H. **Neural compromise** (altered sensation or loss of motor ability) and **vascular compromise** (loss of peripheral pulse) may occur with femoral condylar fractures.

I. **Increased pain with compression** of the side of the joint occurs with tibial plateau fractures.

J. **Patella alta** or **patella baja** are seen with knee flexion in patellar tendon or quadriceps tendon rupture, respectively.

VII. **Laboratory tests.** If examination of a patient with a severe injury is limited by pain and swelling, examination under anesthesia by an orthopedic surgeon should be considered.

A. **Imaging studies.** Radiologic studies should be ordered whenever the severity of injury or physical signs suggest a fracture. Standard x-rays are rarely required in the diagnosis or management of ligamentous and cartilaginous injuries, patellofemoral dysfunction, and bursitis, although patellar subluxation should be evaluated with x-ray because of the possibility of associated fractures.

   1. Three standard views (anteroposterior, lateral, and a 30-degree sunrise view) should be ordered for diagnosis of patellar, tibial plateau, and femoral condylar fractures.
   2. A lateral x-ray of the tibial tubercle will show fragmentation of the apophysis of the tibial tubercle in Osgood-Schlatter disease and will corroborate the diagnosis, but the x-ray is usually not required to support the clinical findings.
   3. The intercondylar notch or tunnel x-ray view is helpful in searching for loose bodies, such as those that may be found in osteochondritis dissecans. The lateral surface of the medial femoral condyle most often shows a fragment of avascular bone.
   4. **Magnetic resonance imaging** is extremely helpful in accurate diagnosis of torn meniscus or cruciate ligaments.
   5. **Arthrography** definitively diagnoses a Baker's cyst.
   B. **Aspiration of effusion** may be done for diagnostic purposes. A tense effusion can be aspirated in order to provide some pain relief.
   1. The anterior knee is prepared with Betadine and covered with a sterile drape. A small area just medial or lateral to the patella is anesthetized with intradermal 1% Xylocaine hydrochloride. A large-bore (16- or 18-gauge) needle is inserted through the anesthetized area, withdrawing the syringe plunger until fluid is obtained. Bloody fluid should be sent to the laboratory in a heparinized test tube if cell counts are desired. The aspiration site is then covered with a Band-Aid or similar dressing.
   2. See Table 42–2 regarding evaluation of findings.
   C. Positive **culture** of synovial fluid is diagnostic of septic arthritis.
   D. **Laboratory testing** for differentiation of the causes of inflammatory arthritis is discussed in Chapter 71.
VIII. **Treatment.** Indications for urgent orthopedic referral are included in Table 42–3. Treatment plans should differentiate those patients who are likely to improve with conservative care from those in whom urgent or eventual orthopedic referral is likely to be necessary.
   A. **Ligamentous injuries.** If the initial examination is limited by pain and swelling, the following regimen can still be followed. An adequate examination will probably be possible after 1 week.
   1. **Collateral and cruciate injuries** with little or no laxity on testing should be managed as follows.
      a. **Immobilization** is accomplished with a compression dressing (cotton batting wrap with firm Ace wrap application), knee immobilizer (Velcro or strap type with lateral stays), or cylindrical cast. The length of immobilization depends on the extent of injury; protected early range of motion is an option after several days for mild sprains.

TABLE 42–2. EVALUATION OF JOINT FLUID

	Appearance	WBC/μL	Glucose	Other
Septic inflammation	Purulent, opaque, poor mucin clot	10,000 to >100,000 50–75% PMNs	< Serum glucose	Positive Gram stain Positive culture (usually)
Aseptic inflammation	Yellow, translucent, poor mucin clot	2000–10,000 50% PMNs	< Serum glucose	Uric acid crystals in gout, positive rheumatoid factor in rheumatoid arthritis
Degenerative change	Yellow, transparent, good mucin clot	200–2000 <25% PMNs	= Serum glucose	
Injury	Bloody, nonclotting	<15,000	= Serum glucose	Fat globules suggest fracture or pad rupture

PMN, Polymorphonuclear neutrophil.

TABLE 42–3. INDICATIONS FOR URGENT ORTHOPEDIC REFERRAL

Neurovascular compromise
Suspected complete ligamentous disruption
Locked knee—unable to be manipulated into place
Fractures
  Patellar (complete)
  Femoral condylar
  Tibial plateau
  Any compound fracture
Severe injury with limited examination (examination under anesthesia may be indicated)

  b. **Weight bearing** is allowed as tolerated. Crutches for aid in ambulation are often initially helpful. **Isometric quadriceps exercises** (tensing of the quadriceps, 10 contractions every few hours while awake) is recommended during immobilization to minimize atrophy.
  c. **Cold application** with an ice pack through the immobilization apparatus is recommended for 24–48 hours after an acute injury. Elevation of the knee above heart level is helpful in decreasing swelling during this period.
  d. **Nonsteroidal anti-inflammatory drugs (NSAIDs)** such as aspirin, 600–1000 mg four times a day, or ibuprofen, 400–800 mg three times a day, are beneficial for treatment of pain and inflammation.
  e. After immobilization, **gradual rehabilitation** to full activity is necessary. The rehabilitation interval should be twice as long as the period of immobilization. For most knee injuries, strengthening of the quadriceps muscle with straight leg lifting, 10 repetitions three times daily, will promote knee stability and minimize the likelihood of reinjury. The use of ankle weights, with progressive increases in 2- to 4-lb increments, will maximize the benefit of this exercise.

2. Iliotibial band syndrome
  a. **Ice** should be applied for 24 hours. **NSAIDs** can also be used (see section VIII,A,1,d).
  b. **Rest** and avoidance of aggravating activities usually for 1–2 weeks until pain and inflammation subside will facilitate the healing process. Resumption of full activity should be gradual. Rehabilitation is recommended (see section VIII,A,1,e).

B. Cartilaginous injuries. Meniscal tears are treated the same as ligamentous injuries (see section VIII,A). After the acute injury, if the knee is persistently locked or if locking or clicking in the knee recurs, orthopedic referral is indicated.

C. Patellofemoral dysfunction
  1. Patellar subluxation is treated like an acute ligamentous injury (see section VIII,A). If the patella is still dislocated, it can be reduced by hyperextending the knee and pushing the patella back into place. Follow-up referral to an orthopedic surgeon within 1 week is necessary.
  2. Chondromalacia patellae (patellofemoral arthralgia). Acute pain is treated with ice, elevation, and NSAIDs, as for ligamentous injuries (see section VIII,A). The knee should be immobilized for 1 week if the patient is in severe pain. Climbing, jumping, running, and squatting should be limited until pain subsides, often for 2–4 weeks. Quadriceps strengthening exercises (see section VIII,A,1,b) are beneficial for this disorder.
  3. Patellar or quadriceps tendon rupture. Complete ruptures require surgical repair; partial tears are treated as are ligamentous injuries (see section VIII,A).

D. Bursitis
  1. Prepatellar, infrapatellar, and anserine bursitis. Ice should be applied for 24 hours and NSAIDs may be used (see section VIII,A,1,d). Aggravating activities should be avoided until pain and inflammation subside (usually several days to several weeks). A tense, inflamed, noninfected bursa can be aspirated, and corticosteroid solution is then injected.
  2. A **Baker's cyst** may be aspirated to relieve pressure and pain. The cyst will reform unless underlying irritation is corrected.

E. Fractures. Most fractures of the patella, femoral condyles, and tibial plateaus require prompt referral to an orthopedic specialist, as noted in Table 42–3.
  1. **Patellar fractures** without complete disruption of the patella can be immobilized (see section VIII,A,1,a), with orthopedic follow-up in 1 week. Cylindrical casting is usually required for 6 weeks.
  2. **Tibial plateau fractures** require immobilization and no weight bearing. Surgical reduction is usually required for fracture displacement >3 mm.
  3. **Femoral condylar fractures** should be stabilized with a splint until a specialist can attend. If a neurovascular deficit is found, a vascular surgeon should be consulted.
F. Osgood-Schlatter disease and **Sinding-Larsen-Johansson syndrome** are treated symptomatically by avoidance of resisted knee extension (running, climbing, jumping, and kicking) until symptoms subside. Consider immobilization of the affected knee, if walking aggravates pain, for 1–2 weeks. **Osteochondritis dissecans** requires limited weight bearing. NSAIDs can be prescribed (see section VIII,A,1,d). Because of the potential for chronic knee pain and the occasional need for removal or fixation of fracture fragments, orthopedic follow-up should be arranged.
G. Inflammatory arthritis (see Chapter 71 for discussion of treatment). Patients with septic arthritis should be hospitalized for parenteral antibiotic therapy to minimize morbidity.
H. Pain referred from the hip (see Chapter 38).

REFERENCES

DeLee JC, Drez D (editors): *Orthopedic Sports Medicine.* Saunders; 1994.
Post WR: Patellofemoral pain—Let the physical exam define treatment. Physician Sports Med 1998;**26:**68.
Smith BW, Green GA: Acute knee injuries: Part I. History and physical examination. Am Fam Physician 1995;**51:**615.
Smith BW, Green GA: Acute knee injuries: Part II. Diagnosis and management. Am Fam Physician 1995;**51:**799.
Steinberg GG, Akins CM, Baran DT, et al (editors): *Ramamurti's Orthopaedics in Primary Care.* 2nd ed. Williams & Wilkins; 1992.
Stuart MJ: Painful knees: When damaged menisci are the cause. Physician Sports Med 1994; **22:**100.
Stull MA, Nelson C: The role of MRI in diagnostic imaging of the injured knee. Am Fam Physician 1990;**41:**489.

43   Lacerations

Jason Chao, MD, MS

  I. **Definition.** A laceration is a cut or tear in the skin or mucosa that extends through the epidermis into deeper, underlying tissues.
 II. **Common diagnoses**
   A. Superficial wounds
   B. Puncture wounds
   C. Clean lacerations
   D. Wounds with extensive tissue loss or injury, including dirty lacerations, compound lacerations, and electrical wounds.
III. **Epidemiology.** Lacerations and open wound injuries occur in 5–10 of every 100 persons each year in the United States. These wounds constitute one quarter of all injuries in this country, occurring mostly in the home environment.
   A. Lacerations are more common among males and happen more frequently during the summer.
   B. There is a bimodal age distribution, with one peak of lacerations occurring in persons under the age of 5 years and a second peak occurring in persons between 18 and 24 years of age.

IV. Pathophysiology

A. Mechanism of injury

1. Lacerations may result in two ways: (1) from a **shearing force** that slices through the skin or (2) from **blunt trauma** that compresses or stretches the skin.
2. A laceration caused by blunt trauma requires greater energy and results in more extensive tissue damage. This creates an increased inflammatory response and contributes to additional scarring. Such lacerations are much more susceptible to infection.

B. Healing process

1. The body begins a **repair response** immediately after a laceration. Red and white blood cells and platelets bind the wound edges, and injured blood vessels contract. Within a few hours, neovascularization begins. Macrophages gradually replace the leukocytes and stimulate epithelialization and fibroplasia. The final maturation phase, involving collagen synthesis, continues for 6–12 months, during which time the disorganized collagen fibers are reorganized.
2. **Tensile strength** of the wound increases most rapidly during the first 3 weeks. Unfortunately, sutures must be removed by 2 weeks to minimize suture scars, and dehiscence may occur at this time.

C. Infection.
All traumatic lacerations are contaminated with bacteria. The presence of more than 100,000 organisms per gram of tissue is associated with clinical infection. Local factors that increase infection rates include poor local blood supply and the presence of any necrotic tissue, foreign bodies, hematoma, or dead space.

V. Symptoms.
Lacerations cause **pain, bleeding,** and **swelling.**

VI. Signs

A. Tissue damage

1. The surface epidermis is left intact by contusions or bruises (see Chapter 60).
2. Underlying tissue is denuded by abrasions.
3. In patients who have sustained puncture wounds, a small surface opening may hide a deeper, serious injury. An electrical or chemical wound with a break in the skin requires special attention, since the patient may have severe soft tissue injury that is not apparent initially.
4. A partial or complete severing of bones, muscles, tendons, ligaments, major blood vessels, or nerves may occur in compound lacerations.
   a. Loss of a pulse or slow capillary refill after the application of pressure distal to wounds may indicate a vascular injury that must be treated.
   b. Sensorineural function distal to wounds should be assessed before anesthesia is administered. Loss of sensation or movement suggests a nerve injury that must be investigated. Poor finger flexion or extension indicative of a tendon injury is common in hand lacerations because the hand lacks subcutaneous fat.

B.
Dirty lacerations are contaminated with foreign matter. In contrast, clean lacerations are free of contamination. The depth and degree of contamination of lacerations and the surrounding tissue must be assessed. Full exploration of wounds is best performed after the administration of anesthesia.

C.
Inflammatory reaction with surrounding erythema begins several hours after the patient sustains a laceration. Marked erythema or pus signifies wounds that are not recent and are probably infected.

VII. Laboratory tests

A.
A **deep wound culture** is usually indicated if the laceration is dirty, more than 24 hours old, or obviously infected. The culture results are helpful as a guide in the treatment of the wound if it does not improve with initial therapy.

B.
X-rays may be appropriate for patients with compound or deep lacerations so the physician can check for a fracture, subcutaneous air, or a foreign body that might be in the laceration. Most glass is visible on x-rays.

C.
Xerograms may be used by the physician to locate nonradiopaque foreign bodies.

VIII. Treatment.
The goals of the physician are to assist the healing process by approximating the wound when possible and to minimize complications, including infection and unsightly scars.

A. Wound preparation.
Most bleeding can be stopped by the application of direct pressure for 10–15 minutes. Hemostasis of active bleeders can be obtained using ligation, electrocautery, or Gelfoam.

1. Thorough cleansing of the wound is performed to ensure that no foreign body is left in the wound.
   a. Gentle rinsing with saline solution is an adequate cleanser for many lacerations. An antiseptic solution such as Betadine or Hibiclens is often used, but laboratory studies have shown that these disinfectants inhibit the wound repair process.
   b. Dirty lacerations should be forcefully irrigated with copious amounts of sterile saline. A 20- to 50-mL syringe and a 19-gauge needle should be used. Sharp debridement with a scalpel or scissors is sometimes necessary to remove the most contaminated tissue. Scrubbing the wound should be avoided if possible in order to prevent additional trauma to the wound.
   c. Areas such as the face or the neck that have a rich blood supply require less debridement than other areas.
2. Hair rarely needs to be shaved. If shaving of hair is indicated, clipping with scissors is preferable to using a straight razor. Eyebrows should never be shaved, since they grow slowly and a defect in the eyebrows is very noticeable.
3. Wound edges should be perpendicular to the skin surface. If they are beveled, skin should be removed to produce a sharp perpendicular edge that will approximate with the other side. Small skin flaps with inadequate blood supply should be excised to ensure that the skin at the margins of the laceration is vascularized.
4. If tissue is missing, so that easy closure of the wound is precluded, the physician may undermine the subcutaneous layers to free the overlying skin, which in turn will allow approximation of the skin margins.

B. **Anesthesia** may be used both for pain relief and to aid in adequate examination, debridement, and repair. Landmarks that need to be approximated should be identified and marked before local anesthesia is administered in order to prevent distortion.
   1. **Local infiltration** of the wound with anesthesia is often sufficient. A slow injection (ie, for more than 10 seconds) of 1% **lidocaine hydrochloride** through a 27-gauge needle is commonly used. Mixing the lidocaine with **sodium bicarbonate** in a ratio of 9:1 will reduce the pain of injection. This procedure provides adequate anesthesia for as long as 2 hours.
   2. **Epinephrine** may be included in an injection with lidocaine except in an area with reduced circulation, such as the fingers, toes, tip of the nose, or earlobes, since it has a vasoconstrictor effect. Contaminated wounds should not be injected with epinephrine because these wounds become easily infected when their blood supply is reduced.
   3. A **regional block** may be suitable for wounds that are very large or involve the distal fingers or toes.

C. **Wound repair**
   1. **Wound closure.** When clean lacerations present within 12–24 hours, they can be closed primarily. Lacerations closed during this "golden period" are likely to heal without infection. Evidence suggests that head wounds with good blood supply may be closed even after 24 hours and still heal well.

   Lacerations with extensive devitalized tissue or evidence of infection require thorough debriding but should not be closed primarily. Delayed closure, 3–4 days later, may be performed if the wound appears free of infection and is adequately supplied with blood.
   2. **Equipment.** The equipment required to repair a laceration includes a needle holder, smooth and toothed small forceps, scissors, small hemostats, a scalpel, sterile gauze, suture material, gloves, and drapes. Skin hooks are optional; they allow less traumatic handling of the skin. Adequate lighting is essential.

   The choice of suture material depends on the location and purpose of the suture (Table 43–1).
   a. **Absorbable sutures** should be used for dermal or fascial layer repair or for ligation of vessels. They lose their tensile strength by gradual degradation over days to weeks. Synthetic absorbable polymers (eg, Dexon, Vicryl, PDS, or Maxon) retain their tensile strength longer than does plain or chromic gut.
   b. **Nonabsorbable sutures** should be used for epidermal repair. Types of nonabsorbable sutures include silk, cotton, synthetic monofilament nylon

TABLE 43–1. WOUND CLOSURE

Site of Wound	Size of Subcutaneous Suture (Absorbable)	Size of Surface Suture (Nonabsorbable)	Time to Removal (Days)
Scalp	#4-0 or #5-0	#3-0 or #4-0	5–7
Face	#5-0 or #6-0	#6-0 or #7-0	3–5
Trunk and extremities	#3-0 or #4-0	#4-0 or #5-0	7–10
Hands, feet, and skin over joints	None	#3-0 or #4-0	7–14

or polypropylene (eg, Ethilon, Dermalon, Prolene, Surgilene, or Deklene), and braided polyester. Nonabsorbable sutures remain strong but induce a cellular reaction and increase the likelihood of infection in dirty wounds. Synthetic monofilament is the most commonly used material for the final epidermal closure.

3. **Placement of sutures.** Tissue should be handled gently to minimize additional trauma to the wound (Figures 43–1 through 43–6).

a. **Dermal sutures** are used to approximate larger wounds and provide tensile strength. Fat and muscle are closed to prevent dead space and to provide hemostasis. An inverted suture will bury the knot deep in the wound.

b. **Skin sutures** should approximate the wound edges and not be tied too tightly. Excessive tightness of sutures restricts blood flow and produces a depressed scar that is more noticeable.

c. **Simple interrupted sutures** are the most commonly used epidermal suture and provide good cosmetic repair. The deep portion of the suture should be wider than the surface to help evert the skin edges and prevent a depressed scar. **Vertical mattress sutures** evert skin edges more than do simple sutures, but they are time-consuming and may lead to increased inflammatory reaction. **Half-buried horizontal mattress sutures** are useful when the patient has skin flaps that appear viable. These sutures are least likely to compromise vascular supply to the flap.

d. **Running simple sutures** provide the fastest repair; however, they are generally not used in cosmetically important areas. **Locked running sutures** are particularly useful when the laceration is in mucosal surfaces, such as the vagina or the rectum. Absorbable suture material should be used. **Subcuticular (buried running) sutures** are time-consuming but

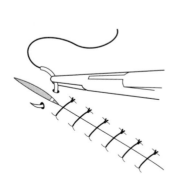
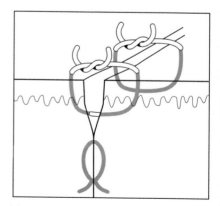

FIGURE 43–1. Simple interrupted suture.

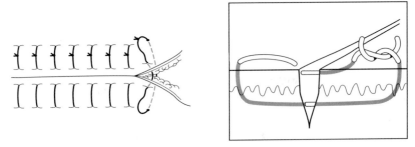

FIGURE 43-2. Vertical mattress suture.

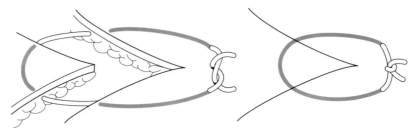

FIGURE 43-3. Half-buried horizontal mattress suture.

produce good cosmetic results without suture marks when used to close small, clean lacerations. Absorbable sutures may be used. If nonabsorbable sutures are used, the ends should be left on the outside of the skin so the suture can be easily removed.

e. In patients with facial lacerations, slight misalignments in repair of the eyebrows and the vermilion border of the lips become very noticeable even at a distance. The first sutures that are placed should align the edges of these structures. Lacerations inside the mouth do not need to be closed

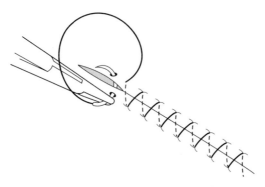

FIGURE 43-4. Running, or continuous, simple suture.

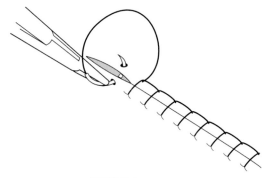

FIGURE 43–5. Locked running suture.

primarily. For through-and-through wounds, the skin and muscle should be closed, and the oral mucosa should be left alone to heal by secondary intention.

f. For patients with scalp lacerations, choosing a suture of a color different from that of the patient's hair helps the physician in repairing the laceration.

g. Discussion of Z-plasty and other plastic techniques is beyond the scope of this chapter. These techniques may be used in patients with long lacerations that do not follow the natural contours of the body or with lacerations over joints that are likely to involve excessive motion during the healing process.

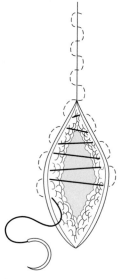

FIGURE 43–6. Subcuticular (buried running) suture. (Adapted with permission from Stillman RM [editor]: *Surgery: Diagnosis & Therapy.* Appleton & Lange; 1989.)

D. Tissue adhesive for closure
1. **Octylcyanoacrylate** (Dermabond) tissue adhesive has been shown to have **comparable cosmetic outcome to suturing** in repair of selected traumatic lacerations. Tissue adhesive closure is **faster** and **less painful** than suturing.
2. Most **facial and selected trunk and extremity lacerations** are suitable for tissue adhesive closure. It should not be used on hands or over joints.
3. When using topical tissue adhesive, care should be taken to **keep adhesive out of the wound,** which would act as a foreign body and inhibit wound healing (Figure 43–7).
4. The patient should be instructed to **avoid washing or soaking** the wound, but may get it wet, as in a shower.

E. Prevention of infection
1. The physician should provide tetanus immunization if it is indicated (Table 43–2).
2. **Prophylactic antibiotics** are not necessary except in selected cases, such as in patients with dirty compound lacerations or with lacerations that involve significant tissue ischemia because of blunt trauma.

F. Patient education. Patients should be given the following advice.
1. **Keep the wound clean and dry** for the first 24 hours, after which the dressing should be removed, and the wound should be cleaned daily.
2. **Contact a physician** if redness, excessive swelling, tenderness, or increased warmth of the skin around the wound occurs; if pus or watery discharge occurs; if there are tender bumps or swelling in an armpit or groin area; if red streaks appear in the skin near the wound; if there is a foul smell from the wound; or if generalized body chills or fever develop.
3. **Elevate an extremity** with a laceration to reduce swelling.
4. **Limit activity** somewhat for 1 week after the sutures are removed to avoid reopening the wound. Wound healing takes several weeks.
5. **Use sunscreen** to protect the scar from sunlight in order to avoid marked pigment changes that occur in lighter-skinned patients. A scar normally appears red and slightly raised or thickened for several months after an injury.

IX. Patient follow-up. See Table 43–1 concerning the timing of suture removal.

A. The physician should see patients with contaminated or deep lacerations 48 hours after the sutures are placed in cases in which infection is likely to present.

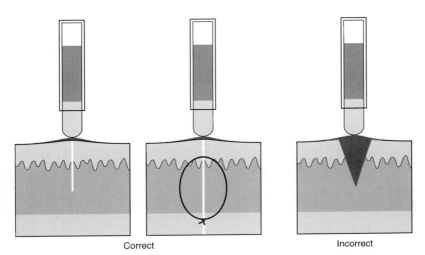

Correct   Incorrect

FIGURE 43–7. Proper tissue adhesive closure (left, center); improper use (right). (Adapted with permission from Quinn J, Wells G, Sutcliffe T, et al: Randomized trial comparing octylcyanoacrylate tissue adhesive sutures. JAMA 1997;**277**:1529. © 1997, American Medical Association.)

TABLE 43–2. GUIDE TO TETANUS PROPHYLAXIS

| Type of Wound | Immunization Status (Doses of Tetanus Toxoid Received) | |
	Uncertain, Less Than 3, or None Within the Last 5 Years	3 or More (Booster Within 5 Years)
Clean wound[1]	Td[1]	No prophylaxis necessary
Dirty wound[2]	Td,[1] and human tetanus immune globulin, at different site	Consider human tetanus immune globulin

[1] Adult tetanus and diphtheria toxoids, 0.5 mL intramuscularly. If the patient is less than 7 years old, diphtheria-tetanus or diphtheria-tetanus-pertussis is given intramuscularly.

[2] A wound that is grossly contaminated, is more than 8 hours old, contains devitalized tissue, or is of a form that prevents adequate irrigation.

Modified with permission from Chesnutt MS, Dewar TN, Locksley RM: *Office & Bedside Procedures.* Appleton & Lange; 1992.

B. When lacerations are in areas of tension, every other suture may be removed initially and replaced by Steri-Strips. The remaining sutures should be removed several days later.

REFERENCES

Quinn J, Wells G, Sutcliffe T, et al: Randomized trial comparing octylcyanoacrylate tissue adhesive sutures. JAMA 1997;**277:**1527.

Singer AJ, Hollander JE, Valentine SM, et al: Prospective, randomized, controlled trial of tissue adhesive (2-octylcyanoacrylate) versus standard wound closure techniques for laceration repair. Acad Emerg Med 1998;**5:**94.

Trott A: *Wounds and Lacerations: Emergency Care and Closure.* Mosby–Year Book; 1991.

---

44   Leg Pain

Richard Viken, MD, & Richard Brunader, MD

I. Definition. Leg pain is a sensation of discomfort in the lower extremities ranging from mild to severe and incapacitating.

II. Common diagnoses

  A. Causes of leg pain in infants and toddlers (aged 0–3 years) that should be considered include septic arthritis of the hip (Chapter 38) and osteomyelitis.

  B. Causes of leg pain in children (aged 4–14 years) that should be considered are injuries, transient synovitis of the hip (Chapter 38), Perthes disease (Chapter 38), and growing pains.

  C. Causes of leg pain in adolescents (aged 11–16 years) that should be considered are slipped capital femoral epiphysis (Chapter 38), knee disorders such as Osgood-Schlatter disease and Sindig-Larsen-Johansson syndrome (Chapter 42), and growing pains.

  D. Causes of leg pain in athletic adolescents and adults that should be considered include shinsplints, stress fractures, chronic compartment syndromes, and patellofemoral dysfunction (Chapter 42).

  E. Causes of leg pain in adults that should be considered are deep venous thrombosis (DVT), peripheral neuropathies (Chapter 53), arterial insufficiency (Chapter 48), osteoarthritis (Chapter 71), gout and other crystal arthropathies (Chapter 71), rheumatoid arthritis (Chapter 71), and nocturnal leg cramps.

III. Epidemiology. The prevalence of leg discomfort in an outpatient practice is difficult to determine and varies depending on the patient's age. A young, physically active population presents with a large proportion of sports-related injuries such as shinsplints and stress fractures. An older population will have more symptoms related to peripheral artery disease, arthritis, and neuropathy.

  A. Osteomyelitis is usually associated with a febrile illness in children. It affects males twice as often as females. The incidence is increased in lower socioeconomic groups. It is more common in immunocompromised children. There is a seasonal variation, with the peak incidence in autumn.

- **B. Growing pains** occur in children of all age groups at an incidence of 15%. They resolve when growth ceases.
- **C. Chronic compartment syndrome** typically occurs in athletic persons in their early 20s.
- **D. Stress fractures** have a peak occurrence in the late teenage to early adult years. In almost every instance, there is an associated increase in physical activity.
- **E. Shinsplints** develop most frequently because of training errors. Usually, an activity is increased too quickly without the body having a chance to adapt. The condition occurs in about 7% of athletic persons.
- **F. DVT.** Risk factors include a past history of DVT; pancreatic, lung, genitourinary, colon, stomach, or breast cancer; exogenous estrogen therapy; heart disease, including congestive heart failure and atrial arrhythmias; paralysis or immobility; pregnancy or puerperium; major surgery; lower extremity trauma; and inherited hypercoagulable states.
- **G. Nocturnal leg cramps.** Although symptoms occur in all age groups, nocturnal leg cramping is most common in elderly persons.

IV. Pathophysiology

- **A. Osteomyelitis** is a bacterial invasion of bone, usually via hematogenous spread, but occasionally secondary to direct contamination (eg, open fracture or nail puncture wound). The organism, usually *Staphylococcus aureus,* sets up local inflammation with associated hyperemia and a cellular response. Pus forms within the medullary cavity of the bone, resulting in bone necrosis and resorption. The metaphysis of long bones is the most common location of osteomyelitis in children, because of the sluggish blood flow at the metaphyseal-physeal barrier, where the vessels make a "U turn." If the metaphysis is intra-articular, as in the hip, pus may spread into the joint.
- **B. Growing pains.** The pathophysiology of growing pains is unknown.
- **C. Chronic compartment syndrome** occurs when high pressure within a closed fascial space decreases capillary perfusion below a level critical for tissue viability. Heavy exercise increases muscle mass approximately 20% due to increased transcapillary filtration. This increase in muscle volume within small unyielding muscular compartments of the leg results in increased soft tissue pressures.
- **D. Stress fractures** are partial or complete fractures of bone caused by repeated, rhythmic, subthreshold stress.
- **E. Shinsplints** are caused by musculotendinous inflammation from repetitive running on hard surfaces or forcible, excessive use of the foot dorsiflexors.
- **F. DVT** occurs in the setting of venous stasis, venous injury, or changes in blood coagulability. Stasis delays the local clearance of activated clotting factors, venous injury causes release of tissue thromboplastin into the circulation, and the preceding two events change blood coagulability. Once formed, DVT requires 7–10 days for fibrinolysis and organization.
- **G. Nocturnal leg cramps** are due to mechanical causes. While the patient is asleep, the feet become passively plantar flexed. A sudden contraction of the plantar muscles in this state of passive flexion results in a painful cramp. They are rarely associated with underlying electrolyte imbalance or denervating neuromuscular disease.

V. Symptoms

- **A. Osteomyelitis** presents with rapid onset of leg pain and refusal to walk. There is a history of a recent (within 2 weeks) skin or respiratory infection in about 25% of cases. Local pain, swelling, tenderness, erythema, and warmth, as well as generalized malaise may all be present.
- **B. Growing pains** consist of intermittent pain, usually in the muscles of the legs and thighs. The joints are rarely involved. The pain is typically bilateral, whereas most serious causes of pain in children's limbs, such as septic arthritis, are unilateral. The pains usually begin in the late afternoon and evening, although they may develop at night and awaken the child from sleep. The discomfort generally resolves by the time the child awakens in the morning.
- **C. Chronic compartment syndrome.** The primary complaint is a sensation of aching or tightness in the affected compartment. Symptoms may begin during exercise or shortly after training ceases. The pain may resolve with cessation of activity or

may persist for a few minutes to days. The problem gradually develops over 1 year or more. How far the patient can walk or run before symptoms occur is usually constant. Symptoms may worsen as the syndrome progresses because of muscle hypertrophy, which further increases the volume of the muscle within the confined fascial space. The location of symptoms depends on which fascial compartment of the leg is involved.

1. **Anterior tibial compartment syndrome** is the most common type of compartment syndrome. Pain occurs on the lateral aspect of the leg. An area of anesthesia may be present in the webbed space between the first and second toes with decreased dorsiflexion strength of the foot.

2. **Superficial and deep posterior compartment syndromes** consist of calf pain and paresthesias within the plantar aspect of the foot.

3. **Lateral compartment syndrome** consists of symptoms localized to the outer lower leg; complaints of ankle instability are common.

D. **Stress fractures.** The early symptoms of stress fractures include the gradual onset of localized pain at the termination of an activity. The pain usually increases over a period of days to weeks, depending on the intensity of physical training. If training is not decreased, the pain eventually occurs during the activity and finally progresses to pain at rest. Stress fractures of the lower extremities most commonly occur in the mid- to lower shaft of the tibia (34%), fibula (24%), metatarsals (20%), femur (14%), and pelvis (6%).

E. **Shinsplints.** The pain is most frequently a dull, aching discomfort along the inner distal two thirds of the tibial shaft. As with stress fractures, the pain of shinsplints increases over a period of days to weeks and may progress to rest pain, depending on the level of activity.

F. **DVT.** The signs and symptoms of DVT are nonspecific in most patients. Patients with relatively minor symptoms may have extensive venous thrombosis, whereas patients with marked symptoms may be entirely free of thrombosis, thus making clinical diagnosis unreliable.

G. **Nocturnal leg cramps.** The calf muscles or the intrinsic muscles of the sole of the foot are generally affected, although the thighs may be involved as well. Symptoms usually occur at night in bed.

VI. **Signs**

A. **Osteomyelitis** is typically associated with fever to 38.0 °C (100.4 °F). The child appears unwell, consistent with septicemia. Tenderness is noted in the involved region. There also may be noticeable redness and warmth. Movement of the adjacent joint is limited, but not to the degree seen in septic arthritis.

B. **Growing pains** are characterized by a paucity of physical findings and are not associated with limping, local tenderness, erythema, or swelling.

C. **Chronic compartment syndrome** is characterized by a lack of physical findings. Pulses are present, and the involved muscles are nontender.

D. **Stress fracture.** Point tenderness over a bony surface is the most important clinical diagnostic sign of stress fractures. However, if there is a significant amount of overlying soft tissue, as over the femur or pelvis, stress fractures usually appear as chronic soft tissue problems that fail to resolve.

E. **Shinsplints.** Most common findings are a 3- to 6-cm area of linear pain and tenderness along the medial edge of the midshaft or distal third of the tibia. The area is often mildly indurated and tender.

F. **DVT** of the lower extremity is characterized by inflammation of the vessel wall that causes local redness, pain, and heat, although these signs are not always extensive enough to be clinically detectable. Venous obstruction predisposes to edema formation. However, incomplete obstruction, obstruction of a small drainage area, or obstruction of an area with collateral drainage may obscure signs of edema. Because the signs and symptoms are so nonspecific, more than 50% of cases of DVT of the lower extremity are not clinically detectable.

G. **Nocturnal leg cramps.** The muscles affected by nocturnal leg cramps are tender and may remain painful the following day. The remainder of the physical examination is normal.

VII. **Laboratory tests**

A. Early in osteomyelitis, **plain x-rays** show loss of the normal fascial planes and fat shadows, due to soft tissue and muscle edema. Bony changes appear 7–10 days after symptoms and include (1) destruction of bone, with or without periosteal elevation; (2) fading cortical margins; and (3) absence of surrounding reactive bone. A stress fracture line may rarely be seen after multiple views; but usually the diagnosis is made by the presence of callus formation at the fracture site 2–4 weeks after the onset of symptoms. Patients with chronic compartment syndrome and shinsplints have normal plain x-ray findings.

B. The **white blood cell (WBC) count** and **erythrocyte sedimentation rate (ESR)** are generally raised in children with osteomyelitis, although the WBC may be normal initially. **C-reactive protein (CRP)** is also raised in osteomyelitis and can be useful for monitoring response to treatment.

C. **Blood cultures** must be obtained in patients with osteomyelitis before antibiotics are given. This test will identify the offending organism in 40–50% of cases.

D. **Tissue pressure measurement** with insertion of a needle-tissue manometer directly into the suspected muscle compartment is the means of diagnosing chronic compartment syndrome. Documentation of the elevated tissue pressures is essential because the treatment is surgical.

E. A **three-phase technetium-99m bone scan** is very sensitive for detecting subacute osteomyelitis, and it is considered essential for making the diagnosis of stress fracture. In osteomyelitis, the test is positive 24–72 hours after onset of infection. There is increased uptake in the affected area in all three phases of the scan. Cold areas indicate bone infarction. A stress fracture shows a discrete area of uptake within several days after the injury occurs. However, the findings may remain positive for up to 2 years, making it difficult to determine a clinical healing point.

F. **Duplex ultrasound** is the most accurate noninvasive test for diagnosing first-time symptomatic proximal DVT. The test is less accurate for symptomatic isolated distal (calf) DVT. **Impedance plethysmography (IPG)** is probably equally as accurate as ultrasound, and it is less operator dependent. Withholding anticoagulant therapy in symptomatic patients who have normal results on serial ultrasound or IPG appears to be safe.

G. **Contrast venography** is the gold standard for diagnosing DVT; however, patient discomfort, technical difficulty, and small risk of morbidity limit its initial diagnostic utility.

H. **Magnetic resonance imaging (MRI)** is the most sensitive test for detecting osteomyelitis in unclear situations. The earliest finding of bone marrow edema is well seen with this test. MRI can also show joint fluid, cartilage damage, and soft tissue sinus tracts.

I. **Aspiration** of pus present in an identified subperiosteal abscess will identify the organism causing osteomyelitis in 60–70% of cases.

VIII. **Treatment**

A. **Osteomyelitis** is initially treated with limb immobilization, hydration, fever control, and intravenous antibiotics. Until culture results are available to guide antibiotic use, a reasonable starting dose for children is nafcillin, 50 mg/kg intravenously every 6 hours, or vancomycin, 10–15 mg/kg intravenously every 6 hours. Oral antibiotics may supervene when warranted by clinical circumstances and improving laboratory parameters. Oral antibiotics should continue for 3–6 weeks. Immobilization should continue for at least 3 weeks to assist the healing process and protect against pathologic fracture secondary to bony destruction.

B. Because the cause of **growing pains** is unknown, treatment consists of supportive measures including heat, massage, and non-narcotic analgesics such as aspirin, 10–20 mg/kg/6 hr, or ibuprofen, 30–40 mg/kg divided into three or four doses. If symptoms persist despite a negative work-up, referral to a rheumatologist or pediatric orthopedic surgeon should be considered.

C. **Chronic compartment syndrome** requires surgical decompression of the affected fascial compartment.

D. **Stress fractures**

1. Running should be discontinued until x-ray evidence of healing is seen and there is no pain on palpation, after which gradual resumption of running may occur.

2. Application of ice and the use of nonsteroidal anti-inflammatory medications such as ibuprofen, 1200–3200 mg divided into three or four doses, or aspirin, 2400–6000 mg divided into four doses, may help relieve pain and swelling.

E. Shinsplints

1. The initial treatment for shinsplints includes rest, application of ice, administration of nonsteroidal anti-inflammatory medications or aspirin (see above), and wrapping or taping the leg for comfort.
2. Once symptoms resolve, a stretching program of toe raises should be initiated, and the patient may gradually return to running on a soft, level surface.

F. DVT

1. Treatment is begun with a 5000-U intravenous bolus of heparin followed by an initial maintenance drip of 1000 U/hr. The activated partial thromboplastin time is checked before treatment and 4 hours postbolus; it should be maintained at 1.5–2.0 times the control.
2. Treatment with heparin should be continued for 5–10 days, and oral anticoagulation with warfarin (Coumadin) should be overlapped with heparin for 4–5 days. Oral anticoagulation should then be continued for at least 3 months, keeping the prothrombin time between an international normalized ratio (INR) of 2.0 and 3.0.
3. Low-molecular-weight heparin (LMWH) may supplant continuous intravenous unfractionated heparin therapy for the initial treatment of DVT. The LMWHs are given subcutaneously and have a predictably high absorption rate and a prolonged duration of action. They can be administered by injection once or twice daily and do not require laboratory monitoring. At least one LMWH, enoxaparin (Lovenox), has been approved for treatment of venous thromboembolism. It should be given subcutaneously at a dose of 1 mg/kg every 12 hours until a stable INR has been achieved with warfarin. Appropriately selected patients may receive outpatient treatment.

G. Nocturnal leg cramps

1. When cramping occurs, the calf muscles should be stretched by dorsiflexion of the foot. This provides prompt relief of the symptoms.
2. Quinine sulfate, 200–300 mg at bedtime, has been used for nocturnal leg cramps since 1940. At least 4 weeks of therapy may be necessary for the medication to work. *The potentially beneficial effects should be balanced with the risk of side effects, which include pancytopenia, visual toxicity, cinchonism, and cardiac effects.*

REFERENCES

Adams RD, Victor M, Ropper AH: *Principles of Neurology.* 6th ed. McGraw-Hill; 1997:1489.
Aguilar D, Goldhaber SZ: Clinical uses of low-molecular-weight heparins. Chest 1999;**115**:1418.
Barnes M: Diagnosis and management of chronic compartment syndromes: A review of the literature. Br J Sports Med 1997;**31**(1):21.
Graham HK: Normal variants: Intoeing, bow legs and flat feet. In Broughton NS (editor): *A Textbook of Paediatric Orthopaedics.* Saunders; 1997:183.
Kearon C, Julian JA, Newman TE, et al: Noninvasive diagnosis of deep venous thrombosis. McMaster Diagnostic Imaging Practice Guidelines Initiative. Ann Intern Med 1998;**128**:663.
Pfeffer GB: Foot and ankle. In Snider RK (editor): *Essentials of Musculoskeletal Care.* American Academy of Orthopaedic Surgeons; 1997:366.
Rock MG: Sports and occupational injuries. In Klippel JH (editor): *Primer on the Rheumatic Diseases.* 11th ed. Arthritis Foundation; 1997:149.
Saxton VJ, O'Sullivan MD: Bone and joint infection. In Broughton NS (editor): *A Textbook of Paediatric Orthopaedics.* Saunders; 1997:149.

---

45   Liver Function Test Abnormalities

James P. McKenna, MD

I. **Definition.** Abnormalities in liver function tests (LFTs) are elevated levels of static biochemical tests, including aspartate aminotransferase (AST) (formerly serum glutamic-oxaloacetic transaminase [SGOT]), alanine aminotransferase (ALT) (formerly serum glutamate pyruvate transaminase [SGPT]), alkaline phosphatase, bilirubin, and albumin. The tests are most frequently obtained as part of LFT panels. Tests other than those mentioned are often included in LFT panels but are less useful in evaluating the spectrum of liver disease, and therefore are not discussed here. Hepatic clearance tests measuring liver metabolism of lidocaine or caffeine may be used by hepatologists to assess liver function in patients with chronic compensated liver disease.

II. Common diagnoses

   A. Elevated aminotransferases (transaminases), AST, or ALT are most indicative of hepatocellular dysfunction (Table 45–1).

   B. Elevated alkaline phosphatase occurs in patients with cholestatic liver disease (eg, intrahepatic or extrahepatic obstruction or medications that induce cholestasis [Table 45–2]) or infiltrative disease (eg, cancer or granulomas).

   C. Elevated bilirubin may signify hepatobiliary disease (eg, hepatitis, cirrhosis, or gallstones) or hemolysis.

III. Epidemiology.
In asymptomatic populations, the frequency of abnormal LFTs on routine screening ranges from 1% to 6%. The prevalence of liver disease is approximately 1%.

   A. Elevated aminotransferases are found to some degree in almost all patients with liver disease.

   1. In asymptomatic populations, as many as 6% of patients have abnormal values of AST.
   2. Alcohol liver damage is the most common cause of aminotransferase abnormality in adults.
   3. Hepatitis A virus is the most common cause of aminotransferase abnormality in children.

   B. Elevated alkaline phosphatase has been found in as many as 4% of asymptomatic patients.

   C. Hyperbilirubinemia

   1. Mild degrees of indirect hyperbilirubinemia may be found in as many as 10% of asymptomatic patients as a result of Gilbert's syndrome.
   2. Prior to age 30, hepatitis causes 75% of cases of hyperbilirubinemia.
   3. After age 60, extrahepatic obstruction causes 50% of the cases of hyperbilirubinemia (eg, gallstones or pancreatic cancer).

IV. Pathophysiology

   A. Aminotransferases

   1. Cellular damage in the liver, heart, kidneys, brain, intestines, or placenta causes release of AST. ALT is predominantly released because of hepatocellular injury and is a more specific indication of liver disease.
   2. Cellular injury may occur because of formation of toxic metabolites, alteration of cellular components causing a secondary immunologic response, disruption of membrane function, or blockage of hepatic uptake processes.

   B. Alkaline phosphatase is associated with cellular membranes, and elevated levels may be caused by injury to the liver, bone, kidneys, intestines, placenta, or

---

TABLE 45–1. CAUSES OF ELEVATED AMINOTRANSFERASES

Alcoholic hepatitis
Viral hepatitis
   Hepatitis A
   Hepatitis B[1]
   Hepatitis C[1]
   Hepatitis D[1]
   Hepatitis E
   Hepatitis G[1]
   Cytomegalovirus
   Epstein-Barr virus
Drug-induced hepatitis[1]
Autoimmune hepatitis[1]
Toxic hepatitis
Metabolic hepatitis[1]
   Hemochromatosis
   α_1-Antitrypsin deficiency
   Wilson's disease

---

[1] These conditions may cause chronic active hepatitis.

TABLE 45–2. MEDICATIONS THAT MAY ADVERSELY AFFECT LIVER FUNCTION TESTS

Cholestatic pattern
Amoxicillin/clavulanic acid
Anabolic steroids
Chlorambucil
Chlorpromazine
Chlorpropamide
Erythromycin estolate
Estrogen (oral contraceptives)
Methimazole
Phenobarbital
Tolbutamide

Cytotoxic pattern
Acetaminophen
Amiodarone
L-Asparaginase
Aspirin and nonsteroidal anti-inflammatory drugs
Carbamazepine
Etretinate
Halothane
Hydralazine
Imipramine
Isoniazid
Ketoconazole
Lovastatin
6-Mercaptopurine
Methotrexate
Methyldopa
Nicotinic acid (especially sustained-release)
Nitrofurantoin
Phenytoin
Propylthiouracil
Rifampin
Sulfonamides
Tetracycline
Valproic acid

leukocytes. In the liver, the enzyme is predominantly located at the microvilli of bile canaliculi. Biliary obstruction induces increased synthesis of alkaline phosphatase and spillage into the circulation.

C. **Hyperbilirubinemia** may be caused by increased production, decreased metabolism, or reduced biliary excretion of bilirubin.

1. Increased production may be secondary to hemolysis, extravasation of blood (hematoma), or ineffective erythropoiesis.

2. Decreased metabolism may be caused by hereditary disease (eg, Gilbert's syndrome) or acquired defects in bilirubin conjugation.

3. Obstruction of bile ducts causes increased pressure and dilated ducts proximal to the obstruction. Serum levels rise secondary to blocked excretion.

V. **Symptoms**

A. Abnormal LFTs in asymptomatic patients may indicate very mild hepatic dysfunction or may represent a more serious illness in its presymptomatic phase. Subsequent testing and follow-up are usually necessary to determine which abnormality exists.

B. Fatigue, nausea, malaise, pruritus, jaundice, anorexia, or right upper quadrant discomfort are common complaints of patients with compensated liver disease and abnormal LFTs. The severity of the complaints is often related to the acuteness and extent of the illness.

C. Fatigue, anorexia, weight loss, abdominal distention, hematemesis, hematochezia, confusion, jaundice, and abdominal discomfort are symptoms of hepatic decompensation in patients with decompensated liver disease and abnormal LFTs.

VI. Signs
A. Hepatomegaly or an unusually firm liver may be present in asymptomatic patients.

B. Fever, jaundice, splenomegaly, and a tender, enlarged liver may indicate compensated liver disease.

C. Ascites, edema, jaundice, vascular spiders, esophageal varices, splenomegaly, hepatic encephalopathy, testicular atrophy, gynecomastia, or loss of pubic and axillary hair may indicate decompensated liver disease.

VII. Laboratory tests
A. A **stepwise approach to evaluating LFT abnormalities** is recommended.

1. **LFTs should be repeated** to confirm any abnormalities in asymptomatic patients. Any offending agents (Table 45–2) should be discontinued, and the test should be repeated in 2–4 weeks.

   If abnormal LFTs persist for more than 6 months, treatable causes of chronic hepatitis should be ruled out. Such causes include hemochromatosis; autoimmune hepatitis; α_1-antitrypsin deficiency; hepatitis B, C, and D; and Wilson's disease (see Chapter 75).

2. A **γ-glutamyltransferase (GGT) test** should be ordered in patients with abnormal alkaline phosphatase levels to confirm the hepatic origin of the enzyme.

3. Direct and indirect **bilirubin fractions** should be obtained if total bilirubin levels are increased. If the indirect (unconjugated) fraction is elevated (>80% of total), a reticulocyte count and a peripheral blood smear should be obtained (see Chapter 6).

4. **Serum albumin** determinations are indicated in any symptomatic patient. Decreased levels reflect decreased synthesis (from poor nutrition or hepatic dysfunction) or increased loss (from the kidneys or the intestines). Serum levels correlate poorly with prognosis in acute liver disease, although patients with decompensated liver disease routinely have low levels.

5. **Prothrombin time (PT)** reflects hepatic synthesis of vitamin K–dependent clotting factors (II, VII, IX, and X) and should be ordered for patients with acute or chronic liver disease or coagulopathy.

   a. Improvement by 30% after a 10-mg intramuscular injection of vitamin K suggests intact hepatocellular function and makes biliary obstruction the likely cause of the abnormal PT.

   b. If the PT fails to improve after administration of vitamin K, significant loss of hepatocellular function exists and the prognosis is poor.

6. If evidence suggests hepatitis, further serologic testing is indicated to confirm the diagnosis (see Chapter 40).

   Liver biopsy should be considered for any patient with abnormal LFTs for 6 months. A biopsy sample should be obtained before the end of the 6-month period if the patient's condition deteriorates. Liver biopsy is the only definitive means of establishing a diagnosis of chronic hepatitis.

B. Interpretation of particular abnormal LFT patterns

1. **Alcoholic liver disease** results in modest elevations of the transaminases. An elevation of ALT >300 IU is not consistent with alcoholic liver damage. The ratio of AST to ALT is useful diagnostically, since a ratio of 2 : 1 or greater suggests a high probability of alcoholic liver disease. Elevated mean corpuscular volume and GGT suggest alcoholic liver disease.

2. **Viral hepatitis** often causes significant elevations of the transaminases, with levels exceeding 1000 IU. ALT is typically elevated more than AST; the AST-ALT ratio is <1.

3. **Medications** causing cholestasis (Table 45–2) may result in transaminase and alkaline phosphatase elevations that are as much as 10 times the normal levels.

4. **Cytotoxic reactions** from medications may cause severe injuries resembling viral hepatitis, with transaminase values as high as 500 times the normal levels.

5. **Intrahepatic or extrahepatic obstruction** cause values of alkaline phosphatase to be five or more times higher than normal. The highest values are found in primary biliary cirrhosis.

6. **Infiltrative diseases** such as neoplasm, granulomas, or amyloidosis may cause moderate to marked elevations of alkaline phosphatase. Bilirubin is minimally elevated, however.

7. **Hemolysis** causes an elevated reticulocyte count and an abnormal peripheral smear, with the bilirubin level generally <5 mg/dL.
8. **Gilbert's syndrome** is characterized by indirect bilirubin levels of 2–3 mg/dL, normal LFTs, and no evidence of hemolysis.

VIII. **Treatment.** For information on the management of the following causes of abnormal LFTs, refer to the chapters indicated.
   A. **Cholelithiasis** (see Chapter 1).
   B. **Hemolysis** (see Chapter 6).
   C. **Hepatitis** (see Chapter 40).
   D. **Cirrhosis** (see Chapter 75).
   E. **Alcohol and drug abuse** (see Chapter 92).

REFERENCES

Aranda-Michel J, Sherman KE: Tests of the liver: Use and misuse. Gastroenterologist 1998; **6**(1):34.

Kamath PS: Clinical approach to the patient with abnormal liver test results. Mayo Clin Proc 1996;**71**:1089.

Moseley RH: Evaluation of abnormal liver function tests. Med Clin North Am 1996;**80**:887.

Scheig R: Acute and chronic viral hepatitis. Lippincotts Prim Care Pract 1998;**2**(4):390.

Younossi ZM: Evaluating asymptomatic patients with mildly elevated liver enzymes. Cleveland Clin J Med 1998;**65**:150.

46   Low Back Pain

David C. Lanier, MD

I. **Definition.** Low back pain is a sharp or aching sensation between the lower rib cage and the gluteal folds, with or without pain or neuromotor deficits in the distribution of lumbosacral (LS) nerve roots.

II. **Common diagnoses**
   A. **Mechanical disorders** of the LS spine, such as those listed below, cause 90% of back pain.
      1. **Back strain,** involving the muscles and ligaments of the LS region.
      2. **Lumbar disk disease,** which at times may be associated with the following conditions.
         a. **Sciatica** (pain radiating below the knee).
         b. **Cauda equina syndrome** (acute urinary or rectal incontinence, with or without paraplegia, usually caused by a massive, centrally herniated disk).
      3. **Osteoarthritis,** which may be associated with **spinal stenosis.**
      4. **Spondylolysis,** with or without **spondylolisthesis.**
   B. Less common but serious or life-threatening causes of back pain include the following conditions.
      1. **Visceral pain** referred to the back from vascular, genitourinary, or gastrointestinal diseases.
      2. **Compression fracture** (traumatic or pathologic).
      3. **Tumor** (metastatic or primary).
      4. **Infection** (eg, LS spine osteomyelitis, diskitis, or epidural abscess).
      5. **Inflammatory diseases** (eg, ankylosing spondylitis, Reiter's syndrome, arthritis of psoriasis, or inflammatory bowel disease).
   C. Social or psychological **distress** may amplify or prolong back pain.

III. **Epidemiology.** Low back pain affects >80% of individuals at some time during their active life and accounts for about 4% of adult primary care visits.
   A. Overall, mechanical disorders of the back affect men and women equally. Men, however, are affected more often by **low back strain** at an earlier age (30–50 years of age) than women, who often report symptoms after the age of 60. Risk factors include repetitive lifting (especially in a twisted position), exposure to mechanical vibrations, static work postures (eg, prolonged sitting), cigarette smoking, and a sedentary lifestyle.

B. Patients under 50 years of age are likely to experience back pain related to the following conditions.

1. **Spondylolysis,** a defect of the vertebral arch, is found in 5% of people over the age of 7. **Spondylolisthesis** occurs when this defect allows slippage of all or part of a vertebra on another. Spondylolisthesis is the most common cause of back pain in patients under the age of 26, especially athletes, but is rarely the sole cause of complaints after the age of 40.

2. The peak incidence of **herniated lumbar disk** is between the ages of 30 and 55 years. Only about 35% of individuals with disk herniation actually develop sciatica, which is seen in <2% of all patients with acute low back pain. Cauda equina syndrome is an extremely rare condition.

3. **Scoliosis,** most commonly found in young females, rarely causes back pain unless the spinal angulation is >40 degrees.

4. **Lumbosacral infections** may occur in children or adults, especially those who have diabetes mellitus, use intravenous drugs, or have a history of septicemia, sickle cell disease, or recent spinal or urinary tract surgery.

5. **Inflammatory diseases.** Ankylosing spondylitis, for example, most frequently affects males between the ages of 15 and 40 (3:1 male-female ratio).

C. Patients over 50 years of age with back complaints are most likely to have the following conditions.

1. **Osteoarthritis of the LS spine.** The prevalence of this condition increases with age and is almost universally present in individuals over 75 years of age.

2. **Compression fractures.** Older patients with osteoporosis, especially postmenopausal women who are inactive and have a low calcium intake, are at greatest risk.

3. **Visceral pain,** especially secondary to abdominal aortic aneurysm or gastrointestinal cancer, may be referred to the back.

4. **Malignant neoplasms** account for <1% of episodes of low back pain. Metastatic lesions (eg, from the breast, prostate, or lung) are 25 times more common than primary bone tumor.

D. Patients with **chronic low back pain** are more likely to have a history of depression, failed previous back treatments, substance abuse, or disability compensation claims. Psychosocial factors, including work dissatisfaction and poor relationships with coworkers, also increase the risk of back complaints.

IV. Pathophysiology

A. Acute mechanical disorders of the LS spine result from overuse of normal musculoskeletal structures or from injury or deformity of an anatomic structure.

1. **Acute back strain** is often related to a specific event (eg, heavy lifting) or continuous mechanical stress on the ligamentous or muscular support of the LS spine.

2. A **herniated lumbar disk** is often preceded by years of recurrent episodes of localized back pain corresponding to repeated damage to the annular fibers of the disk. When herniation of the nucleus pulposus through the annulus fibrosus occurs, leg pain usually overshadows the back pain. Approximately 98% of herniations occur at the L-5 to S-1 (involving the first sacral nerve) or L-4 to L-5 (involving the fifth lumbar nerve) level. Herniations at the L-2 to L-3 and L-3 to L-4 levels are relatively uncommon. **Sciatica** is caused by mechanical compression and/or inflammation of nerve roots.

3. **Osteoarthritis** of the LS spine primarily affects the articular processes of the facet joints. Degenerative changes can result in a decrease in the size of the spinal canal, causing claudication-like symptoms of the lower extremities through mechanical pressure on neural structures (**spinal stenosis**).

4. **Spondylolysis** is the equivalent of a stress fracture of the vertebral arch, although the exact cause of the defect is not clear. It appears to occur at any age in persons who are genetically predisposed, and can also be produced by degenerative changes.

B. The other conditions outlined above (see section II,B) generally cause back pain by direct stimulation of sensory nerves within the LS spine.

V. Symptoms. To differentiate the more common mechanical disorders from other serious causes of back pain, the clinician should carefully evaluate the following symptoms.

A. **Onset.** Mechanical back pain typically has an acute, sudden onset; the pain from a compression fracture may also begin acutely. Medical causes of pain (eg, ankylosing spondylitis, referred pain, or tumor pain) generally have a more gradual or insidious onset.

B. **Frequency and duration.** Most mechanical low back pain occurs in intermittent episodes that last from a few days to a few months. A degenerating disk may cause low-grade, chronic discomfort that is exacerbated during acute attacks. Patients with osteoarthritis, ankylosing spondylitis, or tumor usually develop chronic persistent symptoms.

C. **Time of day.** Mechanical disorders generally cause pain that increases with the day's activities. Inflammatory conditions produce greater pain and stiffness in the morning. Most individuals with spinal tumors complain of back pain that is worse during the night.

D. **Location of pain.** Most mechanical and medical disorders result in pain localized to the LS spine and surrounding areas. Nerve root irritation (eg, from a herniated disk, spinal stenosis, or spondylolisthesis) is signaled by pain that radiates from the back to the lower leg or is felt exclusively in the lower leg. Poorly localized pain along nonanatomic routes suggests the presence of social or psychological distress.

E. **Aggravating and alleviating factors.** Pain caused by mechanical disorders typically improves with recumbency and worsens with activity, while patients with back pain caused by inflammatory diseases or tumor feel worse with bed rest. The pain from nerve root compression is usually increased by any Valsalva's maneuver (eg, coughing or bowel movements). Relief of pain only with absolute immobility is often a sign of acute infection or a compression fracture.

VI. **Signs**

A. While patients with mechanical back pain often exhibit **local tenderness, muscle spasm,** or **limited range of motion** of the back, these signs are neither highly sensitive nor specific for this condition.

B. **Fever, weight loss,** or an **abdominal, rectal, or pelvic mass** may indicate infection, tumor, or aortic aneurysm.

C. **Point tenderness** over bony landmarks is a sensitive but nonspecific sign of infection; it is also commonly seen in patients with arthritis or tumor.

D. **Pain from percussion of the sacroiliac joints** is suggestive but not diagnostic of ankylosing spondylitis.

E. The physical findings listed below are signs of nerve root irritation or compression.

   1. **Antalgic gait** (avoidance of weight bearing on the involved leg).

   2. **Diminished or absent ankle reflex** or **calf weakness or atrophy** (compression of the first sacral nerve root).

   3. **Weakness of dorsiflexors of the great toe** (compression of the fifth lumbar root).

   4. **Diminished knee jerk** (compression of the fourth lumbar nerve root).

   5. Pain during a **straight leg raising test,** in which the examiner raises the affected leg of the supine patient by the heel while keeping the knee fully extended.

      a. Pain below the knee as the leg is raised 30–60 degrees indicates nerve root irritation or compression.

      b. Reproduction of the sciatica when the unaffected leg is elevated increases to 98% the probability that the patient suffers from disk herniation.

      c. A modified straight leg raising test confirms the diagnosis. As the patient sits with both legs dangling, the examiner slowly raises the foot of the affected leg; nerve root sensitivity will cause the patient with true sciatica to bend the trunk back to relieve pressure on the nerve root.

F. **Anatomically "inappropriate" signs** (eg, increased back pain from downward pressure applied to the skull, patient overreaction during the physical examination, or marked discrepancy between the examination and the patient's ability to dress or move about) are helpful in identifying psychological distress as a result of, or as an amplifier of, low back symptoms.

VII. **Testing.** For most patients with acute low back pain, x-rays, imaging studies, and laboratory tests are unnecessary. These are indicated only if clinical signs or symptoms suggest a serious disorder or if significant improvement is not seen after 2–4 weeks of conservative treatment.

A. Radiologic evaluation should be used selectively.

  1. LS spine plain films should be limited to individuals with unrelenting pain at rest, an evolving neurologic deficit, a history of cancer or direct trauma to the back, or failure to respond to conservative therapy.

  a. Oblique projections are rarely indicated, since they add useful information in only 4–8% of cases and more than double the patient's exposure to radiation.

  b. Attributing back pain to radiographic findings of degenerative arthritis, narrowed disk space, vertebral sacralization, mild scoliosis, facet subluxation, or spina bifida occulta may be inaccurate, since these conditions are found with the same frequency in symptomatic and asymptomatic individuals.

  c. A normal plain film series does not rule out significant LS spine disease. This study may give **false-negative results** in as many as 40% of patients with known vertebral cancer.

  2. The **bone scan** appears to be more accurate than plain x-ray for detecting suspected tumor, infection, or occult fractures of the vertebrae, but not for specifying the diagnosis. A positive scan usually needs to be confirmed using other tests.

  3. Computerized tomography (CT) or **magnetic resonance imaging (MRI)** should be used for confirmation of clinical findings, not for primary diagnosis. The major role of CT is the delineation of osseous abnormalities, while MRI is more sensitive in depicting changes in the vertebra resulting from infection or neoplasm. Both techniques have a sensitivity of >90% and a specificity of 88% (nearly identical to those of myelography) in detecting a herniated lumbar disk. MRI has the advantage of involving no radiation exposure, although patients with claustrophobia or implanted metallic objects (eg, surgical clips) may not be candidates for this procedure.

B. Laboratory tests may be useful in evaluating selected patients who have not responded to conservative therapy.

  1. The **erythrocyte sedimentation rate** can be used to screen for malignancy or an acute infectious or inflammatory process.

  2. An elevated **serum alkaline phosphatase** can be associated with metastatic tumors or Paget's disease.

  3. Abnormalities of the routine **urinalysis** are helpful in identifying those patients with referred back pain of urinary origin.

  4. Tests for antinuclear antibodies, rheumatoid factor, and specific human leukocyte antigens (HLA-B27) should not be used for routine screening. The common spondyloarthropathies affecting the back are seronegative conditions. Although HLA-B27 is present in 95% of white patients with ankylosing spondylitis, only about 20% of HLA-B27–positive individuals develop the disease.

C. Electromyography may be useful in evaluating a confusing clinical picture of back-related leg symptoms of more than 3–4 weeks' duration. Test results are not reliable before this time. The accuracy of the test is also highly dependent on the skill of the examiner.

VIII. Treatment

  A. Conservative treatment. When clinical evaluation of the patient with acute low back pain fails to suggest a serious or life-threatening cause, the patient should be made aware that acute back pain is usually self-limited and that in 80–90% of cases, the pain will resolve or improve significantly within 4–6 weeks with conservative management.

  1. Activity modification. Among patients with acute low back pain, continuing ordinary activities within the limits permitted by the pain leads to a more rapid recovery than either bed rest or back-mobilizing exercises. Prolonged periods of sitting and activities stressful to the back (eg, lifting) may need to be limited temporarily. The goal, however, is for the patient to be ambulatory as soon as possible. Neither prolonged bed rest (ie, more than a few days) nor spinal traction has any proven efficacy in the treatment of acute low back pain.

  2. Medication

  a. Nonsteroidal anti-inflammatory drugs (NSAIDs) such as aspirin (2600 mg/day), ibuprofen (1600 mg/day), or naproxen (1000 mg/day), every 4–6 hours for 2–7 days, will provide analgesia for most low back pain. Gastrointestinal bleeding and renal dysfunction are the major toxicities of NSAIDs. Acetaminophen (2600 mg/day, every 4–6 hours) is a reasonably safe and effective alternative for patients who are intolerant of NSAIDs.

   b. Severe or radicular pain not relieved by NSAIDs may require **opioid** analgesics, such as codeine, 30–60 mg every 4–6 hours. Because of the potential for developing tolerance and physical dependence, patients should be prescribed opioids for a fixed period of time (usually a few days). A major problem with opioids is their sedative effect, which may limit the patient's efforts to ambulate or participate in other activities. Constipation may also be a side effect.

   c. While **muscle relaxants,** such as cyclobenzaprine (10–20 mg every 8 hours for 7 days), appear to be as effective as NSAIDs in relieving back symptoms, the clinician should be aware of side effects, including drowsiness in up to 30% of patients.

   d. **Epidural corticosteroid injections** may be useful for leg pain and sensory deficits early in the course of sciatica secondary to a herniated lumbar disk.

3. Spinal manipulation. Defined as manual therapy using lever methods to apply loads to the spine, manipulation has been shown to be effective in reducing low back pain and perhaps in speeding recovery within the first month of symptoms.

4. Other modalities. While some patients appear to have temporary relief of low back symptoms with physical modalities (eg, diathermy, ultrasonography, or massage) or application of hot or cold packs, these treatments have no proven effect on longer-term outcomes.

5. Exercise. The patient should be encouraged to begin low-impact aerobic exercise (eg, short walks, swimming, or cycling) as soon as possible. Exercise programs to improve abdominal and paraspinal muscle tone should be delayed for at least 2 weeks following the onset of symptoms.

6. Patient education

   a. To prevent recurrences, patients should be instructed in body mechanics (eg, appropriate work stance and the best ways to lift and carry objects). As many as 75% of patients with occupationally related acute episodes of low back pain will have recurrent symptoms within 1 year. Job design/redesign to avoid pain-inducing movements may help prevent recurrences.

   b. Improvement of the patient's general physical condition through weight loss, exercise, and cessation of smoking will help prepare the patient for future strain on the LS spine.

   c. The clinician should assist the patient in identifying and addressing significant psychosocial stresses or family dysfunction that may contribute to slow recovery or recurrence of back pain.

B. Surgery

1. The only absolute indication for early lumbar disk surgery is an acute disk herniation associated with either a cauda equina compression or progressive neurologic deficits. Patients with unequivocal but stable disk-related neurologic signs and symptoms may be treated either medically or surgically, depending on individual patient preferences. While no improvement in long-term outcomes has been noted with either approach, surgical diskectomy may substantially improve the short-term quality of life for carefully selected patients with symptomatic herniated lumbar disks.

2. Patients with acute low back pain alone, who have neither sciatica nor evidence of a malignant lesion, infection, or fracture, do not need surgical consultation.

3. Surgical treatment of spinal stenosis or spondylolisthesis should be considered only after an adequate trial of conservative therapy has failed.

C. Chronic back pain. Only about 20% of patients with acute low back pain will have significant symptoms that persist longer than 3 months. Patients with chronic low back pain may require one or more of the following treatments.

1. An **individualized exercise program** aimed at increasing endurance and strength of the back to perform specific tasks required on a daily basis at home or work.

2. Other **medications,** such as tricyclic antidepressants, if the pain is associated with symptoms of depression (see Chapter 95).
3. **Counseling** that includes the patient's family, especially if the pain is associated with secondary gains at home.
4. Referral to a multispecialty pain clinic.

REFERENCES

Borenstein DG: Epidemiology, etiology, diagnostic evaluation and treatment of low back pain. Curr Opin Rheumatol 1998;**10:**104.
Croft PR, Macfarlane GJ, Papageorgiou AC, et al: Outcome of low back pain in general practice: A prospective study. Br Med J 1998;**316:**1356.
Deyo RA: Drug therapy for back pain. Which drugs help which patients? Spine 1996;**21:**2840.
Malmivaara A, Hakkinen U, Aro T, et al: The treatment of acute low back pain—Bed rest, exercises, or ordinary activity? N Engl J Med 1995;**332:**351.
Suarez-Almazor ME, Belseck E, Russell AS, et al: Use of lumbar radiographs for the early diagnosis of low back pain. JAMA 1997;**277:**1782.
Turner JA: Educational and behavioral interventions for back pain in primary care. Spine 1996;**21:**2851.
van Tulder MW, Koes BW, Bouter LM: Conservative treatment of acute and chronic nonspecific low back pain. A systematic review of randomized controlled trials of the most common interventions. Spine 1997;**22:**2128.

47   Lymphadenopathy

Martin S. Lipsky, MD, & Mari E. Egan, MD

I. **Definition.** Lymphadenopathy is lymph gland enlargement >1 cm. Two exceptions are inguinal nodes, which are considered normal up to 1.5 cm in diameter, and epitrochlear nodes, which are considered abnormal if >0.5 cm.

II. **Common diagnoses**
   A. **Generalized lymphadenopathy** is defined as involvement of three or more noncontiguous lymph nodes. It is seen in a wide spectrum of diseases, including infectious, immunologic, metabolic, and malignant disorders.
   1. **Infections.** Generalized lymphadenopathy is caused by viral infections, including infectious mononucleosis, cytomegalovirus (CMV), rubella, rubeola, and human immunodeficiency virus (HIV). Nonviral infectious causes include scarlet fever, brucellosis, tuberculosis, syphilis, histoplasmosis, leptospirosis, tularemia, malaria, toxoplasmosis, typhoid fever, and pyogenic bacterial infections. Most infectious causes produce a short history of lymphadenopathy lasting less than 2 weeks.
   2. **Immunologic disorders** include connective tissue disorders (eg, systemic lupus erythematosus and rheumatoid arthritis), immunologic reactions (eg, serum sickness and drug reactions [eg, to phenytoin or propylthiouracil]), and benign reactive hyperplasia.
   3. **Metabolic disorders** include Gaucher's disease, Niemann-Pick disease, and hyperthyroidism.
   4. **Malignant disorders** include leukemias, lymphomas, metastatic cancers, and malignant histiocytosis.
   5. **Miscellaneous disorders** are those such as Kawasaki disease, sarcoidosis, and chronic pseudolymphomatous lymphadenopathy.
   B. **Regional lymphadenopathy** may be caused by a local infection, growth, or recent immunization in the area drained by an involved lymph node.
   1. **Cervical lymphadenopathy** is usually caused by infections, primarily upper respiratory viral infections. Mononucleosis, CMV, toxoplasmosis, mycobacterial infection, and bacterial infections of the head and neck are infectious causes. Neoplasms, Kawasaki disease, sarcoidosis, Kikuchi disease, Rosai-Dorfmann's disease, and benign reactive hyperplasia can also cause cervical lymphadenopathy.
   2. **Supraclavicular lymphadenopathy** may be caused by tuberculosis, histoplasmosis, sarcoidosis, lymphomas, and metastatic disease, particularly lung

and gastrointestinal cancers. Virchow's node is an enlarged left supraclavicular node. It usually signals a metastasis from a gastrointestinal primary cancer.

3. **Axillary lymphadenopathy** commonly results from upper extremity infections, connective tissue disorders, neoplasms, and cat scratch disease.

4. **Epitrochlear nodes** are usually caused by hand infections or, less commonly, secondary syphilis.

5. **Inguinal nodes** are commonly enlarged by nonspecific benign causes (eg, skin rashes or mild infections). Less frequent causes include syphilis, lymphogranuloma venereum, genital herpes, chancroid, cat scratch disease, lower extremity or local infections, and neoplastic disorders such as vulvar or testicular cancer.

6. **Mediastinal nodes** commonly result from primary lung disorders, infectious mononucleosis, sarcoidosis, tuberculosis, histoplasmosis, lymphomas, and metastatic cancers.

7. **Any region.** Benign reactive hyperplasia, cat scratch disease, lymphomas, leukemia, sarcoidosis, metastatic cancer, and granulomatous diseases may present with localized lymphadenopathy in any region.

C. **Cancer** and **septicemia** should be ruled out in severely ill patients.

III. **Epidemiology.** Palpable lymph nodes are common, particularly in children, and are found in as many as 80% of patients. However, fewer than 1% are found to be malignant.

A. **Generalized lymphadenopathy** is usually caused by systemic viral infections. Risk factors for less common infections include sheep contact (brucellosis), geographic locale (histoplasmosis or coccidioidomycosis), and animal bites (tularemia or pasteurellosis). Syphilis and acquired immunodeficiency syndrome (AIDS) should be considered in patients with a history of multiple sexual partners or intravenous drug abuse. In 1998, there will be more than 44,000 new cases of HIV infections in the United States. Patients having acute HIV infection will present with lymphadenopathy 40–70 % of the time.

B. **Regional lymphadenopathy.** Benign reactive hyperplasia (transient lymphadenopathy from an unknown stimulus) occurs very commonly in children and young adults. Neoplasms are a more frequent cause of local lymphadenopathy in adults than in children.

IV. **Pathophysiology.** The following three mechanisms produce lymphadenopathy.

A. **Proliferation** in response to an antigenic challenge.

B. **Invasion by cells** from outside the node, such as malignant cells.

C. **Transformation of primary nodular tissue** into neoplastic cells that can enlarge the gland as the malignant cells proliferate autonomously.

V. **Symptoms.** The patient's history often provides the direction for clinical evaluation. Information regarding the patient's age, gender, occupation, exposure to pets, travel, sexual behavior, and use of drugs should be obtained.

A. **Onset.** Lymph node enlargement from acute infection becomes less likely as time progresses. As days to weeks pass, the possibility that the patient has sarcoid, a mycobacterial infection, or a neoplastic disorder becomes a greater concern.

B. **Systemic symptoms**

1. **Constitutional symptoms such as fever and weight loss** suggest cancer, systemic infection, or connective tissue disease.

2. **Recent rashes, arthralgias, pharyngeal symptoms,** or **pet exposure** may suggest specific diagnoses such as connective tissue disease, viral illness, or cat scratch disease.

VI. **Signs.** All lymph nodes should be classified by size, texture, and tenderness. Generalized lymphadenopathy is characterized by multiple firm, nontender discrete nodes, frequently accompanied by hepatosplenomegaly. Other key clinical signs may suggest certain diagnoses.

A. **Lymph node characteristics**

1. **Neoplastic:** hard, matted, fixed, nontender, and usually >3 cm.

2. **Infectious:** firm, tender, and warm.

3. **Pyogenic:** warm, red, and fluctuant.

4. **Reactive:** discrete, rubbery, freely movable, and mildly tender.

B. **Key diagnoses and associated disorders**

1. **Thyromegaly:** hyperthyroidism.

2. **Arthritis:** collagen vascular disease and leukemia.

3. **Massive splenomegaly:** cancer, infectious mononucleosis, and storage diseases.

4. **Skin rash:** viral exanthem, collagen and vascular diseases, and Kawasaki disease.

VII. Laboratory tests. If it appears that the patient has a benign cause of lymphadenopathy, either close observation or limited testing (eg, monospot or "strep screen") is indicated to confirm a specific diagnosis. In contrast, an initial assessment that suggests a malignant disorder indicates a need for extensive testing and a bone marrow examination or lymph node biopsy. If the diagnosis is uncertain, stepwise testing, starting with a complete blood cell count (CBC) and serology, is appropriate.

A. **CBC.** A markedly abnormal CBC, revealing severe anemia, thrombocytopenia, or malignant cells, implies cancer and a pressing need for a bone marrow aspiration or lymph node biopsy. A CBC provides clues to the detection of infectious mononucleosis or other viral syndromes (eg, atypical lymphocytes or lymphocytosis), pyogenic infection (eg, granulocytosis), and hypersensitivity states (eg, eosinophilia).

B. A **chest x-ray** is indicated as an initial test in severely ill patients or in the presence of supraclavicular lymphadenopathy or pulmonary symptoms. It is useful as a second-level evaluation for persistent undiagnosed lymphadenopathy. The presence of hilar adenopathy suggests sarcoidosis, lymphoma, fungal infections, tuberculosis, or metastatic carcinoma.

C. **Serologic tests** that are initially helpful are monospot or Epstein-Barr virus (EBV) antibody titers (see Chapter 61). If atypical lymphocytes are present and the EBV titers are negative, serologic testing for CMV and toxoplasmosis is indicated. In acute HIV infections, analysis of the virus's RNA should be measured (viral load) 30 days after acute infection standard serologic tests for HIV antibodies can be performed (see Chapter 70). Additional serologic tests that are helpful in the appropriate clinical setting are VDRL, HIV antibody, antinuclear antibody, and rheumatoid factor.

D. **Skin tests**

1. A positive tuberculin skin test suggests mycobacterial infection.

2. Skin tests for atypical mycobacterial infection and cat scratch disease may be helpful, although the antigens required for these tests are not commercially available and must be acquired from a local infectious disease specialist or a university center.

E. **Cultures**

1. A **strep screen** or throat culture is recommended if the cause of cervical lymphadenopathy is not clinically evident.

2. **Urethral and cervical cultures** are helpful for determining the cause of inguinal lymphadenopathy in the presence of genitourinary infections.

3. **Blood cultures** are required in cases of suspected bacteremia or rare disorders such as plague, tularemia, or brucellosis.

4. **Culturing lymph tissue** or aspirated material may be helpful. Special media for fungus or mycobacterium should be used if these organisms are suspected. Special stains can also detect the presence of cat scratch disease, mycobacterium, or fungi.

F. **Lymph node biopsy** should be considered when simple measures have failed to provide a diagnosis or if there is a clinical suspicion of a therapeutically important cause such as tuberculosis, sarcoidosis, or neoplasm. One algorithm suggests that a biopsy should be done if there is progressive lymph node enlargement over 2–3 weeks, or no diminution in lymph node size in 5–6 weeks.

1. Certain clinical features suggest the need for an early biopsy. These features include a diameter >2 cm; hard texture of the node; lack of pain or tenderness over the node; patient age >40 years; an abnormal chest x-ray (adenopathy or infiltrate); associated signs and symptoms, such as weight loss or hepatosplenomegaly, that suggest a serious disorder; an absence of upper respiratory tract symptoms; an enlargement of a supraclavicular node; or a cervical node in a smoker.

2. Small lymph nodes, an upper respiratory tract infection, positive viral serology, or a normal chest x-ray argue against the need for a biopsy.

3. During follow-up for undiagnosed lymphadenopathy, nodes that remain constant in size in 4–8 weeks or fail to resolve in 8–12 weeks should be biopsied.

   4. If a biopsy is nondiagnostic, careful observation of the patient is still important. As many as 25% of patients with persistent lymphadenopathy who undergo a second biopsy have a form of cancer.
   G. Imaging studies such as ultrasonography or computerized tomography (CT) of
   the involved area may be useful to differentiate lymphadenopathy from non-
   lymphatic enlargements. CT is also useful to evaluate lymphadenopathy or to
   demonstrate the presence of abdominal lymph nodes.
   H. A **bone marrow examination** is indicated for patients with severe anemia, neu-
   tropenia, thrombocytopenia, or a peripheral smear with malignant blast cells.
VIII. Treatment
   A. Viral infections. Treatment of viral infections is primarily limited to symptomatic
   treatment such as warm compresses, analgesics, and the avoidance of trauma
   to the swollen node (see Chapter 59).
   B. Cat scratch disease is usually self-limited, requiring only symptomatic treatment. Aspiration of suppurative glands may reduce swelling and discomfort. Incision and drainage should be avoided to prevent sinus tract formation. Although
   indications for antibiotic therapy are unclear, combination of rifampin, trimethoprim-
   sulfamethoxazole, and gentamicin can be considered for severe disease.
   C. Neoplasm. Neoplastic disease should be referred to an oncologist for treatment.
   D. Mycobacterial infection. Nodes affected with atypical mycobacteria are treated
   by surgical excision. A positive culture or the demonstration of acid-fast bacilli is
   the most direct method of diagnosis, although treatment of *Mycobacterium tuberculosis* can be initiated on the basis of the clinical presentation and a positive skin
   test. Active tuberculosis should be treated with at least three antitubercular drugs
   initially, such as isoniazid, 10 mg/kg/day to a maximum of 300 mg/day, and rifampin, 10 mg/kg/day for 6–12 months and followed up carefully.
   E. Acute lymphadenitis. Initial therapy should be directed toward staphylococcal
   and streptococcal infections. Cephalexin (25–50 mg/kg in divided doses up to
   500 mg four times a day), erythromycin (30–50 mg/kg up to 500 mg four times a
   day), or a semisynthetic penicillinase-resistant penicillin such as dicloxacillin
   (25–50 mg/kg up to 500 mg four times a day for 7–10 days) is useful.

REFERENCES

Chesney PJ: Cervical lymphadenopathy. Pediatr Rev 1994;**15:**276.
Grossman M, Shiramizu B: Evaluation of lymphadenopathy in children. Curr Opin Pediatr 1994;
   6:68.
Kahn JO, Walker BD: Acute human immunodeficiency virus type I infection. N Engl J Med 1998;
   339:33.
Lipsky MS: A systematic approach to evaluating pediatric lymphadenopathy. Fam Pract Recer-
   tification 1987;**9:**23.
Morland B: Lymphadenopathy. Arch Dis Child 1995;**73:**476.
Pangalis GA, Vassilakopoulos TP, Boussiotis VA, et al: Clinical approach to lymphadenopathy.
   Semin Oncol 1993;**20:**570.
Park YP: Evaluation of neck masses in children. Am Fam Physician 1995;**51:**1904.

---

48   Myalgia

Tomás P. Owens, Jr., MD

   I. Definition. Myalgia is defined as generalized or localized pain perceived as origi-
   nating in skeletal muscle tissue, usually characterized as a deep, aching sensation
   but sometimes as a burning or electric sensation.
   II. Common diagnoses
   A. Viral syndromes (and other infectious causes).
   B. Major or minor trauma.
   C. Fibromyalgia and myofascial pain (8–10% of all visits to a primary care out-
   patient practice).
   D. Collagen vascular diseases (about 15% in the general population and over 1 mil-
   lion newly afflicted patients each year).

    E. Vascular insufficiency (less than 1% of patients with myalgia).
    F. Primary muscle malignancy (an extremely rare cause of myalgia in primary care).
    G. Substance-induced (an emerging cause of myalgia).
III. Epidemiology. As many as one third of patients presenting in an ambulatory primary care setting complain of muscle pain in an extremity or in the back. In the general population, as much as 60% of adults have such musculoskeletal pain lasting more than 1 month or caused by identified trauma. In one study, 9% of primary care visits were for myofascial pain syndrome.

    A. Most **viral syndromes** have seasonal variations, with a peak in the winter months in temperate climates. Children are particularly at risk for viral syndromes, but myalgia in children is a less common primary complaint compared with myalgia in adults. A rare form of localized myalgia is staphylococcal myositis, which can accompany cellulitis.

    B. Trauma is ubiquitous but has a strong association with occupational hazards (faulty ergonomics, repetitive acts of a monotonous nature), recreational pursuits ("weekend warrior syndrome," with poor conditioning or inappropriate training), and substance abuse (repetitive accidental or self-inflicted trauma).

    C. Fibromyalgia (former name: fibrositis) affects 5–10% of the US population at some point in their lives. It is more common in women than in men (10:1), particularly in women between the ages of 20 and 50 years (with a peak incidence at age 35). Fibromyalgia is the second most common disorder in American rheumatology practices. It may arise spontaneously, but it is usually preceded by physical or emotional trauma or a viral illness. Fibromyalgia has been associated with a history of sexual abuse during childhood, drug use, and eating disorders, but no causal relationship has been established. Depression, personality disorders, and anxiety are strongly associated with the fibromyalgia syndrome.

    Fibromyalgia and chronic fatigue syndrome are sometimes difficult to differentiate. Less generalized **myofascial pain syndromes** (not fulfilling fibromyalgia syndrome diagnostic criteria) are seen in up to 50% of the population, are equally common in men and women, and have a much better prognosis with appropriate therapy.

    D. Collagen vascular diseases. Inflammatory articular diseases such as rheumatoid arthritis and lupus occur primarily in women between the ages of 20 and 50 years. Inflammatory nonarticular diseases such as polymyositis and dermatomyositis are more common in children and occur equally in men and women, but a particular form occurs in men over the age of 40 years in association with malignancy of other organ systems. Polymyalgia rheumatica occurs equally in men and women, usually over the age of 65 years.

    E. Vascular insufficiency, including arterial and venous insufficiency, occurs in less than 1% of patients complaining of myalgia and has a strong association with older age, smoking, hypertension, hyperlipidemia, and diabetes mellitus.

    F. Primary muscle malignancy has no specific epidemiologic associations.

    G. The **"statins"** class of lipid-lowering agents has rarely been associated with generalized myalgia. The synchronous use of gemfibrozil or cyclosporine potentiates the effect significantly, as does preexisting renal insufficiency. It is believed that lipid-soluble statins are more likely to produce the syndrome. Excipients in some batches of ʟ-**tryptophan** supplements (eg, "peak X") produce the so-called **eosinophilia-myalgia syndrome (EMS).** Other drugs that can cause myopathy or myalgia but are not discussed further here are amphotericin B, chloroquine, cimetidine, clofibrate, glucocorticoids, oral contraceptives, and zidovudine.

IV. Pathophysiology

    A. The cause of muscle pain due to **viral syndromes** is unknown, but the generalized symptoms of viral infections (ie, malaise, weakness, and any combination of the following: headache, nausea, vomiting, diarrhea, and upper respiratory symptoms), including fever, are usually present.

    B. Trauma. The accumulation of metabolic waste products causes muscle pain due to strenuous exercise in a deconditioned patient. Direct blunt trauma or minor repetitive trauma causes hemorrhage within the muscle tissue and muscle fiber or fascial tears. Trauma also causes muscle spasm or cramping.

    C. Fibromyalgia. The cause of muscle pain from fibromyalgia is unclear. Biochemical abnormalities are inconsistent and muscle biopsies are unrevealing. There is clear evidence of abnormalities of regional blood flow in the thalamus and caudate nucleus that are associated with low pain threshold levels (hyperalgesia) and allodynia. These abnormalities may be triggered by neuroimmune responses to viral and/or physical or psychological trauma.

D. Collagen vascular diseases. Muscle pain associated with articular rheumatic conditions results from a systemic inflammatory reaction leading to a localized inflammation of a joint (mediated by prostaglandins and leukotrienes) that affects adjacent muscle or tendon tissue. Pain from nonarticular conditions such as polymyositis or dermatomyositis is caused by intense localized inflammation with muscle fiber destruction.

E. The muscle pain of **vascular insufficiency** is caused by insufficient perfusion and delivery of nutrients and oxygen, and affected muscles may show spasm and edema.

F. The pain caused by **primary muscle malignancy** results from rapid growth of the tumor with local compression and alterations in muscle function.

G. Statin-induced myalgia (SIM) is caused by direct toxicity to the muscle (rhabdomyolysis). **EMS** is caused by a complex immunologic response to L-tryptophan excipients.

V. Symptoms

A. Myalgia from **viral syndromes** is relatively mild, and the time course parallels the course of the illness, with or without fever. The pain is usually generalized but many patients complain of pain in larger, proximal muscle groups and in the back (particularly the upper back, neck, and shoulders). Many experts believe that acute viral infection can precipitate progression to the more chronic form of fibromyalgia, in which case palpable pain can be localized. Patients report a deep, aching discomfort and an inability to be comfortable in any position.

B. Myalgia due to **trauma** is localized and specific to the trauma history. Patients sometimes report the relatively acute onset of localized pain without associated illness or obvious trauma, but further probing usually reveals some new activity or minor repetitive act (eg, lifting furniture, gardening, painting, or new work responsibility). The pain of major trauma (eg, a motor vehicle accident) or overuse usually starts several hours after the event and reaches a peak at 48 hours. The pain may persist for days or weeks, particularly if the offending activity is not identified and stopped. The patient may report some loss of function or pain with a specific movement or position, which sometimes reminds the patient of the precipitating event.

C. The symptoms of **myofascial pain syndrome** include localized muscle pain in such common areas as the paraspinous regions of the upper and middle back, neck, shoulders, arms, and legs. In patients with **fibromyalgia,** pain is worse after even minimal activity and may include generalized symptoms such as diffuse myalgia, fatigue, a low-grade fever, muscle tension, headache, and skin sensitivity. Sleep disturbance is a particularly prominent and nearly universal complaint.

D. The myalgia associated with a **collagen vascular disease** parallels the course of the primary disease.

1. The onset of **polymyositis** may be acute, particularly in children, and may include fever. Polymyositis may be postviral; it is especially common following enteroviral infections, particularly by coxsackie or a parasitic infection such as trichinosis. In polymyositis of any cause, the patient reports loss of muscle function either from pain or loss of functioning neuromuscular units. Primary idiopathic **dermatomyositis** can present with multiple abdominal complaints (eg, pain or dysphagia) and a classic lilac-colored (heliotrope) rash.

2. The pain and stiffness of inflammatory articular disorders such as rheumatoid arthritis or lupus are more severe in the morning upon arising.

3. Patients with **polymyalgia rheumatica** complain of stiffness, weakness, and pain, particularly in the hip and shoulder girdle, along with systemic symptoms such as malaise and fatigue.

E. Vascular insufficiency causes the most severe muscle pain of any of the causes of myalgia.

1. The pain associated with **arterial insufficiency** (intermittent claudication) occurs with exercise of a predictable type and intensity, is almost always in the lower extremity, and can be described precisely by the patient. It resolves shortly after cessation of the activity. With severe ischemia, rest pain may be

present. In **thoracic outlet syndrome** pain, weakness, paresthesias, and claudication occur in one of the upper extremities.

  2. The pain of **venous insufficiency** is more vague in onset, nature, and cessation, but is often related to a dependent position of the affected extremity (almost always the leg). Rarely, a **superior vena cava syndrome** will produce symptoms in the upper extremities.

  F. The pain of **primary muscle malignancy** is gradual in onset and vague in nature, but patients usually report associated weakness and a mass in the muscle.

  G. Generalized, slowly progressive pain and asthenia are characteristic of **SIM.** The onset of **EMS** can be abrupt or insidious. Early manifestations include low-grade fever, fatigue, cough, dyspnea, arthralgias, muscle cramping, and myalgia.

VI. **Signs**

  A. **Viral syndromes** cause diffuse muscle pain that is manifested in generalized, but usually mild, pain or muscle palpation. Neck, upper back, and trapezius muscles are particularly tender. Pyrexia is often present, and the degree of muscle pain often parallels the course of fever and the disease itself. Well-localized inflammation in relation to cellulitis is the hallmark of staphylococcal myositis.

  B. Repetitive minor **trauma** causes pain on palpation of the specific muscle, sometimes with crepitus; decreased active range of motion; and erythema. Blunt trauma may cause ecchymosis, hematoma, superficial abrasions, pain on palpation, or decreased active and passive range of motion of the involved muscle.

  C. **Myofascial pain syndrome** is characterized by trigger points (excruciatingly painful foci of muscle from which diffuse pain and spasm can emanate). The American College of Rheumatology (1990) diagnostic criteria for **fibromyalgia** require the patient to have at least 11 of 18 possible tender points on digital examination and a history of widespread pain. Patients frequently report trigger points in such locations as the trapezius, levator scapulae, lumbar paraspinous, and gluteus muscle groups.

  D. The muscle pain associated with a **collagen vascular disease** is increased with muscle palpation, but the signs of the primary rheumatic disease dominate. These include erythema and swelling of the involved joints, joint effusion, Raynaud's phenomenon, vasculitis, conjunctivitis, urethritis, and uveitis. Polymyositis and dermatomyositis cause pain on muscle palpation, but weakness on active testing is even more prominent. Polymyalgia rheumatica causes particular pain in the hip and shoulder girdle, along with systemic findings such as weight loss, and headache due to temporal arteritis (giant cell arteritis).

  E. **Vascular insufficiency** is intermittent and causes infrequent physical findings in the muscle at the time of examination. In arterial insufficiency, peripheral pulses are delayed, decreased, or absent, and extremity blood pressures are asymmetric, with a decreased leg:arm ratio. Marked hair loss, dry skin, decreased capillary refill, and pronounced pachyonychia are commonly present. In **thoracic outlet syndrome,** abducting the affected arm and externally rotating the shoulder may precipitate pain and/or cyanosis and pulselessness. Venous insufficiency signs may include increased circumference, edema, erythema, brawny hyperpigmentation, and ulceration of dependent areas, particularly the lower legs and ankles ("venous stasis"). In **superior vena cava syndrome,** these findings are accompanied by facial swelling, cyanosis, and neck vein distention.

  F. **Primary muscle tumors** appear as an enlarging, painful, localized mass in the body of the muscle.

  G. Muscle weakness and tenderness of major muscle groups is characteristic of **SIM.** **EMS** can be accompanied early by arthritis, evanescent erythematous rashes. Months later, scleroderma-like skin changes, an ascending polyneuropathy with cognitive impairment and, rarely, pulmonary hypertension can develop.

VII. **Laboratory tests** (see also Chapters 71 and 87). Laboratory evaluation is not usually indicated in cases of trauma or clear-cut fibromyalgia, but tests may be indicated in patients with rheumatoid symptoms or who have impressive systemic symptoms; whose symptoms have been present despite conservative, nonspecific therapy for several weeks; who have joint effusions; or whose disease has caused significant disability.

  A. **Complete blood cell count.** The white blood cell count may show a neutropenic or inflammatory (leukocytosis) reaction if a viral syndrome is present, although the **erythrocyte sedimentation rate (ESR)** is usually normal. A normal ESR may also indicate fibromyalgia by eliminating collagen vascular diseases, in which the ESR would be high (>50 mm/hr). With a high ESR, further testing (eg, ANA, RF, and more comprehensive rheumatologic panels) may be indicated (see Chapter 71). Parasitic infection may cause eosinophilia. Mild anemia and thrombocytosis are common in rheumatic diseases.

B. **Culture of specific infectious lesions** (eg, primary herpes simplex) should be performed only in appropriate clinical situations. Routine throat swabs and blood cultures are usually unrevealing with viral syndromes.

C. **X-rays** may be required to rule out bony pathology as a result of known or unknown trauma (particularly relating to the hip or pelvis in older persons), or they may be helpful in patients with localized muscle or tendon pain that is difficult to differentiate from bone pain (eg, lateral epicondylitis).

D. An empiric trial of a low daily dose (10–20 mg orally) of prednisone usually has a dramatic positive effect on almost all collagen vascular diseases and thus has some diagnostic value pending more definitive studies. Unfortunately, corticosteroid use can produce a sense of well-being in patients with almost any pathology. Therefore, empiric corticosteroid use must be adapted to each clinical situation.

E. **Impedance Doppler studies** are required in patients with evidence of vascular insufficiency. These may be followed or, in some instances, substituted by **arteriography** or **venography.**

F. **Muscle biopsy** should be arranged for any enlarging painful muscle mass not explainable by specific trauma. Abnormal histology on muscle biopsy is the only specific laboratory abnormality in patients with primary muscle tumors.

G. In **SIM,** marked elevations of creatine phosphokinase (CPK) are noted. In **EMS,** the eosinophil count is higher than 1000/mm^3 and biopsies show eosinophilic fasciitis.

VIII. Treatment

A. Myalgia due to **viral syndromes** is relieved by treatment with nonsteroidal anti-inflammatory drugs (NSAIDs). **Aspirin,** 650–1000 mg orally every 4 hours, is as effective as a prescription NSAID. **Ibuprofen,** 600 mg orally every 6 hours, or **naproxen,** 375–500 mg orally every 8–12 hours, is an excellent substitute for the anti-inflammatory effects of aspirin but each is less effective as an antipyretic agent. **Acetaminophen,** 650–1000 mg orally every 4 hours, can be used in addition to the NSAID and, for severe myalgia (particularly associated with severe headache), can be combined with **codeine,** 15–30 mg (eg, Tylenol No. 2 or No. 3), one to two tablets orally every 4 hours.

B. Myalgia due to **blunt trauma** or repetitive minor trauma is best treated with rest of the affected muscle, ice and cold therapy (particularly after use of the muscle injured by overactivity or inappropriate athletic training), heat therapy (particularly for generalized myalgia or for localized myalgia with muscle weakness or dysfunction), and immobilization (for localized myalgia due to trauma with significant dysfunction). Immobilization can be accomplished with either soft (eg, felt) or rigid (eg, commercial plastic or metal) splints for only a few days to prevent atrophy and weakness. A more specific diagnosis of the cause of repetitive overuse injuries (recreational or occupational) may lead to specific exercises, strengthening, or avoidance/modification of certain activities in the workplace (ergonomics evaluation) or during leisure time.

C. Myalgia due to **fibromyalgia.** Prescribed reading may give the patient hope by naming the problem and informing the patient that the problem is manageable, and it may help in controlling health care–seeking behavior for the multitude of associated symptoms. Support groups may have similar benefit.

   1. An **exercise and stretching program** should be similar to that for rehabilitation of a postmyocardial infarction patient, with specific submaximal heart rate targets (70–80% of maximum heart rate), frequency (three to five times weekly), and duration (30–40 minutes with appropriate warm-up and cooldown).

   2. **Antidepressant therapy** (eg, **imipramine** or **amitriptylline,** 75–100 mg orally 1–2 hours before bedtime; SSRIs, heterocyclics, or bupropion) is used in a moderate dosage, primarily for regulation of sleep, rather than in the full dosage used for major depressive disorder (see Chapter 96).

   3. **Trigger point injection** can be performed as often as necessary with local anesthetic, but preferably no more than four or five injections per year should be given if corticosteroids are used. The trigger point should be carefully pal-

pated to determine the point of most exquisite pain. This point is injected intramuscularly using a long 25- or 27-gauge needle that contains 0.5–1.0 mL of a long-acting local anesthetic such as bupivacaine. A corticosteroid, such as 0.5 mL of **triamcinolone**, 40 mg/mL, can be added to the injection, but no evidence exists that the injection will be more effective than any of the local anesthetics or even normal saline.

4. **Cognitive behavioral therapy** is very useful in many patients. Minimal intervention (paradoxical approach) has also been effective, particularly in the outpatient setting. Disability claims, with legal and financial repercussions and tremendous secondary gain, make the management of this syndrome complicated in a subset of patients.

5. **Alternative, integrative, complementary,** or **balanced medicine** approaches, including biofeedback, yoga, meditation, tai chi, qi gong, spray-and-stretch techniques, acupuncture, and acupressure, may be helpful, but strong research supporting their efficacy is scarce.

D. Myalgia due to **collagen vascular diseases** (see Chapter 71).

E. Myalgia due to **vascular insufficiency** (see Chapter 87).

F. Myalgia that results from **primary muscle malignancy** is relieved by excision of the malignant tumor.

G. In **SIM,** a full resolution of symptoms and normalization of laboratories can be expected within days of withdrawal from the drug. Intense hydration and loop diuretics are recommended with CPKs higher than 2000. Chronic renal insufficiency can occur secondary to the myoglobinuria. **EMS** has been successfully treated during the acute phase with prednisone, 1–2 mg/kg/day for days to weeks. In the late phase of the illness, no treatment has been helpful. Most symptoms and signs of the illness are resolved in 2–3 years, except for the cognitive impairment and the peripheral neuropathy.

REFERENCES

Alarcon GS, Bradley LA: Advances in the treatment of fibromyalgia: Current status and future directions. Am J Med Sci 1998;**315**:397.

Belillos E, Carsons S: Rheumatologic disorders in women. Med Clin North Am 1998;**82**:77.

Clauw DJ: Fibromyalgia: More than just a musculoskeletal disease. Am Fam Physician 1995;**52**:843.

Doherty M, Jones A: ABC of rheumatology: Fibromyalgia syndrome. Br Med J 1995;**310**:386.

Goldenberg DL: Fibromyalgia: Why such controversy? Ann Rheum Dis 1995;**54**:3.

Komaroff AL: A 56-year-old woman with chronic fatigue syndrome. JAMA 1997;**278**:1179.

Reiffenberger DH, Amundson LH: Fibromyalgia syndrome: A review. Am Fam Physician 1996;**53**:1698.

Wilke WS: Treatment of "resistant" fibromyalgia. Rheum Dis Clin North Am 1995;**21**:247.

Wolfe F, Smythe HA, Yunus BM, et al: The American College of Rheumatology 1990 criteria for the classification of fibromyalgia. Arthritis Rheum 1990;**33**:160.

49   Nausea & Vomiting

Jay A. Swedberg, MD

I. **Definition. Nausea** is an unpleasant sensation of impending vomiting. **Retching** is a strong, involuntary effort to vomit without bringing up emesis. **Vomiting** is the forceful expulsion of stomach contents in a series of involuntary, spastic movements.

II. **Common diagnoses**

A. **Vomiting in infants** may be associated with acute gastroenteritis or any acute illness (eg, urinary tract infections, otitis media, or asthma), feeding disorders, hypertrophic pyloric stenosis, or intussusception.

B. **Vomiting in women** is common during the first trimester of normal pregnancy. It may occur with hyperemesis gravidarum, hydatidiform molar pregnancy, and extrauterine pregnancy.

C. **Vomiting in adolescents and adults** occurs most commonly in association with the disorders below (listed in the approximate order of frequency).

1. **Acute gastroenteritis,** which is self-limited and often associated with diarrhea.
2. **Reaction to drugs, toxins, or tumor-produced peptides** (Table 49–1).
3. **Gastrointestinal tract inflammation or infection,** for example, peptic ulcer disease, hepatitis, pancreatitis, cholecystitis or cholelithiasis, appendicitis, pyelonephritis, Reye's syndrome, and postgastrectomy states (often associated with bile reflux).
4. **Motility disorders,** such as gastroparesis associated with diabetic autonomic neuropathy and postvagotomy states, as well as intestinal pseudo-obstruction (gastroduodenal motor dysfunction).
5. **Gastrointestinal obstruction,** such as gastric outlet obstruction, small bowel obstruction, incarcerated hernia (femoral or inguinal), volvulus, and achalasia.
6. **Vestibular disorders,** such as motion sickness, Meniere's disease, or labyrinthitis.
7. **Increased intracranial pressure** associated with meningitis or central nervous system space-occupying lesions (eg, tumors or subdural hematomas).
8. **Metabolic disorders,** including severe electrolyte derangements, uremia, diabetic ketoacidosis, hypercalcemia, adrenal insufficiency, and thyrotoxicosis.
9. **Psychogenic vomiting** associated with syndromes of physical or sexual abuse, posttraumatic stress, and eating disorders.

III. **Epidemiology.** Based on estimates from the National Health Interview Survey in 1994, there are 3.7 episodes of nausea or vomiting per 100 persons per year. Sporadic cases are common, but episodic occurrences suggest environmental exposure to infections (viral or bacterial) or food poisoning caused by toxic agents (eg, staphylococcal enterotoxin).

IV. **Pathophysiology.** Vomiting is a reflex under central nervous system control that occurs when pathologic processes stimulate neuroreceptors in the emetic center located in the reticular formation of the medulla oblongata. Histamine (H_1) receptors, muscarinic (M) cholinergic receptors, and serotonin ($5HT_3$) receptors have been identified at this site.

A. The **emetic center** is the final common neurologic pathway mediating the vomiting response when adequate impulses are initiated in peripheral or central sites. Stimuli may be received through the sympathetic nervous system, the cerebral cortex, the limbic system, the vestibular system, the chemoreceptor trigger zone (CTZ), and peripheral afferents via the vagus nerve.

1. **Distention** of the stomach antrum or pylorus, duodenum, colon, or biliary ducts from mechanical obstruction or motility disorders sends impulses to the emetic center via peripheral afferents.
2. **Irritation, inflammation, or ischemia** to the heart, pericardium, or gastrointestinal tract (including the liver, pancreas, and gallbladder) can stimulate the emetic center.

TABLE 49–1. MEDICATIONS ASSOCIATED WITH NAUSEA AND VOMITING

Medication	Probable Mechanism
Aspirin	DI
Nonsteroidal anti-inflammatory drugs	DI
Erythromycin	DI, CNS, CTZ
Tetracycline	CNS
Nitrofurantoin	CNS
Aminophylline/theophylline	CNS, CTZ
Opiate analgesics (codeine, morphine)	CNS, CTZ
Bromocriptine	CNS
L-Dopa	CNS
Chemotherapeutic agents (cisplatin)	CNS, CTZ
Cardiac glycosides (digoxin)	CNS, CTZ
Lithium	CNS
Quinidine	CNS
Phenytoin (anticonvulsant)	CNS

DI, Direct irritant; CNS, central nervous system; CTZ, chemoreceptor trigger zone.

      3. Vestibular dysfunction sends impulses to the emetic center by way of the vestibular connections.

  B. The **CTZ,** an area rich in $5HT_3$ and dopamine (D_2) receptors, is located in the medulla at the area postrema on the floor of the fourth ventricle. The neuroreceptors of the CTZ are sensitive to chemical changes in blood or cerebrospinal fluid. Stimulation of the CTZ is associated with metabolic derangements (eg, electrolyte disorders, diabetic ketoacidosis, and uremia), medications (eg, cardiac glycosides, chemotherapeutic agents, and opiates), and toxins (eg, staphylococcal enterotoxin). The CTZ can be inhibited by D_2 antagonists such as phenothiazines (eg, prochlorperazine or chlorpromazine) or butyrophenones (eg, haloperidol or droperidol), $5HT_3$ antagonists (eg, ondansetron or dolasetron), and prokinetic agents (eg, metoclopramide or domperidone) (Table 49–2).

  C. The **vestibular apparatus** is stimulated through H_1 and M receptors, which provide input to the emetic center. Antihistamines such as cyclizine and meclizine act as antagonists on the H_1 receptors in the emetic center and the vestibular apparatus. Cholinergic antagonists such as hyoscine and scopolamine act on the M receptors in the emetic center and the vestibular apparatus.

V. Symptoms

  A. Duration of symptoms. Nausea and vomiting of acute onset lasting less than 72 hours in a previously healthy individual are usually caused by an acute illness such as **viral gastroenteritis** or **toxin exposure.** Nausea and vomiting lasting more than 72 hours (especially if associated with weight loss and impaired nutritional status) are most often caused by gastrointestinal irritation (eg, **cancer** or **peptic ulcer disease**), a gastrointestinal motility dysfunction (eg, diabetic autoimmune neuropathy), or anticholinergic medications.

  B. Relationship to eating

    1. Repetitive vomiting during or immediately after meals suggests the following causes.

      a. In adults, **psychoneurotic vomiting** is suggested when there is no history of dysphagia and when vomiting can be suppressed long enough to get to the toilet.

      b. In infants or children, a **feeding disorder** associated with overfeeding or too rapid feeding should be considered. Feeding disorders are not associated with weight loss, abdominal distention, or bilious emesis.

    2. Vomiting occurring more than 2 hours after eating, especially if recurrent and not associated with significant abdominal pain, suggests **gastric outlet obstruction** (especially if emesis is food material eaten several hours earlier), **motility disorder** of the stomach (eg, gastroparesis associated with diabetic autonomic neuropathy and postvagotomy states), or **esophageal disorders** (eg, Zenker's diverticulum or achalasia, in which emesis is typically undigested food).

    3. Vomiting in the early morning hours before eating is characteristic of the first 14 weeks of **normal pregnancy** and is also seen with **increased intracranial pressure** (eg, meningitis or space-occupying lesions of the central nervous system).

    4. Nausea and vomiting without any clear relationship to meals can be from any cause but are most likely related to metabolic disorders, vestibular disorders, or drugs and toxins.

VI. Signs. The physical examination is unremarkable in many cases of nausea and vomiting, especially when associated with motility disorders, metabolic disorders, or drugs and toxins.

  A. Vomiting in infants

    1. If there is no fever, no weight loss, and no abdominal distention and the child does not appear ill, the cause may be a **feeding disorder.**

    2. Weight loss, dehydration, and occasionally a palpable "olive" mass in the epigastric area are consistent with **hypertrophic pyloric stenosis,** a problem that usually occurs in male infants under 7 weeks of age.

    3. Stools that are loose, heme-positive, and classically described as currant jelly may indicate **intussusception,** which occurs in infants and young children. Sometimes a sausage-shaped mass is palpable. Intussusception is usually associated with significant abdominal pain.

  B. Gastrointestinal tract obstruction

    1. Emesis with a fecal odor, high-pitched bowel sounds, and occasionally visible peristalsis is often associated with **small bowel obstruction.**

TABLE 49–2. PHARMACOLOGIC TREATMENT FOR NAUSEA AND VOMITING

Agents	Receptor Antagonist[1]	Range of Doses and Routes of Administration			Common Side Effects
		Oral	IM/IV	Rectal	
Antiemetic agents					
Phenothiazines					
Prochlorperazine (Compazine)	D_2	5–10 mg q4–6h	5–10 mg IM q4–6h	25 mg q6h	Drowsiness
Promethazine (Phenergan)		12.5–25 mg q4–6h	12.5–25 mg IM q4–6h	12.5–25 mg q6h	Dizziness, hypotension
Chlorpromazine (Thorazine)		10–50 mg q4–6h	25–50 mg IM/IV	100 mg q6–8h	Extrapyramidal reactions
Thiethylperazine (Torecan)		10 mg q4–6h	10 mg IM/IV q6h	10 mg q6h	
Perphenazine (Trilafon)		4–8 mg q6h	5 mg IM q6h	—	
Butyrophenones					
Haloperidol (Haldol)	D_2	1–3 mg q6–12h	2–3 mg IM q4–6h	—	Less hypotension than with phenothiazines; extrapyramidal reactions more common with higher doses
Antihistamines					
Trimethobenzamide HCl (Tigan)	H_1	250 mg qid	200 mg IV qid	200 mg qid	Drowsiness
Promethazine					Dizziness, hypotension
Prokinetic agents					
Metoclopramide (Reglan)	D_2	5–10 mg 30 min before meals and at bedtime	10 mg IV over 2 min q6h (with chemotherapy, 1–2 mg/kg q6h)		Sedation Marked extrapyramidal reactions, especially in elderly or with higher doses (fewer central nervous system side effects with domperidone than with metoclopramide)

Drug	Receptor	Dose	Side effects
Domperidone (Motilium)	D_2	10 mg q6–8h	Few side effects have been noted in clinical trials; there have been a few reports of abnormal movements or seizures in patients on cisapride therapy
Cisapride	D_2	10 mg q6–8h	
		30–60 mg q6h	
Serotonin (5-HT₃) receptor antagonists	$5-HT_3$		Dizziness, headache
Dolasetron (Anzemet)		100 mg PO once	100 mg IV once (1.8 mg/kg)
Ondansetron (Zofran)		8 mg PO twice	32 mg IV once
Granisetron (Kytril)		2 mg PO once	10 µg/kg IV once
Steroid (adjunct with 5-HT₃) receptor antagonist)			
Dexamethasone		4–8 mg PO with chemotherapy	10 mg IV
Methylprednisolone		4 mg tid for 3 days	
Antimotion sickness agents (use prior to development of symptoms)			
Antihistamines	H_1		Sedation, drowsiness, confusion in the elderly, dry mouth, constipation, vision, urinary retention
Dimenhydrinate (Dramamine)		50–100 mg q6–8h	50–100 mg IM q12h
Meclizine (Antivert, Bonine)		12.5–25 mg q8h	—
Cyclizine		25–50 mg q6–8h	—
			25–50 mg q6–8h
Anticholinergics	M		
Scopolamine (Transderm Scōp)[3]		150–300 µg q8h	
Hyoscine			

[1] Serotonin receptor, 5-HT₃; dopamine receptor, D_2; histamine receptor, H_1; muscarinic chlorinergic receptor. M.
[2] Stimulates acetylcholine receptors in myenteric plexus of the gut via 5HT, receptor stimulation.
[3] Transdermal patch is applied behind the ear every 72 hours (can be removed and reapplied, if necessary).

2. An inguinal hernia, occasionally with bowel sounds in the hernia sac, may indicate an **incarcerated hernia.**

3. Acute abdominal distention and periumbilical tenderness are associated with **volvulus.**

4. Nonspecific physical findings are common with gastric outlet obstruction and achalasia. In patients with **gastric outlet obstruction,** emesis usually consists of old food, and a succussion splash may be present more than 4 hours after the patient has eaten. Undigested food is often present in the emesis of patients with **achalasia.**

C. **Increased intracranial pressure**

1. Focal neurologic signs are usually present with **space-occupying central nervous system lesions.**

2. A change in mental status, fever, and stiffness of the neck occur frequently with **meningitis.**

D. For a discussion of signs associated with the following causes of nausea and vomiting, see the chapters indicated below.

1. Vestibular disorders (Chapter 20).

2. Pregnancy (Chapter 103).

3. Gastroenteritis (Chapter 19).

4. Gastritis (Chapter 22).

5. Appendicitis (Chapter 1).

6. Hepatitis (Chapter 40).

VII. **Laboratory tests.** Laboratory tests should be directed by the history and the physical examination. Many of the causes of nausea and vomiting (eg, gastrointestinal tract inflammation or infection, drugs and toxins, and metabolic disorders) have nonspecific physical findings. The differentiation of these conditions requires additional diagnostic testing.

A. **Initial evaluation** of patients with significant nausea and vomiting, especially if accompanied by abdominal pain, include the following tests.

1. **Serum electrolytes and calcium** to evaluate hydration, hypercalcemia, electrolyte derangements, and evidence of metabolic disorders.

2. **Creatinine and blood urea nitrogen** for evidence of renal failure or increased risk of medication toxicity.

3. **Complete blood cell count** for evidence of infection or blood loss (acute or chronic).

4. **Liver function tests** to evaluate the possibility of hepatitis or Reye's syndrome.

5. **Serum amylase** for evidence of acute pancreatitis. If levels are elevated, the physician should consider confirming pancreatic origin with **serum lipase.**

6. **Urinalysis** to check for evidence of urinary tract infection or suggestion of ureteral calculus or metabolic disorder.

7. **Supine and upright abdominal x-ray series** for evidence of obstruction, perforation, or ileus.

8. **Serum pregnancy test** to evaluate the possibility of ectopic or intrauterine pregnancy in women of childbearing age.

B. **Additional diagnostic testing** may be helpful in selected patients.

1. **Drug levels for digoxin, aminophylline, lithium, or anticonvulsants** in patients who are taking these medications.

2. **Radiologic studies**

a. **Chest x-ray** for evidence of pneumonia, aspiration, pneumomediastinum, or air under the diaphragm.

b. **Barium swallow, upper gastrointestinal series, or barium enema** to investigate the possibility of anatomic obstruction, ulceration, or extrinsic compression of the gastrointestinal tract.

c. **Ultrasonography of the gallbladder and biliary tracts** for evidence of cholelithiasis or extrabiliary obstruction.

d. **Intravenous urography** to identify urinary tract obstruction or **renal scanning** to evaluate renal function.

e. **Computerized tomography (CT)** to evaluate the pancreas for cancer or pseudocyst or **magnetic resonance imaging (MRI)** of the head to diagnose space-occupying lesions of the central nervous system.

C. **Endoscopy.** Sigmoidoscopy, colonoscopy, and esophagogastroduodenoscopy are useful for evaluating anatomic lesions, especially if biopsy is required. In addition, endoscopy is helpful to determine the site and to treat gastrointestinal bleeding. Endoscopy is not reliable in diagnosing physiologic motility disorders of the gastrointestinal tract.

D. Significant **gastric residual** after an overnight fast suggests outlet obstruction.

E. **Labyrinthine function testing.** A **nystagmogram, audiometric testing,** or both may be helpful in the evaluation of the vestibular system.

F. **Specialized testing** may require referral.

    1. **Formal psychiatric assessment** and psychological testing such as the Minnesota Multiphasic Personality Inventory may be helpful in patients in whom psychogenic vomiting is suspected.

    2. **Radionuclide methods** used to assess gastrointestinal motility and gastric emptying may be helpful with recalcitrant, undiagnosed patients in whom there is no evidence of disease on endoscopy and who have been unresponsive to therapeutic trials of prokinetic agents.

VIII. **Treatment.** Initial treatment for nausea and vomiting is usually symptomatic. The underlying disorder should be identified and treated if possible. If appropriate diagnostic tests have been obtained and no specific diagnosis is possible, a therapeutic trial of a prokinetic agent is justified. Symptoms are usually controlled with a combination of nonpharmacologic treatment and the use of antiemetics. If gastrointestinal obstruction is evident, nothing should be given by mouth, nasogastric suction should be considered, and surgical consultation should be obtained.

A. **Nonpharmacologic treatment** consists of clear liquids sipped slowly, foods served cool or at room temperature, bland foods (ie, avoidance of very sweet, fatty, salty, and spicy foods), and minimization of visual, auditory, and olfactory stimulation.

B. **Pharmacologic treatment** (Table 49–2)

    1. **Antiemetics.** These agents (eg, **phenothiazines, butyrophenones,** and **metoclopramide**) are D_2 antagonists and have a central antiemetic effect, probably via D_2 antagonism on the CTZ. Antiemetics are effective for vomiting secondary to drugs (eg, chemotherapy, cardiac glycosides, or opiates), as well as nausea and vomiting associated with radiation therapy, gastrointestinal causes, and postoperative effects. **Ondansetron hydrochloride** (Zofran) and **dolasetron** (Anzemet) are antiemetics used primarily for prevention of nausea and vomiting associated with chemotherapy. Ondansetron is a $5HT_3$ receptor antagonist that probably acts both peripherally on vagus nerve terminals and centrally on the CTZ. When treating nausea and vomiting associated with chemotherapy, ondansetron is often used in combination with steroids (eg, dexamethasone or methylprednisolone).

    2. **Prokinetic agents. Metoclopramide** (Reglan), **domperidone** (Motilium), and **cisapride** are helpful in treating motility disorders, such as gastroparesis associated with diabetic autonomic neuropathy and postvagotomy states (Table 49–2).

        a. **Metoclopramide,** in addition to D_2 antagonism, directly stimulates gastrointestinal smooth muscle, increasing motility through cholinergic effects, probably via the intramural cholinergic neurons. Side effects such as drowsiness, anxiety, motor restlessness, and confusion occur in approximately 20% of patients.

        b. **Domperidone** is a selective peripheral D_2 antagonist that stimulates gastrointestinal motility and is thought to block CTZ D_2 receptors. The agent has been used extensively in Europe and Canada but is currently unavailable in the United States except through investigational protocols. Domperidone causes fewer central nervous system side effects than does metoclopramide.

        c. **Cisapride** is a nondopaminergic agent that has been shown to be effective in the treatment of gastroesophageal reflux, diabetic gastroparesis, and chronic constipation. Like metoclopramide, cisapride appears to enhance the release of acetylcholine in the gut at the nerve endings in the myenteric plexus. Unlike other prokinetic drugs, cisapride has no D_2 antagonistic properties (ie, no central antiemetic effect) and therefore fewer side effects, although it is less effective in suppressing vomiting.

3. **Agents to prevent motion sickness and vertigo** (eg, **meclizine, dimen-hydrinate,** and **scopolamine**) affect the vestibular system, and probably the emetic center, through antagonism of H_1 and M (muscarinic cholinergic) receptors. These agents are most effective if administered prior to the onset of nausea and vomiting.
C. **Patient education** is aimed at increasing understanding of the disease process and factors that are likely to alleviate or worsen the condition. Support is necessary to improve coping skills, maximize function, and promote general well-being.

REFERENCES

Axelrod RS: Antiemetic therapy. Compreh Ther 1997;**23**(8):539.
Benson V, Marano MA: Current estimates from the National Health Interview Survey. National Center for Health Statistics. Vital Health Stat 1994;**10:**189.
Hawthorn J: *Understanding and Management of Nausea and Vomiting.* Blackwell; 1995.
Lichter I: Which antiemetics? J Palliat Care 1993;**9**(1):42.
Sleisenger MH (editor): *The Handbook of Nausea and Vomiting.* Caduceus; 1993.

---

50   Neck Pain

Lynn V. Mitchell, MD, MPH

I. **Definition.** Neck pain is discomfort arising from those structures beginning at the occiput and including the seven cervical vertebrae. The source of the pain may stem from any of the components, including the cervical vertebrae, ligaments, tendons, nerves, vasculature, or muscles. It may also be referred from other areas of the body, most notably the temporomandibular joint, mediastinum, and pleura.
II. **Common diagnoses.** These include cervical strain, self-limited torticollis (ie, "wryneck" or "stiff neck"), acceleration injury (ie, whiplash), myofascial pain, and osteoarthritis. Less frequent causes of pain encountered in the primary care setting include rheumatoid arthritis, neoplasms, fractures, osteomyelitis, and ankylosing spondylitis.
III. **Epidemiology.** In one study, approximately 10% of the adult population reported experiencing some symptoms of neck pain at one time. Thirty-five percent of the population was able to recall one previous episode.
   A. **Cervical strain** is usually the result of an overuse of the musculature of the posterior neck and shoulder region or is a result of an unbalanced force exerted on this area. It is one of the most frequently diagnosed causes of neck pain. This strain may result from flexion, extension, or rotation of the neck beyond the point which the tissues are able to withstand, or from a persistent activity that fatigues the tissues. This condition is commonly seen following a sudden turning of the neck (eg, looking over the shoulder to check traffic).
   B. **Self-limited torticollis,** or stiff neck, occurs predominantly after excessive exposure to the cold or activities requiring unusual or prolonged rotation or twisting of the neck musculature. This condition is the typical "crick of the neck" noted upon awakening.
   C. **Acceleration injury,** or whiplash, is a result of a sudden, abrupt movement of the head in one direction. The most common cause is a motor vehicle accident.
   D. **Myofascial pain** is pain confined to the soft tissues of the neck region. It may be associated with the diagnosis of fibromyalgia but more commonly results from tension and repetitive motion of the neck structures. Sustained muscle contraction, such as that seen in stressful situations or when maintaining an awkward position for a prolonged period, can cause irritation and pain similar to those seen in a muscle tension headache.
   E. **Osteoarthritis** is the most frequent cause of neck pain in older patients, because of the effects of aging on the structures of the neck. Degenerative changes in the cervical spine are present in 40% of the population in the fourth decade of life and 70% of the population by age 65.

IV. Pathophysiology

A. **Cervical strain** is a result of tearing of the musculature and supporting structures.

B. **Self-limited torticollis** causes neck pain resulting from acute muscle spasm. Neck muscles respond to overextension or unusual use by tightening into spasm to prevent further disruption.

C. **Acceleration injury** may range from a minor muscle strain to a more severe injury involving intratissue bleeding or possibly cervical fracture.

D. **Myofascial pain** is not readily identified with any acute trauma but usually results from maintaining the neck in a particular position, which leads to a trigger (tender) point within one particular muscle site or area. These tender muscle areas are a result of local inflammation and, when palpated, produce pain locally that radiates to surrounding structures.

E. **Osteoarthritis** is caused by loss of the normal water content of the cervical disk combined with joint space narrowing, creating pain as a result of irritation of the bone, ligament, or articular cartilage. Osteoarthritis may result in spinal cord or nerve root irritation. Progression of the process may cause osteophyte formation, disk protrusion, or subluxation of apophyseal joints.

V. Symptoms

A. **Pain, discomfort,** and **tightness** in the posterior neck are common with cervical strain, acceleration injuries, and myofascial pain. The pain of cervical strain is most commonly in the paraspinal region, although it may be generalized throughout the upper thoracic and shoulder regions. Flexion of the neck toward the involved side increases the symptoms of cervical strain, and relief from pain may be obtained if the neck is held immobile. Unilateral pain and tightening of the musculature in the neck that is relieved with immobilization occur with self-limited torticollis. Persistent neck pain is common with acceleration injuries.

B. **Referred pain** may be seen with acceleration injuries, in which pain is commonly seen in the interscapular area, shoulders, and arms, and with osteoarthritis, if nerve root involvement is a component.

C. **Tenderness,** or a trigger point, in a particular muscle group may occur with myofascial pain.

D. A **headache** may occur with cervical strain, acceleration injuries, and myofascial pain. Pain caused by cervical strain commonly radiates into the occiput region, and myofascial pain may manifest as a headache beginning in this region.

E. **Stiffness after rest** is a symptom of osteoarthritis. **Decreased range of motion** and **paresthesias** may be seen with cervical strain, acceleration injuries, and osteoarthritis. **Decreased motor strength** may also occur with osteoarthritis (see Chapter 71).

F. **Neurologic sequelae** are not common. These may occur with a severe acceleration injury that causes vertebral fracture or with osteoarthritis as it impinges on surrounding neurologic structures.

VI. Signs

A. **Palpable muscle spasms** may occur with cervical strain, acceleration injuries, myofascial pain, or self-limited torticollis. The spasms of cervical strain may be unilateral or bilateral, while those of self-limited torticollis are usually unilateral. Spasms of the sternocleidomastoid or trapezius area are most common, although any of the neck musculature may be involved. The spasms that sometimes occur with myofascial pain may be either acute or chronic.

B. **Tenderness** in an identifiable area of the posterior musculature on palpation is common with myofascial pain.

C. **Decreased range of motion** is usually noted during physical examination of patients with cervical strain and self-limited torticollis, and it may be present in patients with acceleration injuries and osteoarthritis.

D. **Paresthesias** may be seen with cervical strain and osteoarthritis and occasionally in the upper extremities with acceleration injuries.

E. **Neurologic signs** may occur with osteoarthritis, depending on the progression of the disease (see Table 50–1). The most common levels of involvement are C-5 to C-6 and C-6 to C-7; C-4 to C-5 and C-7 to T-1 are less frequently affected. Arm pain or neurologic findings are relatively uncommon with cervical strain but should be carefully searched for to rule out neurologic compromise.

TABLE 50–1. NEUROLOGIC SIGNS ASSOCIATED WITH CERVICAL OSTEOARTHRITIS

Disk Level	Nerve Involvement	Symptoms	Signs
C-4–C-5	C-5	Pain in shoulder, lateral arm	Paresthesias of shoulder, weakness of deltoid and biceps with decreased biceps reflex
C-5–C-6	C-6	Pain to shoulder, lateral arm, forearm, thumb, index finger	Paresthesias of thumb, index finger; weakness of biceps and wrist extensors with decreased biceps reflex
C-6–C-7	C-7	Pain to forearm, middle and ring fingers	Paresthesias of middle and ring fingers; weakness of triceps, finger flexors, intrinsic hand muscles; decreased triceps reflex
C-7–T-1	C-8	Pain in forearm, ring and small fingers	Paresthesias of ring and small fingers; weakness of finger flexors, intrinsic hand muscles; decreased or normal triceps reflex

VII. Laboratory tests

   A. **Radiographic evaluation** is not routinely needed for uncomplicated diagnoses, but it is useful if symptomatology continues past the time when improvement is expected or if the history suggests significant trauma, infection, tumor, or spinal instability. Additionally, x-rays should be considered in patients over the age of 50 or when pain is severe and increases in the prone position.
   1. A **standard cervical spine series** of x-rays is used to evaluate most neck pain and injuries. This series will detect subluxations, fractures, congenital anomalies, and some components of osteoarthritis.
   2. The most common finding on neck x-ray is a straightening of the normal lordotic curve, usually a sign of acute muscle spasm and pain.
   3. **Magnetic resonance imagining (MRI)** has become the "gold standard" if evaluation beyond a standard cervical spine series is deemed appropriate.
   B. **Blood studies** are usually not useful as a diagnostic tool when neck pain is involved. However, if an infectious cause is suspected, a **complete blood cell count with differential** is in order. If an autoimmune process is in the differential diagnosis, then, at a minimum, an erythrocyte sedimentation rate should be obtained.
   C. **Further diagnostic studies** are listed in Table 50–2.

VIII. Treatment of the first three diagnoses of commonly encountered neck pain (see section II) **is similar:** decreased activity (not inactivity) and pain and inflammation control (see Table 50–3).

   A. **Treatment of myofascial pain** is directed at the cause of the pain if its origin is in the area of tension. Treatment can be accomplished by ergonomic management as well as specifics to address the tender trigger points identified during the physical examination. One commonly used modality is a steroid injection into the tender muscle tissue with a small-gauge needle (or 2% **lidocaine** with 0.5 mL of **triamcinolone acetonide**).
   B. Initially, **osteoarthritis** can be managed like an acute condition, which may slow the progression of symptoms. If symptoms progress, surgical consultation should be considered, especially if neurologic compromise is present.
   C. Alternative treatments (most notably, acupuncture) are readily available for the alleviation of neck pain. The literature suggests sufficient efficacy of acupuncture to merit its consideration as a treatment alternative.

TABLE 50–2. DIAGNOSTIC STUDIES FOR NECK PAIN

Test	Objective
Electromyography	Identification of nerve root compression or myelopathy
Myelography	Identification of spinal cord or nerve root involvement
Computerized tomography	Identification of spinal stenosis and nerve root compression
Bone scan	Identification of osseous involvement
Magnetic resonance imaging	Identification of disk herniation, soft tissue and cord abnormalities

TABLE 50–3. TREATMENT OF COMMON CAUSES OF NECK PAIN

Cause	Treatment	Activity	Physical Therapy/ Manipulation	Alleviating Factors
Neck strain	NSAIDs (eg, naproxen sodium, 375–500 mg PO bid; ibuprofen, 400–600 mg PO tid–qid)	Decreased initially, 24–48 hours, then as tolerated	Helpful if symptoms persist or worsen after 48–72 hours or if initial exam more severe than usual case	Ice for 24 hours, then alternate with heat; use of cervical collar may be helpful
Torticollis	Muscle relaxants (cyclobenzaprine HCl, 10 mg PO tid; chlorzoxazone, 500 mg PO tid–qid), NSAIDs	As above	As above	As above
Acceleration injury	NSAIDs	As above	As above	As above
Myofascial pain	Steroid injection if trigger point identified; NSAIDs if headache present	Normal activities	Helpful if tension-related	Ice packs to painful area
Osteoarthritis	NSAIDs	As tolerated	Conditioning program	Re-education to result in better care of neck

NSAIDs, Nonsteroidal anti-inflammatory drugs; PO, orally.

REFERENCES

Barry M, Jenner JR: Pain in neck, shoulder, and arm. Br Med J, ABC Rheumatol 1995;**310:**183.
Cailliet R: *Neck and Arm Pain.* 3rd ed. Davis; 1990.
Goodman BW Jr: Neck pain. Primary Care 1988;**15:**689.
Rainville J, Sobel JB, Banco RJ, et al: Low back and cervical spine disorders. Orthop Clin North Am 1996;**27**(4):729.
Swezey RL: Chronic neck pain. Rheum Dis Clin North Am 1996;**22**(3):411.
Thorne RP, Curd JG: A systematic approach to disorders of the cervical spine. Hosp Pract (Off Ed) 1993;**28**(6):49.

---

51   Nosebleeds (Epistaxis)

Mitchell A. Kaminski, MD

I. **Definition.** Epistaxis is profuse bleeding from the nose which may be spontaneous or induced.
II. **Common diagnoses**
    A. **Trauma** (accidental or iatrogenic [eg, nose picking]).
    B. **Inflammation** (due to infection, allergy, drug use, environmental irritants, and dryness).
    C. **Foreign body (FB).**
    D. **Coagulopathy** (blood dyscrasias, anemias and leukemia, or drug induced).
    E. **Associated conditions and medications,** including hypertension, atherosclerotic cardiovascular disease, chronic obstructive pulmonary disease, excess ethanol intake, or warfarin (Coumadin) or aspirin use.
III. **Epidemiology.** Epistaxis is a common problem affecting 7–15% of the population. It is a frequent reason for emergency medical visits; 15 persons per 10,000 require physician care annually, and 1.6 per 100,000 require admission to a hospital. Most

cases occur in patients less than 10 years old, and the incidence decreases with age. Nosebleeds are promoted by low humidity, which is more common during the winter and in colder climates. In older patients, in whom there is a greater prevalence of associated conditions (see section II,E), epistaxis is more likely to be posterior and of greater severity.

IV. **Pathophysiology** (see Figure 51–1). Ninety percent of nosebleeds occur at the anterior nasal septum, from a fragile plexus of vessels in Kiesselbach's area. Posterior epistaxis usually arises from a branch of the sphenopalatine artery on the posterior nasal septum (bleeding is seen below and posterior to the middle turbinate).

A. **Trauma** from nose picking or external blunt force causes bleeding through disrupting vascular epithelium.

B. **Inflamed mucosa** from infection or allergy causes hyperemia and increased fragility of the fine vessels in the nose.

C. An **FB** can directly traumatize anterior vessels, especially with attempts at removal.

D. **Blood dyscrasias and clotting disorders,** especially in older patients, can promote anterior or posterior epistaxis through interference with platelet function and/or blood clotting. Normal hemostasis is impaired. Aspirin interferes with platelet function by inhibiting cyclooxygenase and thromboxane A_2 activity, while warfarin (Coumadin) inhibits the synthesis of vitamin K–dependent coagulation factors II, VII, IX, and X.

E. **Miscellaneous.** Hypertension and atherosclerotic cardiovascular disease are associated with more severe posterior bleeds in elderly patients. Sclerotic arterioles in these patients are more prone to rupture and more resistant to normal hemostatic mechanisms. Excess alcohol intake and other conditions that lead to chronic liver disease (see Chapter 75) interfere with hepatic production of the vitamin K–dependent clotting factors important to normal coagulation.

V. **Symptoms**

A. Determining the severity, amount, and duration of bleeding is critical but often difficult. Historical features can suggest whether bleeding is anterior or posterior (see Table 51–1). The amount of blood that is swallowed can be underestimated, while blood lost from anterior epistaxis can be overestimated.

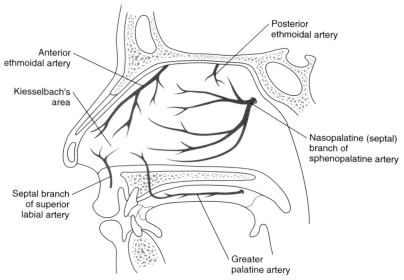

FIGURE 51–1. Blood supply to the nasal septum. (From Pfaff JA, Moore GP: Ear, nose, and throat emergencies. In Rosen P [editor]: *Emergency Medicine—Concepts and Clinical Practice.* 4th ed. Mosby; 1998:2726.)

TABLE 51–1. CLUES TO ANTERIOR VERSUS POSTERIOR EPISTAXIS

	Anterior	Posterior
Spontaneous	+	+++
Induced	+++	+
Initial blood swallowed	+	+++
Initial blood through nares	+++	+
Bilateral bleeding	+	+++

+, Less frequent; +++, more frequent.

    B. History of allergy or infection (Chapter 59) should be sought as contributing factors to epistaxis. The recent use of topical nasal drugs (eg, topical vasoconstrictors, steroids or cocaine) should be determined, as well as exposure to environmental irritants.

    C. FBs should be considered, especially in toddlers.

    D. Easy bruising, bleeding at other sites, or constitutional symptoms such as weight loss and fatigue can signify blood dyscrasias and clotting disorders.

    E. A history of hypertension or atherosclerotic cardiovascular disease (Chapter 87) can suggest causes of epistaxis.

VI. Signs. The patient's blood pressure, pulse, and level of consciousness should be determined. Detailed intranasal examination depends on control of the bleeding (see section VIII). Additional findings may also affect testing and management. These include the following.

    A. Signs of external trauma to the nose and face should be noted. Blood under the fingernails suggests nose picking.

    B. Mucosal edema and hyperemia from chronic allergies or irritation or purulent drainage from infection.

    C. Loss of patency of a nostril is noted with an FB. The FB is usually readily evident on speculum nasal examination.

    D. Multiple or large bruises on other parts of the body, bleeding at other mucosal sites, or prolonged bleeding from venipuncture or intravenous catheter sites could signify coagulopathy.

    E. Besides elevated blood pressure, signs of cardiovascular disease (Chapter 87) should be noted. Jaundice, telangiectasias, hepatomegaly, and/or liver tenderness would all support liver disease and an underlying cause of epistaxis.

VII. Diagnostic tests. Examination and treatment to stop bleeding (see section VIII) should precede consideration of further testing.

    A. Laboratory testing

        1. In a stabilized patient in whom there is concern about significant blood loss, a hemoglobin and/or hematocrit can be ordered, along with a clot tube for a type and hold in case transfusion of blood may be necessary. Acute blood loss may not be reflected in the hematocrit for several hours.

        2. If there is concern about a possible blood dyscrasia or clotting disorder, a complete blood cell count, platelet count, prothrombin time, and partial thromboplastin time should be ordered.

        3. History or signs suggesting liver disease should prompt further laboratory testing (Chapter 75).

    B. Radiologic testing

        1. If facial bone fracture is a concern, the Waters' projection is the single best view for evaluation of the maxilla, maxillary sinuses, floors and inferior rims of orbits, and zygomatic bones. This view is usually combined with a posteroanterior and lateral view of the facial bones. One can get specific views of the nasal bones if nasal fracture is suspected. If posterior packing will be necessary, x-rays should be obtained before the packing procedure.

        2. Other studies, such as computerized axial tomography (CAT) scan or arteriogram, may be required in more cases in which consultation with an otolaryngologic surgeon is required (see section VIII,F).

VIII. Treatment. An algorithm summarizing treatment is presented in Figure 51–7 and is keyed by letter to this text.

A. The patient who is hemodynamically unstable (pulse, >120 beats/min; systolic blood pressure, <90 mm Hg) should be in a recumbent position, and a large-bore intravenous line should be placed for rapid administration of intravenous fluids (0.9% NaCl or Ringer's lactate solution). Unstable vital signs, significant anemia (see Table 6–1 in Chapter 6), or continued bleeding despite procedures discussed below are indications for hospitalization.

B. If there is a history of trauma, or deformity on examination, consider radiologic studies (see section VII,A,4). Consider consultation with an otolaryngologist if facial fracture is disclosed. Nasal fracture with cosmetic deformity will require manipulation, but not acutely unless it is severe.

C. Adequate examination of the nasal mucosa requires the patient to be seated in the "sniffing" position (Figure 51–2), shadow-free lighting, and proper medical equipment (Table 51–2). Clots obstructing examination of the mucosa can be removed with suction with a No. 8 or 10 French Frazier suction tip catheter or by having the patient blow his or her nose. If bleeding is profuse, several minutes' application on a moistened cotton pledget of a topical vasoconstrictor with anesthetic such as cocaine topical solution or 1:1 mixture of oxymetazoline and 4% Xylocaine will allow better visualization. Brisk bleeding from behind the middle turbinate (Figure 51–3) suggests a posterior bleed.

D. Direct pressure on the nostrils to compress the nasal septum blood vessels will stop many nosebleeds. The patient should sit upright, and spit out rather than swallow blood. Pressure should be applied for 5–10 minutes. Ice packs may be applied to the nasal bridge and beneath the upper lip, although benefit of cold application is less clearly documented.

E. After bleeding has stopped, the nose should be reexamined. If the source of **anterior bleeding** is visible, chemical cautery can be applied with a silver nitrate applicator stick, especially if epistaxis is recurrent. Application requires topical anesthesia (Table 51–2). The stick should be held with a rolling motion against the bleeding site for less than 5 seconds. The area cauterized, which turns a dark color, should be kept confined to the nasal mucosa. Electrocautery, which requires special equipment and deeper local anesthesia, is rarely needed for anterior epistaxis.

F. If cautery fails or continued bleeding makes it impractical, anterior packing should be applied. Application of a topical anesthetic, if time permits, makes the packing procedure less uncomfortable. A strip of petrolatum gauze is inserted in layers from the floor of the nose up (Figure 51–4). Alternatively, a prefabricated pack that swells with hydration (eg, Merocel Pope Epistaxis Packing) is quicker and easier to use (Figure 51–5). The packing is left in place for 2–4 days, and antibiotics are prescribed (eg, cephalexin, 250–500 mg orally three or four times a

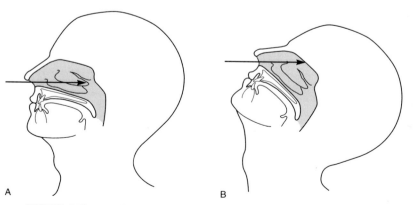

A   B

FIGURE 51–2. The correct **(A)** and incorrect **(B)** positions for examining the nose. In **A**, the head is in the sniffing position, facing forward, allowing better visualization of the structures in the nose.

TABLE 51–2. OFFICE MATERIALS FOR THE EXAMINATION AND MANAGEMENT OF EPISTAXIS

Examination chair with posterior head and neck support for patient
Headlamp or head mirror for examiner
Suction apparatus (No. 8 or 10 French Frazier suction tip catheter)
Gloves, mask, eye shield, and gown for examiner
Nasal speculum (adult or child size)
Tongue depressors
Bayonet forceps
Gauze, cotton pledgets
Silver nitrate ($AgNO_3$) applicator sticks
Cocaine 4% (40 mg/mL) topical solution (total dosage, 2–3 mg/kg in adults), or 1 : 1 mixture of oxymetazoline
    (Afrin) 0.05% or phenylephrine (Neo-Synephrine) 0.5–1.0% and 4% lidocaine
Vaseline petrolatum gauze packing strip ($\frac{1}{2} \times 72$ in. or 1×36 in.)
Antibiotic ointment (eg, Bacitracin)
Merocel Pope Epistaxis Packing (or similar), 10 cm
Nasostat or Epistat II catheter (Xomed-Treace, Jacksonville, Florida) or No. 14 French Foley catheter with
    30-mL balloon
Meperidine hydrochloride (Demerol HCl), 50–100 mg (adult) or 0.25–0.4 mg/kg (child), for intramuscular injection
Intravenous diazepam (Valium), 2–5 mg (adult) for intramuscular or intravenous injection

day) to prevent sinus infection from potentially blocked drainage. The patient
should return to have the packing removed. Packing will be uncomfortable; pain
medicine such as acetaminophen with codeine (Tylenol No. 3), one or two tablets
orally every 4–6 hours as needed, and an anxiolytic agent such as diazepam
(Valium), 5–10 mg orally every 6 hours as needed, should be considered.

G. **Posterior bleeding** should be suspected if examination shows bleeding from
behind the middle turbinate, or if bleeding continues down the posterior pharynx
despite topical vasoconstriction and anterior packing. Urgent otolaryngologic consultation should be considered. Posterior packing or nasal balloon tamponade
should be performed.

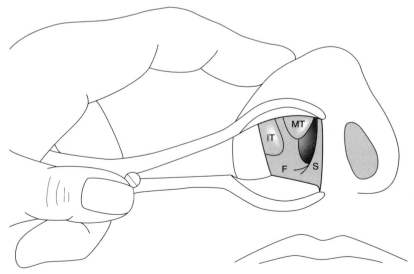

FIGURE 51–3. Structures seen on nasal speculum examination of the right nostril. F, Floor of the nose;
IT, inferior turbinate; MT, middle turbinate; S, septum.

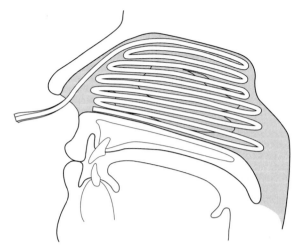

FIGURE 51–4. Anterior packing with a gauze strip. (From Smith JA: Nasal emergencies and sinusitis. In Tintinalli JA [editor]: *Emergency Medicine—A Comprehensive Study Guide.* 4th ed. McGraw-Hill; 1996:1085.)

1. Posterior nasal gauze packing has been the traditional treatment for posterior epistaxis. Because posterior packing is more complicated and uncomfortable than balloon devices, it is now less frequently used.
2. Balloon nasal tamponade can be achieved with a Foley catheter or specialized devices such as the Epistat II catheter. Analgesia with intramuscular meperidine (Demerol), 50–100 mg, or intravenous diazepam (Valium), 5–10 mg, helps the patient tolerate the procedure. Packing and tamponade with the Merocel sponge and the Epistat II catheter are illustrated in Figure 51–6. Posterior packing or tamponade can induce hypoxemia and stimulate the vagus nerve, causing bradycardia and dysrhythmia. Patients with posterior packing or tamponade should be hospitalized for cardiac monitoring and measurement of oxygen saturation.

Merocel nasal pack

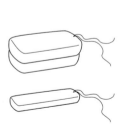 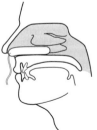 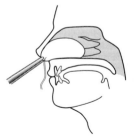

(1) The sponge is compressed and expanded.

(2) The sponge in place, before expansion.

(3) The expanded sponge being removed.

FIGURE 51–5. Merocel nasal pack. (1) The sponge is compressed and expanded. (2) The sponge in place, before expansion. (3) The expanded sponge being removed.

1. Lubrication

Clean blood clots from the nose. Use a topical anesthesia to numb the nose. Liberally apply antibiotic ointment or lubricant to the EPISTAT II Nasal Catheter.

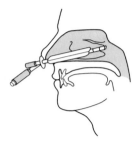

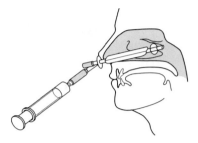

2. Position

Position the EPISTAT II Catheter so the posterior balloon rests in the nasopharynx.

3. Inflation

Using a syringe, inflate the balloon by injecting approximately 10 mL sterile saline into the valve.
After inflation of the balloon, gently pull the catheter outward to position it in the nasopharynx.

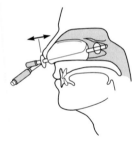

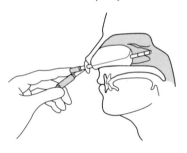

4. Expansion/Adjustment

Hydrate the MEROCEL sponge with sterile saline until fully expanded. Advance the retaining ring until it gently rests against the nose. The 4" x 4" gauze pad can be placed between the nose and retaining ring for added comfort.
Check the catheter periodically. Release or add pressure as needed.

5. Removal

Introduce a syringe firmly into the valve and withdraw the solution. Rehydrate the MEROCEL sponge with sterile saline until saturated (approximately 10 mL). Physicians recommend allowing the pack to rehydrate for 5–10 minutes before removal. Slowly withdraw the catheter from the nose. The sponge can be left in place by removing only the catheter.

FIGURE 51–6. Epistat II nasal catheter instructions. Begin by cleaning blood clots from the nose. Use a topical anesthetic to numb the nose. Liberally apply antibiotic ointment or lubricant to the Epistat II nasal catheter, then proceed with the steps shown. The catheter is usually left in place for up to 3 days and can be used in outpatients. A hollow inner airway tube allows the patient to breathe.

3. The posterior packing and tamponade will require antibiotics, analgesics, and possibly anxiolytic agents (see section VIII,F). Packing and tamponade are left in place for 2–4 days.
4. Posterior bleeding not controlled with packing and tamponade may require more advanced procedures by the specialist, including endoscopic cauterization, arterial ligation, or angiographic embolization.

Initial Evaluation

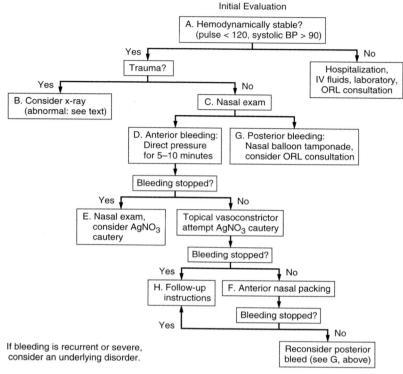

FIGURE 51–7. Algorithm depicting the management of epistaxis. BP, Blood pressure; ORL, otorhino-laryngology.

H. Follow-up instructions

1. The patient sent home with anterior packing or posterior packing and tamponade should return for follow-up within 2–3 days. Antibiotics should be taken as prescribed.
2. The patient who does not require packing should be encouraged to use the preventive measures that follow. Pressure should be applied for recurrent bleeding, and the patient should return if bleeding does not stop within 15–30 minutes.
3. Lubrication with petroleum jelly on cotton swabs twice a day prevents dryness.
4. Bedside humidification also prevents dryness.
5. Nose picking should be discouraged and the fingernails trimmed to minimize mucosal trauma.
6. Forceful nose blowing should be avoided.

REFERENCES

Alvi A, Joyner-Triplett N: Acute epistaxis. Postgrad Med 1996;**99**:83.

Josephson GD, Godley FA, Stierna P: Practical management of epistaxis. Med Clin North Am 1991;**75**:1311.

Pfaff JA, Moore GP: Ear, nose, and throat emergencies. In Rosen P (editor): *Emergency Medicine—Concepts and Clinical Practice.* 4th ed. Mosby; 1998:2725.

Roberts JD, Hedges JR (editors): *Clinical Procedures in Emergency Medicine.* 3rd ed. Saunders; 1998:1135.

Wurman LH, Stack JG, Flannery JV, et al: The management of epistaxis. Am J Otolaryngol 1992; **13**:193.

52   Palpitations

Alison E. Dobbie, MB, ChB MRCGP, & Mark P. Knudson, MD, MSPH

I. **Definition.** Palpitations are sensations perceived by the patient to be an abnormal action of the heart. They may represent a change in action of the heart (eg, forceful, rapid, or slow beats). In some cases, they are noncardiac events mistaken for abnormal cardiac activity.

II. **Common diagnoses**
   A. **Arrhythmias** (Table 52–1) are the most common and dangerous cause of palpitations. Sinus tachycardia and ventricular premature contractions (VPCs) are the most frequent arrhythmic causes of palpitations.
   B. **Nonarrhythmic cardiac abnormalities** causing palpitations (Table 52–2) include congestive heart failure and, less commonly, valvular heart disease.
   C. **Noncardiac abnormalities** (Table 52–2) often create a secondary cardiac effect perceived as palpitations. The most frequent causes include systemic illness, medications, and psychological conditions.

III. **Epidemiology.** Palpitations occur commonly and may be perceived by healthy individuals as normal or not worrisome. A smaller subgroup of patients with palpitations seek medical attention. No accurate estimate exists of how often patients present with palpitations in the ambulatory setting, since most patients are given another diagnosis. While gender and race are not independent risk factors, several populations are at greater risk for occurrence of worrisome palpitations.
   A. **Cardiac disease** (eg, ischemic disease, cardiomyopathies, or valvular disease) frequently precipitates arrhythmias perceived as palpitations. Patients with ischemia are at greater risk of sudden death from the arrhythmias.
   B. **Psychiatric disease** (eg, anxiety, panic disorder, or somatization disorder) is associated with increased incidence of both cardiac and noncardiac palpitations. Although patients with such diseases are not at increased risk of sudden death, they are frequently treated with antiarrhythmic drugs, which may paradoxically increase morbidity.
   C. **Elderly patients** have more arrhythmias and a greater risk of sudden death.
   D. **Other illnesses** (eg, diabetes, thyroid disease, fever, or anemia) may be associated with palpitations, and the majority of patients hospitalized for such illnesses admit to palpitations upon review of the systems.

IV. **Pathophysiology.** With the exception of noncardiac activity (eg, chest wall spasm or intestinal gas) perceived as palpitations, most palpitations are caused by a change in the cardiac rate, rhythm, or force of contraction.
   A. **Arrhythmias** can alter any of the three components: rate, rhythm, or force. The rapid rate resulting from sinus tachycardia may be perceptible. VPCs cause a pause in rate that may be detected, and the forceful contraction following a compensatory pause may be perceived as palpitations.
   B. **Nonarrhythmic cardiac abnormalities** may alter the force of contraction or may have a secondary effect on the heart rate.

TABLE 52–1. COMMON ARRHYTHMIC CAUSES OF PALPITATIONS

Sinus tachycardia
Ventricular premature contractions
Atrial premature contractions
Re-entrant atrial tachycardias
Atrial fibrillation or flutter
Sinus bradycardia
Sick sinus syndrome
Atrioventricular nodal block
Conduction defects
Ventricular tachycardia
Ventricular fibrillation

TABLE 52–2. NONARRHYTHMIC CAUSES OF PALPITATIONS

Noncardiac Origin	Cardiac Origin
Anxiety	Ventricular failure
Fever	Valvular heart disease (eg, aortic stenosis or mitral
Anemia	regurgitation)
Pregnancy (high-output states)	Cardiomyopathy
Hypoglycemia	Pericarditis
Thyrotoxicosis	Cardiac pacemaker
Pheochromocytoma	Mitral valve prolapse
Restrictive diet (ketogenic diet)	
Aortic aneurysm	
Arteriovenous fistula	
Diaphragmatic flutter	
Muscle twitch	
Intestinal flatus	
Drugs (eg, nicotine, ethanol, theophylline, digoxin, nitrates, l-thyroxine, insulin, caffeine, calcium channel blockers, decongestants, ganglionic blockers, epinephrine, dopamine, and isoproterenol)	

1. **Congestive heart failure** may cause a rapid heart rate that is perceived as palpitations.
2. **Valvular heart disease** can result in palpitations by changing the rate or force of cardiac motion.
- C. **Noncardiac abnormalities** may have a secondary effect on the heart rate or force of contraction.
   1. **Systemic illness** such as anemia or hyperthyroidism can increase both the rate and force of cardiac contraction.
   2. **Drugs** can cause palpitations by changing the rate (**beta blockers**) or the force (**digoxin**) of contraction.
   3. **Psychological conditions** (eg, anxiety or panic disorder) may cause patients to experience palpitations because of the increased awareness of normal cardiac activity, the perception of noncardiac sensations as palpitations, and the release of excess catecholamines that increase the rate and force of contraction.
- V. **Symptoms.** An adequate patient history is the key step in the evaluation of palpitations.
   - A. **Presenting complaints.** Patients may describe palpitations as "my heart is racing," "pounding in my chest," or "skipped beats." Less frequently, patients use potentially misleading terms such as "pain in my chest," "feeling short-winded," or "tightness in my chest." Some patients may complain of palpitations when their problem is really shortness of breath or chest pain.
   - B. **Description of rhythm** by the patient, or tapping out the cadence of the rhythm, may be helpful in as many as 30% of patients. Although most patients cannot distinguish between serious and benign rhythms, a patient who describes an erratic rapid rate may have atrial fibrillation.
   - C. **Precipitating factors** that may cause VPCs or sinus tachycardia should be elicited. These factors include exercise, anxiety, stress, fever, menses, occupational chemical exposure, use of tobacco or alcohol, and consumption of caffeine or chocolate. A thorough history of drug use (nonprescription, prescription, and illicit drugs) should be elicited.
   - D. **Terminating events,** such as carotid massage or Valsalva's maneuver, may suggest tachyarrhythmias such as supraventricular tachycardia.
   - E. **Associated symptoms**
      1. **Chest pain, syncope or presyncope,** and **diaphoresis** are often indicative of serious underlying causes and mandate a more thorough evaluation when present. Chest pain with palpitations may represent ischemia and should prompt more aggressive diagnosis and therapy. Most patients with syncope and dizziness in addition to palpitations have arrhythmias.

      2. Other associated symptoms, such as hot flashes or paresthesias, may suggest nonarrhythmic causes of palpitations such as menopause or panic disorder.

VI. Signs

    A. An **irregular rhythm** detected by the physician's palpation of the patient's pulse for a full 60 seconds during the examination is predictive of significant arrhythmias on Holter monitoring >90% of the time. Rarely, a physician may palpate an extra systole and correlate this with symptoms of palpitations.

    B. A **midsystolic click,** or **click-and-murmur,** may indicate valvular heart disease such as mitral valve prolapse. Murmurs may suggest other valvular abnormalities as well.

    C. Noncardiac findings, such as an enlarged thyroid, fever, or orthostatic hypotension, should raise suspicion of thyrotoxicosis, infection, or anemia, respectively. The patient's history should be a guide to the physician in the search for noncardiac causes of palpitations.

VII. Laboratory tests and investigations

    A. Particular blood analyses can occasionally be useful in the diagnosis of a patient's condition.

       1. Electrolyte abnormalities can induce or exacerbate some arrhythmias and should be suspected in patients using diuretics or in those with renal or gastrointestinal disease.

       2. Hemoglobin should be evaluated in the patient with tachycardia.

       3. Renal disease should be evaluated if present (eg, by blood urea nitrogen or creatinine), as worsening renal failure may cause arrhythmias.

       4. Drug levels to detect toxic levels of digoxin, theophylline, and other medications may be helpful.

       5. Thyroid studies (eg, thyroid-stimulating hormone levels) are valuable only if the patient's history or physical examination suggests thyroid abnormalities.

       6. A **toxicology screen** may be helpful if illicit drug use is suspected.

    B. Electrocardiographic (ECG) evaluation, when indicated by a patient history of arrhythmia, ischemia, other cardiac disease, or advanced age, is the mainstay of the laboratory workup of palpitations. The ECG is often normal, however, in patients with cardiac disease. Helpful findings are listed below.

       1. Ischemic changes and old myocardial infarctions may be suspected when ST-segment abnormalities or T-wave inversion is present.

       2. Cardiomegaly should be suspected when left-axis deviation is present or when the Q wave in V_1 or the R wave in V_5 is prominent.

       3. Conduction abnormalities such as atrioventricular nodal block, ventricular conduction defects, or pre-excitation syndromes such as Wolff-Parkinson-White (shortened PR interval or delta waves) may exist.

       4. Arrhythmias such as ventricular ectopy or atrial fibrillation may be detected.

    C. Twenty-four–hour Holter monitoring, which increases the chance that an arrhythmia will be detected, may be the most useful ECG test available.

       1. Indications for Holter monitoring include suspected significant arrhythmia (ie, associated chest pain, diaphoresis, or syncope) and presence of ischemia, cardiomyopathy, or valvular heart disease. In addition, Holter monitors should be used to correlate symptoms and ECG findings.

       2. Limitations of Holter monitoring

          a. Many symptoms perceived during monitoring do not correlate with arrhythmias.

          b. The false-positive rate is high. As many as 77% of individuals in an asymptomatic population may have frequent or complex arrhythmias during 24-hour monitoring.

          c. Not all arrhythmias occur during a single 24-hour period.

       3. Monitoring options for the patient with infrequent but significant symptoms (eg, syncope) include transtelephonic monitors, 48- to 72-hour monitors, and event recorders.

          Exercise ECG may disclose arrhythmias in 15% of patients with normal 24-hour Holter monitor examinations and is warranted for patients with symptoms of ischemia, risk factors for coronary artery disease, or exercise-induced palpitations.

   D. Programmed electrical stimulation may demonstrate the presence of inducible life-threatening sustained ventricular arrhythmias, especially in patients with coronary artery disease.

   E. Echocardiography may be useful for the evaluation of cardiac valves or chamber size. More recent use of "stress echo" to evaluate wall motion may help to detect palpitations associated with ischemia.

   F. Cardiac catheterization may be necessary to determine the presence of coronary artery disease and the need for treatment.

VIII. Treatment. Because palpitations have myriad causes, both cardiac and noncardiac, no treatment is warranted until a diagnosis is made.

   A. Treatment of palpitations with nonarrhythmic causes (Table 52–2)

   1. **General treatment** should include counseling and education. This approach will benefit many patients by treating any underlying psychiatric cause of the palpitations and by decreasing any associated anxiety. Reassurance is most effective after an appropriate evaluation has ruled out serious causes of palpitations.

   2. **Treatment of systemic illness** (eg, infection, thyroid disease, or anemia) will often resolve palpitations.

   3. **Removal of precipitating causes** such as medications or caffeine will often be sufficient to treat palpitations.

   4. **Empiric treatment** with antiarrhythmic drugs should be avoided. Beta blockers are of little use to patients who need counseling and may be dangerous in patients with palpitations from congestive heart failure or valvular heart disease. Other antiarrhythmic agents are contraindicated until an arrhythmia is diagnosed. All antiarrhythmics have arrhythmogenic activity, and their use in a low-risk population may increase morbidity and mortality.

   B. Treatment of palpitations with arrhythmic causes (Table 52–1). Patients whose palpitations have benign arrhythmic causes, such as sinus tachycardia, should be reassured, and precipitating factors should be treated. Most patients with palpitations that are not associated with severe symptoms (eg, syncope or chest pain) are not at risk for cardiac morbidity or mortality. Antiarrhythmic therapy may be instituted when necessary to control a significant arrhythmia (Table 52–3); this therapy has a secondary benefit of symptom relief.

   1. **Benign atrial arrhythmias** such as atrial premature contractions or supraventricular tachycardia (SVT) with minimal symptoms should not be treated.

   2. **Atrioventricular nodal re-entrant tachycardias** and **symptomatic SVT** may be treated with vagal maneuvers (eg, gagging, carotid body massage, or submersion of the face in cold water), adenosine, verapamil, or beta blockers. Cardioversion is effective when the patient is hemodynamically unstable, and radiofrequency catheter ablation may offer a definitive cure.

   3. **Atrial fibrillation.** The goals of treating atrial fibrillation are to prevent stroke, control the ventricular rate, and/or restore sinus rhythm. Risk factors for stroke are previous cerebrovascular accident (CVA), coronary artery disease, hypertension, congestive heart failure, and valvular disease or valve replacement. Current recommendations for anticoagulation for CVA prevention are warfarin for all patients with risk factors as above, regardless of age; aspirin or no treatment for patients <65 years of age with no risk factors; and warfarin or aspirin for patients aged 65–75 without risk factors. For each individual patient, the risk-benefit ratio of treatment should be assessed. For control of ventricular rate, verapamil, diltiazem, or metoprolol may be used. Digoxin is beneficial in patients with reduced systolic function and established atrial fibrillation.

   4. **VPCs and unsustained ventricular tachycardia** (lasting <30 seconds) are an independent risk factor for sudden death in patients with cardiovascular disease, with a 2- to 3-fold risk during the first 6–12 months post–myocardial infarction. Unfortunately, there is no evidence that antiarrhythmic drug treatment reduces risk. The underlying cardiovascular disease should be addressed and high-risk patients may be treated with sotalol, amiodarone, or an implantable cardioverter/defibrillator (ICD) (Figure 52–1). Recent studies suggest that patients without cardiac disease have no increased risk for sudden death.

   5. **Patients with sustained ventricular tachycardia** (>30 seconds) occurring >48 hours post–myocardial infarction or with a history of ventricular fibrillation

TABLE 52–3. COMMONLY USED ANTIARRHYTHMIC AGENTS

Drug	Purpose	Initial Dose	Comments
Digoxin	SVT, A-fib with ventricular dysfunction	0.25–0.375 mg/day or 1.0-mg load over 24 hours	Can increase conduction of accessory path, so avoid in Wolff-Parkinson-White syndrome
Verapamil	SVT, A-fib	5–10 mg slow IV bolus, 80 mg PO tid or qid	Negative inotrope and chronotrope
Propranolol	SVT, A-fib, VPCs from catecholamines	20–80 mg PO q6h, 1–3 mg in NaCl IV slowly	Negative inotrope and chronotrope
Metoprolol	SVT, A-fib	50–200 mg PO bid	Negative inotrope and chronotrope
Diltiazem	A-fib	120–480 mg PO daily	Negative chronotrope
Quinidine	VPCs, V-tach	324 mg PO tid or qid	Decreases digoxin clearance, common gastrointestinal side effects (nausea, diarrhea), hypotension, heart block; QT-interval prolongation; torsades de pointes
Adenosine	Convert PSVT	6 mg rapid IV bolus; may repeat at 12 mg	Avoid in secondary or tertiary AV block or in sick sinus syndrome
Disopyramide	VPCs, V-tach, A-fib	100 mg PO qid	Anticholinergic, AV block, negative inotrope, digoxin clearance reduced; QT-interval prolongation
Amiodarone HCl	A-fib (with CHF), VPCs, V-tach	800–1600 mg/day PO	Initiate in hospital with cardiac monitoring
Sotalol	A-fib (with CAD but without ventricular dysfunction), VPCs, V-tach	80 mg PO bid	Initiate in hospital with cardiac monitoring

A-fib, Atrial fibrillation; AV, atrioventricular node; CAD, coronary artery disease; CHF, congestive heart failure; PSVT, premature supraventricular tachycardia; SVT, supraventricular tachycardia; VPC, ventricular premature contraction; V-tach, ventricular tachycardia.

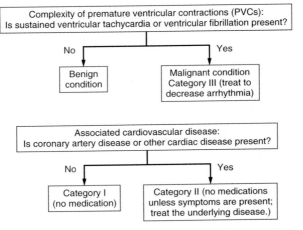

FIGURE 52–1. Classification of palpitations from ventricular premature contractions.

should receive long-term antiarrhythmic drugs (eg, metoprolol or amiodarone) or an ICD to control arrhythmias and to reduce the chance of sudden death. Antiarrhythmic drugs or an antitachycardia pacemaker may be used in conjunction with an ICD to reduce the number of painful shocks administered.

IX. **Follow-up.** The vast majority of patients with palpitations will not suffer mortality from their palpitations. The greatest morbidity is related to the worry and anxiety that come from having palpitations, and this can be effectively decreased through the use of counseling and education.

REFERENCES

Bocker D, et al: Antiarrhythmic therapy—Future trends and forecast for the 21st century. Am J Cardiol 1997;**80**(8A):99G.

Landers MD, Reiter MJ: General principles of antiarrhythmic therapy for ventricular tachyarrhythmias. Am J Cardiol 1997;**80**(8A):31G.

Masoudu FA, Goldschlager N: The medical management of atrial fibrillation. Cardiol Clin 1997; **4**:689.

Shah CP, et al: Clinical approach to wide QRS complex tachycardias. Emerg Med Clin North Am 1998;**16**(2):331.

53　　Paresthesias

Marvin A. Dewar, MD, JD

I. **Definition.** Paresthesias are burning or tingling sensations, cramplike feelings, pain without a known stimulus, or actual numbness.

II. **Common diagnoses**

A. **Myelopathy** appears with spasticity, hyperreflexia, a positive Babinski's sign, and a sensory level.

B. **Polyneuropathy** is characterized by hyporeflexia or areflexia, with varying degrees of sensory defects. The sensory or motor defects are greater distally than proximally.

C. **Nerve entrapment syndromes** result from compression anywhere along the root with paresthesias or weakness in the field served by the involved nerve.

D. **Mononeuritis multiplex.** Simultaneous or successive dysfunction of several peripheral nerves remote from each other is necessary to make the diagnosis of mononeuritis multiplex.

III. **Epidemiology.** Temporary paresthesias are experienced by virtually everyone in his or her lifetime. Persistent paresthesias are common, as they are associated with a large number of common illnesses. For example, 8% of patients with diabetes mellitus have neuropathy at the onset of this disease, and as many as 50% develop neuropathy within 25 years.

A. **Myelopathy** secondary to cord trauma from an automobile or diving accident is the most common type seen in practice. Fracture of the vertebrae is a more common cause of myelopathy than tumor, but occurs less often than cervical spondylosis. Other causes of myelopathy include multiple sclerosis and radiation therapy.

B. **Neuropathy** is usually the result of an underlying disease state such as diabetes mellitus (the most common cause), uremia, or alcoholism (Table 53–1). Specific causes other than underlying disease states are listed below.

1. **Guillain-Barré syndrome** is often preceded by a viral infection. It was also associated with immunization with swine flu vaccine.

2. **Brachial plexus neuropathy** is most often seen following an upper respiratory tract infection, but can also be caused by a stretch injury or by Pancoast's tumor infiltration.

3. Chronic exposure to lead can result in a pure **motor neuropathy.**

4. **Inherited neuropathies** include Charcot-Marie-Tooth disease and Dejerine-Sottas disease, which are dominant inherited diseases, and Refsum disease, which is autosomal recessive.

C. **Entrapment syndromes**

1. Repetitive flexion-extension movements at the wrist can cause **carpal tunnel syndrome.** This disease is frequently seen with pregnancy, hypothyroid-

TABLE 53–1. CLASSIFICATION OF NEUROPATHY

  A. Metabolic
    1. Diabetes
    2. Hypothyroidism
    3. Uremia
    4. Nutritional deficiency (eg, vitamin B_{12} or B_6)
    5. Acute intermittent porphyria
  B. Infectious
    1. Human immunodeficiency virus (HIV)
    2. Lyme disease
    3. Syphilis
  C. Inflammatory
    1. Vasculitis
    2. Acute or chronic inflammatory polyneuropathy
    3. Collagen vascular disease
  D. Toxin related
    1. Alcohol
    2. Heavy metals (eg, arsenic, lead, or mercury)
    3. Industrial agents (eg, acrylamide, carbon tetrachloride, or insecticides)
    4. Medications (eg, gold, amiodarone, hydralazine, phenytoin, metronidazole, isoniazid, cisplatin, or vincristine)
  E. Malignancy
    1. Carcinoma
    2. Lymphoma
    3. Gammopathy related
  F. Other
    1. Guillain-Barré syndrome
    2. Hereditary neuropathy

ism, and rheumatoid arthritis. Women are more frequently affected than men, and the dominant hand is affected first and most severely.

    2. Meralgia paresthetica, caused by entrapment of the purely sensory lateral femoral cutaneous nerve, is more commonly seen in men and in overweight individuals.

    3. Common peroneal nerve entrapment most commonly results from trauma to the peroneal nerve at the level of the fibular head, habitual leg crossing, and pressure on the nerve during operative procedures or from casts used in the treatment of fractures.

    4. Individuals involved in activities with prolonged standing or walking (eg, military recruits) are at risk for developing **tarsal tunnel syndrome.**

  D. Mononeuritis multiplex is vascular in origin, resulting in infarction of nerve trunks anywhere in the body. Therefore, it is seen with diseases affecting small arteries, especially diabetes mellitus, polyarteritis nodosa, and collagen vascular diseases.

IV. Pathophysiology

  A. Myelopathy. Destruction of the gray matter of the cord by compression or inflammation is followed by cavitation or gliosis within the cord with permanent paresthesias and motor loss.

  B. Neuropathy. Afferent (sensory) fibers conduct impulses from cutaneous and subcutaneous receptors via the spinal cord to the brain stem and the parietal cortex. Alterations of sensations can occur anywhere along these pathways, but clinically, the majority of diseases involve peripheral sensory nerves.

    1. Diabetic neuropathy is presently thought to occur because of the abnormal accumulation of sorbitol in the peripheral nerves themselves.

    2. Guillain-Barré syndrome is an autoimmune demyelinating syndrome precipitated by viral infections.

  C. Entrapment syndromes

    1. Disk syndromes. Patients with compression of a cervical or lumbar nerve by herniation of an intervertebral disk present with paresthesias or weakness in the field served by the involved nerve (Table 53–2).

    2. Peripheral entrapment. Compression of a single nerve at a specific site results in impaired neural function over a short segment of the nerve. For

TABLE 53–2. RADICULOPATHIES

	Root	Paresthesia	Sensory Loss	Reflex Change
Cervical radiculopathies	C-5	Shoulder, lateral arm to elbow	Lateral deltoid region	↓ Biceps
	C-6	Lateral arm to thumb and 2nd finger	Thumb and 2nd finger	↓ Biceps
	C-7	Lateral arm to 3rd finger	2nd, 3rd, and 4th fingers	↓ Triceps
	C-8	Medial forearm	4th and 5th fingers	↓ Triceps
Lumbar radiculopathies	L-3–L-4	Medial leg	Knee, medial surface of foot	↓ Knee jerk
	L-4–L-5	Lateral leg	Dorsum of foot	—
	L-5–S-1	Lateral leg, 4th and 5th toes	4th and 5th toes	↓ Ankle jerk

example, **tarsal tunnel syndrome** results from compression of the posterior tibial nerve as it passes through the tarsal tunnel at the level of the ankle.

V. Symptoms

A. **Myelopathy** causes paresthesias of the extremities accompanied by symmetric weakness and difficulties with gait.

B. **Polyneuropathy.** Patients complain of painful or weak extremities with altered sensation. An abrupt onset suggests a metabolic or vascular neuropathy, whereas an insidious onset suggests an inherited neuropathy.

1. **Predominantly motor symptoms**
   a. **Guillain-Barré syndrome** has a rapid onset and results in ascending motor weakness with only mild sensory complaints of distal numbness and pain.
   b. **Brachial plexus neuropathy** is abrupt in onset and causes pain, numbness, and weakness in the shoulder girdle musculature.
   c. **Porphyria** and **lead intoxication** produce painful extremities with major motor deficits.
2. **Sensory symptoms.** Patients with primarily sensory neuropathy complain of burning, numbness, tingling, restless legs, and painful touch.
   a. **Diabetes mellitus** can cause painful extremities and decreased sensitivity to temperature, pressure, and pain.
   b. **Alcoholism** can cause numbness and tingling of the hands and feet; the classic complaint is tender feet.
   c. **Uremia** causes restless legs, a painful sensation causing the patient to move the legs constantly while resting, with relief by ambulation. Eventually, there is severe pain in the lower legs and feet and profound distal sensory loss.
   d. **Tumors, toxins, amyloidosis,** and **vitamin B deficiency** cause painful extremities and distal sensory loss.
3. **Sensorimotor symptoms.** Painful extremities with sensory loss and decreased motor strength characterize the sensorimotor neuropathies.
   a. **Diabetes mellitus** produces a sensorimotor neuropathy frequently associated with autonomic dysfunction (eg, impotence, silent myocardial infarction, or postural hypotension without reflex tachycardia).
   b. **Alcoholism** and **uremia** mimic the symptoms of diabetic sensorimotor neuropathy.
   c. Chronic **inflammatory polyneuropathy,** although idiopathic in origin, is similar in presentation to Guillain-Barré syndrome, except for its relapsing course.
4. **Inherited neuropathies** are characterized by an insidious onset without pain.
   a. **Charcot-Marie-Tooth disease** occurs in the second or third decade with loss of proprioception and touch and motor weakness in the limbs.
   b. **Dejerine-Sottas disease** is noted for its peroneal atrophy with weak foot extensors and palpably enlarged nerves.
   c. **Refsum disease** begins with the onset of progressive night blindness by the second decade, followed by ataxia and limb weakness.

C. **Nerve entrapment syndromes**
   1. **Disk syndromes.** Compression of a cervical or lumbar nerve by a herniated disk causes pain and numbness to the field supplied by the entrapped nerve.
   2. **Peripheral entrapment**
      a. **Carpal tunnel syndrome** causes pain and paresthesias in the thumb and the second and third fingers. Symptoms, which are worse in the morning, frequently cause patients to awaken from sleep and shake their hands to relieve the numbness and pain.
      b. **Cubital tunnel syndrome.** Ulnar nerve entrapment at the elbow can occur at the postcondylar groove, causing aching in the medial arm and paresthesias of the fifth finger and ulnar half of the fourth finger.
      c. **Femoral nerve entrapment** causes local tenderness in the groin with pain below the inguinal ligament and paresthesias of the anteromedial thigh.
      d. **Meralgia paresthetica** results in burning pain and numbness over the anterolateral thigh without motor involvement along the distribution of the lateral femoral cutaneous nerve.
      e. **Common peroneal nerve entrapment** causes paresthesias from the outer side of the lower leg in the anterior tibial area distally and in the footdrop.
      f. **Tarsal tunnel syndrome.** Entrapment of the posterior tibial nerve causes burning and tingling in the toes and the sole of the foot.
D. **Mononeuritis multiplex.** Patients experience a rapidly progressive, painful disability that is often proximal as well as distal. Isolated ocular palsies, footdrop, or painful femoral neuropathy can be the initial clinical symptom.

VI. **Signs**
  A. **Myelopathy.** The findings of increased reflexes along with a circumferential sensory level and positive long tract signs are seen with myelopathic disease.
  B. **Neuropathies.** Areflexia is the hallmark of neuropathy. Decreased distal sensation, often in a stocking-glove distribution, is typical of diffuse polyneuropathies.
  C. **Nerve entrapment syndromes**
   1. **Carpal tunnel syndrome.** Findings are decreased pinprick sensation in the first three digits along with an electric shock sensation by percussing the carpal tunnel (Tinel's sign). Acute flexion of the wrist will produce a tingling sensation in the same sensory distribution (Phalen's sign).
   2. **Cubital tunnel syndrome.** Decreased sensation in the fifth finger and a Tinel's sign is produced by percussion of the ulnar nerve at the elbow.
   3. **Femoral nerve entrapment** produces quadriceps weakness, decreased sensation over the anterior thigh, and a diminished knee jerk reaction.
   4. **Compression of the lateral femoral cutaneous nerve** (meralgia paresthetica) produces sensory changes along the anterolateral and lateral thigh.
   5. **Common peroneal nerve entrapment** findings are loss of dorsiflexion and eversion of the foot with footdrop deformity.
   6. **Tarsal tunnel syndrome** results in sensory changes over the plantar aspect of the foot with symptoms often most marked at night.
  D. **Mononeuritis multiplex.** Loss of motor and sensory function in an asymmetric distribution of more than one peripheral nerve distinguishes mononeuritis multiplex from other causes of paresthesias.

VII. **Laboratory tests.** A comprehensive history and physical examination along with routine laboratory testing are essential in evaluating any patient with paresthesias.
  A. A **complete blood cell count (CBC), blood urea nitrogen (BUN), glucose, erythrocyte sedimentation rate,** and **thyroid functions** make up the basic tests.
  B. **Electromyography (EMG)** remains the mainstay in sorting out the various causes of paresthesias. It is particularly useful in distinguishing a polyneuropathy from a mononeuropathy such as a disk or peripheral entrapment syndrome. EMG results are basically normal in myelopathy but show a predominance of large motor units along with fibrillations and fasciculations in neuropathic diseases.
  C. Supplementary tests such as **heavy metal and toxin screening, vitamin B_{12} levels, antinuclear antibodies, Lyme disease serology,** and **human immunodeficiency virus (HIV) testing** are important in patients without a clear diagnosis.

VIII. **Treatment**
  A. **Myelopathies.** Compressive myelopathies require a surgical approach. Myelopathies induced by multiple sclerosis and radiation sometimes respond to corticosteroids.

B. **Polyneuropathies.** Treatment of the underlying disorder causing the neuropathy remains the first step in alleviating paresthesias, although such treatment is usually inadequate and frequently does not correct the neuropathy.
   1. **Guillain-Barré syndrome.** Hospitalization is required to monitor respiratory function. Plasmapheresis is the present treatment of choice, with pooled infusions of gamma globulin presently being studied as more efficacious.
   2. **Chronic inflammatory polyneuropathy** has been shown to respond to **prednisone,** and plasmapheresis has occasionally produced dramatic improvement.
   3. **Drug-induced neuropathies** respond well to discontinuation of the drug.
   4. **Diabetic neuropathy** often improves with careful glucose control. Other management options include tricyclic antidepressants (eg, **amitriptyline,** 50–150 mg/day divided into one to three oral doses); **capsaicin** (Zostrix) cream, applied to affected areas three or four times daily; mexiletine; carbamazepine; and diphenylhydantoin.
   5. **Inherited neuropathies** are not treatable, except with genetic counseling and symptomatic therapy.
C. **Nerve entrapment syndromes.** Surgical decompression of an entrapped nerve is usually effective, but is reserved for patients who do not respond to more conservative management.
   1. **Carpal tunnel syndrome.** Treatment with wrist splints and steroid injections into the carpal tunnel are often effective for relief of this disease, especially if it is caused by trauma, pregnancy, or rheumatoid arthritis.
   2. **Cubital tunnel syndrome** can usually be controlled with an elbow splint and avoidance of leaning on the elbow.
   3. **Meralgia paresthetica** often resolves spontaneously. If necessary, steroid injection medial to the anterior superior iliac spine provides relief.
   4. **Common peroneal nerve entrapment** responds well to removal of external pressures from the lateral fibular neck along with a footdrop brace.
D. **Mononeuritis multiplex.** Treatment of the underlying causes of the vasculitis responsible for the mononeuritis, along with physical therapy programs, can improve the majority of these cases.

REFERENCES

Asbury AK, et al: A focused workup for neuropathy. Patient Care 1985;**19:**136.
Cohen JA, Gross KF: Peripheral neuropathy: Causes and management in the elderly. Geriatrics 1990;**45:**21.
Ferrante JA: *American Academy of Family Physicians Home Study Self Assessment: Peripheral Neuropathies.* American Academy of Family Physicians; 1989.
Flaggman PD, Kelly JJ: An electrophysiologic evaluation. Arch Neurol 1980;**37:**160.
James JS, Page JC: Painful diabetic peripheral neuropathy. J Am Pod Med Assoc 1994;**84:**439.
Reddy MP: Peripheral nerve entrapment syndromes. Am Fam Physician 1983;**28:**133.
Stuart JD, et al: Nerve compression syndromes of the lower extremity. Am Fam Physician 1989;**40:**101.

54	Pediatric Fever

Sanford R. Kimmel, MD

I. **Definition.** Fever is an elevation of body temperature above the normal range. The normal range for temperature of the body varies according to the age of the child, method of measurement, and time of day. A rectal temperature >37.8 °C (100 °F) in newborns or 38 °C (100.4 °F) in older infants denotes fever, as does an oral temperature of 37.8 °C in older children. Since rectal temperature most consistently reflects the body's core temperature, this is the temperature referred to in this chapter.
II. **Common diagnoses.** Common and significant infectious causes of fever in children are listed below.
   A. **Upper respiratory infections (URIs)** (eg, viral infections, otitis media, pharyngitis, and sinusitis).

B. **Lower respiratory infections (LRIs)** (eg, bacterial and viral pneumonias, bronchitis, bronchiolitis, and epiglottitis).

C. **Bacterial and viral gastroenteritis.**

D. **Bacteremia.**

E. **Urinary tract infections (UTIs).**

F. **Bacterial and viral meningitis.**

G. **Infections of the musculoskeletal system** (eg, osteomyelitis and septic arthritis).

H. **Febrile exanthems** (eg, roseola, measles, varicella, and scarlet fever).

III. **Epidemiology.** During the first 2–3 years of life, children have an average of four to six acute infectious episodes per year. At one family practice center, mild temperature elevations of 37.8 °C (100 °F) to 38.3 °C (101 °F) were present in 20% of infants under 6 months of age who visited the center, while 4% had a fever of at least 38.3 °C.

A. **Viral infections** cause most febrile episodes, but bacterial infections are present in 15–20% of febrile infants <3 months old and in one of four children presenting with a fever of 40 °C (104 °F) or higher.

B. **Bacteremia** occurs in 3–8% of febrile children <36 months of age seen in the emergency room. Additional risk factors for bacteremia include immunodeficiency or immunosuppression, anatomic or functional asplenia, and household or day care contact with invasive bacterial disease.

C. **UTIs** occur in 5–7% of girls under the age of 2 years with fever without localizing signs. Uncircumcised male infants have a 10 times greater incidence of UTIs (1%) during the first year of life than do circumcised infants (0.1%).

D. **Meningitis**

1. **Bacterial meningitis** can occur throughout the year, but *Streptococcus pneumoniae* and *Neisseria meningitidis* usually occur during the winter months. Invasive *Haemophilus influenzae* type b (Hib) disease has significantly decreased due to the Hib vaccine. Hib disease has been more frequent in boys, African Americans, Native Americans, and children attending day care centers.

2. **Viral meningitis** usually occurs during the summer and fall in temperate climates. Enterovirus is the most common cause and is spread from person to person by fecal-oral and respiratory routes and by fomites.

E. **Septic arthritis** frequently occurs in children <3 years old and in sexually active adolescent girls. Although **osteomyelitis** occurs in children at all ages, it is more commonly diagnosed in infants and preadolescents.

F. **Febrile exanthems**

1. **Roseola** usually affects children between the ages of 6 and 24 months and seldom occurs after 3 years of age.

2. **Measles** is transmitted by direct contact with infectious airborne droplets, predominantly during the winter and spring in temperate climates. Measles cases in the United States have declined as a result of a second measles immunization given prior to school entry.

3. **Scarlet fever** is usually associated with group A streptococcal pharyngitis and follows close contact with the respiratory secretions of infected individuals.

4. **Varicella** usually occurs by direct contact with persons with varicella or zoster, and occasionally by airborne spread from respiratory secretions. It is highly contagious among susceptible contacts.

IV. **Pathophysiology.** See the discussions of pathophysiology in Chapter 16, regarding LRIs; Chapter 19, regarding gastroenteritis; Chapter 24, regarding UTIs; Chapter 25, regarding otitis media; Chapter 59, regarding sinusitis; and Chapter 61, regarding pharyngitis.

A. Pathogens gain access to the host through mucosal contact or a break in the skin. Infection of an organ system may then occur directly or by contiguous or hematogenous spread. For example, osteomyelitis and septic arthritis may result from hematogenous spread of organisms or by direct invasion as a result of trauma or spread from a neighboring area of cellulitis.

B. The development of disease following contact depends on the virulence of the organism, the size of the infecting inoculum, and the resistance factors of the host. For example, most invasive *H influenzae* disease is caused by the encapsulated type b strain, while nonencapsulated, nontypeable *H influenzae* is a frequent cause of otitis media. Relatively large numbers of *Salmonella* spp must be ingested to produce an often self-limited illness, but young infants and those with impaired immune systems are prone to systemic invasion and disease such as osteomyelitis or meningitis.

C. The febrile response occurs when exogenous pyrogens such as viruses, bacteria, fungi, toxins, drugs, malignancies, metabolic disorders, and antigen-antibody complexes induce the release of endogenous pyrogens such as interleukin 1. These stimulate the production of hypothalamic prostaglandin E_2 (PGE_2) that raises the "set point" of the body's thermostat. Heat is generated or conserved through shivering or peripheral vasoconstriction. The resulting fever may increase leukocyte migration and antibacterial activity as well as T-cell and interferon production. However, the risk of dehydration also increases, since the body's basal metabolic rate increases 10% for each degree Celsius above normal.

D. Infectious diseases associated with pediatric fever and their causal organisms include the following.

    1. Epiglottitis: Hib.

    2. Bacteremia: *S pneumoniae,* Hib, *N meningitidis, Salmonella* spp, *Escherichia coli,* and group B streptococci.

    3. Bacterial meningitis

        a. Less than 3 months of age: gram-negative enteric bacteria, group B streptococci, and *Listeria monocytogenes.*

        b. Over 3 months of age: *N meningitidis, S pneumoniae,* and Hib.

    4. Viral meningitis: enteroviruses, arboviruses, varicella-zoster virus, mumps, and herpes simplex types 1 and 2.

    5. Osteomyelitis: *Staphylococcus aureus* (most common), Hib, *Salmonella* (sickle cell disease), *Pseudomonas aeruginosa* (eg, a nail puncture through a sneaker), group B streptococci, and *E coli* (in neonates).

    6. Septic arthritis: Hib (ages 2 months to 4 years), *S aureus* (in neonates and children over 5 years old), streptococci, meningococci, gonococci in sexually active or abused children, and *Borrelia burgdorferi* in areas endemic for Lyme disease.

    7. Roseola: human herpesvirus type 6.

    8. Scarlet fever: group A streptococci producing erythrogenic exotoxins.

V. Symptoms. The febrile child will often demonstrate some degree of lethargy, loss of appetite, or irritability.

    A. Respiratory symptoms include sore throat, nasal congestion, otalgia, cough, and wheezing.

    B. Diarrhea and **vomiting** usually indicate a gastrointestinal infection, although these symptoms occasionally occur in acute otitis media or UTI.

    C. Fever may be the only symptom of a UTI in young infants, but older infants and children may **cry with urination or refuse to urinate.**

    D. Persistence of worsening of **lethargy** and **irritability** may indicate meningitis.

    E. Refusal to bear weight or use an extremity may be seen with septic arthritis or osteomyelitis.

    F. A transient red maculopapular **rash appearing after defervescence of several days of high fever** is characteristic of roseola. **Cough, coryza,** and **conjunctivitis** accompany the confluent red rash of measles. A **strawberry tongue may be seen with the characteristic sandpaper-like rash** of scarlet fever. The simultaneous appearance of **macules, papules,** and **vesicles** on the scalp, face, or trunk denotes varicella.

VI. Signs

    A. The **degree of temperature reduction in response to acetaminophen** is generally not helpful in differentiating viral from bacterial infection.

    B. Initial observation of the child's general physical state and **interaction with the parent or caregiver** often determine whether the physician needs to have a high or low index of suspicion of serious underlying disease.

        1. McCarthy and associates (1982) developed six key predictors of serious illness in febrile children based on observation and interaction with the child while the child is seated on the caregiver's lap, prior to antipyretic therapy (Table 54–1).

        2. A serious underlying disease was found in 92% of children with an acute illness observation scale (AIOS) score of 16 or more and in 26% of those with a score of 11–15. Only 2.7% of children with a score of 10 or less had a serious illness.

        3. No child who smiled normally had a serious illness.

TABLE 54–1. ACUTE ILLNESS OBSERVATION SCALES

Observation Item	Normal—1	Moderate Impairment—3	Severe Impairment—5
Quality of cry	Strong cry with normal tone, or contented and not crying	Whimpering or sobbing	Weak cry, moaning, or high-pitched cry
Reaction to parental stimulation	Cries briefly and then stops, or is contented and not crying	Cries off and on	Cries continually or hardly responds
State variation	If awake, stays awake, or if asleep and then stimulated, awakens quickly	Closes eyes briefly when awake, or awakens with prolonged stimulation	Falls asleep or will not arouse
Color	Pink	Pale extremities or acrocyanosis	Pale, cyanotic, mottled, or ashen
Hydration	Normal skin and eyes, moist mucous membranes	Normal skin and eyes, slightly dry mouth	Doughy or tented skin, dry mucous membranes or sunken eyes
Response (talk, smile) to social overture	Smiles, or "alert" (≤2 months)[1]	Smiles briefly, or "alert" briefly (≤2 months)[1]	No smile, anxious face, dull expression, or does not "alert" (≤2 months)[1]

[1] "Alert" applies to children under 2 months of age, since these young infants do not have a social smile.
Adapted with permission from McCarthy PL, et al: Observation scales to identify serious illness in febrile children. Pediatrics 1982;**70**:806, as used in Kimmel SR, Gemmill DW: The young child with fever. Am Fam Physician 1988;**37**:196.

      4. The AIOS is most useful in children 2 months of age or older. In infants 4–8 weeks old, the AIOS detected <50% of those with a serious illness in one study. The sensitivity and positive predictive value of the AIOS also decrease as the prevalence of bacteremia in the population decreases.
   C. Physical findings associated with specific diseases are presented in Table 54–2.
VII. Laboratory tests
   A. Screening laboratory tests help determine whether further diagnostic studies are needed for the child who appears moderately ill (eg, an AIOS score of 11–15) but for whom there is no obvious focus of infection.
      1. In infants >30 days of age, the following conditions suggest an underlying or occult bacterial illness.
         a. White blood cell count (WBC) of ≥15,000 cells/μL.
         b. Absolute band count >1500 cells/μL.
      2. The positive predictive value of the above tests for serious bacterial illness (SBI), such as pneumonia or meningitis, is about 10–25%. Thus, many children who have a positive screening test result will not have an underlying SBI.
      3. The presence of vacuolation or toxic granulation in any one of 100 neutrophils scanned may have a positive predictive value of >50% for bacteremia in febrile children <24 months of age.
      4. No test will detect bacteremia or other serious illnesses in all children. Some children with meningitis may have a WBC of <15,000/μL, and some children with overwhelming sepsis may have a WBC of <5000/μL.
      5. Careful clinical assessment of the child is necessary in interpreting screening tests. A positive test result is more likely to be significant for the child who appears ill or has underlying risk factors than for one who looks well.
   B. Diagnostic studies. Further diagnostic tests (Table 54–3) should be considered in febrile children who appear moderately or severely ill (AIOS score >10) or who have an abnormal screening test result.
VIII. Treatment (Figure 54–1)
   A. Hospitalization is indicated in the following circumstances.
      1. Infants 0–28 days old with a fever of 38 °C (100.4 °F) or higher should have a complete sepsis work-up and begin receiving parenteral antibiotics pending culture results.

TABLE 54–2. PHYSICAL FINDINGS AND CLINICAL CLUES TO ILLNESSES IN FEBRILE CHILDREN

Body Region or System	Physical Findings	Potential Disease(s)
Skin	Petechial rash	Meningococcemia
	Maculopapular rash, followed by petechial rash	Rocky Mountain spotted fever
Head	Bulging fontanelle, nuchal rigidity	Meningitis (later manifestation in child under 2 years of age)
Eyes	Conjunctivitis	Associated otitis media, Kawasaki disease, or measles with cough, coryza
	Redness or swelling around eye	Periorbital cellulitis
Ears	Red, dull, nonmobile tympanic membrane	Otitis media
	Swelling and tenderness behind ear	Mastoiditis
Nose	Purulent rhinorrhea	Sinusitis
	Nasal flaring	Pneumonia or any condition producing respiratory distress
Throat	Stridor	Laryngotracheobronchitis (croup)
	Stridor with drooling, dysphagia, or aphonia	Epiglottitis
	Petechiae on soft palate and uvula	Streptococcal pharyngitis
	Vesicles or ulcers on soft palate and tonsilar pillars	Herpangina
	Vesicles or ulcers on tongue, lips, and buccal mucosa	Herpes stomatitis
	Strawberry tongue	Streptococcal pharyngitis or Kawasaki disease
Chest	Tachypnea, retractions, decreased breath sounds, rales (may not be present)	Pneumonia
	Rhonchi	Bronchitis
	Wheezing	Bronchiolitis, asthma (inhaled foreign body or other causes)
Heart	Murmur	Subacute bacterial endocarditis, rheumatic fever (or normal due to increased cardiac output)
Abdomen	Local tenderness worsening with movement	Appendicitis or condition producing peritoneal irritation
Rectal	Fluctuant mass	Ruptured appendix or perirectal abscess
Musculoskeletal	Refuses to bear weight or use extremity	Septic arthritis or osteomyelitis, especially in the hip

Reprinted with permission from Kimmel SR, Gemmill DW: The young child with fever. Am Fam Physician 1988;**37**:202.

TABLE 54–3. DIAGNOSTIC STUDIES IN FEBRILE CHILDREN WITHOUT AN OBVIOUS FOCUS OF INFECTION

Test	Indications	Comments
Chest x-ray	Fever of sudden onset, tachypnea, decreased breath sounds	Pneumonia may lack usual auscultatory findings
Urinalysis (UA) with culture and sensitivity (C&S)	Male infants under 6 months of age. Female children less than 2 years old	Bladder tap newborn; catheterize older children; negative UA does not rule out infection
Lumbar puncture	Child less than 3 months of age or very irritable or lethargic, feeds poorly, has seizures, bulging fontanelle, or nuchal rigidity	Use needle with stylet; consider hospital admission
Blood culture	Age less than 3 years at high risk of bacteremia, acute illness observation score (AIOS) $\geq 11 \pm$ WBC $\geq 15,000/\mu L$	Draw 0.5–2 mL of blood; one test sufficient for outpatient use
Stool for polymorphonuclear cells (PMNs) with C&S	Abrupt onset or bloody diarrhea, greater than four stools per day, and no vomiting before diarrhea	Positive if ≥ 5 PMNs/hpf

hpf, High-power field.

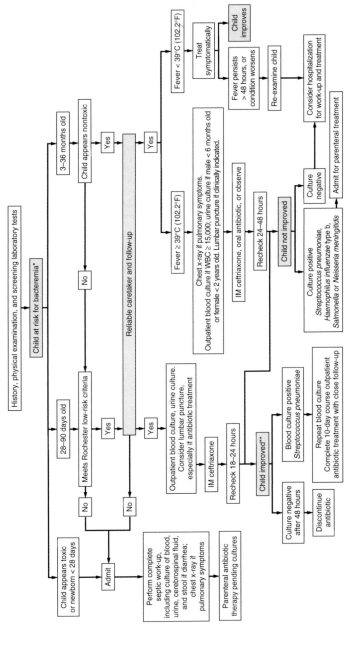

FIGURE 54-1. Guidelines for the management of children with fever without localizing signs. WBC, White blood cell count; IM, intramuscular.

*Children who are immunosuppressed, have undergone splenectomy, or have sickle cell anemia, leukemia, nephrosis, and other conditions placing them at high risk for overwhelming bacterial infection should be managed like toxic children.
**Nontoxic, nonbacteremic, afebrile children with otitis media or urinary tract infection may be treated with outpatient antibiotics.

2. Febrile children 28–90 days of age who do not fulfill the Rochester low-risk criteria (Table 54–4) are at risk for bacteremia or SBI based on their clinical appearance, physical findings, and laboratory studies. These children should be admitted to the hospital for further evaluation and treatment.

3. Any febrile child who is severely ill (eg, AIOS score ≥16), who is immunosuppressed, or who has an underlying condition placing him or her at high risk of overwhelming infection requires hospital admission.

B. Ambulatory management

1. Specific therapy should be initiated for conditions diagnosed and amenable to outpatient treatment as outlined in Chapter 16, for LRIs; Chapter 19, for gastroenteritis; Chapter 24, for UTIs in female patients; Chapter 25, for otitis media; Chapter 59, for sinusitis; and Chapter 61, for pharyngitis.

2. Infants aged 28–90 days old who fulfill **all** of the Rochester low-risk criteria may be managed as outpatients, provided they have reliable caregivers who are able to contact their physician by telephone and obtain medical care within 30 minutes. Parents must be instructed to call or seek immediate medical attention if the child demonstrates worrisome signs such as poor feeding, vomiting, excessive fussiness or sleepiness, skin rash, or color changes.

3. Febrile children without localizing signs who are 3 months of age or older may be followed up as outpatients if their caretakers are reliable and the children can be re-examined within 24–48 hours.

4. Oral amoxicillin improves the clinical appearance in bacteremic children seen 48 hours later but may not prevent major sequelae. Intramuscular ceftriaxone at a dose of 50 mg/kg once daily and amoxicillin–potassium clavulanate appear to be more effective in decreasing the risk of focal infection.

   a. Presumptive antibiotic therapy may be begun after obtaining a blood culture and other appropriate diagnostic studies if the child is between 3 months and 3 years of age, the fever is 38.9 °C (102 °F) or more, the AIOS score is 11–15, or the WBC is ≥15,000/μL.

   b. Therapy should be directed against *S pneumoniae,* which is the most common cause of occult bacteremia, as well as *H influenzae* and meningococcus.

5. Follow-up of the older child who has fever without an obvious focus must occur by re-examination or telephone in 24–48 hours.

   a. If the child is better or cultures are negative after 48 hours, antibiotic therapy should be discontinued.

   b. If the child is improved and blood culture grows *S pneumoniae,* outpatient antibiotic therapy should be continued for 10 days under close observation. A follow-up blood culture should be obtained to confirm clinical cure.

TABLE 54–4. ROCHESTER CRITERIA FOR LOW-RISK INFANTS

1. Infant appears generally well
2. Infant has been previously healthy
   Born at term (≥37 weeks' gestation)
   Did not receive perinatal antimicrobial therapy
   Was not treated for unexplained hyperbilirubinemia
   Had not received and was not receiving antimicrobial agents
   Had not been previously hospitalized
   Had no chronic or underlying illness
   Was not hospitalized longer than mother
3. No evidence of skin, soft tissue, bone, joint, or ear infection
4. Laboratory values
   Peripheral blood WBC count 5.0–15.0 × 10⁹ cells/L (5000–15,000/mm³)
   Absolute band form count ≤1.5 × 10⁹ cells/L (≤1500/mm³)
   ≤10 WBCs per high-power field (×40) on microscopic examination of a spun urine sediment
   ≤5 WBC per high-power field (×40) on microscopic examination of a stool smear (only for infants with diarrhea)

WBC, White blood cell.
Jaskiewicz JA, McCarthy CA, Richardson AC, et al, and the Febrile Infant Collaborative Study Group: Febrile infants at low risk for serious bacterial infection—an appraisal of the Rochester criteria and implications for management. Reproduced with permission from *Pediatrics,* Vol. **94**, page 391, 1994.

    c. If the child is improved and afebrile but the urine culture is positive, the outpatient antibiotic therapy should be continued. A follow-up culture should be obtained and a structural evaluation of the urinary tract should be done in all children in this age group.

    d. If the blood culture grows Hib, *N meningitidis, Salmonella,* or other pathogenic organisms, the child should be hospitalized for parenteral antibiotic therapy and evaluated for focal sites of infection.

    e. If the child is worse or not improved, thorough re-evaluation, including history, physical examination, and laboratory studies, should be performed. Hospital admission is often indicated at this time.

6. The primary reason to treat fever symptomatically is to make the child more comfortable. Parents should be instructed as follows.

    a. Treat fever of 38.9 °C (102 °F) or greater with **acetaminophen,** 10–15 mg/kg every 4 hours up to a maximum of five doses per day. **Ibuprofen,** 5–10 mg/kg every 6–8 hours, may also be used for fever reduction in children aged 6 months or older.

    b. Sponge children with lukewarm water if their temperature exceeds 40 °C (104 °F) and acetaminophen or ibuprofen has been previously administered without effect. Alcohol or cold water should not be used.

    c. Cover children with light blankets and encourage them to drink liquids.

    d. Fever itself is seldom dangerous. It is a symptom of an underlying illness. Observation of children's behavior is even more important than a record of their temperature.

REFERENCES

American Academy of Pediatrics Committee on Infectious Diseases: *1997 Red Book.* 24th ed. American Academy of Pediatrics; 1997.

Baker MD, Avner JR, Bell LM: Failure of infant observation scales in detecting serious illnesses in febrile, 4- to 8-week-old infants. Pediatrics 1990;**85:**1040.

Baraff LJ, et al: Practice guidelines for the management of infants and children 0 to 36 months of age with fever without source. Pediatrics 1993;**92:**1.

Harper MB, Bachur R, Fleisher GR: Effect of antibiotic therapy on the outcome of outpatients with unsuspected bacteremia. Pediatr Infect Dis J 1995;**14:**760.

Jaskiewicz JA, McCarthy CA, Richardson AC, et al, and the Febrile Infant Collaborative Study Group: Febrile infants at low risk for serious bacterial infection—An appraisal of the Rochester criteria and implications for management. Pediatrics 1994;**94:**390.

Kimmel SR: Fever in young children: A complex challenge. Fam Pract Recert 1996;**18:**69.

Kimmel SR, Gemmill DW: The young child with fever. Am Fam Physician 1988;**37:**196.

Mace SE, Le N: Controversies in the evaluation and management of a febrile infant or young child. J Clin Outcomes Manage 1997;**4:**52.

McCarthy PL, et al: Observation scales to identify serious illness in febrile children. Pediatrics 1982;**70:**802.

Narasimhan N, Marks M: Osteomyelitis and septic arthritis. In Nelson et al (editors): *Textbook of Pediatrics.* 15th ed. Saunders; 1996:724.

Teach SJ, Fleisher GR, and the Occult Bacteremia Study Group: Efficacy of an observation scale in detecting bacteremia in febrile children three to thirty-six months of age, treated as outpatients. J Pediatr 1995;**126:**877.

Willoughby RE, Polack FS: Meningitis: What's new in diagnosis and management. Contemp Pediatr 1998;**15:**49.

---

55   Pelvic Pain

David W. Euans, MD

I. Definition. Pelvic pain is pain occurring in the lower abdomen of the female and may originate in the female reproductive system, the lower urinary tract, or the intestinal tract.

II. Common diagnoses

    A. Endometriosis (present in as many as 45–50% of women with chronic pelvic pain).

B. Ovarian cysts (which cause as much as 40% of pelvic pain).

C. Pelvic inflammatory disease (PID) (which accounts for as much as 20% of acute pelvic pain in female patients).

D. Adnexal torsion (which accounts for as much as 16% of acute pelvic pain).

E. Appendicitis (accounting for as much as 10% of acute pelvic pain).

F. Uterine leiomyomata (fibroids) (which cause as much as 5% of chronic pelvic pain).

G. Ectopic pregnancy (which causes 1–2% of acute pelvic pain).

H. Urinary tract infection (UTI).

I. Mittelschmerz.

J. Cancers.

K. Psychogenic pelvic pain.

III. Epidemiology. The complaint of pelvic pain is presented by approximately 1–2% of the patients seen in the primary care practice.

A. Endometriosis is found only in postmenarcheal women. Most of these women are between the ages of 25 and 45 years. Genetic factors may play a role in the development of this problem. Women who are multiparous or who were pregnant early in their reproductive lives may have a lower incidence of this condition.

B. Ovarian cysts are usually found in women of reproductive age.

C. PID. Over 1 million cases of PID occur yearly. Adolescents account for 20% of the total. Sexually active adolescent females are at the highest risk for contracting the condition. Other risk factors include nonwhite race, prior episodes of PID, and, possibly, intrauterine contraceptive device (IUD) use.

D. Adnexal torsion is often the first sign of an ovarian tumor. It is more common with tumors that are small to moderate in size. If the condition is caused by a cyst, it is most common during the reproductive years. Torsion caused by a malignant tumor of the ovary is more common in elderly women.

E. Appendicitis occurs most frequently in the second and third decades of life, the peak being in the midteens. There is a twofold male predominance during this period; the sex ratio is nearly equal in other age groups.

F. Uterine fibroids are present in as many as 50% of women in autopsy series. These fibroids may be associated with obesity and hypertension in black women and are more common in the later reproductive years.

G. Ectopic pregnancy. The frequency of this type of pregnancy increases with age and is more common in lower socioeconomic groups and in women with a past history of PID, pelvic surgery, or, possibly, IUD use. The rate ranges between 5 and 25 per 1000 pregnancies.

H. UTI incidence in women increases with age, beginning at puberty. The incidence increases rapidly after menopause. Approximately 20% of all women have at least one episode of UTI during their lives. UTIs are more common during pregnancy.

I. Mittelschmerz. Pain related to ovulation may be noted by many women at the middle of the menstrual cycle.

J. Cancers. Cancers of the uterus and the ovaries are estimated to represent 11% and 4%, respectively, of all cancers in females.

    1. The mean age for women with invasive **cervical cancer** is 52 years. Risk factors include human papillomavirus and herpesvirus exposure.

    2. The mean age for **endometrial cancer** is 56 years, and the problem is associated with obesity, nulliparity, and estrogen exposure unopposed by progestational agents.

    3. The frequency of **ovarian cancer** increases with age until approximately 70 years. It is more common in whites and in the United States and western Europe.

K. Psychogenic pelvic pain. Women who have difficulty in managing stress in their personal relationships and who have abnormal attitudes concerning their own and their partner's sexuality may experience pelvic pain. Risk factors include depression, past sexual and physical abuse, current sexual dysfunction, and alcoholism.

IV. Pathophysiology. Pain from pelvic organs originates from nerve endings in arterial walls and the peritoneum. For this reason, it may be poorly localized by the patient. Pain of the uterine cervix may be felt in the lumbar and sacral region. Uterine fundal pain may be reported in the hypogastric area. Ovarian pain is extremely variable in its presentation.

A. **Endometriosis** (see Chapter 21).
B. **Ovarian cysts** may develop from a blighted follicle that becomes filled with fluid, rather than being resorbed. Lutein cysts result from bleeding into the corpus luteum with distention of the lutein wall. The blood cells are usually resorbed, leaving a thin, clear fluid. Pain may result from pressure on the ovary or other structures. Rupture of either type of cyst will cause peritoneal irritation and severe pain.
C. **PID** usually begins as an infection of the endocervix. During menses, the cervical mucous barrier thins and may allow an ascending infection from the endometrium to the tubal mucosa. Offending organisms are typically *Neisseria gonorrhoeae* and *Chlamydia trachomatis*. In addition, anaerobes, including *Bacteroides* spp, and enteric bacteria may be involved because of the favorable environment created by the sexually transmitted organisms. Pain results from the acute inflammatory process caused by infection. Healing usually takes place with much scarring and adhesion formation.

Infertility is a frequent complication of PID, in spite of adequate treatment. In one study, the infertility rate ranged from 8% after one episode of PID to 40% after three or more episodes. Evidence suggests that the severity of the tubal inflammation is directly related to infertility.
D. **Adnexal torsion** frequently occurs with medium to small ovarian cysts or solid tumors. The direction of the twist is usually clockwise, and one or more complete twists usually occur. The torsion causes venous stasis and can also bring about total arterial occlusion and gangrene.
E. **Appendicitis** (see Chapter 1).
F. **Uterine fibroids** (see Chapter 21).
G. **Ectopic pregnancy** (see Chapters 1 and 103).

Implantation of the fertilized ovum may take place anywhere along the course of the fallopian tube when the normal transport of the embryo is delayed, frequently because of a scarred tube. The growth of the embryo causes pain and rupture of the tube. There is a potential for fatal hemorrhage unless the embryo is removed.
H. **UTI** (see Chapter 24).
I. **Mittelschmerz.** The cause of pain production in this condition is uncertain, but the pain may result from a small amount of bleeding caused by the rupture of the follicle or from ovarian swelling caused by the growth of the follicle.
J. **Cancers.** Pain from bone, nerve, and pelvic organ invasion is common with cancers of the female reproductive tract in the later stages.
K. **Psychogenic pelvic pain** is a somatic response to unresolved psychosocial issues.

V. **Symptoms** (see Table 55–1).
VI. **Signs** (see Table 55–1).
VII. **Laboratory tests**
   A. **White blood cell counts (WBCs)** are useful in narrowing the differential diagnosis of any abdominal or pelvic pain. An elevated WBC suggests an inflammatory or infectious cause, such as PID, appendicitis, or UTI. A normal WBC does not rule out such possibilities, however.
   B. **Urinalysis (UA).** The presence of pyuria or hematuria suggests that the source of pain may be in the urinary tract. However, inflammation near the bladder or the ureter can also cause pyuria. As for the WBC, the request for a UA is justifiable in most cases of abdominal and pelvic pain, although its specificity is low.
   C. **Gram's stain** of an endocervical discharge may help to make a diagnosis of gonococcal infection in PID. This test is inexpensive and readily available, although its sensitivity, at 68%, is rather low.
   D. **Ultrasonography** is probably the most useful noninvasive test for the diagnosis of pelvic pain. It is especially useful for evaluating adnexal masses and detecting ectopic pregnancy and tubo-ovarian abscesses. In particular, the use of a transvaginal probe allows the imaging of intrauterine pregnancies as early as the fifth week after the last menstrual period. Likewise, it is more sensitive in the detection of extrauterine pregnancies than is the transabdominal probe. Ultrasonography should be considered in any case of pelvic pain that is not clearly diagnosable by less costly means.
   E. **Bacterial cultures** of endocervical discharge using modified Thayer-Martin agar may help the physician make the diagnosis of gonococcal infection. The test is readily available, relatively inexpensive, and more sensitive than Gram's stain.

TABLE 55–1. SIGNS AND SYMPTOMS OF THE VARIOUS CAUSES OF PELVIC PAIN

Etiology	Location and Nature of Pain	Other Symptoms	Physical Signs
Endometriosis	Dysmenorrhea starting prior to menses; dyspareunia; painful defecation	Premenstrual spotting, hematuria, infertility	Often none; rupture of cyst may mimic acute abdomen; endometrial cysts and nodules on the uterosacral ligaments may be palpable on pelvic examination
Ovarian cyst	Dull, pressure-like, on affected side; severe and diffuse if ruptured	Lutein cysts may cause delayed or scanty menses	Smooth, mobile adnexal mass; diffuse abdominal and pelvic tenderness if ruptured; shock and abdominal distention if significant hemorrhage present
Pelvic inflammatory disease	Lower abdomen, usually bilateral	Fever, vaginal discharge, abnormal vaginal bleeding, dysuria	See Table 55–2
Adnexal torsion	Acute, severe, and progressive; may resolve if torsion untwists	Usually none	Mass and tenderness on affected side; examination may be less impressive than symptoms
Appendicitis	Vague epigastric to mid-abdominal early; right lower quadrant, suprapubic, or flank pain late	Anorexia early; nausea and vomiting after pain onset	Low-grade fever; tenderness over McBurney's point; rebound, guarding, psoas, and obturator signs
Fibroids	Pressure; dysmenorrhea, severe cramping with prolapse; moderate to severe pain with torsion or degeneration; back pain; nerve trunk pressure	Menorrhagia, anemia, urinary frequency, constipation	Palpable mass on uterine surface
Ectopic pregnancy	Variable to diffuse or localized, colicky, or dull; shoulder pain with hemoperitoneum	Amenorrhea variable, usually abnormal vaginal bleeding	Abdomen tender, with rebound and guarding if ruptured; uterus slightly enlarged; adnexal mass may be present; tachycardia; shock with hemorrhage
Urinary tract infection	Suprapubic pain; dysuria; low back pain; flank pain (with upper tract infection)	Urinary frequency; fever, nausea, and vomiting (with upper tract infection)	Suprapubic tenderness, sometimes bladder or urethral tenderness, flank or costovertebral angle tenderness (with upper tract infection)
Mittelschmerz	Variable in severity; lasts hours to 3 days	Occurs midcycle (related to ovulation), minimal vaginal bleeding	None
Malignancies			
Ovarian carcinoma	Vague abdominal pain, fullness, or indigestion	Usually none	Adnexal mass; palpable ovary in postmenopausal patients
Endometrial carcinoma	Pain usually not a factor until cancer is far advanced	Postmenopausal vaginal bleeding, abnormal discharge	Uterine enlargement
Cervical carcinoma (invasive)	Sacral pain in advanced disease; hip and leg pain sometimes severe	Vaginal bleeding or discharge	Friable, exophytic growth on uterine cervix; ureteral obstruction; lymphedema of leg; rectal or bladder fistulae may be present in advanced disease
Psychogenic pain	Variable	Depressive symptoms, anxiety	No evidence for organic disease on appropriate workup; signs of depression or anxiety

Because of the polymicrobial nature of infections of the upper reproductive tract, cultures of the endocervix may not give a true picture of the infection.

F. Enzyme immunoassay tests for *N gonorrhoeae* and *C trachomatis* in endocervical discharges are relatively rapid, inexpensive, and technically easy to perform. A positive test result strongly suggests the presence of infection by the appropriate organism. This method has a sensitivity of 92% and a specificity of 97% for *N gonorrhoeae* and a sensitivity of 80% and a specificity of 98% for *C trachomatis.* This test suffers from the same limitations as bacterial cultures.

G. DNA probes for *N gonorrhoeae* and *C trachomatis.* Tests for both organisms can be performed from a single cervical or urethral swab. This test has sensitivities of 86% for *N gonorrhoeae* and 93% for *C trachomatis.* The specificity is 98–99% for both organisms. This test has the advantage of a 24-hour turnaround time and should be available through most hospital laboratories.

H. Pregnancy tests. Monoclonal antibody enzyme-linked immunosorbent assays for urinary human chorionic gonadotropin (hCG) will be positive in as many as 96–100% of all ectopic pregnancies. Quantitative serum β-hCG immunoassay will be positive in 5–7 days postconception. Therefore, ectopic pregnancy is most unlikely if this test is negative.

I. Erythrocyte sedimentation rate (ESR). This test is one of the Centers for Disease Control and Prevention's diagnostic criteria for PID (see Table 55–2). However, the ESR may be normal in 25% of PID cases, and it may not be useful in differentiating PID from other causes of pelvic pain. Other conditions associated with an inflammatory response will also cause an elevation of the ESR, however. The test has the advantage of being low in cost.

J. Culdocentesis. Needle aspiration of fluid from the posterior cul-de-sac is useful in the diagnosis of PID. The presence of nonclotting blood should raise suspicion of a ruptured ovarian cyst or ectopic pregnancy. This test is most appropriate when bleeding into the pelvic cavity is suspected. It has the disadvantage of being an invasive procedure.

K. Laparoscopy is the "gold standard" for diagnosis of pelvic pain. It is invasive and thus carries a degree of risk, although this risk is very low when the test is performed by an experienced physician. Its chief value is in determining treatable causes of previously undiagnosed pelvic pain.

L. Endometrial biopsy should be considered for any woman with pelvic pain and postmenopausal vaginal bleeding. Tissue sampling can be done in the ambulatory setting using instruments such as the Novak curette, the Vabra aspirator, or the Pipelle endometrial curette. The latter instrument has the advantage of usually not requiring cervical dilatation, analgesia, or anesthesia.

M. Papanicolaou (Pap) smears and **colposcopy** should both be used to evaluate a cervix with an abnormal appearance in a woman with pelvic pain. The Pap

---

TABLE 55–2. CRITERIA FOR THE DIAGNOSIS OF ACUTE PELVIC INFLAMMATORY DISEASE

Minimum criteria for clinical diagnosis of PID
1. Lower abdominal tenderness
2. Cervical motion tenderness
3. Adnexal tenderness (may be unilateral)

Additional criteria useful in diagnosing PID (for more specificity when the patient's presentation is more severe)

Routine
1. Oral temperature >38.3°C
2. Abnormal cervical or vaginal discharge
3. Elevated erythrocyte sedimentation rate and/or C-reactive protein
4. Culture or nonculture evidence of cervical infection with *Neisseria gonorrhoeae* or *Chlamydia trachomatis*—**recommended for all suspected cases of PID**

Elaborate
1. Histopathologic evidence on endometrial biopsy
2. Tubo-ovarian abscess on sonography
3. Laparoscopy

PID, Pelvic inflammatory disease.
From the Centers for Disease Control and Prevention recommendations, January 1998.

smear is inexpensive and easy to perform and can detect lesions hidden from the colposcope. It has a significant false-negative rate of 5–10% and has no place in the detection of endometrial carcinoma. Colposcopy, which is the direct visualization of the cervical mucosa and vascular patterns, allows determination of the extent of the abnormal lesion and is used to identify areas for biopsy. The disadvantages of colposcopy are that it cannot detect lesions of the endocervix and special training is required.

N. **CA-125 tests** can be used to detect elevated levels of this antigen, found in ovarian adenocarcinomas. The test is not very specific and can be associated with endometriosis and PID. It is most specific in postmenopausal patients who have a pelvic mass. Its sensitivity is also quite low. Therefore, its utility is not in screening but as an adjunct to other testing in symptomatic patients.

VIII. **Treatment**

A. **Endometriosis** (see Chapter 21).

B. **Ovarian masses** that are mobile on pelvic examination and appear to be cystic and ≤5 cm in diameter on ultrasonography are usually benign cysts and can be observed for one menstrual cycle. Functional ovarian cysts should resolve by that time. Because of the possibility of neoplasia or endometriosis, a cyst that persists longer than 8 weeks should be further evaluated by laparoscopy or laparotomy. Oral contraceptives, of any variety and in the usual dosage, may be used to hasten the cyst resolution by suppressing ovulation (see Chapter 101). Ovarian cysts >6 cm should be treated surgically. Ovarian masses in postmenopausal women should be evaluated surgically because of the higher likelihood of cancer.

C. **PID**

1. **Hospitalization.** Patients with the following conditions should be hospitalized for treatment with parenteral antibiotics and close monitoring: possible surgical emergencies such as appendicitis, a tubo-ovarian abscess, pregnancy, severe illness, inability to tolerate an outpatient regimen, and unresponsiveness to outpatient therapy and immunodeficient states such as HIV infection. Patients in whom reliable follow-up cannot be assured should be treated as inpatients. Hospitalization should also be considered for all nulliparous patients and others desiring future pregnancy.

2. Suggested **outpatient antibiotic therapy** is listed in Table 55–3.

D. **Adnexal torsion** requires immediate hospitalization and operative intervention. Tubal and ovarian function may be preserved if the problem is treated prior to the onset of infarction.

E. **Appendicitis** (see Chapter 1). Patients suspected of having acute appendicitis should be hospitalized and evaluated by a surgeon.

F. **Uterine fibroids** (see Chapter 21).

G. **Ectopic pregnancy** is a surgical emergency, especially if the tube has ruptured. Hemodynamic stabilization and preparation for surgery should be begun as soon as the diagnosis is likely. An unruptured ectopic pregnancy may be effectively treated pharmacologically with methotrexate, with the tube being preserved. Outpatient laparoscopic surgery may also be utilized for unruptured ectopic pregnancy.

H. **UTI** (see Chapter 24).

TABLE 55–3. OUTPATIENT THERAPY FOR PELVIC INFLAMMATORY DISEASE

Regimen A

Ofloxacin, 400 mg orally twice a day for 14 days,
plus
Metronidazole, 500 mg orally twice a day for 14 days

Regimen B

Ceftriaxone, 250 mg IM once
or
Cefoxitin, 2 g IM, plus **probenecid,** 1 g orally in a single dose concurrently once,
or
Other parenteral third-generation cephalosporin (eg, ceftizoxime or cefotaxime),
plus
Doxycycline, 100 mg orally twice a day for 14 days (include this regimen with one of the above regimens)

From the Centers for Disease Control and Prevention recommendations, January 1998.

    I. Mittelschmerz requires no specific therapy except reassurance in mild cases. Oral contraceptives, by inhibiting ovulation, may be of benefit to patients with severe intermenstrual pain.

    J. Cancers are treated often by a combination of surgery, radiation, and chemotherapy. Therapy must be individualized for the stage, tissue type, and patient desires. Such treatment should involve an oncologist familiar with the treatment of female genital cancers.

        1. The 5-year survival rate in patients with **cervical cancer** ranges from 92% for patients with in situ lesions to 70–90% for patients with invasive lesions confined to the cervix to 10% for patients with cancers that have spread beyond the true pelvis.

        2. For **endometrial carcinoma,** 5-year survival rates also vary. For patients in whom the cancer is confined to the uterine corpus, 96% survive 5 years; for patients in whom the cancer has extended outside the true pelvis, 28% survive for 5 years.

        3. The **ovarian carcinoma** 5-year survival rates range from 93% for patients with lesions limited to one ovary to 25% for patients in whom the disease is widely metastatic.

    K. Psychogenic pain. Once physical causes have been eliminated, psychotherapy is helpful to relieve any underlying psychological causes and to prevent unnecessary operative procedures.

REFERENCES

Berek J (editor): *Novak's Gynecology.* 12th ed. Williams & Wilkins; 1998.

Centers for Disease Control and Prevention: 1998 guidelines for treatment of sexually transmitted diseases. MMWR 1998;**47:**RR-1.

DeCherney AH, Pernol ML (editors): *Current Obstetric & Gynecologic Diagnosis & Treatment.* 8th ed. Appleton & Lange; 1994.

Landis SH, Murray T, Bolden S, et al: Cancer statistics, 1998. CA 1998;**48:**6.

Newkirk GR: Pelvic inflammatory disease: A contemporary approach. Am Fam Physician 1998; **53:**1127.

---

56   Proteinuria

William R. Scheibel, MD

    I. Definition. Proteinuria is the presence of urinary protein in concentrations >0.150 g/day in adults and >4 mg/m^2/hr in children. Protein excretion of >3.5 g/day is defined as a nephrotic level of proteinuria.

    II. Common diagnoses

    A. Benign proteinuria is the most common cause of a positive qualitative test result for urine protein.

        1. Functional proteinuria is a transient isolated proteinuria. Other abnormalities of the urine are not present.

        2. Idiopathic transient proteinuria is defined as isolated, self-limited proteinuria. It is found in otherwise healthy patients. Transient proteinuria occurs in 70–80% of young men with isolated proteinuria.

        3. Orthostatic proteinuria appears when a person is upright and accounts for up to 60% of all proteinuria seen in children.

        4. Constant proteinuria occurs in 5–10% of patients with isolated proteinuria. As many as 50% of these patients may develop hypertension during the next 5 years, and as many as 20% may develop renal insufficiency during the next 10 years following the development of constant proteinuria.

    B. Primary renal diseases, including acute glomerulonephritis, acute renal failure, acute tubular necrosis, and anomalies such as polycystic kidneys, may cause proteinuria.

    C. Drugs and **toxins,** including antibiotics, analgesics, anticonvulsants, antihypertensives, and heavy metals, may lead to proteinuria.

    D. Infectious diseases, including bacterial, viral, and parasitic diseases, may cause proteinuria.

E. Systemic illnesses that may give a positive qualitative test result for urine protein include amyloidosis, collagen vascular diseases, hypertension, malignancy, diabetes mellitus, pre-eclampsia, sarcoidosis, dehydration, cryoglobulinemia, and transplant rejection. About one third of type I diabetics and one quarter of type II diabetics develop persistent proteinuria.

F. Nephrotic syndrome is defined as massive proteinuria (>3.5 g/day), hypoalbuminemia (<3 g/dL), hyperlipidemia, and edema.

III. Epidemiology. Proteinuria is found in as many as 4% of men and 7% of women screened with a routine urinalysis. As many as 10% of school-aged children have proteinuria, with a peak prevalence at age 13 years for girls and 16 years for boys.

   A. Benign proteinuria. As many as 1.4% of asymptomatic patients with proteinuria are found to have a significant disease.

      1. Functional proteinuria can occur with fever, strenuous exercise, exposure to cold, emotional stress, congestive heart failure, seizures, or abdominal operations.

      2. Idiopathic transient proteinuria usually occurs in children and young adults.

   B. Primary renal diseases may cause patients to develop isolated proteinuria. This may occur with hematuria and can indicate a pathologic process of the glomerulus.

   C. Drugs and **toxins** likely to cause proteinuria are listed in Table 56–1.

   D. Infectious diseases likely to cause proteinuria are listed in Table 56–2.

   E. Systemic illnesses likely to cause proteinuria are listed in Table 56–2.

      1. Diabetes. Persistent proteinuria in diabetic patients indicates diabetic nephropathy, which causes end-stage renal disease in 26.4 of every 100,000 type II diabetics and 410.5 of every 100,000 type I diabetics annually. The incidence of persistent proteinuria in patients with type I diabetes is rare in the first 5 years of diabetes, rises rapidly and peaks in the second decade of the disease, and then declines.

IV. Pathophysiology

   A. Benign proteinuria results from poorly understood pathogenic mechanisms but may be related to changes in renal blood flow such as renal vasoconstriction or increased renal venous pressures.

TABLE 56–1. DRUGS CAUSING PROTEINURA

Acute interstitial nephritis
Cephalosporins
Penicillins
Sulfonamides

Aminoglycoside toxicity

Analgesic nephropathy
Nonsteroidal anti-inflammatory drugs

Anticonvulsants
Phenytoin
Trimethadione

Antihypertensive agents
Angiotensin-converting enzyme inhibitors

Cyclosporine toxicity

Heavy metals
Gold
Lead
Mercury

Heroin

Lithium

Penicillamine

Probenecid

Sulfonylureas
Tolbutamide

TABLE 56-2. SYSTEMIC ILLNESSES CAUSING PROTEINURIA

Infections	Multisystem diseases
Acute poststreptococcal glomerulonephritis	Amyloidosis
Bacterial	Cryoglobulinemia
Endocarditis	Diabetes mellitus
Syphilis	Goodpasture's syndrome
Tuberculosis	Henoch-Schönlein syndrome
Parasitic	Polyarteritis
Malaria	Pre-eclampsia
Toxoplasmosis	Sarcoidosis
Viral	Systemic lupus erythematosus
Cytomegalovirus	Transplant rejection
Epstein–Barr virus	
Hepatitis B	
Human immunodeficiency virus	
Cancers	
Carcinoma	
Leukemia	
Lymphoma–Hodgkin's disease	
Multiple myeloma	

- B. **Glomerular proteinuria** is caused by increased glomerular capillary permeability to protein because of structural injury. **Primary glomerular diseases** include minimal change disease, focal segmental glomerulosclerosis, membranous glomerulonephropathy, and mesangial proliferative glomerulonephritis. **Secondary glomerular diseases** include infections (acute poststreptococcal glomerulonephritis), systemic illnesses (systemic lupus erythematosus), and drug-induced disorders (lipoid nephrosis).
- C. **Tubular proteinuria** occurs because of tubular dysfunction with decreased reabsorption of proteins in the glomerular filtrate. Congenital anomalies, acute renal failure, tubular necrosis, and interstitial nephritis caused by drugs or infections are examples of this pathologic process.
- D. **Overload proteinuria** is caused by increased production of abnormal proteins, usually low-molecular-weight proteins, which pass freely through the glomerulus in large amounts and exceed the resorptive capacity of the tubules. This condition occurs in patients with multiple myeloma and leukemia.
- E. **Nephrotic syndrome** is the consequence of excessive glomerular leakage of plasma proteins into the urine. Intrinsic glomerular disease is the cause of the nephrotic syndrome in 75% of patients with this syndrome.
- V. **Symptoms.** It is rare to find any symptoms of proteinuria except in patients with the nephrotic syndrome, in whom swelling may be prominent.
    - A. An isolated finding of a positive qualitative test result for urine protein in an asymptomatic patient may indicate benign proteinuria.
    - B. Characteristic symptoms of primary renal disease or systemic illness may appear in a patient with proteinuria that is caused by the pathologic process of an underlying disease.
        - 1. Red or cola-colored urine can be a presenting symptom of acute glomerulonephritis.
        - 2. Polydipsia or polyuria can indicate uncontrolled diabetes.
        - 3. Joint stiffness or pain may be the presenting complaint of lupus erythematosus.
        - 4. Fatigue, weakness, anorexia, and malaise may be associated with chronic renal insufficiency.
- VI. **Signs.** If the patient excretes <2 g of protein daily, signs will usually be absent.
    - A. **Periorbital edema, peripheral edema, ascites,** or **pleural effusions** may result from a decrease in serum albumin level and plasma oncotic pressure from nephrotic levels of proteinuria.
    - B. **Elevated blood pressure** may aggravate proteinuria in patients with primary renal disease.
    - C. A **toxic neuropathy** may indicate heavy metal poisoning.

    D. Fever may be present with infection.

    E. A **heart murmur** may accompany bacterial endocarditis.

    F. Characteristic signs of systemic illness may appear in patients whose proteinuria is caused by such illness.

        1. Adenopathy, organomegaly, and **masses** can occur with cancer.

        2. Malar rash and **joint inflammation** are usually present with lupus erythematosus.

        3. Diabetic retinopathy is strongly associated with proteinuria in diabetics.

VII. Laboratory tests and their use are outlined in Figure 56–1.

    A. The **initial screen** for proteinuria is a qualitative test of protein concentration (by **dipstick**) performed on a random clean-catch urine sample.

        1. Qualitative tests detect urine protein concentrations of >10–30 mg/dL and give positive results if used in relatively concentrated samples. Colormetric reactions are graded from yellow (negative) to green (2+, 100 mg/dL) to blue (4±, 1000 mg/dL). Qualitative tests should be repeated on a second sample if there is a ≥1+ reaction.

            a. False-positive dipstick test results can occur with highly concentrated urines, gross hematuria, contamination with antiseptics, or highly alkaline urines (pH >8.0). Radiographic contrast media, analogs of cephalosporin or penicillin, or metabolites of tolbutamide or sulfonamide can give false-positive tests with turbidimetric assays.

            b. False-negative qualitative test results may occur with dilute urines. Dipstick qualitative urine tests are relatively insensitive to proteins other than albumin and may give a false-negative result for nonalbumin proteins such as Bence Jones proteins. Nonalbumin proteins can be detected by protein precipitation methods (turbidimetric assays).

        2. A **24-hour urine test** for protein and creatinine levels will verify a repeated positive qualitative test result.

            a. A normal 24-hour **urinary protein** level indicates a false-positive qualitative test result or transient proteinuria.

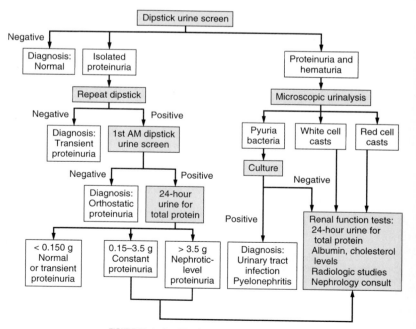

FIGURE 56–1. Algorithm for evaluation of proteinuria.

     b. Urinary creatinine will validate an adequate urinary collection if it is in the normal range (16–26 mg/kg body weight per day for males and 12–24 mg/kg body weight per day for females). A 24-hour urine creatinine test will allow the calculation of a creatinine clearance ($\frac{\text{urine creatinine} \times \text{volume}}{\text{plasma creatinine}}$),

which is a good measure of renal function. Inulin or [^{125}I]iothalamate clearance measures the actual glomerular filtration rate but is not readily available.

     c. A negative qualitative test result on a first-morning specimen (recumbent) followed 2 hours later by a positive test result on a second sample (upright) indicates **orthostatic proteinuria.** This can be confirmed with a separate, timed 12-hour urine collection, supine and ambulatory.

     d. Microalbuminuria is defined as urine albumin levels between 30 mg/24 hr (20 µg/min) and 300 mg/24 hr (200 µg/min) and is used to screen diabetic patients for the development of diabetic nephropathy.

B. Urinalysis of a freshly collected specimen is needed to diagnose primary renal disease. Positive urine cultures indicate infection.

    1. Red blood cell casts indicate glomerulonephritis.

    2. White blood cell casts indicate an inflammatory process such as pyelonephritis or interstitial nephritis.

C. Blood tests should be performed when systemic disease is suspected.

    1. Serum creatinine and **blood urea nitrogen (BUN)** levels should be determined in order to evaluate renal function. Creatinine clearance is more accurate, especially in elderly patients with decreased muscle mass.

    2. Blood glucose or a **glycolysated hemoglobin test** is helpful in the detection of diabetes mellitus.

    3. Protein electrophoresis or **immunoelectrophoresis** of urine and serum may assist in the diagnosis of multiple myeloma or other monoclonal gammopathies.

    4. Complement studies may be helpful in the diagnosis of immune complex diseases.

    5. Antistreptococcal enzyme titers can help the physician diagnose poststreptococcal glomerulonephritis.

    6. Fluorescent antinuclear antibody tests may indicate the presence of systemic lupus erythematosus.

    7. Serum albumin levels will be decreased in patients with nephrotic syndrome.

    8. The **complete blood cell count (CBC)** should be determined to help the physician identify infection or the anemia of renal insufficiency.

D. Radiographic evaluation may detect congenital or malignant disease.

    1. Intravenous pyelography or **computerized tomographic (CT) scans** of the kidney with contrast can show structural or obstructive pathology. There is a risk of contrast-induced acute renal failure in patients with diabetes, renal insufficiency, or multiple myeloma.

    2. Renal ultrasonography can be of value in determining renal size, obstruction, and congenital cysts.

    3. Voiding cystourethrogram is useful in documenting reflux.

E. Renal biopsy is reserved for diagnosing and differentiating the glomerulonephropathies and is usually performed on most patients with nephrotic-range proteinuria.

VIII. Treatment of proteinuria is directed at the underlying cause.

A. Benign proteinuria (<1000 mg/24 hr) usually requires no treatment.

    1. Transient proteinuria requires no further evaluation or follow-up, as no harmful sequelae have been documented.

    2. Intermittent protein excretion often remits, especially in young patients, but in older patients the problem can progress and should be monitored with a yearly urinalysis and blood pressure reading.

    3. Orthostatic proteinuria involves a low risk of progression. Patients with this problem have a 50% chance of remission over 10 years. Follow-up of this problem should occur every 1–2 years, if proteinuria persists, and should involve a blood pressure check as well as urinalysis.

B. Primary renal disease

    1. Supportive therapy, including **sodium,** 2 g/day, and **fluid restriction** may help relieve fluid retention.

2. **Loop diuretics** such as **furosemide,** 20–400 mg/day, can be used to treat circulatory congestion, edema, and hypertension. These agents have not been shown to alter the course of acute renal failure or to improve the patient's chance of survival, however.
3. **Dietary protein restriction** may be of benefit in preventing progression of renal disease and is usually limited to 20–40 g (0.5 g/kg) of protein per day, with 100 g of carbohydrate per day if azotemia is present.
4. **Corticosteroids** such as **prednisone,** 1–1.5 mg/kg/day, and cytotoxic drugs such as **cyclophosphamide,** 1–2 mg/kg/day, may be of benefit to patients with certain types of nephrotic syndrome and primary glomerulonephritis.
5. **Renal dialysis** is indicated for patients with progressive renal failure and should be initiated when any of the following conditions exist: volume overload, severe acidosis, hyperkalemia, or uremia (BUN >80–100 mg/dL or creatinine >8–10 mg/dL).
6. **Renal transplantation** should be considered when a poor quality of life or health exists on dialysis, or with younger patients when a donor is available.

C. **Removal of toxins or medications** can reverse or at least prevent progression of proteinuria.
D. **Appropriate antibiotics** can resolve infectious causes of proteinuria (see Chapter 24).
E. **Specific treatment of the systemic illness** may resolve or improve proteinuria (see Chapters 71, 78, and 80).
1. **Constant proteinuria** is associated with a higher mortality rate and involves a greater risk of death from renal disease. It is therefore recommended that this problem be followed every 6 months to 1 year with urinalysis, blood pressure, and renal function studies.
2. **Hypertensive therapy** in a patient with nephropathy characterized by proteinuria can delay progression of renal failure.
3. **Corticosteroids** and cytotoxic drugs may improve proteinuria from lupus nephritis.

REFERENCES

Ettenger RB: The evaluation of the child with proteinuria. Pediatr Ann 1994;**23**(9):486.
Hricik DE, Chung-Park M, Sedor JR: Glomerulonephritis. N Engl J Med 1998;**339**:888.
Larson TS: Evaluation of proteinuria. Mayo Clin Proc 1994;**69**:1154.
Mahan JD, Truman MA, Mentser MI: Evaluation of hematuria, proteinuria, and hypertension in adolescents. Pediatr Clin North Am 1997;**44**:1573.
Mosre J Jr, Carome MA: Proteinuria. Clin Lab Med 1993;**13**(1):21.
Springberg PD, Garrett LE Jr, Thompson AL Jr, et al: Fixed reproducible orthostatic proteinuria: Results of a 20 year follow-up study. Ann Intern Med 1982;**97**:516.

57   Rectal Pain

Cathryn B. Heath, MD

I. **Definition.** *Rectal pain* refers to irritation, soreness, or discomfort in the anal area between the buttocks. *Tenesmus* refers to painful sphincter contractions with involuntary ineffectual straining efforts.
II. **Common diagnoses.**
   A. **Anal fissures.**
   B. **Hemorrhoids.**
   C. **Proctitis.**
   D. **Infected pilonidal cysts.**
   E. **Pruritus ani.**
   F. **Proctalgia fugax.**
III. **Epidemiology.** Rectal pain is a common outpatient complaint, often brought to medical attention only after home treatments have been ineffective in relieving symptoms. The prevalence of specific disorders is difficult to determine because of frequent misidentification of the source of pain by patients and physicians alike. The most common cause of rectal pain is anal fissures, not hemorrhoids.

    A. Anal fissures are equally common in men and women and can also occur in children of all ages.

    B. Hemorrhoids are found in 4.4% of the US population. They are equally prevalent in men and women and are more common with increasing age.

    C. Proctitis is common in those participating in anal intercourse, including both homosexuals and heterosexuals. It also occurs with inflammatory bowel disease or after radiation therapy for prostate, ovarian, or colon cancer. Proctitis can lead to **abscess** formation.

    D. Pilonidal cysts occur more frequently in those with sedentary occupations.

    E. Pruritus ani affects men more often than women. It is more common in the 40–60 age group, but can be found in individuals of any age. It is most commonly found in individuals with diabetes mellitus, obesity, or sensitive skin. It generally lasts 6 weeks.

    F. Proctalgia fugax occurs most often in adults who are under stress.

IV. Pathophysiology

    A. Anal fissures are related to passage of an abnormal bowel movement. These painful ulcers of the anal mucosa frequently result from consistently high feces volume, explosive diarrhea, or constipation. Increased sphincter tone causes constricted anal blood vessels, which lead to chronic ischemic fissures.

    B. Hemorrhoids. When anchoring and supporting tissues around the anal canal deteriorate, veins in the anorectal mucosal tissues become tortuous and dilated from obstruction of the entrapped blood. These enlarged nonfunctioning veins then bulge and descend in the anal canal lumen, becoming subject to increased pressure from straining and trauma. They can extend so far as to prolapse through an abnormally tight anal sphincter, thus becoming trapped and nonreducible. Thrombosed hemorrhoids cause an inflammatory reaction by activating tissue thromboplastin within the hemorrhoidal blood vessels.

    C. Proctitis. Most causes of proctitis are sexually transmitted through the anal sphincter by direct invasion of the infectious agent through the mucous membrane. The most common infectious agents are herpes simplex virus, *Neisseria gonorrhoeae, Chlamydia trachomatis,* and *Treponema pallidum.* Proctitis can also arise from colitis due to *Shigella* spp, *Campylobacter fetus,* or *Giardia lamblia,* in which case it is referred to as proctocolitis. Herpes simplex and *Condyloma acuminata* infections can occur either above or below the anal sphincter. In human immunodeficiency virus (HIV)–positive patients, herpes simplex virus accounts for 40% of the cases of proctitis. For additional information, see Chapters 55 and 67.

    D. Pilonidal cysts. These dermoid cysts of involuted epithelium are found in the sacral area. Traditionally believed to be an inherited defect, these cysts are now thought to be caused solely by prolonged repetitious irritation about the sacral area. Pilonidal cysts are especially prevalent in individuals with certain sedentary occupations such as truck or bus driving and may result from occult fecal leakage as a result of abnormal internal sphincter relaxation.

    E. Pruritus ani can occur from diarrhea, poor hygiene, or transient sphincter relaxation. These factors result in excessive moisture around the anal canal, causing a breakdown of the epidermal layer of skin into which mycotic infections, *Candida* spp, pinworms, lice, and *Condyloma acuminata* can invade the damaged skin and cause secondary infection. Abnormal transient sphincter relaxation may cause fecal soilage. Environmental factors such as excessive skin cleaning, mucous seepage, perspiration, or tight underclothes, as well as caffeine and spicy foods, may be implicated as causes of pruritus ani. Anal cancer may present as pruritus ani, especially in those with longstanding symptoms refractory to primary treatment.

    F. Proctalgia fugax is attributed to spasm of the levator ani and coccygeal muscles.

V. Symptoms

    A. Anal fissures can cause a tearing rectal pain with evacuation. The pain may cease immediately after the bowel movement or may last for several hours. The pain can be so acute and intense that the patient's fear of having another bowel movement causes severe constipation. Bleeding, pruritus, and the sensation of a mass in the rectal area are common symptoms of anal fissures.

    B. Hemorrhoids do not cause severe pain unless they are thrombosed. More often, patients complain of bright red bleeding mixed with or coating the stool, in the toilet bowl, or on the toilet paper. Bleeding may be accompanied by fecal soilage, pruritus, and prolapse.

    C. Proctitis most commonly causes a rectal discharge, tenesmus, and rectal pain. If the lower colon is involved, the patient may have abdominal pain, cramping, and changing stool consistency. **Abscesses** cause continual pain.

    D. Infected **pilonidal cysts** cause pain in the sacral area, superior to the rectum.

    E. Pruritus ani is an intense itching sensation of the rectal area that may be associated with mucous discharge. By the time most patients arrive at the physician's office, they have tried many over-the-counter treatments that may have exacerbated the condition.

    F. Proctalgia fugax presents as abrupt, sharp, nonradiating pain in the anorectal area. The pain often occurs at night. Relief occurs within seconds to minutes.

VI. Signs

    A. Anal fissures are small, longitudinal ulcers in the anal canal located posteriorly in 95% of patients. In the acute phase, digital examination of the rectum may be impossible because of pain and internal sphincter spasm. Chronic fissures also show hypertrophy of the anal papillae and a sentinel pile or tag at the anal verge. Multiple fissures of varying depth and with ragged edges should raise suspicions of inflammatory bowel disease. Fissures can accompany proctitis, abscesses, or neoplasms.

    B. Hemorrhoids. External hemorrhoids located below the dentate line are covered by anoderm and skin and have cutaneous nerve sensation. Internal hemorrhoids are commonly characterized as (1) first degree (small and nonprolapsing), (2) second degree (prolapsing with defecation but spontaneously reducible), (3) third degree (prolapsing with defecation and manually reducible), and (4) fourth degree (prolapsing and nonreducible).

    C. Proctitis. Findings can range from a mild mucoid exudate to marked infection with spontaneous bleeding, purulent discharge, and erosions. Patients who are HIV positive tend to exhibit the latter condition.

        1. Patients with herpes simplex typically present with papules, vesicles with red areolae, shallow ulcerations, and crusts around the anal and genital areas.

        2. Infection with *Chlamydia trachomatis* causes severe inflammation and fistulae of the rectum.

        3. Infection with *N gonorrhoeae* causes erythema, discharge, and swelling in the anal canal.

        4. Syphilis causes single or multiple pink chancres with a regular surface, covered with discharge.

        5. *Giardia lamblia, Shigella* spp, or *Campylobacter fetus* may cause diarrhea during the rectal examination.

    D. Infected **pilonidal cysts** cause erythema and swelling over the sacrum and are often fluctuant.

    E. Pruritus ani may have no physical signs, although usually a slight mucous discharge, accompanied by a mild erythema but no fluctuance or warmth, is seen at the anal verge. Chronic excoriation with bleeding may also occur.

    F. There are no real signs of **proctalgia fugax.** The anal area looks completely normal.

VII. Laboratory tests

    A. Anoscopy is essential in the evaluation of all patients with anorectal pain, except those with pilonidal cysts. A hand-held anoscope attached to a battery-operated halogen light source leaves the physician with a free hand to obtain cultures or biopsies. Following a gloved digital rectal examination, the anoscope should be warmed with water and eased in slowly while the patient bears down as if having a bowel movement so as to relax the external sphincter. Anoscopy may be impossible initially in those patients who have a fissure, but should be scheduled on a repeat visit in order to detect occult inflammatory bowel disease or rectal cancer.

    B. Flexible fibrosigmoidoscopy is an important procedure for elderly patients and for those with a history of familial polyposis to rule out an occult malignancy. Crohn's disease or ulcerative colitis may appear as fissures or proctitis in younger patients, but if these patients do not respond to a short course of conservative treatment, the physician should perform flexible fibrosigmoidoscopy. This procedure is not necessary in patients with pilonidal cysts.

    C. Additional studies in patients with proctitis. Anoscopy and a gram-stained slide of rectal discharge allow a causative diagnosis in 92% of patients with proctitis. Proctitis is confirmed by finding more than one polymorphonuclear leukocyte per oil immersion field on a gram-stained slide of the rectal discharge.

1. Gram-negative diplococci on a gram-stained slide confirm the diagnosis of gonorrhea.
2. Syphilis can be diagnosed by rapid plasma reagin and, if available, dark-field examination of the rectal discharge.
3. If a diagnosis is not easily discernible, cultures for *N gonorrhoeae,* herpes simplex virus, and *Chlamydia trachomatis* should be obtained.
4. Stool examination for enteric pathogens and ova and parasites should be considered in patients with symptoms of enterocolitis to rule out infection from *Campylobacter fetus, Shigella* spp, *G lamblia,* and *Cryptosporidium* spp. *Cryptosporidium* is common in immunocompromised patients.

VIII. Treatment
A. Anal fissures
1. Most anal fissures can be treated conservatively with increased dietary fiber, bulk laxatives, and sitz baths.
2. Those patients who do not respond to conservative treatment or have chronic fissures require a **lateral internal anal sphincterotomy,** most often performed in a 1-day surgery unit. This method is nearly 100% effective, and patients have few recurrences.
3. Some physicians are treating fissures with **topical nitroglycerin ointment** once daily until healing occurs. This presently needs to be compounded by a pharmacist with 2% nitroglycerin ointment diluted in a waxy substrate in a 1:10 ratio for a 0.2% ointment.

B. Hemorrhoids
1. **General measures** for hemorrhoid reduction.
   a. Patients should be cautioned to avoid straining.
   b. Although there are few studies to prove efficacy, most authorities recommend bran and bulk laxatives in the treatment of first- and second-degree hemorrhoids.
   c. Sitz baths and cool compresses for 15 minutes three times a day can be useful.
   d. A twice-daily application of a steroid-containing suppository (eg, **Anusol HC**) for 10 days can be helpful.
   e. Over-the-counter ointments (eg, Preparation H) have not been proven effective, although they are commonly used.
2. **Rubber band ligation** is the most common procedure and can be performed on second- and third-degree hemorrhoids. A rubber band ligator "gun" and an assistant to hold the anoscope are required. The hemorrhoid is grasped with a clamp and pulled through the barrel of the gun, then the rubber band is forced onto the base of the tissue when the trigger is pulled. The ligation band should be placed 7 mm above the pectinate line or the patient will experience severe discomfort. Since the procedure can be painful, the remaining hemorrhoids may be ligated one at a time at 2-week intervals.
3. **Surgical resection** is reserved for large third- and fourth-degree hemorrhoids. This surgery can usually be accomplished in same-day surgery under local anesthesia; patients are generally able to return to work within 2 weeks.
4. Other, less effective treatments of second- and third-degree hemorrhoids include **infrared photocoagulation, bipolar diathermy** (Bicap), and **laser photocoagulation,** all of which cause localized tissue destruction by increasing the temperature of a 3-mm area very rapidly. Sclerosing with 5% phenol solution in vegetable oil with 2–3 mL injected into the submucosa of the right anterolateral, right posterolateral, and left lateral areas approximately 3 cm above the dentate line is also used. All methods have very few side effects and are most often performed in the general or colorectal surgeon's office.
5. Thrombosed hemorrhoids can be treated conservatively with a **bulk diet** and **bed rest** for 3 days. Complete resolution usually occurs within 3 weeks. If the patient is unable to take time from work, an alternative treatment consists of anesthetizing the area locally and then excising and extracting the clot, using an elliptical incision. This works best if performed within 48 hours of initial pain.

C. Proctitis should be treated with a specific antiviral or antibiotic agent if clinical findings lead the physician to suspect a specific cause.

    1. Empiric therapy of **ceftriaxone,** 250 mg intramuscularly, and 7 days of either **doxycycline,** 100 mg twice daily, or **erythromycin,** 500 mg four times daily, should be given. Follow-up cultures should be done after the antibiotics are finished, as one quarter of patients with proctitis fail to respond to empiric therapy.

    2. If the patient has a primary herpes infection, **acyclovir,** 400 mg orally five times a day for 10 days, is indicated. Patients with acquired immunodeficiency syndrome (AIDS) who have frequent herpes simplex virus infections may benefit from suppressive therapy with **acyclovir,** 200 mg orally two to five times daily.

    3. If a perirectal abscess occurs, surgical drainage is necessary and can be performed under local anesthesia immediately after diagnosis is made.

D. Infected pilonidal cysts should be treated with **cephalexin,** 1 g orally twice daily for 10 days, or **amoxicillin-clavulanic acid,** 500 mg three times daily for 10 days. Surgical excision of the cyst, frequently performed on an outpatient basis, should be postponed for at least 4 weeks to allow for control of abscess inflammation.

E. Pruritus ani

    1. Patients with **pruritus ani associated with hypersensitivity** should be advised to discontinue use of all creams and ointments, keep the anal region clean and dry, avoid the use of toilet paper, pat rather than rub the anus dry after elimination, and wear loose, cotton undergarments. Antihistamines (eg, **Benadryl,** 25–50 mg orally every 4–6 hours) may be useful to break the chronic itch-scratch cycle.

    2. Patients with **infective pruritus ani** should be treated for the appropriate cause.

        a. Tinea and *Candida* respond well to 1% **clotrimazole** cream applied twice daily for up to 4 weeks.

        b. Pinworms are treated with one 100-mg dose of **mebendazole** or a single 1-g dose of **pyrantel pamoate.**

        c. *Condyloma acuminata* can be eradicated by treatments with **liquid nitrogen** or 10% **podophyllin** applied by the physician. Podophyllin should be washed from the treated area 6 hours after application or sooner if the patient experiences burning or swelling of the anal area. **Podofilox** applied by the patient every 12 hours for 3 consecutive days is an alternative. Application may be repeated after 4 days.

F. Reassurance of the benign nature of **proctalgia fugax** is often all that is necessary. Warm baths and massage may correct moderate cases. In severe cases, inhaled **albuterol,** one or two puffs every 3 hours as necessary for pain, or oral **diltiazem,** 2.5–5 mg every 6 hours as necessary, may help.

REFERENCES

Janicke DM, Pundt MR: Anorectal disorders. Emerg Med Clin North Am 1996;**14:**757.

Lund JN, Scholefield JH: A randomised, prospective, double-blind, placebo-controlled trial of glyceryl trinitrate ointment in treatment of anal fissure. Lancet 1997;**349:**11.

MacRae HM, McLeod RS: Comparison of hemorrhoidal treatment modalities. A meta-analysis. Dis Colon Rectum 1995;**38:**687.

Pfenninger JL, Surrell J: Nonsurgical treatment options for internal hemorrhoids. Am Fam Physician 1995;**52:**821.

---

58   The Red Eye

Dana W. Peterson, MD

I. Definition. The red eye is a physical manifestation of inflammation in the eye that causes vasodilation of the conjunctival, episcleral, or scleral vessels.

II. Common diagnoses. These include viral, bacterial, allergic, and irritant conjunctivitis, corneal abrasions and foreign bodies, subconjunctival hemorrhage, episcleritis and scleritis, keratitis, iritis, and acute angle-closure glaucoma.

III. Epidemiology. Two percent to 3% of all ambulatory patients present with ocular symptoms.
   A. Conjunctivitis. Viral conjunctivitis and allergic reactions are more common than bacterial conjunctivitis.
      1. Viral conjunctivitis occurs in epidemics and is most common in young adults.
      2. Bacterial conjunctivitis may be seen in patients of all ages at any time of year and may also occur in an epidemic form known as pinkeye.
      3. Allergic conjunctivitis is sporadic and seasonal and frequently occurs in patients with a history of allergies during times of high pollen counts.
      4. Irritant conjunctivitis is often caused by dust or smoke exposure.
   B. Corneal abrasions and foreign bodies occur most frequently in patients who spend time outdoors or in environments such as metal shops or lumber mills.
   C. Subconjunctival hemorrhage can occur spontaneously, as a result of trauma, or subsequent to recurrent Valsalva's maneuvers such as in coughing or during obstetric deliveries.
   D. Episcleritis and scleritis occur in patients with systemic autoimmune and connective tissue disorders.
   E. Keratitis. Immunocompromised patients may be at increased risk for contracting this disorder.
   F. Iritis. Fifty percent of patients with iritis are positive for HLA-B27, indicating a genetic predisposition.
   G. Acute angle-closure glaucoma is more common in individuals over the age of 50 than in younger patients. Patients frequently have a positive family history of the condition, and women are affected more often than men.

IV. Pathophysiology
   A. Conjunctivitis. Inflammation of the conjunctiva may be caused by bacterial, chlamydial, or viral infection or by allergic or irritant stimuli.
      1. Viral conjunctivitis may be caused by many viruses, especially adenovirus, picornavirus, rhinovirus, and herpesvirus.
      2. Bacterial conjunctivitis is commonly caused by *Staphylococcus aureus, Streptococcus pneumoniae,* group A streptococcus, *Haemophilus influenzae,* and *Neisseria gonorrhoeae. Chlamydia trachomatis* can cause a pathologically unique form of infectious conjunctivitis called **inclusion conjunctivitis.**
      3. Allergic conjunctivitis is caused by a hypersensitivity reaction to a specific antigen.
      4. Irritant conjunctivitis is caused by smoke, irritating fumes, or dust exposure to the eye.
   B. Corneal abrasions and foreign bodies cause irritation, inflammation, and pain. Most corneal foreign bodies are small particles that stick to the anterior surface of the cornea. Subtarsal foreign bodies may become implanted on the palpebral conjunctiva, causing the cornea to become irritated when the patient blinks.
   C. Subconjunctival hemorrhage usually results from rupture of a small blood vessel in the conjunctival tissue and frequently develops after episodes of coughing or straining.
   D. Episcleritis and scleritis are unusual inflammatory conditions that are associated with rheumatoid arthritis and other collagen vascular and autoimmune disorders.
   E. Keratitis. Bacterial, fungal, and viral organisms can cause infection of the cornea primarily or secondary to an event that has compromised corneal integrity. Herpes simplex virus, in particular, may cause keratitis. Alteration in the defense mechanisms of the eye may result from trauma, the use of contact lenses, or steroid eye drops.
   F. Iritis. Inflammation of the iris and the ciliary body, also known as iridocyclitis or anterior uveitis, may be idiopathic or may develop in response to coexistent conjunctivitis, keratitis, or eye trauma. Systemic diseases associated with iritis include ankylosing spondylitis, psoriatic arthritis, Reiter's syndrome, Behçet's syndrome, inflammatory bowel disease, sarcoidosis, and a variety of chronic infections, including syphilis, tuberculosis, toxoplasmosis, and histoplasmosis.
   G. Acute angle-closure glaucoma. In persons predisposed to angle-closure glaucoma, the angle between the corneal surface and the iris is narrowed. In an acute episode, iris tissue bulges anteriorly, closing off the flow of fluid through the trabecular meshwork, resulting in increased pressure in the anterior chamber and an acute rise in intraocular pressure.

V. Symptoms (see Table 58–1)

VI. Signs (see Table 58–2)

VII. Laboratory tests

A. **Culture of eye discharge.** Most cases of conjunctivitis encountered in the ambulatory care setting are self-limited, and the cost-benefit ratio of culture of eye discharge is excessively high. In patients with severe infections and in cases that do not respond to therapy, cultures of the conjunctiva or the cornea may be helpful.

B. **Microscopic examination** of eye discharge or conjunctival scrapings may be helpful in characterizing the cause of conjunctivitis.

1. **Gram's stain examination** should be considered for any patient with a severe conjunctival discharge. It may aid in the choice of topical antibiotics and rapidly identify cases of gonococcal conjunctivitis. Multinucleated giant cells or intranuclear inclusions are highly suggestive of herpetic infection.

2. **Wright-stained smears** may show numerous polymorphonuclear cells in bacterial conjunctivitis, lymphocytes in viral conjunctivitis, and eosinophils in allergic conjunctivitis.

3. **Conjunctival scrapings subjected to Giemsa stain** show large basophilic cytoplasmic inclusion bodies in patients with inclusion conjunctivitis and confirm the diagnosis.

C. **Tonometry** should be performed using a Schiötz' tonometer if acute glaucoma cannot be ruled out by history and physical examination.

D. **Fluorescein staining** of the cornea or examination of the eye with a slit lamp confirms the diagnosis of corneal abrasion and facilitates identification of foreign bodies. Slit lamp examination is also useful in characterizing iritis, keratitis, episcleritis, and scleritis.

VIII. Treatment. Warning signs that indicate a serious ocular disease requiring referral and evaluation by an ophthalmologist include decreased visual acuity, deep eye pain, photophobia, the presence of a ciliary flush, corneal opacification, pupil abnormalities, increased intraocular pressure, or symptoms that fail to improve after 24–48 hours of treatment.

A. **Conjunctivitis.** All patients should be advised of general hygienic measures such as avoiding eye-to-hand contact, washing hands thoroughly, and not sharing face towels. Cool compresses to the eyes may give some relief.

1. **Viral conjunctivitis** generally requires no specific treatment beyond hygienic measures.

2. **Bacterial conjunctivitis.** Topical antibiotic therapy shortens the duration. When bacterial infection is suspected, the preferred therapy is **sodium sulfacetamide ophthalmic solution 10%** (eg, Bleph-10, Cetamide, or Sulamyd),

TABLE 58–1. SYMPTOMS OF COMMON CAUSES OF RED EYE

Condition	Eye Pain	Discharge	Visual Acuity	Other Associated Photophobia	Symptoms
Viral conjunctivitis	Burning, mild	+++	Normal	–	Upper respiratory infection
Bacterial conjunctivitis	Burning, mild to moderate	+++	Normal	–	Exposure history
Allergic conjunctivitis	Burning, mild	+++	Normal	–	Rhinitis
Corneal abrasions and foreign bodies	Moderate to severe	++	Normal decreased	+	History of eye trauma
Subconjunctival hemorrhage	None	None	Normal	–	History of coughing or straining
Episcleritis and scleritis	Mild to moderate aching	+	Usually normal	+	
Keratitis	Moderate to severe	+	Usually decreased	+	
Iritis	Moderate aching	+	Usually decreased	++	
Angle-closure glaucoma	Severe with headache	None	Usually decreased	++	Nausea or vomiting

TABLE 58–2. PHYSICAL FINDINGS IN COMMON CAUSES OF RED EYE

Condition	Eye Discharge	Pupil Size and Reactivity	Ciliary Flush[1]	Corneal Appearance	Redness of Eye	Intraocular Pressure
Viral conjunctivitis	Watery	Equal and normal	–	Normal	++	Normal
Bacterial conjunctivitis	Purulent	Equal and normal	–	Normal	+++	Normal
Allergic conjunctivitis	Watery	Equal and normal	–	Normal	+	Normal
Corneal abrasions and foreign bodies	Watery	Equal and normal	–	Abrasion visible with fluorescent staining	+	Normal
Subconjunctival hemorrhage	None	Equal and normal	–	Normal	+++	Normal
Episcleritis and scleritis	Minimal	Equal and normal	±	Normal	Localized area (+)	Normal
Keratitis	Minimal	Equal and normal	+	Clouded	Diffuse (++)	Normal
Iritis	Minimal	Affected pupil smaller	+	Normal	Central (+)	Normal
Acute angle-closure glaucoma	None	Mid-dilated, decreased reactivity to light	+	Clouded	Diffuse (++)	>21.5 mm

[1] Ciliary flush is an inflammation of deeper vessels in the limbal area of the eye.

one or two drops to each eye every 2–3 hours while the patient is awake, continued for 1 week. If the patient is allergic to sulfa drugs, other broad-spectrum agents, such as **erythromycin ointment,** aminoglycoside antibiotic solutions (eg, **gentamicin** or **tobramycin**), or quinolone solutions (eg, **norfloxacin, ciprofloxacin,** or **ofloxacin**), are alternatives. Follow-up is indicated if the symptoms persist or worsen.

3. **Conjunctivitis from** *N gonorrhoeae* or *Chlamydia* **species.** Systemic and topical antibiotics are required. Current guidelines for the treatment of sexually transmitted diseases should be followed (see Chapter 64).

4. **Allergic conjunctivitis.** When mild symptoms are present, topical antihistamine/vasoconstrictor eyedrops (eg, **Naphcon-A** or **Opcon-A,** one or two drops four times daily) and cool compresses are effective treatment. For more severe symptoms, one or two drops twice daily of **olopatadine hydrochloride 0.1%** (Patanol) will often provide relief. Combination therapy with an oral antihistamine (see Chapter 59) may also be helpful. **Cromolyn sodium 4%** (Crolom) or **lodoxamide tromethamine 0.1%** (Alomide) eye drops, one or two drops in each eye four to six times daily, may prevent symptoms, but this method requires several weeks of therapy before the maximal effect is achieved. **Ketorolac tromethamine 0.5%** (Acular), one drop in each eye four times daily for up to 1 week, or **levocabastime hydrochloride 0.05%** (Livostin), one drop in each eye four times daily for up to 2 weeks, may be useful for short-term treatment of severe symptoms.

5. **Topical corticosteroids and anesthetics** are not recommended in the treatment of conjunctivitis.

B. **Foreign body.** A foreign body on the cornea may be removed with the use of a topical anesthetic. The foreign body may be carefully removed with a sterile needle. Cotton swabs should not be used on the cornea but may be used to remove foreign bodies from the conjunctiva. After removal of the foreign body, an ophthalmic topical antibiotic ointment should be placed in the eye, and the eye may be patched for a period of 24 hours for comfort. If the patient's symptoms have not improved in 24 hours or if the foreign body cannot be easily removed, referral to an ophthalmologist is indicated.

C. **Subconjunctival hemorrhage** requires no treatment and will spontaneously resolve over a period of several days to weeks.

D. **Episcleritis and scleritis.** Referral to an ophthalmologist is indicated for both of these conditions because recurrences are common.

E. **Keratitis.** Urgent referral to an ophthalmologist is indicated. Intensive treatment with topical antibiotics and injections of antibiotics into the subconjunctival space may be necessary. Systemic steroids may be necessary to reduce the local inflammatory changes, but these drugs may be contraindicated, depending on the inciting agent.

F. **Iritis.** The patient should be immediately referred to a specialist. Treatment consists of dilation of the pupil with **homatropine** or **atropine** and the use of topical steroids to reduce inflammation and prevent adhesions within the eyes. Systemic nonsteroidal anti-inflammatory agents also have been shown to be useful.

G. **Angle-closure glaucoma.** Immediate referral to an ophthalmologist is indicated in this case. Definitive treatment of angle-closure glaucoma is surgical. Medications useful in aborting an acute attack while preparing for surgery include **0.5% pilocarpine, acetazolamide, timolol,** and osmotic agents such as **mannitol** or **glycerol.** The use and dosage of these medications should be determined by an ophthalmologist.

REFERENCES

Bertolini J, Pelucio M: The red eye. Emerg Med Clin North Am 1995;**13**:561.
Friedlaender MH: Management of ocular allergy. Ann Allergy Asthma Immunol 1995;**75**:12.
Hara JH: The red eye: Diagnosis and treatment. Am Fam Physician 1996;**54**:2423.
Morrow GL, Abbott RL: Conjunctivitis. Am Fam Physician 1998;**57**:735.
Weiss A: Acute conjunctivitis in childhood. J Pediatr 1993;**122**:10.

59   Rhinitis & Sinus Pain

Pieter J. de Wet, MD

I. **Definition.** Rhinitis is an inflammation of the nasal mucous membrane due to a variety of causes, and frequently resulting in edema of the mucous membranes with profuse watery mucous secretion. The most common cause of sinus pain is sinusitis with numerous other conditions that can mimic this symptom. Sinusitis is an inflammatory process in the paranasal sinuses mainly due to viral, bacterial, or fungal infections or secondary to allergic reactions.

II. **Common diagnoses**
   A. **Common cold.**
   B. **Allergic rhinitis** (seasonal or perennial).
   C. **Vasomotor rhinitis** (perennial nonallergic rhinitis).
   D. **Atrophic rhinitis** (ozena).
   E. **Rhinitis medicamentosum.**
   F. **Sinusitis.**
   G. **Conditions that can mimic sinus pain** include migraine headaches and temporal arteritis (see Chapter 35), periapical dental abscesses of the maxillary teeth, and nasal polyps.
   H. **Other causes** of rhinitis not discussed in this chapter include nonallergic rhinitis with eosinophilia (NARES), nasal foreign bodies, cocaine snorting, endocrine-induced rhinitis including hypothyroidism (see Chapter 91), nasal neoplasms, pregnancy (see Chapter 103), and menstruation-induced rhinitis.

III. **Epidemiology.** Forty to 50 million adults in the United States suffer from chronic rhinitis. The prevalence of acute rhinitis, a very common problem, is unknown.
   A. The incidence of the **common cold** increases in the fall, peaks in the winter, and slowly decreases each spring. Colds occur more commonly in families with children aged 2–7. The average preschool child has six to 10 colds per year; the average adult, two to four. Women are affected more often than men. The virus is spread most readily by wet fomites, transferred by an infected individual to a solid object, which is then touched by another individual, who spreads the virus to his or her eyes or nose.
   B. **Allergic rhinitis** is uncommon before the age of 2 and rarely occurs for the first time after the age of 50. The peak incidence occurs in the late teenage years, with another peak between the ages of 30 and 40. It may be seasonal or perennial, depending on the types of allergens involved. The seasonal allergens are mostly encountered outdoors and include tree, grass, and ragweed pollens and, less commonly, mold spores. The perennial allergens include dust mites, many mold spores, cockroach feces, and animal dander. These allergens are more likely to be encountered indoors, especially in the home.
   C. **Vasomotor rhinitis** occurs most commonly in adults in the third to fifth decades od life, but is occasionally seen in childhood and adolescence.
   D. The majority of patients with **rhinitis medicamentosum** are young to middle-aged adults, although cases have been reported in children as young as 4 years. Both sexes are equally susceptible.
   E. Primary **atrophic rhinitis** occurs mainly in elderly adults. The incidence has declined in developed countries but is still prevalent in some underdeveloped nations, such as China, India, and certain eastern European countries. Secondary atrophic rhinitis develops as a direct result of chronic nasal infections, chronic sinusitis, irradiation, trauma, or radical nasal surgery.
   F. The overall incidence of **sinusitis** is unclear because it is commonly underdiagnosed (especially in children) and is often confused with other conditions, such as the common cold and allergic rhinitis. We know that sinusitis affects as many as 35 million Americans per year. Children are affected by sinusitis almost twice as often as adults. This is apparently because of the far greater incidence of viral upper respiratory infections in children than in adults and the anatomically small sinus ostea in children, which obstruct easily. The diagnosis is also being made more often because of increased physician awareness of the frequency of occurrence

of this disease, especially in children, and the availability of more sophisticated diagnostic tools. The incidence peaks in late fall, winter, and early spring, when viral upper respiratory infections are common.

G. **Dental abscesses** once were a common cause of sinusitis in the United States, but now account for <4% of cases due to improved dental care.

IV. Pathophysiology

A. The majority of cases of the **common cold** are caused by viruses, including rhinovirus (which causes 30–50% of colds), influenza, parainfluenza, respiratory syncytial virus, coronavirus, adenovirus, echovirus, and coxsackievirus. Other infectious agents, such as *Mycobacterium pneumoniae* and *Chlamydia trachomatis,* are occasionally responsible for the symptoms of the common cold. After exposure to a viral agent, replication occurs in the nasopharynx and causes acute inflammation with edema, erythema, and an acute catarrhal response. The nose, pharynx, larynx, and trachea are the anatomic areas most commonly affected.

B. **Allergic rhinitis** is a type I hypersensitivity reaction. Antigens such as those present on pollen initially stimulate production of antigen-specific immunoglobulin E (IgE) antibodies that attach to antibody receptors on the surface of mast cells and basophils in the nasal mucosa. Repeated exposure to the antigen causes release of several mediator substances, including histamine, prostaglandins, kinins, and leukotrienes. These substances cause vasodilatation, increased capillary permeability, smooth muscle contraction, and the migration of other inflammatory cells, such as eosinophils, into the affected mucosa. Two phases of reaction are described: early phase reactions (in which symptoms occur within minutes to 1–2 hours after exposure to an antigen) and late phase reactions (in which symptoms begin 3–11 hours after exposure).

C. The cause of **vasomotor rhinitis** is uncertain, but abnormal autonomic responsiveness resulting in intermittent vascular engorgement of the nasal mucous membrane is believed to play a role. Certain factors, such as a dry atmosphere, changes in temperature, alcohol ingestion, or exposure to irritants such as tobacco smoke, perfumes, and gasoline fumes, can lead to an exacerbation of symptoms. Vasomotor rhinitis of pregnancy occurs most frequently from the second trimester on and resolves spontaneously by the fifth postpartum day.

D. In **rhinitis medicamentosum,** the abuse of topical nasal decongestants causes rebound congestion of the nasal mucosa. Repeated use is thought to cause coagulation in the small vessels, leading to fibrosis. It may occur after the use of nasal decongestants more frequently than every 3 hours or for longer than 3 weeks. In some individuals, a form of rhinitis medicamentosum occurs with the use of certain antihypertensive agents (eg, beta blockers, guanethidine, methyldopa, or reserpine), aspirin, and oral contraceptives.

E. In **atrophic rhinitis,** the mucous membrane changes from ciliated, pseudostratified, columnar epithelium to stratified squamous epithelium, and the lamina propria is reduced in thickness and in vascularity. Bacterial infection, especially by *Klebsiella pneumoniae ozaenae* and other bacteria, is thought to play a role in primary atrophic rhinitis.

F. **Sinusitis.** Five main groups of paranasal sinuses drain into the nasal cavity: the maxillary, frontal, anterior ethmoid, posterior ethmoid, and sphenoid. The maxillary and ethmoid sinuses are present at birth, whereas the sphenoid sinuses develop by age 3 and the frontal sinuses appear by age 5. The maxillary, anterior ethmoid, and frontal sinuses drain into the middle meatus and are most susceptible to infections because of certain anatomic and physiologic characteristics unique to the middle meatus and drainage of these sinuses into this area. This drainage area is commonly called the osteomeatal complex.

The sphenoid sinus is surrounded by a number of important anatomic structures (ie, the apex of the orbital cavity, optic nerve, hypophysis, and cavernous sinus), and serious complications are therefore more common with sphenoid sinusitis than with infections of other sinuses.

Sinusitis is thought to result mainly from obstruction of the sinus ostea secondary to the inflammation and swelling of mucous membranes. This inflammation is most frequently related to infection, viral upper respiratory infections being by far the most common cause. Inflammation caused by allergy, abnormalities such as nasal polyps, or other local anatomic abnormalities can also obstruct the sinus ostea. Inflammation can also drammatically increase mucoid secretions that are unable to drain out of the sinus and can immobilize sinus mucous membrane cilia, leading to stagnation of secretions and potential secondary sinus infection. Causes of sinusitis include bacteria, fungi, and a variety of local and miscellaneous factors.

1. The **bacteria** most frequently isolated from the sinuses in acute sinusitis are *Streptococcus pneumoniae* (41%), *Haemophilus influenzae* (35%), anaerobes (7%), other streptococci (7%), *Moraxella catarrhalis* (4%), *Staphylococcus aureus* (3%), and other bacterial species combined (4%). *Staphylococcus aureus* is more frequently involved with serious complications of sinusitis and (along with anaerobic bacteria such as *Peptostreptococcus, Bacteroides,* and *Fusobacterium*) in cases of chronic sinusitis.

2. **Fungi** (eg, *Aspergillus, Zygomycoses, Phaeohyphomycosis, Pseudallescheria,* and *Hyalohyphomycis*) are found in a small percentage of cases of sinusitis and are more likely in chronic sinusitis than in acute sinusitis. Mucormycosis can cause sinus disease in poorly controlled diabetics and in the immunocompromised.

3. **Local factors** predisposing individuals to sinusitis include **nasal septum deviation, hyperplastic nasal turbinates, nasal polyps, cleft lip and palate, choanal atresia,** and **intranasal foreign bodies** (including nasogastric tubes). Fractures such as Le Fort's type may directly injure the sinuses, hindering normal drainage or leading to direct invasion by infectious agents such as bacteria. Adenoidal hypertrophy (especially in children) predisposes individuals to sinusitis because the adenoids may serve as a bacterial reservoir.

4. **Other factors** predisposing to sinusitis include decreased humidity, irritants such as cigarette smoke, cystic fibrosis (abnormally thick mucus), Kartagener's syndrome (immobile cilia within the respiratory tract), and congenital or acquired immunodeficiency syndrome.

V. Symptoms

A. **Sneezing** occurs with the common cold and with allergic rhinitis. There is no sneezing with vasomotor rhinitis.

B. **Rhinorrhea** and **nasal congestion** are common with colds, allergic rhinitis, vasomotor rhinitis, and sinusitis. Rhinorrhea is very watery in vasomotor rhinitis; it is watery to mucoid in allergic rhinitis and initially with a cold. With colds, the rhinorrhea becomes more mucoid and sometimes mucopurulent after 1–3 days. A mucopurulent discharge is normal in this situation but may raise the suspicion of sinusitis if it continues for more than 7–10 days, especially if associated with other symptoms of sinusitis. Patients with rhinitis medicamentosum commonly complain of intense, unrelenting nasal congestion but mostly without significant rhinorrhea. **Postnasal drip** is often present in patients with allergic rhinitis, the common cold, and sinusitis and can exacerbate cough especially at night in some cases.

C. **General malaise, fatigue, sore throat, hoarseness, cough,** and **headache** are frequent complaints of patients suffering from the common cold and sinusitis.

D. **Nasal and conjunctival itching** are very common with allergic rhinitis and occur occasionally with the common cold, but not with vasomotor rhinitis.

E. **Epiphoria,** or watery discharge from the eyes, is common with allergic rhinitis. The sensation of **nasal congestion** and a complaint of a constant bad smell (**ozina**) in the nose are common symptoms in patients with atrophic rhinitis. **Anosmia** and recurrent severe **epistaxis** may also be seen.

F. The following symptoms occur commonly in **acute sinusitis** (see Table 59–1): nasal secretions (often but not necessarily purulent), cough, sneezing, nasal congestion with poor response to decongestants, anosmia or hyposmia, maxillary toothache (painful mastication), malaise, headache, and/or intrafacial pressure sensation, fever, and halitosis that last more than 3 days but less than 3 weeks. A history of preceding upper respiratory tract infection is often present. The first three symptoms listed here are the most sensitive for this diagnosis but are relatively nonspecific, whereas symptoms such as toothache are highly specific but have very low sensitivity. **Subacute sinusitis** is characterized by the same symptoms but lasts more than 3 weeks and less than 3 months. **Recurrent sinusitis** is repeated bouts of acute sinusitis with apparent complete resolution of symptoms between bouts. Patients with **chronic sinusitis** present with the same symptoms that persist for 3 months or more.

TABLE 59–1. SYMPTOMS OF ACUTE VERSUS CHRONIC SINUSITIS

Symptom	Acute Sinusitis	Chronic Sinusitis
Nasal congestion	Usually present; most often bilateral; occasionally unilateral	Often present; can be bilateral or unilateral; more often unilateral than in acute sinusitis
Nasal discharge Discharge can drain anteriorly (rhinorrhea) and/or posteriorly (postnasal drip)	Usually present; usually a purulent discharge but occasionally mucoid or even watery	Often present; sinuses can be completely occluded with no drainage present; if present, drainage can be purulent, mucoid, or serous
Pain The patient may complain of pain or pressure over the affected sinuses (ie, facial pain with maxillary sinuses, pain between the eyes with ethmoid sinusitis, frontal headaches with frontal sinusitis, and vertex headache with sphenoid sinusitis or more vague tension-type headaches with involvement of any of the sinuses)	Often present; headache, facial pain, and tenderness common	Often present; symptoms such as facial pressure and headache are common; headache is often worse in the morning and with head movement
Generalized malaise	Relatively common; may be persistent until acute sinusitis has resolved	Unusual
Halitosis Thought to result from the purulent drainage and the increased growth of bacteria in the nose and throat associated with this drainage	Often described in adults and children with acute sinusitis	Often present
Loss of smell and taste Caused by edema of the nasal mucosa associated with sinusitis	Very common	Common when bilateral sinuses are involved; less common when unilateral sinuses are involved
Fever	Often present; usually a low-grade fever but occasionally high fever with aggressive sinusitis	Seldom present
Pain in the upper teeth	Sometimes present, mainly when the maxillary sinuses are involved	Occasionally present with chronic maxillary sinusitis
Respiratory symptoms, such as cough and exacerbation of asthma	Frequently present; nighttime and early morning are often the worst times for cough, most likely because of postnasal drip	Often present because of chronic postnasal drip

The symptoms of sinusitis may mimic and overlap those of other diseases, ranging from the common cold to allergic rhinitis. Sinusitis should be suspected, especially when symptoms of these common conditions are prolonged and interfere with daily living or when these symptoms are severe rather than mild or moderate.

Periapical dental abscesses of maxillary premolar and molar teeth can affect the maxillary sinuses and can lead to symptoms of sinusitis. The pain of an uncomplicated dental abscess can also be very hard to differentiate from that caused by maxillary sinusitis.

Symptoms of **nasal polyps** include nasal congestion or complete nasal obstruction in almost all patients, with other symptoms (in decreasing order of frequency) including hyposmia, rhinorrhea, sneezing, postnasal drip, facial pain, and ocular itching.

VI. Signs

A. Erythema, swelling, and rhinorrhea of the **nasal mucosa** and erythema of the **pharynx** are usually present with the common cold. The nasal mucosa appears pale and boggy or bluish with allergic rhinitis. Watery rhinorrhea may be visible. In vasomotor rhinitis, the nasal mucosa varies from bright red to bluish. Marked erythema or even a hemorrhagic appearance and swelling of the nasal mucosa are typical in patients with rhinitis medicamentosum. In sinusitis, marked erythema and swelling of the nasal mucous membranes are seen, especially in acute sinusitis. Nasal discharge on physical examination can be mucoid but is most often thick purulent green or yellow in nature. In chronic sinusitis, the appearance of the mucous membranes depends on the underlying cause—pale or bluish and edematous in allergic rhinitis or even relatively normal with anatomic causes, such as choanal atresia or septal deviation.

B. **Fever** is unusual in adults with the common cold but occurs frequently in children with the same type of infection. In sinusitis, **fever** occasionally occurs and is usually low grade, seldom exceeding 39 °C (101 °F). Fever is more likely with acute sinusitis and is very seldom seen in chronic sinusitis.

C. **Nose wrinkling, nose rubbing** (also known as the allergic salute), and **allergic "shiners"** (dark rings under the eyes) are especially common in children with allergic rhinitis.

D. In patients with allergic rhinitis, the **conjunctiva** may appear inflamed, the palpebral conjunctiva may have an edematous and cobblestone appearance, and nasal polyps may be present.

E. **Nasal crusting,** a shrunken-appearing nasal mucosa, and enlarged nasal cavities suggest atrophic rhinitis. Patients may also present with **epistaxis.** Despite the sensation of nasal congestion, there is no increase in airflow resistance in most of these cases.

F. **External signs** of sinusitis, especially with maxillary sinusitis, include redness of the skin overlying the maxillary sinuses. The bony structures overlying the maxillary, frontal, or ethmoid sinuses may be tender to palpation, and eyelid puffiness (chemosis) may be present, especially with maxillary and ethmoid sinusitis.

G. **Sinus transillumination** is often discussed as an aid in diagnosing maxillary or frontal sinusitis; however, it has very low sensitivity and specificity because of the great variability in sinus anatomy, including asymmetry and underdevelopment. Only negative findings are useful and can be helpful in ruling out the diagnosis of maxillary or frontal sinusitis.

H. **Signs of complications** of sinusitis include periorbital erythema and edema resulting from periorbital cellulitis. Cranial nerve deficits, especially an abducens nerve palsy, can indicate invasion of infection into the surrounding tissues. Meningitis should be considered in patients with signs of severe acute sinusitis (eg, high fever or severe headache), especially if they have additional signs such as mental status changes, neck stiffness, visual disturbance, and an unusually high white blood cell count (>15,000/mL).

VII. Laboratory tests

are not indicated in patients clinically diagnosed with an uncomplicated common cold, or when allergic rhinitis or rhinitis medicamentosum is initially suspected. In these cases, it is appropriate to initiate therapy. Tests might become necessary if symptoms and signs indicate the possibility of a complication of a common cold. If allergic rhinitis becomes perennial, has a significant impact on the quality of life, or does not respond to intermittent, simple medical therapy, further workup may be warranted. A good history and physical examination are the most important aids to diagnosing sinusitis. If four or more major signs or symptoms discussed in section V are present (see also Table 59–1), sinusitis is likely and treatment can be initiated without further testing. When two or three major signs or symptoms are present, symptoms are vague, or recurrent or chronic sinusitis is suspected, further diagnostic work-up may be justified to confirm the diagnosis or find predisposing conditions leading to recurrent or chronic disease. When fewer than two major signs or symptoms are present, acute sinusitis is unlikely to be the diagnosis and further workup is probably unnecessary. It is also important to confirm the diagnosis if serious underlying conditions such as cystic fibrosis, diabetes mellitus, or immunosuppression are present, because of the risk of complications if the wrong diagnosis is made and the patient is treated incorrectly.

A. **Nasal smears** can help distinguish allergic rhinitis from other causes of rhinitis but are usually not necessary to make a diagnosis. Smears can be limited to questionable cases, such as defining the cause of chronic rhinitis. A smear for eosinophils may be especially helpful in distinguishing between allergic rhinitis and vasomotor rhinitis.

   1. Nasal secretions obtained by a cotton swab or superficial nasal scrapings obtained using a plastic probe (eg, a Rhino probe) are placed on a glass slide; stained with Hansel, Wright's, or Giema stain; and examined microscopically.

   2. Eosinophil predominance may suggest the diagnosis of allergic rhinitis, NARES, or nasal polyposis. An abundance of neutrophils supports the diagnosis of infectious rhinitis or sinusitis (viral or bacterial).

B. **Bacterial cultures of nasal secretions** may be helpful in detecting the bacteria responsible for sinusitis or atrophic rhinitis. Cultures are seldom obtained in cases of uncomplicated acute sinusitis and in the initial treatment of many chronic sinusitis cases. However, cultures are indicated when acute sinusitis is resistant to one or, at most, two courses of antibiotic therapy, in cases of chronic refractory sinusitis nonresponsive to medical treatment, in immunocompromised individuals, or in neonates. Cultures are also obtained during most surgical procedures on the sinuses if persistent sinus infection is suspected. Aerobic and anaerobic cultures should be obtained, and fungal cultures should be added if a fungal origin is suspected. Pus obtained at the sinus ostium or infundibulum during rigid or flexible rhinoscopy via the biopsy channel increases the likelihood of a valid culture compared to random nasal pus sampling. However, direct aspiration of the sinuses is often necessary to determine the causative organism(s). This procedure, which is technically difficult and painful, is most often performed by an otorhinolaryngologist. Aspirates are obtained most frequently by aspiration of the maxillary sinuses through their anterior wall or through the inferior meatus in the nasal cavity.

C. A **nasal speculum** and a strong light source can help visualize the anterior chambers of the nose. A **rigid** or **flexible rhinoscope** might give additional information, especially if anatomic or pathologic abnormalities are not clearly visualized on inspection by speculum. These instruments are especially useful to search for sources of nasal obstruction or postnasal drip if the diagnosis is not readily apparent based on physical examination alone. Rhinoscopy frequently reveals **purulent nasal discharge** emanating from the sinus ostea, particularly from the middle meatus in acute sinusitis. Anatomic abnormalities (eg, polyps, choanal atresia, or septal deviation) can often be identified by direct visualization.

D. **Allergen skin testing** is helpful in cases in which allergic rhinitis is suspected and specific allergens might be causing the symptoms. These tests are relatively inexpensive and fairly reliable. They are not useful in children under the age of 3 because the very young produce inadequate amounts of histamine.

   1. Groups of allergens or single allergens are selected for testing based on the most likely causes of the patient's allergy. This is determined by a thorough history that includes geographic information, history of exposure to specific antigens, and recall of symptoms associated with certain exposures.

   2. Allergens are introduced into the skin by intradermal injection (which is most accurate but carries a greater risk of anaphylaxis), skin prick test (the easiest, most widely used, and reasonably accurate), or scratch test. *Note:* Methylxanthines and antihistamines should be discontinued 3–30 days (in the case of astemizole) before skin testing.

E. **Radioallergosorbent (RAST) testing** is the determination of serum allergen-specific IgE levels by immunoassay. This test is useful in young children, who might not tolerate multiple skin pricks; those with skin conditions such as dermatographia and severe eczema; and those receiving medications that might affect the reliability of skin testing (eg, antihistamines). However, it is relatively more expensive, is less sensitive, and can test for fewer antigens than skin testing.

F. **Imaging studies**

   1. **Sinus films** are still frequently used to diagnose sinus disease, but their popularity is waning because of their relatively low sensitivity compared to other modalities, such as computerized tomographic (CT) scans. The sensitivity of sinus films in diagnosing disease in the maxillary and frontal sinuses (90%)

is much better than that in diagnosing disease of the ethmoid and sphenoid sinuses (65%). Four views constitute the sinus series: Water's view (maxillary sinuses), the Caldwell view (ethmoid and frontal sinuses), the submental vertex view (sphenoid sinuses), and the lateral view. A sinus film is read as abnormal if there is mucosal thickening >4 mm, air-fluid levels, or opacification of one or more sinuses on one or more views. Other abnormalities, such as bony erosions (suggesting a sinus tumor) or expansion of the sinus wall (suggesting a mucocele), may be seen in chronic sinusitis.

2. The **CT scan** is being used more frequently, often without preceding sinus films, because of its superior sensitivity (95–98%) and specificity. CT scanning is indicated in the following situations.

   a. When chronic sinusitis is suspected.

   b. In patients with recurrent sinusitis or no response to therapy.

   c. To confirm acute sinusitis in individuals with serious underlying disease.

   d. When complications are suspected.

   e. When a sinus tumor is suspected.

   f. When sinus surgery is being considered.

   The CT scan gives a very accurate picture of all the paranasal structures; the drainage system, including the sinus ostea and the osteomeatal complex; and structures inside the nasal cavity.

3. **Magnetic resonance imaging (MRI)** is restricted to the evaluation of complicated sinusitis (ie, if intraorbital and intracranial complications or sinonasal neoplasms are suspected).

VIII. Treatment

A. **Common cold.** Treatment is largely palliative and may include the following strategies.

1. For fever and headache, **acetaminophen** (eg, Tylenol), 325 mg, one or two tablets orally every 4–6 hours for adults or 8–16 mg/kg every 4–6 hours of suspension, liquid, or elixir for children. **Ibuprofen** (eg, Advil), 200 mg, one or two tablets every 6–8 hours for adults or children's suspension (100 mg/ 5 mL), 5–10 mg/kg every 6–8 hours, or **aspirin,** 325 mg, two tablets every 4–8 hours, can be recommended as needed. These medications may slightly prolong viral shedding and other cold symptoms, but this is probably not clinically significant. Aspirin should be avoided in children and teenagers under the age of 18 years because of its association with Reye's syndrome.

2. For nasal congestion and rhinorrhea, oral decongestants such as **pseudoephedrine** (eg, Sudafed), 30 mg, one or two tablets every 4–6 hours for adults and children over age 12, or 0.5–1 tsp every 4–6 hours of the liquid for children under 12, may be used. Short-term use (up to a maximum of 3–4 days) of topical decongestants such as **phenylephrine hydrochloride** (eg, Neo-Synephrine), 0.125% or 0.25%, two or three sprays in each nostril up to every 4 hours for children and the same dosing schedule of the 0.5% spray for adults, may be helpful.

3. For cough, syrups containing **dextromethorphan** (eg, Robitussin DM) or **codeine** (eg, Robitussin AC), 0.5–2 tsp every 4 hours (the exact dose depends on the patient's age), can be prescribed, with **benzonatate** (eg, Tessalon Perles), 100 mg three times daily for adults, a potentially helpful alternative.

4. **Ipratropium bromide** (eg, Atrovent 0.06%) nasal spray, one or two sprays per nostril four times daily, is an anticholinergic agent that can be helpful in reducing the watery rhinorrhea that is such as prominent symptom in most patients with the common cold.

5. A number of combination products that contain analgesics, decongestants, and cough suppressants in various combinations (eg, **Tylenol Cold Formula,** one or two caplets every 6 hours for adults and children over 6 years) are available over the counter and can be useful. However, antihistamines, alone or in combination, have not been shown to be beneficial, nor are antibiotics indicated or helpful in these patients.

6. **Alternative therapies**

   a. **General supportive measures** in the treatment of **common colds** and **allergies** include adequate sleep and rest, with relaxation strategies, visualization (positive imaging), and meditation possibly also helpful because they reduce stress and may help balance immune function.

Certainly, adequate fluids (especially water, soups, etc) improve mucous membrane and ciliary function and may also enhance immune function which even mild dehydration may negatively impact. Excessive sugar intake even in the form of "natural sugars" may also have a negative impact on the function of the immune system; therefore, even fruit juices, if consumed, should be diluted with water.

b. Vitamin C supplementation may shorten the course of the common cold but does not seem to prevent it. Dosing recommendations vary from 500 mg/day to 1000 mg every 2 hours while awake. The higher dosing levels may be harmful over the long term and should be limited to <1 week. Like vitamin C, zinc possesses direct antiviral activity and may significantly reduce the duration of symptoms. Use of zinc gluconate lozenges, 20–30 mg orally every 2–3 waking hours for up to 1 week, is a reasonable recommendation; longer-term use of >50 mg/day may depress the immune system. Beta carotene, vitamin A, and other carotenoids also enhance the immune system and are available from natural sources such as adequate intake of green and yellow vegetables and fruit.

c. Botanical medicines (herbs) that may boost immune function and shorten the course of the common cold include echinacea, astragalus root, goldenseal, licorice (deglycyrrhizinated form to prevent increased blood pressure and water retention), cat's claw, elderberry, and olive leaf.

d. Homeopathic remedies for the common cold and allergic rhinitis are very popular in Europe and India and are becoming more popular in the United States, but quality research proving their efficacy is somewhat limited.

e. Acupuncture may be helpful and is becoming more popular in the West for this and a multitude of other conditions, although, again, quality research into its use in conditions such as colds and flu and allergic rhinitis is hard to find, except in the Chinese medical literature.

B. Allergic rhinitis

1. Environmental control. If the antigens to which sensitivity exists are known, the patient should minimize exposure to them as much as is feasible.

a. For pollen allergy, patients should keep doors and windows closed, use air conditioners both in the home and in automobiles, use a high-efficiency particle air (HEPA) filter, and avoid being outdoors on sunny, windy days, especially during certain times of the year when particular pollens are present.

b. For dust mite allergy, patients should cover bedding with plastic, zippered covers, eliminate wall-to-wall carpets (especially in bedrooms), use acaricides such as tannic acid solutions regularly to kill dust mites, avoid or regularly wash stuffed animals in hot water (if they are washable), keep home humidity below 40%, and use HEPA filters, especially in the bedroom.

c. Patients with mold allergies should decrease mold exposure in the home by wiping vulnerable surfaces (eg, those in the bathroom) with household bleach, keeping indoor humidity below 40%, using air filters, avoiding piles of leaves in the fall, and cutting grass to reduce exposure outside.

d. Cat dander (saliva) is by far the most frequent cause of allergies to animals. If sensitivity develops, animals should be kept outside, washed at least once every 2 weeks to remove the antigen-containing cat saliva from their coats, or given to new homes.

e. Elimination of food allergens causing delayed reactions may benefit patients with allergic rhinitis, but the impact of these allergens is difficult to assess. Relatively common food allergens include dairy products, chocolate, wheat, citrus fruits, and food additives such as artificial dyes and preservatives.

2. Pharmacologic therapy includes the following.

a. Antihistamines (Table 59–2) are the most commonly prescribed first-line therapy. If economic factors are less important, the newer-generation antihistamines are usually preferred, because they have fewer side effects and especially cause less sedation. These agents include **astemizole** (Hismanal), **loratadine** (Claritin), **fexofenadine** (Allegra), and **cetirizine** (Zyrtec). First-generation antihistamines tend to cause more side effects, such as sedation, mouth dryness, and fatigue. Even more serious

TABLE 59-2. ANTIHISTAMINES USEFUL IN THE TREATMENT OF ALLERGIC RHINITIS

Class	Generic Name	Sample Trade Name	Dose[1]	Sedative Effects	Anti-cholinergic Effects
First generation					
Ethanolamines	Diphenhydramine	Benadryl[2]		Marked	Mild
		Allergy tablets	A: 25–50 mg qid		
		Syrup	C: 12.5 mg/5 mL		
			5–10 mL q 4–6 hours		
	Clemastine	Tavist			
		Tablets	A: 1.32–2.68 mg bid		
		Syrup	C: 0.5 mg/5 mL		
			5–10 mL bid		
Ethylenediamines	Tripelennamine	PBZ SR tablets	A: 50 mg qid	Moderate	Moderate
Alkylamines	Chorpheniramine	Chlor-Trimeton tablets	A: 4 mg qid	Mild	Mild
		Triaminic[2] syrup	C: 1 mg/5 mL		
			1.5–10 mL q 4 hours		
Phenothiazines	Promethazine	Phenergan		Marked	Mild
		Tablets	A: 25–50 mg qid		
		Syrup	C: 6.25 mg/5 mL		
			5–10 mL tid–qid		
Piperidines	Cyproheptadine	Periactin tablets	A: 4 mg qid	Moderate	Mild
			C: 2 mg/5 mL		
			5–15 mL bid–tid		
	Azatadine	Trinalin tablets	A: 1 bid		
Piperazine	Hydroxyzine	Atarax		Moderate	Mild
		Tablets	A: 10–50 mg qid		
		Syrup	C: 10 mg/5 mL		
			5–15 mL tid–qid		
Second generation					
	Astemizole	Hismanal tablets	A: 10 mg qd	None	None
	Cetirizine	Zyrtec		Mild	None
		Tablets	A: 10 mg qd		
		Syrup	C: 5–10 mL qd		
			(1 mg/mL)		
	Fexofenadine	Allegra tablets	A: 60 mg bid	None	None
	Loratadine	Claritin		None	None
		Tablets	A: 10 mg qd		
		Syrup	C: 10 mL qd	None	None
			(1 mg/mL)		

Children's dosages are listed for those medications with available pediatric suspensions. Be aware that a range of dosages are listed. Look up the exact dosages by age before prescribing these medications for children.
[1] A, Adults' dose (mg); C, children's dose (mL).
[2] A decongestant is added to this formulation.

side effects can occur, such as slowed reaction times, which can potentially lead to accidents; urinary obstructive symptoms can also occur, especially in the elderly. However, first-generation agents are very effective and much less expensive than the newer second-generation agents. Terfenadine was recently pulled from the market because of concerns about its potential for causing adverse health effects. **Levocabastine** (Livostin 0.05%), one drop into each affected eye four times daily, can be very helpful in the treatment of allergic conjunctivitis often associated with allergic rhinitis.

b. **Antihistamine-decongestant combinations** such as **Claritin-D 12 Hour, Claritin-D 24 Hour, Tavist-D,** and **Allegra-D** are also useful, especially if nasal congestion is a prominent symptom. The dose is one tablet twice daily for all except Claritin-D 24 hour, which is taken once daily.

c. **Steroid nasal sprays** are useful either in combination with antihistamines or as first-line agents. Available preparations include **beclomethasone** (eg, Beconase or Vancenase), one or two sprays per nostril two or three times daily; **flunisolide** (eg, Nasalide), two sprays per nostril twice daily; **triamcinolone acetonide** (eg, Nasacort), two to four sprays per nostril daily; **budesonide** (eg, Rhinocort), two to four sprays per nostril daily; and **fluticasone** (eg, Flonase), one or two sprays daily. **Dexamethasone** (eg, Decadron Turbinaire), two sprays per nostril two or three times daily, should be used only for short courses of therapy because of potential systemic effects. Other steroid nasal sprays have good long-term safety records. **Oral steroids** should be avoided, except in severe cases of refractory allergic rhinitis, in rhinitis medicamentosum while topical decongestants are discontinued, and in obstructive nasal polyposis. If used in these situations, short-acting steroids should be used (eg, prednisone, 40 mg orally initially, tapered over 7–10 days).

    d. Mast cell-stabilizing agents such as **cromolin sodium** (eg, Nasalcrom), one spray per nostril three or four times per day, can be useful either prophylactically for unavoidable exposures to an antigen or for treatment. **Nedocromil sodium** (eg, Tilade) can be given as two sprays in each nostril two or three times per day and may be a little more effective.

    e. Anticholinergic agents such as **ipratropium bromide** (eg Atrovent 0.03% nasal spray), one or two sprays in each nostril every 6 hours, provide symptomatic relief of rhinorrhea in these patients. They may also relieve sneezing and nasal itching but do not relieve nasal congestion. Ipratropium bromide can also alleviate symptoms of vasomotor rhinitis and cold air–induced rhinorrhea.

3. Immunotherapy is useful especially in severe and/or refractory cases and in those patients with year-round symptoms (perennial allergic rhinitis). Criteria for treatment should include a history of at least moderate symptoms of allergic rhinitis for 2 years or more, or severe symptoms for at least 6 months that are difficult to treat symptomatically. Candidates for treatment should also have a history of positive skin testing for allergens that correlate with their symptomatic history. The purpose of this treatment is to reduce sensitivity to antigens. The patient receives weekly injections of an antigen(s) to which he or she is sensitive. The dose is increased at weekly intervals until a maintenance dose is achieved; injections are then given every 3–6 weeks for 3–5 years. If therapy does not significantly relieve symptoms within 12 months, immunotherapy should be terminated. Even though anaphylaxis occurs infrequently with immunotherapy, resuscitation equipment and drugs such as epinephrine and intravenous steroids should be immediately available, and personnel administering immunotherapy should be trained in basic resuscitation.

4. Patient education should include information about environmental controls to minimize antigen exposure, management options, and complications.

5. Alternative therapies

    a. For more information on **common supportive measures,** see section VII,A,6.

    b. Dietary supplements possibly helpful in allergic rhinitis include antioxidants, such as buffered vitamin C (1000–3000 mg/day in divided doses), vitamin E (100–400 IU/day), selenium (100–200 µg/day), and carotenoids such as beta carotene. Omega-3 fatty acids (fish oil or flax seed oil), evening primrose oil, bee pollen, vitamin B_6 (100–200 mg/day), vitamin B_{12} (1 mg/day), pantothenic acid, and bioflavonoids may also be helpful. Dosages listed above are applicable to adults.

    c. Botanicals (herbs) possibly beneficial in controlling symptoms of allergic rhinitis include ephedra, stinging nettles, Chinese scullcap, angelica, Indian tobacco, chili pepper, skunk cabbage, green tea, onions, garlic, eyebright, Siberian ginseng, elderberry, and licorice.

C. Treatment of **vasomotor rhinitis** consists mainly of symptomatic therapy with oral decongestants such as **pseudoephedrine** (eg, Sudafed), 60 mg three or four times a day. Anticholinergic agents such as **ipratropium bromide** (eg, Atrovent nasal spray) (see section VII,B,2,e) can be very helpful in alleviating profuse watery rhinorrhea. **Intranasal steroids** (see section VII,B,2,c) may be helpful in treating troublesome exacerbations unresponsive to the therapies listed above. Severe nonresponsive cases may require surgical resection of the inferior turbinate. Patients should be educated to avoid irritants that may exacerbate this condition; these include tobacco and fireplace smoke, strong perfumes, chemical and gasoline fumes, and wood dust. Sudden changes in temperature or humidity should also be avoided when possible.

D. In **rhinitis medicamentosum,** topical decongestants should be discontinued. Oral decongestants or a short course of a topical nasal steroid may be helpful (see section VII,B,2,c). A short course of systemic steroids (eg, **prednisone,** 40 mg orally initially, tapered over 7–10 days) may be required if other methods are ineffective. The problem usually resolves in 2–3 weeks without long-term sequelae. Patients should be educated about the causes of the condition and discouraged from further abuse of topical decongestants.

E. Treatment of **atrophic rhinitis** is directed toward reducing the crusting and eliminating the odor. Topical antibiotics such as **bacitracin** ointment, two or three times a day, are useful. Systemic estrogens in menopausal women may alleviate rhinitis symptoms. Surgical reductions of nasal cavity patency are used only as a last resort. Patient education is important (see section VII,B,4).

F. **Sinusitis** can usually be managed in the outpatient setting. Hospital admission is necessary for complicated sinusitis or when there is a high risk of complications from a serious underlying disease and close outpatient monitoring is not feasible.

   1. Antibiotics (Table 59–3)

      a. The current standard is to treat adults and children with uncomplicated acute sinusitis for a minimum of 10–14 days, with an additional 10–14 days

TABLE 59–3. AMBULATORY ANTIBIOTIC REGIMENS IN THE TREATMENT OF UNCOMPLICATED SINUSITIS

Antibiotic	Dose
Amoxicillin (Amoxil)	Adult: 250–500 mg tid Child: 40 mg/kg/day tid
Trimethoprim-sulfamethoxazole (TMP–SMX) (Bactrim, 160 mg of TMP and 800 mg of SMX per DS tablet; Septra, 8 mg of TMP and 40 mg of SMX per tsp)	Adult: one DS tablet bid Child: 6–12 mg/kg/day TMP and 30–60 mg/kg/day bid
Erythromycin; ERYC	Adult: 250 mg qid Child: 30–50 mg/kg/day qid
E-mycin	Adult: 250 mg qid or 333 mg tid Child: 30–50 mg/kg/day qid or tid
EES	Adult: 400 mg qid Child: 30–50 mg/kg/day qid
Clarithromycin (Biaxin)	Adult: 500 mg bid Child: 50 mg/kg/day bid
Amoxicillin-clavulanate (Augmentin)	Adult: 500–850 mg bid Child: 45 mg/kg/day bid
Erythromycin-sulfisoxazole (Pediazole) (200 mg of erythromycin and 600 mg of sulfisoxazole per tsp)	Child: 50 mg/kg/day erythromycin and 150 mg/kg/day sulfisoxazole tid
Cefixime (Suprax)	Adult: 400 mg qd Child: 8 mg/kg/day (100 mg/tsp suspension) qd
Cefuroxime axetil (Ceftin)	Adult: 250–500 mg bid
Cefprozil (Cefzil)	Adult: 500 mg bid Child: 15 mg/kg bid
Cefpodoxime proxetil (Vantin)	Adult: 100–200 mg bid Child: 10 mg/kg/day bid
Azithromycin (Zithromax)	Adult: 500 mg day 1, 250 mg days 2–5 Child: 10 mg/kg day 1, 5 mg/kg days 2–5
Loracarbef (Lorabid)	Adult: 400 mg bid Child: 30 mg/kg/day (100 mg/tsp or 200 mg/tsp suspension) bid
Cloxacillin (Tegopen)	Adult: 500–1000 mg qid Child: 50–100 mg/kg/day qid
Dicloxacillin (Dynapen, Pathocil)	Adult: 250–500 mg qid Child: 25–50 mg/kg/day qid
Levofloxacin (Levaquin)	Adult: 500 mg qd
Sparfloxacin (Zagam)	Adult: 200-mg tablets, two tablets day 1, one tablet days 2–10

if symptoms are improving but not yet completely resolved after initial therapy. Antibiotics should be changed if there is no improvement after 5–7 days of therapy. As little as 3 days of antibiotic treatment (ie, with **trimethoprim-sulfamethoxazole [TMP-SMX]**) may be as effective as 10 days' treatment, but the standard of care still seems to be to treat for a minimum of 10 days.

b. Appropriate first-line therapy in otherwise healthy patients with uncomplicated acute sinusitis includes amoxicillin-clavulanate, cefuroxime axetil or TMP-SMX, or amoxicillin, but **amoxicillin** should be used only in areas where the incidence of β-lactamase–producing pathogens is <20%.

c. If the response is poor to first-line therapy, if there is relatively high incidence of β-lactamase–producing pathogens, or if the patient is immunocompromised, reasonable alternative antimicrobials include **cefprozil, cefpodoxime proxetil, erythromycin, clarithromycin, cefixime, loracarbef, cefaclor, ceftibuten, azithromycin,** and **erythromycin-sulfisoxazole** (in children). **Levofloxacin** or **sparfloxacin** is also appropriate but should be used only in individuals 18 years or older.

d. For chronic or complicated sinusitis, antibiotic therapy should continue for at least 3–6 weeks. Antibiotics with good staphylococcal coverage are often preferred; these include **cloxacillin, dicloxacillin, cephalexin, cefadroxil monohydrate, erythromycin, clarithromycin, amoxicillin-clavulanate,** and **cefuroxime axetil.** With complicated sinusitis, hospital admission for parenteral antibiotics is indicated.

2. Pain and **malaise** may respond to bed rest and oral analgesics (see Section VII,A,1). For more severe pain, **acetaminophen with codeine** (eg, Tylenol 2, 3, or 4), one or two tablets three or four times per day for adults, or **Tylenol with codeine** liquid, 1–2 tsp every 6–8 hours for children can be used (the exact dose depends on the patient's age).

3. Humidification with cool vapor steam and increased oral intake of water helps thin nasal secretions.

4. Decongestants (see section VII,A,3) are commonly used to decrease nasal congestion and may also promote drainage from the sinuses by shrinking edematous mucous membranes blocking the sinus ostea (see section VII,A). **Oral decongestant–antihistamine combinations** (section VII,B,2,6) are also very popular and may be helpful in patients with underlying allergic rhinitis. However, in the absence of allergic rhinitis, antihistamines are of little use in the treatment of sinusitis, because of their drying effect on the respiratory mucosa and their thickening effect on secretions.

5. Mucolytics containing **guaifenesin** (eg, Robitussin, 0.5–2 tsp every 4–6 hours, depending on age; or Humibid-LA, one-half to one tablet twice daily) may thin tenacious secretions and therefore promote sinus drainage.

6. Nasal irrigation with a normal saline solution can facilitate removal of thickened or dry secretions from the nose that cause discomfort and possibly inhibit sinus drainage. Saline irrigation is especially helpful in infants and young children in improving nasal patency. The easiest technique in infants and young children is to instill 5–10 drops of **saline solution** (eg, Nasal or Ocean drops) into the child's nose while he or she is recumbent with the head tilted slightly backward, and then to suction the thinned secretions out with a bulb syringe. This should be repeated three or four times or until no more mucoid or purulent secretions can be suctioned out.

7. Other therapies

a. Topical and/or systemic **corticosteroids** should not be used except where evidence indicates allergic disease. Corticosteroids (topical or systemic) are very helpful for the treatment of nasal polyps. Direct injection of polyps with steroids, on the other hand, is controversial because of a few reported cases of unilateral loss of vision after this procedure. If polypectomy is planned, a 10- to 14-day tapering dose of oral prednisone, starting at 60 mg/day in adults, is usually given preoperatively; topical intranasal steroids are used postoperatively to reduce the risk of recurrence. This regimen—a 10- to 14-day tapering dose of oral prednisone followed by topical intranasal steroids—is also a reasonable medical approach even if surgery is not immediately planned.

    b. Surgery should be considered for patients who suffer frequent recurrences of sinusitis (ie, three or more attacks in 1 year) despite adequate medical treatment, who have chronic sinusitis responding inadequately to medical therapy alone, or who have an anatomic obstruction amenable to surgery. Functional endoscopic surgery is now the most popular, least destructive, and most physiologically sound surgical procedure being performed on these patients, especially when the CT scan confirms that the osteomeatal complex is the site of obstruction. Other surgical drainage procedures, such as the Caldwell-Luc procedure, are still occasionally performed but are becoming less popular. When polyps are present and cause marked mechanical obstruction, particularly when this condition is associated with sinusitis, polypectomy may be indicated. Simple polypectomy is controversial because of the very high incidence of recurrence. Functional endoscopic sinus surgery in which the tissue source of the polyps is removed seems far more successful in reducing recurrence rates. Adenoidectomy may be indicated primarily in younger children with moderate to severe nasal obstruction secondary to adenoidal hyperplasia and may decrease recurrence of sinusitis.

8. Dental referral is indicated in patients in whom a tooth abscess is suspected as the underlying cause of maxillary sinusitis.

9. Patient follow-up

    a. There are no clear recommendations for follow-up of acute sinusitis; however, it is reasonable to see a patient 10–14 days after therapy is initiated to establish whether symptoms and signs of sinusitis have completely resolved. If symptoms of sinusitis persist, antibiotic therapy should be extended an additional 10–14 days, or a different antibiotic should be substituted if very little or no improvement has occurred.

    b. Complications of sinusitis are infrequent but occur more frequently in children and in patients with immunodeficiency disorders; they must therefore be diagnosed promptly and treated emergently. Patients should be instructed to return to the physician immediately if symptoms such as fever, headache, or cough become worse or if new symptoms such as visual disturbance, neck stiffness, or lethargy develop. Complications of sinusitis can be **local, orbital, or intracranial.**

        (1) Local complications include mucoceles or mucopyoceles. Mucoceles occur most frequently in the frontal sinus, and patients often present complaining of diplopia because the affected eye is displaced.

        (2) Orbital complications are the most common, and children with acute ethmoid sinusitis are the most prone to this complication. Preseptal or postseptal cellulitis can occur; the latter is more severe because it involves orbital structures. Signs of septal cellulitis include swelling and inflammation of the eyelids and proptosis of the affected eye. Complete ophthalmoplegia, impairment of vision, and chemosis indicate likely orbital abscess.

        (3) Intracranial complications include cavernous sinus thrombosis (signs include bilateral orbital involvement, ophthalmoplegia, progressive and severe chemosis, retinal engorgement, fever, and prostration), meningitis, subdural empyema, and brain abscess.

REFERENCES

Clement PA, Bluestone CD: Management of rhinosinusitis in children: Consensus meeting, Brussels, Belgium. Arch Otolaryngol 1998;**124**(1):31.

Durham S: ABC of allergies. Summer hay fever. Br Med J 1998;**316**:843.

Guarderas JC: Rhinitis and sinusitis: Office management. Mayo Clin Proc 1996;**71**(9):882.

Incaudo GA, Wooding LG: Diagnosis and treatment of acute and subacute sinusitis in children and adults. Clin Rev Allergy Immunol 1998;**16**:157.

Jordan AJ, Mabry RL: Geriatric rhinitis: What it is and how to treat it. Geriatrics 1998;**53**(6):76.

Kankam CG, Sallis R: Acute sinusitis in adults. Difficult to diagnose, essential to treat. Postgrad Med 1997;**102**(2):253.

Lemanske RF: A review of current guidelines for allergic rhinitis and asthma. J Allergy Clin Immunol 1998;**101**(2):S392.

Low DE, Desrosiers M: A practical guide for the diagnosis and treatment of acute sinusitis. Can Med Assoc J 1997;**156**:(6S):1S.

Mackay IS, Durham SR: ABC of allergies. Perennial rhinitis. Br Med J 1998;**316**:917.
Newton DA: Sinusitis in children and adolescents. Primary Care 1996;**23**(4):701.
Rachelefsky GS: Pharmacologic management of allergic rhinitis. J Allergy Clin Immunol 1998;
   101(2):S367.
Slavin RG: Nasal polyps and sinusitis. JAMA 1997;**278**:1849.

---

60   Soft Tissue Injury

Marvin A. Dewar, MD, JD

I. Definition. Soft tissue injuries include injuries to skin skeletal muscle, tendons, or ligaments as a result of the application of external force or excessive internal loading.

II. Common diagnoses. Soft tissue injuries include **contusions, muscle strains, ligament sprains, burns, overuse injuries,** and **lacerations** (see Chapter 43).

III. Epidemiology. Soft tissue injuries are responsible for 2.7% of all ambulatory patient encounters. Family physicians provide the care for 52% of patients with soft tissue injuries.

    A. Contusions, sprains, strains, and overuse injuries are most commonly seen in athletes and manual workers, particularly those whose work involves heavy lifting and repetitive motions. In one study, sprains and strains made up 90% of the injuries on a professional soccer team and 80% of the injuries on a professional football team.

    B. Burns. Burns most commonly occur in males between the ages of 18 and 35. The most common cause of major burn injuries is residential fires.

IV. Pathophysiology

    A. Contusions result from the application of excessive external force to soft tissues, producing tissue bleeding and edema. Contusions range from mild bruising to significant hematoma formation.

    B. Strains result from sudden excessive muscle loading, producing disruption of musculotendinous units with bleeding and edema. Strains are classified as (1) **first-degree** (microscopic musculotendinous disruption), (2) **second-degree** (partial disruption of musculotendinous units), or (3) **third-degree** (complete disruption of musculotendinous units).

    C. Burns. Thermal injury involves varying degrees of soft tissue coagulation, vascular stasis, and hyperemia. Burns are classified as outlined below.

        1. First-degree burns (eg, most sunburns) are characterized by epidermal hyperemia without tissue destruction.

        2. Second-degree burns (partial-thickness burns) often result from hot liquid spills or flash burns and involve both epidermal and dermal injury. Deep dermal structures (eg, hair follicles and sweat glands) survive, and skin regeneration occurs.

        3. Third-degree burns (full-thickness burns) often result from contact with open flames, steam, or hot oil and produce epidermal, dermal, and subcutaneous tissue destruction. Skin regeneration is minimal or absent.

    D. Sprains result from sudden excessive ligament loading, producing bleeding and edema (see Chapters 7 and 42 for further discussion of ankle and knee sprains). Sprains are classified as (1) **first-degree** (microscopic ligament injury), (2) **second-degree** (partial ligament disruption), or (3) **third-degree** (complete ligament disruption).

V. Symptoms. Contusions, sprains, strains, and overuse injuries produce **pain** localized to the region of the injury. The degree of pain is usually related to the severity of the injury. First- and second-degree burns also produce localized pain, but third-degree burns are often painless. Severe sprains and strains may produce weakness or instability of the involved musculotendinous unit.

VI. Signs. Signs of soft tissue injury are usually localized to the injury site (see Chapters 7 and 42).

    A. Local tenderness, edema, ecchymosis, muscle spasm, and functional impairment are common in sprains, strains, and contusions. The severity of findings is usually proportional to the extent of injury.

B. Signs associated with burn injuries vary depending on the depth and severity of the injury.

    1. Painful erythema that blanches with pressure is common in first- and second-degree burns. Third-degree burns do not blanch and may be anesthetic due to destruction of nerve endings.

    2. Blistering is common with second-degree burns but is absent in most first- and third-degree burns.

    3. Dry, leathery, charred skin with visible thrombosed blood vessels characterizes third-degree burns. Second-degree burns often appear **raw and moist.**

VII. Laboratory tests

  A. **A thorough history and physical examination** are adequate for evaluation of most soft tissue injuries.

  B. X-ray evaluation is indicated in the following situations.

    1. To rule out associated fractures in particularly severe injuries characterized by marked pain (particularly when over bony prominences), edema, and/or functional impairment.

    2. To rule out the development of myositis ossificans in patients with quadriceps contusions ("charley horses") who remain symptomatic after 2–6 weeks of treatment. The history of injury is important in helping to distinguish x-ray changes of myositis ossificans from juxtacortical osteosarcoma.

    3. To rule out associated fractures and avulsions in third-degree and selected severe second-degree strains and sprains.

    4. To rule out apophyseal avulsions in children and adolescents with second- or third-degree strains and sprains.

VIII. Treatment (see Chapters 7, 8, 30, 34, 42, and 44 for additional information about treatment of specific injuries).

  A. Contusions and strains

    1. General management includes rest, ice, compression, elevation (**RICE**) and analgesia.

      a. Rest. In all but the mildest injuries, rest of the injured extremity for 24–48 hours is recommended to limit tissue hemorrhage and facilitate earlier return to normal function. In general, gradual return to activity should be permitted after 24–48 hours within the reasonable limits of pain.

      b. Ice should be applied for 48–72 hours after the injury to limit pain, swelling, and tissue hemorrhage. Ice chips enclosed in a plastic bag may be applied to the injury for 10–20 minutes two to four times per day. The risk of frostbite is eliminated by limiting exposure to the recommended duration and by placing a damp cloth between the ice bag and the skin.

      c. Compression. Posttraumatic swelling may be diminished by external compression with an Ace bandage for 24–72 hours after injury.

      d. Elevation of the injured extremity for 24–72 hours after injury decreases swelling by decreasing hydrostatic pressure and promoting lymphatic drainage.

      e. Analgesia. Nonsteroidal anti-inflammatory drugs (NSAIDs), for example, **ibuprofen** or **indomethacin,** are frequently used for posttraumatic analgesia. In addition, NSAIDs may limit the acute inflammatory response in the immediate postinjury period. **Acetaminophen,** 325–650 mg every 4 hours, is also useful in the management of posttraumatic pain. Severe pain may require a **combination of acetaminophen and codeine,** 15–60 mg, or **oxycodone,** 5 mg every 4–6 hours.

    2. Rehabilitation involves early mobilization and progressive strengthening of injured tissue.

      a. Active range-of-motion exercises can begin 48–72 hours after injury in most mild to moderate injuries. Early activity minimizes deconditioning and loss of muscle strength caused by prolonged immobilization. The presence of a large muscle hematoma, especially of the quadriceps, is a contraindication to early mobilization because of the risk of myositis ossificans. Once activity is begun, **progressive muscle strengthening** should be undertaken within the limits of the patient's pain tolerance.

      b. Physical modalities, including the use of warm whirlpools moist heat packs, contrast baths (hot and cold), and therapeutic ultrasonography, facilitate early mobilization and may enhance healing.

   c. **Protective padding** over muscle contusions often facilitates early return
      to activity.
   d. **Strengthening and endurance exercise** targeted at the injured site are
      important to decrease the risk of recurrent injury.
3. **Orthopedic referral** is helpful in the management of third-degree strains and
   sprains, apophyseal injuries in children, and contusions and second-degree
   strains and sprains that are unresponsive to conservative treatment.
4. **Prevention.** The risk of soft tissue injury can be diminished by adequate
   warm-up and stretching before vigorous activity. Balanced stretching of agonist and antagonist muscle groups is optimal.

B. **Burns.** General management of burns requires assessment of the extent and
   severity of the burn injury. Anatomic charts may be used to estimate the percentage of body surface area (BSA) burned (Figure 60–1). Knowledge that the palm
   represents approximately 1% of the BSA is also helpful.

   1. **Hospitalization** should be considered in the following cases.
      a. Second-degree burns involving more than 18% BSA in an adult or 12%
         BSA in a child.
      b. Third-degree burns involving more than 5% BSA.
      c. Burns involving the hands, feet, face, eyes, or perineum.
      d. Inhalation or airway injuries.
      e. Burn wound infections not responding rapidly to outpatient management.
      f. General conditions warranting admission. A lower threshold for hospital-
         ization is necessary in children, the elderly, and patients with other signif-
         icant medical conditions.
   2. **Cold, wet compresses** applied soon after injury may reduce pain and limit the
      extent of burn injury. This is adequate treatment for most first-degree burns.

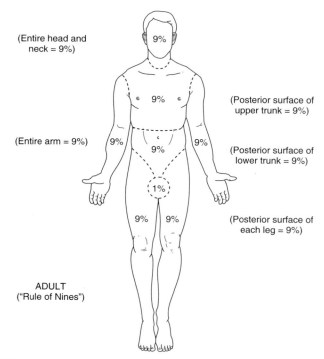

FIGURE 60–1. Estimation of body surface area in burns. (Reprinted with permission from Schroeder
SA, et al: *Current Medical Diagnosis & Treatment.* Appleton & Lange; 1992.)

3. **Asepsis.** Burned skin should be cleaned with mild soap and irrigated with sterile saline. Debris, necrotic tissue, and broken blisters should be carefully removed under aseptic conditions. Intact blisters should be left unbroken until re-epithelialization occurs to provide a sterile biologic wound dressing. Outpatient whirlpool treatment may facilitate burn asepsis and debridement in patients having difficulty with personal wound care.

4. **Analgesia** (see section VIII,A,1,e).

5. **Tetanus immunization** (see Chapter 43).

6. **Wound dressing.** Most second- and third-degree burns should be covered with an occlusive sterile dressing such as course mesh gauze. Wound dressings should be changed daily if topical antibiotics are not used and twice daily if topical antibiotics are used. Some burns, particularly those around the face, neck, hands, and perineum, may be left open without dressings.

7. **Antibiotics**
   a. **Oral antibiotics** are required in patients with evidence of burn wound infection (eg, erythema at burn margins) or patients at particularly high risk of burn wound infection (eg, patients with "dirty" wounds). Early burn wound infections, primarily caused by β-hemolytic streptococci, are best treated with the following drugs.
      (1) **Penicillin V potassium**
         (a) Adults: 500 mg every 6 hours.
         (b) Children: 30–50 mg/kg/day in four divided doses.
      (2) **Erythromycin** is an acceptable alternative for patients allergic to β-lactam antibiotics.
         (a) Adults: 500 mg every 6 hours.
         (b) Children: 30–50 mg/kg/day in four divided doses.
   b. **Topical antibiotics** are frequently utilized in patients with second- and third-degree burns to reduce the incidence of burn wound infection. **Silver sulfadiazine** 1% cream (Silvadene) may be applied twice daily with sterile gloves or a sterile tongue depressor to a depth of $\frac{1}{16}$ inch.

8. **Skin grafting.** Third-degree and deeper second-degree burns often heal with scarring and may require referral for skin grafting.

REFERENCES

Bhatia X, Hill X, Macpherson X, et al: Myositis ossificans conscripta. Arch Fam Med 1997;**6**:316.

Baumert PW: Acute inflammation after injury. Postgrad Med 1995;**97**:35.

Dyment PG: Initial management of minor acute soft-tissue injuries. Pediatr Ann 1988;**17**:99.

Peck DM: Apophyseal injuries in the young athlete. Am Fam Physician 1995;**51**:1891.

Phillips LG, Robson MC, Heggers JP: Treating minor burns. Postgrad Med 1989;**85**:219.

Rivenburg DW: Physical modalities in the treatment of tendon injuries. Clin Sports Med 1992; **11**:645.

Stanitski CL: Management of sports injuries in children and adolescents. Orthop Clin North Am 1988;**19**:689.

Wachtel TL: Major burns. Postgrad Med 1989;**85**:178.

61   Sore Throat

L. Peter Schwiebert, MD

I. **Definition.** Sore throat is a scratchy sensation or pain in the throat, usually made worse by swallowing.

II. **Common diagnoses.** Causes of sore throat commonly encountered in the ambulatory primary care setting are listed below.
   A. **Irritants,** such as cigarette smoke, dust, or allergens; low humidity; gastroesophageal reflux disease (GERD); and postnasal drainage. In up to 40% of patients with sore throat, no pathogen can be isolated. In an undetermined number of these cases, the pharyngitis is caused by an irritant.
   B. **Common cold viruses,** including rhinovirus, coronavirus, respiratory syncytial virus, and parainfluenza (25–30% of cases).

    C. Group A β-hemolytic streptococci (GABHS) (15–30% of cases).

    D. Other viral infections, including coxsackieviruses A and B, herpesviruses, adenovirus, and influenza viruses A and B (5–10% of cases).

    E. Viruses that cause infectious mononucleosis, including Epstein-Barr virus and cytomegalovirus (CMV) (1–2% of cases).

    F. Other causes. The role of *Chlamydia trachomatis* and *Mycoplasma pneumoniae* in pharyngitis is controversial. One study reported serologic evidence of *C trachomatis* in 20% of patients with pharyngitis, but subsequent research using cultures in pediatric and adult patients has failed to confirm these results. In another study of adults with pharyngitis, *M pneumoniae* was found in 9% of patients.

III. Epidemiology. In the ambulatory primary care setting, up to 8% of patient visits per year are for sore throats.

    A. The **most common environmental irritant** is tobacco smoke, but exposure to dust or low humidity is another risk factor. Patients with allergies may report that their symptoms regularly follow seasonal patterns and may be associated with a past or family history of similar problems (see Chapter 59). Patients with sore throat due to GERD may give a history of heartburn or sour eructations, worsening of symptoms after a large meal or lying down, and relief with antacids.

    B. Common cold viruses cause sore throats most frequently during the colder months of the year.

    C. Streptococcal pharyngitis is most common in children between the ages of 5 and 15 years. In one study of 106 febrile children with exudative tonsillitis, no children under 3 years of age had streptococcal pharyngitis. The prevalence of streptococcal pharyngitis increases from 10% during the summer and fall to approximately 40% during the winter and early spring.

    D. Adenoviral infection is a relatively common cause of exudative pharyngitis in children. In the study of pediatric patients with exudative pharyngitis mentioned above, 19% of patients had adenoviral infection. **Influenza** usually occurs in epidemics between December and April. **Coxsackievirus** infections occurs most frequently in young children.

    E. Infectious mononucleosis occurs most frequently in patients who are not exposed to the Epstein-Barr virus until their second decade of life. These individuals are chiefly adolescents from higher socioeconomic groups in industrialized societies. The Epstein-Barr virus is a ubiquitous agent of low contagion. The majority of infections require intimate contact between susceptible individuals and symptomatic shedders of the virus.

    F. *Neisseria gonorrhoeae* is a rare cause of pharyngitis, but should be considered in high-risk patients, such as individuals who have a history of oral-genital sexual relations.

IV. Pathophysiology

    A. Irritants. Chemical irritants, cigarette smoke, postnasal drainage, refluxed gastric contents, and low humidity may cause sore throat through irritant effect, and allergies cause sore throat via a type I hypersensitivity reaction (for further information, see Chapter 59).

    B. Common cold viruses. Rhinoviruses produce pharyngeal irritation through invasion of the nasal epithelium.

    C. GABHS. These organisms invade the pharyngeal epithelium, where they multiply and cause an intense immune response.

    D. Other viruses invade and destroy respiratory tract columnar epithelial cells, causing desquamation of these cells. Coxsackieviruses are transmitted by respiratory droplets and directly seed the oral mucosa, invading the epithelium and causing cell lysis.

    E. Infectious mononucleosis viruses. The Epstein-Barr virus infects B lymphocytes of the pharynx with subsequent dissemination and replication throughout the lymphoreticular system, resulting in an immune response (heterophile antibodies). CMV causes infectious mononucleosis in 5% of cases.

V. Symptoms

    A. Sore throat. A scratchy, dry throat is caused by respiratory irritants, common cold viruses, and streptococcal pharyngitis. A more painful sore throat accompanied by dysphagia typically occurs with streptococcal pharyngitis, infectious mononucleosis, coxsackievirus, herpesvirus, or adenoviral infection.

B. Cough, rhinorrhea, hoarseness, conjunctivitis, or **diarrhea** decreases the likelihood of streptococcal pharyngitis. In studies correlating these symptoms with a positive streptococcal culture, cough and rhinorrhea make streptococcal infections less likely and other causes (eg, the common cold, influenza, allergies, or irritants) more likely. Among febrile pediatric patients with exudative pharyngitis, 45% of patients with cough had viral sore throat and 10% had streptococcal pharyngitis.

C. Gastrointestinal symptoms. Pediatric and geriatric patients with influenza may present with nausea, vomiting, and diarrhea. Ten percent to 20% of patients with infectious mononucleosis complain of anorexia and nausea.

D. Other symptoms

1. Patients with **allergies** classically complain of paroxysms of sneezing, watery, itchy eyes, and rhinorrhea associated with exposure to the allergen, although these symptoms often are absent (see Chapters 58 and 59).

2. With **influenza,** symptoms typically occur in three phases: abrupt onset of fever and systemic symptoms (eg, myalgias and headache) that last about 3 days; followed by 3–4 days of cough, rhinorrhea, and pharyngitis; and then 1–2 weeks of convalescence with symptoms of cough and malaise.

VI. Signs

A. Pharyngeal hyperemia occurs with influenza, respiratory irritants, and the common cold.

B. Tonsillar exudate. A marked tonsillar exudate is characteristic of streptococcal pharyngitis.

C. Pharyngeal exudate

1. Viruses (principally adenovirus) cause a majority (53% of cases in one study) of exudative pharyngitis in children under the age of 6 years.

2. Fifty percent of patients with infectious mononucleosis present with exudative pharyngitis.

D. Fever

1. A temperature of >38.3 °C (101 °F) is one of a combination of physical findings correlating with a positive streptococcal culture. Other findings include a marked tonsillar exudate and enlarged tender anterior cervical nodes.

2. In 56% of cases, pediatric patients with adenoviral infection typically present with a temperature of >40 °C (104 °F). Moderate to high fever is also associated with coxsackievirus and initial herpesvirus infections.

3. Children with Epstein-Barr virus have a lower-grade fever than with adenoviral or streptococcal infections. In one study, 43% of patients had a fever for 5 days or more.

4. Influenza is characterized by abrupt onset of temperature in the range of 37.8–40 °C (100–104 °F).

E. Conjunctivitis is associated with adenoviral infections. In 22% of cases, otitis media may also occur.

F. Lymphadenopathy is a cardinal sign of infectious mononucleosis. In addition, over 90% of patients with this disease have enlarged posterior cervical nodes. Enlarged tender anterior cervical nodes are one of a combination of findings correlating with positive streptococcal culture (see above).

G. Other findings. Coxsackievirus infections are associated with erythematous-based small vesicles or ulcers in the pharynx and may be associated with similar papulovesicles on the palms and soles. The shallow, erythematous-based vesicles and ulcers of herpesvirus can occur anywhere on the pharynx, gingiva, or vermilion border.

VII. Laboratory tests. For patients whose clinical picture is consistent with influenza, the common cold, or exposure to respiratory irritants, no further laboratory work-up is indicated (for further information on the evaluation of suspected allergies, see Chapters 58 and 59; for evaluation of GERD, see Chapter 22).

A. Streptococcal screen. A decision on which patients with pharyngitis should have a streptococcal screen depends on the physician's goals—minimizing total cost, minimizing risks associated with a missed diagnosis, or minimizing the cost of a missed diagnosis and unnecessary use of antibiotics. The following strategy, which is more cost-effective than mass screening but minimizes chances of missing a case of streptococcal pharyngitis, is recommended. A rapid streptococcal screen should be performed on patients with a sore throat and an intermediate pretest likelihood of streptococcal pharyngitis (Table 61–1). In obtaining the screen or culture, the swab should contact both tonsils or tonsillar fossae and the posterior pharyngeal wall.

1. A **rapid streptococcal screen** is a 10-minute test for streptococcal antigens. These screens have a sensitivity of 80–90% and a specificity of >90% for detecting streptococcal pharyngitis. Therefore, with appropriate test selection (Table 61–1), therapeutic decisions can confidently be based on a positive result. However, a negative screen in the context of clinical suspicion of streptococcal pharyngitis should be followed up with blood agar plate (BAP) culture.

2. A large multicenter study found that a rapid antigen detection test using **optical immunoassay (OIA)** had higher sensitivity and slightly lower specificity compared to BAP. If these results are confirmed and if cost and test time improve, OIA could become the standard for diagnosis of GABHS.

3. A **follow-up screen** to test for cure is not recommended or indicated in patients who respond clinically to antibiotic therapy within 5 days.

4. The **carrier state** (positive strep screen or BAP with low pretest likelihood or without GABHS antigenemia) usually represents low infectivity. In certain situations, the carrier state warrants treatment; these include a history of rheumatic fever, community outbreak of rheumatic fever or nephritogenic streptococcal infection, or "Ping-Pong" spread of GABHS in a family or other closed community, such as military barracks, prison, or college dormitory.

B. **Throat culture.** The BAP culture is approximately 95% sensitive and has a low false-positive rate in diagnosing streptococcal pharyngitis, but requires 24 hours' incubation. A culture should be performed in the high-risk, low-prevalence situations outlined in Table 61–1.

C. **Heterophile antibody test.** The Monospot test, which rapidly detects heterophile antibodies, compares favorably with the sensitivity and specificity of older heterophile antibody tests. It is used to diagnose infectious mononucleosis. A complete blood cell count (CBC) with differential smear showing at least 50% lymphocytes and at least 10% atypical lymphocytes also confirms this diagnosis.

D. **Other tests**

1. Pharyngeal, endocervical, and urethral cultures for gonorrhea should be performed in high-risk patients (see section III,F).

2. Chlamydial culture or serology is not recommended. In one recent study, investigators concluded that *C trachomatis* and *M pneumoniae* were not significant causes of pharyngitis in children. In another study of 95 college students with pharyngitis, *C trachomatis* was not found.

TABLE 61–1. TESTING PATIENTS WITH SORE THROAT BASED ON PRETEST LIKELIHOOD OF STREPTOCOCCAL PHARYNGITIS

Signs	Season	
	Winter/Spring	Summer/Fall
Temperature >38 °C (101 °F), enlarged erythematous tonsils with exudate, enlarged tender anterior cervical nodes	No testing necessary; begin treatment[1]	Rapid streptococcal screen[2]
Patient with two of the above signs, or all three signs with cough, rhinorrhea, or hoarseness	Rapid streptococcal screen[2]	Blood agar plate culture (BAP)
Patient with one of the three signs or with no signs but in a high-risk group[3]	BAP[4]	No testing necessary unless in a high-risk group[3]

[1] High pretest likelihood (>50%).
[2] Intermediate pretest likelihood (20–50%).
[3] Such patients include those who have diabetes mellitus, have a history of rheumatic fever, or present during a community outbreak of nephritogenic streptococcal infection.
[4] Low pretest likelihood (<20%).

3. Liver function tests, including serum aspartate aminotransferase (AST) and serum alanine aminotransferase (ALT) as well as serum bilirubin, CBC, platelet count, and Coombs' test, should be performed if infectious mononucleosis is suspected. Patients with this disease are at risk for developing hepatitis, hemolytic anemia, granulocytopenia, and thrombocytopenia (see Chapter 45). Severe hepatitis is indicated by an ALT or AST of >1000 U/L or a serum bilirubin of >10 mg/dL.

VIII. Treatment

A. Environmental irritants should be avoided if possible. In particular, patients should be encouraged to stop smoking, avoid allergens or dusty environments, and humidify low-humidity environments. Treatment of allergies is discussed in Chapter 59, and management of GERD is discussed in Chapter 22.

B. Viral infections (eg, common cold, adenovirus, coxsackievirus, and herpesvirus). These infections are self-limited, lasting from a few days to 2 weeks. Patients may obtain symptomatic relief from the following regimens.

1. Topical pain relief may be provided by as-needed lozenges (eg, Cepastat or Chloraseptic) or saline nasal spray or gargles, made by mixing 1 tsp of salt in 1 pint of warm water. Oropharyngeal lesions of coxsackievirus or herpes simplex virus may benefit from viscous Xylocaine 2% or benzocaine 15%, applied to lesions every 3–4 hours with a cotton-tipped applicator; soothing rinses (1 tsp of baking soda in 32 oz of water or saline, swished orally then expectorated three or four times daily); or a variety of coating agents (eg, diphenhydramine elixir, 12.5 mg/5 mL, mixed with an equal volume of either kaolin and pectin [Kaopectate] or aluminum-magnesium hydroxide antacid [Maalox], 1 tsp swished intraorally for 2 minutes every 2 hours).

2. Fluid intake should be increased to up to 2–3 quarts of water or juice per day.

3. Analgesic drugs include either aspirin, 650 mg every 4–6 hours orally in teenagers or adults, or acetaminophen, 5–10 mg/kg/day every 4–6 hours orally in children. Codeine relieves more severe discomfort; the dosage is 30–60 mg orally every 4–6 hours in adults or 3 mg/kg/day orally every 4–6 hours in children.

4. Decongestants (see Chapter 59).

C. Streptococcal infections. Antibiotic therapy has been shown to decrease the duration of fever, sore throat, and adenopathy. Such treatment also reduces suppurative complications (eg, peritonsillar abscess, otitis media, or cervical adenitis) and autoimmune sequelae, chiefly rheumatic fever.

1. Indications

a. Patients with a positive rapid streptococcal screen, throat culture, or both.

b. Patients with a high probability of having streptococcal infection (Table 61–1).

c. Some clinicians initiate antibiotic therapy in high-risk patients pending throat culture results (see section VII,B), although studies have demonstrated that delaying therapy for 48 hours does not interfere with the antibiotic's reduction of the risk of rheumatic fever.

2. Initial regimens

a. Penicillin is the drug of choice for streptococcal pharyngitis. Adults should receive **penicillin V potassium,** 500 mg orally two or three times daily for 10 days, and children should receive 30–50 mg/kg/day in two or three divided doses for 10 days. **Penicillin G benzathine** intramuscularly may be preferred for patients in whom compliance with the oral regimen or follow-up is questionable. Adults and children weighing >27 kg (60 lb) should receive 1.2 million U intramuscularly, and those weighing <27 kg should receive 600,000 U. A mixture of 900,000 U of benzathine and 300,000 U of procaine penicillin (**Bicillin C-R**) is also effective and causes less local reaction than penicillin G benzathine alone.

b. Erythromycin (eg, Ery-Tab, Eryc, or E-Mycin) is the drug of choice for those allergic to penicillin. Adults should receive 500 mg orally twice daily for 10 days. The pediatric dosage is 30–50 mg/kg/day, given in two to four divided doses daily. **Azithromycin** (Zithromax), 500 mg orally on day 1 and 250 mg on days 2–5, is also effective for those 15 years or older; pediatric patients take 10 mg/kg of the suspension on day 1 and 5 mg/kg on days 2–5.

    c. The following **short regimens** have been proven comparable to 10 days' penicillin V: azithromycin (see above); amoxicillin (Amoxil), 20–50 mg/kg divided into two or three doses daily or 375–750 mg divided into three doses for 6 days; cefpodoxime proxetil (Vantin), 100 mg or 5 mg/kg every 12 hours for 5 days; or cefixime (Suprax), 400 mg or 8 mg/kg daily for 5 days. Disadvantages of these agents include higher cost than penicillin and broader spectrum, which may foster bacterial resistance.

3. Further treatment (if necessary). Patients should feel better within 12–24 hours of initiation of antibiotic therapy. Failure to improve within 1 week may result from noncompliance with the drug regimen, penicillin tolerance, destruction of penicillin by β-lactamase–producing organisms, missed diagnosis, or an undiagnosed second cause of pharyngitis, particularly infectious mononucleosis. The following guidelines should be observed.

    a. Appropriate tests for infectious mononucleosis should be performed (see sections VII,C and D).

    b. Antibiotic regimens for penicillin tolerance should be instituted. **Amoxicillin-clavulanate potassium** (Augmentin), 40 mg/kg/day orally in three divided doses, or a cephalosporin (eg, **cefadroxil,** 30 mg/kg/day orally in one dose) has been shown to be effective in eradicating streptococci in those patients who do not respond to repeated courses of oral penicillin.

4. Recurrent episodes of acute pharyngitis raise the issue of whether **acute streptococcal pharyngitis** or **acute viral pharyngitis with streptococcal carrier state** is occurring. **Viral pharyngitis** is suggested by clinical or epidemiologic findings consistent with viral infection, failure to improve on antistreptococcal antibiotics, no rise in antistreptolysin O (ASO) titers, or positive throat cultures between episodes of pharyngitis. **Acute recurrent streptococcal infection** is suggested by appropriate clinical or epidemiologic findings, dramatic response to antibiotic therapy, a rise in ASO titers, or negative throat cultures between episodes of acute pharyngitis.

5. When eradication of the carrier state is appropriate (see section VII,A,4), the following regimens are effective: clindamycin (Cleocin), 20 mg/kg/day orally in three doses for 10 days, *or* rifampin (Rifaden), 20 mg/kg/day orally in two doses for 4 days, *plus* the standard regimen of phenoxymethyl *or* penicillin G benzathine.

D. Influenza symptoms may be alleviated within 48 hours of onset by giving **amantadine,** 100 mg orally twice a day (once a day in elderly patients). This drug may cause insomnia, dizziness, drowsiness, or difficulty concentrating.

E. Infectious mononucleosis

1. Ninety-five percent of patients with infectious mononucleosis recover uneventfully, and supportive treatment will suffice. Such therapy includes avoidance of contact sports or heavy lifting in the first 2–3 weeks of illness (especially if the patient has splenomegaly), adequate rest, and analgesics (see section VIII,B,3).

2. Corticosteroids may be necessary in the following circumstances: impending airway obstruction, severe hepatitis, thrombocytopenia, hemolytic anemia, or granulocytopenia. Treatment should be initiated with **prednisone** (or an equivalent), 60–80 mg/day orally in divided doses, tapered over 1–2 weeks.

REFERENCES

Bailey RE: Diagnosis and treatment of infectious mononucleosis. Am Fam Physician 1994;**49:**879.

Gerber MA: Treatment failures or carriers: Perception or problems? Pediatr Infect Dis J 1994; **13:**576.

Gerber MA, Tanz RR, Kabat W, et al: Optical immunoassay test for group A beta-hemolytic streptococcal pharyngitis. JAMA 1997;**277:**899.

Kiselica D: Group A beta-hemolytic streptococcal pharyngitis: Current clinical concepts. Am Fam Physician 1994;**49:**1147.

Perkins A: An approach to diagnosing the acute sore throat. Am Fam Physician 1997;**55:**131.

Pichichero ME, Cohen R: Shortened course of antibiotic therapy for acute otitis media, sinusitis, and tonsillopharyngitis. Pediatr Infect Dis J 1997;**16:**680.

62 Syncope

Ted D. Epperly, MD, & John P. Fogarty, MD

I. **Definition.** Syncope is a sudden transient loss of consciousness and motor control. Syncope must be differentiated from presyncope or near syncope, which is a feeling of lightheadedness or dizziness not associated with loss of consciousness or motor control.

II. **Common diagnoses.** There are five major causes of syncope.

A. **Reflex syncope** (60–65% of cases) includes vasodepressor, vasovagal, orthostatic, and vagotonic causes.

B. **Neurologic or psychogenic syncope** (15–20% of cases) includes seizures and hysteric causes.

C. **Cardiac syncope** (10% of cases) includes dysrhythmias and obstructive and ischemic causes.

D. **Vascular syncope** (2–3% of cases) includes cerebrovascular accidents (CVAs), transient ischemic attacks (TIAs), migraines, and subclavian steal syndrome.

E. **Metabolic syncope** (2–3% of cases) includes hypoglycemia, hypoxia, and hyperventilation.

III. **Epidemiology.** Syncope is a common medical problem and accounts for approximately 3% of emergency room visits and 1–6% of hospital admissions. The prevalence of syncope increases with age from 0.7% in men aged 35–44 to 5.6% in men over the age of 75. In long-term care institutions, the annual incidence is approximately 6%. In the Framingham cohort of patients, approximately 3% of men and 3.5% of women experienced syncope. The elderly represent the population at greatest risk for most of the causes of syncope. The young and middle-aged populations can have syncope from any of the listed causes, but reflex syncope is the most common cause in the pediatric age group. There appears to be no gender, occupational, or racial predilection. Underlying cardiac, seizure, vascular, or metabolic problems are potential risk factors. Medications that produce hypotension or increased vagal tone may also be associated with an increased incidence of syncope and account for about 11% of the episodes of syncope in the elderly.

IV. **Pathophysiology.** The interruption of blood flow to the brain for longer than 8–15 seconds can lead to loss of consciousness. Similarly, a drop in systolic blood pressure below 70 mm Hg (or a mean drop of 30–40 mm Hg) for the same period can lead to syncope.

A. **Reflex syncope.** The underlying mechanism in reflex syncope—transient decreases of venous return to the heart—may be exacerbated by an associated bradycardia with increased vagal tone. This further decreases cardiac output and cerebral perfusion.

1. **Vasovagal syncope** results from vagal stimulation that leads to bradycardia, reduced cardiac output, and eventually decreased cerebral perfusion.

2. **Orthostatic or postural syncope** results from a decrease in blood pressure with change to the upright position, usually with a compensatory increase in pulse rate. This drop may be due to drugs, especially diuretics, vasodilators, antihypertensives, antidepressants, antipsychotics, and many sedative-hypnotics that lower intravascular volume and peripheral resistance. Intravascular volume depletion secondary to blood or fluid losses such as diarrhea, sweat, polyuria, or third space loss can also lead to orthostatic syncope. A peripheral neuropathy (eg, diabetes mellitus) causing decreased vascular tone and other miscellaneous conditions, including pregnancy, severe varicose veins, prolonged bed rest, and postsurgical sympathectomy, can result in orthostatic syncope.

3. **Vasodepressor syncope** (the common faint) occurs in response to distress. The "fight or flight" reflexes are only partially mobilized, resulting in peripheral venous and arterial pooling. This pooling decreases cardiac preload, cardiac output, and cerebral perfusion.

4. **Vagotonic syncope** is seen in several situations, most commonly posttussive, postmicturition, and following a Valsalva's maneuver. Typically, vagally mediated venous pooling and a corresponding decrease in cardiac output,

coupled with increased intrathoracic pressure from coughing or Valsalva's maneuver, further decrease cardiac output and lead to reduced cerebral perfusion.

B. Neurologic or psychogenic syncope
   1. **Epilepsy** (see Chapter 89).
   2. **Hysteria,** or the "swoon," produces syncope-like symptoms without true changes in the cardiovascular, central, or autonomic nervous system.

C. Cardiac syncope
   1. **Dysrhythmias.** Bradyarrhythmias, tachyarrhythmias, heart block, and sick sinus syndrome cause syncope through a decrease in cerebral perfusion.
      a. **Bradyarrhythmias** are usually sudden or abrupt in onset with transient asystole or severe bradycardia and profound decreases in cerebral perfusion.
      b. **Tachyarrhythmias.** The onset of syncope in cases of tachycardia depends on the rate (usually symptomatic at >160 beats per minute) in addition to how well the cardiac output is maintained.
      c. **Heart block** and **sick sinus syndrome** can lead to syncope if there is 5 seconds or more of ineffective systoles.
   2. **Obstructive syncope.** The structural abnormalities of aortic stenosis, asymmetric septal hypertrophy, atrial myxoma, and mitral valve prolapse interfere with effective cardiac output and are often worsened with exercise. To produce syncope, a pulmonary embolus must be large enough to decrease effective pulmonary circulation and oxygenation.
   3. **Cardiac ischemic events.** Syncope may occur with acute myocardial infarction (MI) secondary to dysrhythmias or pump dysfunction. Coronary vasospasm or severe angina with resultant transient dysrhythmias or hypotension can also lead to syncope.

D. Vascular syncope is not a common finding in transient cerebral ischemia or cerebral vascular accidents unless severe bilateral disease or coexistent brain stem ischemia occurs. In subclavian steal syndrome, the proximal subclavian artery is occluded. Arm exercise decreases the muscle bed's peripheral resistance and shunts blood from the vertebral artery, leading to cerebral ischemia and eventual syncope.

E. Metabolic syncope. Metabolic entities are more prone to alter consciousness than to cause true syncope, but they must be kept in mind, as they are treatable.

V. Symptoms
A. Reflex syncope is heralded by vague nausea, warmth, sweating, clamminess, blurred vision, and lightheadedness. Syncope occurs within seconds to minutes following these symptoms. Associated with these symptoms may be a history of recent bad news, emotional distress, heavy coughing, urination, or a Valsalva-like maneuver. In orthostatic syncope, the patient often gives a history of these symptoms when assuming the upright position.

B. Neurologic or psychogenic syncope
   1. **A seizure is associated with an abrupt loss of consciousness.** There may be associated warning symptoms (aura) involving certain smells, sounds, or visual cues. The patient will often be confused and disoriented for up to 30 minutes after the seizure (see Chapter 89).
   2. **Hysteria often produces a graceful fall or swoon** to the couch or the floor and usually an emotionally detached description of the event.

C. Cardiac syncope
   1. **Dysrhythmias usually cause an abrupt loss of consciousness.** Warning symptoms seldom occur, unless associated with angina or MI. Bradyarrhythmias usually produce syncope within 12–15 seconds when the patient is supine but within 5–6 seconds when the patient is upright. Patients who are experiencing tachyarrhythmias usually present with a sensation of palpitations, chest pain, or pressure; a gradual "graying out," rather than abrupt loss of consciousness, results. The physician should consider cardiac syncope as a possible cause of unexplained falls in the elderly.
   2. **Obstructive syncope is usually associated with exertion,** which may be abrupt or gradual, depending on the cause. The exception is pulmonary embolism, which can occur at any time.

      3. Syncope in the setting of ischemia usually has preceding symptoms of **acute angina** or MI.

  D. Vascular syncope. It is rare for a CVA or TIA to cause syncope, unless there is significant bihemispheric or reticular activating system involvement. Subclavian steal syndrome, on the other hand, can lead to significant posterior brain stem ischemia with symptoms consisting of **diplopia, dysarthria, dysphagia, dysesthesia,** and **dizziness** during peak arm exercise activities.

  E. Metabolic causes of syncope (eg, hypoxia or hypoglycemia) can lead to symptoms of **restlessness, confusion,** and **anxiety.** In hyperventilation, the patient often relates a sensation of smothering or shortness of breath in conjunction with circumoral, facial, and extremity paresthesias.

VI. Signs

  A. Reflex syncope

    1. The patient may be **pale, confused, restless,** or **diaphoretic,** and the **pulse, which is initially rapid, is usually slow** or unobtainable. Pupillary dilation, yawning, sighing, and hyperventilation also may occur.

    2. Unconsciousness is usually brief (seconds to a few minutes) once the patient reaches the supine position. Brief tonic-clonic movements can accompany syncopal episodes.

    3. In **orthostatic syncope,** pallor or weakness does not usually occur. A **drop in blood pressure** upon assuming the upright position is seen; however, there is no corresponding increase in heart rate. The failure of the pulse to rise often indicates autonomic dysfunction as the cause of the orthostatic hypotension. Near syncope is often reported by these patients with changes in position.

    4. Residual signs postsyncope often consist of weakness and diaphoresis. Bowel and bladder control is not lost.

  B. Neurologic or psychogenic syncope

    1. In **seizure disorders,** eyewitness accounts are important and usually consist of the classic **tonic-clonic movement disorder, incontinence,** and **postictal phase.** The patient is often groggy, fatigued, or confused and may smell of urine.

    2. Patients with **hysterical syncope** often present with signs of normal pulse, skin color, and blood pressure.

  C. Cardiac syncope. Signs are consistent with **poor perfusion** and **rapid or slow pulse,** depending on the underlying dysrhythmia. The syncopal episode is usually rapid in onset and may occur in any position. A murmur may or may not be present. If a pulmonary embolus is responsible, the patient may be dyspneic and tachypneic.

  D. Vascular syncope. Focal neurologic deficits may or may not be present following CVA, TIA, or migraine. A murmur over the proximal subclavian artery may be present in subclavian steal syndrome.

  E. Metabolic syncope. Restlessness, confusion, and **anxiety** may occur in these patients prior to syncope. Syncope can occur in any position. Pupils may be dilated in hypoxemia, and carpopedal spasm may accompany hyperventilation.

VII. Laboratory tests. The evaluation of patients with syncope should distinguish cardiac from noncardiac causes. Studies have shown that cardiac syncope has a 33% mortality rate compared to a 5% rate of mortality for noncardiac syncope and an 8% mortality rate in patients with an unknown cause when followed up over 5 years. Multiple investigators have found that the history, physical examination, and electrocardiogram (ECG) establish the diagnosis in 65–85% of cases in which a cause is determined. Although the cause of syncope remains undetermined in 38–47% of patients, their prognosis is generally excellent. Recurrences of syncope in these patients require reevaluation, as a causative factor may be determined. Patients with recurrent syncope (more than five episodes in 1 year) are more likely to have psychiatric than cardiac causes.

  A. Reflex syncope. No single laboratory test will diagnose a common faint. If the **history** suggests reflex syncope and the **physical examination** is normal, no diagnostic studies are needed. A careful drug history, a search for underlying diseases, and a carefully taken set of vital signs in the recumbent, sitting, and standing positions will often confirm orthostatic syncope. **Tilt table testing** may help demonstrate these blood pressure changes and help reproduce near syncopal or syncopal symptoms. In this test, the table is tilted at 60–80 degrees for 15–60 minutes in an effort to create a vasovagal-like reaction. If this response is not seen, an infusion of isoproterenol (Isuprel) can be added. A positive test is the occurrence of a syncopal episode with associated bradycardia, hypotension, or both. Addition of sublingual nitroglycerin (400 μg) has been shown to increase the total positivity rate to 70% with a specificity of 94%.

B. Neurologic or psychogenic syncope (see Chapter 89). Electroencephalography (EEG) and computerized tomography (CT) are useful studies in patients with new-onset seizure disorders.

C. Cardiac syncope. Patients believed to have cardiac syncope should be hospitalized and undergo **cardiac monitoring,** especially elderly individuals with a prior history of cardiac disease (ie, coronary artery disease, congestive heart failure, valvular heart disease, obstructive cardiomyopathy, bundle branch block, or bifascicular block) or those persons who experience sudden syncope without warning. All of these patients should receive an ECG. Patients with a normal initial ECG are unlikely to have an underlying dysrhythmia or experience sudden death.

    1. Ambulatory cardiac monitoring with continuous-loop ECG recorders and **echocardiography** may be utilized if subtle or infrequent dysrhythmias or obstructive lesions are suspected. The optimal duration of ambulatory cardiac monitoring is unclear; however, the benefit of extending monitoring beyond 24 hours is questionable. The continuous-loop ECG recorder is useful for evaluating recurrent syncope and can be worn for extended periods, with an average monthly charge of less than $300.

    2. An **exercise stress test** may help identify dysrhythmias not seen on ambulatory cardiac monitoring. Stress tests should not be performed on individuals suspected of having an obstructive cardiac condition (eg, aortic stenosis, asymmetric septal hypertrophy, or atrial myxoma).

    3. Cardiac angiography may be needed to help clarify ischemic or anatomic abnormalities.

    4. Intracardiac electrophysiologic studies are not widely available and should be considered only in patients with recurrent life-threatening syncope to rule out a specific cardiac diagnosis. Such a specific diagnosis is more likely in patients with known underlying cardiac disease who are over age 60.

D. Vascular syncope. Head CT and **carotid and vertebral artery studies** can be helpful in patients suspected of having a vascular cause for their syncope. Subclavian vascular studies are warranted if subclavian steal is suspected.

E. Metabolic syncope. Arterial blood gas and **blood sugar** can be obtained if the physician suspects hypoxia or hypoglycemia as the cause of the patient's syncope.

VIII. Treatment. The prognosis for the patient who has idiopathic syncope is excellent. Therefore, if a thorough history, physical examination, ECG, and other tests as deemed appropriate fail to suggest a known cause, the patient can be so counseled and needs no further evaluation or work-up unless the syncope becomes recurrent.

A. Reflex syncope

    1. General measures. Once syncope has occurred, cerebral perfusion can usually be restored by placing the patient supine with the legs elevated. The upright position (fainting in a phone booth) is theoretically potentially fatal.

    2. Prevention. Reflex syncope can usually be prevented by removing or avoiding precipitants (eg, a hot, close environment or the upright position during painful procedures), by lying down, or by placing the head between the knees during the presyncopal period.

    3. Treatment of orthostatic syncope depends on the underlying cause. Drug-induced syncope requires modification or withdrawal of the agent, volume depletion requires fluid replacement, and metabolic neuropathies often respond to treatment of the underlying cause.

        a. Nonpharmacologic measures such as careful assumption of the upright position, pressure stockings, alcohol abstention, avoidance of prolonged bed rest, contracting the leg muscles before rising or standing for prolonged periods, and increasing salt intake (if no contraindications exist) are helpful.

        b. Pharmacologic measures are used if the above measures fail, and should be individualized.

(1) **Fludrocortisone** (Florinef), a sodium-retaining steroid, reduces the vasodepressor response and relieves the symptoms of vasodepressor carotid sinus syndrome. Therapy should begin with 0.1 mg orally daily and can be increased to 0.3–0.4 mg daily over several weeks. This therapy is contraindicated in patients with congestive heart failure.

(2) **Indomethacin** (eg, Indocin), 25–50 mg three times a day with meals, can also be tried. This medication may improve symptoms by opposing the vasodilatory effect of endogenous prostaglandins.

(3) A number of other agents have had success, including **beta blockers** such as **metoprolol** (Lopressor), 50 mg orally twice daily; **transdermal scopalamine** (Transderm Scōp), one 0.5-mg disk applied to the skin every 3 days; **disopyramide** (Norpace CR), 100 mg, two capsules orally twice daily (Norpace CR can be carefully adjusted upward to a dose of 800 mg/day); **theophylline** (Slo-Bid), 200 mg orally twice daily; **dextroamphetamine** (Dexedrine Spansule), one 5-mg capsule orally each morning, with the dosage titrated upward as needed; and **fluoxetine** (Prozac), 20 mg orally daily. Disopyramide works through a combination of negative inotropic, anticholinergic, and direct peripheral vasoconstrictive actions. Fluoxetine may help prevent recurrent syncope when other therapies have failed.

(4) In patients with vasovagal syncope associated with bradycardia asystole, drug therapy (eg, **metoprolol, theophylline,** or **disopyramide**) is often effective in preventing syncope, whereas pacing is not.

B. **Neurologic or psychogenic syncope.** If hysteria is suspected, counseling or psychiatric referral is recommended. Treatment of the underlying seizure disorder should control further seizures.

C. **Cardiac syncope.** Drug therapy or withdrawal may suffice for many bradyarrhythmias and tachyarrhythmias (see Chapter 52), and surgery may be indicated for structural or ischemic conditions. A **demand pacemaker** is indicated only when heart block or severe bradycardia has been proven responsible for the syncope. Dual-chamber pacing is clearly superior to single-chamber pacing when used for this purpose.

D. **Vascular syncope.** If test results indicate a stenotic lesion of 70% or greater in the carotid system, surgery should be contemplated. If the posterior circulation is involved or if there is a nonsurgical carotid lesion, aspirin, 300–1300 mg/day, or anticoagulants may be necessary (see Chapter 90 for dosages). Migraine prophylaxis should be instituted, if appropriate, for migraine-related syncope (see Chapter 35). Surgery is indicated for symptomatic proximal subclavian artery occlusion.

E. **Metabolic syncope.** Hypoglycemia should be treated immediately with one or two ampules of 50% dextrose in water intravenously; the underlying cause must then be determined and treated. Reasons for underlying hypoxia and hyperventilation should be investigated as appropriate and treatment should be instituted.

REFERENCES

Del Rosso A, Bartoli P, Bartoletti A, et al: Shortened head-up tilt testing potentiated with sublingual nitroglycerin in patients with unexplained syncope. Am Heart J 1998;**135**:564.

Gutgesell HP, Barst RJ, Humes RA, et al: Common cardiovascular problems in the young: Part I. Murmurs, chest pain, syncope, and irregular rhythms. Am Fam Physician 1997;**56**:1825.

Hart GT: Evaluation of syncope. Am Fam Physician 1995;**51**:1941.

Kapoor WN: Diagnostic evaluation of syncope. Am J Med 1991;**90**:91.

Kapoor WN: Syncope in older persons. J Am Geriatr Soc 1994;**42**:426.

Linzer M, Yang EH, Estes NA, et al: Diagnosing syncope. Part 1. Value of history, physical examination, and electrocardiography. Ann Intern Med 1997;**126**:989.

Linzer M, Yang EH, Estes NA, et al: Diagnosing syncope. Part 2. Unexplained syncope. Ann Intern Med 1997;**127**:76.

Shaw FE, Kenny RA: The overlap between syncope and falls in the elderly. Postgrad Med J 1997;**73**:635.

Sra JS, Jazayeri MR, Boaz A, et al: Comparison of cardiac pacing with drug therapy in the treatment of neurocardiogenic (vasovagal) syncope with bradycardia or asystole. N Engl J Med 1993;**328**:1085.

63   Urinary Incontinence

Barry D. Weiss, MD

I. **Definition.** Urinary incontinence is the involuntary leakage of urine at undesired or inappropriate times.

II. **Common diagnoses**
   A. **Transient (reversible) incontinence.**
   B. **Urge incontinence** resulting from uncontrolled contractions of the detrusor muscle.
   C. **Stress incontinence** associated with structural or neuropathic conditions affecting the ability of the urethral sphincter to hold urine in the bladder.
   D. **Overflow incontinence** caused either by obstruction of urinary outflow or impaired detrusor contractility.
   E. **Mixed incontinence** resulting from the simultaneous presence of two or more of the above causes.

III. **Epidemiology.** Urinary incontinence becomes more frequent with advancing age and is associated with poor general health and functional status. Among ambulatory, community-dwelling persons over age 65, urinary incontinence of varying severity occurs in 17–55% of females and 11–34% of males. About 14% of older women and 4% of older men are incontinent on a daily basis.
   A. **Reversible incontinence** may be present in as many as 20% of incontinent patients and is more likely when incontinence is of recent onset.
   B. **Urge incontinence** accounts for approximately 50–75% of irreversible incontinence in older individuals. Although most cases are idiopathic, patients with neurologic disorders (including dementia) are at particularly high risk.
   C. **Stress incontinence** is most commonly found in parous women, but a similar syndrome can occur in nulliparous women, in patients with neuropathic disorders that denervate the urethral sphincters, or in postprostatectomy patients whose sphincter mechanisms have been surgically damaged.
   D. **Overflow incontinence** accounts for <5% of incontinence in women but, because of the prevalence of prostate disorders, is found in 30–50% of older male patients with incontinence.
   E. **Mixed incontinence** is very common and may occur in as many as 50% of incontinent patients. Most often, urge incontinence is present in combination with another type of incontinence.

IV. **Pathophysiology.** Bladder detrusor contractions are under control of the "brain stem micturition center." Cortical and subcortical centers inhibit the brain stem micturition center, preventing it from stimulating detrusor contractions. The urethral sphincters are under both voluntary and autonomic adrenergic control (α-adrenergic stimulation causes sphincter contraction and β-adrenergic stimulation causes sphincter relaxation). Pelvic anatomic structure also facilitates sphincter control.
   A. **Reversible incontinence** (Table 63–1).
   B. **Urge incontinence,** also referred to as overactive bladder, occurs when pathologic disorders (eg, Parkinson's disease, Alzheimer's disease, or cerebrovascular insults) or idiopathic age-related cerebral degeneration causes the central inhibitory centers to function inadequately so that they fail to prevent detrusor muscle contractions. This leads to detrusor overactivity or irritability.
   C. **Stress incontinence** can result from prolapse or weakness of pelvic musculature or from neuropathic, surgical, or other damage to the urethra or its innervation.
   D. **Overflow incontinence** may be caused by obstruction of urethral outflow because of cancer, urethral stricture, or sphincter-detrusor dyssynergia (ie, loss of the synergistic urinary sphincter relaxation that normally occurs simultaneously with bladder detrusor contraction). Overflow bladder may also occur when detrusor contractility is impaired (eg, by neuropathic, vascular, or neoplastic damage to the bladder's innervation).
   E. **Mixed incontinence** occurs when multiple factors coexist, each of which independently causes or contributes to urinary incontinence.

TABLE 63–1. CONDITIONS COMMONLY ASSOCIATED WITH TRANSIENT (REVERSIBLE) URINARY INCONTINENCE

Obstructions of bladder outflow
Fecal impaction
Prostate enlargement
Medications that increase sphincter tone
α-Adrenergic agonists
β-Adrenergic antagonists
Decreased contractility of the bladder detrusor muscle
Medications that decrease detrusor tone
Anticholinergics
Prostaglandin inhibitors
Calcium channel-blocking agents
Narcotic analgesics
Irritability of the bladder detrusor muscle
Acute urinary tract infection
Atrophic vaginitis or urethritis
Bladder neoplasms and stones
Excessive urine production
Diuretic medications
Glycosuria or hypercalciuria
Excessive fluid intake
Impairment of urethral contraction
Medications (α-adrenergic blockers)
Central nervous system depression
Medical or psychiatric illness (eg, hypoxia, delirium, or depression)
Medications (eg, sedative-hypnotics or narcotics)
Temporary impairments of mobility
Injury, medical illness

V. Symptoms

A. **Urgency** is the primary symptom of uncontrolled bladder contractions (ie, urge incontinence). The sensitivity of the symptom of urgency in identifying patients with true urge incontinence, in comparison to formal urodynamic testing, is approximately 80%.

B. **Loss of urine with coughing,** descending stairs, sneezing, and so on is a classic symptom of stress incontinence. The positive predictive value of these symptoms exceeds 85% for identifying patients with true stress incontinence and exceeds 95% when accompanied by physical examination findings typical of stress incontinence. However, symptoms similar to those of stress incontinence can occur in patients with urge incontinence (pseudo-stress incontinence), because in urge incontinence the bladder is "irritable" and may contract when stimulated by repetitive increases in intra-abdominal pressure, such as from repetitive coughing.

C. **Dribbling** is a symptom of overflow incontinence, and it may occur with sphincter weakness, especially when it is caused by sphincter denervation. It usually increases with postural change or with Valsalva's maneuver.

D. **Abdominal discomfort** may be present in patients with overflow incontinence because of bladder distention, particularly if urinary retention and overflow are of recent onset.

VI. Signs

A. **Abnormal reflex, motor, or sensory function** suggests the presence of a neurologic disorder such as neuropathic sphincter or detrusor denervation, or cerebral dysfunction associated with urge incontinence.

B. **Abnormal mental status** (eg, dementia) indicates decreased function of cerebral inhibitory centers associated with urge incontinence.

C. **Abdominal distention** or **palpable bladder** is suggestive of urinary retention caused by overflow.

D. **Atrophic vaginitis** indicates the possibility of urge incontinence due to estrogen-responsive irritable bladder.

E. **Prolapse of pelvic organs** is frequently associated with stress incontinence.

F. **Prostate enlargement or masses** suggest the possibility of overflow incontinence secondary to bladder outflow obstruction.

G. **Impacted rectal stool** points toward overflow incontinence caused by obstruction of urethral outflow by the fecal impaction.

VII. **Laboratory and other tests.** Note that some patients may have pre-existing conditions that warrant specialized evaluations not discussed in this chapter (Figure 63–1).

A. **Basic evaluation** (for all incontinent patients)

1. **Urinalysis.** Pyuria or bacteriuria suggests infection, and a culture can confirm the diagnosis. Hematuria may indicate neoplasm or calculi, necessitating further evaluation with cystoscopy, renal ultrasound, and/or radiography.

2. **Postvoid residual urine (PVR)** volume should be measured to exclude overflow incontinence. Normal PVR is <50 mL. PVR of 200 mL or more is abnormal and indicates outflow obstruction or detrusor contractility problems. PVRs between 50 and 200 mL are equivocal, and the test should be repeated on another occasion.

   a. **Postvoid catheterization** is the most common method for determining PVR. A sterile catheter is inserted into the patient's bladder immediately after the patient voids, and the volume of collected urine is recorded. Inability to pass the catheter suggests obstruction from urethral stricture, prostate enlargement, etc.

   b. **Ultrasound** measurement of bladder volume is a noninvasive method for determining the presence of residual urine. Where it is available, ultrasonography may be preferable to catheterization, especially in men with

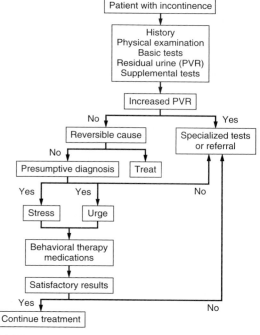

FIGURE 63–1. Urinary incontinence—diagnostic and management strategy for primary care physicians. Note that patients with certain conditions may need specialized evaluation and should not be diagnosed and managed exclusively according to this algorithm. Such patients are those with (1) hematuria or pyuria in the absence of infection, (2) recent (within 2 months) onset of irritative voiding symptoms, (3) previous anti-incontinence surgery or radical pelvic surgery, (4) severe pelvic prolapse, (5) suspicion of prostate cancer, or (6) neurologic abnormalities. PVR, Postvoid residual urine.

suspected prostate enlargement, because ultrasound involves no risk of infection or urethral trauma, both of which sometimes occur after catheterization.

3. A **cough stress test** should be performed on all female patients. With the patient in the lithotomy position and with a full bladder, the patient coughs while gauze or a menstrual pad is held over the perineum. Instantaneous leakage onto the pad during coughing suggests stress incontinence. Delayed leakage suggests urge incontinence. If there is no leakage, the test should be repeated with the patient in the standing position.

B. **Supplementary basic tests** can be performed if a presumptive diagnosis cannot be reached with a history, physical examination, and basic tests.

1. **Office cystometrography** (Table 63–2) is a simple office procedure that is useful for detecting the presence of uncontrolled bladder contractions associated with urge incontinence. Cystometrography is safe; urinary infection develops in <5% of patients who undergo this test. Compared to that of formal urodynamic testing, several studies have shown that the sensitivity of simple office cystometry for diagnosing detrusor instability is between 75% and 100%, the specificity is 69–89%, and the positive predictive value is 74–91% in patients for whom reversible causes of incontinence have been excluded.

2. **Urinary flow determination** can be useful in male patients suspected of having prostate enlargement causing outflow obstruction. Decreased flow is indicated by either straining or an interrupted stream, or abnormally low flow measurement with a commercially available urine flowmeter. Flow rates in geriatric-aged men are usually >20 mL/s; rates <10–15 mL/s are abnormal.

C. **Specialized tests** can be performed in selected patients with specific indications or in those for whom a presumptive diagnosis cannot be reached after history, physical examination, and basic and supplemental tests.

1. **Complete urodynamic testing** (including full cystometrography, perineal electromyelography, urethral pressure profilimetry, and other measurements) is commonly performed when a presumptive diagnosis cannot be made, when patients do not respond to treatments for the presumptive diagnosis, when the PVR is increased, and when surgical interventions are being considered.

2. **Endoscopic and imaging studies** of the urinary tract may be indicated in patients with hematuria, sterile pyuria, or recent onset of irritative voiding symptoms (ie, symptoms of urge incontinence that developed within the previous 2 months). In such patients, these tests may detect neoplasms, stones, diverticuli, etc.

VIII. **Treatment.** After the basic and supplemental evaluations described above, in most cases a presumptive diagnosis can be made as to the cause and type of incontinence. Treatment, as outlined below, can be administered based on the presumptive diagnosis. If treatment is unsuccessful, the diagnosis should be re-evaluated, and more specialized tests may be indicated to better define the cause of incontinence. The patient can keep a **voiding diary,** in which symptoms and information on the frequency and circumstances of incontinent episodes are recorded. The diary is useful for defin-

---

TABLE 63–2. PERFORMANCE OF OFFICE CYSTOMETROGRAPHY

1. Have the patient empty his or her bladder by voiding in the toilet, and then have him or her assume the dorsal lithotomy position.
2. Insert a sterile nonballooned No. 12–14 French catheter, and empty the patient's bladder. Measurement of postvoid residual and collection of urinalysis may be performed at this time.
3. Insert the syringe (50 mL, with the plunger removed) into the end of the catheter, and position it 15 cm above the urethra.
4. Fill the bladder by pouring sterile water through the open end of the syringe in 25- to 50-mL aliquots.
5. Record the cumulative total fluid instilled into the bladder, and note the volume at which the patient first reports having the urge to void. Severe urge to void at <300–350 mL is suggestive of detrusor overactivity (urge incontinence).
6. Continue adding fluid slowly until the fluid level (meniscus) in the syringe rises, indicating contraction of the detrusor muscle with transmission of intrabladder pressure to the syringe.
   a. The rise in fluid level may be either gradual or explosive.
   b. Detrusor contractions at <300–350 mL of bladder volume are generally indicative of urge incontinence.

ing the patient's symptoms and for determining the baseline frequency of incontinence as a reference by which to judge the effect of therapy.

A. Transient causes of urinary incontinence are managed by treating the identified cause. If incontinence does not resolve, other causes of transient incontinence should again be considered. If none are found, the patient is then treated for the type of irreversible incontinence (eg, urge or stress) presumptively diagnosed based on the testing described above.

B. Urge incontinence

  1. Behavioral therapies are the first-line treatment because they are safer and generally more effective than drug therapy.

   a. Bladder training is the treatment of choice for urge incontinence. It involves progressively lengthening the interval between voiding and encouraging the patient to postpone voiding for increasing lengths of time. Several randomized controlled studies have demonstrated bladder training to be effective. At least one study found it superior to drug therapy in cognitively intact women. The majority of patients experience improvement in their incontinence symptoms, and most studies indicate cure rates exceeding 50%.

   b. Pelvic muscle exercises (ie, Kegel exercises) can also improve symptoms of urge incontinence (see section VIII,C,1,a), especially when supplemented with biofeedback.

  2. Medications are a second-line treatment for urge incontinence.

   a. Anticholinergic medications decrease uncontrolled bladder detrusor contractions. **Oxybutynin** is the traditional anticholinergic agent for urge incontinence. It is used at doses ranging from 2.5 mg at bedtime to 5 mg four times per day. An extended-release preparation is also available. **Tolterodine** is a new anticholinergic drug that appears to have fewer anticholinergic side effects (especially xerostomia). The dose of tolterodine ranges from 0.5 mg at bedtime to 2 mg twice a day. **Propantheline** is another alternative drug, but many patients cannot tolerate its anticholinergic side effects. Flavoxate has no proven efficacy for urge incontinence. In older patients, drugs must be used with caution because anticholinergic medicines can "overshoot," causing complete relaxation of the detrusor (atonic bladder) with urinary retention and overflow. For this reason, it is advisable to begin with a low dose, make dosage changes infrequently, and re-evaluate patients often to detect urinary retention.

   b. Tricyclic antidepressants with anticholinergic side effects (eg, **imipramine** and **doxepin**) can be used for urge incontinence, but only limited research supports their use.

   c. Calcium channel blockers inhibit detrusor contractions and may be useful for urge incontinence. Limited research supports their effectiveness, but they may be appropriate if another indication for calcium blockers exists in a patient with urge incontinence.

  3. Other treatments

   a. Electrical stimulation with both implantable and nonimplantable electrodes may improve urge incontinence in some patients. This therapy is used in many centers but is considered investigational.

   b. Surgical treatment of urge incontinence with procedures such as augmentation cystoplasty is effective, but is used only in selected patients. Bladder denervation, which reduces detrusor contractility, can be accomplished with subtrigonal phenol injections and a variety of other methods. Cure rates with bladder denervation are low.

C. Stress incontinence

  1. Behavioral therapies are effective in some patients with stress incontinence.

   a. Pelvic muscle (Kegel) exercises may lessen the severity of sphincter weakness in stress incontinence. Patients are instructed to contract the pelvic muscles for 10 seconds at a time, 30–80 times per day, and continue the exercises indefinitely. On average, incontinence is improved in about 75–85% of patients and eliminated in about 10–15%.

   b. Adjuncts to pelvic muscle exercises include **biofeedback** and **vaginal cones.** Each may further improve the effectiveness of treatment, although further research is necessary to quantitate the additional improvement.

   c. Bladder training (as described in section VIII,B,1,a for urge incontinence) can result in additional improvement in symptoms of stress incontinence.

2. **Medications**
    a. **α-Adrenergic agonists,** which cause urethral sphincter contraction, may be tried if no contraindication (eg, hypertension) exists. **Phenylpropanolamine** (25–100 mg sustained release, twice daily) and **pseudoephedrine** (30 mg up to four times a day) are the a-agonists of choice. Up to 50% of patients are improved, and about 10% are cured.
    b. **Estrogen,** either oral, vaginal, or transdermal, can be administered in conjunction with alpha blockers and may result in more improvement than alpha blockers alone. Estrogen alone improves symptoms of stress incontinence to about the same degree as alpha blockers alone.
3. **Surgery** is the most effective treatment for women with stress incontinence. The appropriate surgical treatment is dictated by whether the patient's symptoms are caused by hypermobility (ie, descent) of the urethra or by intrinsic weakness of the sphincter muscle (intrinsic sphincter deficiency). Surgery can eliminate incontinence in 70–85% of patients with stress incontinence. For men with stress incontinence, such as sometimes occurs after prostatectomy, injections of periurethral bulking agents (eg, collagen) or surgical implantation of an artificial urethral sphincter can improve or eliminate incontinence in some patients. When men are treated with periurethral bulking injections or artificial sphincters, cure (ie, complete elimination of incontinence) occurs in 20% and 50%, respectively.
4. **Devices** are also available for treating stress incontinence. For women, these include pessaries, suction devices that occlude urethral outflow, and ballooned inserts that lie within the urethral orifice. For men, penile clamps are sometimes used on a temporary basis; clamps sometimes result in injury to the urethra or penile skin.
D. **Overflow incontinence** must be treated by draining the bladder. Failure to drain retained urine may result in hydronephrotic distention of the urinary tract and subsequent renal damage.
    1. **Herbal medications.** Some patients use saw palmetto, a palm tree extract that blocks binding of dihydrotestosterone in prostate tissue, to relieve urinary symptoms caused by prostate enlargement. Limited evidence suggests that treatment with saw palmetto can reduce symptoms of prostatism and residual urine by 40–50%. However, the specific role of saw palmetto for treating urinary incontinence has not been determined.
    2. **Intermittent catheterization,** performed by patients or their caretakers, is the treatment of choice. The catheter must be clean, but not necessarily sterile, although sterile catheters are recommended for immunocompromised patients. The interval between catheterization varies, depending on how often the individual patient's bladder becomes distended.
    3. **Chronic indwelling catheterization** (ie, Foley catheter) is generally used if intermittent catheterization is not possible.
        a. **Urinary infection** is universal among chronically catheterized patients. Antibiotic treatment results in selection of antibiotic-resistant organisms, so infection should generally not be treated unless the infection is symptomatic (eg, pyelonephritis or sepsis).
        b. **Leakage around the catheter** is generally caused by encrustation of the catheter lumen and orifice with calculo-proteinaceous debris, with subsequent drainage of urine around the sides of the catheter. A larger catheter should not be used in an attempt to prevent leakage. Instead, the catheter should be replaced at a frequency dictated by the development of encrustation and leakage.
            (1) **Acidification of urine** decreases build-up of encrusted material and lengthens the interval between catheter changes. Several medications can acidify urine, for example, **methenamine hippurate** (1 g orally twice a day), **ascorbic acid** (500 mg orally every day), and **acetic acid** (0.25% or less) lavage of catheter and bladder, performed anywhere from once per week to every other day, as needed to prevent encrustation.
            (2) **Mortality** from septic complications is increased among patients who require chronic bladder catheterization.
    4. **Suprapubic catheterization** is useful in selected patients for whom neither intermittent nor chronic urethral catheterization is appropriate.

E. Intractable incontinence exists when incontinence from any cause cannot be adequately controlled by the above measures. As noted above, irreversible overflow incontinence always requires catheter drainage. When other forms of incontinence are intractable, the following treatment options are available.

1. **Behavioral techniques** may be sufficient to decrease incontinence episodes and improve hygiene in some chronically incontinent patients.
   a. **Habit training** involves identification of the patient's natural voiding schedule and ensuring that toilet facilities are available at that time. This technique is used at nursing homes and is superior to placebo and as effective as drug therapy in reducing episodes of incontinence.
   b. **Prompted voiding** involves asking patients whether they need to void and providing them with toilet facilities if they answer affirmatively. It also is used for institutionalized patients and is effective at reducing the frequency of incontinence.
   c. **Routine or scheduled toileting** involves bringing the patient to the toilet on a fixed schedule. It also reduces the frequency of incontinent episodes.
2. **Incontinence underpants** and absorbent pads are useful for collecting and absorbing incontinent urine. The absorbent garment or pad is changed at intervals dictated by the frequency of incontinence.
3. **Condom catheters** may sometimes be useful in male patients, especially on a short-term basis. Condom catheters increase the risk of skin problems and urinary tract infections.
4. **Intermittent catheterization,** if logistically feasible, can be used to control intractable incontinence from any cause.
5. **Chronic bladder catheterization** may be used in patients whose incontinence cannot be managed by other means.
6. **Diverting ureteroileostomy** may be appropriate for controlling incontinence in carefully selected patients.

REFERENCES

Abrams P, Freeman R, Anderstrom C, et al: Tolterodine, a new antimuscarinic agent: As effective but better tolerated than oxybutynin in patients with an overactive bladder. Br J Urol 1998; **81**:801.

Burgio KL, Locher JL, Goode PS, et al: Behavioral vs drug treatment for urge urinary incontinence in older women: A randomized controlled trial. JAMA 1998;**280**:1995.

Coombes GM, Millard RJ: The accuracy of portable ultrasound scanning in the measurement of residual urine volume. J Urol 1994;**152**:2083.

Fantl JA, Newman DK, Colling J, et al: *Urinary Incontinence in Adults: Acute and Chronic Management.* Clinical Practice Guideline No. 2, 1996 Update; AHCPR Publ. No. 96-0682. US Department of Health and Human Services, Public Health Service, Agency for Health Care Policy and Research; 1996.

Thom D: Variations in estimates of urinary incontinence prevalence in the community: Effects of differences in definition, population characteristics, and study type. J Am Geriatr Soc 1998; **46**:473.

Videla FLG, Wall L: Stress incontinence diagnosed without multichannel urodynamic studies. Obstet Gynecol 1998;**91**:965.

Weiss BD: The diagnostic evaluation of urinary incontinence in geriatric patients. Am Fam Physician 1998;**57**:1675.

---

64   Urinary Symptoms in Men

Linda L. Walker, MD, & Steven E. Reissman, DO

I. **Definition.** Urinary symptoms in men include voiding pain or discomfort, abnormal urinary flow, hematuria, or urethral discharge.
II. **Common diagnoses**
   A. **Genitourinary infectious and inflammatory disorders**
   1. **Urethritis**
   2. **Prostatitis**

      a. **Acute bacterial prostatitis.**
      b. **Acute nonbacterial prostatitis.**
      c. **Chronic prostatitis.**
      d. **Prostatodynia.**

  B. **Neoplasms**
     1. **Benign prostatic hypertrophy (BPH).**
     2. **Prostate cancer.**
     3. **Bladder cancer.**

III. Epidemiology

  A. **Urethritis** affects more than 4 million men each year. It is primarily a disease of sexually active younger men with multiple partners. As gonococcal urethritis case numbers decline, nongonococcal urethritis (NGU) cases continue to increase. One factor for the rising incidence of NGU is the high rate of transmission from asymptomatic partners who harbor the responsible organisms. NGU has been cited as the most common sexually transmitted disease in men, and recurrence is very common.

  B. One quarter of men who present with genitourinary symptoms have **prostatitis.** This disease results in more than 100,000 hospitalizations each year. Up to 50% of all men experience symptoms of prostatitis sometime during their adult years. **Nonbacterial prostatitis** is most common, usually occurring in younger men. In contrast, **chronic prostatitis** is a common condition of aging men. **Bacterial prostatitis** and **prostatodynia** are less frequently diagnosed.

  C. **BPH** is the most common neoplastic and urologic disorder of older men. By age 80, at least one quarter of men will seek medical attention for BPH symptoms. Annually, BPH causes close to 2 million patient visits.

  D. **Prostate cancer** has surpassed lung cancer during the 1990s as the most common cancer in men, accounting for one third of all cancer diagnoses in men, with over 200,000 new cases each year and nearly 40,000 deaths. This rise is partially due to more widespread screening. Since the incidence increases with age, more cases will emerge as the life span of men continues to rise. The lifetime risk of acquiring prostate cancer is now 1 in 6, with black men having up to a three-fold increased incidence compared to whites. Having a first-degree relative with prostate cancer also increases risk. No definitive causation has been proved for pre-existing BPH, smoking, high-fat diet, or cadmium exposure. Although the exact role of androgen exposure in stimulating prostate cancer is not clear, eunuchs are known to be invulnerable to this cancer. The role of prior vasectomy remains controversial. Nutritional factors that protect against prostate malignancy include a low-fat diet, selenium supplementation, use of soy products, eating cooked tomato products (high content of lycopene, an antioxidant carotenoid), and daily intake of 800 IU of vitamin E.

  E. **Bladder cancer** is diagnosed in more than 50,000 individuals each year, in a 3 : 1 male-female ratio. About 11,000 people die each year from this form of cancer. The incidence increases with age—approximately 80% of bladder cancer occurs in individuals over age 50. Known carcinogens for transitional bladder carcinoma include tobacco use and occupational exposure to aniline dyes and chemicals in metal and leather workers. Bladder calculi, chronic infection, and long-term catheter use are associated with squamous cell carcinoma of the bladder.

IV. Pathophysiology

  A. **Infectious and inflammatory disorders**
     1. **Urethritis** is caused by gonococcal and nongonococcal infections, which often coexist. NGU is more often diagnosed than is gonorrhea, and known causative agents include *Chlamydia trachomatis, Mycoplasma genitalium,* and *Ureaplasma urealyticum.* Up to 30% of cases of NGU have no causative agents identified by culture.
     2. **Acute prostatitis** may result from spread of infection from urethritis, reflux from a chronically catheterized bladder, direct migration of rectal bacteria, pelvic lymphatic dissemination, or hematogenous seeding. Microorganisms are generally gram negative.
     3. **Nonbacterial prostatitis** is an inflammatory process without known causative organisms. Autoimmune theories exist, but the condition remains a diagnosis of exclusion.

   4. **Chronic prostatitis** is occasionally a sequela of acute bacterial prostatitis. However, most cases are insidious and account for the underlying disease in most men with recurrent urinary tract infections (UTIs).
   5. **Prostatodynia** is an ailment in which the prostate is irritated by refluxed urine when functional urethral hypertonicity increases voiding pressure. Spasm and pain of the pelvic floor muscles is an alternative basis for this diagnosis.
B. **Neoplasms**
   1. **BPH** development is dependent on continued exposure to androgens, which enlarge the prostate first periurethrally and later peripherally. Urinary obstructive symptoms result from urethral compression and increased tone in prostatic smooth muscle.
   2. Most **prostate cancers** are adenocarcinomas. Tumors are graded histologically based on the degree of anaplasia and aneuploidy. Clinical staging is based on tumor size, local extension, spread to pelvic lymphatics, and metastases to bone, the lungs, or the liver. Poorly differentiated cell types are more often found in widespread and metastatic disease.
   3. Ninety percent of **bladder cancers** are transitional cell carcinomas; the remainder of cases are usually squamous cell carcinomas or adenocarcinomas. Transitional cell carcinoma is multicentric, often arising in multiple areas of uroepithelium at differing time intervals. It usually presents in a papillary exophytic growth, but can be ulcerated or sessile. Carcinoma in situ presents as a flat epithelial lesion adjacent to or separate from more advanced tumors. Poorly differentiated cell types are found in tumors that have a much stronger tendency to invade, recur, or metastasize.
V. **Symptoms**
A. **Voiding pain and discomfort**
   1. **Dysuria** is the most common symptom of urethral or bladder infection. Although it is usually painless, bladder cancer can present as dysuria and should be suspected when there is no response to antibiotic therapy. Dysuria can be very disabling in **acute bacterial prostatitis.** In chronic and nonbacterial prostatitis, this symptom is less distressing.
   2. **Urgency** is the sensation that the bladder must be emptied immediately to relieve symptoms of fullness or pressure. It is characteristic of infection or bladder distention in **obstructive** or neurologic abnormalities.
   3. The **pelvic pain** accompanying acute bacterial prostatitis may be referred to the abdomen, back, flank, or perineum and can be quite severe. Milder discomfort with voiding or ejaculation is found in **chronic prostatitis, nonbacterial prostatitis,** and **prostatodynia,** and often radiates to the thighs, rectum, and genitals.
B. **Abnormalities of urinary flow**
   1. The **urinary stream may be split or slow** because of urethral scarring from prior infection. In prostatic enlargement caused by **acute infection** or **BPH,** the stream is decreased in force and caliber because of encroachment on the prostatic urethra.
   2. **Hesitancy** and **dribbling** signify the inability to abruptly initiate or terminate urinary flow, and both are common in **BPH.** Together with an abnormal stream and sensation of incomplete emptying, this symptom complex is known as prostatism. **Prostatodynia** may present similarly, with a flow sometimes described as pulsing in nature, perhaps because of smooth muscle spasm.
   3. **Nocturia** occurs when there is increased residual urine volume in an obstructed bladder, necessitating more frequent voiding of smaller volumes of urine. Daytime frequency usually indicates irritation of the genitourinary tract from inflammation or infection.
   4. **Urinary retention** can be partial or complete. Mechanical blockage results from **BPH, inflammation,** or **cancer.** Many drugs, such as alcohol, antihistamines, anticholinergics, tranquilizers, or adrenergic medications, can lead to complete obstruction and inability to void. Overflow incontinence of small amounts of urine occurs when a distended bladder exerts enough pressure to overcome obstruction.
C. **Gross or microscopic hematuria** is the most common presentation of bladder cancer in the minority of patients who have any warning symptoms at all. It also results from ruptured vessels in **BPH.**

D. **Urethral discharge** is copious, purulent, and yellow-green in **gonococcal infection,** developing 2–7 days after exposure. In **NGU,** the incubation period is 1–3 weeks, and the discharge is scantier and more mucoid. Swabbing the infected urethra can cause significant distress because of apprehension and pain. It is important to realize that both infections may be asymptomatic.

VI. **Signs**

A. Abdominal examination of men with **prostatitis** may show **suprapubic tenderness. Acute infections** can cause generalized tenderness in the lower abdomen, as can **urinary retention.** A completely obstructed bladder may hold more than 1 L of urine, palpable as a mass distending the lower abdomen, percussable as proximally as the umbilicus.

B. **Digital rectal examination** of the prostate should be omitted in obvious cases of acute bacterial prostatitis to avoid unnecessary pain for the patient and progression to bacteremia and sepsis. For other suspected diagnoses, careful palpation reveals prostate size, consistency, symmetry, and masses. **Mild tenderness, sponginess,** or **induration** may be noted in **chronic prostatitis.** In **nonbacterial prostatitis** and **prostatodynia,** the examination may show only **slight tenderness** in an otherwise normal gland. **BPH** can present as a **normal or enlarged gland** that has a firm and smooth texture. **Carcinoma** may be palpable as lobular **asymmetry** of size or texture, diffuse or localized **induration,** or a palpable **mass.**

C. **Anal sphincter tone** may be somewhat **increased in prostatodynia.** Decreased tone may be a clue to **neurologic causes** of urinary symptoms.

VII. **Laboratory tests**

A. **Urinalysis.** Dipstick testing of urine indicates that UTI is likely when positive for nitrite or strongly positive for leukocyte esterase. Microscopic findings of pyuria (>10 white blood cells [WBCs] per high-power field) or bacteriuria also support the diagnosis of UTI. Hematuria exists when there are more than five red blood cells per high-power field.

B. **Urine culture** has traditionally been reported to be indicative of infection only when the colony count exceeds 100,000 per milliliter. However, when a midstream collection in a patient with pyuria grows 10,000 colonies per milliliter of a known urinary pathogen, the diagnosis of UTI is confirmed. Even lower counts are diagnostic in specimens collected by catheterization.

C. A **"three-glass urine test"** aids in the diagnosis of **chronic prostatic infection.** The first 10 mL of urine is collected as a urethral sample. A midstream collection constitutes bladder urine. The prostate is then massaged, and secretions are expressed from the urethra into a sterile container. Finally, 10 mL of urine is voided as a prostatic specimen. Chronic prostatitis is diagnosed when prostatic secretions exhibit >15 WBCs per high-power field and yield heavy culture growth while the urine specimens show only light growth and few WBCs. In **nonbacterial prostatitis,** secretions show no growth of urinary pathogens—despite the presence of WBCs.

D. **Urine flow studies** objectify voiding time, rate, and pattern. Uroflowmetry is helpful in detecting the degree of **obstruction** present. **Neurogenic dysfunction** can also be detected, but detrusor and contractility problems may be difficult to distinguish from obstruction.

E. **Postvoid residual urine volume** can be measured by catheterization to detect incomplete emptying. A volume of 100 mL or more is diagnostic of retention.

F. **Urine cytology** of the first morning voided specimen may be helpful in diagnosing **bladder cancer,** but is often omitted when urethrocystoscopy is part of the evaluation. Flow cytometry assists in detecting malignant cells. False-negatives are common, but positive results correlate well with transitional cell carcinoma. Tumor markers show promising results for clinical use.

G. **Serum chemistries** should include **creatinine** and **blood urea nitrogen** in patients with **BPH, prostate cancer,** or **recurrent UTI.** Monitoring can determine renal impairment from infection or obstruction, guiding intervention decisions. When prostate cancer is known to exist, elevations of **prostatic acid phosphatase or alkaline phosphatase** imply bone metastasis.

H. **Prostate-specific antigen (PSA)** can be used as a screening test for **prostate cancer.** However, men should be carefully counseled because its use is very controversial. False-positives from benign conditions are common when mild elevations (4–10 ng/mL) are found. Evaluation by ultrasound and biopsy may show no disease, or early disease in which treatment by surgery and radiation may cause morbidity from incontinence and impotence without affecting mortality overall. In mild elevations, a **free PSA** (non–protein-bound) level of <25% strongly favors a diagnosis of true malignancy. **PSA velocity** of >0.7 ng/mL/yr and elevated **PSA density** (adjustment for prostate size) can be used to refine cancer detection, as can modifications for aging and race. Marked elevations of PSA usually indicate advanced disease and are best utilized as follow-up markers after treatment. Many other tumor markers are under investigation in clinical trials.

- I. **Gram staining of a urethral smear** denotes **gonococcal infection** when gram-negative intracellular diplococci are seen. More than five WBCs per high-power field are diagnostic of **NGU** if no gonococci are seen. A culture of the discharge specimen on appropriate media confirms the diagnosis of gonorrhea more definitively. *Chlamydia* is detectable only when cellular material is obtained from a urethral scraping or swab placed several centimeters into the meatus. Studies can include direct **fluorescent antibody testing, culture, DNA probe assay,** or en-zyme **immunoassay;** DNA probe assay is preferred, as it is 99% sensitive and inexpensive. *Ureaplasma* can be cultured from a similarly obtained specimen.
- J. **Urethrocystoscopy** and **ureteroscopy** evaluate the anatomy of the urinary tract and visualize defects seen in imaging studies. In conjunction, biopsy of abnormal mucosa and suspicious lesions is performed.
- K. **Ultrasonography** of the abdomen provides structural information. It detects renal position and size and can discover hydronephrosis caused by **chronic obstruction.** Abdominal ultrasonography can evaluate the bladder for masses and post-void volume. A **rectal ultrasound probe** is useful in the evaluation of **prostatic masses** or **elevated PSA** to help guide biopsy decisions. When a rectal ultrasound scan is abnormal in a man with a prostatic mass and elevated PSA, the likelihood of finding carcinoma is almost 50%.
- L. **Intravenous urography** evaluates upper urinary tract function and anatomy and demonstrates bladder emptying. The lower urinary tract can also be evaluated with retrograde dye studies to find urethral and bladder anatomic abnormalities.

VII. Treatment

- A. **NGU** can be treated with a multitude of acceptable regimens. The most commonly used is oral **doxycycline,** 100 mg twice daily for 7 days. **Azithromycin,** 1 g in one oral dose, is a more expensive option with increased patient compliance. Alternatives for drug allergy or resistant organisms are **erythromycin,** 500 mg orally four times daily for 7 days, or 5- to 7-day oral courses of various fluoro-quinolones.

    Gonorrhea is effectively treated with either one dose of **ceftriaxone,** 125 mg intramuscularly, or **cefixime,** 400 mg by mouth. Single oral doses of **fluoroquinolones** such as ofloxacin, 400 mg, are also effective. Concurrent treatment for NGU is normally given.

- B. **Prostatitis**
    1. **Acute prostatitis** can be treated on an outpatient basis with oral **trimethoprim-sulfamethoxazole (TMP-SMX),** 160 mg/800 mg twice daily. A 30-day course is recommended to prevent relapse or chronic infection. An alternative treatment includes 10 days of therapy with an oral **fluoroquinolone** such as **cipro-floxacin** (Cipro), 500 mg twice daily, or **ofloxacin** (Floxin), 200 mg twice daily. These agents achieve a high concentration in prostatic tissue. Dosage should be adjusted for patients with decreased renal function. Patients should be hospitalized for intravenous antibiotics when systemic symptoms predominate. Acute urinary retention may require suprapubic drainage, since the urethral route may cause pain and bacteremia. **Oral anti-inflammatory agents,** such as **ibuprofen** (Motrin), 400–800 mg three times daily, or **naproxen** (Naprosyn), 250–500 mg twice daily, provide pain relief. In severe cases, the use of narcotics may be required.
    2. **Chronic prostatitis** is treated similarly, with a 30-day course of **TMP-SMX** as above, repeated for a 14- to 21-day course if evidence of infection recurs. Lower-dose therapy can be used for several months to suppress recurrent symptoms. **Fluoroquinolones** (see the previous section for agents and dosing) are also effective, but very costly when used for the 6-week period recommended in chronic infection. The relapse rate remains high, despite ad-

vances in treatment. Acupuncture may be helpful for chronically symptomatic patients.

3. **Nonbacterial prostatitis** is treated symptomatically with sitz baths and nonsteroidal anti-inflammatory agents (see the previous section). Avoidance of spicy foods and caffeine may help. Normal sexual activity should not be prohibited, as ejaculation may relieve overall symptoms. Prostate massage is an old, unproven therapy that is again being tried by some practitioners. Irritative symptoms may respond to oral **anticholinergic medications** such as **oxybutynin** (Ditropan), 5 mg two or three times daily, or **hyoscyamine** (Levsin), 0.125 mg, one or two tablets every 4–6 hours. Anxiety and depression often coexist in this sometimes chronic and frustrating condition and should be elicited and treated accordingly. A prolonged course of antibiotics as for chronic prostatitis may be offered but is usually ineffective.

4. **Prostatodynia** may respond to the regimen for nonbacterial prostatitis, and oral **α-adrenergic blockers** such as **terazosin** (Hytrin), 1 mg at bedtime titrated slowly to 10 mg, or **doxazosin** (Cardura), 1 mg titrated slowly to 8 mg once daily, have been tried as well. **Prazosin** (Minipres) has also been used. These drugs were first used for hypertension but do not typically affect blood pressure in normotensive men. Symptoms may be refractory and chronic despite treatment.

C. BPH

1. **Watchful waiting** is often appropriate in the care of men with BPH. Surveillance for urinary retention, increased postvoid bladder residual, rising serum creatinine, development of bladder calculi, or worsening symptoms is necessary to determine when other treatment options should be recommended.

2. **Lifestyle changes** that can help to lessen symptoms include restriction of caffeine and bedtime fluids and use of anticholinergic medications. Establishment of frequent, regular voiding habits may also help in the management of BPH.

3. **Drug therapy**
   a. **α-Adrenergic blockers** are initiated in low doses and titrated slowly, as described in section VIII,B,4.
   b. **5α-Reductase inhibition** with **finasteride** (Proscar) blocks testosterone conversion in the prostate, leading to gradual shrinkage of the gland. Dosed at 5 mg orally once daily, it can replace or supplement α-adrenergic blockers. Symptoms may gradually improve over months or even years of therapy. Long-term use is safe and effective; the cost is more than that of α-adrenergic blockers but considerably less than that of surgical intervention.

4. **Dietary supplements**
   a. **Saw palmetto** alleviates voiding symptoms in approximately 50% of users, although prostate size is not decreased, PSA levels are unaffected, and objective voiding measurements do not change. This dried palm fruit (also known as *Serenoa repens* or Permixon) exerts its effects by blocking androgen sites, and is well tolerated. A typical oral dose of extract is 160 mg twice daily.
   b. **Multiple-ingredient herbal and supplement preparations** have no benefit and can be hazardous because of contaminants and unknown active substances.

5. **BPH** can be treated **surgically** by transurethral resection of the prostate (TURP) and by alternate procedures such as transurethral incision of the prostate (TUIP), placement of prostatic stents, balloon dilatation, or ablation by microwave, radio waves, heat, focused ultrasound, or cryotherapy. TURP is effective in relieving symptoms, but retrograde ejaculation ensues in a majority of patients. Less frequent complications include impotence, UTIs, and incontinence.

D. Prostate cancer management should be based on the individual's symptoms and expected longevity. The 10-year survival rate for localized disease is approximately 85%, and survival for several years is not uncommon in metastatic disease. Localized disease may be treated with radical prostatectomy or radiation. Surgical methods can relieve obstruction, and radiation therapy ameliorates urinary

and metastatic symptoms. Widespread or metastatic disease is often treated palliatively. Endocrine therapy is often utilized to induce a state of androgen deprivation and subsequent tumor regression. This can be done by several methods.
1. **Surgically,** by performing an **orchiectomy.**
2. **Drug therapy**
   a. **Exogenous estrogen** such as **diethylstilbestrol.**
   b. **Luteinizing hormone–releasing hormone (LHRH) analogs** such as injections of **leuprolide** (Lupron), which inhibits the release of pituitary gonadotropins after a transient rise.
   c. **Androgen receptor competitors (antiandrogens)** such as **flutamide** (Eulexin) block the effect of androgens on target organs. This oral agent is usually used in combination with an LHRH analog.
   d. **Other antiandrogens** blocking testosterone synthesis include oral **ketoconazole** (Nizoral), which inhibits steroid hydroxylation, and oral **finasteride** (Proscar), which blocks the conversion of testosterone in prostatic tissue. Hormone-refractory prostate cancer remains incurable, and no chemotherapy agents prolong survival. Median survival is 40–60 weeks.
E. **Bladder cancer** may be treated with resection or fulguration for localized disease. **Intravesicular chemotherapy** with **mitomycin, thiotepa, bacille Calmette-Guérin (BCG),** or **doxorubicin** is commonly used. For advanced disease, **cystectomy, radiation,** and **systemic chemotherapy** with **cisplatin-based combination therapy** are available. The 5-year survival rate with localized tumor is 75%, but in metastatic disease the prognosis is very poor.

REFERENCES

Droller MJ: Bladder cancer: State-of-the art care. CA Cancer J Clin 1998;**48:**269.
Gilbert DN, Moellering RC Jr, Sande MA: *The Sanford Guide to Antimicrobial Therapy.* Antimicrobial Therapy; 1999.
Gleich P: Prostatitis: A state-of-the-art review of diagnosis and therapy. Consultant 1998; **February:**345.
Gunby P: Prostate detection possibility. JAMA 1999;**281:**2274.
Lipsky BA: Prostatitis and urinary tract infection in men: What's new; what's true? Am J Med 1999;**106:**327.
Naitoh J, Zeiner RL, Dekernion J: Diagnosis and treatment of prostate cancer. Am Fam Physician 1998;**57:**1531.
Saw palmetto for benign prostatic hypertrophy. Med Lett 1999;**41:**18.
Tanagho EA, McAninch JW (editors): *Smith's General Urology.* 14th ed. Appleton & Lange; 1995.
Tomatoes: A healthy indulgence. Great Life 1998;**August:**55.
Wynder EL, Fair WR: Prostate cancer—Nutrition adjunct therapy. Clin Urol 1996;**156:**1364. (Editorial.)

---

65   Urticaria

Charles F. Margolis, MD

I. **Definition.** Urticaria are transient, circumscribed, raised skin lesions, which are usually intensely pruritic and characterized by areas of erythema and edema of varying size and duration.

II. **Common diagnoses.** The characteristic appearance of urticaria is usually readily apparent, making the diagnosis obvious. Edema is sometimes transient, leading the clinician to suspect other erythematous rashes. **Angioedema** ("giant hives") is caused by the same pathophysiologic process as urticaria, but occurs deeper in the skin, is more commonly nonpruritic, and is characterized by nonpitting edema and often involves oral and respiratory mucosae. Urticarial vasculitis presents with lesions that have the appearance of urticaria but are persistent (individual lesions last longer than 24 hours), are more intensely syptomatic, and may leave residual bruising. Often there is associated immune complex–mediated disease in other parts of the body.

Uncovering the cause of urticaria is more difficult than diagnosing it. In 60–70% of cases of urticaria, the origin is not apparent after a careful history, physical examination, and full laboratory investigation. While reports of the relative incidence of specific causes of urticaria vary significantly, most list **physical causes** occurring in 5–10% of cases, **infectious causes** in 10–15% of cases, and **medications** in 5–10% of cases. A specific cause is more likely to be identified in patients with acute urticaria than in those with chronic urticaria, which is recurrent urticaria lasting longer than 6 weeks.

Specific causes of urticaria are discussed below.

A. **Physical factors** can induce urticaria at the site of the stimulus in the suscepti- ble patient (Table 65–1).

    1. **Dermographism** ("skin writing") is the occurrence of whealing and erythema within minutes of exposure to pressure or mechanical irritation such as stroking or scratching. It occurs in about 5% of the general population, although wheals may occur in anyone if the pressure stimulus is great enough. Patients with **symptomatic dermographism** develop urticaria in sites where minor pres- sures associated with activities of daily living have been applied. Common sites are the waist and the neck, where tight-fitting garments are the pres- sure source. Scratching wheals already present may lead to the formation of additional wheals. Symptomatic dermographism accounts for two of every three cases of urticaria caused by physical factors.

    2. Other physical causes are more unusual. **Cold urticaria,** which may be rec- ognized in the patient who urticates on the face and the extremities in cold weather, can be demonstrated by the application of an ice cube to the skin. **Cholinergic urticaria,** induced by heat, emotional stress, or exercise, results in 2- to 3-mm scattered wheals surrounded by large erythematous flares.

B. **Infections** also cause urticaria (Table 65–2). Streptococcal infection is considered a common cause in children.

C. **Medications** may cause urticaria, especially penicillins, cephalosporins, and sulfa drugs. **Aspirin** and nonsteroidal anti-inflammatory drugs, which may facilitate ur- ticaria caused by other factors, and **codeine,** which may cause direct degranula- tion of mast cells, deserve special mention. **Angiotensin-converting enzyme in- hibitors** may cause urticaria and angioedema, which may occur months or years after initiation of treatment, or with long symptom-free intervals between multiple epidodes.

D. **Foods** and **food additives** used for color, preservation, and taste may also cause urticaria. Nuts, seafood, eggs, and strawberries are among the foods implicated. Penicillin is commonly fed to livestock and may appear in small quantities in milk and meat.

E. Urticaria can uncommonly be a sign of **collagen vascular disease, cancer, hyperthyroidism,** and **familial, hereditary conditions.** Inhalant allergens and insect bites or stings may also cause urticaria. Contact with substances such as foods, fibers, radiocontrast media, chemicals, and cosmetics may induce urticaria by direct degranulation of mast cells in the skin. **Papular urticaria** is a hyper- sensitivity reaction to the bites of fleas, mosquitos, chiggers, and mites. The ap- pearance of the lesions is papular, and they are more persistent than typical urticaria.

F. Physicians and patients have felt that many cases of urticaria are strongly influ- enced by **emotional and psychogenic factors.** While case studies support the significance of psychogenic factors, it has been difficult to prove that these fac- tors are the sole cause of urticaria in individual patients.

III. **Epidemiology.** Urticaria is among the most common skin conditions encountered by family physicians. The annual incidence of urticaria in an urban US family practice

TABLE 65–1. TYPES OF PHYSICAL URTICARIA

Symptomatic dermographism
Cold urticaria
Cholinergic urticaria
Heat urticaria
Solar urticaria
Vibratory urticaria
Aquagenic urticaria
Decompression urticaria

TABLE 65–2. INFECTIONS ASSOCIATED WITH URTICARIA

Streptococcal infections
Sinusitis
Hepatitis B infection
Infectious mononucleosis
Coxsackie and other viral infections
Parasitic infections
Fungal skin infections

center was found to be 0.27%, and the lifetime incidence is 15–20% of the population. Acute urticaria is more than twice as common as chronic urticaria. Females are three times as likely as males to present with this skin condition. While urticaria and angioedema may occur at any age, the incidence is highest in young adults.

IV. **Pathophysiology.** Urticaria and angioedema are caused by localized vasodilation and transudation of fluid from capillaries and small blood vessels. The locus of vascular permeability is deeper in the skin in angioedema and more superficial in urticaria. Urticaria and angioedema often occur at the same time in patients and differ little in demographic features or apparent cause.

The increased vascular permeability is due to chemical mediators released by mast cells and basophils. Histamine is the most prominent mediator, but substances such as leukotrienes, prostaglandins, kinins, and others also play a role. The presence of various mediators may account for different clinical patterns of urticaria and for varying responses to medications in individuals. A number of factors result in the release of the mediators, including physical and immunologic factors and certain substances that result in the direct release of histamine by degranulation of mast cells. Immunologic mechanisms are probably involved more often in acute than in chronic urticaria.

V. **Symptoms.** Pruritis is usually present with urticaria in varying degrees of severity. The intensity of the pruritus, like urticaria itself, is affected by external factors such as temperature, alcohol, and emotional distress.

VI. **Signs.** The characteristic skin lesions of urticaria are evanescent, well demarcated, and raised. Erythema surrounds edematous central areas. Where the skin has been scratched, lesions are more prominent. While examining the patient, the physician should test for dermographism by stroking the patient's skin and should test for other causes of physical urticaria when the patient's history indicates that further testing would be appropriate.

VII. **Laboratory tests.** Extensive laboratory evaluation usually provides little information beyond that suggested by the patient's history and physical examination.
- A. When patients are seen initially with urticaria, laboratory evaluation should include testing children for streptococcal infection and evaluating all patients for causes suggested by the history or the physical examination.
- B. If urticaria persists, the tests shown in Table 65–3 may be helpful.

VIII. **Treatment.** Removal of the offending agent or management of the underlying cause is the treatment of choice when possible.
- A. **Patient education.** If the cause of urticaria cannot be established during the office visit, the patient should be educated about possible offending agents, ideally with the help of a printed handout. The patient can be asked to think about possible associations after the office visit. The patient's observations and additional insights are one of the physician's best sources of information in determining the cause of this condition.
- B. **General measures**
  1. The patient should avoid vasodilating influences such as heat, emotional stress, exertion, or alcohol.
  2. Cool compresses, Aveeno baths, and antipruritic lotions may provide some relief.
  3. Aspirin use probably should be discontinued.
  4. Urticaria and angioedema, like other skin conditions, are highly visible to the patient. The visibility of the condition contributes to the patient's anxiety, which can aggravate the condition. The physician should **reassure the patient** that the condition usually resolves in a few days or weeks and that it is usually associated with a benign outcome.

TABLE 65–3. LABORATORY EVALUATION OF URTICARIA

Initial tests
Complete blood cell count and sedimentation rate
Urinalysis
Multichemistry screening panel
Thyroid function tests
Throat and urine cultures[1]

Further tests to be considered if urticaria persists
Stool for ova and parasites
Vaginal smear for *Candida* and *Trichomonas* spp
Sinus or chest radiographs
Serum complement, antinuclear antibody, and immunoglobulin analysis
Hepatitis B tests
Elimination diets and skin tests
Skin biopsy

---

[1] Testing for streptococcal infection, either culture or rapid antigen testing, should be performed on children upon initial presentation with urticaria.

5. Follow-up care is required when the condition is prolonged, when the condition intensifies rather than improves, or when new symptoms supervene.
C. **Medications**
  1. **Antihistamines** such as **hydroxyzine, diphenhydramine, chlorpheniramine, loratadine,** and **cetirazine** are commonly used. There is some individual variation in response. The use of antihistamines may be limited by their sedating side effects.
      a. **Hydroxyzine** and **cetirazine** are often more effective than other antihistamines. Cetirazine is less likely to cause sedation. The usual dose of hydroxyzine is 25 mg every 4–6 hours, and cetirazine's usual dose is 10 mg once daily, but higher doses may be used to control symptoms if the patient can tolerate them. In children, the starting dose of diphenhydramine is 2 mg/kg/day, dosed every 4–6 hours, and cetirazine may be prescribed at doses of 5 mg once daily for ages 2–5 and 10 mg for children 6 years and above.
      b. Newer antihistamines, such as **loratadine** (10 mg once daily for adults and children 6 years of age and older) and **fexofenadine** (60 mg twice daily) are especially useful because they are generally nonsedating. *Note:* Terfenadine and astemizole are no longer used because drug interactions with erythromycin, ketoconazole, and itraconazole and dosage increases beyond recommended amounts have resulted in serious cardiac arrhythmias.
      c. **Diphenhydramine** (25 mg four times a day) and **chlorpheniramine** (4–12 mg twice a day) are available without a prescription, which may represent an advantage for some patients.
  2. **Other medications** that are occasionally used include the following.
      a. **Systemic corticosteroids** are useful in severe and poorly responsive cases of urticaria. **Prednisone** may be given for 10 days, starting at 40–60 mg and tapering to 5–10 mg on the last day, and should be added to antihistamine therapy.
      b. Topical steroids have very little value in the treatment of urticaria.
      c. The subcutaneous injection of **epinephrine** (0.3 mL) may be used to confirm the transient nature of the lesions, to provide temporary relief to the acutely symptomatic patient, and in cases of anaphylaxis.
      d. Cimetidine and other H_2 antihistamines provide benefit when added to H_1 antihistamine treatment but are of little value when used alone. The use of **ephedrine, terbutaline, doxepin, nifedipine, colchicine,** and **dapsone** has been reported to benefit some patients.

REFERENCES

Cooper KD: Urticaria and angioedema: Diagnosis and evaluation. J Am Acad Dermatol 1991; **25:**166.
Mahmood T: Physical urticarias. Am Fam Physician 1994;**49:**1411.

Pollak CV, Romano TJ: Outpatient management of acute urticaria: The role of prednisone. Ann Emerg Med 1995;**26**(5):547.

Soter NA: Acute and chronic urticaria and angioedema. J Am Acad Dermatol 1991;**25**:146.

66 Vaginal Bleeding

Clark B. Smith, MD

I. **Definition.** Abnormal vaginal bleeding is any vaginal bleeding that is not the result of normal menstruation.

II. **Common diagnoses** (Table 66–1)

A. **Dysfunctional bleeding resulting from ovulatory and anovulatory causes.**

B. **Pregnancy and its complications** (see Chapters 103 and 104).

C. **Contraceptive complications** (see Chapter 101).

D. **Pelvic inflammatory disease (PID)** (see Chapter 55).

E. **Benign and malignant neoplasms of the vagina, cervix, uterus, and ovaries.**

F. **Trauma and foreign bodies** (including rape, sexual abuse, and incest) (see also Chapter 100).

G. **Blood dyscrasias.**

III. **Epidemiology.** The incidence of consultation for abnormal vaginal bleeding in the primary care office is quite variable. In one family practice residency center (primarily indigent care), it is the primary reason for 4% of all visits. A review of the literature suggests that 10–20% of women have abnormal uterine bleeding at some time in their lives.

A. **Dysfunctional bleeding**

1. **Anovulatory bleeding** accounts for 95% of dysfunctional uterine bleeding in women less than 20 years of age. This incidence falls to less than 20% in women between 20 and 40 years of age, then rises again to about 90% beginning 2–3 years prior to menopause.

2. Not all abnormal bleeding for which a specific cause is not apparent is anovulatory. **Ovulatory bleeding** occurs in about 10% of patients with dysfunctional bleeding.

B. **Pregnancy and its complications.** The highest incidence of pregnancy-related abnormal vaginal bleeding is in the 18- to 35-year age group. Although the liter-

TABLE 66–1. CAUSES OF ABNORMAL UTERINE BLEEDING

Anovulatory dysfunctional uterine bleeding	Marked weight changes
Ovulatory dysfunctional uterine bleeding	Endocrinopathies
Blood dyscrasias	Chronic illness
Complications of pregnancy	Major organ failure
Disorders of the cervix	Cardiac
Disorders of the vagina	Renal
Disorders of the uterus	Liver
Neoplasia	Medications
Congenital anomalies	Oral contraceptives
Endometritis	Antidepressants
Adenomyosis	Antihypertensives
Endometriosis	Anticoagulants
Foreign bodies (eg, intrauterine contraceptive devices)	Anticholinergics
Disorders of the ovary	Digitalis
Polycystic ovary syndrome	Phenothiazines
Persistent corpus luteum	Steroids
Neoplasm	Tamoxifen
Adrenal disorder	Vitamins
Central nervous system neoplasm	Illegal drugs
Pelvic inflammatory disease	Emotions
	Sexual abuse

ature is unclear regarding the exact frequency, it is the author's experience that bleeding occurs in about 1 in 5 pregnancies.

C. Contraceptive complications. Oral contraceptives are the source of irregular (although usually not excessive) bleeding in about 10% of users.

D. PID. Risk factors for PID include multiple sexual partners and failure of the male to use a condom.

E. Benign and malignant neoplasms

    1. Uterine leiomyomas, benign endometrial polyps, and **adenomyomas** (adenomyosis) are the most common benign tumors of the uterus and are usually seen in the 25- to 45-year age group.

    2. Ten percent to 15% of postmenopausal bleeding is caused by **endometrial carcinoma,** and **endometrial hyperplasia** occurs with similar frequency. Populations at increased risk include those who are obese, diabetic, or hypertensive and, perhaps most important, those patients who are taking tamoxifen for breast cancer. Endometrial carcinoma is three times more common in women who are chronically anovulatory than in those who are ovulatory, but seven times more common in women who take tamoxifen.

        In a British study, 20% of abnormal vaginal bleeding in girls under age 11 was the result of a malignant genital tract tumor. **Vaginal adenosis** and **adenocarcinoma,** although uncommon, must be considered in patients who had intrauterine exposure to diethylstilbestrol (DES).

    3. Condyloma acuminata of the cervix, vagina, or vulva, a sexually transmitted disease caused by the human papillomavirus, may occasionally result in bleeding.

F. Trauma and **foreign bodies** are not uncommon causes of bleeding in children. **Sexual abuse** of children and young teens frequently presents as abnormal bleeding. **Foreign bodies,** particularly in younger girls, may include objects that can cause abrasions or lacerations.

G. Blood dyscrasias, most commonly thrombocytopenic purpura or von Willebrand's disease, although not frequent causes, can cause vaginal bleeding.

    1. Ten percent of women with blood dyscrasias will have abnormal uterine bleeding. Twenty-five percent of patients with a hereditary coagulation disorder give a negative family history.

    2. One study of adolescents hospitalized to control their bleeding reported that coagulation disorders caused 19% of the cases of acute menorrhagia in adolescents. Twenty-five percent of those adolescents with severe menorrhagia (hemoglobin <10 g/dL), 33% of those requiring a transfusion, and 50% of those presenting at menarche with heavy bleeding had coagulation disorders.

IV. Pathophysiology of abnormal vaginal bleeding depends on the cause. Some causes are obvious (eg, lacerations and trauma); others are less apparent.

A. Dysfunctional bleeding. In the normally cycling patient, the amount of tissue shed and blood lost at menstruation is dependent on the length of time the endometrium is stimulated by estrogen. Since in regular menstrual cycles that time is nearly constant, the amount of bleeding and tissue shed will be similarly constant.

    1. Anovulatory dysfunctional bleeding usually results from continuous estrogen stimulation, causing growth of the endometrium until it has reached the point at which the available estrogen can no longer support it or at which the stroma is not adequate to support the excessively vascular endometrium, and the endometrium sloughs. The bleeding that occurs can be anything from light and infrequent to severe menorrhagia.

    2. Ovulatory dysfunctional bleeding. Because of a 25% decrease in circulating estrogen at ovulation, over one half of ovulating women will have at least microscopic midcycle spotting. This condition is usually self-limited and requires no treatment. **Prolonged production of progesterone,** as in persistent corpus luteum, may produce irregular endometrial shedding. Corpus luteum insufficiency or luteal phase defect may produce inadequate amounts of progesterone for endometrial maturation.

B. Benign and malignant neoplasms

    1. Uterine leiomyomas produce abnormal bleeding in two ways: (1) by deforming the endometrial cavity so that normal hemostatic mechanisms of intrauterine pressure are inhibited and (2) by deforming the myometrium so that normal uterine contractile forces are impaired.

2. **Benign endometrial and endocervical polyps** usually bleed secondary to trauma, although they occasionally outgrow their blood supply and become necrotic.

3. **Endometrial hyperplasia** is usually associated with prolonged unopposed estrogen stimulation of the endometrium.

4. **Condyloma acuminata** bleed from trauma or occasionally because the lesions become so large they outgrow their blood supply and become necrotic.

V. **Symptoms.** The history should include age at onset, frequency, duration (ie, number of days of bleeding), date of the last menstrual period, and an estimate of the amount of bleeding. Normally, <80 mL of blood is lost during menstruation; loss of >80 mL is considered menorrhagia. Pad counts are not very accurate for estimating blood loss but provide at least a rough guide—soaking more than 25 pads or 30 tampons per menstrual period is probably abnormal.

A. **Premenstrual symptoms** (eg, breast tenderness, mood swings, and bloating) tend to be associated with ovulatory cycles.

B. **Amenorrhea** preceding the abnormal bleeding, without other signs or symptoms of pregnancy, or recent oral contraceptive use suggests anovulatory bleeding, particularly in the adolescent or perimenopausal patient. In the perimenopausal or postmenopausal patient, a period of amenorrhea preceding abnormal bleeding suggests endometrial atrophy or endometrial carcinoma.

C. **Fever,** particularly if associated with pelvic or abdominal pain or dyspareunia, may suggest a sexually transmitted disease, PID, or sepsis associated with abortion.

D. A **history of easy bruising** may indicate coagulation defects, drug or medication use, or dietary extremes. **Multiple injuries** may indicate trauma, which can include spouse or child abuse (physical or sexual).

E. **History of maternal drug use during pregnancy** (eg, DES), particularly in adolescents with abnormal bleeding, suggests congenital anomalies of the genitourinary tract, including carcinoma of the upper vagina.

F. **Headaches** and **visual changes** may suggest a central nervous system cause such as pituitary neoplasia.

VI. **Signs.** The physical examination should include a pelvic examination, which, in very young girls or in girls who have not used tampons, may require anesthesia. Rectal bimanual examination is not a substitute for pelvic examination, since the rectal examination fails to reveal most vaginal or cervical causes or to allow for adequate evaluation of the uterus or adnexal structures.

A. **Pallor** not associated with tachycardia or signs of hypovolemia suggests chronic excessive blood loss such as that found in anovulatory bleeding, adenomyosis, uterine myomas, or blood dyscrasia.

B. If **signs of shock** or impending shock are present, the blood loss is likely to be related to pregnancy (including ectopic pregnancy), trauma, sepsis, or neoplasia.

C. **Pelvic masses** may represent pregnancy, uterine or ovarian neoplasia, or pelvic abscess or hematoma.

D. **Fever, leukocytosis,** and **pelvic tenderness** strongly suggest PID.

E. **Fine, thinning hair** and **hypoactive or slow-reactive reflexes** suggest hypothyroidism.

F. **Ecchymoses** or **multiple bruises** may indicate trauma (including sexual abuse or incest), coagulation defects, drug or medication use, or dietary extremes.

VII. **Laboratory tests** should be directed by history and physical findings. For detailed evaluation of the following causes of vaginal bleeding, see the chapters indicated: PID, Chapter 55; child abuse, Chapter 95; contraceptives, Chapter 101; and pregnancy and complications, Chapter 103.

A. All patients should have a complete blood cell count (CBC), platelet count, urinalysis, Pap smear, and pregnancy test (unless outside the childbearing age group *and* there is *no* suspicion of pregnancy). Determination of partial thromboplastin time, prothrombin time, and bleeding time, thyroid function testing, and screening for sexually transmitted diseases should be performed on all patients.

B. **Endometrial sampling**

1. **Indications.** The need for endometrial sampling in patients with abnormal uterine bleeding depends on the age group. *Under the age of 20, it is rarely necessary.* Endometrial sampling should precede hormonal therapy in all women over 30, in women younger than 30 at increased risk for endometrial cancer (ie, diabetic, hypertensive, or obese women), and in women over age

20 who have frequent or exceptionally heavy or prolonged bleeding and have failed a course of management with cyclic hormonal therapy. Ideally, the endometrial biopsy should be performed on the presumed first or second day of menstruation. If bleeding is continuous, it may be done at any time.

Hysteroscopy prior to endometrial sampling will show abnormalities in up to 30% of patients who would be missed by endometrial sampling or dilatation and curettage (D&C) alone. Hysteroscopy is easier to perform when the patient is not bleeding, but it can be done at any time.

2. **Contraindications** and **complications** are listed in Table 66–2.
3. **Patient preparation.** Premedication with a nonsteroidal anti-inflammatory drug (NSAID) such as **ibuprofen** (Motrin), 1600 mg (or comparable), taken orally about 2 hours before the procedure is performed, is usually adequate for pain relief. Paracervical block is usually not necessary for endometrial biopsy but is frequently done for office hysteroscopy. **Antibiotic prophylaxis** is unnecessary for endometrial sampling or hysteroscopy.
4. **Procedure.** The Novak curette has been replaced as the standard instrument for endometrial biopsy by newer instruments such as the Vabra aspirator, the Pipelle, the Explora, Vakutage, and others that have been shown to be excellent for endometrial histologic sampling.
5. **Interpretation of results.** In addition to providing information regarding ovulation, appropriate cycling of endogenous or exogenous hormones, infection, and polyps and other neoplasms, the biopsy may reveal endometrial hyperplasia. Endometrial hyperplasia with cytologic atypia progresses to endometrial carcinoma in about 25% of cases; without atypia, fewer than 2% progress to carcinoma. Some patients with the diagnosis of adenomatous endometrial hyperplasia will already have a superficial endometrial cancer.
C. **Transabdominal and transvaginal ultrasonography** may help delineate pelvic masses and can provide information regarding endometrial thickness, uterine size, and the presence of small ovarian cysts that may be of significance, such as persistent corpus luteum cysts.
D. In addition to the basic laboratory work-up, patients with pelvic masses require **pelvic ultrasonography, computerized tomography,** or **magnetic resonance imaging.** These patients frequently require **laparoscopy** or **laparotomy** as well.
VIII. **Treatment** of abnormal bleeding should be directed at the underlying cause, when possible. Symptomatic treatment depends on the amount of bleeding.
A. **Infrequent bleeding.** If the CBC is within normal limits, reassurance and an explanation of the physiology of the cause are sufficient.
B. **Frequent heavy bleeding.** If the patient has frequent heavy bleeding or the patient's hemoglobin is <12 g/dL, the following treatments may be necessary.
1. **Acute bleeding phase.** If the hemoglobin is <7 g/dL, the patient should be hospitalized for control and possible transfusion; if the hemoglobin is <10 g/dL, hospital admission should be considered for treatment with parenteral conjugated estrogens and oral or parenteral progestins. If the hemoglobin is 10 g/dL or higher, the patient may be treated with one of the oral regimens described below.

TABLE 66–2. COMPLICATIONS AND CONTRAINDICATIONS OF ENDOMETRIAL SAMPLING

Complications	Contraindications
Pain	Pregnancy
Vasovagal syncope	Acute vaginitis
Uterine perforation	Acute pelvic inflammatory disease
Bleeding	Known intrauterine hemangioma
Intraperitoneal	Clotting disorder
Cervical	
Uterine	
Infection	
Endometritis	
Pelvic inflammatory disease	
Bowel or bladder injury	
Anesthetic complications	

    a. **Progestins** such as medroxyprogesterone acetate (Provera), 20 mg orally to start, followed by 10 mg twice daily for 7 days, or aqueous medroxyprogesterone acetate (Depo-Provera), 200 mg intramuscularly, will usually stop the acute bleeding.

    b. **Oral contraceptives** such as Lo-Ovral, four times daily for 4 days, then tapered over 7–10 days, are also effective.

  2. Subsequent hormonal therapy

    a. **Provera,** 10 mg orally each day for the first 10 days of each calendar month (or from days 16–25 of the menstrual cycle) for 3–6 months, should be given. Alternatively, **oral contraceptives** can be used for a period of 3–6 months. However, if the cause is anovulation, oral contraceptives may prolong the problem.

    b. **Estrogen replacement therapy.** In the menopausal patient, once endometrial or other pelvic malignancy has been excluded, estrogen replacement therapy can be considered (see Chapter 82).

  3. Other therapies

    a. An **oral iron supplement** should be used for anemia until there is good evidence of recovery of iron stores (see Chapter 6).

    b. **D&C** is curative in over 40% of all patients with menorrhagia but is less useful in known ovulatory patients.

    c. **NSAIDs,** such as naproxen (Naprosyn), 500 mg initially, then 750 mg daily, in divided doses with meals for 5 days, effectively reduce blood loss in chronic menorrhagia but are ineffective for acute bleeding episodes or in regulating noncyclic bleeding.

    d. **Hysterectomy** or **other surgical treatment** may be appropriate in patients with neoplasms, endometriosis, adenomyosis, or chronic PID or in patients with abnormal bleeding and symptomatic uterine prolapse in whom childbearing is completed.

REFERENCES

Barbieri RL, Ryan KJ: The menstrual cycle. In Ryan KJ, Berkowitz RS, Barbieri RL (editors): *Kistner's Gynecology: Principles and Practice.* 6th ed. Mosby; 1995.

Claessens EA, Cowell CA: Acute adolescent menorrhagia. J Obstet Gynecol 1981;**139:**277.

Fisher B, Costantino JP, Redmond CK, et al: Endometrial cancer in tamoxifen-treated breast cancer patients: Findings from the National Surgical Adjuvant Breast and Bowel Project (NSABP). JNCI 1994;**86:**527.

Goldstein SR, Zeltser H, Horan CK, et al: Ultrasonography-based triage for perimenopausal patients with abnormal uterine bleeding. Am J Obstet Gynecol 1997;**177:**102.

Rosenfeld JA: Treatment of menorrhagia due to dysfunctional uterine bleeding. Am Fam Physician 1996;**53:**165.

Smith CB: The why, when, and how of endometrial sampling and hysteroscopy. Consultant 1995; **35:**451.

Van Eijkeren MA, Christiaens JJ, Sixma JJ, et al: Menorrhagia: A review. Obstet Gynecol Surv 1989;**44:**421.

---

67   Vaginal Discharge

L. Peter Schwiebert, MD

I. Definition. Vaginal discharge is discharge from the vagina that is unusual in amount or odor or causes symptoms such as itching or burning.

II. Common diagnoses

  A. Bacterial (anaerobic) vaginosis (BV), formerly known as nonspecific vaginitis (33% of cases).

  B. Cervicitis caused by *Chlamydia trachomatis, Neisseria gonorrhoeae,* and herpes simplex virus (20–25% of cases).

  C. *Candida* vaginitis (20% of cases).

  D. *Trichomonas* vaginitis (10% of cases).

E. **Physiologic discharge** due to normal increase in either cervical mucus or vaginal epithelial discharge (10% of cases).

F. **Atrophic vaginitis** due to estrogen deficiency (frequency of occurrence not known).

G. **Allergic vaginitis** due to vaginal irritants or sensitizers (frequency of occurrence not known).

III. **Epidemiology.** In the ambulatory primary care setting, vaginal discharge is the 10th to 15th most common problem encountered, and two thirds of patients with genitourinary symptoms present with vaginal discharge. These figures underestimate the true prevalence of the problem, however, since many women with discharge or odor do not seek medical attention.

A. The risk of developing **bacterial vaginosis, *Trichomonas* vaginitis, or cervicitis** is increased in unmarried women less than age 25 with a history of more than one sexual partner in the past 3 months, a partner who has had other partners in the past 3 months, or other sexually transmitted diseases (STDs). Most of the pathogenic organisms (anaerobic bacteria, *Trichomonas, N gonorrhoeae,* or *C trachomatis*) that cause vaginal discharge are spread during sexual intercourse with an infected partner.

B. The risk of ***Candida* vaginitis** increases with history of recent use of oral antibiotics (especially penicillin, tetracycline, or cephalosporins), oral contraceptives, or systemic glucocorticoids and the conditions of pregnancy, poorly controlled diabetes mellitus, obesity, and immunocompromise. Recent reports indicate that up to 35% of vaginal candidiasis is non-*albicans*. Risk factors for non-*albicans* infections include immunocompromise, recurrent infection (more than four microscopically or culture-documented episodes per year), and long-term treatment for vaginal candidiasis.

C. **Vaginal infections often coexist.** Twenty-three percent of patients with *Trichomonas* vaginitis have a coexistent and often clinically silent *N gonorrhoeae* infection; 45% of patients with *N gonorrhoeae* also have *C trachomatis*.

D. **Atrophic vaginitis** occurs primarily after the menopause, but also occasionally in lactating or prepubertal patients.

E. **Allergic vaginitis** appears to be associated with topical sensitizers or irritants, such as synthetic tampons, spermicides, hygenic sprays, soaps, perfumes, povidone-iodine solution, latex condoms, or douches.

IV. **Pathophysiology**

A. **Normal vaginal environment.** During the childbearing years, estrogen causes vaginal squamous epithelial cells to proliferate and produce glycogen, which lactobacilli convert to lactic acid, resulting in a vaginal pH of <4.0.

The amount of normal discharge may vary considerably among women, and different women tolerate varying amounts of discharge. The amount of normal discharge may vary with the stage of the menstrual cycle. Normal cervical discharge is clear to slightly opaque.

B. **Abnormal vaginal environment**

1. **Little or no estrogen.** This condition, found in prepubertal girls and postmenopausal women, leads to a thinner vaginal epithelium and diminished levels of glycogen. The vaginal flora is mixed, and the pH is >5.0.

2. **Pathogenic organisms** (eg, anaerobic bacteria or *Trichomonas*). These organisms increase vaginal pH. Douching can also alter the pH, thus increasing susceptibility to infection.

3. **Immunocompromised states or suppression of normal flora by antibiotics** permit overgrowth of opportunistic organisms (eg, *Candida*). *Candida* also grows well in the glycogen-rich vaginas of women in the childbearing years, but has no such substrate in premenarchal children or postmenopausal women and is therefore rare in these populations.

4. **Inflammation.** Endocervical inflammation produces a cloudy, mucoid secretion. Inflammation also causes friability, which produces intermenstrual and postcoital spotting.

V. **Symptoms and signs** (Table 67–1)

VI. **Laboratory tests** (Table 67–2)

A. A **wet preparation** is made by adding a drop of normal saline to a drop of vaginal discharge on a glass slide, and then examining the slide with a microscope.

TABLE 67–1. SYMPTOMS AND SIGNS OF VAGINAL DISCHARGE

Condition	Complaint	Appearance of Discharge and Mucosa
Bacterial vaginosis	Odor or vaginal discharge	Thin, watery, grayish discharge; minimal mucosal erythema
Candida vaginitis	Vulvar itching or burning (50% specificity), external dysuria	Curdy white discharge; sometimes erythematous vaginal epithelium
Cervicitis	Mucoid discharge, intermenstrual spotting, dyspareunia	Yellow, mucoid endocervical discharge; inflamed cervix with focal hemorrhage
Trichomonas vaginitis	Discharge, vulvar itching	Typically copious, frothy; green or yellow discharge; punctate cervical hemorrhage sometimes present; vulvar and vaginal erythema
Physiologic discharge	Discharge without itching or odor	Clear to slightly opaque cervical discharge
Atrophic vaginitis	Discharge, burning, or dyspareunia, or all three	Thin and inflamed with loss of rugal folds; discharge, if present, is watery and may be foul-smelling

B. A **potassium hydroxide (KOH)** preparation is made similarly using a drop of 10% KOH solution instead of saline.

C. **Nitrazine paper** changes color in response to changes in the pH of vaginal discharge. A 1- to 2-inch strip of Nitrazine paper is applied to secretions on the vaginal walls or pooled in the posterior fornix.

D. The **Hansel stain** is a modified Wright-Giemsa stain that enhances eosinophils. This test should be considered in women with persistent discharge in whom the usual tests are normal and no other diagnosis is obvious. In one unpublished study of 50 patients with vaginal discharge, 12% had no evidence of infection and also had more than 25% eosinophils in their discharge using the Hansel stain.

E. **Cultures.** Because of the fairly low sensitivity of wet and KOH preparations in diagnosing *Candida* vaginitis, *Trichomonas* vaginitis, and cervicitis, cultures for *Candida, Trichomonas, N gonorrhoeae,* and *C trachomatis* should be performed in high-risk patients (see sections III,A–C) if KOH and wet preparations show negative results. In addition, all pregnant women should be screened for *C trachomatis* and *N gonorrhoeae.*

   1. Culture results for *C trachomatis* are unavailable for 4–7 days. Recently, direct immunofluorescence and enzyme immunoassays have become available.

TABLE 67–2. OFFICE LABORATORY FINDINGS IN VAGINAL DISCHARGE

Condition	pH (From Vaginal Walls, Not Cervix)/ Color of Nitrazine Paper	Wet and Potassium Hydroxide (KOH) Preparations
Bacterial vaginosis	>4.5/green to purple	Clue cells (bacteria obscuring epithelial cell border in 90% of cases), few WBCs on wet preparation amine "fishy" odor on addition of KOH (>90% sensitive)
Candida vaginitis	3.5–4.5/yellow to green	Spores and hyphae on KOH preparation (21% sensitive)
Cervicitis	>4.0/yellow to purple	Mature squames, >10 WBCs (50–70% sensitive) on wet preparation
Trichomonas vaginitis	>4.5/green to purple	Mature squames with many WBCs on wet preparation, motile protozoa can be seen in 60% of cases
Physiologic discharge	<4.0/yellow	Normal superficial epithelial cells, lactobacilli, no WBCs or spores on wet preparation
Atrophic vaginitis	>5.0/green to purple	Wet preparation shows many WBCs, small round epithelial cells (parabasal cells) which are immature squames unexposed to sufficient estrogen

WBCs, White blood cells.

The predictive positive value (PPV) depends on the prevalence of *C tracho-matis* studied in the population. So far, studies indicate that direct immuno-fluorescence has a better PPV than the enzyme immunoassay in populations at intermediate risk. The PPV of neither test has been adequately studied in populations with a low prevalence of *C trachomatis* infection.

    2. Culture for cure following treatment of cervicitis with a recommended regi-men (see section VII,D,2) is not necessary. However, cultures should be re-peated 1–2 months after finishing treatment to detect reinfection.

F. Serologic **syphilis test (eg, VDRL), human immunodeficiency virus (HIV) test-ing (eg, enzyme-linked immunosorbent assay [ELISA]),** and counseling should be offered to patients with a documented *N gonorrhoeae* infection.

VII. Treatment

  A. General measures. The patient should be instructed to observe the following guidelines.

    1. Discontinue irritating agents (eg, sprays or bubble baths).

    2. Wear nonocclusive, absorbent clothing (cotton rather than nylon under-clothing).

    3. Use barrier contraceptives (eg, condom or diaphragm) to prevent recurrence.

    4. Restore a normal vaginal environment (ie, pH and flora). Some clinicians rec-ommend the use of lactobacillus suppositories or oral yogurt.

    5. Practice good perineal hygiene (ie, wiping from front to back).

  B. Bacterial vaginosis is diagnosed if three of the following five signs are present: (1) pH >4.5, (2) homogeneous gray discharge adherent to the vaginal walls, (3) "fishy" odor upon addition of 10% KOH, (4) clue cells, and (5) absence of vagi-nal lactobacilli, which are long rods microscopically. In addition, a gram-stained slide is 100% sensitive and specific in diagnosing bacterial vaginosis. Therapeu-tic measures are outlined below.

    1. Metronidazole (Flagyl or Protostat), 500 mg orally twice a day for 7 days, has been the standard therapy. Single-dose therapy (2 g) is the least expensive treatment and an effective option when compliance is a problem. Other ef-fective regimens are metronidazole vaginal gel 75% (Metrogel), 5 g vaginally twice daily for 5 days; and clindamycin (Cleocin), 300 mg twice a day orally or applied vaginally as a 2% cream for 7 days.

    2. Recent research has linked bacterial vaginosis to such adverse pregnancy outcomes as premature rupture of membranes, premature labor, neonatal sepsis, and chorioamnionitis. Treatment with oral agents reduces pregnancy-associated morbidity, while intravaginal treatment does not.

  C. Candidiasis (Table 67–3)

    1. Uncomplicated infection (healthy host, infrequent occurrences, and mild to moderate symptoms)

      a. Imidazole creams, ointments, or suppositories share similar efficacy (>80%) in curing uncomplicated vaginal candidiasis.

      b. Several imidazoles are available over the counter (Table 67–3); potential problems with self-treatment include misdiagnosis (at least 33% of cases) and possible emergence of resistant *Candida* strains.

      c. Tioconazole and terconazole are effective against a broader spectrum of *Candida* species than butoconazole, clotrimazole, or miconazole.

      d. Single-dose fluconazole (Diflucan) is less expensive, better tolerated, and equally efficacious as standard 3- to 7-day intravaginal regimens.

    2. Recurrent candidiasis (more than four microscopically or culture-documented infections per year) or complicated infection (moderate to severe symptoms or risk factors listed in section III,B). Effective approaches include the following.

      a. Extension of standard intravaginal regimens to 10–14 days for acute symptoms.

      b. With recurrent infections, 6 months' treatment with one of the following reg-imens: ketoconazole (Nizoral), 100 mg orally daily; itraconazole (Spora-nox), 50–100 mg orally daily; fluconazole (Diflucan), 100 mg orally weekly; or clotrimazole, one 500-mg vaginal suppository weekly. *Note:* Chronic daily use of the foregoing oral medications can interact with other med-ications (eg, theophylline, anticonvulsants, anticoagulants, astemizole, and oral contraceptives), can be hepatotoxic, and may be teratogenic.

TABLE 67–3. TREATMENT OF VULVOVAGINAL CANDIDIASIS

Medication	Proprietary Name	Formulation	Dosage[1]
Clotrimazole	Gyne-Lotrimin[2]	100-mg vaginal suppository	1 daily for 7 days
	Gyne-Lotrimin[2]	1% vaginal cream	1 applicatorful hs for 7 days
	Gyne-Lotrimin 3[2]	200 mg vaginal suppository, 1% cream	Insert/apply daily for 3 days
	Mycelex-7[2]	1% vaginal cream	1 applicatorful daily for 7 days
	Mycelex-G	500-mg tablet	1 tablet for 1 day
	Mycelex-7 vaginal insert[2]	100-mg tablet	1 daily for 7 days or twice a day for 3 days
	Mycelex Thin Pack	500-mg tablet, 1% cream	1 tablet for 1 day; cream twice a day for 7 days
Miconazole	Monistat 7[2]	2% vaginal cream	1 applicatorful daily for 7 days
	Monistat 7[2]	100-mg vaginal suppository	1 daily for 7 days
	Monistat 3	200-mg vaginal suppository	1 daily for 3 days
	Monistat 3 Combination[2]	200-mg suppository, 2% cream	1 suppository daily for 3 days; cream prn
Butoconazole	Femstat 3[2]	2% cream	1 applicatorful daily for 3 days
Tioconazole	Vagistat-1[2]	6.5% ointment	1 applicatorful for 1 day
Terconazole	Terazol 3	0.8% cream	1 applicatorful daily for 3 days
	Terazol 7	0.4% cream	1 applicatorful daily for 7 days
	Terazol 3 suppository	80-mg vaginal suppository	1 daily for 3 days
Nystatin	Mycostatin	100,000-U vaginal tablet	1 daily for 14 days
Fluconazole	Diflucan	150-mg tablet	1 orally for 1 day
Ketoconazole	Nizoral	400-mg tablet	1 orally twice a day for 5 days
Itraconazole	Sporanox	200-mg tablet	1 orally either twice a day for 1 day or daily for 3 days

[1] Unless otherwise indicated, the route of administration is intravaginal; for daily doses, the preferred administration time is at bedtime.
[2] Available over the counter.

    c. Repopulating vaginal lactobacillus using yogurt douches (possibly effective).

D. Cervicitis. Empiric therapy for *C trachomatis* and *N gonorrhoeae* can be instituted in high-risk individuals while awaiting culture results.

    1. Because of the coprevalence of *N gonorrhoeae* and *C trachomatis* infections, patients with *N gonorrhoeae* should be treated for presumptive chlamydial infection with **ceftriaxone,** 250 mg intramuscularly one time, plus either **doxycycline,** 100 mg orally twice daily for 7 days, *or* azithromycin (Zithromax), 1 g orally one time, *or* ofloxacin (Floxin), 300 mg orally twice daily for 7 days. Pregnant or breastfeeding women should receive **ceftriaxone** plus **erythromycin** (erythromycin ethylsuccinate, 800 mg, or erythromycin base, 500 mg), four times daily for 7 days.

    2. Acyclovir, 200 mg orally five times daily for 10 days, should be given for treatment of herpes simplex. Patients with acute urethral syndrome (see Chapter 24) or endometritis/salpingitis (see Chapter 55) should be evaluated for coexisting cervicitis.

E. *Trichomonas* **vaginitis**

    1. Standard regimen. Metronidazole, 500 mg orally twice daily for 7 days, or a single 2-g dose for both the patient and her sexual partner.

    2. Treatment of pregnant patients. Metronidazole should be avoided during the first trimester. The safety of treatment during the second and third trimesters is controversial. However, a 2-g single dose may be considered for patients with severe symptoms after the first trimester. Clotrimazole vaginal suppositories, 100 mg at bedtime or twice daily for 7 days, are about 30% effective in relieving symptoms.

    3. Recurrent *Trichomonas* **vaginitis.** Metronidazole-resistant *Trichomonas* has been documented. As of yet, there is no proven effective treatment for this condition; however, metronidazole, 500 mg orally twice daily for 14 days or 2 g orally for 3 days, may be effective.

   F. No treatment is necessary for **physiologic discharge.**

   G. The treatment for **atrophic vaginitis** is **estrogen replacement** (for treatment regimens, see Chapter 82).

   H. The treatment for **allergic vaginitis** is elimination of likely sensitizers (see section III,D).

VIII. Patient follow-up. The recurrence of cervicitis, *Trichomonas* vaginitis, or bacterial vaginosis following appropriate treatment for vaginal discharge and a symptom-free interval makes reinfection from a new or untreated partner likely. The patient and her partner should be treated with an appropriate regimen and the patient should be educated about improved sex partner referral.

REFERENCES

Desai PC, Johnson BA: Oral fluconazole for vaginal candidiasis. Am Fam Physician 1996;**54**:1337.
Majeroni BA: Bacterial vaginosis: An update. Am Fam Physician 1998;**57**:1285.
Majeroni BA: Chlamydial cervicitis: Complications and new treatment options. Am Fam Physician 1994;**49**:1825.
Reed BD, Eyler A: Vaginal infections: Diagnosis and management. Am Fam Physician 1993;**47**:1805.
Sobel JD: Vaginitis. N Engl J Med 1997;**337**:1896.

---

68   Wheezing

Benjamin W. Chaska, MD, CAQG, RPh

   I. Definition. Wheezes are high-pitched sounds produced by the lungs when the airways become narrowed.

  II. Common diagnoses

    A. Acute viral respiratory infection (up to 50% of wheezing).

    B. Acute bronchitis and pneumonia (33–50% of wheezing).

    C. Asthma (hyperactive airways diseases) (10–15% of wheezing).

    D. Chronic obstructive pulmonary disease (COPD) (emphysema and chronic bronchitis) (5–20% of wheezing).

    E. Congestive heart failure (CHF) (<5% of wheezing).

    F. Bronchiolitis (<5% of wheezing).

    G. Aspiration (eg, resulting from a foreign body or gastroesophageal reflux).

    H. Hypersensitivity or anaphylactoid reaction.

    I. Cystic fibrosis.

    J. Pulmonary embolism (a rare cause of wheezing).

  III. Epidemiology. As many as one of five patients seen by primary care physicians have a respiratory disorder. Up to 15% of children and 10% of adults have wheezing.

    A. Acute viral respiratory infection. Risk factors include young age (under 2 years), fall or winter season, atopy, older siblings, hospitalization, day care, passive smoking, bottle feeding, and previous lower respiratory infection. Epidemics occur frequently.

    B. Acute bronchitis and pneumonia. Common risk factors include smoking or passive smoking, extremes of age, concomitant viral respiratory infection, impaired gag reflex, and COPD.

    C. Asthma (hyperactive airways disease) (see Chapter 72). Viral respiratory infections, family history of asthma, environmental pollutants, passive cigarette smoking, young age, and atopy are risk factors. Asthma is usually recurrent. An environmental trigger can often be identified.

    D. COPD (emphysema and chronic bronchitis) (see Chapter 74). Risk factors are cigarette smoking or passive smoking, air pollution, α_1-antitrypsin deficiency, advanced age, and family history of COPD.

    E. CHF (see Chapter 76). Risk factors include hypertension, obesity, glucose intolerance, smoking, cardiomegaly, atrial fibrillation, electrocardiographic abnormalities, arteriosclerotic heart disease, cardiomyopathy, valvular heart disease, congenital heart disease, pulmonary embolism, infection, anemia, and thyrotoxicosis.

F. Bronchiolitis. Young age (under 2 years), concomitant upper respiratory viral infection, and fall or winter season are risk factors.

G. Aspiration. Risk factors include extremes of age, diminished gag reflex, diminished level of consciousness, and structural abnormalities in the tracheobronchial tree or the esophagus.

H. Hypersensitivity or anaphylactoid reaction. The only risk factor for hypersensitivity or anaphylactoid reaction is a previous reaction to the inciting agent.

I. Cystic fibrosis. Risk factors for cystic fibrosis include white race and a family history of cystic fibrosis. This disease occurs in 1 in 1600 to 1 in 2500 live births, and it is unusual in nonwhite individuals. The incidence in African Americans is 1 in 17,000 live births.

IV. Pathophysiology

A. Acute viral respiratory tract infection, acute bronchitis and pneumonia, and bronchiolitis (see Chapter 16).

B. Asthma (see Chapter 72).

C. COPD (see Chapter 74).

D. CHF (see Chapter 76).

E. Aspiration. A foreign body in the airways may act as a ball valve, causing localized inspiratory and expiratory wheezing. Chronic aspiration, gastroesophageal reflux, and toxic fume inhalation cause cytolysis, edema, inflammation, bronchoconstriction, and wheezing. Wheezing is absent with complete occlusion of the airway.

F. Cystic fibrosis is an inherited defect of epithelial chloride transport. It affects the pancreas, lungs, liver, gut, and exocrine glands. Defects of the cystic fibrosis transmembrane regulation gene on chromosome 7 are related to the causation of this disease. These defects lead to abnormally thick mucus secretions. Wheezing results from poorly cleared, abnormally thick mucus that obstructs airways and predisposes the patient to infectious agents, especially *Staphylococcus, Pseudomonas,* and *Haemophilus influenzae.*

V. Symptoms. Onset of symptoms of viral lower respiratory tract infections, asthma, and CHF may be either acute or gradual. Acute bronchitis, pneumonia, and bronchiolitis usually develop gradually over a period of days. In early life, gastrointestinal symptoms may predominate in patients with cystic fibrosis.

A. Fever may be present in patients with asthma. Low-grade fever is common with viral lower respiratory tract infections, acute bronchitis and pneumonia, and bronchiolitis.

B. Coryza is often seen with viral lower respiratory tract infections and bronchiolitis. **Rhinorrhea** may be present with asthma and bronchiolitis.

C. Sore throat is common with viral lower respiratory tract infections. **Pharyngitis** may be present with bronchiolitis. **Hoarseness, discomfort, chest tightness,** or a **lump in the throat** may suggest chronic aspiration or a hypersensitivity or anaphylactoid reaction. **Angina** may be seen in patients with CHF.

D. Cough is common with viral lower respiratory tract infections, asthma, bronchiolitis, and cystic fibrosis. **Hemoptysis** may occur in patients with cystic fibrosis. A productive cough may be present with acute bronchiolitis, pneumonia, and COPD. A "croupy" cough may suggest a laryngeal foreign body.

E. Wheezing may be present in patients with viral lower respiratory tract infections, acute bronchitis and pneumonia, and asthma. High-pitched wheezing, or **stridor,** may accompany acute aspiration or a hypersensitivity or anaphylactoid reaction. Wheezing is the most common pulmonary symptom in infants with cystic fibrosis.

F. Dyspnea often develops with acute bronchitis, pneumonia, and bronchiolitis and may be present with chronic aspiration. Paroxysmal dyspnea is common with asthma, and paroxysmal nocturnal dyspnea or exertional dyspnea may occur in CHF. Perennial dyspnea is the hallmark of COPD. **Orthopnea** may be seen in patients with CHF.

G. Reduced food intake may occur with bronchiolitis. Either **voracious appetite** or **failure to thrive** may indicate cystic fibrosis.

H. Restless sleep, conjunctivitis, and **otitis media** may be present with bronchiolitis. **Nocturia** and **edema** may occur with CHF.

     I. Sudden choking, gagging, dysphonia, or **complete aphonia** may occur with acute aspiration.

     J. Hives, flushing, and **pruritus** may be caused by a hypersensitivity or anaphylactoid reaction.

     K. Nausea and vomiting may be present with bronchiolitis and a hypersensitivity or anaphylactoid reaction. **Diarrhea** may be present with bronchiolitis. **Constipation, steatorrhea, flatulence, gas pain, meconium ileus,** and **recurrent rectal prolapse** are symptoms of cystic fibrosis.

VI. Signs

     A. Coughing with increased expiratory phase and **generalized rhonchi** are found in acute viral respiratory infection, acute bronchitis, pneumonia, asthma, COPD, bronchiolitis, and cystic fibrosis.

     B. Signs of consolidation, including bronchial breath sounds, rales, and egophony, may be present in patients with pneumonia. **Fever, tachycardia,** and **tachypnea** usually also occur.

     C. Jugulovenous distention, a **gallop,** and **bibasilar rales** are often found in patients with CHF.

     D. Wheezing localized to the right lung is common with aspiration.

     E. Patients with an anaphylactoid reaction present with **urticaria.**

     F. Poor growth, recurrent rectal prolapse, and meconium ileus are common findings in patients with cystic fibrosis.

VII. Laboratory tests. History and physical examination reveal the diagnosis in most patients. Laboratory examination is usually only confirmatory but occasionally may assist with the diagnosis.

     A. Peak expiratory flow rate (PEFR) is indicated in all patients with wheezing, unless physical incapacitation interferes. This test may be difficult to perform in patients under age 6. It is most useful as an indicator of the severity of airway obstruction.

          1. The PEFR may be reduced in patients with bronchospasm or airway obstruction caused by acute viral respiratory infection, acute bronchitis and pneumonia, asthma, COPD, CHF, aspiration, and hypersensitivity or anaphylaxis.

          2. Severe obstruction is indicated by a PEFR of <150 L/min in an adult.

     B. A **complete blood cell count with or without differential** and a **white blood cell count (WBC)** are indicated in patients with fever, tachypnea, cyanosis, or productive cough. The WBC is frequently elevated in patients with acute pneumonia or anaphylaxis and may be elevated in any patient in acute severe respiratory distress.

       Lymphocytosis is often seen with viral infections, and a left shift with increased polymorphonuclear neutrophils frequently accompanies bacterial infections.

     C. Chest radiography is useful in patients with wheezing and fever, tachypnea, productive cough, dyspnea, signs of consolidation or CHF, first episode of wheezing, undiagnosed chronic dyspnea, or history of aspiration. Chest x-rays are not indicated by wheezing alone in patients with recurrent asthma or cystic fibrosis.

          1. Hyperinflation is visible in asthma, bronchiolitis, acute viral respiratory infection, cystic fibrosis, and COPD. Air trapping is evident in foreign body aspiration on inspiratory and expiratory views in adults and on bilateral lateral recumbent views in small children. Perihilar peribronchial infiltration and hilar adenopathy are visible in acute viral respiratory infection and bronchiolitis.

          2. Lobar atelectasis is seen in severe bronchiolitis and foreign body aspiration.

          3. "Dirty lungs" may indicate chronic bronchitis.

          4. Blebs are visible in emphysema.

          5. Infiltrates are frequently seen in acute pneumonia. Local consolidation is present with bacterial pneumonia, while diffuse infiltrates are seen with infections by viruses, *Mycoplasma,* and *Chlamydia.*

          6. Pulmonary venous cephalization, Kerley's B lines, and cardiomegaly are signs of CHF.

     D. Pulmonary function tests are indicated in patients with abnormal PEFR results and in those with persistent, severe, or recurrent wheezing (see Chapters 72 and 74).

     E. Sweat sodium and chloride are indicated when cystic fibrosis is suspected. An elevated sweat sodium is >90% sensitive for the diagnosis of cystic fibrosis.

F. Arterial blood gases are rarely useful in the office setting but are indicated in patients with severe dyspnea or cyanosis.

   1. A normal Po_2 and a normal or depressed Pco_2 are seen in mild asthma, and a depressed Po_2 and a normal Pco_2 are seen in moderately severe asthma. Patients with severe asthma have depressed Po_2 and elevated Pco_2.

   2. Hypoxia and hypercarbia may be seen in patients with aspiration, pneumonia, COPD, CHF, pulmonary embolus, and bronchiolitis.

G. Genetic testing has proved useful in identifying gene carriers, in prenatal diagnosis, and in establishing a definitive diagnosis of cystic fibrosis. An abnormality in the D F508 region of chromosome 7 has been associated with pancreatic insufficiency.

VIII. Treatment

A. Acute viral respiratory tract infection, acute bronchitis, pneumonia, and **bronchiolitis** (see Chapter 16).

B. Asthma (see Chapter 72).

C. COPD (see Chapter 74).

D. CHF (see Chapter 76).

E. Aspiration of stomach contents can be prevented by elevating the head of the bed and by avoiding evening snacks or large evening meals, alcohol, sedating drugs, and drugs that reduce lower esophageal sphincter tone (eg, theophylline). **Acute foreign body aspiration** requires immediate bronchoscopy and removal of the foreign body.

F. A comprehensive discussion of the **management of cystic fibrosis** is beyond the scope of this book; however, basic management principles include a team effort that involves the primary care physician and a regional cystic fibrosis center. There is no specific treatment for cystic fibrosis, although daily therapeutic and prophylactic postural drainage and cupping to the chest followed by coughing to mobilize mucus are recommended. Exercise may also mobilize mucus. Genetic therapy is being actively investigated but has not shown clinical utility yet.

   1. **Antibiotics** are indicated for acute upper respiratory infections, wheezing, and the prevention of recurrent pneumonia. Early aggressive use of antibiotics is recommended. Antibiotics should be selected to cover *Staphylococcus aureus, Streptococcus pneumoniae,* and *Haemophilus influenzae* in mild cases, and in advanced infections, *Pseudomonas* spp. Acute exacerbations are usually treated with combination antibiotic therapy such as a penicillin derivative and an aminoglycoside. Subsequent therapy should be guided by culture and sensitivity testing. Aerosolized tobramycin has been used.

   2. **Pancreatic enzyme replacement** can be given to patients with steatorrhea, azotorrhea, and maldigestion. Initial dosage is one to three capsules of pancreatic enzyme replacement (eg, Cotazym) with each meal or snack; the dosage can then be adjusted as indicated. Chronic high-dose therapy has been associated with fibrosing colonopathy in some patients.

   3. Bronchodilator use may be appropriate and should be individualized.

   4. Lung transplantation may be considered for patients with advanced lung disease.

REFERENCES

Eisenberg JD: Antibiotic use in cystic fibrosis. Curr Opin Pulmon Med 1996;**November**(6):439.

Fiel SB: Aerosol delivery of antibiotics to the lower airways of patients with cystic fibrosis. Chest 1995;**107**(suppl 2):615.

Foster WL Jr, Gimenez EI, Roubidoux MA, et al: The emphysemas. Radiologic-pathologic correlations. Radiographics 1993;**13**:311.

Goldman J: All that wheezes is not asthma. Practitioner 1997;**241**(1570):35.

Jackson A: Clinical guidelines for cystic fibrosis care. Summary of guidelines prepared by a working group of the Cystic Fibrosis Trust, the British Paediatric Association and the British Thoracia Society. J R Coll Physicians Lond 1996;**30**(4):305.

Kennedy DT, Chang Z, Small RE: Selection of peak flowmeters in ambulatory asthma patients: A review of the literature. Chest 1998;**114**:587.

Mamlok R: A cost-effective approach to the diagnosis and treatment of the wheezing infant. Allergy Asthma Proc 1997;**18**(3):149.

Milla PJ: Cystic fibrosis: Present and future. Digestion 1998;**59**(5):579.

69   Acne Vulgaris

Martin Quan, MD

I. **Definition.** Acne vulgaris is a chronic, polymorphic skin disease of pilosebaceous units located on the face, chest, and back. It is generally a self-limited condition that begins during adolescence; however, acne can persist into adulthood.

II. **Common diagnoses.** Clinical manifestations of acne vulgaris follow the pathophysiologic progression described below and include obstructive, inflammatory, and severe acne.

A. **Obstructive acne**
  1. The **closed comedo,** or **"whitehead,"** is a flesh-colored or whitish, slightly palpable lesion that is approximately 1–3 mm in diameter.
  2. The **open comedo,** or **"blackhead,"** is a flat or slightly raised, brownish or black lesion that measures up to 5 mm in diameter.

B. **Inflammatory acne**
  1. **Acne papules** are red, tender, elevated lesions that are as large as 5 mm in diameter. Pustules are superficial papules containing visible pus.
  2. **Acne nodules** are solid, inflammatory lesions that exceed 5 mm in diameter and are situated deeper than papules in the dermis.
  3. The **acne "cyst"** is actually a large nodule that has suppurated and become fluctuant.
  4. **Acne scars** are sequelae of inflammatory acne and may appear as small, deep, punched-out pits ("ice pick" scars), atrophic macules, hypertrophic scars, or broad, sloping depressions.

C. **Severe acne variants**
  1. **Acne conglobata** is a disfiguring, highly inflammatory form of acne found predominantly in males. It is characterized by the presence of multiporous comedones, nodules, cysts, abscesses, and draining sinus tracts on the face, upper trunk, and posterior neck.
  2. **Acne fulminans** is an uncommon systemic disease characterized by sudden eruptions of large, highly inflammatory, encrusted, ulcerative acne lesions on the trunk, accompanied by other systemic features, including fever, polyarthritis, leukocytosis, anemia, and weight loss.

III. **Epidemiology**
A. An estimated 17 million Americans are affected by acne vulgaris. The National Health Survey has found the prevalence of significant acne vulgaris to be as follows: in the 12- to 17-year age group, 250 per 1000; in the 18- to 24-year age group, 191 per 1000; in the 25- to 34-year age group, 84 per 1000; in the 35- to 45-year age group, 25 per 1000; and in the 45- to 54-year age group, 9 per 1000.
B. The incidence and severity of acne vulgaris are lower in Asians than in whites, and severe acne is less common in blacks than in whites.
C. Acne vulgaris tends to be familial, although its exact genetic pattern remains undetermined.

IV. **Pathophysiology**
A. Although the cause of acne remains unknown, its manifestations arise from the interaction of the following four pathogenic events.
  1. **Increased sebum production** caused by androgenic stimulation of sebaceous glands.
  2. **Outlet obstruction** of the pilosebaceous follicle caused by retention hyperkeratosis, an abnormal keratinization process characterized by increased cohesiveness and turnover of follicular epithelial cells.
  3. **Proliferation of *Propionibacterium acnes,*** an anaerobic diphtheroid residing in the pilosebaceous follicle.
  4. **Inflammation** mediated by the irritant action of sebum leaking into the dermis, as well as the production of chemotactic factors and enzymes produced by *P acnes*.
B. **Impaction of the pilosebaceous follicle** is the primary pathologic event in acne vulgaris, giving rise to the microcomedo. When this obstruction occurs, the continued production of sebum and keratin gives rise to visible lesions, which include

373

closed and open comedones. Leakage or rupture of the contents of closed comedones into the dermis causes inflammatory acne lesions, including papules, pustules, nodules, and cysts.

V. Treatment. Scarring is an important physical and psychosocial sequela of acne that
occurs in a small percentage of patients with severe inflammatory acne. The treatment of acne is directed toward minimizing scarring and providing the patient with the
best appearance possible by reducing the frequency and severity of exacerbations.
Attempts at scar revision should be limited to patients with significant scarring whose
acne is quiescent or well controlled. Scars should be permitted to evolve to their final
appearance for at least 1 year before revision is considered.

  A. Obstructive acne. The treatment of patients with predominantly obstructive acne
  includes applying topical comedolytic agents, extracting comedones, and avoiding comedogenic products.

    1. Comedolytic agents and exfoliating agents

      a. Benzoyl peroxide is an antibacterial, oxidizing agent that possesses mild
      comedolytic properties and is available in a variety of concentrations (2.5%,
      5%, or 10%) and formulations, including lotions, creams, and gels. A thin
      film of a low-strength (2.5% or 5%) preparation is applied once or twice
      daily. Preparation strength is increased as needed every 1–2 months. Mild
      redness and scaling frequently develop during the first few weeks of ther-
      apy but usually diminish with continued use. The liquid and cream prepa-
      rations are less irritating, but the gel formulation is more effective. Con-
      tact allergy occurs in 1–2% of patients.

      b. Tretinoin (topical retinoic acid) is commercially available as Retin-A
      gel (0.01% or 0.025%), Retin-A cream (0.025%, 0.05%, or 0.1%), and
      Retin-A liquid (0.05%). It is applied lightly once a day at bedtime; patients
      must take care to avoid the eyes, nose, and mouth. The most effective
      topical comedolytic agent available, tretinoin accelerates follicular epithe-
      lial cell turnover and reduces the cohesiveness of epidermal cells. Ben-
      eficial effects may not be seen for up to 12 weeks. Skin irritation is the
      major side effect of tretinoin, and an apparent exacerbation of inflamma-
      tory lesions may occur during the early weeks of therapy. Treatment for
      patients with fair or sensitive skin should be initiated with the cream
      preparation (0.025%) on an every other day or twice-weekly basis, since
      this preparation is the least irritating. The liquid preparation is the most
      irritating and therefore should be reserved for patients with recalcitrant
      lesions. The skin should be completely dry before tretinoin is applied, and
      the patient should minimize sun exposure and use a protective sun-
      screen (sun protection factor >15).

      c. Combined benzoyl peroxide and tretinoin. Combination therapy may
      be tried in patients who continue to form comedones despite monother-
      apy with either benzoyl peroxide or tretinoin. Benzoyl peroxide is gener-
      ally applied in the morning and tretinoin in the evening. It is best to initi-
      ate therapy by using each medication on alternating days and advancing
      to day and night applications in accordance with the patient's tolerance.

      d. Adapalene is a new synthetic retinoid analogue that is commercially
      available as Differin gel (0.1%). In addition to providing comedolytic activ-
      ity comparable to that of tretinoin, adapalene possesses anti-inflammatory
      activity and appears to be less irritating. It is applied once a day (at bed-
      time) as a thin film, to affected areas, avoiding the eyes, lips, and mucous
      membranes. Its therapeutic effect is typically seen 8–12 weeks after the
      initiation of treatment, and patients should be advised that their acne may
      actually worsen during the first few weeks of therapy. Skin irritation is
      seen in 10–40% of patients, and the use of sunscreen and the avoidance
      of excessive sun exposure should be recommended.

      e. Azelaic acid is a naturally occurring dicarboxylic acid that possesses a
      combination of antimicrobial and comedolytic properties. Although a less
      potent comedolytic than the retinoids, it may be useful in patients with ob-
      structive acne who are unable to tolerate these agents. It is commercially
      available as Azelex cream (20%) and is approved by the Food and Drug
      Administration (FDA) for the topical treatment of mild to moderate inflam-

matory acne. It is applied as a thin film that is massaged into the affected areas twice daily, after the skin is thoroughly washed and patted dry. Azelaic acid is not associated with photosensitivity and causes minimal skin irritation in 1–5% of patients. Clinical improvement in inflammatory lesions is typically seen by the fourth week of therapy.

    f. Exfoliating agents, such as salicylic acid, elemental sulfur, and resorcinol, are less effective than benzoyl peroxide or tretinoin and are best used only in cases in which patients are unable to tolerate the latter preparations.

  2. Comedo extraction. Both open and closed comedones can be extracted manually by applying gentle pressure with a comedo extractor or with the opening of an eye dropper. Prior to extraction, the pore may be enlarged with a 25-gauge needle.

B. Inflammatory acne. Antibiotics are the mainstay of treatment of inflammatory acne. Topical antibiotics are generally favored as first-line therapy for patients who have mild to moderate acne or as maintenance therapy during the tapering and withdrawal of systemic antibiotics. Systemic antibiotics are indicated for patients who have moderate to severe inflammatory acne as well as for those who fail topical therapy. Tretinoin and benzoyl peroxide, either singly or in combination, and intralesional steroid injections are important ancillary measures.

  1. Topical antibiotics. These antibiotics work by inhibiting the growth and activity of *P acnes* within the follicle.

    a. Commonly used preparations include **clindamycin** (Cleocin T 1%, available as a solution, lotion, or gel formulation), **erythromycin** (eg, A/T/S 2% gel and solution, Akne-mycin 2% ointment, Emgel 2% gel, Erycette 2% solution, or Theramycin 2% solution), **tetracycline** (Topicycline 0.22%), and **meclocycline** (Meclan 1%). Benzamycin is a topical gel combining 3% erythromycin and 5% benzoyl peroxide.

    b. The usual dosage is applied twice daily to affected areas.

    c. The most common side effects of topical antibiotics are skin dryness and irritation. Antimicrobial-associated colitis is a rare complication resulting from topical clindamycin use. Topical tetracycline can produce a yellow fluorescence in the skin (most visible under a black light).

  2. Systemic antibiotics. Clinical experience of nearly four decades has shown such therapy to be effective in the treatment of acne.

    a. The antibiotics most commonly prescribed for acne are **tetracycline** and **erythromycin.**

    b. The initial daily dosage is 1–2 g in two to four divided doses, continued until beneficial effects occur (generally 1–2 months). This dose is then gradually reduced over 2–4 months to the lowest maintenance dose sufficient to maintain control. Patients should increase their dose to 1–2 g at the first sign of a flare-up.

    c. Side effects are infrequent, consisting primarily of gastrointestinal upset and vaginal candidiasis. Gram-negative folliculitis is a superinfection seen in 1–4% of patients on long-term antibiotic therapy.

    d. Tetracycline is contraindicated in pregnant patients and in children less than 9 years of age because it may stain developing teeth.

    e. Antibiotics less frequently prescribed in acne include minocycline and trimethoprim–sulfamethoxazole. Minocycline (Minocin), in a daily dosage of 100–200 mg, is a second-generation tetracycline agent usually reserved for inflammatory acne unresponsive to conventional oral antibiotic therapy. Side effects limiting its use include dizziness and, rarely, pigmentary changes in the skin. Trimethoprim–sulfamethoxazole (eg, Bactrim or Septra), administered as a double-strength tablet once or twice a day, is usually prescribed for severe cases refractory to other antibiotics and for gram-negative folliculitis.

  3. Intralesional corticosteroid injection is an important adjunct in the management of nodulocystic acne lesions. It often produces a rapid reduction in inflammation and reduces the likelihood of scarring.

    a. A 30-gauge needle is used to inject a solution containing **triamcinolone acetonide** (0.63–2.5 mg/mL), formed by diluting the preparation with either normal saline or lidocaine. Approximately 0.05–0.3 mL is injected into the cavity of the acne lesion so as to slightly distend it. Injections can be repeated after 3 weeks.

b. The risk of steroid-induced skin changes (eg, atrophy, telangiectasia, and pigmentary changes) can be reduced by using the dilute solution and injecting the minimum amount required. Adrenal suppression can be avoided by administering no more than 20 mg at a time.

4. Combined oral contraceptives. Birth control pills that combine ethinyl estradiol with a progestin agent with low androgenicity (ie, norgestimate, desogestrel) can improve acne by raising sex hormone–binding globulin and lowering serum free testosterone levels in females.

a. Birth control pills represent a particularly valuable option in female patients with acne who need an effective contraceptive method and have no medical contraindications to their use.

b. Ortho Tri-Cyclen is the first birth control pill to have FDA approval for use in the treatment of acne.

C. Severe inflammatory acne. Patients with severe nodulocystic acne refractory to standard therapy as well as patients with severe acne variants are generally best managed by a dermatologist. Treatment options include oral isotretinoin, dapsone, estrogens, and systemic corticosteroids.

1. Oral isotretinoin. Isotretinoin (Accutane), a highly effective treatment for acne that often produces prolonged remissions following a successful course of therapy, is the only acne treatment that can alter the natural history of the disease. It is indicated for patients with acne that is unresponsive to conventional therapy who have either severe nodulocystic acne or moderate to severe noncystic, inflammatory acne that has the potential for scarring. Isotretinoin causes an involution of sebaceous glands, lowers intrafollicular bacterial counts, reverses retention hyperkeratosis, and directly decreases inflammation.

a. The recommended daily dosage of isotretinoin is 0.5–1.0 mg/kg. A dose of 2 mg/kg should be used in resistant cases. During treatment, the dose can be modified according to the clinical response, the appearance of side effects, or both; most of these are dose related. The drug should be taken once or twice daily for 15–20 weeks.

b. Adverse reactions to isotretinoin are frequent. Mucocutaneous side effects, which include cheilitis, conjunctivitis, dry mucous membranes of the nose and mouth, xerosis, and photosensitivity, are the most common and can generally be managed by the use of topical emollients, artificial tears, or dose reduction. Other side effects include arthralgias and myalgias as well as central nervous system side effects such as headache, nyctalopia, and pseudotumor cerebri. Laboratory changes associated with isotretinoin include hypertriglyceridemia, elevated total cholesterol, and reduced high-density lipoprotein levels, as well as abnormalities in liver function tests and hematologic parameters.

c. Isotretinoin is a teratogen, resulting in a 25-fold increase in major fetal malformations (eg, hydrocephalus, microcephalus, external ear abnormalities, facial dysmorphia, and cardiovascular abnormalities). It is imperative that female patients of reproductive age understand the risk of these severe birth defects and observe **strict contraceptive precautions** during therapy and for at least 1 month following completion of therapy. A pregnancy test should be performed prior to starting therapy as well as monthly during therapy.

2. Estrogen

a. A minimum dose of 80–100 μg of **ethinyl estradiol** is required to suppress sebum production. This large dose precludes the use of estrogen in male patients.

b. The risk of thromboembolic disease associated with this dosage limits the use of estrogen therapy to selected female patients with particularly severe, treatment-resistant, nodulocystic acne.

3. Other agents. Although **dapsone** (diacetyl diaminodiphenylsulfone) and systemic **corticosteroids** have been used in patients with severe inflammatory acne because of their powerful anti-inflammatory properties, these agents are rarely prescribed because of significant side effects associated with long-term use.

VI. **Management strategies.** Successful acne management has its roots in patient education and compliance. Sufficient time should be allotted at the initial visit to explain the pathogenesis of acne and the rationale behind its treatment. It is important that the patient be involved as an active participant in his or her own care and that the physician be viewed as a caring and interested ally. Follow-up visits should be routinely scheduled at regular intervals and used to monitor therapy and to respond to questions or concerns that may arise. Important points of information that warrant discussion include the following items.

A. Acne vulgaris is a **chronic skin disorder** likely to run a waxing and waning course. Although treatment generally controls acne, it does not cure it.

B. **Long-term therapy** is required to control acne. Therefore, therapy must be continued even after the patient's skin clears. **Topical therapy** should be applied to all affected areas, not just individual lesions. **Oral antibiotics** (particularly tetracycline) should generally be taken on an empty stomach, either 1 hour before or 2 hours after meals.

C. Significant improvement of the patient's appearance may not be apparent for 3–6 weeks after the initiation of therapy, and maximum benefit may not be seen for several months.

D. Acne is not caused by poor **hygiene.** Obsessive scrubbing can actually exacerbate the condition. Picking and popping pimples serve only to increase inflammation and the likelihood of scarring.

E. There is no relationship between acne and **masturbation, sexual activity,** or **venereal disease.**

F. **Oil-based cosmetics and moisturizers** can be comedogenic and should be avoided.

G. Research studies have failed to substantiate the need for rigid **dietary restrictions** in acne management. Patients are advised to eat a healthy diet, avoiding only those foods that have consistently resulted in aggravation of acne.

REFERENCES

American Academy of Dermatology: Guidelines of care for acne vulgaris. J Am Acad Dermatol 1990;**22:**676.

Gibson JR: Rationale for the development of new topical treatments for acne vulgaris. Cutis 1996;**57:**13.

Habib TP: *Clinical Dermatology: A Color Guide to Diagnosis and Therapy.* Mosby; 1996.

Layton AM, Cunliffe WJ: Guidelines for optimal use of isotretinoin in acne. J Am Acad Dermatol 1992;**27**(6, part 2):S2.

Leyden JJ: New understanding of the pathogenesis of acne. J Am Acad Dermatol 1995;**32:**S15.

Leyden JJ: Therapy for acne vulgaris. N Engl J Med 1997;**336:**1156.

Redmond G, et al: Norgestimate and ethinyl estradiol in the treatment of acne vulgaris: A randomized, placebo-controlled trial. Obstet Gynecol 1997;**89:**615.

Sykes NL Jr, Webster GF: Acne: A review of optimum treatment. Drugs 1994;**48**(1):59.

---

70   Acquired Immunodeficiency Syndrome (AIDS)

Wendy O. Buffett, MD, Cristina I. Gruta, PharmD,
& Ronald H. Goldschmidt, MD

I. **Definition. Human immunodeficiency virus (HIV) disease** is a chronic progressive disease caused by a retrovirus, the **human immunodeficiency virus.** Clinical **acquired immunodeficiency syndrome (AIDS),** as defined by characteristic opportunistic infections (eg, *Pneumocystis carinii* pneumonia [PCP]), cancers (eg, Kaposi's sarcoma), neurologic conditions (eg, HIV-related encephalopathy), and/or a CD4$^+$ lymphocyte count below 200 cells per microliter, is the advanced stage of HIV disease.

A. **Acute syndrome.** This syndrome, which usually occurs about 2–4 weeks following HIV infection, is difficult to identify because of its nonspecific nature. The symptoms and signs are similar to those of infectious mononucleosis and can include fever, lymphadenopathy, sore throat, headache, malaise, arthralgias, myalgias, and a maculopapular rash. Sometimes abdominal cramps and diarrhea are present. (Aseptic meningitis, encephalopathy, and neuropathies rarely occur.) The acute HIV syndrome usually resolves spontaneously within 1–2 weeks.

B. Asymptomatic HIV infection. After infection, an asymptomatic phase lasting 5–10 years occurs. Although infection persists and the virus continues to proliferate, the immunologic system remains relatively intact.

C. Symptomatic HIV infection. Conditions such as oral candidiasis (thrush), oral hairy leukoplakia, generalized lymphadenopathy, thrombocytopenia, and weight loss generally precede the development of clinical AIDS. Some of these conditions, when found in persons who are HIV positive, have been termed **AIDS-related complex.** These conditions can also occur in persons who are not infected with HIV, however, so their presence alone does not define HIV infection.

D. AIDS. Clinical AIDS is characterized by advanced immunodeficiency with specific opportunistic infections, wasting, cancers, and encephalopathy. AIDS is also defined by the finding of a CD4$^+$ (T helper) lymphocyte count of <200 cells per microliter.

E. AIDS in children

1. Infants and children with AIDS present with recurrent bacterial infections, lymphadenopathy, pneumonia, failure to thrive, loss of developmental milestones, or behavioral problems. Consultation with pediatric AIDS specialists is generally necessary to guide therapy and arrange for clinical trials.

2. Immunization schedules for children with HIV differ from the standard schedules found in Chapter 107. Oral polio vaccine should not be used in children with AIDS or in families with children who are either infected or suspected of being infected with HIV.

II. Epidemiology

A. Prevalence. An estimated 750,000 to 1 million Americans are infected with HIV; more than 650,000 of these persons have developed clinical AIDS. As of December 1997, more than 8000 children were infected through vertical transmission in the United States.

B. Transmission of HIV requires the exchange of body fluids. HIV, which is not spread by casual contact, can be transmitted in the following ways.

1. **Intimate sexual contact.**
2. **Intravenous drug use involving sharing of needles.**
3. **Transfusion of HIV-infected blood products.** Since the introduction of HIV antibody screening in 1985, blood products have become extremely safe (approximately 1 in 40,000 units is infected). Organ transplantation, once a means of HIV transmission, is also very safe.
4. **Perinatal transmission from mother to child.**
5. **Occupational exposures from needlesticks.**

C. The **average period between initial infection and development of clinical AIDS** has been estimated to be about 8–11 years among homosexual males. AIDS takes less time to develop in children and among intravenous drug users.

D. Prior to the use of Highly Active Antiretroviral Therapy (HAART), the **average length of survival** depended on the case-defining condition. Now in the era of HAART it seems that the average length of survival is increasing, but data are pending.

E. The **distribution of AIDS cases by population groups** is shown in Figure 70–1.

III. Pathophysiology

A. HIV, a retrovirus, invades CD4$^+$ lymphocytes, macrophages, monocytes, and certain other tissue cells, causing their destruction and dysfunction. Immunodeficiency results from the destruction of the CD4$^+$ lymphocytes and associated abnormalities of the immune system.

B. Opportunistic infections and cancers can occur in virtually any organ system during this state of impaired immune function.

IV. Differential diagnosis. Advanced AIDS, with the combination of wasting, infections, and cancers, is rarely confused with other diseases. Early stages of AIDS can be similar to diseases of specific organ systems or nonspecific illnesses such as influenza. AIDS complications can be confused with other disorders, so risk assessment, counseling, and HIV testing must be considered for diseases such as the following.

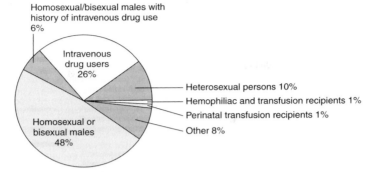

FIGURE 70–1. Distribution of adult and adolescent AIDS cases by population groups in the United States. "Other" category includes persons perinatally infected but diagnosed with AIDS after age 13, those with occupational transmissions, and cases still under investigation. Information from Centers for Disease Control and Prevention, 1998 Surveillance Report, Table 5.

A. Respiratory diseases. Bacterial pneumonia, asthma, or a viral illness accompanied by mild shortness of breath or cough can be mistaken for early PCP.

B. Lymphatic cancers. Cancers of lymphoreticular or histocytic tissue (eg, Hodgkin's disease, non-Hodgkin's lymphoma, lymphocytic leukemia, or multiple myeloma) may resemble the lymphadenopathy or lymphomas of AIDS (for further information, see Chapter 47).

C. Weight loss. This condition may result from causes other than AIDS.

D. Skin lesions. Other skin lesions may resemble those of Kaposi's sarcoma. Common dermatologic conditions (eg, seborrhea, fungal infections, or allergic rashes) can occur in HIV-infected persons.

E. Oral candidiasis (thrush). Patients with diabetes mellitus and patients receiving antibiotic therapy can also have thrush. The disorder is considered an incidental finding in healthy persons.

F. Neurologic conditions. Changes in mental status can be caused by drugs, depression, or other factors.

G. Immunodeficiencies. Disorders of the immune system may result from immunosuppressive or cytotoxic therapy (eg, high-dose or long-term treatment with systemic corticosteroids) or a congenital immunodeficiency syndrome.

V. Diagnosis
  A. Symptoms and signs
   1. Nonspecific symptoms such as weakness, anorexia, fever, and weight loss are most commonly caused by HIV or opportunistic infections and cancers. Such symptoms can also be caused by bacterial or fungal sepsis or *Mycobacterium avium–intracellulare* complex (MAC) disease or tuberculosis. Cultures can help determine the cause of significant fevers. Treatment of infections caused by MAC can relieve associated fever and other symptoms, although treatment can be more toxic than helpful in some cases.
   2. Common opportunistic infections and cancers
      a. Skin conditions
         (1) Kaposi's sarcoma of the skin, oral mucosa, or both appears as red to purple lesions, usually >0.5 cm in diameter.
         (2) Maculopapular rashes are exceedingly common and are often associated with drug treatment (either prescription or over-the-counter drugs).
      b. Eye diseases. Yellow–white or hemorrhagic patches on the retina can indicate sight-threatening **cytomegalovirus (CMV) retinitis.**
      c. Oral cavity
         (1) White plaques or erosive (erythematous) areas suggest **oral candidiasis.** Thrush is common in advanced symptomatic HIV infection and is seen almost universally in clinical AIDS.

  (2) Painless, white, somewhat hairlike lesions on the lateral borders of the tongue indicate **hairy leukoplakia.** This condition, which is caused by the Epstein–Barr virus, will disappear and may recur. It requires no treatment.

d. Lymph nodes. Lymph nodes are frequently enlarged, usually reflecting a generalized response to HIV infection. Hard, asymmetrical, or extremely prominent nodes may require biopsy to exclude fungal infection or cancer.

e. Pulmonary involvement is the most common condition in patients with AIDS. *P carinii* is the most common pathogen, and PCP is the most common pulmonary disease. Bacterial pneumonias, fungal and mycobacterial infections, and Kaposi's sarcoma are also important causes of pulmonary diseases.

  (1) Patients with pulmonary disease may present with symptoms that range from mild shortness of breath or nonproductive cough to severe respiratory distress. Acute PCP is most commonly characterized by shortness of breath, dry cough, and fever. Chest x-rays usually show patchy infiltrates or diffuse interstitial disease, although 5% of chest x-rays of patients with pulmonary disease may be normal. Sputum production is uncommon unless bacterial pneumonia is present.

  (2) Evaluation of pulmonary disease generally requires examination of induced sputum, bronchial washings, or biopsies. Careful microscopic examination and cultures for *P carinii, Mycobacterium tuberculosis,* bacteria, and fungi are essential.

f. Gastrointestinal conditions

  (1) Esophagitis. Dysphagia, odynophagia, and substernal burning pain are symptomatic of esophagitis. Esophagitis can be caused by *Candida albicans,* CMV, or herpes simplex virus. When an empiric trial of anticandidal medications for patients with concurrent oral candidiasis fails, endoscopy with biopsies and cultures is essential to establish a diagnosis and direct treatment.

  (2) Diarrhea, often copious and frequently associated with malabsorption, can be caused by *Isospora belli, Cryptosporidium, Entamoeba histolytica, Campylobacter,* and other enteric pathogens. Diarrhea from HIV infection alone can occur and requires symptomatic treatment. Diarrhea can also be a complication of HIV medications.

  (3) Liver disease. Increased alkaline phosphatase levels commonly indicate (1) liver infection by *M avium–intracellulare* or *M tuberculosis* or (2) liver involvement by Kaposi's sarcoma or lymphoma. Acute and chronic viral hepatitis and drug-induced hepatitis can also occur. Biopsy, although rarely helpful, can be considered in some cases in which *M tuberculosis* infections or other treatable conditions may be present.

g. Neurologic problems

  (1) Peripheral neuropathies can result in painful dysesthesias of the feet and the legs. Cranial neuropathies can also occur. Presumably, HIV involvement of neural tissue causes this condition.

  (2) AIDS dementia complex is characterized by behavioral changes, deficits in cognitive function, and lack of coordination. Although HIV appears to be the principal cause, other pathogenic conditions (eg, cryptococcal meningoencephalitis or cerebral toxoplasmosis) can also be involved.

  (3) Meningoencephalitis, most often caused by *Cryptococcus neoformans* infection, is characterized by headache (usually slight, although at times severe), fever, and decreased mental functioning. Neck pain and nuchal rigidity can be present. Cryptococcal antigen determination from serum and cerebrospinal fluid is positive in most cases.

  (4) Mass lesions in the central nervous system may result in encephalopathic symptoms, seizures, or focal neurologic deficits. These lesions can be caused by *Toxoplasma gondii* infection, lymphomas, and, rarely, other opportunistic infections.

B. Laboratory tests
   1. **Screening for HIV.** A reactive screening test (eg, enzyme-linked immuno-absorbent essay [ELISA]) plus a positive specific test (eg, Western blot or immunofluorescent antibody) confirm HIV infection. Generally, these tests become positive within 1 month of infection; almost all infected persons display positive HIV tests within 3–6 months of infection. In most cases, these tests will remain positive indefinitely.
   2. **Indicators of progression of HIV disease**
      a. A person with advanced HIV disease usually has a CD4$^+$ count of <200 cells per microliter. Normal levels of CD4$^+$ cells usually exceed 800 cells per microliter.
      b. Quantitative plasma HIV RNA (viral load) testing is used for staging and monitoring response to therapy. Current tests can now detect viral particles down to 20–50 copies/mL. After a baseline test is obtained (2 tests 2 weeks apart), viral load testing should be checked every 3–4 months. A significant change in viral burden is measured as greater than a 0.5 log increase and can be caused by disease progression, failure of antiretroviral therapy, active infection, or immunizations. Conversely, a 0.5 log decrease from baseline is considered a significant drop in viral burden when therapy is instituted.
   3. **Laboratory evaluation of specific organ systems** includes hematologic tests, examinations of body fluids, invasive diagnostic tests to obtain cultures and tissues, and imaging studies.
   4. **Drug resistance testing** may be useful for individual patient management.
   5. **Genotypic and phenotypic testing assays** are currently under development and need standardization and a clearer definition of their clinical roles.
VI. **Treatment** *Note: Drug therapy for HIV disease is rapidly changing and is increasingly complex. Starting or changing regimens may have far-reaching implications that may affect the availability and efficacy of future therapy. Before one prescribes any medications, consultation with an HIV expert is recommended.*
   A. HIV. All patients with AIDS and patients symptomatic with any level of viremia should be offered therapy. The best time to initiate antiretroviral therapy for asymptomatic patients is uncertain. Current standards recommend that antiretroviral therapy be initiated when CD4$^+$ cell counts fall below 350–500 cells/mm^3 *or* when the viral load is above 10,000–20,000 copies/mL. Patients whose viral load is below 10,000–20,000 copies/mL and whose CD4+ count is above 500 cells/mm^3 have the option to delay therapy. First-line therapy consists of a combination of two nucleoside analogues (NA) and one protease inhibitor (PI). A combination of two NAs plus a non-nucleoside reverse transcriptase inhibitor (nnRTI) is a reasonable alternative regimen for patients who cannot tolerate or adhere to first-line therapy. Potent regimens should not be a random selection of agents from different antiretroviral classes. Clinically proven combinations should be considered in conjunction with potential for toxicities, drug–drug interactions, and cross-resistance patterns.
      1. **Nucleoside analogues (NAs)**
         a. **Zidovudine** (AZT or Retrovir)
            (1) **Dosage and administration.** Zidovudine is usually given either as 200 mg three times daily or 300 mg twice daily by mouth. A formulation that combines 300 mg of zidovudine with 150 mg of lamivudine (Combivir) is also available and is dosed 1 tablet orally twice daily.
            (2) **Adverse effects.** Anemia, myositis, headache, and gastrointestinal (GI) intolerance can occur. Macrocytosis is a normal response to zidovudine treatment and does not indicate drug toxicity.
         b. **Didanosine** (dideoxyinosine [ddI] or Videx)
            (1) **Dosage and administration.** Didanosine, 200 mg, should be taken by mouth twice daily. For patients who weigh <60 kg, the dosage should be reduced to 125 mg twice daily.
            (2) **Adverse effects.** Pancreatitis and peripheral neuropathy are the most common adverse effects.
         c. **Zalcitabine** (dideoxycytidine [ddC] or Hivid)

  (1) Dosage and administration. Zalcitabine, 0.75 mg, should be taken orally three times daily. For patients who weigh <30 kg, the dosage should be reduced to 0.375 mg three times daily.
  (2) Adverse effects. Peripheral neuropathy and stomatitis are the most common adverse effects.
d. Stavudine (d4T or Zerit)
  (1) Dosage and administration. Stavudine, 20 mg, should be taken orally twice daily. For patients who weigh 40–60 kg, the dosage should be reduced to 15 mg twice daily.
  (2) Adverse effects. Peripheral neuropathy is most common.
e. Lamivudine (3TC or Epivir)
  (1) Dosage and administration. Lamivudine, 150 mg, should be taken orally twice daily. For patients weighing <50 kg, the dosage should be reduced to 2 mg/kg twice daily. A formulation that combines 150 mg of lamivudine with 300 mg of zidovudine (Combivir) is also available and is dosed 1 tablet orally twice daily.
  (2) Adverse effects. Headache, fatigue, and insomnia are the most common side effects.
f. Abacavir (Ziagen)
  (1) Dosage and administration. The normal adult dose of abacavir is 300 mg by mouth twice daily.
  (2) Adverse effects. Nausea, vomiting, and diarrhea were reported most frequently in clinical trials. Approximately 5% of patients have manifested a hypersensitivity reaction to abacavir that consists of fever and other symptoms such as fatigue, GI symptoms, or rash. Patients should NOT be re-challenged with abacavir if they experience this hypersensitivity reaction.
g. Adefovir (Preveon). *Note:* As of this writing, this antiretroviral agent has not yet been approved by the Food and Drug Administration. However, approval is thought to be imminent.
  (1) Dosage and administration. Adefovir is dosed at 60 mg orally once daily given with L-carnitine 500 mg daily.
  (2) Adverse effects. Renal dysfunction has been observed in >40% of patients, usually after 20 weeks of treatment. Monitor electrolytes and renal function.
2. Protease inhibitors (PI)
  a. Saquinavir (Invirase = hard gel capsule [HGC] or Fortovase = soft gel capsule [SGC]). *Note: As of this writing, both the HGC and SGC are available, but the manufacturer of saquinavir plans to phase out Invirase.*
    (1) Dosage and administration. Fortovase should be given 1200 mg three times daily with food when used with two nucleoside analogues (NAs) as a lone PI. In combination with ritonavir (Norvir), Invirase or Fortovase can be dosed 400 mg twice daily. Invirase is no longer recommended for use as a lone PI in an antiretroviral regimen.
    (2) Adverse effects. Headache, confusion, and nausea are the most common side effects.
    (3) Drug interactions. Saquinavir is both a substrate and inhibitor of the p450 hepatic enzymes. Consult package insert for further information.
  b. Indinavir (Crixivan)
    (1) Dosage and administration. The usual dose of indinavir is 800 mg every 8 hours orally on an empty stomach or with a light meal. The patient should be well hydrated, with at least 1.5 L of noncaffeinated fluid daily. Separate administration by 1 hour from antacids or didanosine.
    (2) Adverse effects. GI intolerance, nephrolithiasis, and increased indirect bilirubin are the main complications of indinavir.
    (3) Drug interactions. Indinavir is both a substrate and inhibitor of the p450 hepatic enzymes. Its dose may need adjustment when combined with certain enzyme inhibitors or inducers. Consult the package insert for more information.

    c. Ritonavir (Norvir)
- **(1) Dosage and administration.** The usual dose of ritonavir is 600 mg twice daily by mouth when given with 2 NAs. If given in combination with saquinavir, the dose is decreased to 400 mg twice daily.
- **(2) Adverse effects.** Nausea, vomiting, diarrhea, circumoral paresthesias, increased triglycerides (>200%) are the most common adverse effects.
- **(3) Drug interactions.** Ritonavir is a potent inhibitor of liver enzymes. There are numerous agents contraindicated for use with it. Consult the package insert for complete prescribing information.

    d. Nelfinavir (Viracept)
- **(1) Dosing and administration.** Nelfinavir can be given either as 750 mg three times a day orally or 1250 mg twice daily by mouth in combination with NAs.
- **(2) Adverse effects.** Diarrhea is the most common side effect of nelfinavir.
- **(3) Drug interactions.** Nelfinavir is both a substrate and inhibitor of the p450 hepatic enzymes. Consult the package insert for further information.

    e. Amprenavir (Agenerase)
- **(1) Dosage and administration.** The usual adult dose of amprenavir is 1200 mg by mouth twice daily. Each dose is equivalent to eight 150-mg capsules.
- **(2) Adverse effects.** The most frequently reported adverse effects were rash, nausea, vomiting, depression, and perioral paresthesias.
- **(3) Drug interactions.** Amprenavir is both a substrate and an inhibitor of the p450 enzymes. Consult the package insert for information about agents that need dose adjustments or are contraindicated for co-administration with amprenavir.

3. Non-nucleoside reverse transcriptase inhibitors (NNRTI)

    a. Nevirapine (Viramune)
- **(1) Dosing and administration.** In combination with other antiretrovirals, nevirapine is dosed 200 mg once daily by mouth for the first 2 weeks and then 200 mg twice daily thereafter.
- **(2) Adverse effects.** The most common complications include rash and increased transaminase levels.
- **(3) Drug interactions.** Nevirapine can induce the p450 hepatic enzymes. Consult the package insert for information for affected agents.

    b. Delavirdine (Rescriptor)
- **(1) Dosing and administration.** Delavirdine is usually given 400 mg orally three times a day in combination with other antiretroviral agents. Separate administration by 1 hour from antacids or didanosine.
- **(2) Adverse effects.** Rash and headaches are the most common adverse effects.
- **(3) Drug interactions.** Delavirdine is an inhibitor of p450 hepatic enzymes. Consult the package insert for information for affected agents.

    c. Efavirenz (Sustiva)
- **(1) Dosing and administration.** The recommended dose of efavirenz is 600 mg orally once daily (usually at bedtime) in combination with other antiretroviral agents.
- **(2) Adverse effects.** Sedation, dizziness, bizarre dreams, and rash are the most common side effects.
- **(3) Drug interactions.** Efavirenz is both a p450 enzyme inducer and inhibitor. Consult the package insert for complete prescribing information.

4. Regimens NOT recommended. Due to poor virological outcomes or overlapping toxicities, certain regimens should be avoided. These include all monotherapies and the following NA combinations: stavudine (d4T) + zidovudine (AZT); zalcitabine (ddC) + didanosine (ddI); zalcitabine (ddC) + stavudine (d4T); or zalcitabine (ddC) + lamivudine (3TC).

5. Adherence. Optimal adherence to antiretroviral therapy is key in achieving and maintaining durable viral suppression. Patients should be counseled on the risks of developing resistance if adherence is less than excellent. Many aids such as pill boxes or watch alarms can be used to help enhance adherence.

B. Kaposi's sarcoma of the skin and oral mucosa does not require treatment unless the lesions are uncomfortable or cosmetically disturbing. Widespread disease can be treated with chemotherapeutic agents. Radiation therapy and direct injection with chemotherapeutic agents are effective for some localized disease. Treatment does not appear to prolong life.

C. CMV retinitis. Ganciclovir, foscarnet, or **cidofovir** given intravenously for an induction period followed by lifelong intravenous maintenance therapy is effective in retarding the progression of CMV retinitis. The dosage schedule and the choice of drug depend on clinical toxicity variables and availability of supportive care.

D. Oral candidiasis is readily treated with standard antifungal troches or solutions. **Clotrimazole** troches, 10 mg five times daily, or vaginal suppositories, 100 mg once or twice daily, or **nystatin,** 5 mL swish-and-swallow every 6 hours or 500,000-U vaginal tablets dissolved in the mouth every 6 hours, are quite effective. **Fluconazole,** 50–100 mg by mouth daily, or **ketoconazole,** 400 mg by mouth daily (induction) followed by 200 mg once or twice daily, is a suitable alternative therapy.

E. PCP

1. **Acute PCP.** Three weeks of uninterrupted treatment is successful in most episodes of acute PCP. Clinical and radiologic evidence of response to therapy usually takes 3–7 days. Acute PCP can be treated on an inpatient or outpatient basis. Outpatient therapy is preferred when the disease appears mild and adequate home support is available.

   a. **Trimethoprim–sulfamethoxazole (TMP–SMZ),** administered intravenously or orally, is the drug of choice in treating acute PCP. TMP–SMZ has the advantage of providing additional treatment against most bacterial pulmonary pathogens. The dosage is 15 mg of TMP and 75 mg of SMZ per kilogram daily, divided into four equal doses. Two- to 3-week therapy is recommended. Skin rashes are common; when the rash is mild and does not involve the mucous membranes, TMP–SMZ treatment can usually be continued with the addition of antihistamine therapy. Nephrotoxicity and hepatotoxicity can also occur.

   b. **Pentamidine,** administered intravenously, is effective against PCP. Switching to oral therapy with other agents is necessary to complete 3-week therapy in the outpatient setting. Nephrotoxicity, hepatotoxicity, and hypoglycemia are the most important side effects. Inhaled pentamidine is not reliably effective against acute PCP.

   c. **Other agents can be effective against mild to moderate PCP.** These include clindamycin plus primaquine; trimetrexate; and possibly atovaquone.

   d. **Oral dapsone–trimethoprim** is a suitable alternative treatment choice for patients with mild PCP. The toxic effects of this drug are similar to those of TMP–SMZ. In addition, methemoglobinuria may occur.

2. **Prophylaxis.** Any patient with a CD4$^+$ lymphocyte count <200 cells per microliter is a candidate for primary PCP prophylaxis. Patients who have had previous episodes of PCP also should receive prophylaxis. Pharmacologic agents used for prophylaxis include the following.

   a. **TMP–SMZ** is the drug of choice. The dosage is one double-strength tablet twice daily, or three times per week.

   b. **Dapsone,** 50–100 mg orally daily, is a suitable alternative to TMP–SMZ.

   c. **Atovaquone** dosed at 750 mg twice daily is another reasonable alternative to TMP–SMZ or to dapsone.

   d. **Aerosolized pentamidine,** 300 mg given once monthly, is a second-line agent for patients unable to take TMP–SMZ or dapsone.

F. Esophagitis is most often caused by *C albicans* and can be treated with oral **fluconazole,** 100–200 mg daily, or **ketoconazole,** 400 mg daily. Failure to respond necessitates endoscopic evaluation for herpes esophagitis or CMV esophagitis. Intravenous **acyclovir,** 5 mg/kg every 8 hours, followed by oral acyclovir suppression, is effective against herpes simplex esophagitis. **Ganciclovir** or **foscarnet** can be used to control CMV esophagitis.

G. Diarrhea caused by specific bacterial or parasitic organisms may respond to standard therapy (see Chapter 19). Symptomatic treatment should be offered when antimicrobial therapy is not effective or when no causative organisms can be identified.

H. Peripheral neuropathies may respond to **tricyclic antidepressant drugs** (eg, amitriptyline, 25–150 mg orally daily) or may require **narcotic analgesics.**

I. Cryptococcal meningitis and other cryptococcal infections should be treated acutely with **amphotericin B,** 0.7–1 mg/kg daily, in combination with **flucytosine (5-FC)** at 75–100 mg/kg/day. If the patient is clinically well after receiving 7.5 mg/kg of amphotericin B, **fluconazole** at 400 mg by mouth daily can be given to complete a 10- to 12-week course. Long-term suppressive therapy with fluconazole should be given.

J. Toxoplasmosis of the central nervous system can be treated with **pyrimethamine,** 25 mg by mouth daily, plus **sulfadiazine,** 1 g by mouth four times daily. **Clindamycin,** 600–900 mg by mouth four times daily, can be substituted for sulfadiazine in patients who are allergic to sulfa drugs.

K. Mycobacterium avium complex (MAC) can cause a wide range of localized or systemic problems, including hepatic or other GI disease, fevers, weight loss, and anemia. Treatment with ethambutol, 15 mg/kg by mouth daily, plus either clarithromycin, 500 mg by mouth twice daily, or azithromycin, 500 mg by mouth daily, can be effective. Some clinicians prescribe prophylaxis against MAC disease, with clarithromycin at 500 mg orally twice daily, azithromycin at 1200 mg by mouth once weekly, or rifabutin (Mycobutin), 300 mg by mouth daily, for patients with fewer than 75 or 50 CD4+ cells per microliter.

L. Unapproved drugs are available for many HIV-related conditions. Some are available from pharmaceutical companies via compassionate-use protocols or in the context of clinical trials. Others are available "underground." The physician must exercise caution in the use of untested drugs.

VII. Management strategies. Patients with HIV infection require comprehensive primary care. A team of physicians, public health or visiting nurses, social workers, hospice workers, and family members that is organized around the care of the patient is essential to the treatment of patients with HIV disease.

    A. Psychosocial problems. Special attention to the psychosocial impact of HIV disease is essential to the development of therapeutic strategies. Especially important interventions include discussions about transmission of HIV, treatment strategies, and consideration of the quality of life. Aftercare for the family of a patient who has died of AIDS is also very helpful.

    B. Ideally, one primary physician who is responsible for health care maintenance, early intervention, and treatment of common opportunistic infections should be identified. Consultation with specialists for specific problems can augment primary care.

REFERENCES

Bartlett JG: *1998 Medical Management of HIV Infection.* John Hopkins University School of Medicine; 1998. Carpenter CC, et al: Antiretroviral therapy for HIV infection in 1998. JAMA 1998; **280**(1):78.

Centers for Disease Control: Report of the NIH Panel to Define Principles of Therapy of HIV Infection and Guidelines for the Use of Antiretroviral Agents in HIV-Infected Adults and Adolescents. MMWR 1998;**47**(RR-5):1.

Centers for Disease Control and Prevention: Public Health Service Task Force Recommendations for the Use of Antiretroviral Drugs in Pregnant Women Infected with HIV-1 for Maternal Health and for Reducing Perinatal HIV-1 Transmission in the United States. MMWR 1998; **47**(RR-2):1.

Centers for Disease Control and Prevention: USPHS/IDSA guidelines for the prevention of opportunistic infections in persons infected with human immunodeficiency virus: A summary. MMWR 1997;**46**(RR-12):1.

Goldschmidt RH, Dong BJ: Treatment of AIDS and HIV-related conditions—1999. J Am Board Fam Pract 1999;**12**(1).

Goldschmidt RH, Legg JJ: Counseling patients about HIV test results. J Am Board Fam Pract 1991;**4**:361.

Powderly WG, et al: Recovery of the immune system with antiretroviral therapy. JAMA 1998; **280**(1):72.

Sande MA, Volberding PA (eds): *The Medical Management of AIDS.* Saunders; 1997.

71   Arthritis

Richard J. Ham, MD

I. **Definition.** Arthritis includes numerous conditions that produce inflammation or at least pain and stiffness, in the joints and their supporting structures. The most common type is osteoarthritis (OA), recognized as the most prevalent chronic condition in the world. Rheumatoid arthritis (RA), the most common primary inflammatory arthritis, is more rare, but its inflammatory nature must be identified, since different treatment approaches are required. Other arthritides are gout and arthritis associated with autoimmune diseases such as systemic lupus erythematosus (SLE), psoriasis, and other inflammatory conditions.

II. **Prevalence**

  A. **Degenerative joint changes,** which are frequently associated with arthritis, are found in more than 80% of men and women in the 55- to 64-year age group; however, symptoms occur in only 15–20%.

  B. **OA,** which often begins in midlife, becomes much more common with increasing age. RA generally begins earlier in life, with onset characteristically between 20 and 60 years and affecting women two to three times more frequently than men.

  C. At least 1 in 20 ambulatory visits to physicians are for some form of arthritis.

III. **Pathophysiology**

  A. **OA,** which is not entirely synonymous with degenerative joint disease, is more than a "wear and tear" phenomenon. OA involves all the tissues that form the synovial joint. Probably the earliest change is in the articular cartilage, where the surface becomes irregular, roughened, and fissured, and fragments break off into the joint space. Tissue responses only partially repair this. Simultaneously, there is degeneration of the subchondral bone, with cyst-like cavities and formation of new layers of bone of increased density. It is not clear whether the cartilage or the bone changes come first. Ultimately, breakdown in the bone architecture, with microfractures, combines with the loss of articular cartilage to cause actual shortening if a limb is involved, with deformity, instability, and pain.

  Osteophytes start to form peripherally in the joints on cartilaginous or bony prominences. These can be palpable and tender and can restrict movement and in certain sites (eg, the vertebral column) can cause symptoms from nerve root pressure. The end results are the classic changes seen on x-ray: loss of joint space, changes in the adjacent bone, and osteophytes.

   1. Secondary changes of OA include inflammatory reactions in response to the articular cartilage fragments in the joint and changes in the supportive ligaments, with contracture. Joint painfulness leads to local muscular atrophy, which reduces the joint support, thus further reducing joint stability.

   2. Menisci are cartilaginous projections from the margin of the joints, interposed between the bone ends; they occur, for example, in the knee joints. Fragmentation of degenerated menisci, with symptoms such as "locking" or abrupt inflammatory reactions, can occur.

   3. The sites of OA are many, but the most frequently involved joints are the hips, knees, and lumbar and cervical spine. In the hand, the distal and proximal interphalangeal joints, particularly the first carpometacarpal joint, are most commonly involved; in the foot, the first metatarsophalangeal joint is the most common site of OA.

  B. **RA,** in common with the many other inflammatory arthritides, has a very different pathophysiology from that of OA. It primarily involves an inflammatory reaction in the joints. This inflammation can be so persistent that eventually erosion of the cartilage and contraction of the ligaments occur, with calcification, local muscle wasting, and degenerative changes in the joints. The early joint findings are inflammatory. Initially, the pattern of joint involvement is variable; RA is ultimately and characteristically a symmetric polyarthritis.

  C. **Gout** produces a more dramatic inflammatory arthritis than RA, with episodes of acute joint pain due to the deposition of urate crystals, which are secondary to disordered purine metabolism. Persistent elevation of the uric acid level can lead to more chronic deposition of the crystals in the joints and in other tissues, particularly the kidneys. Persistent hyperuricemia thus leads to renal failure.

D. Pseudogout, a more rare condition than gout but more common in the elderly, produces an inflammatory arthritis similar to gout but with a different chemistry—the crystals are calcium pyrophosphate.

E. Other inflammatory arthritides include those associated with psoriasis and with the spectrum of autoimmune diseases, such as SLE, in which autoantibodies induce inflammatory reactions. Characteristically, inflammation is present in multiple sites, with the joints being but one of many systems involved.

IV. Diagnosis
A. Symptoms and signs

1. In **OA,** the findings from the history and physical examination are key to the diagnosis and guide the intensity and nature of therapy.

    a. OA characteristically produces pain and stiffness in the joints, with the stiffness worsened by immobilization and resolving quickly with movement (generally in less than 30 minutes after arising in the morning). The pain is typically aggravated by the weather and by increased activities. If activity-associated pain is present, it usually starts quickly when the joint is used, but may last for hours after the activity has stopped. Often the history is of some minor injury leading to exacerbation of symptoms. Eventually, the pain becomes constant and wakes the patient from sleep.

    b. On examination of a normally mobile joint, crepitus may be noted when the joint is passively moved, and there may be localized tenderness. The range of movement of an osteoarthritic joint is limited. In testing the range of motion, the patient should move the joint actively first, because passive joint movement can be painful. In weight-bearing joints, it is important to assess joint stability and the status of the supporting musculature, which has therapeutic significance.

    c. In the hip, manifestations include changed gait, with a characteristically flexed, externally rotated hip, with the gait "sparing" the painful side. There may well be limb shortening due to subluxation of the head of the femur. Note that the pain from OA of the hip is often referred, with pain being felt in the groin, the buttocks, or even the knee, thus distracting the clinician from the true source of the pain. The first sign of OA in the hip is loss of rotation (since the hip is a ball-and-socket joint); this loss should be tested for in all older patients. Ultimately, there is limitation of all movement of the joint.

    d. In the knees, in which the normal movement is in one plane only, crepitus may be marked, with limitation of flexion and extension. Osteophytes are sometimes actually palpable in the knee, and commonly there are effusions. Limb circumference is a useful measure to assess muscular atrophy.

    e. When OA is in the cervical spine, movement of the neck can lead to compromised flow through the vertebral arteries (probably only if there is pathologic change in them), causing symptoms such as visual impairment and dizziness or vertigo (the **vertebrobasilar syndrome).** Osteophytes in the spinal vertebrae can produce nerve root pressure, with radicular symptoms.

    f. In the hands, **Heberden's nodes** are the characteristic finding; these are firm and tender nodes on the dorsal aspect of the distal interphalangeal joints. **Bouchard's nodes** may also be seen; they occur over the proximal interphalangeal joints.

2. In **RA,** joint pain and tenderness are more marked, and characteristically the stiffness after being immobilized lasts much longer—generally more than 30 minutes. When RA is particularly active, the joints are hot, tender, and swollen, and any movement is clearly painful. Subcutaneous nodules and other more general manifestations of RA may be present.

    The severity of RA ranges from transient inflammatory joint disease to prolonged progressive crippling disease, ultimately with marked and generalized muscle wasting and weakness and the characteristic hand deformities, with ulnar deviation and wasting of the intrinsic muscles of the hand. At this late stage, RA may "burn out," leaving the patient with problems mostly associated with the residual degenerative changes from the prior inflammatory phase, the disability generally being worsened by the associated muscle wasting.

3. **Gout** is characteristically an acute monoarthritis; during acute exacerbations, the pain is intense. Gout of new onset is common in the elderly. Polyarthritic and more chronic arthritic changes can also occur; such patterns are more common in the elderly. About 50% of patients with an acute attack are taking a diuretic. Tophi (subcutaneous deposits of urate) can occur.

4. **Pseudogout** also produces acute monoarthritis, mostly in the knee, but also in the wrist, shoulder, and ankle. Ten percent of patients have differing patterns, sometimes involving several joints over weeks or months. There are also associated chronic arthritic changes.

5. **Other arthritides,** associated with systemic disorders, are generally polyarticular and inflammatory in nature.

B. **Investigations**

1. **Blood tests** are required in the initial diagnostic phase, and during acute exacerbations; results must be cautiously interpreted in terms of diagnosis, since false positives frequently occur.

   a. Particularly in RA, **tests** such as rheumatoid factor, antinuclear antigen (ANA), erythrocyte sedimentation rate (ESR), and other acute-phase reactants may be positive or elevated. Although changes in these results in the individual patient parallel the clinical status and therefore can be useful in management (particularly in attempting to judge the subjectivity of the patient's symptoms), caution must be observed. For example, less than one-third of patients with a positive rheumatoid factor actually have RA, and rheumatoid factor is increasingly positive in old age, regardless of the presence of pathology. In RA, it is important to look for associated anemia.

   b. In a patient with OA, there are no characteristic laboratory changes. However, in the more inflammatory polyarthritic type of OA, which characteristically starts in midlife in women and also occurs during inflammatory episodes associated with fragmentation of menisci or cartilages, hotness, tenderness, and swelling may be found, as well as a raised white blood cell count and ESR.

   c. In gout, the uric acid is generally elevated, although it is normal in about 10% of people with acute attacks.

   d. The antinuclear antibody test can be useful if autoimmune disorders such as SLE are suspected, since it is positive in over 95% of patients with SLE. Hematuria and proteinuria, as well as anemia, leukopenia, and thrombocytopenia, are commonly found. High levels of anti–double-stranded DNA and low C3 are found in severe disease; the ESR is a poor guide to severity.

   e. Because of the potential side effects of treatments for arthritis, ongoing monitoring of the CBC and other laboratory parameters will often be required. It is especially important to monitor patients receiving nonsteroidal anti-inflammatory drugs (NSAIDs) because these drugs tend to cause gastrointestinal bleeding, especially in the elderly.

2. **X-rays**

   a. OA changes are frequently seen on x-ray in the absence of significant symptoms. X-rays can be useful to confirm or assess narrowing of the joint space and to see changes in the subchondral bone and osteophytes; they also give information about joint position. For weight-bearing joints, it is recommended that the x-rays be taken with the patient standing in order to assess the joint space during use.

   b. In RA, x-rays can show characteristic changes with blurring of the joint margins and soft tissue swelling; however, they generally add little to the clinical assessment.

3. **Magnetic resonance imaging (MRI)** is increasingly used, but has little place in primary care practice. It provides good visualization of soft tissues and subchondral bone changes, as well as of ligament and meniscal damage.

4. When joint effusion is present, **joint aspiration** is usually desirable in order to obtain a sample of fluid. Doing a joint aspiration will prevent a physician from being occasionally misled by the patient with a septic joint. Suspecting a septic joint is clinically easy in an ill, febrile patient with marked tenderness and swelling, so the clinical diagnosis is strongly suspected. However, patients

with septic arthritis may have no systemic symptoms and merely a moderately inflamed, tender, and swollen joint with effusion.

Definitive diagnosis of gout is established by tapping the synovial fluid and demonstrating the urates, which are present in most patients with gout. If this procedure is carried out, it will distinguish gout from pseudogout, in which different crystals (pyrophosphate) are present.

5. **Arthroscopy** also has a place in the diagnosis of arthritis, particularly in a joint that is "locking." Through the arthroscope, fragments of tissue can be removed, and the fibrillar changes in the cartilages, which can contribute to early symptoms, can be planed off. The primary care physician should establish professional rapport with an orthopedic surgeon to ensure appropriate use of this invasive but useful procedure. The arthroscopic procedure itself is temporarily disabling and should not be undertaken lightly.

V. **Treatment.** Physical therapy, medication, and surgery all play a role in the management of the patient with arthritis.

A. **Physical therapy.** Common sense dictates that the acutely tender, swollen painful joint must be rested, treated initially with cooling and ice packs, and then more chronically with heat, to disperse the injured tissue and cells. Even in OA, such techniques are occasionally indicated for inflammatory episodes or following trauma to an arthritic joint. However, in general, resting an osteoarthritic joint is contraindicated in the absence of acute symptoms. Indeed, steps must be taken to maintain mobility in a person who has been immobilized for other reasons and is known to have OA.

1. It is crucial to increase the muscular support around the joints where possible. The knees can be supported by increasing bilaterally the strength and capability of the muscular and ligamental support. Exercise can increase strength and range of movement both in OA and in inflammatory joint conditions. It is best to exercise when the joint is least stiff, for example, after a warm shower. The patient or therapist must note whether exercise produces pain. For example, if the pain is persistent for more than 2 hours after exercise or if there is pain or swelling the next day, then the intensity of exercise should be reduced and wise judgment used. Damage by overuse of a currently inflamed joint must obviously be avoided.

2. In inflammatory arthritis such as RA, especially when the inflammation is marked, immobilization in a splint may be necessary to allow the inflammation to settle and to avoid damage to the joint during the episode. If there is related muscle spasm or nerve root pain from cervical OA, a collar or, in extreme cases, traction may be helpful.

3. When the feet are affected, attention to the shoes and to podiatric health is vital. Orthotic devices can be of considerable help in correcting chronic foot deformities, which predispose to other musculoskeletal pain, not only in the feet themselves, but also in the knee, hip, or lumbar spine. Remember that many older women have used high heels and that moving rapidly to "flatties" (including sneakers) may produce Achilles' tendinitis and other problems.

4. In all forms of arthritis of the hand, it is important to pay attention to the person's routine tasks. Devices can assist in opening containers that require torsion strength and grip, functions that can chronically exacerbate and acutely precipitate arthralgia.

5. Other methods of reducing joint stress and improving functionality, such as a raised toilet seat, grab-bars, and tub seats or shower seats, can also reduce accidents.

6. Persistent pain, particularly nerve root pain, may be relieved from other pain-relieving methods such as transcutaneous electrical nerve stimulation (TENS), ultrasonography, and other physical therapy techniques.

7. In the obese, weight must be reduced, if possible, where weight-bearing joints are involved.

8. Exercise of weight-bearing joints must be of low impact, with avoidance of torsion, prolonged standing, and kneeling. Impact on the knees can be spared by shoes and surfaces that cushion the limb while walking; an indoor skiing machine can be very helpful in OA of the knees.

9. General care of the patient, noting the functional impact of the arthritis, is vital. Counseling about sexuality including sexual position; about posture, toileting,

and especially exercise and activity habits; and about attention to chair heights and positions in the home, at work, and in the car are all vital elements in reducing the symptoms and impact of the disease itself.

B. Medication

1. Many patients with OA are reluctant to initiate medication, because they fear that dosages will have to be increased to "merely" control pain. It is necessary to emphasize to the patient, and to the caregiver if appropriate, that the objective of pain relief is to allow exercise and the maintenance of function and is not merely to create comfort. In addition, NSAIDs are therapeutic in potentially reducing damaging inflammatory processes in the joints when these are part of the pathology.

2. In OA, analgesics such as acetaminophen, which are not anti-inflammatory in nature, can be very useful. Acetaminophen, taken on a regular basis, is a good pain reliever for much osteoarthritic pain, is inexpensive, and is safe for almost any patient. The starting dosage is 650 mg every 4–6 hours, increasing to 1 g four times a day (some patients can tolerate more). Acetaminophen can have an adjunctive effect when taken with NSAIDs and can also be very useful with rest pain or pain at night. For continual pain, the patient should be encouraged to take analgesics regularly, so that the pain is prevented. In addition, other palliative methods, including surgical treatment, may be helpful.

   If acetaminophen is insufficient, more potent analgesics such as codeine and other narcotics may be necessary, but should be used with caution, especially in the elderly because of the tendency of these agents to cause both constipation and impaired cognition. (Start low: eg, acetaminophen with codeine 15 mg, such as Tylenol #2). Before one escalates a patient's regimen to such drugs, adjunctive treatment with antidepressants, even if the patient does not appear depressed, may be helpful (see section V,B,5).

3. NSAIDs, which include aspirin and other salicylate preparations, over-the-counter ibuprofen, and prescription NSAIDs like naproxen and piroxicam, are widely used to relieve the pain and stiffness in OA, RA, and other arthritides and thus to allow exercise (Table 71–1). Since inflammation is often present, even in patients with OA, it is logical to use these medications. Individual patients may respond to one type of NSAID and not to another, and side effects can cause problems. For example, indomethacin is not recommended because of its gastric side effects and its central nervous system effects on brain function in the elderly; also, it has been shown to accelerate degeneration in human hip joints. Naproxen is associated with diminishing sexual (orgasmic) response. In fact, since the introduction of the COX-II antagonists, celecoxib and others, "fast-tracked" by the Food and Drug Administration because of the widespread interest in having available NSAIDs active only in inflamed tissue, any patient who is at increased risk for peptic ulceration, and the elderly in particular, should be considered for these agents rather than the traditional NSAIDs. Indeed, any patient receiving long-term treatment

TABLE 71–1. SELECTED ANTI-INFLAMMATORY ANALGESICS[1]

Generic Name	Relative Cost Index[2]	Usual Effective Dose (mg)
Aspirin[3]	1	650–1000 q4–6 h
Ibuprofen[3]	1	400–800 tid
Piroxicam	1	20 once daily
Salsalate[4]	1	1500 bid
Naproxen	2	250–500 bid
Sulindac	2	150 bid
Nabumetone[5]	4	1000 once daily
Celecoxib	3	100–200 daily

[1] The cost index of acetaminophen is 1 in its usual dose of 650–1000 mg every 4–6 hours; it is omitted because it is not an anti-inflammatory analgesic. Misoprostol, the gastric ulcer protective agent, has a cost index of 3 in the usual doses.

[2] Cost index: 1 = among the lowest-cost (generic) drugs; 5 = the most expensive.

[3] Available over-the-counter without prescription.

[4] The dose should be reduced in the elderly.

[5] Not available generically.

should also be considered for these drugs, because of the reduced likelihood of chronic renal changes. The initial dose of celecoxib in OA is 100 mg daily. Traditional NSAIDs affect the chemistry in many organs, particularly the stomach and kidneys, as well as the liver and bone marrow. Except for salsalate and the COX-II antagonists, all NSAIDs prolong the bleeding time because they impair platelet aggregation (which may be useful in patients with cerebrovascular disease). Thus, the uncontrolled availability of some over-the-counter medications, although good in some ways, should be accompanied by careful monitoring by the primary physician.

In highly ulcer-prone patients who need the benefit of NSAIDs, concurrent use of misoprostol (Cytotec) gives some protection; the usual dose is 200 μg four times daily with food, but 100 μg is almost as effective and is associated with less diarrhea.

4. Another medication treatment sometimes used for arthritis is corticosteroid by intrajoint injection; the effect lasts only a few weeks. Various corticosteroid preparations are available and can be combined with local anesthetics for relief of acute pain. This technique requires that the primary physician be specially trained. The medications and doses are beyond the scope of this text (see Pfenninger, 1994).

5. Antidepressants have an important role in the management of chronic arthritis. Patients with chronic pain are at increased risk of developing a true major depression and must be identified and treated accordingly (see Chapter 96). Even nondepressed persons with chronic pain can benefit from the analgesic effects of adjunctive antidepressant medications. In younger patients, and in older patients who can tolerate the anticholinergic side effects, inexpensive generic medications in relatively low doses, such as imipramine, 25 mg at bedtime, increasing as tolerated to 50 mg or even 100 mg or more in younger patients, can be very effective. The newer antidepressants, such as the selective serotonin reuptake inhibitors ([SSRIs] eg, paroxetine and sertraline), with their considerably better side-effect profile, can also be used. An adequate trial of antidepressants as adjunctive analgesics is not complete until the agents have been titrated to normal antidepressant doses and sustained for at least 8 weeks. Most clinicians feel that the adjunctive effect can be achieved at doses below that which would normally be required for a major depressive episode.

6. In RA, NSAIDs are used first, with aspirin as the mainstay for those who can tolerate it. High doses of aspirin can be used in otherwise healthy younger patients. In older patients, ototoxicity limits the upper dose, and the dose frequency (generally every 4–6 hours) is problematic in chronic use and does not last through the night. As noted earlier, the COX-II antagonists represent an advance in patient safety: the recommended initial dose in RA is double that recommended for OA (ie, celecoxib 200 mg a day either as a single or a divided dose).

Corticosteroids (eg, prednisone) have their place in RA and in the other autoimmune arthritides, both locally and systemically. Depending on the severity and the response, a common starting dose is 60–80 mg/day, tapering rapidly, if possible, to a lower maintenance dose and discontinuing as soon as practicable. The long-term side effects of corticosteroids (osteoporosis as well as gastrointestinal bleeding) limit their use to those whose symptoms justify it.

When the latter measures are failing or patients have severely progressive disease, several medications have the potential to induce remissions and change the course of the disease itself. Antimalarial drugs and gold are both first choices for attempting disease remission, although methotrexate is often used first in severe situations. Sulfasalazine and penicillamine also have the power to induce remission. All these agents require intensive monitoring and a physician experienced in their use and, in general, rheumatological referral is appropriate. Table 71–2 summarizes initial doses of four of these agents.

7. In acute gout, the treatment of choice is an NSAID, given at the high end of the normal dosage range for a few days, then tapering off over the next 5 days or so. Between acute episodes, some physicians recommend keeping the attacks at bay with maintenance colchicine (which can also be used to abort

TABLE 71-2. REMISSION-INDUCING MEDICATIONS IN RHEUMATOID ARTHRITIS

Generic Name	Relative Cost Index[1]	Initial Dose (mg)
Azathioprine	3	50–100 once daily, titrating upward after the initial 6–8 weeks
Hydroxychloroquine	3	400–600 once daily, reducing by 50% when remission obtained
Methotrexate	3	5–15 once weekly, with intensive monitoring
Auranofin	4	6 once daily, increasing after 6 months if remission not obtained

[1] For cost index, see Table 71–1.

acute attacks) or indomethacin. However, most recommend reducing the hyperuricemia by the long-term use of allopurinol or probenecid, and generally continuing indefinitely. The goal is to keep the uric acid level within the normal range both to reduce the chance of acute attack and to reduce the chronic deposition of uric acid in joints and other organs. Allopurinol blocks the formation of uric acid, whereas probenecid is a uricosuric agent; therefore, probenecid can be used only in patients with adequate renal function and who are underexcretors of uric acid in a 24-hour period (<500 mg of uric acid in 24 hours) (Table 71–3). Both allopurinol and probenecid should be avoided if the patient is in, or still recovering from, an acute attack of gout, since these agents can prolong an acute attack.

8. In pseudogout, NSAIDs and sometimes intra-articular corticosteroid injections are used; prophylaxis in those with frequent attacks can be achieved with oral colchicine, approximately 0.6 mg twice daily.

9. In the inflammatory arthritides associated with autoimmune disorders, salicylates and NSAIDs, corticosteroids, and chloroquine are all mainstays of treatment.

C. **Surgical management**

1. In general, surgical management of OA should be initiated before too much contraction, muscular atrophy, deformity, and joint instability occur, and while the older, frailer patient is still capable of cooperating with rehabilitation efforts. If any of these physical reactions are present, it is necessary either to prepare for surgery with formal physical therapy or to consider whether surgery is in the patient's best interest. Especially in older women, it is essential to assess bone density and do what one can to optimize bone density medically (estrogen, calcitonin, and alendronate, etc).

2. Knee or hip joint replacement is now well established, in fact nearly "routine" for orthopedic surgeons. It is inappropriate now to wait months and years until the patient virtually "earns" a replacement. By that time, deconditioning of the patient may have taken place, and it is likely that muscular support will have diminished. Relatively early surgery, while the patient is as fit as possible, should now be the aim.

3. As the joint space in weight-bearing joints is diminished and bone grates against bone, medical treatment becomes hopeless in relieving pain, and palliative surgery has an important place. A number of techniques, which are basically osteotomies, can immobilize the joint. This type of procedure can be extremely useful in an older patient with a persistently painful joint, especially one who can tolerate the limping or stiffness that the procedure often produces, and in a patient who could not rehabilitate from full joint replacement.

TABLE 71-3. AGENTS FOR TREATMENT OF HYPERURICEMIA

Generic Name	Relative Cost Index[1]	Initial Dose
Allopurinol	1	200 mg/day in mild disease; up to 800 mg/day in severe disease
Probenecid	2	0.5 g qid, reducing the dose in the elderly
Colchicine[2]	1	0.6 mg/h for 4–8 doses during acute attack; 0.6 mg twice daily after acute attack for several weeks

[1] See Table 71–1 for cost index.
[2] Not usually used for long-term prophylaxis.

   4. Lesser surgical procedures through the arthroscope have been described above, especially in the knee when cartilaginous changes and fragmentation are producing symptoms.

   5. Surgery is not indicated for the inflammatory arthritides; however, later in the burned-out phase of chronic degeneration, certain joint-stabilizing procedures are often justified in persistently painful or weak joints.

VI. Clinical management. It is very important to go beyond medications and formal physical therapy in educating the patient (and the caregiver if relevant) in the many techniques that can reduce symptoms by reducing the stress on diseased joints. These techniques thus reduce the impact of the arthritis on the patient's life.

   A. Patients and families must be educated about the pathology of the type of arthritis and should be able to identify significant symptoms and recognize inflammatory phases and other symptoms that may necessitate modifications in management. Patients and families should be directed toward such organizations as the Arthritis Foundation, which has local chapters and extensive educational and support activities.

   B. Since even the most acute of arthritides have the potential for chronic symptomatology, scheduled rather than "as needed" follow-up visits are desirable. In older patients, arthritis and its many consequences (which can be devastating to the person's overall health and function) are often tolerated as "normal" accompaniments of aging.

   C. Depression often accompanies chronic joint pain, and then interferes with motivation and compliance, as well as increasing the patient's awareness of the pain itself. Good clinical management thus involves seeing patients and their families in the entire context of their lives, functionality, and the rest of their health, since movement and everyday activities are inevitably affected by these illnesses.

VII. Prognosis. Even with an accurate diagnosis, a prognosis for the arthritides cannot be made with confidence.

   A. In OA, worsening of symptoms over time can be anticipated, although improving muscular support and general fitness and continual attention to mobility and range of motion can keep symptoms at bay for years. Major interventions in OA, such as joint replacement (particularly the knee or hip), can be seemingly "curative" of that particular joint, provided that the patient can fully collaborate in the necessary rehabilitative process.

   B. In RA, the spectrum of disease is very wide: RA ranges from a relatively acute inflammatory arthritis which settles and never returns, to a severe, progressive, crippling disorder, in which potentially hazardous remission-inducing medications must be considered. RA can be a slight or a crippling disease.

   C. The prognosis in gout and pseudogout can certainly be improved by maintenance treatment, with prevention of acute attacks and of the chronic effects on the renal tract and other organs.

   D. The prognosis in the other joint diseases varies widely and depends on the prognosis of the underlying or associated disease process.

REFERENCES

Brandt KD: Osteoarthritis. In: Fauci AS, et al, eds. *Harrison's Principles of Internal Medicine,* 14th ed. McGraw-Hill, 1998; 1935.

Buckwalter JA, Martin J: Degenerative joint disease. Ciba Found Symp 1995;**47**(2):1.

Calkins E, Reinhard JD, Vladutiu AO: Rheumatoid arthritis and auto-immune rheumatic diseases in the older patient. In: Hazzard WR, et al, eds. *Principles of Geriatric Medicine and Gerontology,* 3rd ed. Health Professions Division, McGraw-Hill, 1994; 965.

Fife RS: Osteoarthritis. In: Hazzard WR, et al, eds. *Principles of Geriatric Medicine and Gerontology,* 3rd ed. Health Professions Division, McGraw-Hill, 1994; 981.

Flynn JA, Wigley FM: Musculoskeletal and rheumatic disease common to the elderly. In: Reichel W, ed. *Care of the Elderly: Clinical Aspects of Aging,* 4th ed. Williams & Wilkins, 1995; 308.

Lipsky PE: Rheumatoid arthritis. In: Fauci AS, et al, eds. *Harrison's Principles of Internal Medicine,* 14th ed. McGraw-Hill, 1998; 1880.

Murphy JB: Dysmobility and immobility. In: Ham RJ, Sloane PD, eds. *Primary Care Geriatrics: A Case-Based Approach,* 3rd ed. Mosby–Year Book, 1996; 313.

Pfenninger JL: Joint and soft tissue aspiration and injection. In: Pfenninger JL, Fowler GC, eds. *Procedures for Primary Care Physicians.* Mosby–Year Book, 1994; 1036.

72 Asthma

Paul W. Wright, MD

I. **Definition.** Asthma is a disease of the airways; manifested by recurrent or persistent inflammatory and obstructive processes, or both, secondary to multifactorial stimuli, and may eventuate in irreversible loss of lung function and major disability. The terms describing the severity of asthma are mild intermittent, mild persistent, moderate persistent, and severe persistent.

II. **Epidemiology**

    A. **Onset** is before age 5 in 75–90% of cases, with a peak prevalence between 10 and 12 years of age.

    B. **Risk factors** include a family history of asthma or atopy, parental smoking, ambient air pollution, and viral respiratory infections, especially bronchiolitis from respiratory syncytial virus. Males and blacks are at greater risk.

    C. The **prevalence** of asthma has increased during the last two decades, and the condition currently affects 14 to 15 million persons including 4.8 million children in the United States. Five percent to 10% of all children experience the disease during childhood. Asthma is second only to acute respiratory infection as a cause of pediatric hospital admissions and illness-related school absenteeism.

III. **Pathophysiology**

    A. **Expiratory airflow obstruction** is initiated by bronchial wall inflammation, resulting in bronchospasm, bronchial gland mucus exudation, airway edema, and airway remodeling.

    B. **Resultant pathophysiologic changes** include increased airway resistance and hyperinflation.

        1. **Increased airway resistance** results in increased work of breathing and dyspnea.

        2. **Hyperinflation** with ventilation or perfusion abnormalities gives rise to hypoxia, even in mild cases, and to profound hypercapnia, respiratory acidosis, and death in severe cases.

    C. The **etiology** is not completely understood but encompasses the following.

        1. **Genetic factors** (as noted above) may contribute to the development of asthma. Concordance studies in twins and in first-degree relatives indicate a genetic predisposition.

        2. **Immunologic factors** play a major role in some patients with asthma and may be associated with elevated immunoglobulin E (IgE) levels and hyperreactivity to environmental stimuli. Atopy, the genetic predisposition for the development of elevated immunoglobulin E (IgE) levels in response to common environmental allergens, may be present in 30–50% of the general population and is very strongly related to the development of asthma.

        3. **Infectious factors** include viral infections such as respiratory syncytial virus, influenza and parainfluenza virus, and rhinovirus as well as bacterial infections, such as *Mycoplasma pneumoniae.*

        4. **Environmental factors** include cold air, hyperventilation, occupational chemicals and allergens, perfume, and inhaled antigens such as animal danders, house dust mite antigen, cockroach allergens, mold, pollen, and particulate matter in smoke.

        5. **Foods** and their associated chemicals, such as tartrazine, a yellow azo dye used in food coloring, can provoke asthma. Sulfites, found in such foods as fresh fruits and vegetables, dried fruits, shellfish, beer, and wine, can induce asthma in sulfite-sensitive persons.

        6. **Drugs** such as β blockers as well as aspirin and other nonsteroidal antiinflammatory drugs can trigger asthma.

        7. **Psychological or emotional factors** such as laughter or crying may precipitate asthma.

        8. **Endocrinologic factors** include hyperthyroidism and menses.

        9. **Exercise-induced asthma (EIA)** may affect as many as 19% of conditioned athletes; it is often unrecognized and, like other forms of asthma, includes both early and late phases.

        a. Early phase (EIA) bronchospasm occurs within 3–15 minutes after exercise.

        b. Late-phase (EIA) bronchospasm typically occurs 4–12 hours after exercise.

        c. A **postexercise refractory period** occurs in 50% of patients with EIA, during which time additional symptoms may not recur.

D. Inflammatory processes are now considered the key factors in the pathogenesis of asthma. These processes result from complex inflammatory responses involving both resident and migratory cells and their chemical mediators. While asthma may be classified into various types (eg, extrinsic, allergic, intrinsic, postinfective, exercise induced, or occupational), the pathogenetic mechanisms of each type of asthma are probably similar but not identical. While much of the pathophysiology of asthma has been well studied, it still remains complex and incompletely understood. The following processes are proposed as a model of the inflammatory process of asthma:

    1. Antigens, viruses, chemicals (oxidants), and other agents activate mast cells, eosinophils, epithelial cells, alveolar macrophages, T lymphocytes, and neutrophils.

    2. Mediators (both preformed and synthesized) are secreted from these cells that affect airway function through local or neural action. These mediators include histamine, tryptase, leukotrienes, bradykinin, prostaglandins, platelet-activating factor, and granulocyte-macrophage colony-stimulating factor.

    3. T lymphocytes subpopulations and mast cells secrete cytokines, including interleukin (IL)-3, IL-4, IL-5, which augment the process and establish chronicity. Fibroblasts, epithelial cells, and endothelial cells may add to the process by releasing chemokines and more cytokines.

    4. Acute inflammatory changes may result from the early infiltration of cells. The subacute phase of inflammation may result from the inflammatory activity of activated cells, both recruited and resident. Chronic inflammation may occur when cellular damage and repair persist and give rise to permanent airway damage. This results in deposition of interstitial collagens into the basement membrane, producing subbasement membrane fibrosis.

IV. Diagnosis. The patient's history is most important. Although patients with asthma typically present with recurrent episodes of wheezing, not all asthma is characterized by wheezing—and not all wheezing indicates asthma. Undiagnosed asthma is a common reason for referral to pediatric and adult pulmonary outpatient departments.

A. Symptoms and signs

    1. Symptoms usually include wheezing, coughing, dyspnea, chest tightness, and sometimes sputum production. Most patients report symptom-free intervals, but a rapidly changing and variable clinical picture is common.

        a. Coughing may be the initial symptom of asthma and is essentially the only symptom in cough-variant asthma.

        b. Recurrent pneumonia, usually misdiagnosed as atelectasis, is a common clue to undiagnosed asthma.

        c. A **patient history of atopy** or a family history of atopy or asthma supports the diagnosis.

    2. Signs may be absent in the asthmatic patient, especially early in the disease and during asymptomatic intervals. Forceful expiration occasionally uncovers otherwise unnoticed end-expiratory wheezing.

        a. Severe asthma may be characterized by both expiratory and inspiratory wheezing, prolongation of the expiratory phase, thoracic cage retractions, tachypnea, cyanosis, accessory muscle recruitment, and apprehension.

        b. Pulsus paradoxus (a pulse pressure that markedly decreases in size during inspiration), a silent chest, or chest wall crepitus caused by subcutaneous emphysema may signify severe airway obstruction requiring emergent care.

        c. Chronic changes may include such chest wall deformities as pectus carinatum or an increased anterior-posterior diameter. Clubbing is rarely associated with asthma and should suggest a diagnosis of cystic fibrosis or cancer.

B. Diagnostic tests

    1. A **peripheral blood smear** and a **sputum examination** showing eosinophilia may suggest allergic asthma.

2. **Allergy skin tests, allergen-specific IgE,** and the **radioallergosorbent test (RAST)** can be used to test specific allergens. These tests may identify specific allergens that can be avoided or treated with immunotherapy desensitization. Skin tests are the least costly of the three tests. RAST and IgE blood tests are usually reserved for patients who cannot undergo skin testing because of a history of severe reaction or other intolerance. Positive tests should be correlated with the patient's history of allergies. Total IgE levels are usually elevated in atopic asthma.

3. The **chest x-ray** is useful for selected patients in ruling out other diseases. It may show hyperinflation, atelectasis, pneumonia, or, rarely, pneumomediastinum. Criteria for ordering chest films include tachypnea (>60 breaths per minute), tachycardia (>160 beats per minute), localized rales, localized decreased breath sounds, or cyanosis. Lateral chest films are helpful in acute pediatric pulmonary disease and should be ordered when the posterior-anterior view requires clarification, such as when the physician suspects that a posterior-inferior lung infiltrate is concealed behind the cardiac silhouette.

4. **Pulmonary function tests (PFTs)**
   a. **Indications** for PFTs include confirmation of the diagnosis of asthma, objective measurements of the response to therapy, and measurement of pulmonary dysfunction.
   b. **Forced expiratory volume in 1 second (FEV_1)** is very useful in assessing acute asthma, but the **peak expiratory flow rate (PEFR)** parallels the FEV_1 and is usually easier to obtain. Devices that measure PEFR are inexpensive and can be prescribed to allow patients with asthma to monitor their progress at home. Patients with a PEFR below 70% of their baseline value should be carefully evaluated. An FEV_1 or PEFR below 40% after aggressive therapy indicates severe obstruction, and the patient should be hospitalized. The accuracy of peak flowmeters varies, however, and can deteriorate over time.
   c. The **peak flow-zone system** allows patients to monitor the PEFR and make clinical decisions about their asthma—under the physician's supervision.
      (1) The **green zone** (PEFR = 80–100% of the patient's best score) indicates that the patient can continue the usual course of medicine.
      (2) The **yellow zone** (PEFR = 50–80%) is a warning to the patient to take additional medicine or call the physician.
      (3) The **red zone** (PEFR <50%) indicates that the patient should both use the inhaler and call the physician immediately.

5. **Provocative testing** with either methacholine or histamine is indicated for the rare patient for whom a definitive diagnosis is sought when the clinical picture is unclear. These tests carry a minimal risk of producing life-threatening bronchospasm. They must be performed under experienced supervision with resuscitative support immediately available.

6. **Arterial blood gases** are indicated for patients who have poor respiratory status or a poor response to therapy. Impending respiratory failure should be suspected—even when the PCO_2 is normal or slightly elevated (>40 mm Hg) in the presence of hypoxia (PO_2 <70 mm Hg). Pulse oximetry monitoring is noninvasive and very useful in monitoring the oxygenation of asthmatic patients.

C. **Differential diagnosis**
   1. **Common diseases** to be excluded are bronchiolitis, cystic fibrosis, foreign bodies, chronic bronchitis, and congestive heart failure.
   2. **Less common diseases** to be considered are vocal cord dysfunction, bronchopulmonary dysplasia, allergic bronchopulmonary mycoses, and bronchiolitis obliterans.

V. **Treatment.** Goals include maintenance of normal activities (including exercise) and optimal pulmonary function values while minimizing symptoms, exacerbations, and adverse drug effects. Long-term therapy directed at suppressing inflammation early in the course of illness is now felt to be necessary to modify the disease process and prevent irreversible lung dysfunction.

A. **Environmental control** can provide significant relief by avoiding the triggers identified in the clinical history and known to produce deleterious effects.

1. **Inhaled allergens** can be totally avoided only rarely, but much of the exposure can be eliminated.
    a. **Tobacco smoke** should be banned from the home and automobile. The use of nonsmoking hotel rooms, rental cars, and restaurants is very beneficial.
    b. **House dust mites** are difficult to eradicate. Frequent household cleanings can help reduce their numbers.
        (1) **Rooms,** when practical, should be free of carpets, stuffed toys, and other dust-collecting items.
        (2) **Central air-conditioning systems** should have frequently cleaned mechanical or electrostatic air filters. Portable electrostatic air filters can be used in patients' bedrooms.
        (3) **Nonallergenic mattress covers** should be used.
    c. **Other irritants** to be avoided include pets, flowering plants, molds, perfumes, hair sprays, paints, and aerosolized chemicals.
2. **Emotional factors** may play a significant role in triggering asthma in some patients and must be minimized.
    a. **Parents** should avoid overcompensating behavior that can create opportunities for manipulation by the asthmatic child. They should also avoid the other extreme of ignoring the child's plight.
    b. The **home** should offer the child support, consistency, and loving parental guidance.
3. **Exercise** and exposure to cold air frequently aggravate asthma. Acute exacerbations resulting from exercise may be lessened by appropriate premedication and by restricting activities to participation in such sports as water sports, which typically cause less bronchial irritation than do other athletic activities.

B. **Drug therapy** involves two groups of drugs: long-term-control and quick-relief medications.
    1. **Long-term-control medications** are usually given daily over the long term to control persistent asthma. They include corticosteroids, cromolyn and nedocromil, long-acting bronchodilators, leukotriene modifiers, and theophylline.
        a. **Corticosteroids** are very effective anti-inflammatory drugs for treating acute and chronic asthma, but can cause many serious adverse effects. In children, suppression of linear growth and adverse effects on the hypothalamic–pituitary–adrenal axis are of major concern. In adults, bone demineralization, cataract formation, gastrointestinal hemorrhage, and psychiatric problems sometimes occur with systemic usage. Corticosteroids should be initiated early in the course of treatment and in adequate doses for patients with severe asthma. The mode of action of corticosteroids is unclear, but the current consensus suggests that they improve airflow by decreasing inflammatory activity in the arachidonic acid, leukotriene, prostaglandin, and inflammatory cell systems and by increasing smooth muscle responsiveness to β-agonists.
            (1) **Inhaled corticosteroids** are first-line drugs and are often prescribed with inhaled β-agonists. Inhaled corticosteroids available in metered-dose inhalers (MDIs) include budesonide (Pulmocort), fluticasone (Flovent), beclomethasone (Vanceril or Beclovent), triamcinolone (Azmacort), and flunisolide (AeroBid).
                (a) **Administration** is by MDI and dosages are listed in Table 72–1. These preparations are not available in nebulized solutions.
                (b) **Significant adverse effects** of inhaled corticosteroids are "typically" much less than that of systemic corticosteroids, but data concerning how many inhalations are necessary to produce systemic adverse effects are pending for the newer and more potent ones, budesonide and fluticasone. These two drugs are reported to be more topically potent and have less gastric absorption and less-active metabolites than the older drugs. Minor adverse effects include oropharyngeal candidiasis, cough, and, rarely, dysphonia, but they are seldom severe enough to warrant

TABLE 72–1. COMMONLY PRESCRIBED ASTHMA DRUGS

Drug	Mode of Administration	Adult Dosage	Relative Cost per Month[2]
Beta₂-agonists			
Albuterol	MDI 90 µg/puff	1–2 puffs q4–6 h prn	+
	Rotocaps 200 µg/cap	1 cap q4–6 h prn	++
Salmeterol	MDI 21 µg/puff	1–2 puffs bid	++
	Dry powder 50 µg/puff	1 puff bid	++
Mast cell stabilizers			
Cromolyn sodium	MDI or nebulizer 800 µg/puff	3–4 puffs tid to qid	++++++
Nedocromil soidum	MDI 1.75 mg/puff	2 puffs qid	+++
Inhaled corticosteroids			
Beclomethasone	MDI 42/84 µg/puff	6/12 to 10/20 puffs per day	++
Budesonide	MDI 200 µg/puff	1 puff bid to tid	+++
Flunisolide	MDI 250 µg/puff	4–8 puffs per day	++++
Fluticasone	MDI 44/110/220 µg/puff	2–6 puffs per day	+++
	Dry-powder inhaler 50/100/250 µg/puff	2–6 puffs per day	+++
Triamcinolone	MDI 100 µg/puff	4–20 puffs per day	++++
Methylxanthines			
Theophylline	Extended-release Tablets or capsules	300–600 mg/day	+
Leukotriene modifiers			
Montelukast	Tablets	5 mg–10 mg daily	+++++
Zafirlukast	Tablets	20 mg bid	+++
Zileuton	Tablets	600 mg qid	+++

[1] Cost per month per average dose: + less than or equal to $25; ++ less than or equal to $40; +++ less than or equal to $60; ++++ less than or equal to $80; +++++ less than or equal to $80; ++++++ >$100.
MDI, Metered-dose inhaler.

discontinuation. The use of spacer devices and oral rinses after inhalation can lessen these side effects. Budesonide and fluticasone are available also in powder MDI preparations. The overall effect of these new powder delivery systems is being studied.

    (2) Systemic steroids are indicated when other modes of therapy fail to control severe asthma.

        (a) Oral steroids—prednisone, methylprednisolone, and prednisolone—are given in doses of 1–2 mg/kg/day (usually 20–80 mg/day) and gradually reduced over 1–3 weeks, depending on disease severity.

        (b) Liquid preparations of prednisolone include Prelone (15 mg/5 mL) and Pediapred (5 mg/5 mL). Liquid preparations of prednisone include Liquid Pred Syrup (5 mg/5 mL) and Prednisone Intensol (5 mg/1 mL)

  b. Cromolyn sodium and nedrocromil

    (1) Cromolyn sodium, an anti-inflammatory medication used prophylactically to control chronic asthma and EIA, inhibits both early- and late-response allergic reactions. Although cromolyn's mechanism of action is not fully understood, it probably stabilizes mast cells, preventing their degranulation and release of inflammatory mediators.

        (a) Adverse effects are few, but cromolyn requires dedicated patient compliance, since an adequate therapeutic response may not occur until after 4–6 weeks of therapy. Children appear to respond to cromolyn better than adults do.

        (b) Preparations of cromolyn (Intal) include an MDI, an aerosolized solution that can be combined in an aerosol with a β_2 drug, and an inhaled powder capsule. The recommended dosage is two inhaled metered sprays (800 µg per spray) four times a day at regular intervals. It seems more effective in children with asthma.

(2) Nedocromil (Tilade) is an anti-inflammatory drug available as an MDI. Its action is similar to cromolyn in that it stabilizes mast and other inflammatory cells, but it provides significant clinical improvement within 2–4 days. Similar to cromolyn, its adverse side effect profile is very low. It is considered first-line therapy along with β_2-agonist agents in mild and moderate asthma in children 6 years of age and older. Up to 20% of patients experience an unpleasant taste with nedocromil.

c. Long-acting β_2-agonists

(1) Salmeterol (Seravent), available as an MDI and inhaled powder, is a longer-acting (every 12 hours) β-agonist indicated for maintenance therapy and contraindicated for acute treatment. It is approved for children 6 years and older. Salmeterol acts as a bronchodilator, relaxing smooth muscle by adenylate cyclase activation and increase in cyclic AMP production. Its onset of action is 15–30 minutes and duration of action is greater than 12 hours. It is especially useful for controlling nocturnal symptoms.

(2) Albuterol, sustained-release (Proventil Repetabs) is an oral sustained-release form of albuterol that tends to have more side effects than the inhaled long-acting β_2-agonists.

d. Theophylline is a methylxanthine bronchodilator that is usually well absorbed from the gastrointestinal tract. Theophyllines are considered second-line agents and are used as adjuncts with anti-inflammatory and other bronchodilator drugs.

(1) Dosage requirements of theophylline vary considerably with age and the individual patient. Blood levels should be monitored and maintained between 5 and 15 μg/mL. When possible, therapy should be initiated slowly to minimize side effects. Children tend to clear the drug significantly more rapidly than adults do.

(2) Adverse effects are similar to those of caffeine and include nervousness, anorexia, irritability, nausea, vomiting, enuresis, insomnia, poor school performance, and behavioral problems. Factors that may increase serum levels of theophylline and give rise to toxicity include impaired liver function, age over 55 years, chronic heart and lung disease, sustained high fever, viral illnesses, and drug interactions, including those with cimetidine, allopurinol, ciprofloxacin, erythromycin, rifampin, propranolol, oral contraceptives, phenytoin, clarithromycin, and lithium carbonate.

(3) Overdosage usually manifests as nausea and vomiting but also can cause arrhythmias, seizures, and, very rarely, death. Patients and their family members should be taught to recognize signs of theophylline toxicity.

(4) Oral preparations of theophylline include liquid, tablets, and capsules. Capsules (Theo-Dur Sprinkle, Slo-bid, Slo-Phyllin, and others) can be given to young children by sprinkling the medication on food to facilitate administration and accurate dosing.

e. Leukotriene modifiers indicated for the treatment of mild to moderate nonacute asthma by modifying the inflammatory effects of leukotrienes.

(1) Preparations include orally administered zafirlukast (Accolate) 20 mg twice daily for those over 12 years of age, zileuton (Zyflo) 600 mg four times daily for those over 12 years of age, and montelukast (Singulair) 5 mg for those over 6 years of age and 10 mg daily for those over 12 years of age. These drugs are less effective than inhaled corticosteroids, but easier to take.

(2) Adverse effects include drug–drug interactions, hepatic toxicity with zileuton, and rare Churg–Strauss vasculitis with zafirlukast.

f. Other drugs used to treat asthma.

(1) Antihistamines, which formerly were believed to have adverse effects on asthma, are now considered safe. These agents act as weak bronchodilators.

(2) Antiviral agents, such as ribavirin for respiratory syncytial virus, may be helpful.

    (3) Antibacterial drugs are useful for the treatment of patients with pneumonia, bacterial sinusitis, and other specific bacterial infections. Antibiotics are frequently misused in the treatment of patients with asthma, especially when atelectasis is confused with pneumonia.

    (4) Expectorants and **mucolytics** (eg, guaifenesin and iodides) have not been proven effective. Aerosolized acetylcysteine (Mucomyst) is contraindicated in asthma, since it may cause severe bronchospasm. Sedatives and anxiolytic agents are also contraindicated.

g. Immunotherapy, also called desensitization, allergy injection therapy, or allergen immunotherapy, remains controversial, inconvenient, and expensive but may benefit a few selected patients with allergic asthma. Immunotherapy also involves a small but significant risk of anaphylaxis and even death.

h. Complementary alternative medicine includes relaxation techniques, herbal medicines, vitamin supplements and diet, acupuncture, homeopathy, and chiropractic spinal manipulation. Although these alternative healing processes are not recommended as substitutes for conventional pharmacologic therapy, they are commonly used and growing in popularity.

    (1) Herbal remedies sometimes use the herb Ma huang (ephedra), which contains ephedrine, the drug formerly included in several asthma prescriptions. However, ephedrine is no longer recommended to treat asthma due to its adverse effects including nephrolithiasis, sudden death, high blood pressure, and hyperglycemia. Other herbs used to treat asthma are touted to boost the immune system and include echinacea, Asian mushrooms, and ginseng.

    (2) Acupuncture is very popular, especially in Europe, and has been investigated in a number of controlled studies. It has not been shown to be as effective as conventional therapy, but may be helpful, especially for quick relief of asthma. However, avoidable deaths have been reported in patients with asthma who relied only on acupuncture and refused conventional therapy. Furthermore, acupuncture carries some risk, including organ puncture or infection from contaminated needles.

    (3) Relaxation techniques are designed to relieve stress, which is believed to aggravate asthma. These include yoga and biofeedback training, especially emphasizing breathing techniques.

2. Quick-relief medications

a. Short-acting inhaled β_2-agonists are most frequently delivered as aerosols through MDIs and, less commonly, as solutions via compressed-air nebulizers (Pulmo-Aide, among others). The MDI delivery system should be enhanced by the use of reservoir spacer devices (eg, AeroChamber, Inhal-Aid, InspirEase, or Brethancer). Some spacers have masks that allow for infant and toddler use. Inhaled β_2-agonists are most commonly prescribed as needed, rather than with firm dosage times, because of concerns about tachyphylaxis and adverse side effects.

    (1) Preparations include albuterol (Ventolin, Proventil), bitolterol (Tornalate), pirbuterol (Maxair), and terbutaline (Brethine, Bricanyl).

        (a) Albuterol (Ventolin or Proventil) is available in syrup, tablets, MDI, nebulizer solutions, and powdered capsules for inhalation.

        (b) Terbutaline (Brethaire, Brethine, or Bricanyl) is available in tablets, MDI, nebulizer solution, and an aqueous solution for subcutaneous injection. It is classified as a Food and Drug Administration category B drug in pregnancy and is thus the β_2-agonist of choice for the pregnant patient.

    (2) Indications include the rapid relief of acute bronchospasm and prevention of exercise-induced bronchospasm. These drugs are generally recommended to be administered on a need basis rather than on a regularly scheduled daily basis. The inhaled route is preferred because of faster onset of action, fewer adverse effects, and greater effectiveness.

    (3) Adverse effects include tachycardia, nervousness, irritability, tremor, headache, hypokalemia, and hyperglycemia. The less selective β_2-

agonists (epinephrine, metaproternol, isoproterenol, isoetharine) are no longer recommended for therapy. Patients should be warned against overuse of these drugs (eg, >200 puffs of albuterol per month) and encouraged to use more of their anti-inflammatory medications.

    b. Ipratropium bromide (Atrovent), an anticholinergic quaternary derivative of atropine, is indicated for the relief of acute cholinergically mediated bronchospasm. This drug is frequently used with a β_2 -agonist but has a slightly slower onset of action. It is the treatment of choice for bronchospasm due to the effects of β-blocker therapy.

    c. Systemic corticosteroids (methylprednisolone, prednisolone, prednisone) are indicated in doses of 1–2 mg/kg for patients with acute exacerbations of moderate or severe asthma. They are usually given for 3–10 days and are continued until the patient's PEFR is 80% of his personal best value. Prolonged therapy, greater than 1–2 weeks, requires tapering of dosage to prevent pituitary-adrenal-corticol dysfunction, but tapering per se does not prevent relapse of symptoms of asthma.

VI. Management strategies

A. Education is a critical tool in the care of the patient with asthma. Family members, teachers, and athletic coaches must understand the disease process. Asthma support groups and camps for asthmatic children can be very helpful also.

    1. Patient compliance is much better when patients are given the opportunity to acquire an adequate understanding of both the disease process and the prescribed medications.

    2. Office counseling should be provided to patients and their families, especially to those patients with special educational or behavioral problems.

    3. Referral to an outside counselor may occasionally be necessary to provide parents with additional help in the management of the troubled asthmatic child.

B. Treatment guidelines

    1. Patients with **mild intermittent asthma** have acute episodes of illness separated by symptom-free intervals occurring no more than twice weekly. These patients have normal PEFR and no symptoms between exacerbations. They can usually be managed with inhaled β_2-agonists given on an as-needed (prn) basis.

    2. Patients with **mild persistent asthma** have symptoms greater than twice weekly but less than daily. Their exacerbations may affect their daily activities, but their PEFR is at least 80% of predicted. They are usually managed with one inhaled anti-inflammatory drug or oral leukotriene modifier and augmented with a inhaled β_2-agonist for quick relief.

    3. Patients with **moderate persistent asthma** have daily symptoms requiring daily use of inhaled short-acting β_2-agonists. They have exacerbations at least twice weekly, which affect their activities and may last for days. Their PEFR values may vary >30% of predicted. They are typically managed with medium-dosed inhaled corticosteroids or two daily long-term medications (eg, salmeterol plus low- to medium-dose inhaled corticosteroid) in addition to quick-acting relief, prn short-acting β_2-agonists.

    4. Patients with **severe persistent asthma** have continual symptoms, limited physical activity, frequent exacerbations, and PEFR varying >30%. They usually require high-dose inhaled corticosteroids, long-acting bronchodilators, and sometimes augmentation with oral corticosteroids in addition to quick relief with prn short-acting β_2-agonists.

    5. Nocturnal asthma is now easier to manage with the use of longer-acting agents such as inhaled salmeterol, sustained-release preparations of theophylline or albuterol tablets, or the leukotriene modifiers. Nocturnal asthma may be associated with gastrointestinal reflux disease, even with minimal symptoms of the latter. In patients with nocturnal asthma who respond poorly to therapy, diagnosis and therapy for gastrointestinal reflux should be considered.

VII. Natural history and prognosis

A. Total remission of symptoms occurs in as few as 16% of patients with asthma by late adolescence or early adulthood. Most patients retain airway hyperreactivity (as demonstrated by provocative testing).

B. Onset of disease is not a reliable factor in predicting either the length or the severity of symptoms.

C. **Initial severity** of the illness, especially the length of the episode and the need for hospitalization, is a more reliable factor than the time of onset in predicting whether the child's asthma will persist into adulthood.

D. **Persistence of reduced pulmonary function** and the presence of atopy (eczema, allergic rhinitis, and skin test reactivity to antigens) are associated with continued and more severe disease.

E. **Control** of the disease process through good pharmacotherapy is not a known predictor of future disease. The relationship of childhood asthma and adult emphysema is unclear.

F. **Mortality** of patients with asthma is relatively low but increased from 1982 to 1991 by 40%, from 13.4 to 18.8 per 1 million population. Mortality rates are higher in blacks, males, and patients with coexistent chronic obstructive pulmonary disease. Historical events of concern for potential fatal outcome include previous history of respiratory acidosis with or without intubation, history of episodes of cyanosis, frequent hospitalizations, multiple emergency room visits during a short period, episodes of loss of consciousness, minimal response to a major therapeutic regimen, and presence of severe anxiety and depression.

REFERENCES

Adkinson NF Jr, Eggleston PA, Eney D, et al: A controlled trial of immunotherapy for asthma in allergic children. N Engl J Med 1997;**336:**324.

Barnes PJ, Brunstein MM, Leff AR, et al: *Asthma.* Lippincott-Raven; 1997.

Gross KM, Ponte CD: New strategies in the medical management of asthma. Am Fam Physician 1998;**58:**89.

Kamada AK, Szefler SJ, Martin RJ, et al: Issues in the use of inhaled glucocorticoids: The Asthma Clinical Research Network. Am J Respir Crit Care Med 1996;**153**(6, pt 1):1739.

Montelukast for persistent asthma: Med Lett Drugs Ther 1998;**40:**71.

Nadel JA, Busse WW: Asthma. Am J Respir Crit Care Med 1998;**157:**S130.

National Asthma Education and Prevention Program: Expert Panel Report II (EPR-II): Guidelines for the diagnosis and management of asthma. National Heart, Lung, and Blood Institute. National Institutes of Health. NIH publication No. 97-4051, July 1997. http://www.nhlbi.nih.gov/nhlbi/lung/asthma/prof/asthgdln.htm Sly MR: New guidelines for diagnosis and management of asthma. Ann Allergy Asthma Immunol 1997;**78:**427.

---

73   Cancer Pain Management

David R. Grube, MD

I. **Definitions**

A. **Cancer and other terminal illnesses** are common problems that primary care providers encounter frequently. Although no clinician can perfectly predict the exact course of an illness, experience and knowledge can often approximately assess the dying patient's length of life. This information, though inexact, can be helpful not only for the patient but also for caregivers and family. When it is believed that the patient has less than 6 months of life remaining, the treatment plan often changes from "cure" to "care," and frank discussions of prognoses and end-of-life decisions assume paramount importance.

B. **Suffering** is a consequence of many disease states, not just terminal illness. It is not always possible to prevent pain completely; and pain itself is not the only form of suffering. However, pain and suffering can and must be recognized, continuously reassessed, and appropriately treated. It is medically unethical to undertreat the dying patient's symptoms, whether they are physical or spiritual. Comfort for and respect of the terminal patient's condition must always remain the primary care provider's first priority.

C. The physician is often able, in caring for patients, to direct the treatment plan, ordering appropriate tests and medications as the need arises. In caring for the terminally ill, it is important to remember that it is the patient who is experiencing the pain and that only the patient can know whether that pain is under control. Chronic terminal pain is often underestimated and hence undertreated. Control of pain is always best managed if patients know that they will be allowed to titrate analgesics or use "breakthrough" dosages whenever necessary.

D. In almost no other situation is the primary care provider better able to assist her or his patient than in the care of the dying patient. Because of the primary care provider's knowledge of the patient, the patient's family and resources, and the intimate interactions of the patient with his or her environment, the primary care provider is best able to provide that level of pain relief that each person needs. The primary care provider's recognition of the dying person's pain and suffering in the context of that person's life, and not just as symptoms of disease, not only allows but also obligates that provider to manage this important problem adequately.

II. Epidemiology. The problem of pain management in the care of the terminally ill is not limited to cancer patients. Any condition in which the patient's life expectancy is thought to be about 6 months or less should be considered terminal. Acquired immunodeficiency syndrome (AIDS), chronic obstructive pulmonary disease (COPD), congestive heart failure (CHF), stroke, and numerous other disease states may be included as terminal care diagnoses. Numerous studies have shown that pain in these patients is underdiagnosed and undertreated. There are treatment strategies for terminal pain management that have been recognized as highly effective, but patients continue to suffer unnecessarily.

III. Pathophysiology. Terminal pain may be either acute or chronic. It may be a consequence of the patient's condition or a side effect of treatment. Acute pain usually subsides when bodily injury heals; it is often associated with objective symptoms such as rapid heart rate, elevated blood pressure, sweating, and pallor. Chronic pain may be less readily observable; lack of objective signs, therefore, may result in inadequate assessment and treatment.

The International Association for the Study of Pain has defined pain as "an unpleasant sensory and emotional experience associated with actual or potential tissue damage or described in terms of such damage." Pain is the perception of noxious central nervous system stimulation (nociception) in the context of the patient's environment (eg, physical awareness, psychologic state). Understanding and appreciating the many factors that affect pain are necessary in appropriate pain management.

It is also important to understand the difference between pain and suffering. Suffering and pain are often intertwined, but suffering is the subjective experience of all the harmful factors that make a negative impact on pain. Analgesics may therefore control pain without affecting suffering. Because of this phenomenon, all pain management must take suffering into account; appropriate responses to suffering always enhance pain control.

IV. Diagnosis. The astute clinician, in recognizing the possibility that a patient's condition is terminal, will correctly diagnose the causes of the patient's pain. An adequate physical assessment, relevant laboratory tests, and appropriate radiologic examinations are important, but a complete patient history is most important in the evaluation of pain. Furthermore, continuous reassessment is the hallmark of good pain management.

A. Symptoms and signs of pain in the chronic or terminal patient may differ from those of patients with acute pain. The usual signs of sympathetic nervous system arousal may not be present; the clinician must ask the patient about the pain and listen to the patient's response. Five specific characteristics of the pain are very important to note.

1. The **intensity of the pain** determines (1) the urgency with which appropriate treatment should be given, (2) the choice of analgesic, (3) the route of administration, and (4) the rate of titration. Intensity may also help to characterize the mechanism of the pain.

2. Distribution of the pain symptoms can be helpful in diagnosis and subsequent appropriate care. Focal pain may be associated with a single lesion, systemic pain may be related to systemic metastases or drug reactions, and referred pain may signify tissue destruction at a distant site. The physician should be familiar with the referral patterns of pain to plan diagnostic and therapeutic treatment regimens.

3. Pain quality is usually related to pathophysiology. When pain is described as "sharp," "aching," or "throbbing," it is often related to somatic nociceptors. Pain described as "crampy" or "gnawing" may be visceral and related to mesentery or hollow organs. Descriptions of "burning" or "tingling" sensations may mean that the pain is neuropathic.

4. **Temporal relationships in pain descriptions** can be helpful in diagnosis and treatment. Pain associated with eating or elimination can direct the physician to appropriate evaluation of the gastrointestinal or urologic organ systems. Musculoskeletal damage may be associated with painful movement, but also with resting pain.

5. **Rating pain** (on a scale of 1–10) and subsequently documenting that number can assist clinicians and caregivers in assessing, reassessing, and treating pain. The clinician should consider recording this rating number as carefully as the other vital signs.

B. The **physical examination** of a terminal patient in pain may have originally been completed months before the person requires final care. It is important to update that examination when needed. Just as ongoing reassessment of physical complaints allows caregivers to adjust treatment strategies, so, too, does repeated physical examination contribute to completeness of care. Examinations should include any problem described by the patient, not the terminal condition alone.

C. **Laboratory and radiologic examinations** should be confined to those concerns that might alter the treatment plan. If the result of the examination will contribute to a therapeutic choice that decreases the patient's pain or suffering, the test should be considered. It is most important to remember that a given test may be uncomfortable or expensive, and that in this patient population, care rather than cure is the goal. If, in the care provider's estimation, pain or suffering can be decreased or eliminated by ordering any examination, that test is appropriate.

V. **Treatment.** The goals of treatment in terminally ill patients are primarily the provision of comfort and respect for the patient's wishes. Drug therapy is the basis of pain management in the terminally ill. The World Health Organization (WHO) has developed a standard WHO Analgesic Ladder to standardize appropriate care (Figure 73–1). The ladder is based on increasing potency of medication, titration, and continuous reassessment. Mild pain can be managed with nonopioid medications; moderate pain should be treated with an opioid, a nonopioid, or a combination; severe pain should be managed with potent opioids with or without nonopioids. At each level, adjuvant therapies may be beneficial as well.

A. **Nonopioid analgesics** include acetaminophen, salicylates such as aspirin, and nonsteroidal anti-inflammatory medications. These agents can be helpful with acute and chronic pain, and they represent the first step on the WHO ladder. They are not habituating, are often readily available in over-the-counter preparations, and may have beneficial side effects such as antipyresis. Unlike the opioids, nonopioid agents have a *ceiling effect,* a dose above which there is no increased benefit. Even when pain increases in severity to the point of requiring the addition of opioids, this class of medications can be maintained.

1. **Nonsteroidal anti-inflammatory drugs (NSAIDs)** can be beneficial in pain management, but care must be taken to monitor side effects and to avoid using NSAIDs in patients with contraindications. These contraindications are renal dysfunction, intestinal ulcers, or bleeding disorders; and concomitant steroid therapy. NSAIDs may be more efficacious than aspirin, but are more

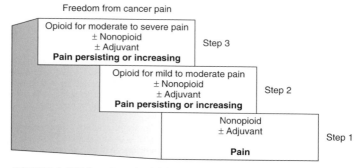

FIGURE 73–1. WHO three-step analgesic ladder. (World Health Organization, 1990.)

expensive and less readily available. A number of NSAIDs are now available without prescription. Side effects may include bleeding, gastrointestinal upset, renal dysfunction, and dermatologic problems. Nevertheless, NSAIDs should not be overlooked in the treatment of cancer patients because their anti-inflammatory properties may be very beneficial. Ibuprofen (600–800 mg/8 hr) or naproxen (500 mg/12 hr) are effective and available without prescription. Piroxicam (20 mg/day) is long-acting; and nabumetone (1000–1500 mg/day) may be helpful if the patient is prone to gastric upset. When using NSAIDs, the patient should be monitored for significant side effects (gastritis, rashes, pruritus); however, if the NSAID is effective in controlling the terminally ill patient's pain, this benefit should outweigh concern for nonsymptomatic risks (eg, elevated liver enzymes).

B. **Narcotic (opioid) analgesics** should be prescribed for patients for whom non-narcotic (opioid) medications have been unsuccessful in adequately managing pain. Pure agonist opioids are of greatest benefit in the treatment of moderate to severe pain. Agonist-antagonist preparations (pentazocine, nalbuphine, and butorphanol) and preparations in combination with other analgesics (aspirin, acetaminophen) are less effective. The antagonists may have a ceiling effect, may precipitate withdrawal reactions, may have a high incidence of limitation by the nonnarcotic component, and are generally more expensive than the pure narcotics. Opioid analgesics are by convention compared with 10 mg of morphine sulfate (given parenterally) to determine potency equivalencies. Knowledge of equipotent doses is useful when changing medications (Table 73–1).

C. In choosing an **agonist opioid** for a patient with pain who does not have any organ system failure and who has not received narcotics, initial consideration should be given to an opioid with a short half-life (morphine, hydromorphone, or oxycodone) because they are more easily titratable. The route of administration depends on the patient's level of consciousness, ability to swallow, presence of nausea, and so on. If an analgesic has been associated with significant side effects, an alternative opioid should be considered.

D. The **route of administration** should be the least invasive, least expensive, and most convenient route possible. Generally, oral medications are preferable, but alternatives include rectal, sublingual, and transdermal preparations. Intramuscular routes of administration should be avoided because of discomfort, inconvenience, and unreliability of absorption. Often, a pharmacist knowledgeable about medication preparation can be helpful in individualizing analgesics if standard dosages are not available. Continuous infusions are ordinarily much more expensive routes of administration, but may circumvent problems associated with bolus effects. It may be necessary to change routes of administration in the course of a given patient's care; in these cases, it is important to pay close attention to titration and relative potency.

E. **Continuous pain relief** depends on regular (not prn [as needed]) analgesic dosing. A close approximation exists between the duration of the action of the opioid and the plasma half-life if the narcotic has a short half-life. The clinician should

TABLE 73–1. OPIOID ANALGESICS[1]

Drug	Equianalgesic Dose (mg)	Starting Oral Dose (mg)	Duration of Action (hr)
Morphine	10 IM, 30 po	15–30	3–4
Oxycodone	15 IM, 30 po	15–30	2–4
Hyromorphone	1.5 IM, 7.5 po	2–4	2–4
Levorphanol	2 IM, 4 po	4–8	4–8
Methadone	10 IM, 20 po	5–10	4–8
Morphine	90–120 q12h	N/A	N/A
Fentanyl	100 mg/h = morphine 2 mg/h	N/A	N/A

[1] Agents not recommended in terminally ill patients with moderate to severe pain include meperidine, pentazocine, combination preparations, and mixed agonist-antagonists.
Continuous reassessment of the patient is necessary when treating pain and especially when titrating medications or changing opioids. There is no complete cross-tolerance among narcotics, and it may be beneficial to use slightly less than equipotent dosages of analgesics when changing drugs.

be familiar with the dose and time course of several strong opioids (Table 73–1). Continuous pain relief requires continuous reassessment.

1. An initial narcotic dose of 5–10 mg of morphine sulfate or equivalent is given every 3–4 hours. This will often control pain in the opioid-naive patient.
2. If adequate pain control is established but unacceptable side effects occur, changing analgesics to 50–75% of the equipotent dose is appropriate.
3. For patients with inadequate analgesia and also intolerable side effects, the starting dose of the new equipotent narcotic should be 75–100% of the original opioid.
4. **Continuous assessment and reassessment of pain control** are essential components of compassionate, appropriate care. Monitoring pain relief and the symptomatology of side effects is an ongoing process that must be done on a routine basis.
5. **Titration of the analgesic** is necessary whenever the pain escalates, whether minimally or significantly. Titration must be done in adequate dosages of analgesic, which is generally 35–50% of the current dose. Inadequate titration is often the problem in management of patients with terminal disease. Extremely large doses of opioid may be needed to control pain, but as long as the benefits of the dosage outweigh side effects, the amount of pain medication used is immaterial.
6. The **frequency of titration** is determined by the severity of the pain. Titration can occur every few days when pain is moderate or every 15 minutes when pain is severe. The frequency of the titration, like the amount of medication used, depends on the magnitude of the symptoms.
7. **Tolerance of pain medications** is not usually the reason for the need for titration of analgesics; rather, the reason is most often progression of the illness. Addiction to narcotics is almost never a question in the terminally ill patient. When increasing analgesics, the clinician's primary concern should be control of pain, not tolerance and addiction.
8. Infants and children also require adequate analgesia. Infants may quickly become opioid-resistant, and very large opioid doses may be required for the infant with ongoing severe pain.
9. **Long-acting opioids** are available to assist the clinician in the management of terminal pain. Morphine sulfate and **oxycodone** can be used in forms that release the drug over a period of 8–12 hours. When changing to long-acting preparations, divide the total daily amount of narcotic required for adequate pain relief by two or three to determine dosages for twice daily (bid) or three times daily (tid) administration. Fentanyl is also now available in a transdermal preparation. It is 80 times as potent as morphine and can provide pain relief for 3 days per transdermal patch. Fentanyl has a 12-hour delay in onset of action against pain, and fever increases its dose rate, but it may have fewer gastrointestinal side effects.

F. **Adjuvants to nonopioid and opioid narcotics** can be helpful and should be considered routinely, especially if pain management is difficult or unsuccessful.
   1. **Tricyclic antidepressants** have been shown to have analgesic properties, especially in neuropathic conditions. This characteristic has been proved to be separate from the antidepressant effects. Amitriptyline may be started in low doses (10–25 mg/hr) and increased to 150 mg per day. Doxepin (25–150 mg/day) is also effective. Orthostatic hypotension, sedation, and anticholinergic side effects must be monitored. Doxepin is especially effective for anxious patients.
   2. **Antihistamines** have antiemetic, sedative, and analgesic effects. Parenteral administration of antihistamines is more beneficial for pain relief; oral administration should be considered for nausea or sedation. Hydroxyzine (25 mg/6–8 hr) and promethazine (25 mg/6 hr) are equipotent; but if one is not effective, the other should be considered.
   3. **Benzodiazepines** are useful as anxiolytics and as muscle relaxants, helpful because anxiety and muscle tension are two commonly recognized problems in terminal patients in pain. Diazepam (2–10 mg/6–8 hr) may be given orally or parenterally; lorazepam (1–10 mg/4–8 hr) is also highly effective. Before considering the benzodiazepines, the clinician should titrate opioids to effective dosages, because anxiety is often relieved by larger amounts or more frequent narcotic administration.

    4. Steroids may be very helpful in the management of severe pain. They often decrease edema and can relieve tissue pressure, especially in central nervous system conditions. Dexamethasone (0.75–9 mg/day) is helpful in the management of cerebral edema and spinal cord compression.

    5. Caffeine may be a helpful agent when used with aspirin or aspirin-like medications. Children can also benefit from single doses (1 mg/kg).

    6. Dextromethorphan (DM) has been shown to enhance the analgetic properties of opioids. Combining DM with morphine sulfate in equal doses may double the potency of the narcotic while decreasing constipation and other side effects, as well as decreasing the cost of the medications.

G. Agents to be avoided include meperidine, mixed agonist-antagonist preparations (especially pentazocine), cocaine, and combination preparations.

    1. Meperidine has a short duration (2–3 hours of action), and repeated administration may lead to central nervous system toxicity (confusion, seizures). In general, high oral doses are required to relieve severe pain.

    2. Mixed agonist-antagonist opioids (pentazocine, butorphanol, nalbuphine) are associated with unfavorable psychomimetic effects, such as hallucinations. Furthermore, the use of these agents risks precipitating withdrawal in opioid-dependent patients.

    3. Cocaine has not been shown to have any efficacy as an analgesic in combination with opioids. Its potential for adverse side effects also precludes its use in the terminally ill.

    4. Combination preparations (Brompton's cocktail, DPT-meperidine, promethazine, and chlorpromazine) offer no significant benefits over single-opioid analgesics and have a higher incidence of side effects.

    5. Anxiolytics alone, sedatives alone, hypnotics alone, and especially placebos have no place in pain management in the terminally ill.

VI. Management strategies

A. Alternatives to analgesics and their adjuvants can be helpful in the management of pain in the terminally ill. The clinician should use any modality that can enhance the relief of suffering.

    1. The **application of heat or cold** can relieve pain in many conditions. Care to prevent tissue injury from the source of heat is important. Heat is not recommended for previously irradiated areas. Cold should also be avoided for irradiated tissue, and care must be taken in its use in patients with peripheral vascular disease. Heat and cold should be used intermittently (20 minutes per treatment episode).

    2. Massage and frequent movement are often beneficial in patients with severe pain. Repositioning can prevent pressure ulcers; physical rubbing and massage can promote relaxation and distraction from noxious stimuli. Massage may initially increase pain before relief occurs.

    3. Exercise should be encouraged whenever possible. Activity can assist in promoting flexibility, muscle strength, cardiovascular fitness, and a general sense of well-being. In acute and severe pain, range-of-motion exercise can be helpful.

    4. Transcutaneous electrical nerve stimulation (TENS) is of some benefit in pain management, especially if the pain is not severe. It may be used in concert with opioid analgesia, but is rarely effective alone when pain is judged to be moderate or severe.

    5. Cognitive-behavioral approaches should not be overlooked in the care of the patient with severe pain. These should be used early in treatment regimens so that patients can learn them while they are strong and able to practice. These approaches also allow the patient and the family to develop a sense of empowerment in coping with the pain. Cognitive-behavioral interventions include relaxation techniques, guided imagery, prayer, meditation, distraction exercises, patient education, and occasionally psychotherapy. Pastoral counseling and support groups can be very beneficial to the dying patient and especially to his or her family.

B. Dealing with **side effects** is a universal dilemma in the management of patients with moderate and severe pain. Continuous reassessment and appropriate anticipation can prevent untoward side effects, as well as improve patient care when side effects are promptly recognized.

1. **Nausea and vomiting** are common problems during pain management. Antiemetics can be given orally, rectally, or parenterally. Promethazine (25–50 mg/6–8 hr) and perphenazine (2–16 mg tid) are effective in many cases. Metoclopramide (10 mg before meals three times daily) is especially beneficial if delayed gastric emptying is suspected. Scopolamine (transdermal every third day) is effective if injections or suppositories are felt to be too uncomfortable. Meclizine (25 mg/8 hr) is helpful in cases of significant vertigo. Droperidol, 2.5–10 mg intramuscularly every 6 hours, can be used in cases of severe nausea.

2. **Constipation** is best treated prophylactically. It occurs universally with opioid analgesia. Supplemental fiber and regularly scheduled doses of stool softeners or mild laxatives are prudent. In the case of severe constipation, stimulating cathartics, enemas, or an osmotic laxative (lactulose 15–30 mL/day) should be considered. In the rare case of refractory constipation, oral naloxone in small doses (1.0 mg once or twice daily) has been beneficial. Naloxone should never be used if bowel obstruction is suspected. Colchicine is also effective.

3. **Sedation** is often a problem in the terminally ill patient receiving opioids. If it is not possible to reduce the dosage of the narcotic, central nervous system stimulants may be effective. Methylphenidate (5–20 mg/6 hr before meals), dextroamphetamine (5–20 mg/6 hr), and even caffeine are useful, but should be given early in the day only. If sedation persists, addition of an adjuvant analgesic (such as DM) or nonopioid analgesic may permit a reduction of the narcotic dose. In the rare instance in which these changes are unsuccessful, referral to a subspecialist in pain management should be considered (section VI,D,4).

4. **Respiratory depression** is uncommon in patients receiving chronic opioids; subacute overdose is more likely. Patients with subacute overdose may present with increasing somnolence in association with depressed respirations; it occurs in the span of a few hours to a few days. If it is suspected, the clinician should withhold one or two opioid doses until the symptoms have cleared, then resume the opioid at a lower dosage (75% of previous prescription).

C. **Barriers to appropriate pain management** have repeatedly been shown to result in inadequate pain management in the terminally ill. Understanding and recognizing the potential for any of these obstructions can improve patient care. These barriers can be divided into three areas.

1. **Barriers related to the health care provider** include improper or infrequent assessment of pain, fear of patient addiction to chronic narcotic administration, and incomplete knowledge of pain management strategies (opioids, their effects, and side effects).

2. **Barriers related to the patient** are fear of addiction, reluctance or inability to adequately report or describe pain, and inability to take (or receive from their caregiver/family) opioids. Patients may also fear side effects or not understand their treatment plan.

3. **Barriers related to the health care system** include lack of insurance and financial resources, restrictive regulations regarding controlled substances (narcotics), and problems of access and accessibility.

D. **Additional considerations** in the management of the terminally ill patient with severe pain include the following.

1. **Hospice care** is dedicated to assisting the terminally ill. Early involvement in a hospice can improve patient care and decrease suffering. Many hospices can provide resources that include home nursing services, bath aides, social services, pastoral counseling, physical therapy, and attendants. Hospices can also assist in providing appropriate beds, commodes, supplies, and other durable medical equipment. Hospice services may be covered by Medicare and other insurance programs. The clinician should be aware of local hospice services and include them in the care of the terminally ill if it is appropriate. A template for orders for hospice patients can be helpful in treatment, prevention of side effects, and completeness (Figure 73–2).

2. **The house call** is the most valuable tool available to any health care professional who is treating the terminally ill. Just as a picture is worth a thousand words, so is a house call worth a thousand office visits. The clinician should consider making a house call on any patient who is receiving terminal

Diet _____

Constipation _____
(stool softener, laxative, enema, suppository)

Diarrhea _____

Urinary care _____

Nausea _____

Dyspnea _____

Agitation _____

Fever _____

Skin care _____

Mild pain adjunct to opiate _____
(acetaminophen, ibuprofen)

Opiate analgesics _____

Titration of analgesics _____

Other _____

FIGURE 73–2. Template for orders for terminally ill patients.

care at home. Not only does it provide improved assessment of the clinical situation, but, more important, it demonstrates to the patient that he or she is receiving the full support and attention of the care provider. Abandonment is a great fear of dying persons; a house call clearly shows the patient that he or she is not being abandoned.

3. **Advance directives** (living will, durable power-of-attorney for health care) are indispensable documents for all patients, but especially for those with predicted terminal conditions. Advance directives can be helpful for the patient, the caregivers and the family, and especially for the health care professional when defining treatment options in the event that the patient is unable to express his or her wishes. Advance directives should be completed as early as possible for all patients.

4. **Compounding pharmacies** are playing a greater role in the care of the terminally ill. A compounding pharmacist can prepare medications in special delivery systems (transdermal preparations, vaginal and rectal suppositories, nasal sprays, etc) and in dosages that commercial preparations are unable to offer. The family physician should become acquainted with the local compounding pharmacist for new approaches when current medication regimens fail.

5. **Referral to subspecialists** for "high-tech" interventions should be considered whenever the patient requests nonambulatory procedures or when the physician determines that such treatment options might benefit the patient in preventing suffering and managing care. Patient-controlled analgesia (PCA) can now be delivered in the home setting, but is expensive and requires more sophisticated nursing care. Invasive interventions are not usually necessary to control severe pain in the terminally ill, but may be considered in uncommon cases. They include radiation, surgery, nerve blocks, and neurosurgery.

REFERENCES

American Pain Society: *Principles of Analgesic Use in the Treatment of Acute Pain and Cancer Pain,* 3rd ed. American Pain Society; 1992.

Angell M: The quality of mercy. N Engl J Med 1982;**306:**98.

Chemy NI, Portenoy RK: Cancer pain management. CA 1994;Sept/Oct:259.

Lema M: A compassionate approach to pain management in the terminally ill patient. Hosp Med; May 1998.

US Department of Health and Human Services, Agency for Health Care Policy and Research. Clinical Practice Guideline, No. 9, Management of Cancer Pain. March 1994.

Wanzer SH, et al: The physician's responsibility toward hopelessly ill patients: A second look. N Engl J Med 1989;**320:**844.

74   Chronic Obstructive Pulmonary Disease

Kenneth R. Bertka, MD

I. **Definition. Chronic obstructive pulmonary disease (COPD)** is a respiratory disease characterized by airway obstruction caused by chronic bronchitis, emphysema, or both.
   A. **Chronic bronchitis** is clinically defined as daily cough and sputum production for 3 consecutive months in 2 successive years.
   B. **Emphysema** is anatomically defined as destruction of alveolar walls, resulting in dilation of terminal air spaces.
II. **Epidemiology**
   A. **COPD** affects 14 million Americans. The diagnosis of COPD is usually made between the ages of 55 and 65.
   B. The major cause of COPD is cigarette smoking (usually at least a 20 pack-year history). Approximately 15–20% of smokers develop clinically significant COPD. Although it is more common in men, the incidence of the disease in women has risen with the increased prevalence of smoking in women. Passive smoking is a risk factor for the development of COPD in nonsmokers.
   C. Alpha$_1$-antitrypsin deficiency accounts for less than 1% of COPD cases and is the only known genetic abnormality that leads to COPD. Screening for alpha$_1$-antitrypsin deficiency should be considered for patients with chronic bronchitis who have never smoked or for patients with premature onset of COPD before age 50.
III. **Pathophysiology**
   A. **Development of COPD.** COPD begins as a disease of the medium and small airways, with increased mucus production and destruction of lung parenchyma. Bronchospasm may be present but is usually not the major abnormality.
      1. Mucous obstruction of the airways and increased lung compliance from loss of lung tissue result in **air trapping** and **expiratory airway collapse.** Tachypnea induced by hypoxia or hypercapnia contributes to air trapping by decreasing available expiratory time.
      2. Patients with COPD have **decreased respiratory muscle strength and endurance.** Endurance is compromised more than strength and is the major determinant of respiratory failure. Metabolic abnormalities such as hypokalemia, hypophosphatemia, and hypomagnesemia contribute to muscle weakness.
   B. **Protease–antiprotease theory.** In the absence of COPD, a balance between these two types of enzymes exists. In COPD, proteases from neutrophils (PMNs) and pulmonary alveolar macrophages (PAMs) destroy alveolar structures. Smoking contributes to COPD by increasing the numbers of PMNs and PAMs in the lungs and stimulating PAMs to release proteases and chemotactic factors that attract more PMNs. Smoking decreases the concentration of antielastases, slows tissue repair, and inactivates antiproteases by oxidation.
IV. **Diagnosis**
   A. **Symptoms and signs.** Progressive dyspnea is the most frequent presenting complaint of patients with COPD. Other symptoms include cough, wheezing, weight loss, and recurrent respiratory infection. Many patients report a productive "smoker's cough" in the morning. Table 74–1 compares the diagnostic features of chronic bronchitis and emphysema.
      1. In early or mild COPD, the physical examination may be relatively normal. Wheezing, if present, may be noticeable during forced expiration. In emphysema, auscultation of the chest may reveal distant breath sounds.
      2. In advanced or severe COPD, breathing may be labored, even though there is little or no exertion. Cyanosis and dependent edema may develop. The patient often breathes through pursed lips and leans forward, resting on his or her elbows while sitting, to increase use of the accessory muscles of respiration (*tripoding*).
      3. **Cor pulmonale** is usually present to some degree in patients with severe COPD, but diagnosis by physical examination, chest x-ray, and electro-

TABLE 74–1. CHARACTERISTICS OF EMPHYSEMA AND CHRONIC BRONCHITIS

Diagnostic Approach	Characteristics of	
	Chronic Bronchitis	Emphysema
Clinical presentation		
Dyspnea	Insidious onset, intermittent during infection	Early onset, severe, progressive
Cough	Onset before dyspnea	Onset after dyspnea
Sputum	Copious and purulent	Scant and mucoid
Respiratory infection	Frequent	Rare
Body weight	Normal or overweight	Thin, weight loss
Respiratory insufficiency	Frequent episodes	Late manifestation
Physical examination		
Cyanosis	Often present	Absent
Plethora	Absent	Present
Chest percussion	Normal	Hyperresonant
Chest auscultation	Rales, rhonchi, wheezes	Distant breath sounds, end-expiratory wheezing
Cor pulmonale	Common	Often terminal
Laboratory evaluation		
Hematocrit	Occasional erythrocytosis	Normal
Chest x-ray	Increased bronchovascular markings with normal to enlarged heart and evidence of previous inflammatory disease	Hyperinflation with increased anteroposterior diameter and flat diaphragm; attenuated vascular markings, bullous changes, small vertical heart
Physiologic evaluation		
Spirometry	Expiratory obstruction, reversible component	Irreversible expiratory obstruction, airway closure
Total lung capacity and residual volume	Mild increase	Marked increase
Lung elastic recoil	Near normal	Marked reduction
Diffusion capacity	Normal or slight reduction	Marked decrease
Pao_2 at rest	Marked decrease (45–65 mm Hg)	Slight decrease (65–75 mm Hg)
Pao_2 during exercise	Variable (decrease to increase)	Often falls
$Paco_2$	Normal or elevated (40–60 mm Hg)	Normal or low (35–40 mm Hg)
Pulmonary hypertension	Moderate to severe variable exercise response	None to mild, worsens during exercise
Pathology	Chronic bronchitis with or without mild emphysema	Widespread emphysema, may be panlobular

Adapted with permission from Bleecker ER, Smith PL: Obstructive airways disease. In: Barker LR, Burton JR, Zieve PD, eds. *Principles of Ambulatory Medicine.* 2nd ed. Williams & Wilkins; 1986:659.

cardiogram (ECG) is difficult. Central cyanosis, peripheral edema, hepatomegaly, and increased jugular venous distention are indicative of cor pulmonale. A left parasternal heave or a right-sided S_4 suggests right ventricular hypertrophy. An S_3 may be heard with inspiration over the right ventricle.

  B. Diagnostic tests

    1. Office spirometry. Dynamic pulmonary functions such as forced vital capacity (FVC), forced expiratory volume in 1 second (FEV_1), forced expiratory flow rate over the interval from 25% to 75% of the total FVC ($FEF_{25-75\%}$), $FEF_{75-85\%}$, and calculated FEV_1/FVC ratio are most useful in the diagnosis and treatment of obstructive lung diseases. **Static pulmonary functions** such as functional residual capacity (FRC), total lung capacity (TLC), and residual volume (RV) are not used in the office management of COPD. Static values are needed for accurate diagnosis of restrictive lung diseases such as collagen vascular disease, interstitial pneumonitis, pulmonary fibrosis, pulmonary edema, tumors, pneumothorax, pleural effusions, and obesity.

      a. Indications. Office spirometry should be performed in the initial evaluation of symptomatic patients and in the monitoring of response to treatment. This procedure should also be used to evaluate preoperative patients with COPD.

    b. Contraindications. Patients with active hemoptysis, unstable angina, a recent myocardial infarction, or an active pulmonary infection are poor candidates for spirometry.

    c. Interpretation. Pulmonary function tests (PFTs) are interpreted as percentages of predicted values based on age, height, sex, and race. In adults, 80% of a predicted value is considered normal for FVC, FEV_1, $FEF_{25-75\%}$, and $FEF_{75-85\%}$. A normal FEV_1/FVC ratio is $\geq 75\%$.

      (1) Table 74–2 compares PFTs in **obstructive and restrictive types of respiratory disease.** If FEV_1/FVC indicates obstructive lung disease but FEV_1 is normal, small airway obstruction may be present. In this case, $FEF_{25-75\%}$ should be decreased. A low $FEF_{25-75\%}$ or $FEF_{75-85\%}$ with normal FVC and FEV_1/FVC, which indicates small airway dysfunction, is the first abnormality detected in COPD.

      (2) If initial results indicate **airway obstruction,** a short-acting inhaled bronchodilator should be administered. Spirometry should be repeated after 10 minutes. A substantial reversible component is present if FEV_1 increases by at least 15% or $FEF_{25-75\%}$ improves by at least 30%.

      (3) For **long-term monitoring,** the peak expiratory flow rate (PEFR) is easy to measure at each office visit and correlates well with FEV_1 for an individual patient. There is less intersubject variability with FEV_1, however. Complete office spirometry is better than PEFR alone for the initial evaluation.

      (4) There is no correlation between FEV_1 and Po_2. Therefore, spirometry does not replace arterial blood gas or oxygen saturation determination when hypoxia is suspected.

      (5) The American Thoracic Society has developed a staging system for the severity of COPD based on FEV_1 (Table 74–3).

2. A **complete blood cell count** is indicated when the patient is febrile or fails to respond to empiric antibiotic treatment for pulmonary infection. Eosinophilia suggests a reversible airway component.

3. A **chest x-ray** is useful as a baseline study for future evaluation of changes and to exclude other pulmonary diseases. In early COPD, the chest x-ray may be normal. Lung hyperinflation, flattening of the diaphragms, and increased retrosternal airspace are characteristic of severe emphysema.

4. An ECG is indicated when cor pulmonale or concurrent heart disease is suspected. Changes that may be present with cor pulmonale include right axis deviation, early R waves in V_1 and V_2 and S waves in V_5 and V_6, and peaked P waves in V_1 (P pulmonale). These findings, however, are not always present in patients with cor pulmonale.

5. **Arterial blood gas** analysis is usually normal in early or mild COPD. A partial pressure of oxygen (Pao_2) of <60 mm Hg or an oxygen saturation of <90% indicates hypoxia. The partial pressure of carbon dioxide ($Paco_2$) defines the adequacy of ventilation. A $Paco_2$ of >45 mm Hg indicates hypoventilation and respiratory acidosis. This test is indicated in the following situations.

    a. As part of the initial assessment of the severely symptomatic patient.

    b. When there is acute deterioration of cardiovascular or respiratory status.

    c. For patients with cor pulmonale, polycythemia, dysrhythmias, or altered mental status.

    d. In the initial and periodic evaluations of O_2 therapy.

TABLE 74–2. PULMONARY FUNCTION TESTS IN OBSTRUCTIVE AND RESTRICTIVE DISEASES

Test	Obstructive	Restrictive
FVC	Normal or decreased	Decreased
FEV_1	Decreased	Decreased
FEV_1/FVC	Decreased	Normal or increased
$FEF_{25-75\%}$	Decreased	Normal

$FEF_{25-75\%}$, Forced expiratory flow rate over the interval from 25% to 75% of the total FVC; FEV_1, forced expiratory volume in 1 second; FVC, forced vital capacity.

TABLE 74–3. AMERICAN THORACIC SOCIETY (ATS) STAGING SYSTEM FOR CHRONIC OBSTRUCTIVE PULMONARY DISEASE

Stage	Percentage of Predicted FEV$_1$
I	≥50%
II	35–49%
III	<35%

FEV$_1$, Forced expiratory volume in 1 second.

        e. For preoperative evaluation.

        f. Pending air travel by patients with severe COPD.

V. Treatment goals include correcting reversible bronchoconstriction and increasing respiratory muscle function, along with controlling respiratory infections and cough and sputum production. Many medications used in COPD act on bronchial smooth muscle, which is controlled by the two components of the autonomic nervous system. The sympathetic, or adrenergic, component causes bronchodilation while the parasympathetic, or vagal, component causes bronchoconstriction. These effects are mediated through cyclic nucleotides. β-Adrenergic agents, theophylline preparations, and corticosteroids increase cyclic adenosine monophosphate, which causes bronchodilation. Anticholinergic agents decrease bronchoconstriction mediated by cyclic guanosine 3,5-monophosphate. A typical regimen for treating COPD is outlined in Figure 74–1.

    A. Anticholinergic agents reduce parasympathetic-mediated bronchoconstriction. Increased resting bronchial tone appears to be a major factor in emphysema and

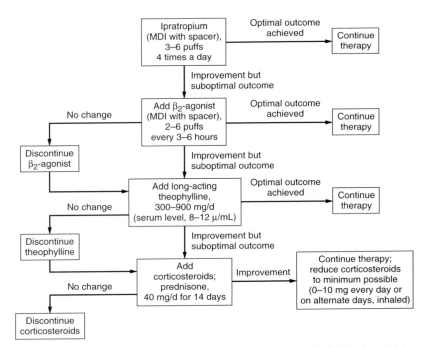

FIGURE 74–1. A typical regimen for treating chronic obstructive pulmonary disease. MDI, Metered-dose inhaler. (Adapted with permission from Ferguson GT, Cherniak RM: Management of chronic obstructive pulmonary disease. N Engl J Med 1993;**328:**1017.)

chronic bronchitis. **Ipratropium** (Atrovent) is the drug of choice for patients with these conditions. Reduced vagal tone with ipratropium use leads to improvement of FVC. Bronchodilation in patients treated with ipratropium begins more slowly but is often greater and longer lasting than that seen in patients treated with β-adrenergic agents.

    1. Dosage. Ipratropium is available in a metered-dose inhaler (MDI). Two puffs (36 μg) four times a day is the dose approved by the Food and Drug Administration. This dose, however, may not achieve optimal bronchodilation. Three to six puffs four times a day may improve therapeutic response without notable side effects. Administration 5–10 minutes after use of a selective adrenergic agent may increase penetration of ipratropium into the smaller airways. A reservoir or spacer is helpful for patients who have difficulty using an MDI. Ipratropium aerosol delivery (500 μg) is beneficial for patients who are acutely short of breath. Ipratropium does not lose its effectiveness with continued use. Ipratropium can be given with β-adrenergic agents and theophylline without adverse interactions. (A combination MDI of ipratropium and albuterol is available.)

    2. Side effects. Ipratropium administered by an MDI does not have the major systemic side effects associated with atropine, although dry mouth and metallic taste have been reported. Blurred vision may result if the agent is inadvertently sprayed into the eyes.

B. β-Adrenergic agents are available in oral, inhaled, and injectable forms (Table 74–4). Selective or β2-adrenergic agents are preferred over nonselective agents that also stimulate cardiac β1-adrenergic receptors, causing tachycardia (see Chapter 72 for more information).

    There is no definite advantage of one β2-adrenergic agent over another. Individual response and cost should be considered when choosing a therapy. MDIs should always be used with a spacer to maximize drug delivery. Administration by an MDI or aerosol is preferable to oral delivery, because inhalation rapidly delivers high concentrations of the drug to target receptors with minimal systemic effects. A β2-adrenergic agent may be used as a single-drug regimen for patients with only mild intermittent symptoms. In severe exacerbations, aerosol administration can deliver high doses of medication; however, repeated puffs of an MDI can have equivalent effect. For long-term control, many patients receive more benefit using four puffs three or four times a day than the conventional two puffs.

C. Theophylline reduces dyspnea in patients with COPD through improvement of diaphragmatic function and through bronchodilation. Theophylline is not used as a first-line drug in patients with stable COPD because of its narrow therapeutic

TABLE 74–4. SELECTIVE β-ADRENERGIC AGENTS

Drug	Route of Administration	Dose	Dose Intervals (hr)
Albuterol (Proventil, Ventolin)	MDI	2–4 puffs	3–6
	Aerosol[1]	0.5 mL	6–8
	Oral	2–4 mg	6–8
Bitolterol (Tornalate)	MDI	2–3 puffs	4–8
Isoetharine (Bronkosol, Bronkometer)	MDI	2–4 puffs	3–6
	Aerosol[1]	0.25–0.5 mL	3–6
Metaproterenol (Alupent, Metaprel)	MDI	2–4 puffs	3–6
	Aerosol[1]	0.2–0.3 mL	3–6
	Oral	10–20 mg	6–8
Pirbuterol (Maxair)	MDI	2 puffs	4–6
Salmeterol[2] (Serevent)	MDI	2 puffs	10–12
Terbutaline (Brethaire, Brethine)	MDI	2–4 puffs	4–8
	Oral	2.5–5 mg	6–8
	SC	0.25–0.5 mg	4–8

[1] Agents used in aerosol machines are usually mixed in 2–3 mL of normal saline.
[2] Salmeterol is indicated for the stable patient with chronic obstructive pulmonary disease. A shorter-acting agent with more rapid onset should be used for acute exacerbations.
MDI, Metered-dose inhaler; SC, subcutaneous.

window. Theophylline should be considered for long-term use in patients who remain symptomatic despite maximal inhalation therapy. Theophylline is not recommended for acute exacerbations.

   1. **Dosage.** The usual starting dose, based on lean body weight, for a nonsmoking patient is 10–12 mg/kg/day of a long-acting preparation that is made to be given twice a day. Many factors may modify this recommended starting dose (Table 74–5). Therefore, a conservative approach is to start with 400 mg/day (Theo-Dur), given as 200 mg twice a day, and to increase the dose every 3–5 days. The use of a long-acting preparation in the evening reduces both overnight declines in FEV_1 and morning dyspnea.
   2. **Monitoring.** Serum levels should be checked on a regular basis, since theophylline has a narrow therapeutic window. Subjective improvement, clinical judgment, and spirometry changes are more important than theophylline levels. Some patients may require levels under or over the normal therapeutic range of 8–15 mg/mL to attain maximum improvement with minimal side effects. Patients with daily fluctuations in symptoms may benefit from peak-and-trough theophylline levels. Rapid metabolizers, such as smokers, who require 900 mg/day or more, may benefit from doses given three times a day in order to achieve steady levels.
   3. **Side effects** (Table 74–6). Patients with a history of gastrointestinal intolerance to medications may benefit from starting at a lower dose and gradually increasing the dose.
   D. **Corticosteroids** are used in patients with COPD who do not respond adequately to β-adrenergics, theophylline, and ipratropium. They are most beneficial in patients whose COPD has an asthmatic component or who have a 15% improvement in FEV_1 with a $β_2$-adrenergic agent. Steroids enhance responsiveness to bronchodilators, inhibit the release of proteases from leukocytes, and reduce mucosal edema.
   1. **Dosage and monitoring**
      a. **Oral administration.** For acute episodes, **prednisone** can be started at as much as 60 mg/day for 5 days and discontinued or tapered by 5–10 mg/day over 2-week periods until discontinued. For long-term use, prednisone at 60 mg/day or 0.5–1 mg/kg/day for a 2- to 4-week trial can be used. If FEV_1 improves by 20–25%, steroids should be tapered to the lowest dose that maintains the improvement. Alternate-day administration may be sufficient. If FEV_1 does not improve, steroids should be tapered and discontinued.

TABLE 74–5. ESTIMATED MAINTENANCE DOSES FOR THEOPHYLLINE[1]

Factors That Increase Need	Dose (mg/kg/day)	Factors That Decrease Need	Dose (mg/kg/day)
Age 10–15 yr	14–18	Hepatic insufficiency	<5
Age 16–20 yr	12	Heart failure	4–7
Smoking	12–18	Cor pulmonale	4–7
Marijuana use	12–15	Viral upper respiratory infection	6–8
Therapy with		Sustained fever	6–8
Sucralfate (Carafate)	10–15	Therapy with	
Phenytoin (Dilantin)	12–14	Cimetidine (Tagamet)	5
Rifampin	12–14	Ranitidine (Zantac)	5
Barbiturates	12	Ciprofloxacin (Cipro),	6–8
Isoniazid	12–14	other quinolones	
Carbamazepine (Tegretol)	12–14	Estrogens	6–8
High-protein diet	12–14	Erythromycin	4–7
Charcoal-broiled meat	12–14	Allopurinol	6–8
		Furosemide	6–8
		Verapamil	6–8
		Nifedipine	6–8

[1] The average adult patient needs 10 mg/kg/day of theophylline. In obese patients, the dosage should be based on ideal body weight. For aminophylline, increase dosages by 20%.
Adapted with permission from Ziment I: Pharmacologic therapy of COPD. In: Hodgkin JE, Petty TL, eds. *Chronic Obstructive Pulmonary Disease: Current Concepts.* Saunders; 1987:75.

TABLE 74–6. RELATIONSHIP BETWEEN SERUM THEOPHYLLINE CONCENTRATION AND TOXIC EFFECTS

Serum Theophylline Concentration (mg/L [μmol/L])[1]	Toxic Effects
15–25 (83–139)	Abdominal cramps
	Agitation
	Diarrhea
	Gastrointestinal disturbances
	Headache
	Nausea
	Tremors
	Vomiting
25–35 (139–194)	Occasional premature ventricular contractions
	Sinus tachycardia (heart rate >120 beats per minute)
>35 (>194)	Frequent premature ventricular contractions
	Ventricular tachycardia
	Gastrointestinal bleeding
	Grand mal seizures

[1] Ranges given are generalizations. Toxic effects have been observed at higher and lower serum theophylline concentrations.
Adapted with permission from Beck BW: Pharmacologic approaches to obstructive airway disease. Primary Care 1985;**12**:239.

    b. MDI administration. This route allows the use of smaller dosages, since
       the medication is delivered directly to its site of action. The usual dosage
       range is two to four puffs administered two to four times a day. Four to
       eight weeks of use may be needed before subjective or objective benefits
       are noted. Available preparations include **beclomethasone** (Beclovent
       or Vanceril), **flunisolide** (AeroBid), **fluticasone** (Flovent, Flovent Rota-
       disk) and **triamcinolone** (Azmacort).
  2. Side effects. Oral corticosteroids have serious short- and long-term effects
       (Tables 74–7 and 74–8). The use of these drugs should therefore be limited
       to patients who do not respond to other therapies. The risk of significant side
       effects is low if the equivalent of 10 mg/day or less of prednisone is used or
       if higher-dose treatment is limited to 2 weeks. Steroids provided in MDI form
       do not result in systemic side effects unless abused. Oral candidiasis is the
       most common side effect reported with use of an MDI and can be prevented
       by use of a spacer and by rinsing the mouth with water after use.
 E. Antimicrobial therapy for exacerbations of COPD has been shown to decrease
    dyspnea, improve peak flow rates, and decrease hospitalization rates. Treatment
    is usually empiric and directed against the most likely pathogens: *Haemophilus
    influenzae, Streptococcus pneumoniae,* and *Moraxella (Branhamella) catarrhalis.*
    Viruses have been isolated in 20–40% of patients with exacerbation of COPD,
    with rhinovirus as the most common isolate. Influenza A is an important factor in
    morbidity. Amantidine prophylaxis for unvaccinated patients should be consid-
    ered during periods of high risk of contracting the virus. There are no good data
    to support the intermittent or chronic use of prophylactic antibiotics.

TABLE 74–7. SIDE EFFECTS OF SHORT-TERM HIGH-DOSE STEROID THERAPY

Cerebral edema
Diabetes mellitus
Glaucoma
Hyperosmolar nonketotic coma
Hypertension
Hypokalemic alkalosis
Mood disorders
Pancreatitis
Peptic ulceration and gastrointestinal hemorrhage
Proximal myopathy
Sodium and water retention

TABLE 74-8. SIDE EFFECTS OF LONG-TERM HIGH-DOSE STEROID THERAPY

Aseptic necrosis of bone
Centripetal obesity
Growth failure
Hyperlipidemia
Impaired wound healing
Mood disorders
Osteoporosis
Posterior subcapsular cataracts
Seizure disorders
Suppression of immune response

F. **Mucokinetic and antitussive agents** are used to control cough and sputum production that persist after other causes of coughing, such as congestive heart failure or occult malignancy, have been excluded.
   1. **Oral expectorants** such as **guaifenesin** are often given to improve cough frequency, cough severity, chest discomfort, dyspnea, and sputum clearance. Subjective improvement usually follows. Secretions may be mobilized by use of a humidifier, systemic hydration, and saline aerosols, although the last can cause bronchospasm in some patients.
   2. **For cough suppression,** a nonnarcotic agent such as **dextromethorphan** should be tried first. If a narcotic agent is used for an acute episode of uncontrolled coughing, the patient should avoid both driving and drinking alcoholic beverages.
G. **Other treatments**
   1. **Respiratory stimulants** are not currently recommended for use in the United States.
   2. **Antiproteases** for aerosol or MDI administration may eventually be available to restore the protease–antiprotease balance, which may retard the progression of COPD. Human α_1-proteinase inhibitor is available for patients with emphysema from a congenital deficiency of this enzyme. The efficacy of human α_1-proteinase inhibitor administered intravenously on a weekly basis is being studied; treatment is very expensive.
   3. **Morphine** has been found to decrease dyspnea and to increase exercise tolerance duration by as much as 20% in end-stage COPD. The duration of action, the optimal dose, and the preferred route of administration have not been established.
   4. **Nitric oxide (NO)** is being studied for its pulmonary vasodilation effect in patients with severe COPD. Inhaled NO has relatively low toxicity, with its activity limited to the lung; its use is still experimental.
   5. **Psychoactive agents** to treat depression, insomnia, or anxiety can be helpful to improve the quality of life for patients with COPD. Benzodiazepines are generally safe to use in patients with mild or moderate COPD. Their use must be closely monitored in patients with severe COPD to prevent suppression of respiration, especially during sleep. Sedating antihistamines and chloral hydrate are safer hypnotics for use in insomnia. In addition to their intended use, antidepressants can help improve sleep and relieve chronic pain.
   6. **Lung volume reduction surgery (LVRS)** in select patients with severe, diffuse emphysema is a promising technique currently being studied. LVRS involves bilateral resection of 30–40% of the worst areas of emphysematous change. Improvements in symptoms, exercise performance, FEV_1, FVC, and arterial blood gases have been encouraging.
VI. **Management strategies.** The primary care physician should develop an individualized plan and coordinate the care given by others.
   A. **Smoking cessation.** This is often the most difficult challenge faced by the patient with COPD. Smoking cessation is the best way to change the course of COPD. Benefits of cessation include a decrease in cough and sputum production, a slowing of the rate of decline of pulmonary function, and a reduction of the risk of respiratory failure. Smoking cessation can also lower the patient's risk of contracting other smoking-related illnesses. The physician needs to be persistent in educating patients about the benefits of cessation (see Chapter 106).

B. Hospitalization. The physician should consider hospitalization for the patient during an acute episode of COPD under such circumstances as the following:

1. Failure to improve symptomatically or objectively with aggressive treatment in the office or emergency department.
2. New or more severe cor pulmonale.
3. New-onset (noncompensated) respiratory acidosis or marked deterioration of blood gases from the patient's baseline levels.
4. Pneumothorax, pleural effusion, pneumonia, rib fractures, or pulmonary contusion.
5. Gradual decline in pulmonary function not responsive to outpatient management or rapid decline that results in a loss of independence.

C. Environmental control

1. Patients with COPD should avoid exposure to secondhand tobacco smoke and should remain indoors during air pollution or smog alerts.
2. Patients who are sensitive to extremes of humidity and temperature may find that use of a humidifier in the winter and a dehumidifier or air conditioner in the summer improves symptoms.
3. Patients with chronic hypoxia generally should not travel to altitudes above 4000 feet. Studies have shown decreased survival rates among patients who live at altitudes above 3500 feet. Commercial aircraft are usually pressurized to between 5000 and 7000 feet. Patients with severe COPD may require supplemental oxygen during flights; this can usually be arranged with a note from the physician and 48-hour notice to the airline. Patients should avoid flying in unpressurized aircraft.

D. Home oxygen therapy. Reversing hypoxia improves the patient's survival, decreases hospitalization, increases exercise capacity and endurance, enhances neuropsychological function, increases cardiac output, and decreases pulmonary vascular resistance. Oxygen is the most potent treatment for cor pulmonale.

1. **Guidelines** (Table 74–9).
2. **Delivery systems** are outlined in Table 74–10.
3. **Monitoring.** The goal of home oxygen therapy is to maintain PaO_2 at 60–65 mm Hg or O_2 saturation at 90–94% with the smallest amount of oxygen that maintains these parameters. The patient should be monitored by arterial blood gases or oxygen saturation tests periodically for worsening symptoms. These tests should also be performed after changes in oxygen dose. A patient who continues to have symptoms at night should be monitored by pulse oximetry or formal sleep laboratory evaluation.

   Historically, oxygen was thought to be dangerous in hypoxic COPD patients because of concern that it would lead to dangerous CO_2 retention by suppression of the hypoxic drive. It has now been shown that the minute ventilation changes very little in COPD patients on low-flow oxygen (24–28% FIO_2, 1–2 L/min by nasal cannula). Oxygen therapy is the only intervention that has been demonstrated to improve survival in patients with severe COPD.
4. **Regular education** on the proper use of equipment and supervision during the first 3 months of use increase patient acceptance of home oxygen therapy.

TABLE 74–9. GUIDELINES FOR PRESCRIBING HOME OXYGEN THERAPY

Criteria for patient selection

1. Stable course of disease with optimal medical therapy, eg, bronchodilator, antibiotics, or corticosteroids (if indicated)
2. At least two arterial blood gas determinations while breathing air for at least 20 minutes
3. Room-air PaO_2 consistently ≤55 mm Hg (oxygen saturation ≤88%) or consistently 56–59 mm Hg plus clinically diagnosed cor pulmonale, hematocrit ≥55%, or both
4. Normoxic patients who demonstrate less dyspnea and increased exercise with oxygen therapy

Oxygen dosage

1. Use continuous flow by single or double nasal cannula or on demand with demonstration of adequate oxygen saturation.
2. Use lowest oxygen flow rate (L/min) that raises PaO_2 to 60–65 mm Hg or oxygen saturation to 90–94%.
3. Increase baseline oxygen flow rate by 1 L/min during exercise and sleep.

Adapted with permission from Petty TL: Respiratory therapy techniques. In: Hodgkin JE, Petty TL, eds. *Chronic Obstructive Pulmonary Disease: Current Concepts.* Saunders; 1987:91.

TABLE 74–10. ADVANTAGES AND DISADVANTAGES OF HOME OXYGEN SYSTEMS

System	Advantages	Disadvantages
Liquid oxygen tank	Lightweight Portable Valuable for pulmonary rehabilitation Provides 100% oxygen at all flow rates	Expensive Not available in small or rural communities

Oxygen concentrators	Less expensive than liquid oxygen
	  tanks
	Convenient for home use
	Attractive equipment
	Widely available
		Requires electricity
		
		May need back-up tank system
		Not portable; does not assist in ambula-
		  tion or pulmonary rehabilitation
		Noisy

Compressed-gas oxygen
  tank
	Less expensive (cost may equal
	  liquid in continuous-use situation)
	Widely available
		Multiple tanks necessary for ambulation
		  unless filling from a large tank can be
		  done at home
		Frequent deliveries needed
		Heavy, unsightly tanks
		Not as effective as liquid in pulmonary
		  rehabilitation

Adapted with permission from Petty TL: Respiratory therapy techniques. In: Hodgkin JE, Petty TL, eds. *Chronic Obstructive Pulmonary Disease: Current Concepts.* Saunders; 1987:91.

    E. Pulmonary rehabilitation is a multidisciplinary team approach to treating patients with chronic respiratory diseases with the goal of achieving the individual's maximum level of independence and functioning in the community (Table 74–11). Documented benefits include symptomatic improvement, increased exercise tolerance, less depression, and a reduction in sick days. A major factor may be that patients with the same disease work together and discuss their condition and feelings with other patients and family members.

       1. Participation. Patients with COPD who are most likely to benefit from rehabilitation are those under optimal medical management, without cardiac disease, who are symptomatic at rest or with mild exertion. Family support increases the likelihood of success.

       2. Therapy should emphasize proper breathing techniques, such as pursed-lip breathing, and exercise training at home, concentrating on activities of daily living, such as climbing stairs. Contraindications to exercise include persistent tachycardia (>110 beats per minute), frequent or symptomatic premature ventricular contractions, $Paco_2$ >55 mm Hg, and FEV_1 <0.5 L.

TABLE 74–11. COMPONENTS OF PULMONARY REHABILITATION

Patient education
Knowledge of the disease process
Family education
Avoidance of smoking
Medication instruction
Proper use of metered-dose inhalers
Maintenance of home oxygen equipment
Normal weight attainment and maintenance
Avoidance of infection
Sexual counseling
Discussion of extraordinary life support measures

Exercise training
Evaluation of activities of daily living
Work simplification techniques
Pursed-lip breathing
Development of a safe exercise routine
Stair climbing
Inspiratory muscle training

TABLE 74–12. MORTALITY RATE IN RELATION TO POSTBRONCHODILATOR FEV₁

Percent of Predicted FEV₁	Mortality Rate (%)	
	5 Years	10 Years
<20	90	>95
20–39	60	90
40–49	10	60
>50	4	5

FEV_1, Forced expiratory volume in 1 second.
Adapted with permission from Celli BR: Chronic obstructive pulmonary disease. In: *Family Practice Annual 1985*. American Academy of Family Physicians; 1985:49.

    F. Personalized patient education improves compliance with the therapeutic regimen and reduces the consumption of health services by patients with COPD.

    G. Vaccinations, both influenza (yearly) and pneumococcal (usually once), are recommended in all COPD patients. For patients who receive a pneumococcal vaccine before the age of 65, revaccination after age 65 and at least 5 years after the initial vaccination is recommended.

VII. Natural history and prognosis

    A. COPD is the fourth leading cause of death in the United States. Mortality statistics from COPD have increased in the last 10 years to more than 95,000 deaths each year. Only heart disease and schizophrenia rank ahead of COPD as major causes of chronic disability in older individuals. In severe COPD, death is related to recurrent episodes of hypoxia, leading to the development of pulmonary vascular hypertension and cor pulmonale. Chronic bronchitis is responsible for an average of 12 disability (restricted activity) days per patient per year. Emphysema results in an average of 68 disability days per patient per year.

    B. Although variable, FEV_1 decreases by 50–75 mL per year in patients with COPD, compared with 20–30 mL per year in nonsmokers. Dyspnea with moderate exertion is usually noticeable when FEV_1 falls to about 1.5 L. Dyspnea with any exertion is usually present at a FEV_1 of 1 L. Patients with a FEV_1 of 0.5 L or less are usually invalids. Increased mortality rates are associated with decreasing FEV_1. Besides age, FEV_1 is the best predictor of mortality (Table 74–12). Other indicators of poor prognosis include resting tachycardia, severe atrial hypoxia, severe hypercapnia, hypoalbuminemia, and cor pulmonale.

    C. Complications of COPD include poor nutrition, respiratory infections, congestive heart failure, cor pulmonale, dysrhythmias, gastroesophageal reflux, psychological dysfunction, and sexual dysfunction. About half of all patients with COPD have nutritional abnormalities. About 40% of patients with severe COPD have significant depression when assessed using the Beck depression inventory. Psychosocial factors are closely correlated with hospitalization in patients with decompensated COPD.

    D. The primary care physician should encourage patient and family discussion about resuscitation and life support before an emergency occurs. Knowledge of the patient's wishes about life support can prevent anguish and guilt when a life-threatening complication arises. Decisions about life support should be routinely reviewed in the office and documented in the medical record.

REFERENCES

American Thoracic Society: Standards for the diagnosis and care of patients with chronic obstructive pulmonary disease. Am J Respir Crit Care Med 1995;**152:**S77.

British Thoracic Society: BTS guidelines for the management of chronic obstructive pulmonary disease: The COPD guidelines group of the standards of care committee of the BTS. Thorax 1997;**52:**S1.

Madison JM, Irwin RS: Chronic obstructive pulmonary disease. Lancet 1998;**352:**467.

O'Brien GM, Criner GJ: Surgery for severe COPD. Postgrad Med 1998;**103:**179.

Senior RM, Anthonisen NR: Chronic obstructive pulmonary disease. Am J Respir Crit Care Med 1998;**157:**S139.

75   Cirrhosis

Martin S. Lipsky, MD, & Mari E. Egan, MD

I. **Definition.** Cirrhosis is a chronic, irreversible liver disease characterized by diffuse hepatic fibrosis and nodule formation.

II. **Epidemiology.** Cirrhosis is a common chronic gastrointestinal disorder, ranking 129th among the most common diagnoses seen by family physicians. Cirrhosis is most prevalent in the 36- to 54-year-old age group.

   A. **Alcoholic cirrhosis** is the most common type of cirrhosis in the United States. Between 8% and 20% of chronic alcoholics develop cirrhosis. The typical patient with alcoholic cirrhosis drinks at least 1 pint of whiskey per day or its equivalent for 10 years. Women are more susceptible to this alcohol-induced injury than men.

   B. **Viral hepatitis,** particularly types B and C, is the leading cause of cirrhosis worldwide. In countries where hepatitis B is endemic, children acquire the infection early in life and cirrhosis may advance in one-fourth of them. However, hepatitis C infection is self-limited in only 10–15% of cases and is the most common cause of chronic viral hepatitis in the United States. Chronic infection leads to cirrhosis in at least 20% of patients within 20 years after the onset of infection. It is now the leading cause of liver transplantation, accounting for 30% of the cases.

   C. **Cryptogenic cirrhosis** is any cirrhosis with an unknown cause (approximately 10% of all patients with cirrhosis). Drugs (eg, methotrexate, isoniazid, acetaminophen, and estrogen) or toxins (eg, industrial cleaning solvents) may produce liver damage leading to cirrhosis.

   D. **Other types** include primary biliary cirrhosis, secondary biliary cirrhosis, cardiac cirrhosis, and metabolic diseases such as α-antitrypsin deficiency, hemochromatosis, and Wilson's disease.

III. **Pathophysiology.** The pathologic process of cirrhosis may be viewed as the end result of many types of chronic liver injury. As a result of these injuries, the liver parenchyma is replaced with fibrous tissue and regenerating nodules.

   A. **Alcoholic cirrhosis.** Ethanol is a direct hepatotoxin, although its exact mechanism of action is not completely understood. Since not all drinkers develop cirrhosis, genetic, nutritional, and environmental factors probably act in concert to cause liver disease.

   B. **Primary biliary cirrhosis** is believed to be an immunologic disorder that causes progressive destruction of the small and intermediate-sized intrahepatic bile ducts.

   C. **Secondary biliary cirrhosis** is a result of long-standing obstruction of the biliary tree because of gallstones, strictures, carcinoma, or sclerosing cholangitis.

   D. **Cardiac cirrhosis** is a complication of severe, prolonged right-sided heart failure.

   E. **Metabolic diseases**

      1. **Hemochromatosis** is a disease produced by excessive iron deposition in parenchymal liver tissue.

      2. **Wilson's disease** is a rare disease characterized by excessive copper storage.

   F. **Postnecrotic cirrhosis** is the histologic result of many types of advanced liver injury, although it is usually caused by a viral infection.

IV. **Diagnosis.** Cirrhosis has great variability in its clinical manifestations. Some patients may be virtually asymptomatic for many years, while others may present with a full spectrum of cirrhotic complications. When one is evaluating patients for liver disease, it is important to assess risk factors (ie, prior blood transfusions, hemodialysis, hemophilia, organ transplants, sexual practices, multiple sexual partners, problem drinking, hepatotoxic drugs [prescription and over-the-counter drugs and vitamins, and herbal remedies], occupation, family history, and other systemic disease).

   A. **Symptoms and signs** of cirrhosis can be separated into three major groups, as described below.

      1. **Hepatocellular dysfunction,** including jaundice, nausea and vomiting, coagulopathy, weakness, palmar erythema, gynecomastia, testicular atrophy, spider angiomas, and parotid hypertrophy.

      2. **Sequelae of cirrhosis,** including ascites, edema, splenomegaly, bleeding varices, and encephalopathy.

3. **Systemic symptoms and signs** resulting from the specific cause of cirrhosis. Examples include the following conditions.
   a. **Dupuytren's contractures** from alcoholic cirrhosis.
   b. **Pruritus or asymptomatic abnormal liver functions** from primary biliary cirrhosis in a female patient between 30 and 50 years of age.
   c. **Arthritis, bronze skin, and diabetes mellitus** from hemochromatosis.
   d. **Neurologic symptoms and cornea deposits** (Kayser–Fleischer ring) from Wilson's disease.

B. **Laboratory tests.** Common laboratory findings, in addition to those listed below, include anemia, normal or slightly decreased white blood cell count, elevated serum globulins, and moderate thrombocytopenia.

1. **Liver enzymes** are usually moderately increased in cirrhosis, although they may be minimally elevated or normal in as many as 10% of patients. Paradoxically, the enzymes may be virtually normal in severe liver disease, since so many of the normal liver cells have been replaced by fibrous tissue. Alanine aminotransferase (ALT) is found predominately in the liver and may be a more sensitive indicator of liver damage. An aspartate aminotransferase (AST)-alanine aminotransferase (ALT) ratio (equivalent to a serum glutamic-oxaloacetic transaminase [SGOT]-serum glutamate pyruvate transaminase [SGPT] ratio) of more than 2 is suggestive of alcoholic liver disease (see Chapter 45).

2. **Bilirubin** may be increased, particularly in biliary cirrhosis because of obstruction or in severely damaged livers.

3. **Alkaline phosphatase** is indicative of injury to the bile ducts. It is elevated disproportionately higher to AST or ALT in primary and secondary biliary cirrhosis as well as primary sclerosing cholangitis.

4. **Serum albumin** is often depressed and the **prothrombin time** is elevated because of the reduced synthetic capabilities of the liver. Low albumin or a prolonged prothrombin time uncorrected by parenteral vitamin K (10 mg subcutaneously every day for 3 days) suggests severe liver damage.

5. A **radionucleotide scan of the liver and spleen** will show decreased, patchy uptake in the liver and increased uptake in the spleen and bone marrow. This noninvasive test is useful in clinically equivocal cases of cirrhosis and is also useful for measuring liver function.

6. An **ultrasound examination or computerized tomography** of the abdomen is helpful in detecting the presence and cause of secondary biliary cirrhosis. Ultrasonography is very sensitive for detecting ascites and can detect as little as 100 mL of peritoneal fluid.

7. Some **laboratory abnormalities** may suggest specific disorders, and appropriate tests should be ordered when suggested by the clinical history or physical examination or when the cause of cirrhosis is not apparent. Examples of such tests are listed below.
   a. To assess for chronic hepatitis B infection, diagnostic tests of HbsAg, IgG anti-HBc, HbeAg, and hepatitis B virus DNA should be done.
   b. Chronic hepatitis C infection will have a positive ELISA and radioimmunoblot assay (RIBA) for hepatitis C virus (HCV). A HCV RNA should also be measured to assess for the need for treatment as well as success of treatment.
   c. Hemochromatosis is suggested by elevated ferritin >900 ng/dL, elevated serum iron >150 pg/dL, and increased transferrin saturation >50%.
   d. Wilson's disease is suggested by decreased ceruloplasmin <29 mg/dL and increased urinary copper secretion.
   e. Primary biliary cirrhosis is suggested by a positive antimitochondrial antibody in 95% of patients.

8. **Liver biopsy.** A liver biopsy provides information on the grade (inflammatory severity) and stage (degree of fibrosis) of liver disease. A liver biopsy is indicated if a treatable cause of cirrhosis, such as Wilson's disease, is suspected. This procedure may also be used to help establish a prognosis or to determine whether a patient with antibody evidence of hepatitis B and C infection would benefit from interferon therapy.

V. **Treatment.** The treatment of cirrhosis consists of managing the complications, preventing further liver damage, and, if possible, treating the underlying cause.

A. **General measures.** Activity should be allowed to the level of the patient's tolerance. The use of alcohol or other hepatotoxic agents is prohibited.
  1. **Diet.** A nutritious low-salt diet is desirable. Protein restriction is necessary only when there are signs of encephalopathy.
  2. **Tranquilizers and sedatives** should be avoided.
  3. **Vitamins and folic acid supplementation** (1 mg/day) may be desirable, particularly in alcoholics. Patients with cholestatic forms of cirrhosis are at risk for deficiencies of fat-soluble vitamins (A, D, E, and K).
B. **Ascites and edema**
  1. **Restriction of sodium intake** is the cornerstone of therapy. Sodium intake should be limited to less than 2 g/day.
  2. **Diuresis** can be initiated with spironolactone, 100 mg as a single dose, if salt restriction alone is ineffective. If there is no effect after 1 week, the daily dose of spironolactone may be increased by 100 mg every 3–5 days until a total dose of 400–600 mg/day is reached.
  3. If diuresis is inadequate, **furosemide** can be added in gradually increasing doses, starting with 20 mg/day. Care must be taken to avoid intravascular depletion. Weight loss should be limited to no greater than 0.5 kg/day for patients with ascites and 1 kg/day for patients with both ascites and edema.
  4. **Repeated large-volume therapeutic paracentesis** is safe and useful for patients with diuretic-resistant ascites. If more than 5 L of fluid is withdrawn, giving 25–50 g of albumin intravenously is helpful to avoid intravascular depletion.
  5. **Restriction of fluid intake to 1500 mL/day** may be necessary for treating ascites in patients with sodium levels less than 125 mEq/L.
  6. **Potassium supplements** should be provided if potassium levels are low because of secondary hyperaldosteronism. Care must be taken to avoid hyperkalemia when using potassium supplements and spironolactone.
C. **Hepatic encephalopathy**
  1. **Protein** should be limited to approximately 30 g/day. Vegetable protein may be tolerated better than animal protein.
  2. **Lactulose,** 30 mL every 4–6 hours, with subsequent adjustment to allow for two or three soft stools a day, is indicated for encephalopathy that is incompletely controlled by diet alone.
  3. **Neomycin,** 1 g orally two to four times per day, alone or in combination with lactulose, may be helpful. However, chronic usage may result in ototoxicity and nephrotoxicity.
D. **Coagulopathy** may be improved by vitamin K, 10 mg subcutaneously every day for 3 days.
E. **Variceal bleeding** requires consultation with a gastroenterologist for management. Endoscopic sclerotherapy is the treatment of choice for acute hemorrhage.
F. **Spontaneous bacterial peritonitis** is one of the major potential treatable complications of cirrhosis. It should be considered in any patient with worsening liver failure and ascites. Ascitic fluid with a total white blood cell count of >500/mL or an absolute count of >250/mL suggests infection. Hospitalization and treatment with broad-spectrum antibiotics are required.
G. **Special measures** may be helpful for cirrhosis with an underlying condition.
  1. The **pruritus of primary biliary cirrhosis** may be improved by cholestyramine, 4 g mixed with food or juice with each meal. Some patients may also need vitamin supplementation. All drug therapy aimed at slowing the disease process is experimental.
  2. **Secondary biliary cirrhosis** may be treated by relieving the obstruction to biliary flow surgically or endoscopically.
  3. **Cardiac cirrhosis** may be improved by treating the underlying cardiac condition.
  4. **Hemochromatosis** is treated with phlebotomies.
  5. **Wilson's disease** responds to chronic D-penicillamine, 500 mg orally three times daily.
  6. **Alcoholic liver disease** may have progression slowed and increased longevity by using colchicine 0.6 mg orally twice daily.
  7. **Chronic hepatitis B** responds to antiviral therapy with alpha interferon for a 4-month duration. Recent research has suggested using lamivudine (an

oral nucleoside analogue) alone or in combination with interferon for chronic infection.

   8. **Chronic hepatitis C** therapy is recommended as 3 million units of interferon alpha three times weekly for 12 months. If patients fail to respond to therapy (by evaluating ALT/HCV RNA) after 3 months, interferon should be discontinued. New research has shown promising results for combination therapy with interferon and ribavirin.

VI. **Management strategies.** The goal of management not only consists of treatment but also involves monitoring for complications, deciding whether hospitalization is required, providing education for the patient, and, if needed, referring the patient for liver transplantation.

   A. **Monitoring**
      1. **Laboratory parameters** to be followed include liver function tests, prothrombin times, serum albumin, and bilirubin. The patient should be checked clinically for ascites, signs of volume depletion, bleeding, and encephalopathy.
      2. **Hospitalization** is indicated for gastrointestinal bleeding, worsening encephalopathy, increasing azotemia, or intractable ascites.
      3. **Diagnostic paracentesis** should be considered for new-onset or worsening ascites.
      4. A **hepatoma** should be considered in patients with an unexplained clinical deterioration of chronic cirrhosis.
      5. Patients with cirrhosis from **hepatitis B** and **C infection** require regular screening every 6 months with ultrasonography and tests of α-fetoprotein levels because of the high incidence of hepatoma in this group.

   B. **Patient support for adherence to diet is essential.** Abstinence from alcohol is also essential; most patients will require considerable skill and support from the primary care physician in order to abstain (see Chapter 92).

   C. **Liver transplantation**
      1. A physician should consider referring a patient for a liver transplant when death from cirrhosis is expected in 3–6 months, no alternative therapy is available, and the patient is otherwise in reasonably good health. Primary biliary cirrhosis is the most common reason for liver transplantation today.
      2. **Absolute contraindications** include portal vein thrombosis, severe medical illness, malignancy, hepatobiliary sepsis, or lack of patient understanding. Among the **relative contraindications** are active alcoholism, human immunodeficiency virus (HIV) positivity, hepatitis B surface antigen positivity, extensive previous abdominal surgery, and lack of a family or personal support system.

VII. **Natural history and prognosis.** Cirrhosis is the eighth leading cause of death among males and the 10th leading cause of death among females. The prognosis for cirrhosis is determined by the cause and the presence of complications. Complications of cirrhosis include portal hypertension, variceal bleeding, splenomegaly, ascites, edema, and hepatic encephalopathy.

   A. **Pathophysiology of complications**
      1. **Portal hypertension.** Increased vascular resistance because of the distortion of the intrahepatic architecture leads to portal hypertension. Portal hypertension contributes to the development of splenomegaly, varices, and ascites.
      2. **Ascites** is the presence of excess fluid in the peritoneal cavity. It develops from increased portal pressure, hypoalbuminemia, secondary hyperaldosteronism, and impaired free water clearance. The same processes can lead to peripheral edema.
      3. **Hepatic encephalopathy** is a complex neuropsychiatric disorder most likely caused by one or more substances of intestinal origin that are not metabolized because of hepatocellular dysfunction and portal systemic shunting.

   B. **Patients without gastrointestinal bleeding,** encephalopathy, low albumin, and ascites have a better prognosis than those with such complications.

   C. **The prognosis of alcoholic cirrhosis** is dependent on abstinence. The 5-year survival rate is 60% or greater for patients who abstain, compared to 40% for patients who continue to drink alcohol.

   D. **In a 20-year prospective study** of cirrhotic individuals, liver failure, hepatoma, and gastrointestinal hemorrhage accounted for three-quarters of the deaths. The 5-year survival rates were 14% for cryptogenic cirrhosis and 60% for chronic active hepatitis.

REFERENCES

Gross JB: Clinician's guide to Hepatitis C. Mayo Clin Proc 1998;**73**:355.
Lai CL, et al: A one year trial of lamivudine for chronic hepatitis B: Asia Hepatitis Lamivudine Study Group. N Engl J Med 1998;**339**:61.
Management of Hepatitis C. NIH Consensus Statement. 1997;Mar 24–26;**15**(3):1.
Moseley RH: Evaluation of abnormal liver function tests. Med Clin North Am 1996; **80**:887.
Podolsky DK, Isselbacher KJ: Cirrhosis of the liver. In: Wilson JD, et al, eds. *Harrison's Principles of Internal Medicine*, 14th ed. McGraw-Hill; 1998:1704.
Prevention, Diagnosis and Management of Viral Hepatitis: A Guide for Primary Care Physicians. American Medical Association; 1995.
Runyon BA: Refractory ascites. Semin Liver Dis 1993;**13**:343.

---

76   Congestive Heart Failure

Douglas R. Smucker, MD, MPH, & Philip M. Diller, MD, PhD

I. **Definition. Heart failure (HF)** is a clinical syndrome of symptoms and signs that may include fatigue, exercise intolerance, dyspnea, peripheral edema, and pulmonary congestion. Heart failure signs and symptoms result when the heart is unable to generate cardiac output sufficient to perfuse body tissues and meet metabolic demands. The commonly used term "congestive heart failure" (CHF) may be misleading since up to one-third of ambulatory patients with HF do not manifest pulmonary or systemic congestion.

II. **Epidemiology**

  A. **Prevalence.** Close to 5 million people in the United States have HF, with 400,000 new cases diagnosed each year. HF is the primary reason for over 1 million hospital admissions each year and is the most common reason for hospital admission among persons over the age of 65. Approximately 200,000 HF-related deaths occur each year in the United States. HF prevalence is 1% among persons aged 50–59 and rises to 10% in persons over age 80.

  B. **Etiology.** Underlying the signs and symptoms of HF are diverse causes that lead to an inability of the heart to perfuse tissues and meet the metabolic demands of the body. Some of the most important predisposing factors include the following:

    1. **Hypertension.** From the Framingham study, 5143 adults without HF at baseline were followed up for an average of 14 years. Of 392 persons who developed HF, 357 (91%) had hypertension that antedated initial HF diagnosis. Hypertension accounted for 39% of new HF cases in men and 59% of new cases in women. Chronic hypertension that leads to left ventricular hypertrophy (LVH) is a common pathway in the development of HF.

    2. **Coronary artery disease (CAD).** CAD and myocardial ischemia are common causes for left ventricular (LV) systolic dysfunction. Measurable decreases in systolic function may be present for months or years before overt HF symptoms develop. Acute myocardial ischemia and myocardial infarction can result in sudden changes in systolic and diastolic ventricular function and acute HF with systemic congestion.

    3. **Other causes of cardiomyopathy.** Many diseases, infections, and toxins can cause ventricular dysfunction through direct effect on the myocardium. Viral infections, diabetes mellitus, and excessive alcohol intake are associated with cardiomyopathy and ventricular dysfunction.

    4. **Valvular disease.** Significant valvular stenosis, regurgitation, or both, particularly in the mitral or aortic valves, are well-documented factors that contribute to ventricular dysfunction.

    5. **Cardiovascular changes that occur with normal aging** help explain why HF incidence and prevalence increase with age. Arterial stiffening with increased afterload and peripheral resistance occurs with advancing age even in normotensive individuals. An increase in left ventricular mass that often occurs with aging may lead to impaired ventricular diastolic filling.

  C. **Prevention of HF.** The common etiologic factors leading to HF suggest potentially useful strategies to prevent HF. Preventive measures include adequate blood pressure control using medications known to limit or reverse LVH, smoking cessation and reversal of other treatable CAD risk factors, alcohol abstention, surgical valve replacement when appropriate, and angiotensin-converting enzyme inhibitors (ACEIs) for patients with asymptomatic LV systolic dysfunction.

III. Pathophysiology

A. The HF syndrome is a heterogeneous condition caused by various combinations of central and peripheral pathophysiologic mechanisms. These mechanisms are often dynamic, leading to wide fluctuations in measured ventricular function and physical impairment that may be observed over time in individual patients.

B. Central/cardiac factors. HF begins with impaired ventricular function that results in inadequate cardiac output, first only with exercise and eventually at rest in advanced HF. LV dysfunction may occur during systole, diastole, or both and is significantly influenced by noncardiac peripheral factors.

   1. Left ventricular systolic dysfunction

      a. Definition. A practical measure of systolic function is left ventricular ejection fraction (LVEF). LVEF is the ratio of LV stroke volume to LV end-diastolic volume. LVEF less than 45% is consistent with systolic dysfunction. LVEF less than 25–30% is considered severe systolic dysfunction.

      b. Etiology. Common causes described above lead to decreased ejection fraction and systolic dysfunction. A given patient with HF may have multiple etiologic factors. Systolic function is negatively affected by peripheral factors that cause increased afterload.

      c. Systolic dysfunction results in elevated left atrial pressures and increased left ventricular end-diastolic pressures. Right ventricular failure may develop in patients with severe LV systolic dysfunction or in those with chronic pulmonary disease. Many patients with LV systolic dysfunction also have a component of LV diastolic dysfunction.

   2. HF with normal systolic function. The typical image of HF is one of a dilated cardiomyopathy with decreased LVEF, the end-stage of which is the patient with a "big baggy heart." Approximately 40% of HF patients seen in primary care practice do not fit this "typical picture" and instead present with HF signs and symptoms and normal systolic function.

      a. Definition. Patients who meet diagnostic criteria for the HF syndrome with normal LVEF have HF with normal systolic function. There is no universally accepted cutoff for defining normal LVEF, but most experts agree that LVEF greater than 45–50% should be considered normal.

      b. Causes. Not all HF patients with normal LVEF have isolated LV diastolic dysfunction. A number of other causes for HF and normal LVEF are shown in Table 76–1. Attention should be given to rule out noncardiac causes of dyspnea, exercise intolerance, and other HF symptoms in patients with normal LVEF.

      c. Isolated LV diastolic dysfunction.

         (1) Definition. If other causes of HF with normal LVEF have been excluded, then HF is presumed to be caused by LV diastolic dysfunction. Diastolic dysfunction is characterized by decreased ventricular filling rate and volume during diastole and high end-diastolic intraventricular pressure.

         (2) Etiology. Inability of the myocardium to properly relax during diastole or conditions that lead to a "stiff" ventricle with altered passive elastic properties can impair diastolic filling of the left ventricle and greatly increase end-diastolic pressures at relatively low filling volumes. Changes in the left ventricle that occur with normal aging may predispose elderly persons toward developing diastolic dysfunction.

   3. Cardiac compensatory responses to ventricular dysfunction include chamber dilatation and hypertrophy, which often precede a measurable decrease in LVEF. Initially dilatation creates a mechanical advantage for maintaining stroke volume and cardiac output. Increases in myocardial oxygen demand and ventricular wall stress during systole (Laplace's law) that accompany ventricular dilatation and hypertrophy eventually outweigh the initial mechanical advantage of these compensatory changes.

C. Peripheral factors. Peripheral compensatory responses to diastolic or systolic LV dysfunction or both may initially help maintain cardiac function and organ perfusion, but eventually they lead to worsening HF signs and symptoms.

TABLE 76–1. COMMON CAUSES OF HEART FAILURE WITH NORMAL LVEF

Inaccurate diagnosis of HF (eg, COPD)
Inaccurate measurement of LVEF
LV systolic function overestimated by LVEF (eg, mitral regurgitation)
Episodic LV systolic dysfunction, normal at the time of evaluation (severe hypertension, ischemia, tachycardia, infection, volume overload, spontaneous variability of EF)
Obstruction of LV inflow (mitral stenosis)
Diastolic dysfunction due to:
    Abnormal LV relaxation
    Ischemia
    Hypertrophy
    Cardiomyopathies
    High-output states
    Volume overload
    Aging
    Diabetes mellitus
    Amyloidosis
    Pericardial disease

COPD, Chronic obstructive pulmonary disease; EF, ejection fraction; HF, heart failure; LV, left ventricular; LVEF, left ventricular ejection fraction.
Adapted from Dauterman KW, Massie BM, Gheorghiade M: Heart failure associated with preserved systolic function: A common and costly clinical entity. Am Heart J 1998;**135**:S310.

1. **Renin-angiotensin system (RAAS).** In response to LV dysfunction, the RAAS is activated, resulting in increased levels of angiotensin II, increased preload and afterload, and sodium and water retention. Initially, RAAS activation may help maintain or even improve LV function, but continued increases in intravascular volume and peripheral resistance become detrimental to LV function and lead to volume overload.
2. The **sympathetic nervous system** is also activated in response to LV dysfunction in order to maintain blood pressure and organ perfusion. Prolonged sympathetic activation causes chronic elevations in afterload and eventual worsening of LV function. Elevated resting plasma norepinephrine levels are independent predictors of clinical outcomes and mortality among patients with severe HF.
3. In response to RAAS and sympathetic activation, **counterregulatory hormones** are produced. Atrial natriuretic peptide (ANP) and brain natriuretic peptide (BNP) are produced from myocytes in response to increased pressures in the cardiac chambers. These peptides initially promote natriuresis and diuresis, but resistance occurs to these effects over time in chronic HF. Endothelins are endogenous peptides with strong vasoconstrictor and vasopressor activities and are found at high levels in patients with HF. Elevated levels of the natriuretic and endothelin peptides correlate with worsening HF and higher mortality rates among HF patients.

D. **Other noncardiac factors** lead to a level of exercise intolerance perceived by HF patients that has little correlation with objective measures of circulatory, ventilatory, or metabolic function during exercise.
1. Skeletal muscle underperfusion, deconditioning, altered metabolism, and impaired arteriole vasodilatation during exercise lead to easy muscle fatigue with activity.
2. HF patients show an exaggerated ventilatory response to low-level physical activity. At low work levels, HF patients are quicker than normal controls to experience subjective feelings of dyspnea, showing greater respiratory effort than would be expected for a given level of CO_2 production.

IV. **Diagnosis** HF diagnosis is based on recognition of a constellation of symptoms and clinical signs. Clinical criteria used to aid in the diagnosis of HF include the Framingham Criteria and the Boston Criteria (Table 76–2). These criteria may not identify individuals with LV dysfunction who have mild or intermittent symptoms. Some of the criteria are not readily obtainable in the ambulatory setting.

TABLE 76–2. CRITERIA USED FOR DIAGNOSIS OF CONGESTIVE HEART FAILURE (CHF) IN CLINICAL STUDIES

The Framingham Heart Study Criteria	The Boston Scale Criteria
Major criteria • Paroxysmal nocturnal dyspnea • Neck vein distension • Rales • Cardiomegaly • Acute pulmonary edema • S3 gallop • Increased venous pressure (> 16 cm) • Circulation time ≥ 25 s • Hepatojugular reflux positive **Minor criteria** • Ankle edema • Night cough • Hepatomegaly • Pleural effusion • Vital capacity reduced by one-third from predicted • Tachycardia (≥ 120) **Major or minor criterion** • Weight loss of more than 4.5 kg over 5 days in response to treatment **Definite CHF** • Two major criteria or one major and two minor criteria	**Category I: History** • Rest dyspnea (4 points) • Orthopnea (4 points) • Paroxysmal nocturnal dyspnea (3 points) • Dyspnea climbing (1 point) **Category II: Physical examination** • Heart rate: 91–110 (1 point): > 110 (2 points) • Jugular venous pressure elevation: > 6 cm H_2O plus hepatomegaly or leg edema (3 points) • Lung rales: Basilar (1 point); more than basilar (2 points) • Wheezing (3 points) • Third heart sound (3 points) **Category III: Chest radiography** • Alveolar pulmonary edema (4 points) • Interstitial pulmonary edema (3 points) • Bilateral pleural effusion (3 points) • Cardiothoracic ratio ≥ 0.50 (3 points) • Upper zone flow redistribution (2 points) **Determine score** • Point value within parentheses and no more than 4 points from each category allowed. The maximum possible is 12 points. **Definite CHF** • 8–12 points **Possible CHF** • 5–7 points

Adapted from McKee PA, Castelli WP, McNamarra PM, et al: The natural history of congestive heart failure: The Framingham study. N Engl J Med 1971;**285**:1441; and Remes J, Miettenen H, Rennanen A, et al. Validity of clinical diagnosis of heart failure in primary health care. Eur Heart J 1991;**12**:315; and Young JB: The heart failure syndrome. In: Mills RM, Young JB (eds): *Practical Approaches to the Treatment of Heart Failure.* Williams & Wilkins; 1998.

A. Symptoms

1. **Shortness of breath** can range from mild to severe.
    a. **Exertional dyspnea** may occur with any level of activity, depending on the severity of the HF syndrome.
    b. **Orthopnea.** Patients will report feeling short of breath while lying flat, may be using pillows to prop themselves up at night, or may need to sleep sitting up if HF is severe.
    c. **Paroxysmal nocturnal dyspnea (PND) or night-time cough.** Waking from sleep because of dyspnea or experiencing dry cough only while lying down are suggestive of HF.
    d. **Dyspnea at rest** occurs in advanced HF or during acute exacerbations and volume overload.
2. **Fatigue and weakness.** These symptoms are nonspecific and are in part due to abnormal autoregulation of blood flow to the extremities and muscle deconditioning.

B. Clinical signs

1. **Tachycardia** is present in many patients with HF and reflects increased adrenergic activity. Other symptoms related to increased adrenergic activity are pallor and coldness of the extremities and cyanosis of the digits (peripheral vasoconstriction).
2. **Moist crackles,** usually heard in both lung bases, are a consequence of transudation of fluid into the alveoli. Pleural effusion collecting in the bases may lead to dullness on percussion. If the bronchial mucosa are congested, then bronchospasm and associated high-pitched wheezes may also be present.

3. **Systemic venous hypertension** is suggested by a jugular venous pressure level higher than 4 cm above the sternal angle when the patient is examined sitting at a 45° angle. In advanced cases, venous pressure is so high that peripheral veins on the dorsum of the hand are dilated and fail to collapse when elevated above the shoulder.

4. **Hepatojugular reflux** is helpful in differentiating hepatomegaly resulting from HF from other conditions. The neck veins are observed, and then the right upper quadrant of the abdomen is compressed continuously for 1 minute. The patient is instructed to breathe normally. This maneuver increases venous return to the heart. In HF patients, the jugular veins expand during and immediately after compression, because of the inability of the heart to respond to the increased venous supply.

5. **Hepatomegaly** is due to congestion of the liver. If this occurs acutely, the liver may be tender to palpation. With advanced HF, the liver is still enlarged, but typically nontender.

6. **Peripheral edema** is a nonspecific yet very common sign in HF. A corresponding symptom of weight gain may often be elicited from patients. The edema is typically bilateral and symmetrical in the dependent portions of the body. For ambulatory patients, the edema worsens as the day progresses and resolves after a night's rest.

7. **Cardiomegaly** is also a nonspecific yet very common sign in HF patients. A normal apical impulse is located in the 4th or 5th intercostal space and is a brief tap. It is only palpable in about 50% of HF patients. If the apical impulse involves more than one intercostal space, cardiomegaly is present. Precordial percussion is more sensitive than the apical impulse for detecting abnormal LV size. A percussion dullness distance greater than 10.5 cm in the 5th intercostal space has a sensitivity of 91% and a specificity of 30% for increased LV size.

8. **The presence of an S_3 gallop** occurs from ventricular vibration with rapid diastolic filling. It is a low-pitched sound that is best heard with the bell of the stethoscope over the apical impulse. Having the patient in the 45° left lateral decubitus position doubles the yield.

C. **Chest roentgenogram.** Findings in HF patients may include the following:

1. **Cardiomegaly.** A cardiothoracic ratio ≥0.5 on an anteroposterior chest x-ray.

2. **Pulmonary edema** marked by equalization of the caliber of blood vessels in the apex and the lung bases, interstitial edema (development of Kerley's B lines, sharp linear densities of interlobular interstitial edema), and alveolar edema (central butterfly or cloud-like appearance of fluid around the hili).

D. **Laboratory testing in a patient with a new HF diagnosis** should include an electrocardiogram (ECG); a complete blood count; a urinalysis; tests of levels of serum creatinine, potassium, and albumin; and thyroid studies (T4, thyroid-stimulating hormone). Screening evaluation for arrhythmias using Holter monitoring is not routinely warranted.

E. **Diagnosing the type of HF and assessing the level of HF severity** are important steps in determining prognosis, outlining physiologic goals of treatment, and individualizing pharmaceutical therapy.

1. **Measuring LVEF** by echocardiography or radionuclide ventriculography determines whether the cardiac mechanism for HF is primarily systolic or diastolic dysfunction. Physiologic goals and the evidence base for specific therapeutic decisions differ for patients with LV systolic dysfunction and those who have normal LVEF and isolated diastolic dysfunction. Doppler flow measures of diastolic filling may have limited practical usefulness, since they are often abnormal in healthy elderly patients without HF and may be deceivingly normal in patients with progressively restrictive filling patterns.

2. **The level of physical impairment** from HF is a strong prognostic marker, allows the physician to monitor the effects of treatment, and determines whether patients will benefit from certain therapies (see section V). **The New York Heart Association (NYHA) Functional Classification** is the simplest and most widely used tool for assessing physical functioning (Table 76–3).

V. **Treatment.** The heterogeneous nature of HF mandates an individualized approach to treatment.

TABLE 76–3. NEW YORK HEART ASSOCIATION FUNCTIONAL CLASSIFICATION

Class I	No limitation of activity.
	Ordinary activity does not cause undue fatigue, palpitation, dyspnea or anginal pain.
Class II	Slight limitations of physical activity.
	Patient is comfortable at rest. Ordinary activity results in fatigue, palpitation, dyspnea, or anginal pain.
Class III	Marked limitation of physical activity.
	Patient is comfortable at rest, but less than ordinary activity causes fatigue, palpitation, dyspnea, or anginal pain.
Class IV	Inability to carry out physical activity without symptoms.
	Symptoms of heart failure often present at rest. Increased symptoms or discomfort with even minor physical activity.

Adapted from Criteria Committee, New York Heart Association: *Nomenclature and Criteria for Diagnosis of Diseases of the Heart and Great Vessels*, 9th ed. Boston: Little, Brown; 1994:253–256.

A. Treatment of specific underlying cardiac factors may significantly improve ventricular function and HF symptoms. Special attention should be given to surgical correction of significant valvular disease when appropriate and reversal of myocardial ischemia with transluminal angioplasty, stent placement, or surgical bypass when indicated. Ventricular rate control and conversion to sinus rhythm may improve ventricular function for patients with atrial fibrillation and HF.

B. A number of **noncardiac comorbid conditions** may affect the proper diagnosis and clinical course of HF and should be carefully assessed and treated:

1. **Chronic obstructive pulmonary disease.** Dyspnea, exercise intolerance, night-time cough, and other symptoms of chronic pulmonary disease may be misinterpreted as HF symptoms.
2. **Diabetes mellitus** may predispose patients to silent myocardial ischemia that worsens LV function, "stiff" ventricles, and diastolic dysfunction.
3. **Renal insufficiency** will influence fluid and electrolyte problems in HF and may limit usefulness or lead to changes in dosing for HF medications, particularly ACEIs and diuretics.
4. **Significant arthritis** may further limit physical activity and worsen the skeletal muscle changes that occur in HF patients.
5. **Depression and poor social support** have been shown to be important predictors of clinical outcomes, hospitalizations, and deaths among patients with ischemic heart disease.
6. **Substance abuse.** Smoking cessation should be encouraged. Patients with a component of LV dysfunction resulting from alcohol abuse may show significant functional improvement with abstention from alcohol.
7. **Hypothyroidism or hyperthyroidism** may aggravate HF symptoms.
8. **Nephrotic syndrome, hypoalbuminemia, or both** may worsen volume overload in HF.

C. Treatment of systolic dysfunction HF. Most of the large clinical trials that have influenced the treatment of HF have only included patients with systolic dysfunction. Many of these trials have supported the acceptance of ACEIs as the most effective life-saving treatment in the long-term management of HF resulting from systolic dysfunction. There is growing evidence that "triple therapy" with diuretics, ACEIs, and digoxin provides the best outcomes for HF patients with systolic dysfunction. The physiologic goals of treatment for systolic dysfunction HF include the following:

1. **Achieving and maintaining optimal volume status.** Although ACEIs should be considered first-line therapy for chronic HF resulting from systolic dysfunction, the initial presentation of the HF patient with pulmonary and systemic congestion dictates acute treatment with diuretics to lessen fluid overload and rapidly improve symptoms.

   a. **The loop diuretic furosemide** is the most frequently prescribed diuretic for treatment of volume overload in HF. Initial oral doses of 10–40 mg once a day should be administered to patients with dyspnea on exertion and signs of volume overload who do not have indications for acute hospitalization. Severe overload and pulmonary edema are indications for hospitalization and intravenous furosemide. Other considerations for prescribing diuretics in HF include the following:

(1) Some patients with mild HF can be treated effectively with thiazide diuretics. Those who have persistent volume overload on 50 mg of hydrochlorthiazide per day should be switched to an oral loop diuretic.

(2) Oral absorption of furosemide is diminished by physiologic changes in HF, particularly if the oral dose is taken on a full stomach. Torsemide is an alternative loop diuretic that is extremely well absorbed from the gastrointestinal tract in HF patients.

(3) HF patients with poor oral absorption, renal insufficiency, or both may require much higher doses of a loop diuretic to reach a threshold level for diuresis, up to a maximum of 240 mg twice a day of furosemide.

(4) Patients should be aware that nonsteroidal anti-inflammatory drugs, including frequently used over-the-counter preparations, may significantly decrease the effect of diuretics and cause volume overload.

(5) Important adverse effects of diuretics that require periodic monitoring include orthostatic hypotension, prerenal azotemia, hyponatremia, hypomagnesemia, and hypokalemia. Most patients taking 40 mg or more of furosemide daily should supplement their oral potassium intake through dietary changes, prescribed potassium supplements, or both.

(6) Once volume overload is corrected and an ACEI is initiated, the diuretic dose can often be carefully decreased or even eliminated. Some patients may only need intermittent diuretic therapy when symptoms and increases in daily weights signal a return of excess fluid volume.

b. **Adding a second diuretic** is sometimes necessary to maintain optimal fluid balance. Adding **metolazone** 2.5–10 mg per day to a daily furosemide dose can significantly increase diuresis for outpatient treatment of moderate volume overload. Prolonged combined therapy with metolazone should be avoided because of the increased risk of electrolyte depletion. **Spironolactone** can also be added to standard regimens to increase diuresis and may improve survival for patients with moderate to severe systolic dysfunction HF.

c. **Sodium restriction.** Patients should limit sodium intake to 2–3 g per day or less by avoiding salty-tasting foods, not adding salt at the table, and reading nutritional labels to choose lower-sodium food options. A sudden increase in dietary sodium intake is a frequent cause of acute fluid overload, pulmonary congestion, and hospitalization.

d. Patients should **weigh themselves daily,** record their weight, and report any gain or loss of more than 3 lbs from their baseline weight. Baseline weight is determined when the patient is at optimal fluid balance on a stable medical regimen. Reliable patients may be instructed to increase daily diuretic dose for 2–4 days when they see an increase in daily weights.

2. **Decreasing preload and afterload by blunting the exaggerated peripheral compensatory response** has, as its foundation, treatment with ACEIs, which should be considered first-line therapy for HF resulting from systolic dysfunction.

a. **Angiotensin-converting enzyme inhibitors (ACEIs).** Many clinical trials have provided consistent evidence that ACEIs result in decreased symptoms, improved quality of life, fewer hospitalizations, and reductions in mortality for patients with NYHA class II–IV HF. In addition, ACEIs slow the progression to HF among patients with asymptomatic LV systolic dysfunction. No other class of medication can claim the same strength of evidence or range of positive outcomes for HF.

(1) Contraindications to ACEI use include pregnancy, bilateral renal artery stenosis, angioedema or other allergic responses, or documented persistent intolerance to ACEI (symptomatic hypotension, severe renal dysfunction, hyperkalemia, or cough).

(2) The positive effects of ACEI probably apply to all available drugs in this class, but preference should be given to drugs with the most

evidence for improved clinical outcomes. Enalapril, captopril, lisino-pril, and ramipril have the strongest evidence for mortality reductions.

(3) To minimize the risk of symptomatic hypotension, one-half the nor-mal starting dose should be given to patients with hyponatremia (<135 meq/L), recent increase in diuretic dose, serum creatinine lev-els >1.7 mg/dL, and patients over 75 years of age. Patients at high risk for symptomatic hypotension should be given a test dose of a short-acting ACEI (captopril 6.25 mg) and be observed in the physi-cian's office for 2 hours before starting daily ACEI therapy.

(4) Blood urea nitrogen (BUN), serum creatinine and potassium con-centrations, and blood pressure should be determined before start-ing ACEI therapy, 1–3 weeks after initiating therapy, after changes in dose, and every 3–4 months thereafter. The average increase in creatinine is 0.4 mg/dL, with most of the change observed in the first 6 weeks. The reversible renal function caused by ACEIs may resolve with a careful decrease in diuretic dose. As long as creatinine sta-bilizes at approximately 3.5 or less, and hyperkalemia or sympto-matic hypotension are not persistent, ACEIs should be continued and titrated up to target doses (Table 76–4). Systolic blood pressure of 90–100 should not deter the physician from titrating to target doses unless hypotension becomes symptomatic.

(5) Nonproductive cough is a common adverse effect of ACEIs, sec-ondary to increased bradykinin levels. Cough may not be attribut-able to ACEIs in a given HF patient, since it is a common HF symp-tom. Only 1–2.5% of patients in clinical trials discontinued ACEI because of cough. For patients with cough on an initial ACEI trial, switching to an alternative ACEI may diminish cough symptoms.

b. For patients unable to use ACEIs, a trial of **hydralazine and isosorbide dinitrate (HYD-ISDN)** should be initiated to decrease preload and after-load (Table 76–4). Patients at high risk for symptomatic hypotension should receive lower initial doses and be monitored for adverse effects. The HYD-ISDN combination has shown decreased mortality in HF clini-cal trials.

c. **Angiotensin II receptor antagonists (A II)** are another promising alter-native therapy for patients who cannot use ACEIs. Current clinical trials will help clarify the role of these drugs alone or in combination with ACEI. A II drugs do not affect bradykinin levels and thus do not induce angio-edema and cough to the same extent as ACEIs.

d. The first- and second-generation **calcium channel blockers** such as nifedipine, diltiazem, and nicardipine may worsen systolic dysfunction

TABLE 76–4. TARGET DOSES-FOR ACEIs AND HYD-ISDN COMBINATION

	Initial Dose (mg)	Target Dose (mg)	Recommended Maximum Dose (mg)
Preferred ACEIs (see text)			
Captopril[1]	6.25–12.5 tid	50 tid	100 qid
Enalapril	2.5 bid	10 bid	20 bid
Lisinopril	5 qd	20 qd	40 qd
Ramipril	1 bid	5 bid	10 bid
Other ACEIs indicated for heart failure			
Fosinopril	5 qd	20 qd	40 qd
Quinapril	5 bid	20 bid	20 bid
Hydralazine-ISDN combination			
Hydralazine (HYD)	25 tid	75 qid	150 qid
Isosorbide dinitrate (ISDN)	10 tid	40 tid	80 tid

ACEIs, Angiotensin-converting enzyme inhibitors.
[1] Give a single dose of captopril 6.25 mg with observation of the patient for 2 hours for patients at high risk for symptomatic hypotension.

symptoms because of their negative inotropic effects. Amlodipine is better tolerated, with evidence of a neutral if not beneficial effect on HF survival. Amlodipine can be considered for patients with continued hypertension who take ACEI and diuretics, or those with symptomatic ischemia not controlled by nitrates, beta blockers, or both.

   e. Exercise training is an effective intervention that reverses some of the exaggerated peripheral compensatory changes in patients with stable mild to moderate (class I–III) systolic dysfunction HF. A series of randomized trials have shown improvements in a number of peripheral hemodynamic parameters, with diminished symptoms and improved physical functioning. Most trials have used supervised aerobic exercise on treadmills or stationary cycles. The long-term effect of exercise training on HF mortality has not been studied.

3. **Delaying the clinical progression of systolic dysfunction HF** and further improving symptoms may be accomplished with two other pharmaceutical interventions. One has been a part of HF treatment for some 200 years (cardiac glycosides/digoxin), while the other has gained acceptance only in recent years (beta blockers/carvedilol).

   a. Digoxin is considered the preferred agent among a number of available cardiac glycoside preparations. Digoxin neither improves nor worsens HF survival but does decrease symptoms, increase exercise capacity, and decrease the need for hospitalization in systolic dysfunction HF. Digoxin is particularly appropriate for patients who remain symptomatic on ACEI and diuretics, and for patients with atrial fibrillation and rapid ventricular response.

      (1) Loading doses are generally unnecessary. A daily oral dose of 0.125–0.25 mg will lead to steady-state serum levels in 1–2 weeks.

      (2) Once a steady state is reached, a serum digoxin level, an ECG, BUN/creatinine levels, and serum electrolytes should be obtained.

      (3) Results of the Digitalis Investigation Group (DIG) trial suggest that a serum concentration in the lower therapeutic range (0.7–1.2 ng/mL) retains the clinical benefit of digoxin while avoiding toxicity. Levels should be checked yearly and at the time of significant changes in HF symptoms or renal function.

   b. Until recent years, HF was considered an absolute contraindication for prescribing **β-adrenergic blockers.** Recent clinical trials have demonstrated improved symptoms, increased LV function, and prevention of HF progression when beta blockers are added to standard HF therapy. Metoprolol and bisoprolol have shown promise in initial trials. **Carvedilol** is a unique nonselective beta blocker with alpha-blocker vasodilation activity and antioxidant qualities and is the first beta blocker approved by the Food and Drug Administration for treatment of HF.

      (1) Carvedilol prescription requires proper patient selection and careful monitoring during dose titration (Table 76–5). It should be considered only for patients with stable, moderate HF (class II, III) who are already taking standard HF therapy. It is not indicated for advanced HF. Primary care physicians not familiar with dose titration should consult with a cardiologist before prescribing carvedilol.

      (2) Patients will frequently experience worsening symptoms, dizziness, and fatigue resulting from the initial vasodilation from carvedilol. With reassurance and persistence, most patients will have improved symptoms with further up-titration of the drug. Only 5% of patients in carvedilol trials stopped the drug because of adverse effects.

      (3) Some patients may have difficulty affording carvedilol at a wholesale cost of approximately $3 per day.

D. **Isolated diastolic dysfunction.** In comparison to the large evidence base for treating systolic dysfunction, there are minimal data available to guide the treatment of HF resulting from diastolic dysfunction. Treatment is largely empiric and directed toward reversing presumed underlying pathophysiology.

   1. The methods for achieving and maintaining optimal fluid balance are similar to those described for systolic dysfunction. Rapid or over-diuresis should be avoided since small changes in intravascular volume may cause significant decreases in diastolic filling and cardiac output.

TABLE 76–5. INITIATION AND TITRATION OF CARVEDILOL FOR PATIENTS WITH HF

1) Become familiar with the manufacturer's printed drug information
2) Indicated for clinically stable NYHA class II–III already on standard HF therapy
3) Contraindications: asthma, Class IV HF, hepatic impairment, severe bradycardia, second- or third-degree AV block, sensitivity to carvedilol
4) Give a single dose of 3.125 mg followed by 1-hour observation for adverse symptoms
5) Inform patient of potential adverse effects
6) Instruct patient for daily weights, to call if weight gain of 2–3 lbs
7) Begin 3.125 mg bid to be taken with food
8) Return visit in 2 weeks; monitor symptoms, weight, volume status, blood pressure
9) Reassure the patient that symptoms from initial vasodilation often diminish with time (fatigue, dizziness)
10) Double the daily dose at every 2-week follow-up visit as tolerated to maximum dose:
    Patients weighing <85 kg (187 lbs): 25 mg bid maximum
    Patients weighing >85 kg (187 lbs): 50 mg bid maximum
11) Continue to monitor for adverse symptoms, change in volume status, symptomatic hypotension
12) Monitor for possible effects on lipid and blood sugar levels

AV, Atrioventricular; HF, heart failure; NYHA, New York Heart Association.
Adapted from Vanderhoff BT, Ruppel HM: Carvedilol: The new role of beta-blockers in congestive heart failure. Am Fam Physician 1998;**58**:1627.

2. Treatment of cardiac ischemia may improve diastolic function. Nitrates, beta blockers, and calcium channel blockers may all be useful, but there is little direct evidence for their effectiveness in treating diastolic dysfunction.
3. Effective treatment of hypertension is indicated with drugs that may limit or even reverse LVH and thus improve the compliance of the ventricle. Beta blockers are attractive in this regard in addition to their anti-ischemic and rate-limiting properties, all of which may improve diastolic filling. ACEIs are often appropriate, but compared with systolic dysfunction there is no evidence for specific indications for diastolic dysfunction HF.
4. Conversion of atrial fibrillation to sinus rhythm will restore the atrial component of diastolic filling and may improve cardiac output. If conversion to sinus rhythm is not feasible, then ventricular rate control with a rate-limiting calcium channel blocker or digoxin may allow more complete ventricular filling in diastole.
5. Theoretically digoxin would not be indicated for patients with diastolic dysfunction; however, a subgroup analysis of the recent DIG clinical trial showed surprising improvement in clinical outcomes for the small number of patients in the study who had normal LVEF. Until more evidence is available, however, digoxin should be reserved for diastolic dysfunction patients who have a separate indication such as atrial fibrillation.

VI. **Management strategies**
   A. **Patient education and self-care** are important components of maintaining clinical stability. Suggested topics for patient, family, and caregiver education and counseling are outlined in the Agency for Health Care Policy and Research guidelines for heart failure treatment. Topics include explanation of symptoms, causes, and prognosis; activity recommendations including exercise prescription when appropriate; proper use of medications; sodium restriction; daily weights; and instructions for monitoring symptoms and when to contact the patient's physician (Table 76–6).
   B. **Case management strategies** such as the MULTIFIT program have been shown to improve quality of life and decrease the need for hospitalization. Nurse case managers work with patients to improve patient education, promote adherence to medication and dietary regimens, improve home-based self monitoring, and co-ordinate, medical, community, and social support resources.
   C. **Consultation or referral** to a cardiologist or HF specialty clinic should be considered for patients who remain symptomatic on standard HF therapy, have underlying valvular or pericardial infiltrative disease, or have potentially reversible ischemic heart disease. Patients may also benefit from co-management with a cardiologist to ensure reaching target doses of an ACEI or to initiate a new therapy such as carvedilol. Those with symptomatic atrial or ventricular tachyarrhythmias should also be assessed by a cardiologist. Evaluation for possible cardiac transplantation includes exercise evaluation with measurement of maximal oxy-

TABLE 76–6. SPECIFIC INSTRUCTIONS FOR PATIENTS ABOUT WHEN TO CONTACT A PHYSICIAN'S OFFICE

Weight gain $\geq$ 3 lbs, not responding to predesignated diuretic change
Uncertainty about how to increase diuretics
New swelling of the feet or abdomen
Worsening shortness of breath with mild exercise
Onset of inability to sleep flat in bed or awakening from sleep because of shortness of breath
Worsening cough
Persistent nausea/vomiting or inability to eat
Worsening dizziness or new spells of sudden dizziness not related to sudden changes in body position
Prolonged palpitations
If you, the patient, experience any sudden severe symptoms, you may need to call 911 or the equivalent emergency phone number to arrange a trip to the emergency room. (These sudden severe symptoms may include **but are not limited to** chest pain, severe shortness of breath, loss of consciousness not due to sudden standing, new cold or painful arm or foot, sudden new visual changes, or impairment of speech or strength in an extremity.)

Note: This is only a sample list and is not intended to include all potential problems for which a patient with heart failure should seek urgent medical advice.
Reprinted with permission from Goldman L, Braunwald E: *Primary Cardiology.* Philadelphia: Saunders; 1998:326.

gen uptake (VO_2max). Patients with VO_2max <14 mL/kg/min and no severe co-morbid conditions may be candidates for transplantation.

VII. Natural history and prognosis

A. Exacerbations and hospitalization frequently occur in HF. More than 40% of hospitalized HF patients require readmission to the hospital within 6 months of discharge. Patients often experience a fluctuating clinical course marked by periods of fluid overload and diminished exercise tolerance. Common preventable reasons leading to hospitalization include poor adherence to sodium restriction or medication regimens, inadequate social support systems, or failure to seek medical attention when symptoms worsen or daily weights increase. Hospital rates are similar for patients with systolic and diastolic dysfunction HF.

B. Mortality risk for HF patients is substantial, with annual rates as high as 50% mortality for patients with advanced disease (NYHA class IV). LVEF is one of the most consistent predictors of mortality, with a marked increase in mortality risk for patients with LVEF less than 20%. Hyponatremia, elevated plasma norepinephrine levels, and significant ventricular arrhythmias are also independent markers for increased mortality risk. Mortality rates are lowest for HF patients with normal LVEF.

REFERENCES

Dauterman KW, Massie BM, Gheorghiade M: Heart failure associated with preserved systolic function: A common and costly clinical entity. Am Heart J 1998;**135**:S310.

D.I.G. (The Digitalis Investigation Group): The effect of digoxin on mortality and morbidity in patients with heart failure. N Engl J Med 1997;**336**:525.

Goldman L, Braunwald E: *Primary Cardiology.* Saunders; 1998.

Konstam M, Dracup K, Baker D, et al: *Heart Failure: Evaluation and Care of Patients with Left-Ventricular Systolic Dysfunction.* Clinical Practice Guideline No. 11. AHCPR Publication No. 94-0612. Agency for Health Care Policy and Research, Public Health Service, US Department of Health and Human Services; 1994.

McKelvie RS, Teo KK, McCartney, et al: Effects of exercise training in patients with congestive heart failure: A critical review. J Am Coll Cardiol 1995;**25**:789.

Vanderhoff BT, Ruppel HM: Carvedilol: The new role of beta-blockers in congestive heart failure. Am Fam Physician 1998;**58**:1627.

Vasan R, Larson MG, Benjamin EJ, et al: Left ventricular dilatation and the risk of congestive heart failure in people without myocardial infarction. N Engl J Med 1997;**336**:1350.

West JA, Miller NH, Parker KM, et al: A comprehensive management system for heart failure improves clinical outcomes and reduces medical resource utilization (MULTIFIT). Am J Cardiol 1997;**79**:58.

Wilson JR, Mancini DM: Factors contributing to the exercise limitation of heart failure. J Am Coll Cardiol 1993;**22**(suppl A):93A.

Young JB, Gheorghiade M, Uretsky BF, et al: Superiority of "triple" drug therapy in heart failure: Insights from the PROVED and RADIANCE trials. J Am Coll Cardiol 1998;**32**:686.

77   Dementia

Richard J. Botelho, MD, & William J. Hall, MD

I. **Definition.** Dementia is defined as an acquired decline in mental function, which affects memory, cognition, language, judgment, visual-spatial skills, and personality.

II. **Differential diagnosis.** Dementia must be differentiated from other causes of cognitive impairment, such as depression, delirium, and normative aging. Older persons with age-related memory impairment have difficulties with memory (eg, difficulty with immediate recall of specific information such as telephone numbers and names), but recognition of other important areas of cognition are not affected. These changes are not associated with a disability.

   A. **Common causes.** Composite findings from 25 studies have revealed that dementia is commonly caused by the following conditions: Alzheimer's disease (56.8%), multi-infarct dementia (13.3%), depression (4.5%), excessive consumption of alcohol (4.2%), and drugs (1.5%). Other conditions account for 19.7% of dementia cases.

   B. **Nonreversible types of dementia.** Other diagnoses are frontal lobe dementia, Wernicke–Korsakoff encephalopathy (80% nonreversible), Parkinson's disease, Huntington's chorea, AIDS dementia, dementia associated with Down syndrome, Creutzfeldt–Jakob disease, chronic renal failure, multiple sclerosis, supranuclear palsy, and Pick's disease.

   C. **Reversible or arrestable types of dementias.** In 11 studies, reversible causes of dementia were identified in 11% of patients. Treating the reversible causes resulted in partial (27%) to full (73%) resolution of dementia on follow-up. The most common causes of reversible dementia were drugs (28.2%), depression (26.2%), and metabolic factors (15.5%) (Table 77–1).

   D. **Distinguishing between depression and dementia.** Patients with depression may present with a dementia, so-called *depressive pseudodementia*. Ten percent of all patients with an initial diagnosis of dementia have a primary depressive illness, and less commonly, dementia may appear as depression. Coexisting depression should be treated to improve mood as well as functional and cognitive abilities. Table 77–2 lists the typical differences between these two conditions.

III. **Epidemiology.** Some degree of dementia affects about 1% of persons aged 60–64. Data from studies of dementia prevalence and age from Europe and North America indicate that rates double about every 5 years, so that 35–40% of persons age 85 and above will have some degree of dementia.

   In aggregate:

   A. In the United States, 1.2 million persons have severe dementia, and 2.7 million have moderate dementia.

   B. People over the age of 85 make up the fastest-growing segment of the population. Patients over the age of 80 have an annual 4% prevalence of dementia. Fifty percent of nursing home patients have dementia, and 70% of patients with dementia are community residents. Dementia is the fourth leading cause of death in the elderly.

IV. **Pathophysiology.** The pathology of Alzheimer's dementia and multi-infarct dementia is described below. These two types account for 70% of all cases of dementia.

   A. **Alzheimer's disease.** The two principal histologic changes are neurofibrillary tangles and neuritic plaques in the hippocampus and cerebral cortex. Amyloid filaments are found in the extracellular deposits in the center of neuritic plaques. Alzheimer's disease is not simply a cholinergic deficit but involves deficiency of a number of other neuropeptides and neurotransmitters. Other changes include loss of neurons, decreased number of synapses, and granular vascular degeneration, which may lead to memory loss. Considerable interest has focused on the discovery of the prominent presence of apolipoprotein in amyloid plaques and neurofibrillary tangles. One gene allele, known as *apolipoprotein E4* (apo E4) with a locus on chromosome 19, is a risk factor for late-onset sporadic Alzheimer's disease. Despite the potential pathogenetic significance of these findings, population-based screening for apo E4 to identify Alzheimer's disease is not recommended by most authorities.

TABLE 77–1. CAUSES OF REVERSIBLE DEMENTIA

Drugs
  Anticholinergics
  Antihypertensives
  Digitalis and its derivatives
  Psychotropic drugs
  Analgesics
  Antihistamines
  Antiparkinsonian drugs
Depression
Endocrine and metabolic conditions
  Hypothyroidism
  Hypopituitarism
  Parathyroid disorders
  "Silent" hyperthyroidism of late onset
  Wilson's disease
  Hypoxia secondary to pulmonary disease
  Hyponatremia
Vascular conditions
  Cranial arteritis
  Subacute bacterial endocarditis
Nutritional problems
  Thiamine deficiency
  Vitamin B_{12} deficiency
  Niacin deficiency
  Folate deficiency
Space-occupying brain lesions
  Particularly frontal and temporal lobes tumors
  Subdural hematoma
  Brain abscesses
Chronic central nervous system infections
  Syphilis
  Cryptococcus
  Whipple's disease
  AIDS
Normal pressure hydrocephalus

TABLE 77–2. DISTINGUISHING DEMENTIA FROM DEPRESSION

Dementia	Depression
Insidious onset	Abrupt onset
Long duration	Short duration
No psychiatric history	Often previous psychiatric history (including undiagnosed depressive episodes)
Conceals disability (often unaware of memory loss)	Highlights disabilities (in particular, complains of the memory loss)
"Near-miss" answers	"Don't know" answers
Day-to-day fluctuation in mood	Diurnal variation in mood, but mood generally more consistent
Stable cognitive loss	Fluctuating cognitive loss
Tries hard to perform but is unconcerned by losses	Often does not try so hard but is more distressed by losses
Memory loss greatest for recent events	Equal memory loss for recent and remote events
Memory loss occurs first	Depressed mood (if present) occurs first
Associated with unsociability, uncooperativeness, hostility, emotional instability, confusion, disorientation, and reduced alertness	Associated with depressed or anxious mood, sleep disturbance, appetite disturbance, and suicidal thoughts

From Gall CM, Black PMC: Dementia. Am Fam Physician 1989;**39**:241.

B. Vascular dementias. Vascular dementias arise from cerebral ischemia resulting from hypoxia or vascular insufficiency from specific arterial occlusions and hemorrhage. The five types of vascular dementia are described below:

1. Multi-infarct, usually associated with lesions of the major (anterior, middle, posterior) cerebral arteries, are characterized by specific cortical dysfunction, such as aphasia and apraxia.
2. Lacunar states, usually involving the lenticulostriate vessels, are manifested by psychomotor slowing.
3. Strategic infarcts involve specific areas, commonly branches of the middle cerebral arteries, and may be associated with right–left disorientation, anomia, and selected agnosia states.
4. Binswanger's disease, related to ischemia of the medullary white matter arteries, is associated with psychomotor slowing and prominent memory defects.
5. Mixed patterns involving both cortical and subcortical arteries are manifested by mixed clinical presentations.

V. Diagnosis. The history, physical examination, and laboratory tests should rule out the possibility of reversible causes for dementia and identify exacerbating factors such as confusional states (see Chapter 14), drug effects, or depression.

A. Symptoms and signs

1. The symptoms of dementia include memory disturbance; impaired judgment and reasoning; lack of insight; aphasic-agonistic-apraxic deficits; and changes in behavior, motivation, affect, and personality.
2. Alzheimer's disease and multi-infarct dementia have heterogeneous presentations, but their characteristics help the physician clinically differentiate these two conditions. Clinical observations and laboratory tests are nearly 90% accurate in diagnosing Alzheimer's disease, although this condition can be definitively diagnosed only by brain biopsy or autopsy. The Hachinski score can be used to differentiate clinically between Alzheimer's disease and multi-infarct dementia (Table 77–3). This scoring system is more useful in cases of moderate to severe dementia.

B. Tests. Although Alzheimer's disease cannot be diagnosed solely by the use of simple office-based tests of global cognitive function, several well-standardized tools are suitable for screening for dementia.

1. Mental status examination

a. The short portable mental status questionnaire has a specificity greater than 90% but a sensitivity as low as 50% for dementia (Table 77–4). More than three errors identifies a person as impaired. The final score takes into consideration educational level; one point is subtracted from

TABLE 77–3. HACHINSKI SCORE

Feature	Possible Score
1. Abrupt onset	2
2. Stepwise deterioration	1
3. Fluctuating course	2
4. Nocturnal confusion	1
5. Emotional lability	1
6. Relative preservation of personality	1
7. Depression	1
8. Somatic complaints	1
9. History of hypertension	1
10. History of stroke	2
11. Evidence of associated arteriosclerosis	1
12. Focal neurological symptoms	2
13. Focal neurological signs	2

A score of 4 or less is indicative of a high probability of Alzheimer's disease. A score of 7 or more is indicative of multi-infarct dementia.

Reproduced, with permission, from Hachinski VC, Iliff LD, Zinka E, et al: Cerebral blood flow in dementia. Arch Neurol 1975;**32**:632.

TABLE 77–4. THE SHORT PORTABLE MENTAL STATUS QUESTIONNAIRE

1. What is the date today?
2. What day of the week is it?
3. What is the name of this place?
4. What is your telephone number?
   If the patient does not have a phone: What is your street address?
5. How old are you?
6. When were you born?
7. Who is the president of the United States now?
8. Who was the president just before that?
9. What was your mother's maiden name?
10. Subtract 3 from 20 and keep subtracting 3 from each new number you get, all the way down.

Reproduced, with permission, from Pfeiffer E: A short portable mental status questionnaire for the assessment of organic brain deficit in elderly patients. J Am Genet Soc 1975;**23**:433.

the error score if the patient has only a grade school education, and one point is added to the score if the patient has had education beyond a high school level. Although this questionnaire can conveniently be used by primary care physicians, its usefulness is limited by its low sensitivity.

  b. The Mini-Mental State Questionnaire (MMS) also tests memory, use of written and spoken language, and construction ability (Table 77–5). A score below 24 indicates cognitive impairment. The MMS questionnaire, which may have a sensitivity of 90%, is easily administered in the primary care setting.

  c. Neuropsychological tests may be indicated in special cases, although such tests have some limitations in the diagnosis of earlier stages of dementia. For example, since the dementing process may be characterized by changes in motivation, judgment, or behavior while the other intellectual functions remain relatively intact, highly gifted persons may still score in the normal or superior range. Nevertheless, these standardized

TABLE 77–5. THE MINI-MENTAL STATE QUESTIONNAIRE

	Maximum Score
Orientation	
What is the (year) (season) (date) (day) (month)?	5
Where are we (state) (county) (town) (hospital) (floor)?	5
Registration	
Name three objects. Patients have 1 second to name each one. Then ask the patient to name all three after you have said them. Give one point for each correct answer. Repeat them until he or she learns all three. Count trials and record number.	3
Attention and Calculation	
Begin with 100 and count backward by 7 (stop after five answers). Alternatively, spell "world" backward.	5
Recall	
Ask for the three objects learned above.	3
Language	
Show the patient a pencil and a watch and ask the patient to name them.	2
Have the patient repeat the following statement: "No 'ifs,' 'ands,' or 'buts.' "	1
Have the patient obey the following three-stage command: "Take a paper in your right hand, fold it in half, and put it on the floor."	3
Have the patient read and obey the following written command: "Close your eyes."	1
Have the patient write a sentence.	1
Have the patient copy a design (eg, complex polygon).	1

tests may lead to more appropriate and comprehensive treatment and management. They have the added advantage of quantitating not only deficiencies, but also residual strengths, and they are standardized for age and educational attainment.

2. **Laboratory tests.** The use of routine tests may be modified according to the individual circumstances of the patient. The depth of the dementia work-up should be determined by the extent to which a reversible cause is suspected on the basis of the history and physical examination. A low probability of reversible causes does not warrant an elaborate work-up. Tests listed for the exhaustive work-up may be reserved for diagnostic dilemmas. However, many authorities recommend a head computed tomography (CT) scan for all patients presenting with dementia. CT scanning may have the greatest usefulness in confirming a diagnosis of vascular dementia. However, small lacunar infarcts on a head CT scan do not confirm the diagnosis of multi-infarct dementia, and it has been suggested that multiple cerebral infarcts must exceed 150–200 mL in volume to cause dementia.

   a. **Routine tests** to be ordered on all patients with dementia are complete blood (CBC) count to rule out anemia (a raised white blood cell [WBC] count may indicate infection), an electrolyte panel to rule out electrolyte imbalance and diabetes mellitus, screening metabolic panel to rule out renal failure, thyroid function tests to rule out hypothyroidism, tests for levels of vitamin B_{12} and folate to rule out vitamin deficiency, a VDRL to rule out syphilis, and urinalysis to rule out urinary tract infections.

   b. **Optional tests** include an electrocardiogram (ECG) to rule out silent myocardial infarction and arrhythmias, a chest x-ray to rule out occult pneumonia, and HIV tests to rule out AIDS dementia.

   c. An **elaborate work-up** involves a CT scan or magnetic resonance imaging (MRI) to rule out subdural hematoma, neoplasm, infarcts, and so on; an electroencephalogram (EEG) to rule out delirium; formal psychiatric assessment to rule out depression; neuropsychological assessment; and speech and language analysis.

   d. **Other tests** that have specific indications are MRI for suspected AIDS dementia, lumbar puncture for possible active central nervous system infection or vasculitis, and carotid studies for suspected carotid stenosis causing multi-infarct dementia.

VI. Treatment

A. Disease-specific treatments

1. **Alzheimer's dementia.** Donepezil hydrochloride (Aricept) is a selective acetylcholinesterase inhibitor developed for the treatment of Alzheimer's disease. The dose is 5–10 mg once a day. Acetylcholinesterase inhibitors increase the acetylcholine available at cortical synapses, thereby offering the potential for improved memory and cognitive function. About 50–60% of patients experience clinically apparent improvement after 9–12 weeks of treatment. Some cholinergic symptoms (nausea, diarrhea) limit the drug's effectiveness in some patients, but side effects are much less frequent compared with those of other available agents. No hepatotoxicity has been observed. In addition, vitamin E supplementation (400–800 IU twice daily), estrogen therapy in women, and gingko biloba (80–250 mg two to three times a day) are promising neuroprotective agents.

2. **Multi-infarct dementia.** Treatment should be aimed at conditions causing the infarctions (such as carotid stenosis, cardiac embolization, cerebral vasculitis, and hypertension) to arrest the progression of the dementia. In selected cases, aspirin (81–325 mg qd) or ticlopidine (250 mg twice a day) may be useful. In hypertensive multi-infarct dementia, slight improvement in cognition and clinical course has been shown to correlate with control of systolic blood pressure within the range of 135–150 mm Hg. If systolic blood pressure was reduced below this level, patients with multi-infarct dementia deteriorated. Normotensive patients had improved cognition associated with cessation of cigarette smoking.

B. Treatment of behavioral symptoms

1. **Agitation** includes inappropriate verbal, vocal, or motor behaviors. Medical conditions that cause agitation such as pain, delirium, reversible dementias,

environmental changes, and family conflicts must be identified. Simple non-pharmacologic treatments such as simplifying tasks presented to the patient, one-on-one nursing, behavior modification, and family education may reduce the level of agitation. All these measures should be exhausted before pharmacologic therapy is attempted. Demented patients are especially prone to the side effects of psychotropic drugs, such as falls, sedative effect, and increased confusion. Agitation that fails to respond to these measures may require the kinds of drugs described in the following sections.

   a. **Antipsychotic drugs** appear to benefit irritability, suspiciousness, and paranoia, but are less likely to affect wandering, calling out, and inappropriate behavior. Antipsychotics may give a favorable response in only one-third of cases. The starting dose of antipsychotic drugs should be small, eg, 0.25–0.5 mg of **haloperidol,** one to four tablets per day. The choice of antipsychotics should be individualized based on the risks of side effects (see Chapter 98). When extrapyramidal side effects are of concern, high-potency antipsychotics, such as haloperidol, should be avoided. Low-potency antipsychotics, such as **thioridazine,** 10–20 mg up to 100–200 mg daily, may be used in single or divided doses depending upon when symptoms are most problematic. However, these drugs have greater anticholinergic side effects, such as orthostatic hypotension. There are specific indications for the general use of neuroleptics cited by OBRA (Omnibus Budget Reconciliation Act) governing the use of these agents. The following are three important guidelines for the use of antipsychotic agents in demented patients:

   (1) There should be evidence that the agitated behavior is harmful to the patient (versus an inconvenience to staff).

   (2) Types of behavior must be specifically described and quantitated. The designation "agitation" is not sufficient.

   (3) There should be documentation of attempts to periodically taper or withdraw the medication.

   b. **Other medications** have been advocated for particular symptoms of agitation. β-Adrenergic blockers such as propranolol, 60–120 mg in divided doses, may be effective in selected patients. Carbamazepine is an anticonvulsant that may control impulsivity and aggression, with initial doses of 50–100 mg twice daily and maintenance doses up to 1000 mg daily. Patients who exhibit manic-like symptoms with pressured speech, hyperactivity, and decreased sleep may respond to lithium and carbamazepine. Lithium should be started at 50 mg twice daily. Patients with negativistic irritable behavior or anxious mood may respond to antidepressants. Patients with panic episodes (catastrophic reactions) may respond to benzodiazepines such as **lorazepam,** beginning at 0.5 mg twice daily to a maximum of 6 mg, or **oxazepam,** starting at 10 mg two or three times daily up to a maximum of 120 mg. A family physician may need to consult a geriatric or psychiatric specialist before using these drugs.

2. **Depression.** All demented patients must be assessed for depression. Drug treatment may be necessary. Antidepressants should be selected for their low anticholinergic effects. Initial dosages of **nortriptyline** (10 mg daily), **desipramine** (10 mg daily), or trazodone (25 mg daily) have been suggested. These dosages should be increased in 10- to 25-mg increments every fourth day until a therapeutic effect is achieved, usually in 4–8 weeks. The maximum daily dosage for nortriptyline is 150 mg, for desipramine 300 mg, and for trazodone 600 mg. The serotoninergic antidepressants, such as fluoxetine, seem to have fewer central nervous system side effects than tricyclic agents and may ultimately have greater usefulness in the adjunctive treatment of demented states. However, there is no evidence that these newer agents are more effective nor have less risk for potential injurious falls.

3. **Sleep disturbance.** The use of **benzodiazepines** should be minimized, but may be helpful in treating insomnia for short-term purposes. Short-acting benzodiazepines should be given at bedtime in dosages that are as low as possible. Examples are **temazepam** (15 mg), **lorazepam** (0.5 mg), and **alprazolam** (0.25 mg).

VII. Management strategies. The family physician should schedule family conferences to present the diagnosis and to collaborate with the family in developing goals for managing the dementing illness.

  A. Management goals for the patient. The goals for the patient are to maintain a safe physical and emotional environment, to preserve functional abilities, and to identify and treat factors exacerbating the dementing illness. In early dementia, the physician can advise the family when the patient should stop working and driving. As the disease progresses, the family physician needs to monitor for dental and foot problems, adequacy of nutrition, and visual and hearing impairments. Families should encourage the patient to stop drinking alcohol and smoking cigarettes.

  The family physician is well advised to clarify treatment guidelines early in the course of the illness while the patient is still competent. A living will, a health care proxy, or a designated power of attorney can help to determine treatment guidelines, which can assist the physician in providing appropriate levels of medical care to the patient.

  B. Management goals for the family. The goals for family and caregivers are to learn how to manage specific behavioral problems (Table 77–6), how to cope with the consequences of caregiving (see references), and how to plan home placement. The physician can also advise the family when medications may be necessary to manage these behavioral problems.

  1. Problems for caregivers. Patients with dementia stress the economic and psychological resources of the family. During this process, family and caregivers often become socially isolated and emotionally distressed. Table 77–7 lists problems often identified by caregivers.

  a. The National Alzheimer's Disease and Related Disorders Association (ADRDA) is an advocacy organization for families. Families can subscribe to ADRDA's newsletter and obtain educational materials from local chapters. Local chapters organize self-help groups; can advise families how to coordinate family, informal, and professional resources, such as aide service and respite care; and may be able to advise families about financial planning regarding the care of their relative.

  b. Relatives of the demented patient sometimes express concerns about whether they themselves will inherit the same condition. First-degree relatives of patients with Alzheimer's disease are four times more likely to develop the disease than members of the general population. The cumulative incidence of Alzheimer's disease in first-degree relatives reaches 50% by age 87. Rarely is the disease inherited as an autosomal dominant gene.

  2. Nursing home placement. Most families strive to keep their loved ones at home and often resist entertaining the idea of nursing home placement. The physician can help the family keep their relative out of an institution. Concurrently, the physician can also encourage the family to gather information about nursing homes, even though it is at present thought to be unnecessary.

TABLE 77–6. BEHAVIORAL PROBLEMS IN DEMENTED PATIENTS

Memory disturbance (100%/45%)[1]	Hitting (32%/50%)[1]
Night waking	Demanding critical behavior
Hiding things	Smoking
Suspiciousness (63%/48%)[1]	Catastrophic relations (87%/55%)[1]
Meals	Communication difficulties
Bathing	Making accusations (60%/50%)[1]
Delusions	Daytime wandering
Incontinence (40%/61%)[1]	Hallucinations
Driving	Physical violence (47%/75%)[1]
Inappropriate sexual behavior	Cooking

[1] Behavioral problems causing serious problems for caregivers (percent of families experiencing this problem/percent of families citing this problem as serious).
From Rabins PV, Mace NL, Lucas MJ: The impact of dementia on the family. JAMA 1982;**248**:333.

TABLE 77-7. PROBLEMS IDENTIFIED BY CAREGIVERS

Problem	Percent
Chronic fatigue, anger, depression	87
Family conflict	56
Loss of friends, hobbies and little time for self	55
Worried that the caregiver will become ill	31
Difficulties assuming new roles and responsibilities	29
Guilt	25

Modified from Rabins PV, Mace NL, Lucas MJ: The impact of dementia on the family. JAMA 1982;**248**:333.

A physician can use the argument that it is better to anticipate a crisis that does not occur than not to anticipate a crisis that does occur. An early referral from a social worker is well advised because nursing homes usually have long waiting lists. Many local chapters of ADRDA provide financial and legal advice about nursing home placement.

REFERENCES

Physician Readings

Clarfield AM: The reversible dementias: Do they reverse? Ann Intern Med 1988;**109**:476.

Copeland JRM: Assessment of dementia. Lancet 1988;**351**:769.

Cummings JL: Dementia: The failing brain. Lancet 1995;**345**:1481.

Froelich TE, Robinson JT, et al: Screening for dementia in the outpatient setting: The time and change test. J Am Geriatr Soc 1998;**46**:1506.

Gallo JJ, Reichel W, Andersen L: Mental Status Testing. In: Gallo JJ, ed. *Handbook of Geriatric Assessment*. Aspen Publishers; 1995.

Jorm AF, Korten AE, Henderson AS: The prevalence of dementia: A quantitative integration of the literature. Acta Psychiatr Scand 1987;**76**:465.

LeBars PL, Katz MN, et al: A placebo-controlled, double-blind, randomized trial with a special extract of gingko biloba in dementia. JAMA 1997;**278**:1327.

Mayeux R, Saunders AM, et al: Utility of the apolipoprotein E genotype in the diagnosis of Alzheimer's disease. N Engl J Med 1998;**338**:506.

Peisah C, Brodaty H: Practical guidelines for the treatment of behavioural complications of dementia. Med J Aust 1994;**161**:558.

Rabins PV, Mace NL, Lucas MJ: The impact of dementia on the family. JAMA 1982;**248**:333.

Rebok GW, Folstein MF: Dementia. J Neuropsych Clin Neurosci 1993;**5**:265.

Rigler SK, Studenski S: Pharmacologic treatment of geriatric depression: Key issues in interpreting the evidence. J Am Geriatr Soc 1998;**46**:106.

Rogers SL, Doody RS, et al: Donepezil improves cognition and global function in Alzheimer's disease. Arch Intern Med 1998;**158**:1021.

Rogers SL, Farrow JT, et al: A 24 week, double-blind, placebo-controlled trial of donepezil in patients with Alzheimer's disease. Neurology 1998;**50**:136.

Rossor MN: Management of neurological disorders: Dementia. J Neurol Neurosurg Psychiatry 1994;**57**:1451.

Yeager BF, Farnett LE, Ruzicka SA: Management of the behavioral manifestations of dementia. Arch Intern Med 1995;**155**:250.

Reading Materials That Physicians Can Recommend to Families

Aronson MK (ed): *Understanding Alzheimer's Disease*. Scribner; 1988.

Heston LL, White JA: *Dementia: A Practical Guide to Alzheimer's Disease and Related Illnesses*. WH Freeman, 1983.

Jarvik LF, Winograd CH (eds): *Treatment for the Alzheimer's Patient*. Springer; 1988.

Mace N, Rabins PV: *The 36-Hour Day: A Family Guide to Caring for Persons with Alzheimer's Disease, Related Dementing Illnesses, and Memory Loss in Later Life*. Johns Hopkins Univ Press; 1981.

Managing the person with intellectual loss (dementia or Alzheimer's disease) at home. Report by The Burke Rehabilitation Center, White Plains, New York; 1980.

National Alzheimer's Disease and Related Disorders Association: *Understanding and Caring for the Person With Alzheimer's Disease: A Practical Guide*. Atlanta Area ADRDA Chapter; 1985.

Powell LS, Courtice K: *Alzheimer's Disease: A Guide for Families*. Addison-Wesley; 1983.

78   Diabetes Mellitus

Mark B. Mengel, MD, MPH

I. **Definition.** Diabetes mellitus, a heterogeneous group of disorders caused by a relative or absolute insulin deficiency, results in abnormalities of carbohydrate and fat metabolism. The American Diabetes Association (ADA) has divided diabetes mellitus into seven diagnostic categories. The two principal forms of diabetes mellitus, insulin-dependent diabetes mellitus (IDDM, or type I) and non–insulin-dependent diabetes mellitus (NIDDM, or type II), are the focus of this chapter.

II. **Epidemiology.** Diabetes mellitus is the ninth most common outpatient diagnosis. In the United States, 2.4% of people consider themselves diabetic. A similar number are felt to be undiagnosed.

  A. **Type I diabetes (IDDM).** This type of diabetes mellitus occurs in 10–15% of people with diabetes in the United States. The peak incidence of IDDM occurs between ages 10 and 15 (11.5 per 100,000 children per year).

  B. **Type II diabetes (NIDDM).** In the United States, 85–90% of people with diabetes have NIDDM. This type of diabetes mellitus affects 22.7 of every 10,000 persons per year, with the peak incidence between ages 50 and 55. **Risk factors for NIDDM include increased age, higher prediabetic fasting plasma glucose levels, a family history of NIDDM, and obesity.** The prevalence of NIDDM in American blacks, Hispanics, and Native Americans is much higher than it is in American whites.

III. **Pathophysiology**

  A. **Type I diabetes (IDDM).** Destruction of pancreatic beta cells is the primary etiologic event in IDDM. This destruction results from multiple factors, including genetic susceptibility, viral infections, and autoimmune phenomena. Beta-cell destruction produces insulin deficiency and hyperglycemia.

  B. **Type II diabetes (NIDDM).** Although patients with NIDDM are hyperglycemic, they often have elevated fasting insulin levels and beta-cell hypertrophy. Two theories attempt to explain this paradox: (1) peripheral insulin resistance, which causes increased basal insulin secretion and eventually pancreatic exhaustion and (2) defective postprandial insulin secretion, which produces increased basal insulin secretion, insulin resistance, and eventually pancreatic exhaustion.

IV. **Diagnosis**

  A. **Symptoms and signs**

    1. **Type I diabetes (IDDM).** Polyuria, polydipsia, weight loss, fatigue, and irritability are typical presenting complaints of IDDM patients. Many IDDM patients are also in frank diabetic ketoacidosis at the time of diagnosis.

    2. **Type II diabetes (NIDDM).** Many patients with NIDDM are relatively asymptomatic initially. Physicians should suspect NIDDM in patients with risk factors (see section II,B), recurrent infections, visual difficulties, and unexplained peripheral neuropathies.

  B. **Laboratory tests**

    1. **Urinalysis.** Most patients with diabetes "spill" sugar into their urine at the time of diagnosis. Many substances, aging, and pregnancy affect the amount of glucose in the urine, however. Thus, urine testing for glycosuria is not useful in diagnosing and following up on patients with diabetes. Urine testing for ketones in patients with diabetes is still advisable, however, particularly when the patient becomes ill, to monitor for the onset of diabetic ketoacidosis.

    2. **Plasma glucose measurement.** This is the preferred method of diagnosis. Meeting any one of the following criteria establishes the diagnosis in nonpregnant adults:

      a. One random plasma glucose measurement of over 200 mg/dL (11.1 mmol/L) in a patient with classic diabetic signs and symptoms.

      b. Two fasting plasma glucose (FPG) levels of over 126 mg/dL (7.0 mmol/L).

      c. A glucose tolerance test (75-g load) in which the blood glucose value at 2 hours and one other blood glucose value taken between time zero and 2 hours exceeds 200 mg/dL.

V. Treatment. The goals of treatment of diabetes mellitus are (1) reduction of diabetic symptoms, (2) prevention of acute complications (eg, diabetic ketoacidosis, hyperosmolar nonketotic coma, hypoglycemia), (3) encouragement of normal growth and development in children with diabetes, and (4) prevention of chronic complications. Current therapeutic options (see following text) can easily achieve the first three goals; controversy still exists about whether all the chronic complications of diabetes mellitus can be prevented.

A. Dietary therapy
   1. Consultation with a dietitian is recommended for all patients with IDDM to achieve a balance between food consumption and insulin administration. Recent research indicates that a high-carbohydrate diet combined with a high fiber intake actually improves diabetic control.
   2. In NIDDM, dietary therapy is often ineffective, since few patients are able to maintain significant weight loss. Obesity contributes to the insulin resistance found in NIDDM patients; 80% of patients with NIDDM are overweight. Even modest reductions in weight can significantly improve diabetic control. Enrollment in behavior modification programs or support groups and involvement of the patient's family are necessary to increase the chances of success.

B. Exercise. Although long-term, well-controlled studies of the effects of exercise on diabetic control are lacking, exercise does have a glucose-lowering effect and is recommended for the improvement of diabetic control. Patients with NIDDM who engage in an exercise program that is integrated with dietary therapy may lose weight, with subsequent improvement in diabetic control. Guidelines for planning an exercise program include the following:
   1. An exercise program should begin at low intensity and increase gradually. Consultation with a physician is recommended to integrate exercise with the other aspects of the therapeutic regimen. Patients with diabetes whose plasma glucose values are over 300 mg/dL (16.7 mmol/L) should not exercise until their control has improved and their blood glucose levels have decreased. Self-monitoring of blood glucose (see section VI,B) is useful during exercise.
   2. When possible, a patient with diabetes should exercise after meals to reduce postprandial hyperglycemia.
   3. Patients with diabetes should avoid exercise during peak insulin actions and should avoid exercising extremities in which insulin has recently been injected.

C. Oral hypoglycemic agents (Table 78–1). In patients with NIDDM, oral hypoglycemic agents have become the mainstay of therapy. *These agents have no place in the treatment of patients with IDDM.*
   1. **Oral sulfonylureas** act either by enhancing basal and postprandial insulin secretion by decreasing insulin resistance in muscle, liver, and adipose tissue or by both actions. There is little cost difference among first-generation agents, although generic brands are less expensive.
   2. **Second-generation oral sulfonylureas** are far more potent than first-generation agents and have a longer half-life allowing once- or twice-daily dosing; thus, these agents have become the agents of choice for treating patients with NIDDM. Second-generation agents lower hemoglobin A_{1c} levels by 1 to 2 percentage points on average, but can cause hypoglycemia and weight gain. All the sulfonylureas undergo hepatic metabolism and should be used with caution in patients with liver abnormalities. Glipizide is preferred in patients with renal abnormalities. Generic glipizide, glimepiride (Amaryl), and Glucotrol XL are the most cost-effective alternatives.
   3. **Acarbose** (Precose) is an oral α-glucosidase inhibitor that reduces the rate of complex carbohydrate digestion, lowering postprandial glucose levels. To be effective, it needs to be given 30 minutes before meals. On average, acarbose lowers hemoglobin A_{1c} by 0.5 to 1.0 percentage points. Patients taking acarbose will have trouble treating hypoglycemic attacks with complex carbohydrates and so should have oral glucose tablets or gel readily available. Acarbose should be avoided in patients with bowel disease or renal failure. Acarbose can be used in combination with other hypoglycemic agents.
   4. **Metformin** (Glucophage) is a biguanide hypoglycemic agent that acts by stimulating glucose uptake. Endogenous insulin is required for metformin to work, and metformin does not stimulate insulin secretion. Clinical trials suggest that metformin is as effective as other oral agents in the treatment of

TABLE 78–1. ORAL HYPOGLYCEMIC AGENTS

Agent	Starting Dose	Maximum Daily Dose	Side Effects	Cost[1]
First-generation sulfonylureas				
Acetohexamide (Dymelor)	250 mg bid	1500 mg	Hypoglycemia, weight gain, rash, and increased LFTs	$ generic, $$ brand
Chlorpropamide (Diabinese)	100–250 mg qd	750 mg		$ generic, $$ brand
Tolazamide (Tolinase)	100–250 mg qd to bid	1000 mg	Disulfiram-like reactions and hyponatremia with chlorpropamide	$ generic, $$ brand
Tolbutamide (Orinase)	250 mg qd to bid	300 mg		$ generic, $$ brand
Second-generation sulfonylureas				
Glimepiride (Amaryl)	1–2 mg qd	8 mg	Hypoglycemia, weight gain, rash, and increased LFTs	$
Glipizide (Glucotrol)	5 mg po qd to bid	40 mg	Hypoglycemia, weight gain, rash, and increased LFTs	$ generic, $$ brand
Glucotrol XL	5 mg po qd	20 mg	Hypoglycemia, weight gain, rash, and increased LFTs	$
Glyburide (Diabeta, Micronase)	2.5 mg po qd	20 mg	Hypoglycemia, weight gain, rash, and increased LFTs	$$
Glynase	1.5–3 mg po qd	12 mg	Hypoglycemia, weight gain, rash, and increased LFTs	$$
Non-sulfonylureas				
Acarbase (Precose)	25 mg tid before meals	300 mg	Bloating, flatulence, diarrhea	$$$
Metformin (Glucophage)	500 mg po qd to bid with meals	2550 mg	Lactic acidosis, nausea, cramps	$$$
Repaglinide (Prandin)	0.5 mg tid before meals	4 mg	Hypoglycemia, weight gain	$$$
Rosiglitazone (Avandia)	4 mg po qd or 2 mg po bid	4 mg po bid	Dizziness, nausea, abnormal LFTs, anemia	$$$$
Pioglitzone (Actos)	15 mg po qd	45 mg po qd	Dizziness, nausea, abnormal LFTs	$$$$

[1]Cost: $, AWP, $0–$10; $$, AWP, $10–$25; $$$, AWP, $25–$75; $$$$, AWP, $75–$150.
AWP, Average wholesale price; LFTs, liver function tests.

patients with NIDDM, with less weight gain noted when compared with patients taking other medications.

Adverse effects are mainly gastrointestinal and include nausea, vomiting, anorexia, diarrhea, and a metallic taste. Lactic acidosis occurs rarely, but is potentially fatal. Since lactic acidosis usually occurs in the setting of renal failure, the drug should not be prescribed in patients susceptible to this condition. Metformin can be added to sulfonylureas if those agents do not achieve optimal diabetic control.

5. **Repaglinide** (Prandin) is a meglitinide compound that stimulates postprandial insulin secretion. Like the sulfonylureas, repaglinide requires the presence of insulin to be effective. It is rapidly absorbed and short-acting and should be given 30 minutes before each meal. It lowers hemoglobin A_{1c} by 1 to 2 percentage points and can be used with other oral agents. It should be used cautiously in patients with liver abnormalities.

6. **Thiazolidinedione** agents enhance insulin action via direct stimulation of receptors in the nucleus of hepatic and skeletal muscle cells. On average, thiazolidinediones lower hemoglobin A_{1c} by 0.5 to 1.0 percentage points, at starting dosages. They can be used as monotherapy or in combination with other oral agents. Liver function tests should be monitored every 2 months for the first 12 months, and periodically thereafter because of the chance of severe liver toxicity when using rosiglitazone or pioglitazone.

D. **Insulin therapy**
   1. **Indications**
      a. **All patients with IDDM require insulin therapy.**
      b. Patients with NIDDM may require insulin therapy if diet and oral hypoglycemic agents do not control their diabetes sufficiently. Depending on the clinical situation, insulin may be added to oral hypoglycemics (eg, as a low dose of NPH insulin at bedtime [0.1 U/kg of body weight]), or oral hypoglycemics may be stopped and insulin started. Nocturnal insulin is then adjusted, based on the results of FPG values. Insulin may also be indicated as initial therapy in patients with NIDDM if the patient's initial FPG value is greater than 400 mg/dL, particularly in young, nonobese, symptomatic patients. Premixed insulin preparations, such as 70/30 (70% NPH, 30% Reg) insulin, work particularly well in type II patients, with improvements in diabetic control due to decreased mixing errors.
   2. **Characteristics of insulin preparations.** Selection from available insulin preparations is based on **concentration** (90% of prescribed insulin is U-100); **species source** (human insulin developed using recombinant DNA technology is less antigenic than pig or beef insulin); **purity** (patients should use the purest preparations of insulin available in hopes of reducing formation of insulin antibodies), and **type** (Table 78–2). A new quicker-acting, short-duration insulin, lispro insulin (Humalog), has recently been released; it allows patients to inject themselves 15 minutes before meals, rather than the usual 30–45 minutes.

TABLE 78–2. INSULIN TYPES

Type	Onset of Action (hr)	Maximal Action (hr)	Duration of Action (hr)
Short-acting			
Regular	0.5–1	2–4	4–6
Semilente	1–2	3–6	8–12
Intermediate-acting			
Neutral protamine Hagedorn (NPH)	3–4	10–16	20–24
Lente	3–4	10–16	20–24
Long-acting			
Protamine zinc insulin (PZI)	6–8	14–20	>32
Ultralente	6–8	14–20	>32

3. **Initiating insulin therapy.** Patients newly diagnosed with IDDM either receive education and begin their insulin regimen while hospitalized, or, if they do not have ketoacidosis, receive it as outpatients. One injection of insulin per day rarely normalizes the glycemic response in such patients and often leaves patients hyperglycemic at night and in the morning. Therefore, patients with IDDM typically receive a "split-dose" insulin regimen consisting of a mixture of regular and NPH insulin before breakfast and in late afternoon before supper. The two methods generally used to initiate insulin therapy are described below.

   a. Patients with IDDM may first receive prandial and night-time injections (four injections per day) of regular insulin based on the prandial blood glucose values given in Table 78–3. When glucose values have stabilized, the daily insulin requirement is totaled and split into two injections, with two-thirds of the total amount of insulin given in the morning and one-third in the evening. The morning and evening dosages can then be split into 75% NPH insulin and 25% regular insulin.

   b. Patients with IDDM may begin insulin therapy by receiving two injections of intermediate-acting insulin per day, with two-thirds of the total administered in the morning and one-third in the evening, starting with a total daily dose of 0.6 U/kg of body weight. Regular insulin may be added and intermediate-acting insulin adjusted depending on results of glucose testing during the day (Table 78–4).

4. **Intensive insulin therapy.** See section VI,C.

5. **Honeymoon period.** Soon after insulin therapy is instituted, a "honeymoon period" of 12–18 months occurs in nearly all patients with IDDM. During this time, patients' insulin requirements usually are drastically reduced.

VI. **Management strategies.** With publication of the Diabetes Control and Complication Trial, a large study of 1441 diabetic patients randomized to intensive versus conventional insulin therapy, which showed a clinically significant reduction in microvascular complications over the 6.5 years of follow-up, many physicians now feel comfortable achieving optimal diabetic control, near-normal hemoglobin A_{1c} levels, while minimizing hypoglycemic episodes. Efforts should be made not only to improve the treatment regimen (see section V), but also to assess and correct other factors known to affect diabetic control. Such factors include recurrent chronic infections, malignancy, insulin resistance, noncompliance, poor adjusting, poor coping skills, and dysfunctional family dynamics.

A. **Hemoglobin A_{1c} (glycosylated hemoglobin)** is one of several forms of hemoglobin A that results from the nonenzymatic attachment of glucose to hemoglobin A. Since the percentage of hemoglobin A_{1c} depends on the average glucose concentration over the life of a red blood cell (120 days), hemoglobin A_{1c} is a good measure of diabetic control over the preceding 2–3 months. Hemoglobin A_{1c} levels that are 1 percentage point above the upper range of normal for a particular reference laboratory indicate that the patient is not in optimal diabetic control and runs the risk of microvascular complications. Falsely elevated levels of hemoglobin A_{1c} occur in the presence of uremia, fetal hemoglobin, alcoholism, and aspirin (acetylsalicylic acid) usage.

B. **Self-monitoring of blood glucose (SMBG).** This technique developed as the poor correlation between blood glucose values and glycosuria became clear.

TABLE 78–3. TYPICAL SLIDING SCALE USED TO INITIATE INSULIN THERAPY

Blood Glucose Value[1] (mg/dL)	Amount of Regular Insulin To Be Given (U)
150–200	8
200–250	12
250–300	16
>300	20

[1] Blood glucose values should be checked before each meal and at bedtime. The sliding scale may be adjusted upward (eg, giving 8 U of regular insulin for a blood glucose value between 200 and 250 mg/dL) if a person is particularly sensitive to insulin or if hypoglycemia occurs. Close monitoring of blood glucose is essential when initiating insulin therapy.

TABLE 78–4. ADJUSTMENT OF INSULIN DOSAGES BY SELF-MONITORING WITH A SPLIT-DOSE REGIMEN[1]

Measurement Time	Dosage to Adjust If Blood Glucose Out of Target Range
0700	Afternoon NPH
1200	Morning regular
1700	Morning NPH
2200	Afternoon regular
0300	Afternoon NPH

Protocol for all insulin dosages

If blood glucose < 60 mg/dL, decrease appropriate dose by 2 U
If 60 mg/dL < blood glucose < 120 mg/dL, no adjustment
If 120 mg/dL < blood glucose < 150 mg/dL, increase appropriate dose by 2 U
If 150 mg/dL < blood glucose < 180 mg/dL, increase appropriate dose by 4 U
If blood glucose > 180 mg/dL, increase appropriate dose by 6 U

[1] Rules may be liberalized if hypoglycemia occurs frequently.
NPH, neutral protamine Hagedorn.

1. SMBG is a reliable technique, providing patients receive proper instruction in the procedure and potential problems. It is expensive, however, with costs averaging over $1000 per year. Fortunately, many insurance companies and programs such as Medicare are beginning to pay for SMBG.

2. Patients with diabetes who use SMBG determine their glucose values before meals, at bedtime, and occasionally in the middle of the night. They then adjust insulin dosages by using simple rules (Table 78–4). In addition, physicians can use the results of SMBG to adjust insulin dosages during regular follow-up visits.

3. Although the ADA recommends using SMBG at least twice daily in all diabetic patients, because of cost and side effects associated with frequent fingersticks (eg, infection and pain), most physicians compromise with their patients. Patients are typically asked to do SMBG only once daily but to vary the time so that over a 2- to 3-week period values have been obtained before all meals and at bedtime. Another option is to ask patients to do SMBG intensively four times daily for 3–5 days before seeing the physician. Frequent SMBG, however, is mandatory in those patients receiving intensive insulin therapy.

C. **Treatment guidelines.** Most authorities now recommend tight glucose control in order to reduce the risk of complications, with goals for FPG being set at less than 140 mg/dL and goals for hemoglobin A_{1c} being set at less than 8% or less than 1 percentage point above the normal range. Goals can be relaxed if attacks of hypoglycemia are common or if patients are not invested in the effort to achieve tight control. Additionally, excess weight gain, particularly in the type II patient, should be avoided.

1. **Type I diabetes.** Intensive patient education, meal planning, exercise counseling, initiation of split-dose insulin therapy, and SMBG all are part of the initial treatment of the patient with IDDM. If split-dose insulin treatment does not achieve optimal glucose control, more intensive methods of insulin therapy should be initiated in the following stages:

   a. **Three injections of insulin per day.** Two choices exist when this stage is reached. The patient with type I diabetes can either move the afternoon NPH dose to bedtime, which will reduce the dawn phenomenon (fasting hyperglycemia due to nocturnal hepatic gluconeogenesis), or replace NPH insulin with Ultralente insulin in the morning and afternoon with an injection of regular or lispro insulin added before lunchtime.

   b. **Four injections of insulin per day.** If three injections of insulin per day are not effective in producing optimal glucose control, then two options exist. If the afternoon NPH dosage is moved to bedtime, then an injection of regular or lispro insulin can be added before lunch, along with injections of NPH and regular or lispro insulin before breakfast and regular insulin before dinner. On the other hand, if the Ultralente option was elected, then an injection of regular or lispro insulin can be added prior to the evening snack.

    c. The continuous subcutaneous insulin infusion (CSII) pump. If four injections of insulin per day are not effective in achieving optimal glycemic control, then the patient should be referred to an endocrinologist who specializes in use of the CSII pump.

2. Type II diabetes. Patients with type II diabetes mellitus can be divided into three categories based on their initial FPG values: (1) those with FPG values less than 200 mg/dL, (2) those with FPG values between 200 and 400 mg/dL, and (3) those with FPG values over 400 mg/dL. Often, type II patients with FPG values over 400 mg/dL have ketones in their urine and significant symptoms.

    a. Stage I, FPG < 200 mg/dL. A well-balanced calorie-restricted meal plan, enough to maintain ideal body weight, and aerobic exercise should be begun. To support the patient through this lifestyle change, frequent follow-up visits, every other week, should be initiated, and SMBG should be considered if target values of FPG are not met in 1–2 months. Stage II should be entered after 3 months if target values are still not met.

    b. Stage II, 200 mg/dL < FPG < 400 mg/dL. In this stage, meal planning and exercise should be continued. The lowest dose of a second-generation oral hypoglycemic agent should be started and adjusted monthly. After 50% of the maximal dose is reached, the dose should be split into a twice-daily schedule. If optimal diabetic control is not reached within 3 months, two options are available. Either the oral agent should be reduced to 50% of the maximal dose and given in the morning or at lunch and NPH insulin (0.1 U/kg of body weight) should be added in the evening, or a second or even a third oral agent, such as acarbose, metformin, or athiazolidinedione, can be added (see section V,C). Stage III should be entered in 6 months if target values are not met.

    c. Stage III, FPG > 400 mL/dL or if urine ketones or severe symptoms are present. This stage begins with split-dose insulin therapy (see section V,E,3). If the patient has previously received oral agents, these should be stopped at this time, since continuing oral agents would just add to the costs of care and would not be able to achieve better glucose control than insulin alone. If optimal control is not achieved with split-dose insulin treatment, then more intensive methods of insulin therapy can be used (see section VI,C,1).

D. Prevention and early detection of diabetes and its complications

    1. Screening. Because many adults with type II diabetes remain undiagnosed, screening all individuals over age 45 every 3 years with an FPG is now recommended. Screening should begin earlier and be more frequent if risk factors are present.

    2. Achieving near-normal diabetic control. The design of an effective treatment regimen and the assessment and correction of other factors associated with poor diabetic control constitute the first step in preventing the onset of both microvascular and macrovascular complications of diabetes. Risk factor reduction, including smoking cessation, hypertension control, and treatment of hyperlipidemia, are also central management strategies needed to prevent the development of complications. Aspirin, 325 mg orally daily, to prevent macrovascular complications in patients with adult type II diabetes, is also important.

    3. Diagnosing complications as early as possible. Periodic ophthalmologic, neurologic, vascular, renal (measurement of microalbuminuria), and foot examinations aid early diagnosis of diabetic complications. The exact frequency of examinations, except for annual ophthalmologic examinations and tests for microalbuminuria, has not been well studied. Most physicians follow up on patients with diabetes at least quarterly, with more frequent visits as necessary.

    4. Treating complications when they develop. Once complications are diagnosed, risk factor reduction and symptomatic treatment remain the mainstays of complication management. Painful peripheral neuropathies can often be treated with a low dose of a tricyclic antidepressant, such as amitriptyline, 50 mg orally at bedtime (qhs), whereas the progression of diabetic nephropathy can be slowed with an angiotensin-converting enzyme inhibitor (even if the patient is not hypertensive) such as captopril, 25–50 mg orally twice daily or lisinopril, 10 mg orally daily.

VII. Prognosis. The outcome of diabetes mellitus in a particular patient depends on several factors. These include the nature and severity of the disease in that patient, the simultaneous occurrence of other diseases, the presence of risk factors for diabetic complications (disease duration is the most important), genetic susceptibility to specific complications, and how well the patient responds to treatment. The patient's ability to adapt constructively to the disease also influences the course of the disease.

Patients with diabetes may experience acute complications, which develop over days to weeks and result in serious disturbances of fluid and electrolytes (diabetic ketoacidosis, nonketotic hyperosmolar coma, and hypoglycemia) and chronic complications, which develop gradually over months to years and involve nearly every organ system of the body, particularly the eyes, kidneys, vascular system, and nervous system.

A. The mean survival of patients with IDDM diagnosed before age 30 is currently 10–15 years less than that of the general population. Death usually results from end-stage renal disease (40–50%) or coronary artery disease, although ketoacidosis and hypoglycemic coma continue to cause significant mortality.

B. Life expectancy in NIDDM patients is roughly one-third less than that of age-matched nondiabetic patients. Cardiovascular disease accounts for 75% of the deaths in NIDDM patients after age 60. Except for ketoacidosis, all the complications associated with IDDM occur in patients with NIDDM. Macrovascular complications are more common in NIDDM patients, however. Hyperosmolar non-ketotic coma, an acute complication, is seen almost exclusively in patients with NIDDM.

REFERENCES

American Diabetes Association: *Medical Management of Type I Diabetes,* 3rd ed. American Diabetes Association; 1998.

American Diabetes Association: *Medical Management of Type II Diabetes,* 4th ed. American Diabetes Association; 1998.

Gaster B, Hirsch IB: The effects of improved glycemic control on complications in type 2 diabetes. Arch Intern Med 1998;**158:**134.

Kahn CR, Weir GC (eds): *Joslin's Diabetes Mellitus,* 13th ed. Lea & Febiger; 1994.

Susman JL, Helseth LD: Reducing the complication of type II diabetes: A patient-centered approach. Am Fam Physician 1997;**56:**471.

White JR: The pharmacological reduction of blood glucose in patients with type 2 diabetes mellitus. Clin Diabetes 1998;**16:**58.

---

79   Dyslipidemias

Michael A. Crouch, MD, MSPH

I. Definition of dyslipidemia types
   A. Hyperlipidemia refers to elevated total blood cholesterol, low-density lipoprotein (LDL) cholesterol, or triglyceride (TG) levels.
   B. Hypercholesterolemia is elevated total blood cholesterol (cutpoints below).
   C. Hyperbetalipoproteinemia is elevated LDL cholesterol (cutpoints below).
   D. Hypoalphalipoproteinemia is low high-density lipoprotein (HDL) cholesterol (below 35 mg/dL or 0.90 mmol/L).
   E. Hypertriglyceridemia is elevated fasting TGs (above 200 mg/dL or 1.7 mmol/L).

II. Epidemiology. The prevalence of hypercholesterolemia increases with age, peaking at age 55–65. Approximately 50% of adults in the United States have hypercholesterolemia if 200 mg/dL (5.2 mmol/L) is used as the cutoff value for total cholesterol. Most patients in this total cholesterol range have an LDL cholesterol level above 130 mg/dL (3.35 mmol/L). If the 200–239 mg/dL (5.2–6.2 mmol/L) level is considered borderline and 240 mg/dL (6.2 mmol/L) is used as the cutoff for elevated total cholesterol, 5–15% of adults have hypercholesterolemia. Most patients in the higher total cholesterol range have an LDL cholesterol level above 160 mg/dL (4.1 mmol/L). Five to 10% of adults have low HDL cholesterol levels and 20–25% have elevated TG levels.

  A. Lipid disorders are most prevalent in populations that consume excessive amounts of saturated fat, cholesterol, sugars, and refined starches; lead sedentary lives; and tend to become obese with advancing age.

  B. Blood lipid levels may fluctuate seasonally. In colder climates, cholesterol and TG levels tend to be somewhat higher in winter because of dietary variation.

  C. Blood lipids change acutely in response to food intake. The TG level is lowest in the fasting state, rises by an average of 50 mg/dL postprandially, and peaks 3–6 hours after a meal. As the TG level rises, total and LDL cholesterol each fall by an average of 5–15 mg/dL. Thus total and LDL cholesterol tend to be higher when fasting. HDL cholesterol varies little between the fasting and postprandial states, averaging 45 mg/dL (1.16 mmol/L) for men and 55 mg/dL (1.42 mmol/L) for women.

  D. Blood lipids can also fluctuate within minutes, days, or weeks, sometimes in response to illness, emotional stress, or malnutrition.

III. Pathophysiology. Lipid disorders are familial problems, transmitted across generations by both genetic factors and learned behaviors.

  A. Genetic predisposition. Several lipid disorders display a mendelian inheritance pattern, including familial hypercholesterolemia, familial combined hyperlipidemia (elevated cholesterol and TGs), and familial hypoalphalipoproteinemia. Most cases of hypercholesterolemia, however, involve a polygenic predisposition.

  B. Lipid metabolism. Lipid disorders can involve abnormalities in one or more of the many steps in lipid metabolism.

    1. Saturated fat and cholesterol are absorbed from the gut and packaged into TG-rich particles called chylomicrons. These chylomicrons are broken down into very low density lipoprotein (VLDL) particles that are rich in TGs.

    2. VLDL particles are metabolized into cholesterol-rich LDL particles. The enzyme lipoprotein lipase catalyzes VLDL metabolism.

    3. LDL particles attach to LDL receptors on cell membranes. Cholesterol from the LDL particles passes into cells.

    4. Influx of cholesterol into cells suppresses the activity of the rate-limiting enzyme in cholesterol synthesis, 3-hydroxy-3-methylglutaryl coenzyme A (HMG-CoA) reductase.

    5. HDL particles facilitate LDL metabolism, which results in cholesterol being carried back to the liver from peripheral tissues.

  C. Dietary influences. Saturated fat intake raises LDL cholesterol levels more than does cholesterol intake. **Polyunsaturated fat** lowers LDL cholesterol and HDL cholesterol values. **Monounsaturated fat** lowers LDL cholesterol and does not affect HDL cholesterol. **Trans fatty acids** present in hydrogenated vegetable oil products appear to be particularly atherogenic. Excessive intake of **sugars** and rapidly absorbed, highly processed **starches** elevate TGs.

  D. Physical inactivity elevates TGs and VLDL cholesterol, and it decreases HDL_2 cholesterol.

  E. Being overweight elevates TGs and decreases HDL_2 cholesterol.

  F. Cigarette smoking decreases HDL_2 cholesterol.

  G. Alcohol in moderation raises HDL_3 cholesterol but not HDL_2 cholesterol. Excess alcohol raises TGs.

  H. Psychosocial factors. Stress and coronary-prone (Type A) behavior can markedly elevate LDL cholesterol and total blood cholesterol in susceptible persons.

  I. Secondary causes

    1. Iatrogenic causes of lipid problems are common.

      a. Diuretics raise LDL cholesterol transiently but seldom have significant long-term effects.

      b. Beta blockers without intrinsic sympathomimetic activity (propranolol, etc) lower HDL cholesterol and may raise LDL cholesterol.

      c. Chenodiol, a gallstone dissolver, lowers both HDL cholesterol and LDL cholesterol.

      d. Oral contraceptives with strong androgen/progestin effect lower HDL cholesterol, raise TGs, and sometimes raise LDL cholesterol.

      e. High-dose steroids and disulfiram (Antabuse) raise TGs.

      2. Other conditions that cause hyperlipidemia include diabetes mellitus, hypothyroidism, pregnancy, nephrotic syndrome, obstructive jaundice, chronic renal failure, dysgammaglobulinemia, anorexia nervosa, porphyria, and glycogen storage disease.

IV. Diagnosis
  A. Symptoms and signs. Lipid problems are usually asymptomatic for several decades.
    1. Arcus senilis, xanthelasma, tendon xanthomas, and eruptive xanthomas are uncommon physical signs of lipid problems.
    2. Retinal arteriovenous crossing changes signal atherosclerosis.
    3. Angina pectoris, intermittent claudication, and impotence are warning symptoms of advanced atherosclerosis.
    4. Myocardial infarction, cerebrovascular accident (stroke), or sudden death is often the first sign of a lipid problem, in the absence of lipid screening.

  B. Laboratory tests
    1. Screening is recommended by the National Cholesterol Education Program (NCEP) every 3–5 years for most adults below the age of 70. Adults with LDL cholesterol levels below 130 mg/dL (3.4 mmol/L) and HDL levels above 50 mg/dL (1.3 mmol/L) probably do not need to be rescreened this often unless they experience major changes in weight, diet, or physical activity. Children and adolescents with a family history of severe dyslipidemia or early atherosclerotic disease should also be screened.
      a. A **random or fasting lipid profile** (with total, LDL, and HDL cholesterol and TGs) should be obtained initially to detect elevated LDL cholesterol or TGs and low HDL cholesterol. The more convenient random lipid profile increases compliance with screening, and it gives useful information about the extent of postprandial hyperlipemia (considered to be a serious atherogenic factor).
      b. If a patient is at **high risk** for coronary artery disease (CAD) and random LDL cholesterol levels are marginally or mildly elevated, a **fasting lipid profile** should be obtained to more accurately categorize the severity of elevated LDL cholesterol.
    2. Interpreting cholesterol results. Although 240 mg/dL (6.20 mmol/L) is the current cutoff point for defining high blood cholesterol, persons in the United States in the 200–239 mg/dL (5.17–6.20 mmol/L) range have 40% of the acute myocardial infarctions. Figures 79–1 and 79–2 show ranges of total blood

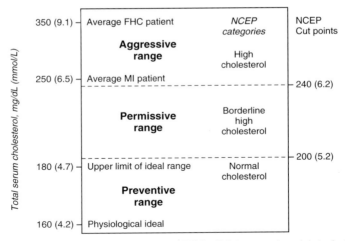

FIGURE 79–1. Prognostic range for total cholesterol. FHC, Familial heterozygous hypercholesterolemia; MI, myocardial infarction; NCEP, National Cholesterol Education Program.

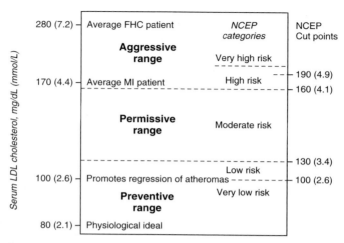

FIGURE 79–2. Prognostic range for low-density lipoprotein (LDL) cholesterol. FHC, Familial heterozygous hypercholesterolemia; MI, myocardial infarction; NCEP, National Cholesterol Education Program.

cholesterol and LDL cholesterol that are preventive, permissive, or aggressive with respect to their risk for promoting atherosclerosis.

3. **Diagnosing lipid disorders**
   a. If a screening lipid profile shows elevated LDL cholesterol, low HDL cholesterol, or high TGs, a **second lipid profile** should be obtained (fasting) before starting treatment, to confirm elevation and establish an accurate baseline.
   b. To maximize accuracy and precision of lipid laboratory values, all specimens should be sent to a laboratory that uses rigorous quality control procedures and participates in standardization testing.

4. **Excluding secondary causes.** If symptoms or signs are suggestive, the physician should consider ordering thyroid, renal, or liver function tests to rule out secondary causes of dyslipidemia.

5. **Prognosis categorization** identifies those patients at highest risk. **Lipid ratios** summarize two or more lipid values into one number that correlates strongly with long-term prognosis; however, these ratios predict outcome only marginally better than absolute HDL cholesterol and LDL cholesterol values.
   a. At **highest risk** are patients who **smoke** or have **diabetes mellitus** along with elevated LDL cholesterol or low HDL cholesterol.
   b. Patients who have **low HDL** cholesterol levels are at some increased risk even if their LDL cholesterol levels are not elevated. Of the lipid values, HDL cholesterol is the best single predictor of adverse outcome. Above average or high HDL cholesterol levels do not, however, guarantee a low likelihood of developing CAD.
   c. Patients with markedly elevated LDL cholesterol levels (above 190 mg/dL, or 4.9 mmol/L) are at increased risk even if they have HDL cholesterol levels at or above average.
   d. Patients with high fasting TG levels are also at increased risk, especially obese females with diabetes mellitus.

6. **Additional tests**
   a. **Apolipoprotein levels** predict outcome more accurately than does LDL cholesterol or HDL cholesterol, but their clinical usefulness has not been proved. Apolipoprotein levels can sometimes help the physician to decide how aggressively to treat patients with LDL cholesterol levels of 130–189 mg/dL (3.35–4.90 mmol/L) and patients with HDL cholesterol less than 35 mg/dL (0.90 mmol/L) whose LDL cholesterol is less than 130 mg/dL (3.35 mmol/L).

       (1) Prognosis is poor if the level of apolipoprotein B, the main apolipoprotein in LDL, is elevated.

       (2) A low level of apolipoprotein A-I, the main apolipoprotein in HDL, also indicates a poor prognosis.

    b. Lipoprotein(a) is a modified LDL moiety similar to plasminogen. Lipoprotein(a) elevation signals a bad prognosis, even if LDL cholesterol is less than 130 mg/dL (3.35 mmol/L). The test may be more useful than apolipoprotein levels for clarifying prognosis.

V. Treatment. Treatment goals should be set and adjusted according to the patient's clinical status and other risk factors (Table 79–1). With **no known CAD and less than two CAD risk factors,** the treatment goal is to lower LDL cholesterol to less than 160 mg/dL (4.15 mol/L). With **2 or more CAD risk factors,** the **treatment goal** is to lower LDL cholesterol to less than 130 mg/dL (3.35 mmol/L). With **clinical CAD or diabetes, treatment goals** are to lower LDL cholesterol to less than 100 mg/dL (2.60 mmol/L) and to lower fasting TG to less than 200 mg/dL (1.7 mmol/L).

    A. Hygienic approaches often improve lipid levels effectively. It is appropriate to encourage lifestyle changes in anyone with LDL cholesterol greater than 130 mg/dL or HDL cholesterol less than 35 mg/dL (0.90 mmol/L). Women with HDL cholesterol levels below 45 mg/dL (1.16 mmol/L) may also be appropriate candidates for lifestyle change.

       1. Dietary modification. Depending on baseline diet, eating less saturated fat and cholesterol can often lower total blood cholesterol by 10–20%. Key dietary changes for lowering elevated cholesterol are listed below.

          a. Eat **less beef and pork** (especially fatty cuts).

          b. Eat **more fish, chicken, and turkey** (white "skinless" meat) or **soy protein.**

          c. Drink **nonfat, 1/2%, or 1% fat milk, instead of 2% or whole milk (3.5% fat).** Eat minimal amounts of other whole-milk dairy products such as cheese, butter, ice cream, and sour cream.

          d. Use **polyunsaturated oil products** (safflower, corn, soybean) or **monounsaturated oil products** (olive) for margarine and cooking oil (desired ratio of polyunsaturated to saturated fat is > 1.5:1). **Avoid hydrogenated oils** present in **stick margarines;** instead use **tub margarines** (preferably small amounts).

          e. Eat oat bran as cereal or muffins, three to six servings per day. Oat bran can reduce total cholesterol and LDL cholesterol an average of 5–10% in some patients with elevated LDL cholesterol.

          f. Fish oil high in omega-3 fatty acids (ie, eicosapentanoic [EPA] and decahexanoic [DHA]) has not been shown to have beneficial effects on LDL or HDL cholesterol at a dose of six capsules a day.

       2. Exercise. Regular aerobic exercise, at least 30 minutes at a time, three or more times a week, raises HDL cholesterol by 5–15 mg/dL, lowers TG and VLDL cholesterol, and sometimes lowers LDL cholesterol. Walking daily for several miles has been shown to have smaller favorable effects on lipids.

TABLE 79–1. RISK FACTORS FOR CORONARY ARTERY DISEASE

Factors cited by the National Cholesterol Education Program
Male gender
Cigarette smoking
Diabetes mellitus
Hypertension
Low HDL-cholesterol
Obesity
Personal history of atherosclerotic disease
Family history of lipid disorder
Family history of atherosclerotic disease (especially men < 55 and women < 65 y.o.)

Other factors (not cited by the National Cholesterol Education Program)
Postmenopausal status for females
Coronary-prone (Type A) behavior or personality
Old age (risk rises with increasing age)

   3. **Weight loss** lowers TG and VLDL cholesterol, raises HDL cholesterol by
      5–10 mg/dL, but lowers LDL cholesterol only transiently during the weight
      reduction period.
   4. **Smoking cessation** increases HDL cholesterol by 5–10 mg/dL but does not
      affect LDL cholesterol, VLDL cholesterol, or TGs.
   5. **Behavioral modification** for coronary-prone (Type A) behavior may lower
      LDL cholesterol in the absence of other interventions.
B. **Medications.** The 1993 NCEP Adult Treatment Panel II recommendations suggest medical treatment if LDL cholesterol remains above 190 mg/dL (4.9 mmol/L)
   despite hygienic management, regardless of the patient's clinical status and other
   CAD risk factors. If the patient has two or more CAD risk factors, a trial of medication is recommended to lower LDL cholesterol that stays above 160 mg/dL. If
   the patient has CAD, medication is recommended if LDL cholesterol stays above
   130 mg/dL. A cost-effective regimen should effectively lower elevated LDL cholesterol and TGs, raise HDL cholesterol if it is low, be convenient and promote
   good long-term patient cooperation and acceptance, have minimal adverse effects,
   and be affordable.
   1. **Over-the-counter (OTC) drugs** are sometimes the preferred choice for med-
      ical treatment because they are inexpensive and relatively safe, and some are
      fairly effective (Table 79–2).
      a. **Psyllium hydrophilic mucilloid** (Metamucil and other brands). Psyllium,
         which lowers LDL cholesterol and total cholesterol an average of 5–10%,
         is a logical choice to treat mildly elevated LDL cholesterol (130–159 mg/dL)
         when HDL cholesterol is above 45 mg/dL, especially in elderly patients.
         It promotes bowel regularity and sometimes causes flatulence, but causes
         no serious adverse effects.
      b. **Niacin.** Niacin is a logical first choice for treating the healthy patient with
         moderately elevated LDL cholesterol who also has either low HDL cho-
         lesterol (<35 mg/dL) or high TGs. Niacin has demonstrated value for pre-
         venting myocardial infarction and CAD death.
         (1) When taken in a dose of 1–3 g/day, niacin lowers LDL cholesterol
             by 15–20%, markedly lowers elevated TGs, and raises HDL cho-
             lesterol by 5–15 mg/dL. Patients should begin with a low dose of
             100–200 mg of the regular release form or 250–500 mg of the sus-
             tained-release form; then the dose should be gradually increased to
             a maximum of 2–3 g/day based on patient tolerance.
         (2) Most patients experience minimal flushing and itching when taking
             sustained-release niacin. Patients who experience flushing and itch-
             ing can block much of the adverse symptoms by taking 325 mg of
             aspirin daily before the first dose.
         (3) Although it is usually well tolerated and safe, niacin can worsen di-
             abetic hyperglycemia, exacerbate gout, precipitate serious arrhyth-
             mias in patients with heart disease, or cause severe reversible liver
             toxicity.
   2. **Prescription drugs for modifying lipids** (Table 79–2) all are relatively ex-
      pensive, especially higher doses. The balance of potential benefit versus ad-
      verse effects and cost should be weighed carefully before prescription drugs
      are used.
      a. **Cholestyramine** (Questran). This resin sequesters bile acids in the gut.
         It is available as a powder to be mixed with water or food. Questran Light
         may be sufficiently palatable for long-term compliance. Cholestyramine is
         a logical choice for the patient with severe LDL cholesterol elevation and
         HDL cholesterol levels above 45 mg/dL who will tolerate its inconvenient
         format.
            When 2 scoops or packs are taken two to three times a day, cholestyr-
         amine lowers LDL cholesterol and total cholesterol by 15–20%. Because
         doses higher than 3 to 4 packs per day cause constipation, the maximal
         dose is poorly tolerated.
      b. **Colestipol** (Colestid) is very similar to cholestyramine in form, dose, effi-
         cacy, cost, and patient tolerance, with no advantages.
      c. **Gemfibrozil** (Lopid) changes the hepatic metabolism of lipoproteins. Gem-
         fibrozil is a logical choice for the patient with low HDL cholesterol and

TABLE 79–2. HOW TO RECOMMEND AND PRESCRIBE LIPID-ALTERING MEDICATIONS

Medication	Retail Cost[1]
Over-the-counter medications	
Psyllium hydrophilic mucilloid (PHM)	$7–10/mo unsweetened/with sugar
Metamucil or equivalent	artificially sweetened $15–21/mo
1 heaping tsp (tbsp if with sugar) in 8 oz water/liquid,	Orange/lemon-lime $11–21/mo
tid with meals	Metamucil Instant Mix $25/mo
Fiberall Fruit & Nut Fiber Wafer	$35–40/mo if sole PHM source
One to two 3.4-gm wafers, tid with 8 oz+ of liquid	convenient lunchtime substitute
Niacin/nicotinic acid, 500-mg SR tab	
Initial dose: 1 tab bid	$8–14 for 100 tab; max 3 g/d
Increase to 2 tab bid in wk 2	$10–12/mo for 2 g/d
Prescription medications	
Atorvastatin (Lipitor), 10/20/40-mg tab	$165/270/315 for 90 tab of 10/20/40 mg
Sig: 5 mg qd evening (½ of a 10-mg tab) (low dose)	$27/mo
10 mg qd evening (usual starting dose)	$55/mo
20 mg qd evening (medium dose)	$90/mo
40 mg qd evening (high dose)	$105/mo
80 mg (two 40-mg tabs) qd evening (very high dose)	$210/mo
Cholestyramine (Questran), powder (1 can contains 378 g)	$138 for 3 cans
Sig: one 9-g scoop bid (starting dose)	$69/mo
two 9-g scoops bid (usual maint dose)	$138/mo
two 9-g scoops tid (max maint dose)	$207/mo
Cholestyramine (Questran Light), powder	$294 for 3 cartons (180 pks)
Sig: one 5-g pack bid (starting dose)	$98/mo
two 5-g packs bid (usual maint dose)	$196/mo
two 5-g packs tid (max maint dose)	$240/mo
Cerivastatin (Baycol), 0.2/0.3-mg tab	$136/131/131/131 for 90 tab of 0.2/0.3/0.4/0.6 mg
Sig: 0.2 mg qd evening (low dose)	$45/mo (unclear why more)
0.3 mg qd evening (usual dose)	$44/mo
0.4 mg qd evening (high dose)	$44/mo
0.6 mg qd	$44/mo
Fenofibrate (Tricor), 67-mg tab	$130 for 180 tab
one tab, bid (usual dose)	$43/mo
Fluvastatin (Lescol), 20/40mg tab	$115/115 for 90 tab of 20/40 mg
Sig: 20 mg qd evening (low dose)	$38/mo
40 mg qd evening (medium dose)	$38/mo
80 mg qd evening (high dose)	$76/mo
Gemfibrozil (Lopid), 600-mg tab	$252 for 180 tab
Gemfibrozil (generic), 600-mg tab	$60 for 180 tab
Sig: 1 tab bid with meals (usual dose)	$20/mo (gen) $84/mo (Lopid)
Lovastatin (Mevacor), 10/20/40-tab	$105/185/345 for 90 tab of 10/20/40 mg
Sig: 10 mg qd evening (low dose)	$35/mo
20 mg qd evening (usual starting dose)	$62/mo
40 mg qd evening (medium dose)	$115/mo
80 mg qd evening (high dose)	$230/mo
Nicotinic acid/niacin	
Nicolar, 500-mg tab	$278 for 360 tab
Sig: 2 tab bid with meals (usual dose)	$93/mo
Pravastatin (Pravachol), 10/20/40-mg tab	$167/183/325 for 90 tab of 10/20/40 mg
Sig: 10 mg qd evening (low dose)	$56/mo
20 mg qd evening (usual starting dose)	$61/mo
40 mg qd evening (medium dose)	$108/mo
80 mg (two 40-mg tabs) qd evening (high dose)	$216/mo
Probucol (Lorelco), 500-mg tab	$205 for 180 tab
Sig: 1 tab bid with meals (usual dose)	$70/mo
Simvastatin (Zocor), 5/10/20/40/80 mg	$140/170/302/302/302 for 90 tab of 5/10/20/40/80 mg
Sig: 5 mg qd evening (low dose)	$47/mo
10 mg qd evening (low dose)	$57/mo
20 mg qd evening (usual starting dose)	$101/mo
40 mg qd evening (medium dose)	$101/mo
80 mg qd evening (high dose)	$101/mo

[1]Quoted by least expensive community pharmacy, June 1999 survey, Houston, TX. Maint, maintenance dose; SR, sustained release.

moderately elevated LDL cholesterol or severely elevated TGs who has not tolerated or responded well to niacin. The drug is well tolerated and appears to be relatively safe for long-term use.

  (1) Gemfibrozil lowers LDL cholesterol by 5–15%, markedly lowers TGs, and raises HDL cholesterol by 5–15 mg/dL. The usual dose is 600 mg twice a day; the maximum dose is 900 mg twice a day or 600 mg three times per day.

  (2) Gemfibrozil has been shown to lower CAD morbidity and mortality by 40% in patients with elevated LDL cholesterol, TGs, or both. It is most beneficial in patients with HDL cholesterol of <45 mg/dL. It may be used cautiously in combination with an HMG-CoA reductase inhibitor.

 d. Fenofibrate (Tricor) is similar to gemfibrozil and is appropriate for the same patients. Its long-term safety is unknown.

 e. HMG-CoA reductase inhibitors (statins). This category is the rational choice for patients with severely elevated LDL cholesterol (>190 mg/dL) and high-risk patients with any LDL elevation who do not reach target treatment levels with diet and other medications. These agents lower LDL cholesterol by 30–60%—more than any other medication. In controlled trials, they have demonstrated benefit for preventing heart attack, stroke, coronary heart disease (CHD) death, and total mortality. Cost-effectiveness analyses of this class of agents have shown favorable cost–benefit ratios. The cost-effectiveness of treatment can be greatly improved by prescribing twice the intended dose and having the patient take one-half of a tablet. Table 79–3 shows recommended medications and doses for cost-effectively treating patients with different baseline LDL-C levels and different treatment goals. All of the agents in this category are very well tolerated. Because of the possibility of liver toxicity at higher doses, it is prudent to obtain baseline and periodic liver enzyme levels when using higher doses. Myopathy occurs rarely, but somewhat more often when these agents are used along with niacin, gemfibrozil, or fenofibrate.

  (1) **Lovastatin** (Mevacor) was the first available HMG-CoA reductase agent.

    (a) The 20-mg starting dose is well tolerated and often produces good results, lowering LDL cholesterol an average of 25–30%.

    (b) Newer, more effective agents, including some with more favorable outcome data, have displaced lovastatin as a medication of choice.

TABLE 79–3. COST-EFFECTIVE MEDICATION REGIMENS FOR TREATING ELEVATED LDL-C

	LDL-C Treatment Goal	
Baseline LDL-C	**<130 mg/dL**	**<100 mg/dL**
130–159 mg/dL	fluvastatin, one-half a 40-mg tab, qd Lescol $20/mo or atorvastatin, one-half a 10-mg tab, qd Lipitor $28/mo or simvastatin, one-half a 10-mg tab, qd Zocor $28/mo or cerivastatin, one 0.3-mg tab, qd Baycol $44/mo	atorvastatin, one-half a 20-mg tab Lipitor $42/mo or simvastatin, one-half a 40-mg tab Zocor $50/mo or cerivastatin, one 0.4-mg tab, qd Baycol $44/mo
160–189 mg/dL	atorvastatin, one-half a 20-mg tab Lipitor $45/mo or simvastatin, one-half a 40-mg tab Zocor $50/mo	atorvastatin, one-half a 20/40-mg tab Lipitor $45/53/mo or simvastatin, one-half a 40/80 mg tab Zocor $50/mo
≥190 mg/dL	atorvastatin, one-half to one 40-mg tab Lipitor $53–105/mo or simvastatin, one-half to one 80-mg tab Zocor $50–100/mo	atorvastatin, one to two 40-mg tabs Lipitor $105–210/mo

LDL-C, Low-density lipoprotein cholesterol.

(2) Pravastatin (Pravachol) is similar to lovastatin but is less costly.

    (a) The usual dose of 20–40 mg/day, taken 2–3 hours after the evening meal, lowers LDL cholesterol an average of 25–35%.

    (b) Pravastatin has reduced CHD events by 24–40% in primary and secondary prevention trials.

(3) Simvastatin (Zocor) has a higher potency. (10 mg of simvastatin is equivalent to 20 mg of lovastatin or pravastatin.) It can be taken anytime in the evening.

    (a) Simvastatin 20–80 mg/day lowers LDL cholesterol by 35–50%.

    (b) Simvastatin reduced acute myocardial infarction or death from CHD by 42% and reduced total deaths by 30% in a large secondary prevention trial.

    (c) Higher doses of simvastatin tend to be more expensive than other similar agents.

(4) Fluvastatin (Lescol) costs substantially less than the other agents, except for cerivastatin. Higher doses (40–80 mg/d) lower LDL cholesterol by 23–33% (Tables 79–2 and 79–4). Outcome studies are lacking.

(5) Atorvastatin (Lipitor) is the most effective "statin" for lowering elevated LDL cholesterol and the most cost-effective for those with severely elevated LDL cholesterol.

    (a) Atorvastatin in the usual dose of 10–20 mg/day lowers LDL cholesterol by an average of 38–45% and TGs by 20–35%. Higher doses of 40–80 mg lower LDL cholesterol an average of 50–55% and TGs by 35–50%.

    (b) Elevated liver enzymes are no more common than with other statins.

    (c) Although results from outcome studies are not yet available, atorvastatin is becoming the drug of choice for severely elevated LDL cholesterol.

TABLE 79–4. RETAIL COST[1] OF THERAPEUTIC EQUIVALENT DOSES OF HMG-CoA-REDUCTASE INHIBITORS

atorvastatin (Lipitor)		cerivastatin (Baycol)		fluvastatin (Lescol)		simvastatin (Zocor)		pravastain (Pravachol)
	=		=		=		=	
5 mg $27		0.3 mg $44		40 mg $38		10 mg $50–57		20 mg $54–61
atorvastatin (Lipitor)		cerivastatin (Baycol)		fluvastatin (Lescol)		simvastatin (Zocor)		pravastatin (Pravachol)
	=		=		=		=	
10 mg $45–55		0.4 mg $44		80 mg $76		20 mg $50–100		40 mg $108
atorvastatin (Lipitor)		cerivastatin (Baycol)				simvastatin (Zocor)		pravastatin (Pravachol)
			=				=	
20 mg $57–90		0.6 mg $44				40 mg $50–100		80 mg $216
atorvastatin (Lipitor)						simvastatin (Zocor)		
				=				
40 mg $105						80 mg $100		
atorvastatin (Lipitor)								
			No comparable dose for any other statin					
80 mg $210								

[1] Quoted by least expensive community pharmacy, June 1999 survey, Houston, TX. HMG-CoA, 3-Hydroxy-3-methylglutaryl coenzyme A.

      (6) Cerivastatin (Baycol) is similar to fluvastatin—less costly than others.

         (a) Cerivastatin in the usual dose of 0.3–0.6 mg/day lowers LDL cholesterol by 30–45%—sufficient for many patients to reach treatment goals.

         (b) Cerivastatin lacks outcome studies; its only advantage is price.

    f. Probucol (Lorelco). This antioxidant acts systemically to prevent (1) the oxidation of LDL cholesterol into atherogenic forms and (2) the transformation of macrophages into foam cells, which are the building blocks for fatty streaks and atheromas. Probucol increases reverse cholesterol transport from peripheral tissues to the liver. This drug regresses tendon xanthomas effectively despite its lowering HDL cholesterol by 5–10 mg/dL. The HDL cholesterol particles become smaller and possibly more efficient in facilitating reverse cholesterol transport.

      Although probucol may be a logical choice as an adjunctive medication for patients at highest risk for atherosclerosis or with proven atherosclerotic disease, it is seldom prescribed because of wariness about its lowering HDL cholesterol. Its antioxidant properties might be particularly useful with elderly patients. The results from controlled studies examining its preventive effect on atherosclerosis have not yet been published.

      (1) A standard dose of probucol at 500 mg twice a day lowers LDL cholesterol an average of 15%.

      (2) Probucol is tolerated well and has demonstrated good long-term safety.

C. Partial ileal bypass surgery, in conjunction with a low-fat diet, lowers LDL cholesterol by 40–50%. The operative and postoperative morbidity and mortality are low. This surgery is a reasonable option for patients with severely elevated LDL cholesterol that cannot be managed satisfactorily with any tolerable combination of lipid-altering medications.

VI. Management strategies

  A. Patient education and discussions with family members are vital in order to foster a thorough understanding of the importance of a lifelong commitment to hygienic and medical management of lipid problems. Explanations of key concepts need to be expressed in lay terms, accompanied by memory devices to help people remember them, such as drawing a "happy face" and characterizing HDL cholesterol as "healthy" cholesterol, and a "frown face" symbolizing LDL cholesterol as "lousy" or "lethal" cholesterol. Many good educational materials are available from the American Heart Association, the NCEP, and commercial sources.

  B. Family-oriented care entails screening as many family members as possible and educating nuclear and extended families who have a member with an identified lipid problem. It is particularly important to work with the persons who buy and prepare the family's food, so that they thoroughly understand how to select and prepare "heart-healthy" foods.

  C. Elderly patients are at a greatly increased risk for myocardial infarction or sudden death. Although no evidence exists on the value of modifying blood lipids in the elderly (>65 years), it seems reasonable to recommend at least hygienic approaches to lowering LDL cholesterol and TGs and raising HDL cholesterol. The use of benign inexpensive medications such as psyllium also seems prudent. Whether elderly patients should be treated aggressively with more costly agents, perhaps having greater potential for adverse effects, remains controversial.

  D. Children and adolescents with dyslipidemias should receive ongoing family-oriented education about diet, exercise, and weight control, as indicated. Extreme low-fat diets should be avoided in children younger than 6 years because of the risk of essential fatty acid malnutrition having deleterious effects on nervous system development. No information is available on the cost-effectiveness and long-term safety of lipid-altering medication treatment in children and adolescents. Children and adolescents with severe dyslipidemias should be treated with lipid-altering medications only with considerable caution and preferably with written parental informed consent detailing the limitations of what is known about the benefits and risks.

  E. Secondary prevention focuses on identifying and treating persons who have already developed clinical atherosclerosis. Many times the lipid problems of these patients are ignored or discounted, based on the faulty logic of "it is too late now to prevent atherosclerosis complications by modifying lipids." Persons with atherosclerosis have clearly demonstrated their high vulnerability to CAD death. They are the most likely to benefit from treatment to prevent further atheroma progression, prevent atheroma rupture, and regress existing atheromas. The lowering of LDL cholesterol has clearly demonstrated substantial benefit in secondary prevention trials.

   F. Systematic follow-up at regular intervals is essential for effective long-term management of lipid problems. Initially monthly visits are advisable to monitor progress and sustain motivation. The interval can be gradually lengthened to every 6–12 months for dietary management and every 6 months for medication treatment. A patient flow chart documenting blood lipid results, dietary and exercise modifications, and medication regimens facilitates the evaluation and alteration of treatment for best results.

VII. Natural history and prognosis. The clinical course of lipid problems depends on the type and severity of lipid disorder and on other risk factors for atherosclerosis, especially cigarette smoking, diabetes mellitus, and hypertension. Other factors thought to be detrimental include lipoprotein(a) and small dense oxidized LDL particles, and perhaps homocysteine and other factors yet to be discovered. In childhood and adolescence, fatty streaks form on the lining of susceptible arteries and subsequently develop into atheromas. In adulthood, accumulation of cholesterol and fibrotic tissue causes atheromas to progress at variable rates.

   A. Atherosclerotic progression, plaque rupture, and thrombus formation may eventually block off crucial arteries, causing ischemic symptoms and necrosis in the tissue supplied by the arteries.

   1. **Coronary artery disease** manifests as angina pectoris, nonfatal myocardial infarction, arrhythmias, or sudden death.
   2. **Peripheral vascular disease** with high-grade occlusion of the ileofemoral arteries causes intermittent claudication or impotence.
   3. **Cerebrovascular disease** with occlusion or atheromatous emboli from the carotid or vertebrobasilar arteries causes transient ischemic attacks or stroke.
   4. **Acute pancreatitis** can occur with severe TG elevation greater than 1000 mg/dL (11 mmol/L). This serious lipid problem requires urgent treatment with intravenous heparin.

   B. The **prognosis** for patients with lipid problems can be greatly improved by systematic patient education, lasting lifestyle changes, good compliance with long-term lipid-altering medication, and diligent follow-up care. Other valuable measures for curtailing atherosclerosis or minimizing its damage include smoking cessation, good control of hypertension and diabetes, daily aspirin (optimal dose still unclear), supplemental intake of the antioxidant vitamin E (400–800 IU/d), and perhaps supplemental folate intake (0.4–1.0 mg/d) to lower elevated homocysteine levels.

REFERENCES

Johannesson M, Jonsson B, Kjekshus J, et al: Cost effectiveness of simvastatin treatment to lower cholesterol levels in patients with coronary heart disease: Scandinavian Simvastatin Survival Study Group. N Engl J Med 1997;**336:**332.

Nawrocki JW, et al: Reduction of LDL cholesterol by 25% to 60% in patients with primary hypercholesterolemia by atorvastatin, a new HMG-CoA reductase inhibitor. Arterioscler Thromb Vasc Biol 1995;**15:**678.

Sacks FM, Pfeffer MA, Moye LA, et al: The effect of pravastatin on coronary events after myocardial infarction in patients with average cholesterol levels: Cholesterol and Recurrent Events Trial Investigators. N Engl J Med 1996;**335:**1001.

Scandinavian Simvastatin Survival Study Group: Randomised trial of cholesterol lowering in 444 patients with coronary heart disease: The Scandinavian Simvastatin Survival Study (4S). Lancet 1994;**344:**1383.

Shepherd J: The cost-effectiveness of preventing initial coronary events with pravastatin: Results of the West of Scotland Coronary Prevention Study Economic Analysis. West of Scotland Coronary Prevention Study Economic Analysis Group. J Am Coll Cardiol 1997;**29:**168A.

Shepherd J, Cobbe SM, Ford I, et al: Prevention of coronary heart disease with pravastatin in men with hypercholesterolemia: West of Scotland Coronary Prevention Study Group. N Engl J Med 1995;**333:**1301.

Stein JH, McBride PE: Benefits of cholesterol screening and therapy for primary prevention of cardiovascular disease: A new paradigm. J Am Board Fam Pract 1998;**11:**72.

Stephens NG, Parsons A, Schofield PM, et al: Randomised controlled trial of vitamin E in patients with coronary disease: Cambridge Heart Antioxidant Study (CHAOS). Lancet 1996;**347**:781.

Summary of the second report of the National Cholesterol Education Program (NCEP) Expert Panel on Detection, Evaluation, and Treatment of High Blood Cholesterol in Adults (Adult Treatment Panel II). JAMA 1993;**269**:3015.

---

80   Hypertension

Evan W. Kligman, MD

I. **Definition.** The Joint National Committee (JNC) on Detection, Evaluation, and Treatment of High Blood Pressure has defined hypertension as a diastolic blood pressure greater than or equal to 90 mm Hg or systolic blood pressure greater than or equal to 140 mm Hg (Table 80–1). About 5% of patients have a specific cause for elevated blood pressure or "secondary" hypertension; the remaining 95% have "primary" or essential hypertension. Sixty million Americans have hypertension or are taking antihypertensive medications. Hypertension is the most common outpatient diagnosis and specific abnormality identified by physicians.

II. **Epidemiology**

   A. **Primary (essential) hypertension**

   1. **Onset** is usually between ages 25 and 55. Diagnosis is uncommon before the age of 20, although children under the age of 16 years with blood pressure readings in the 90th percentile have three times the relative risk of normotensive children for developing primary hypertension. Prevalence increases with age.

   2. Persons with first-degree relatives (parents, siblings) with hypertension have more than three times the relative risk for developing the disorder. Other risk factors for primary hypertension are age, male sex, lower socioeconomic status, environmental influences (salt intake), obesity, black race, alcohol use, and tobacco use.

   3. Lower intakes of calcium, potassium, and vitamins A and C appear to be more common among hypertensive patients compared with normotensive subjects. Primary hypertension is rare in non-Western societies.

   B. **Secondary hypertension.** About 5% of hypertension in the United States is due to a secondary cause (see following text for specific causes).

III. **Pathophysiology.** Individual patients have different pathophysiologic mechanisms that lead to elevated blood pressure. Age and race are major variables determining individual pathophysiology and hemodynamic differences (Figure 80–1).

   A. **Blood pressure** is determined by cardiac output and total peripheral resistance and is regulated by several physiologic feedback loops: (1) vasomotor central mechanisms that affect the sympathetic autonomic nervous system; (2) natriuresis, which regulates extracellular fluid volume and sodium intake; (3) intracellular sodium and calcium exchange; and (4) the renin–angiotensin–aldosterone and the sympathoadrenal systems. Changes in pressure that result in increased

TABLE 80–1. JNC-V CLASSIFICATION OF BLOOD PRESSURE

Category	Systolic (mm Hg)	Diastolic (mm Hg)	Recommended Follow-Up
Normal	<130	<85	Recheck within 2 yr
High normal	130–139	85–89	Recheck within 1 yr
Hypertension			
Stage 1 (mild)	140–159	90–99	Confirm within 2 mo
Stage 2 (moderate)	160–179	100–109	Evaluate and treat within 1 mo
Stage 3 (severe)	180–209	110–119	Evaluate and treat within 1 wk
Stage 4 (very severe)	>210	>120	Evaluate and treat immediately

Adapted from The Fifth Report of the Joint National Committee on Detection, Evaluation, and Treatment of High Blood Pressure. Department of Health and Human Services (NHLBI), NIH Publication No. 93-1008, 1993.

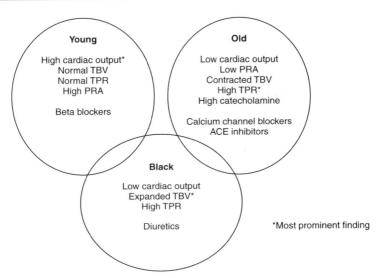

FIGURE 80–1. Matching patient characteristics with antihypertensive agents. ACE, Angiotensin-converting enzyme; PRA, plasma renin activity; TBV, total blood volume; TPR, total peripheral resistance.

activity in any one of these mechanisms are sensed by baroreceptors throughout the circulation.

B. Stage 1 (mild) is considered a result of augmented central sympathetic activity at rest or in response to physical or psychological stressors, especially in young adults. Mental stress activities appear to increase total peripheral resistance and arterial blood pressures. Both physical and mental stress appear to activate the sympathetic nervous system and catecholamine release.

C. Numerous independent processes are responsible for **secondary causes of hypertension,** including oral contraceptives (most common cause), other medications (Table 80–2), renal or renovascular disease (renal artery stenosis accounts for 1–2% of cases of hypertension), primary hyperaldosteronism (0.5%), increased intracranial pressure, Cushing's syndrome, pheochromocytoma, coarctation of the aorta, pregnancy, and primary hyperparathyroidism.

TABLE 80–2. MEDICATIONS CAUSING HYPERTENSION

Prescription medications
Corticosteroids
Epinephrine
Estrogen
Monamine oxidase inhibitors
Nonsteroidal anti-inflammatory drugs
Oral contraceptives
Theophylline
Thyroid supplementation
Topical mineralocorticoids
Tricyclic antidepressants
Other α- or β-adrenergic agonists

Over-the-counter medications
Appetite suppressants
Decongestants with pseudoephedrine, racinephine, phenylpropanolamine, or phenylephrine; cough drops; nasal sprays; cold preparations
Licorice

IV. Diagnosis

A. Symptoms. Patients with hypertension usually remain asymptomatic until they have experienced severe blood pressure elevations (eg, >220 systolic blood pressure or >130 diastolic blood pressure).

    1. Symptoms of hypertension include fatigue, occipital and pulsating headaches in early morning, light-headedness, flushing, epistaxis, chest pains, visual and speech disturbances, and dyspnea.

    2. Specific symptoms of secondary causes can often aid in the diagnosis of hypertension: leg claudication from lower extremity ischemia (coarctation of the aorta); hirsutism; easy bruising (Cushing's syndrome); excessive perspiration; sustained or intermittent hypertension, paroxysmal headaches, palpitations, anxiety attacks, pallor, tremor, nausea or vomiting (pheochromocytoma); hypokalemia, muscle weakness, cramps, polyuria, paralysis, nocturia (primary hyperaldosteronism); and flank pain (renal or renovascular disease).

B. Signs

    1. Blood pressure measurement should be performed while the patient is sitting or supine and standing on more than two occasions to obtain an average for both systolic and diastolic readings. The patient should rest for 5 minutes and not smoke or ingest caffeine for 30 minutes before measurement. The blood pressure cuff should be more than two-thirds the circumference of the arm and placed at heart level. The cuff should be inflated 30 mm Hg above where the radial pulse can no longer be felt. The systolic reading is made at the onset of Korotkoff sounds (phase I), and the diastolic reading is taken when the sounds completely disappear (phase V). The blood pressure should be measured in both arms and if there is a discrepancy in reading, the higher reading should be used. However, in elderly individuals, one reading may be abnormally elevated because of arterial atherosclerosis, causing "pseudohypertension," or medial sclerosis and calcification markedly decreasing arterial collapsibility.

    2. The initial **physical examination** of the hypertensive patient should include an assessment of end-organ damage and identification of signs suggesting a specific secondary cause.

        a. Signs of end-organ damage include arteriolar narrowing, arteriovenous compression, hemorrhages, exudates, or papilledema on fundoscopic examination; carotid bruits and distended jugular veins in the neck; loud aortic second sound, precordial heave, arrhythmia, or early systolic click on cardiac examination; diminished or absent peripheral arterial pulses, peripheral edema of the extremities; aneurysm of the abdominal aorta; and abnormal neurologic assessment.

        b. Signs suggestive of secondary hypertension include abdominal or flank masses (polycystic kidneys); absence of femoral pulses (aortic coarctation); tachycardia, diaphoresis, orthostatic hypotension (pheochromocytoma); abdominal bruits (renovascular disease); truncal obesity, ecchymoses, pigmented striae (Cushing's syndrome); and enlarged or nodular thyroid gland (hyperthyroidism).

C. Laboratory tests. Baseline screening is important to assess end-organ damage, to identify patients at high risk for developing cardiovascular complications, to determine whether other cardiovascular risk factors exist, and to screen for possible secondary causes of hypertension.

    1. Routine tests on all newly diagnosed hypertensive patients include hemoglobin and hematocrit, potassium, creatinine, fasting glucose, calcium, uric acid, total and high-density lipoprotein plasma cholesterol, triglyceride, urinalysis, and electrocardiogram.

    2. The following laboratory tests are recommended when specific secondary causes are suspected based on history, physiologic evaluation, and routine laboratory evaluation.

        a. Chest x-ray (coarctation of aorta)

        b. Dexamethasone suppression test (Cushing's syndrome)

        c. Urinary metanephrine and vanillylmandelic acid levels (pheochromocytoma)

  d. **Intravenous pyelogram, renal scan, or angiography** (renovascular disease)
  e. **Plasma renin activity levels** (primary aldosteronism or renovascular disease)
V. **Treatment** of patients with hypertension is directed toward preventing morbidity and mortality associated with sustained elevated blood pressure and controlling blood pressure by the least obtrusive means possible without producing significant side effects. The presence of other cardiovascular risk factors lowers the threshold at which hypertensive patients should be treated.
  A. **Lifestyle modifications,** including vigorous dietary and behavioral interventions, should be considered as definitive or adjunctive therapy. Such changes may prevent hypertension, as well as reduce other risk factors for premature cardiovascular disease. Lifestyle modifications can also complement pharmacologic treatment to reduce the amount of antihypertensive medication required. One study showed that 39% of subjects who made lifestyle changes sustained normal blood pressure 3 years after discontinuation of medications.
    1. **Dietary therapy.** Dietary recommendations should be given to all hypertensive patients. Recent JNC-VI recommendations include weight reduction (over 60% of hypertensive patients are overweight), moderation of alcohol, and dietary sodium intake. Weight loss improves insulin sensitivity and decreases plasma norepinephrine and aldosterone levels and renin activity. Other recommendations that may be helpful are potassium supplementation, calcium supplementation, avoidance of coffee and tobacco, magnesium supplementation, and a decrease in fat intake. Table 80–3 provides a list of foods high in potassium and magnesium and low in sodium. The recent Dietary Approaches to Stop Hypertension (DASH) Study found that eight to ten servings of fruits and vegetables and two to three servings of low-fat dairy foods per day significantly decreased both systolic and diastolic blood pressures in patients with hypertension, with results in only 2 weeks. Elevated serum homocysteine levels may be an independent risk factor for hypertension in those over age 60, and studies are in progress to determine if folate and vitamin B_6 and B_{12} supplementation will effectively control elevated levels and prevent hypertension.
    2. **Physical activity.** Sedentary and unfit people with normal blood pressure have a 20–50% increased risk of developing hypertension when compared with physically active peers.
       Following 3 months of exercise (eg, walking or running 2 miles a day), blood pressure will increase if the patient returns to a sedentary lifestyle, but the subsequent blood pressure readings will still be lower than the pre-exercise levels. Exercise significantly lowers blood pressure in blacks more dramatically than in whites. In older patients (mean age of 64), low-intensity training has resulted in a decrease in diastolic pressure of 12 mm Hg and a decrease in systolic pressure of 20 mm Hg.

TABLE 80–3. DIETARY CONSIDERATIONS IN TREATING HYPERTENSION (FOODS HIGH IN POTASSIUM OR MAGNESIUM, LOW IN SODIUM)

Food	Serving Size	Sodium (mg)	Potassium (mg)	Magnesium (mg)
Sunflower seeds	1 oz	1	196	100
Soybean nuts	½ cup	2	1173	196
Almonds	1 oz	0	179	86
Black beans, boiled	1 cup	1	611	121
Wheat germ, toasted	1 cup	1	268	91
Orange juice	8 oz	2	474	24
Grapefruit juice	8 oz	2	400	30
Banana	1 medium	1	451	33
Oats, cooked	¾ cup	1	99	42

    3. Stress management. Stress management techniques have been shown to decrease catecholamine release, oxygen consumption, respiratory rate, heart rate, and acute blood pressure. Biofeedback seems to be effective in patients with borderline hypertension. A combination of biofeedback and stress management techniques has fared better than either technique alone.

    4. Other complementary and alternative therapies. Other mind–body interventions such as deep breathing exercises, transcendental meditation, guided imagery, progressive muscle relaxation, yoga, tai chi, and hypnotherapy have proven benefit in treating hypertensive patients. Certain supplements and botanicals such as coenzyme Q10, carnitine, taurine, and hawthorn are currently under investigation. Most patients with hypertension are deficient in Co-Q10 levels; Co-Q10 may have an inhibitory effect on plasma catecholamine levels and functions as an antioxidant at 100–300 mg/day, with effect seen after 8–12 weeks of therapy. Statin drugs to decrease hyperlipidemia may decrease intrinsic levels of Co-Q10, increasing blood pressure. The herbal hawthorn is a flavonoid and functions as a mild diuretic, antioxidant, and positive inotrope; it can increase coronary blood flow. Typical doses are 100–250 mg a day, with mild decreases in blood pressure seen after 2–4 weeks of therapy. Hawthorn potentiates the effectiveness of digitalis and if used concurrently, doses of the latter should be reduced and monitored.

B. Pharmacologic agents. Large clinical trials have documented decreased mortality with pharmacologic treatment of patients with moderate to severe hypertension. Such agents should be prescribed if lifestyle modifications fail to decrease blood pressure to under 140/90. These studies could not document overall reduction in mortality of patients with mild hypertension under age 50, although decreased mortality could be documented with treatment of mild hypertension in patients over age 50, in patients of the black race, and in patients with target-organ damage. Other studies have identified risk from certain pharmacologic agents in the treatment of mild hypertension, especially in elderly individuals for whom the benefit of treating mild hypertension seems to disappear after age 80. However, results from the Systolic Hypertension in the Elderly Program indicated that stepped care with antihypertensive drugs can reduce the incidence of major cardiovascular events and stroke by 36%.

    Rigidly controlled hypertension (eg, diastolic <85 mm Hg) might result in more cases of fatal myocardial infarction. The goal of treatment should be a diastolic pressure between 85 and 95 mm Hg and a systolic pressure between 140 and 155 mm Hg to realize the greatest reduction in mortality and morbidity consistent with the patient's safety and tolerance. If goals are not reached in 3–6 months using nonpharmaceutical therapy, pharmacologic agents should be instituted.

    For stage 1 and stage 2 hypertension, if blood pressure remains at or above 140/90 after a 3- to 6-month period of vigorous lifestyle modifications, antihypertensive medications should be started, especially if the person has other risk factors for cardiovascular disease.

    1. Initial drug therapy is monotherapy for stage 1 and stage 2 hypertension. Both diuretics and beta blockers are indicated for uncomplicated hypertension and have been shown to reduce morbidity and mortality in controlled studies when used as initial single agents. Other classes of antihypertensive drugs are equally effective in reducing blood pressure, but have been less extensively used to demonstrate efficacy in reducing morbidity and mortality. Approximately 50% of patients will respond successfully to monotherapy.

    2. Drug regimens should be tailored based on several factors: age, race, cost, safety, effectiveness, disease severity, general lifestyle including diet and exercise patterns, impact on quality of life (physical state, emotional well-being, sexual and social functioning, and cognitive acuity), convenience, dosage frequency, possibility of other drug interactions, consideration of pathophysiologic mechanisms, concurrent risk factors and diseases, history of previous responses to other agents, and the potential use of the agent or agents for other medical problems. For instance, heart failure or hypertension complicated by diabetes mellitus with proteinuria can be treated with angiotensin-converting enzyme (ACE) inhibitors. Hypertensive patients with a myocardial infarction can be treated with beta blockers (non–intrinsic sympathomimetic activity), ACE inhibitors, or both in the presence of systolic dysfunction. Table 80–4 provides a list of commonly prescribed antihypertensive agents by class and criteria.

3. **Effectiveness of drug regimens.** Even the most effective single agents are less than 70% effective on a long-term basis; however, 80% of compliant patients eventually achieve adequate control on one or two agents. Only a minority of patients require more than two pharmacologic agents.

If the initial agent does not control blood pressure sufficiently, a second agent of a different class may be added. Keeping both agents at low doses will decrease side effects. Combination treatment can be very effective, especially when a diuretic is added to monotherapy; for instance, in elderly patients, the use of an ACE inhibitor with a diuretic can be effective for up to 85% of patients. Common combinations include diuretic plus beta blocker, diuretic plus ACE inhibitor, diuretic plus calcium antagonist, calcium antagonist plus ACE inhibitor, and diuretic plus sympatholytic agent. Resistant hypertension is defined as blood pressure remaining at 140/90 or higher despite an optimal two-drug regimen given at least for 1 month and occurs in less than 10% of patients.

4. **Follow-up tests.** Serum potassium, sodium, blood urea nitrogen and creatinine, uric acid, and glucose levels should be measured periodically, especially if the patient has chronic renal disease or diabetes mellitus or is taking a diuretic agent. The type and frequency of repeated laboratory tests should be based on the severity of target-organ damage and the effectiveness of treatment. A periodic urinalysis is also indicated.

VI. **Management strategies** need to be individualized to take into consideration the severity of the patient's hypertension, the class or classes of pharmacologic agents being used for treatment, patient compliance, and cardiovascular risk factors or disease processes concurrent with hypertension. The three most common causes of uncontrolled hypertension are patient noncompliance (responsible for 50% of treatment failure), inadequate therapy, and inappropriate therapy.

A. **Patient education** is an important part of the physician's management strategy. Education begins with the initial measurement of blood pressure. For a patient who has elevated pressures after three readings, the diagnosis of hypertension should be explained clearly, concisely, and completely. The beliefs of the patient regarding hypertension should be identified with respect to the effectiveness of treatment, the seriousness of the disease if not treated, and personal susceptibility to morbidity and mortality complications. Drug instructions should be written clearly and succinctly. Lifestyle barriers to compliance should be identified as early as possible. Family education should be provided when appropriate.

B. **Initial follow-up.** Monthly check-ups are recommended for the first 6 months and should include an interval history to identify symptoms that may have developed, a discussion of health concerns and compliance problems, an evaluation of drug effects and possible drug reactions (Table 80–5), and measurement of blood pressure and weight. The patient should be instructed to periodically measure blood pressure at home, record the readings, and bring them to the physician's office at regular intervals. Attempts should be made at calibrating home units (automatic or semiautomatic devices using acoustic, oscillometric methods, or digital displays) with office-based mercury sphygmomanometers.

The **trough-peak ratio** is an index of how well an antihypertensive effect is sustained over the dose interval. It is calculated as the ratio of blood pressure reduction at trough, or the end of the dose interval and before the next dose is administered, relative to blood pressure reduction at the time of the peak drug effect. A 50% ratio should be the minimum required of an effective drug.

Compliance can sometimes be improved by changing to an agent with a longer half-life, thereby reducing the number of doses. A memory-assist device, such as Medi-Set, is appropriate for patients receiving complex regimens or with a memory disturbance. Only 7% of people with hypertension are adequately controlled.

C. **Early detection of complications** is an important management strategy to identify potential morbidity from hypertension (retinopathy, coronary artery disease, renal disease, cerebrovascular disease, or nephropathy). Furthermore, people

TABLE 80–4. ANTIHYPERTENSIVE AGENTS

Drug	Usual Starting Dosage	Maximum Daily Dosage	Cost ($)[1]	Common Adverse Effects	Effectiveness	Comments
ANGIOTENSIN-ENZYME CONVERTING (ACE) INHIBITORS				Severe hypotension following first dose if volume-depleted (previous diuretic treatment or if ↓ plasma renin activity); chronic nonproductive cough (14%); pruritus or skin rash (10%)	40–50% as single agents; with diuretic, 85–90% effective	May increase insulin sensitivity by 11%, beneficial effect on left ventricular hypertrophy (LVH); should calculate creatinine clearance to initiate dosing; take captopril on empty stomach; do not use salt substitutes; contraindicated in renal arterial stenosis
Benazepril (Lotensin)	10 mg qd–bid	40 mg	$$			
Fosinopril (Monopril)	10 mg qd–bid	80 mg	$$			
Captopril (Capoten)	25 mg bid–tid	450 mg	$$$$			
Enalapril (Vasotec)	5 mg qd	40 mg	$$$			
Lisinopril (Prinivil, Zestril)	5 mg qd	40 mg	$$			
Quinapril (Accupril)	5 mg qd–bid	80 mg	$$$			
Ramipril (Altace)	1.25 mg qd–bid	20 mg	$$			
ANGIOTENSIN II RECEPTOR ANTAGONISTS						
Valsartan (Diovan)	80 mg qd		$$$			
Losartan (Cozaar)			$$$			
CALCIUM CHANNEL BLOCKERS (SUSTAINED-RELEASE VERSIONS MAY INCREASE PATIENT COMPLIANCE)				Diltiazem: bradycardia, erythema, syncope, constipation	50% as single agent; 70–80% when used with ACE inhibitor or beta blocker	Least affected by sodium intake: ↑ HDL, ↓ cholesterol and (TC)/HDL ratios; negative inotropic effects leading to heart failure in susceptible patients; contraindicated in liver dysfunction
Diltiazem (Cardizem)	30 mg tid–qid	360 mg	$$$	Nifedipine: flushing, nausea, peripheral edema, headache, fatigue, tachycardia, dizziness, constipation		
Nifedipine (Procardia)	10 mg tid–qid	180 mg	$$	Verapamil: similar to diltiazem		
Verapamil (Calan, Isoptin)	80 mg tid–qid	480 mg	$$$			
Felodipine (Plendil)	5 mg qd	20 mg	$$$			

DIURETICS

Thiazides

Drug	Dosage	Cost	Adverse effects		Comments
Hydrochlorothiazide (HydroDIURIL)	12.5–25 mg qd	$	Ventricular irritability; glucose intolerance; impotence; skin rashes; hyperuricemia; orthostatic hypotension; nausea; alkalosis; weakness; $\uparrow$ plasma insulin concentration; $\downarrow K^+$; $\downarrow Mg^{2+}$; $\downarrow Na^+$; $\uparrow Ca^{2+}$; $\uparrow$ LDL, $\uparrow$ triglycerides, $\uparrow$ TC	50–60%	Daily dosing convenient and inexpensive; most widely used agent, indapamide, has no adverse effects on lipids or glucose levels and has beneficial effect on LVH
Chlorthalidone (Hygroton)	12.5–25 mg qd	$			
Indapamide (Lozol)	2.5 mg qd	$$			
Metolazone (Zaroxolyn)	2.5 mg qd	$$			

Loop diuretics

Drug	Dosage	Cost	Adverse effects		Comments
Bumetanide (Bumex)	0.5 mg qd–bid	$	More rapid electrolyte depletion; otherwise, same as thiazides		
Ethacrynic acid (Edecrin)	200 mg bid	$			
Furosemide (Lasix)	20 mg qd–bid	$			

Potassium-sparing diuretics

Drug	Dosage	Cost	Adverse effects		Comments
Spironolactone (Aldactone)	25 mg tid	$	Sexual dysfunction; nausea; gynecomastia; $\uparrow K^+$	50%	Less potent than thiazides alone; magnesium-sparing triamterene may cause renal calculi
Triamterene (Dyrenium)	50 mg qd	$			
Amiloride plus hydrochlorothiazide (Moduretic)	1 tab qd	$			
Spironolactone plus hydrochlorothiazide (Aldactazide)	1 tab qd–bid	$			
Triamterene plus hydrochlorothiazide (Dyazide Maxzide)	1 cap qd–bid	$			

BETA BLOCKERS

Cardioselective agents

Drug	Dosage	Cost	Adverse effects		Comments
Acebutolol (Sectral) (has intrinsic sympathomimetic activity)	200 mg qd–bid	$$	Bronchial asthma, bradycardia; $\downarrow$ exercise capacity; atrioventricular conduction defects; left ventricular (LV) failure; nasal congestion; Raynaud's phenomenon (female); central nervous system symptoms (nightmares, excitement, confusion, fatigue, lethargy, impotence); paradoxical $\uparrow$ blood pressure in pregnancy; volume dependent hypertension; 10–15% of patients will have short-term change in lipids; glucose intolerance; no change in HDL	Over 75% if < age 40; 50% age 40–49; 25% age 50–59	Minimal beneficial effect on LVH; contraindicated in 2nd- or 3rd-degree heart block, congestive heart failure, reactive airway disease, peripheral vascular disease
Atenolol (Tenormin)	25 mg qd	$$			
Metoprolol (Lopressor)	50 mg bid	$$$			

(continued)

469

TABLE 80–4. (*continued*)

Drug	Usual Starting Dosage	Maximum Daily Dosage	Cost ($)[1]	Common Adverse Effects	Effectiveness	Comments
Noncardioselective agents						
Nadolol (Corgard)	40 mg qd	320 mg	$$$$			
Pindolol (Visken) (has intrinsic sympatho-mimetic activity)	10 mg bid	120 mg	$$$			
Propranolol (Inderal) (may be most cost-effective for patients aged 35–64 with mild to moderate hypertension)	40 bid–qid	640 mg	$			
Timolol (Blocadren)	20 mg bid	160 mg	$$			
Beta- combined with alpha-blockers						
Labetalol (Normodyne, Trandate)	200 mg bid	1200 mg	$$$	Vascular insufficiency; dose-dependent orthostatic hypotension and dizziness from alpha blocker; bronchospasm, ↓ myocardial contractility from beta blocker		Add diuretic if dosage 800 mg/d; no adverse lipid effects

VASODILATORS

Alpha

Drug			Cost	Side effects/Comments
Doxazosin (Cardura)	1 mg qd	16 mg	$$$	Drowsiness; dizziness; headaches; hypotension and syncope following first dose (less so with Terazosin); weakness; depression; palpitations; tachycardia; impotence, nausea; diarrhea; constipation; nervousness; dry mouth	Tachyphylaxis develops with long-term use; short term ↑ in TC
Prazosin (Minipress)	1 mg bid–tid	40 mg	$$		
Terazosin (Hytrin)	1 mg qd	20 mg	$$$$		

Central-acting

Drug			Cost	Side effects/Comments	
Clonidine (Catapres)	0.1 mg bid	2.4 mg	$	Fluid retention; transient drowsiness; depression; ↓ alertness; orthostatic hypotension; sedation; fatigue; impotence: rebound hypertension with abrupt withdrawal of clonidine; methyldopa associated with hepatitis, hemolytic anemia	Add to diuretic or ACE inhibitor; contraindicated in stroke patients; methyldopa may lower LDL
Clonidine patch (Catapres TTS)	0.1 mg weekly	0.3 mg	$$		
Guanabenz (Wytensin)	4 mg bid	64 mg	$$$		
Guanfacine (Tenex)	1 mg qhs	3 mg	$$$		
Methyldopa (Aldomet)	250 mg qd–tid	3000 mg	$		

Peripheral-acting

Drug			Cost	Side effects/Comments
Reserpine (Serpasil, Sandril)	0.1–0 mg qd	1 mg	$	Depression; sedation; nasal stuffiness; sleep disturbances; peptic ulcers

Potent vasodilators

Drug			Cost	Side effects/Comments	
Hydralazine (Apresoline)	50 mg bid–qid	300 mg	$	Reflex tachycardia; headaches; angina; palpitations; fluid retention	May increase LV mass; usually added to diuretic or beta blocker to decrease side effects of headache, palpitations, fluid retention
Minoxidil (Loniten)	5 mg bid	100 mg	$$	Hydralazine: gastrointestinal upset, lupus-like syndrome with doses >200 mg/day	
				Minoxidil: hirsutism with hypertrichosis; sodium retention; pleural and pericardial effusions	

[1] Average wholesale cost per month for a generic brand. $, least expensive; $$$$, most expensive.

HDL, High-density lipoprotein; LDL, low-density lipoprotein; TC, total cholesterol.

TABLE 80–5. COMMON ANTIHYPERTENSIVE DRUG INTERACTIONS

Antihypertensive Drug	Other Agent	Action
Diuretic	Lithium	↑ lithium level
Diuretic	NSAID, aspirin	↓ natriuresis
Potassium-sparing diuretic	ACE inhibitor	↑ K+
Thiazide diuretic	ACE inhibitor	Less ↓ K+
Clonidine	Tricyclic antidepressants	↓ effectiveness of clonidine
Propranolol	Cholestyramine, cholestipol	↓ propranolol plasma level
Beta blockers	Cimetidine	↓ bioavailability of beta blockers
Beta blockers	Hydralazine	↑ plasma concentration of beta blocker
Beta blockers	Lidocaine, chlorpromazine, coumarin	↓ plasma clearance of other agents
Beta blockers	Calcium antagonists	↑ negative inotropic effects
Beta blockers	Reserpine	Bradycardia syncope
ACE inhibitor	NSAID, aspirin	↑ K+
Calcium antagonist	Quinidine	Hypotension (especially in IHSS)
Calcium antagonist	Digoxin	↑ digoxin level
Nifedipine	Cimetidine	↑ nifedipine level

ACE, angiotensin-converting enzyme; IHSS, idiopathic hypertrophic subaortic stenosis; NSAID, nonsteroidal anti-inflammatory drug.

Adapted with permission from 1988 Joint National Committee on Detection, Evaluation, and Treatment of High Blood Pressure; The 1988 report. Arch Intern Med 1988;**148**:1023.

with hypertension may be at increased risk of having vascular disease, target-organ damage, dyslipidemias, diabetes mellitus, obesity, arthritis, and liver and renal problems. Prevention, early identification, and treatment of these associated problems are important.

VII. **Natural history and prognosis** are directly related to the effectiveness of treatment, patient compliance, the presence of coexisting diseases, the age of the patient at diagnosis, and the ability of the patient to follow adjunctive therapy recommendations to make lifestyle and behavioral changes.

Studies completed prior to the discovery of antihypertensive drugs revealed that 70% of hypertensive patients died of congestive heart failure or coronary artery disease, 15% from cerebral hemorrhage, and 10% from uremia. Left ventricular hypertrophy (LVH) is a significant complication of hypertension. Progression of LVH can be prevented and reversed by good hypertension control. Development of LVH with strain is an ominous complication with a four- to eightfold increase in mortality from hypertension. Within 5 years of the development of LVH with strain, one-third of patients have a major cardiovascular event. Agents that are most effective in reversing or preventing LVH are central sympatholytics, ACE inhibitors, alpha blockers, and calcium antagonists. Minoxidil and hydralazine may increase LVH.

Patients with concurrent diabetes mellitus and hypertension are at greater risk for developing diabetic nephropathy. However, effective antihypertensive treatment (eg, ACE inhibitors) can reduce proteinuria and the rate of decline of the glomerular filtration rate and postpone end-stage renal failure.

The likelihood of cardiovascular complications in elderly patients can best be predicted by systolic blood pressure. Treatment has been shown to decrease cardiovascular events in patients up to the age of 80.

REFERENCES

Kvasnicker J, Flack JM, Grimm RH: Treatment of hypertension in the presence of coexisting medical conditions (Review). Drugs Aging 1994;**4**(4):304.

Oparil S, Calhoun DA: Managing the patient with hard-to-control hypertension. Am Fam Physician 1998;**57**(5):1007.

The Sixth Report of the Joint National Committee on Prevention, Detection, Evaluation, and Treatment of High Blood Pressure. Arch Intern Med 1997;**157**:2413.

Sutherland J, Castle C, Friedman R: Hypertension: Current management strategies (Review). J Am Board Fam Pract 1994;**7**(3):202.

Wilson MD, Weart CW: Hypertension: Are beta blockers and diuretics appropriate first-line therapies? Ann Pharmacol 1994;**28**(5):617.

81   Ischemic Heart Disease

Jim Nuovo, MD, & Allen Hixon, MD

I. **Definition. Ischemic heart disease (IHD)** results from the effects of atherosclerosis of the coronary arteries. Significant stenosis, along with newly discovered mechanisms that help regulate constriction and relaxation of the coronary arteries, often with superimposed coronary thrombosis, results in a variety of signs and symptoms. It is important for clinicians to recognize the many manifestations of this disease.

II. **Epidemiology**
   A. Cardiovascular disease is the leading cause of death in both men and women, accounting for approximately 25% of all deaths. Eleven million people in the United States have coronary artery disease. Fifty percent of postmenopausal women die of coronary artery disease or its sequelae.
   B. IHD has an enormous impact on medical care in this country. The cost of treatment exceeds $56 billion annually and is expected to rise with the aging of the US population. In industrialized nations, economic loss, disability, and death from coronary artery disease exceeded any other cluster of illnesses.

III. **Pathophysiology.** The heart muscle functions almost exclusively as an aerobic organ, with little capacity for anaerobic metabolism. At rest the heart extracts approximately 80% of the oxygen it receives, leaving it more susceptible to effects of decreased perfusion. Chest pain is the foremost manifestation of myocardial ischemia and results from a disparity between myocardial oxygen demand and coronary blood flow. The mechanisms for ischemia include coronary atherosclerosis (most common), vasoconstriction, and coronary thrombosis.

IV. **Diagnosis.** Chest pain is one of the common reasons for patients to visit primary care physicians. The major diagnostic considerations for chest pain are addressed in Chapter 12. The highest priority is generally given to distinguishing cardiac from noncardiac chest pain. Studies have demonstrated that 10–30% of patients with chest pain who undergo coronary arteriography have no arterial abnormalities. Of the many noncardiac causes of chest pain, gastrointestinal (esophageal), bronchopulmonary, and psychiatric (panic attacks and major depression) are common. Less common causes include chest wall (herpes zoster, costochondritis), aortic dissection, and referred pain from the abdomen.
   A. **Risk factors.** Hyperlipidemia, cigarette smoking, hypertension, diabetes, older age, and male gender are commonly recognized risk factors for IHD. Obesity and lack of postmenopausal hormone replacement therapy are included by some experts. In addition, elevated homocysteine levels are an independent risk factor for IHD.
   B. **Symptoms and signs**
      1. **Angina** is not simply one type of pain; it is a constellation of symptoms related to cardiac ischemia. The description of angina may fit several patterns.
         a. **Classic angina** presents as an ill-defined pressure, heaviness (feeling like a weight), or squeezing sensation brought on by exertion and relieved by rest. The location of classic anginal pain is most often substernal and left-sided. It may radiate to the jaw, interscapular area, or down the arm. Angina usually begins gradually and lasts only a few minutes. It is important to appreciate that the qualitative description of pain may be greatly influenced by socioeconomic status, education, culture, and personality.
         b. **Atypical angina.** The patient either experiences pain that is anginal in quality or has pain with exertional features. For example, this may be a sense of heaviness that is not consistently related to exertion or relieved by rest. Conversely, the pain may have an atypical character—sharp or stabbing—but the precipitating factors are anginal. This is the category of chest pain that is most prone to a diagnostic error. All presentations of chest pain should be taken seriously until proven to be benign.
         c. **Anginal equivalent.** The sensation of dyspnea may be the sole or major manifestation.

    d. Nonanginal pain. The pain has neither the quality nor precipitating characteristics of angina. Chest pain quality not consistent with IHD includes the following descriptive terms: needlelike, shooting, tingling, stabbing, jabbing, knifelike, and cutting.

    e. Diabetics. IHD is the leading cause of death in adult diabetic patients. Hypertension, obesity, and hyperlipidemia cluster in patients with diabetes who have accelerated development of atherosclerotic vascular disease. Atypical clinical presentations have been thought to occur more frequently in diabetics; however, whether diabetic patients experience more "silent MIs" than the general population has recently been challenged.

    f. Women. Women are twice as likely as men to present with angina and less likely to present with infarction or sudden death.

  2. Probability of IHD based on history. Despite the well-known problems experienced in determining the cause of chest pain, the clinical history remains critical in the evaluation of each patient. From the information gathered in the history, the physician should strive to categorize the patient's symptoms as nonanginal, atypical angina, or typical angina. Table 81–1 provides a guideline as to the likelihood of whether a patient has significant IHD based on the history.

  3. Use of nitrate and response to nitroglycerin. Response of the chest pain to sublingual nitroglycerin (NTG) may be used (with caution) as an adjunct for determining whether a patient's chest pain is from IHD. For example, a prompt response of less than 3 minutes increases the probability of IHD; however, esophageal spasm and biliary colic may also respond favorably to nitrate administration. Failure to respond to NTG should not be used to exclude the possibility of IHD.

  4. Signs. There are no reliable, consistent physical signs found on examination for IHD. The main purpose of the examination is to assess the patient for evidence of complications from atherosclerotic disease (eg, peripheral vascular disease, cerebrovascular disease, congestive heart failure). The physician should pay attention to the vascular examination, such as peripheral artery bruits, retinal arteriolar changes, and the presence of an S_3 or S_4, and for the consequences of diminished myocardial contractility, such as lower extremity edema.

C. Diagnostic tests

  1. 12-Lead electrocardiogram (ECG) and serial cardiac enzymes are frequently used to rule out an MI. Several new molecular markers and their sampling schedule are noted in Table 81–2.

  2. The standard provocative test for IHD is the **exercise treadmill test (ETT).** In 1986, the American College of Cardiology and the American Heart Association Task Force on Assessment of Cardiovascular Procedures set guidelines for exercise treadmill testing. The recommendations are as follows:

    a. As a diagnostic test in patients with symptoms suggestive of IHD

TABLE 81–1. LIKELIHOOD OF SIGNIFICANT IHD BASED ON SYMPTOMS

Age (yrs)	Nonanginal Chest Pain	Atypical Angina	Typical Angina
30–39	5% M	22% M	69% M
	0.8% F	4% F	26% F
40–49	14% M	46% M	87% M
	3% F	13% F	55% F
50–59	21% M	59% M	92% M
	8% F	32%F	79% F
60–69	28% M	67% M	94% M
	18% F	54% F	90% F

F, female; M, male.

Adapted from Diamond GA, Forrester JS: Analysis of probability as an aid in the clinical diagnosis of coronary-artery disease. N Engl J Med 1979;**300**:1350.

TABLE 81–2. MOLECULAR MARKERS USED OR PROPOSED FOR USE IN THE DIAGNOSIS OF ACUTE MYOCARDIAL INFARCTION

Marker	Range of Times to Initial Elevation (h)	Mean Time to Peak Elevations (Nonthrombolysis)	Time to Return to Normal Range	Most Common Sampling Schedule
Myoglobin	1–4	6–7 h	24 h	Frequent; 1–2 h after CP
CTnI	3–12	24 h	5–10 d	Once at least 12 h after CP
CTnT	3–12	12 h–2 d	5–14 d	Once at least 12 h after CP
MB-CK	3–12	24 h	48–72 h	Every 12 h × 3[1]

[1] Increased sensitivity can be achieved with sampling every 6–8 hours.
CP, Chest pain; cTnI, cardiac troponin I; cTnT, cardiac troponin T; MB-CK, MB isoenzyme creatine kinase (CK).

    b. To assist in identifying those patients with documented IHD who are at increased risk for higher-grade stenosis or degree of left ventricular dysfunction

    c. To quantify a patient's functional capacity or response to therapies

    d. To follow the natural course of the disease at appropriate intervals

3. Many protocols exist; however, the **Bruce protocol has become the most widely used.** In the standard Bruce protocol, a patient is exercised on a motorized treadmill. Every 3 minutes the speed or elevation of the treadmill is increased. The patient is monitored for symptoms of chest pain, heart rate, and blood pressure response to exercise, arrhythmias, and ST-segment changes. A significant test includes an ST-segment depression of at least 1.0 mm below the baseline. A variety of factors may produce misleading results. Those that can produce false-positive results include the use of medications such as digoxin and estrogen, conditions such as hyperventilation, cardiomyopathy, and mitral valve prolapse. Factors leading to a false-negative result include the use of medications such as nitrates, beta blockers, and calcium channel blockers and the failure to attain a vigorous heart rate response to exercise. For example, approximately 20% of patients with an abnormal ETT have significant ST-segment changes occurring only at maximum or near-maximum heart rate changes. Therefore, if a family physician is reviewing the report of an ETT on a patient and the maximum predicted heart rate was less than 85%, the results should be interpreted more cautiously.

    There are patients who should not undergo the standard ETT for a number of reasons. These include the inability to exercise because of gait or instability problems and underlying ECG abnormalities that make the standard ETT unreadable, such as left ventricular hypertrophy with strain, left bundle branch block, and ST-segment baseline abnormalities in the lateral precordial leads. If the patient is able to exercise and has the noted ECG baseline abnormalities, a thallium ETT is preferred. If the patient is unable to exercise, a persantine/thallium test or dobutamine echocardiogram is indicated. The sensitivity and specificity of ETT in women are less than for men. Although some advocate the use of a persantine/thallium or dobutamine echocardiography for women needing a diagnostic evaluation, these studies, which are not dependent on ECG interpretation, are limited by breast attenuation artifact and provide less functional data than an ETT. Women with a moderate probability of IHD based on age and type of symptoms who have a normal baseline ECG may undergo a standard ETT.

4. Prognostic value of an ETT. In addition to the diagnostic implications of an ETT, there are prognostic implications. The following are considered to be parameters associated with a poor prognosis or increased disease severity: failure to complete stage II of a Bruce protocol, failure to achieve a heart rate greater than 120 beats per minute (off beta blockers), onset of ST-segment depression at a heart rate of less than 120 beats per minute, ST-segment depression greater than 2.0 mm, ST-segment depression lasting more than 6 minutes into recovery, ST-segment depression in multiple leads, poor systolic blood pressure response to exercise, angina with exercise, and exercise-induced ventricular tachycardia.

5. **Resting ECG.** A resting ECG, while important to do on all patients with suspected IHD, must be interpreted with caution. The ECG will be normal or show nonspecific changes in more than 50% of patients with IHD. A normal resting ECG may not be used to rule out IHD. The classic ECG changes of acute ischemia are peaked, hyperacute T waves, T-wave flattening or inversion with or without ST-segment depression, horizontal ST-segment depression, and ST-segment elevation.

6. **Ambulatory Holter monitoring.** Among patients with stable angina who undergo 24-hour Holter monitoring, 40–72% of the episodes are painless. For Holter monitoring when ST-segment changes that meet strict criteria are seen in a patient with known IHD, these episodes are generally considered to represent episodes of myocardial ischemia. Ischemic criteria include at least 1 mm of horizontal or downsloping ST-segment depression that lasts for at least 1 minute and is separated from other discrete episodes by at least 1 minute of normal baseline. This methodology has limitations, including difficulty reading ST-segment changes in patients with an abnormal baseline (left ventricular hypertrophy with strain) or in those with a left bundle branch block. This method is not thought to be superior to the ETT.

7. **Angiography.** Cardiac catheterization is not routinely recommended for initial evaluation of patients with stable angina. Patients who warrant such an evaluation are those who exhibit evidence of severe myocardial ischemia on noninvasive testing or who have symptoms that are refractory to antianginal medications. In patients who undergo catheterization, the most important determinant of survival is left ventricular function followed by the number of diseased vessels. Patients with left main artery disease or three-vessel disease with diminished left ventricular function are candidates for a coronary artery bypass graft procedure. Others (those with one- or two-vessel disease) are managed medically or considered for percutaneous transluminal coronary angioplasty (PTCA).

V. Treatment

A. **Stable angina.** Stable angina is characterized by no change in frequency, severity, duration, or precipitating factors for at least the past 2 months. The treatment of patients with stable angina includes identification and management of specific cardiovascular risk factors, low-dose aspirin, and antianginal drug therapy.

1. **Risk factor modification.** Dietary modification, smoking cessation, and physical conditioning programs should be instituted.

2. **Treatment of associated disease.** Thyroid disease, hypertension, anemia, diabetes, hyperlipidemia, congestive heart failure, valvular disease, and arrythmias should be aggressively identified and managed.

3. **Aspirin.** Most experts recommend a range of 80–300 mg of aspirin per day to decrease platelet aggregability.

4. **Antianginal drug therapy.** The goals are to abolish or reduce anginal attacks and myocardial ischemia and to promote a more normal lifestyle. The three classes of antianginal drugs commonly used are nitrates, beta blockers, and calcium channel blockers (Table 81–3). Each reduces myocardial oxygen demand and may improve blood flow to ischemic areas. No greater efficacy in relieving chest pain or decreasing exercise-induced ischemia has been shown for one or another group of these drugs, although specific clinical indications may favor one over another (diastolic dysfunction, left ventricular hypertrophy, hypertension, asthma, depression, diabetes mellitus, etc).

a. **Nitrates.** The most significant issue for this class of drugs is tolerance. Most studies show that tolerance develops rapidly when long-acting nitrates are given. Tolerance can develop within 24 hours. When prescribing a patch, the usual initial dose of transdermal nitroglycerin is 0.2 mg/hour. It is important to have patch-free intervals of 10–12 hours to retain the antianginal effect. Oral nitroglycerin (isosorbide dinitrate) in the sustained release form is usually started at 40 mg every 8–12 hours.

b. **Beta blockers.** All beta blockers, regardless of their selective properties, are equally effective in patients with angina. About 20% of patients do not respond to beta blockers. Those who do not are more likely to have severe IHD. The dose of the beta blocker should be adjusted to achieve a heart rate of 50 to 60 beats per minute. Examples of starting

TABLE 81–3. ANTIANGINAL MEDICATIONS

Drug	Usual Starting Dosage	Maximum Daily Dosage	Cost	Common Adverse Effects	Comments
BETA BLOCKERS					
Noncardioselective				Fatigue (dose-related), exacerbation of bronchospasm, bradycardia, AV conduction defects, left ventricular failure, Raynaud's phenomenon, impotence, nightmares, mild increase in lipids; may block symptoms of hypoglycemia in diabetics.	Beta blockers are particularly useful in treating the following conditions that occur with IHD: hypertension, ventricular arrhythmia, supraventricular arrhythmias. There is no advantage in using a beta blocker with ISA or alpha₁-sympathomimetic blockade. Cardioselectivity will be overcome as the dose is raised. Abrupt discontinuation may exacerbate angina.
Propranolol	20 mg qid	320 mg	$		
Nadolol	40 mg bid				
	40 mg qd	240 mg	$$$		
Cardioselective					
Atenolol	50 mg qd	200 mg	$$$		
Metoprolol	50 mg bid	400 mg	$$$		
Intrinsic Sympathomimetic Activity (ISA)					
Acebutolol	200 mg bid	1200 mg	$$$		
Pindolol	5 mg bid	60 mg	$$		
Alpha₁ and Beta Blockade					
Labetolol	100 mg bid	2400 mg	$$		
CALCIUM CHANNEL BLOCKERS				Edema, headache, nausea, dizziness, constipation, left ventricular failure, AV conduction defects. Use caution with combined use of beta blockers or digitalis (may experience exacerbation of congestive heart failure or conduction delays). All calcium channel blockers have the potential to induce hypotension; it is important to titrate the dose especially in the elderly.	Calcium channel blockers are useful in treating the following conditions: IHD, hypertension, and supraventricular arrhythmias
Diltiazem sustained-release	60 mg bid	360 mg	$$		

TABLE 81–3. (continued)

Drug	Usual Starting Dosage	Maximum Daily Dosage	Cost	Common Adverse Effects	Comments
Long-acting formulation					
Diltiazem	120 mg qd	480 mg	$$$		
Nifedipine	30 mg qd	90 mg	$$$		
Verapamil	120 mg bid	480 mg	$$$		
SECOND-GENERATION CALCIUM CHANNEL BLOCKERS					
Amlodipine	2.5–5 mg qd	10 mg	$$$	Edema hypotension, flushing, headache.	Plasma T½ 36 hours, little negative inotropic effect, may be useful in treatment of angina associated with hypertension.
NITRATES					
Short-acting nitroglycerin					
Nitrostat	0.4 mg q 5 min × 3 1/150 grain		$	Headache and hypotension. Potential for hypotension greater when used in combination with a calcium channel blocker.	Tolerance is the most significant issue in the use of nitrates. Oral nitrates are more effective given twice daily at a high dose than frequently at a low dose. Nitroglycerin patches should be removed at night to prevent tolerance. Nitrates work well with either beta or calcium channel blockers.
Nitrospray	1–2 sprays q 5 min × 3		$$		
Long-acting nitroglycerin					
Transderm NTG	0.2 mg/hr	0.8 mg/hr	$$		
ISOSORBIDE DINITRATE					
Immediate-release					
Isordil	5 mg qid	160 mg	$		
Longer-acting					
Isordil SR	40 mg bid–tid	240 mg	$		

$, least expensive; $$, moderately expensive; $$$, most expensive.
AV, atrioventricular.

regimens include the following: propranolol, 20 mg four times daily (qid) or 40 mg twice daily (bid); metoprolol, 50 mg bid; and atenolol, 50 mg qd (every day).

C. **Calcium channel blockers.** These are a diverse group of compounds that have different effects on the atrioventricular node, heart rate, coronary arteries, diastolic relaxation, cardiac contractility, systemic blood pressure, and afterload. Most studies show equal effects between beta blockers and calcium channel blockers. Calcium channel blockers may be preferred in patients with obstructive airway disease, peripheral vascular disease, or supraventricular tachycardia. The most troublesome side effects are constipation, edema, headache, and aggravation of congestive heart failure. Examples of starting regimens include the following: nifedipine sustained-release, 30 mg qd; and diltiazem sustained-release, 120 mg qd. A recent case-control study reported an increased rate of MI among a group of hypertensive patients treated with short-acting calcium channel blockers. There is no evidence of a similar effect with long-acting calcium antagonists.

5. **Antioxidants.** Oxidized low-density lipoprotein (LDL) particles are implicated in the development and progression of atherosclerosis. In observational studies, vitamin E 100–400 IU daily has been associated with a decrease in coronary events and shown to slow progression of atherosclerotic lesions in patients who have undergone coronary artery bypass grafting. Further studies are under way to clarify the many questions that remain about the role of antioxidants.

6. **Vitamins B_6, B_{12}, and folate.** Elevated homocysteine levels are associated with IHD. Although the mechanisms are not well understood, alteration in coagulation profile or endothelial damage are postulated to play a role. Supplementation with B_6, B_{12}, and folate reduce plasma homocysteine levels.

7. **Hormone replacement therapy.** Estrogen replacement therapy in postmenopausal women is a major risk modifier for IHD. It has a favorable effect on vascular reactivity, coagulation profile, and both high-density lipoprotein (HDL) and LDL cholesterol. Current estimates suggest that less than 20% of women who could benefit from this therapy receive hormone replacement therapy.

B. **Unstable angina.** Unstable angina manifests clinically as an abrupt onset of ischemic symptoms at rest or as an intensification or change in the pattern of ischemic symptoms as well as an increasing ease of provocation (symptoms at rest or with minimal effort). The most important recent development in the management of unstable angina has been the 1994 report of the Agency for Health Care Policy and Research (AHCPR). The guidelines allow physicians to consider outpatient management for a select group of patients, specifically, those who are felt to be low-risk for MI. Low-risk patients may be treated with aspirin, NTG, or beta blockers. Follow-up should be no later than 72 hours. High- or moderate-risk patients should be admitted for intensive medical management. Clinical features consistent with high-risk include the following:

1. Prolonged rest pain (>20 minutes).
2. Pulmonary edema.
3. Angina with new or worsening mitral regurgitation murmurs.
4. Rest angina with dynamic ST changes >1 mm.
5. Angina with S_3 or rales.
6. Angina with hypotension.

C. **Percutaneous transluminal coronary angioplasty (PTCA).** Although there remains no consensus on definitive indications for PTCA, there has been a marked increase in its use. It is generally chosen for patients with angina who have failed maximum medical management. It is used for single- or double-vessel disease, excluding the proximal left anterior descending coronary artery. Among patients with unstable angina, PTCA is recommended for those who do not show an adequate response to medical treatment. Restenosis continues to be a complication; however, the long-term outcome after successful angioplasty has been reported to be excellent even when compared with patients undergoing bypass surgery. Further research is needed in the areas of long-term outcome for multiple lesions, extensive disease, and avoidance of complications.

D. Coronary artery bypass graft (CABG) surgery. Large randomized trials have shown that surgical revascularization is more effective than medical therapy for at least several years for controlling symptoms. Development of atherosclerosis in the graft resulting in angina generally occurs within 5–10 years. Improved survival with surgical versus medical therapy is seen only in the "sicker" subset of patients who are older and have more severe symptoms, particularly left main coronary artery disease or left ventricular dysfunction.

VI. Management strategies. It is important to maximize therapy with any one class of antianginal drug before considering it a failed trial. Generally, the drug classes complement each other. There is no literature to support one class of antianginal drugs as superior to another. It is a common practice to first use nitrates as needed (prn) for patients with infrequent symptoms. For more frequent symptoms, a long-acting beta blocker or calcium channel blocker in addition to the prn nitrate is often used. With increasingly frequent symptoms, combination or "triple therapy" (nitrate + beta blocker + calcium channel blocker) may be used. Calcium channel blockers and beta blockers should be used in combination with caution because of the greater risk of extreme bradycardia or heart block. Aggressive measures targeted at risk factor modification should be included for all patients with IHD.

VII. Prognosis and natural history

A. Prognosis. The three major factors that determine the prognosis of patients with angina include the amount of viable but jeopardized left ventricular myocardium, the percentage of irreversibly scarred myocardium, and the severity of underlying coronary atherosclerosis. ETT has been used to establish prognosis in patients with symptomatic IHD. The exercise parameters associated with poor outcome have been described above. Comparing medical management and PTCA, one randomized study of male patients with single-vessel disease found PTCA to be superior to medical management at 6 months, although 15% of patients required a second procedure. PTCA is superior to medical management in multivessel disease. CABG is superior to both medical management or PTCA for proximal left anterior descending coronary artery lesions or multivessel disease.

B. Natural history. Based on current information, the following is known regarding the natural history and prognosis of IHD:

1. IHD is the leading cause of premature, permanent disability in the US labor force, accounting for 19% of disability, according to the Social Security Administration.

2. A substantial number of patients with IHD have moderate to severe limitations in their usual activities.

3. Unrecognized MIs are common and as lethal as symptomatic infarcts. At least 25% of MIs are silent and another 25% present with atypical chest pain. Only 20% of MIs are preceded by angina. Most MIs occur at rest and nearly as many occur during sleep as during heavy physical activity. Distressing life events reportedly occur with increased frequency in the months preceding an MI.

   Women are often overlooked as having significant IHD. Women over 65 years are as vulnerable to IHD mortality as men. There is a precipitous increase in IHD in women after the menopause (whether natural or surgical).

5. Hypertension, tobacco abuse, diabetes, hyperlipidemia, sedentary lifestyle, and estrogen-deficient states are modifiable risk factors for IHD that should be aggressively managed.

REFERENCES

Braunwald E, et al: Diagnosing and managing unstable angina. Quick reference guide for clinicians, Number 10. US Department of Health and Human Services, Public Health Service, Agency for Health Care Policy and Research (AHCPR) and National Heart, Lung, and Blood Institute. March 1994; AHCPR Publication No. 94-0603.

Braunwald E: *Heart Disease: A Textbook of Cardiovascular Medicine,* 5th ed. Saunders; 1997.

Ellestad MH: *Stress Testing: Principles and Practice,* 3rd ed. Davis; 1996.

Graboys TB, Blatt CM (eds): *Angina Pectoris: Management Strategies and Guide to Interventions.* Professional Communications; 1994.

Villablanca A: Coronary heart disease in women: Gender differences and effects of menopause. Postgrad Med 1996;**100:**191.

82   Menopause

Mary Kay Mroz, MD

I. **Definition. Menopause** is the permanent cessation of menstruation caused by a loss of ovarian function. This condition can be diagnosed after no menses have occurred for 12 consecutive months. **Perimenopause** is the transitional period immediately prior to menopause. The **climacteric** is a term used to encompass the physiologic changes and symptoms surrounding the transition from reproductive to nonreproductive status.

II. **Epidemiology**
   A. Between 0.2% and 1% of visits made to primary care physicians are for menopausal symptoms.
   B. The mean age of menopause is 51.4 years, with a range of 41–59. This age is not affected by the patient's age at menarche, race, parity, socioeconomic status, or the patient's mother's age at menopause.
   C. Disabling symptoms attributable to decline in estrogen production for which medical therapy is sought are estimated to occur in 10–15% of perimenopausal women. There are no proven risk factors to assist in the identification of women who might experience disabling symptoms of menopause.

III. **Pathophysiology.** Menopause is associated with ovarian, hormonal, and target-organ changes.
   A. **Ovarian changes.** A progressive decrease in the number of ovarian follicles occurs from the 20th week of gestation in utero until the ovary is depleted of follicles at menopause. Ovarian atrophy or hypertrophy occurs during the postmenopausal period. Loss of reproductive ability results from cessation of ovarian function.
   B. **Hormonal changes**
      1. **Gonadotropins.** Levels of follicle-stimulating hormone (FSH) dramatically increase during the perimenopausal period. With the cessation of menses, luteinizing hormone (LH) levels also rise, and prolactin levels sharply decline.
      2. **Estrogen.** Levels of plasma estradiol (the principal ovarian estrogen) decline at rates corresponding to the rise in FSH levels. Estrogen metabolism also changes with aging. Conversion of androstenedione (a circulating androgen) to estrone (an estrogen precursor) occurs in the adipose tissue of postmenopausal women. Consequently, obese women may be less estrogen deficient than their thinner counterparts.
      3. **Androgens.** Production of precursor androgens (eg, androstenedione, testosterone) may increase in the immediate postmenopausal period with ovarian stromal proliferation.
   C. **Target end-organ changes.** Many organs have specific receptors for particular circulating steroid. Many end-organ changes occur as a result of declining or absent circulating estrogen levels (Table 82–1).

IV. **Symptoms.** Most women in their late 40s experience a progressive lengthening of the menstrual cycle with lighter menses. Irregular periods, caused by anovulation, are also common in the perimenopausal period.
   A. **Vasomotor symptoms.** The hot flash and the flush are the two principal components of vasomotor symptomatology. Researchers believe that alterations in the neurotransmitters of the hypothalamus are responsible for the flush. Patients with such disorders as pheochromocytoma, hyperthyroidism, and carcinoid syndrome usually present with vasomotor symptomatology in combination with other conditions, such as hypertension, tachycardia, and diarrhea. This association suggests a nonmenopausal origin.
      1. The **hot flash** is the sudden onset of warmth lasting 2–3 minutes. Experienced by 75–85% of menopausal women, the hot flash begins about 1 minute before the flush and lasts about 1 minute after its onset.
      2. The **flush** consists of visible redness of the upper chest, face, and neck and is followed by profuse sweating in these areas. The flush also lasts 2–3 minutes and is associated with a mean temperature elevation of 2.5 °C (4.5 °F).

TABLE 82–1. END-ORGAN CHANGES RESULTING FROM ESTROGEN DEFICIENCY

Target Organ	Change or Symptom
Neuroendocrine organs (hypothalamus)	Hot flushes, flashes, or both
	Atrophy, dryness, pruritus
Skin/mucous membranes	Dry hair or loss of hair
	Facial hirsutism
	Dry mouth
Skeleton	Osteoporosis with related fractures
	Backache
Vocal cords	Lower voice
Breasts	Reduced size
	Softer consistency
	Drooping (loss of ligamentous support)
Heart	Coronary artery disease
Vulva	Atrophy, dystrophy, or both
	Pruritus vulvae
Vagina	Dyspareunia
	Vaginitis
Uterus/pelvic floor	Uterovaginal prolapse
Bladder/urethra	Cystoureteritis
	Ectropion
	Frequency and/or urgency
	Stress incontinence

Adapted with permission from Utian WH: Overview on menopause. Am J Obstet Gynecol 1987;**156:**1280.

When left untreated, hot flushes are usually most severe in the first 1 or 2 years, after which severity gradually declines. Twenty-five percent of women report a duration of hot flushes of more than 5 years, and occasionally symptoms persist into the seventh or eighth decade.

   3. **Associated symptoms** commonly reported with the above vasomotor phenomena are heart palpitations, headache, throbbing in the head or neck, and nausea.

   B. Psychological symptoms. The following symptoms all have been reported during the perimenopausal period: fatigue, insomnia, anxiety, and depression.

   C. Atrophy of the lower genital tract

   1. **Vulvar pruritus** is common, especially in fair-skinned women.

   2. **Vaginitis and dyspareunia** from atrophy of vaginal mucosa are experienced by about 10–20% of women. Symptoms include dryness, burning, leukorrhea, itching, and bleeding.

   3. **Atrophy of the urethral mucosa,** which leads to frank urethritis, dysuria, urgency, and frequency, is less common.

V. Signs. The physical examination is usually normal during the early perimenopausal period, with characteristic findings evident after the onset of menopause.

   A. The **breasts** appear less firm and smaller, with a regression of glandular tissue and an increase in fibrous tissue.

   B. The **pelvic examination** is most revealing in the postmenopausal period.

   1. The **labia majora** are smaller, and hair in the perivulvar area is thin.

   2. The **vaginal epithelium** appears pale, thin, and dry, with a loss of rugae and secretions.

   3. The **cervical os** is often smaller and may be stenotic. The cervical epithelium is thinner and more easily traumatized.

   4. **Uterine size** is diminished. Reduced collagen in the supporting ligamentous structures of the pelvis can lead to uterine prolapse and pelvic relaxation. This relaxation occurs especially when there is a history of multiparity, prior birth trauma, a family history of uterine prolapse or pelvic relaxation, or chronic pelvic stress from coughing, constipation, or heavy work.

   5. The **ovaries** should not be palpable on pelvic examination after menopause. Palpable ovarian enlargement in a menopausal woman suggests ovarian carcinoma until proven otherwise.

C. Urethral prolapse can occur because of atrophy of the urethral mucosa. A prolapsed urethra or caruncle appears as a red, friable mass within the urethra itself.

D. Dry, wrinkled, and more easily traumatized skin is attributable to both menopause and age. Thinning of scalp hair and increased facial hair (hirsutism) may also be evident.

VI. Laboratory tests. The presence of vasomotor symptoms, oligomenorrhea, and atrophy of the lower genital tract in women in their mid- to late 40s almost certainly confirms the onset of the perimenopausal period. Diagnostic testing (eg, circulating estrogen and gonadotropin levels) is rarely, if ever, indicated.

Determination of FSH and LH levels is warranted in any woman under age 35 experiencing signs and symptoms of menopause. Specific causes of premature ovarian failure include genetic abnormalities, autoimmune disorders, and rare hormonal defects (see Chapter 5). Both FSH and LH levels are elevated during menopause, but elevation in FSH levels is the most sensitive indicator of ovarian failure.

VII. Treatment. Exogenous estrogen is the cornerstone of pharmacologic treatment of perimenopausal and postmenopausal symptoms as well as of osteoporosis. Estrogen deficiency has never been proved in randomized controlled trials to cause the diverse psychological symptoms reported during the perimenopausal period. Consequently, estrogen replacement therapy cannot guarantee relief from these symptoms. In women with an intact uterus, addition of a progestin reduces the risk of endometrial hyperplasia, which is a precursor of endometrial carcinoma. The usefulness of progestational agents for women following a hysterectomy remains controversial.

A. Indications for estrogen replacement therapy

    1. Patients at high risk for postmenopausal osteoporosis. Treatment with estrogen and **selective estrogen-receptor modulators,** such as raloxifene, is the only proven prophylaxis against osteoporotic fractures. About 60% of women do not develop symptomatic osteoporosis, so treatment of all women is unnecessary. Women who have a history of tobacco or alcohol use, who have a family history of osteoporosis, and who have experienced premature or surgical menopause at age 40 or sooner are at particular risk for osteoporosis and thus are good candidates for estrogen replacement therapy.

    2. Patients experiencing moderate to severe symptoms of estrogen deficiency (vasomotor symptoms, lower genital tract atrophy).

B. Estrogens. Some of the many available formulations of estrogen are described in the following text.

    1. One oral regimen is **conjugated estrogens** (Premarin), 0.625 mg daily from day 1 through day 25 of each month. Randomized placebo-controlled studies have shown that regimens of less than 0.625 mg of estrogen per day are ineffective in preventing bone loss. Higher doses must be balanced against the still to be determined risk of breast and endometrial cancer.

    2. Transdermal patch application of **estradiol** (Estraderm, Climara; 0.05 mg/day) results in prolonged blood levels and has a limited effect on hepatic function with subsequent clotting and lipid abnormalities while relieving vasomotor symptoms and preventing osteoporosis. Permeable adhesive disks are applied to the skin every 3–7 days. A progesterone/estrogen combination patch (CombiPatch) is now available for those women with an intact endometrium who prefer a transdermal delivery system. Dosage strengths are **estradiol/norethindrone acetate** 0.05/0.14 mg and 0.05/0.25 mg applied twice weekly. About 24% of women who use this method have some form of skin irritation, which can be managed by rotation of application site.

    3. Intramuscular injections of estrogens (**estradiol valerate,** 10, 20, 40 mg/mL) can be administered. Drawbacks include discomfort of administration, variability in absorption and metabolism, and the necessity of monthly injections.

    4. Vaginal therapy. Many peri- and postmenopausal women experience mild vasomotor symptoms but have more severe symptoms of atrophic vaginitis. For such women, an introital vaginal water-soluble lubricant may suffice. Intravaginal estrogen cream, such as **conjugated estrogens** (Premarin), 0.625 mg/g, and **estropipate** (Ogen), 1.5 mg/g, is useful for more resistant symptoms. The physician must keep in mind that systemic absorption does occur. Daily administration of 1.2–2.4 g is typically recommended on days 1–21 of the month, although continuous therapy on weekdays only is increasingly popular. Even when oral replacement therapy is used, there still may be a need for vaginal lubrication during intercourse.

Vulvar pruritus responds poorly to topical estrogens. Regular application of a testosterone ointment (**testosterone propionate** cream, 2.5% per day), however, maintains thickness of the vulvar epithelium, thereby relieving dryness and itching.

C. **Progestins** have been shown to relieve vasomotor symptoms in postmenopausal patients either alone or in combination with estrogens. They are useful also in preventing endometrial hyperplasia.

    1. **Progestin-only regimens. Medroxyprogesterone acetate** (Provera), 20 mg orally daily, is especially appealing for women for whom estrogen therapy is contraindicated (Table 82–2) or who experience intolerable side effects (breast tenderness, breakthrough bleeding, nausea) even on low-dose estrogen therapy.

    2. **Combination of estrogen and progestin.** Estrogen replacement alone may lead to endometrial hyperplasia which, in a small number of women, progresses to endometrial carcinoma. Maximal protection against endometrial hyperplasia occurs when progestin is prescribed for at least 10–12 days (days 14 through 25) of each calendar month. The newest approach to hormone replacement involves continuous daily oral administration of both estrogen and progestin. This combination allows for eventual cessation of withdrawal bleeding experienced by many women receiving cyclic therapy and the reduction of side effects that can occur with high-dose progestin therapy. The regimen of conjugated estrogens (Premarin), 0.625 mg daily, plus medroxyprogesterone acetate (Provera), 2.5 or 5 mg daily, is well accepted by patients. The cyclic treatment of 21–25 days of an oral estrogen with the concurrent administration of a progestin during the last 10–14 days of estrogen treatment is the most common type of hormone replacement therapy. The daily dose of progestational agent to achieve endometrial protection is small: **norethindrone** (Micronor), 0.7 mg every day, **medroxyprogesterone acetate** (Provera), 5 mg every day, or **micronized progesterone** (Prometrium), 400 mg every day. Additional support for a minimum progestin dose comes from the known effect of progestin, either alone or in combination with estrogens, to increase low-density lipoprotein levels (LDL) and decrease high-density lipoprotein (HDL) levels. Whether these changes in lipoprotein levels translate to an increased risk of coronary artery disease and whether the risk is worth the benefits gained by adding progestin to estrogen therapy have not been established.

    Progestin use for women who have had a hysterectomy and are receiving estrogen replacement remains controversial. In this situation, the uncertain cardiovascular risk attributable to unfavorable lipoprotein profiles may outweigh any known beneficial effect of adding a progestin

D. **Selective estrogen-receptor modulators.** The newest entry into the medical pharmacopeia for the treatment of menopausal sequelae is raloxifene, a benzothiophene. It is a member of the nonhormonal class called selective estrogen-receptor modulators (SERMs). This drug has both estrogen-agonist effects on bone, liver, and heart and estrogen-antagonist effects on breast and uterus in studies conducted to date. Studies in small numbers of women have shown strengthening of bone, lowering of LDL-C cholesterol, no effect on HDL choles-

TABLE 82–2. CONTRAINDICATIONS TO ESTROGEN REPLACEMENT THERAPY

Absolute	Relative
Estrogen-dependent neoplasia (breast, endometrium)	Endometrial hyperplasia
	Past history of vaso-occlusive disease (thrombosis)
	Diabetes mellitus
	Hypertension
	Cholelithiasis
	Family history of estrogen-dependent neoplasia (breast, endometrium)

Adapted with permission from Whitehead MI: The menopause. Practitioner 1987;**231**:42.

terol, no increased incidence in breast cancers, and no proliferation of endometrial lining. These effects make raloxifene an attractive alternative for those women concerned with estrogen's potential for cancer potentiation. No effects are seen for anxiety, depression, or vaginal atrophy. Hot flashes and sweats may actually get worse temporarily when raloxifene treatment is initiated. Like estrogen, the incidence of thrombophlebitis is increased compared with placebo.

VIII. Management strategies

A. Patient education. For many women, the worst thing about menopause is not knowing what to expect. Thorough evaluation of the woman's understanding of menopause and accurate education directed at identification of symptoms and management options will greatly reduce anxiety. Many myths surround menopause, including that menopause signals the end of a women's sexual interest and participation and that menopause is associated with a high incidence of depression, psychosis, and cancer. A review of the patient's sexual activity along with the patient's medical history is the best starting point for addressing these concerns (Table 82–3). Myths should be dispelled with accurate information emphasizing menopause as a normal physiologic event.

B. Patient follow-up

1. Although there is no convincing evidence that maintenance exogenous estrogens significantly alter weight and blood pressure, it is prudent to monitor the patient undertaking estrogen replacement therapy at least once a year.

2. **Endometrial biopsy.** Most women using cyclic combined estrogen–progestin regimens experience regular withdrawal bleeding, but a few women do not bleed at all. Both patterns are normal, and the optimal frequency of endometrial biopsies in the absence of breakthrough bleeding is unknown. For women receiving continuous combined hormonal therapy, irregular bleeding in the first 3–8 months is not uncommon. Biopsies every 2–3 years for women at particularly high risk for endometrial carcinoma have been suggested. Any bleeding that occurs before the 10th day of progesterone therapy should prompt endometrial sampling, since this suggests excessive estrogen stimulation.

C. Duration of therapy. The duration of therapy is determined by the type of symptoms experienced and by the initial reasons for instituting treatment.

1. **Vasomotor symptoms** are usually self-limiting, and many women can terminate therapy after 2–5 years. A few women, however, require long-term treatment for persistent severe symptoms or experience a recurrence of symptoms after therapy has been discontinued.

2. **Atrophy of the lower genital tract** may be effectively treated with topical estrogen cream for many years. Since systemic absorption of topically administered creams through the vaginal epithelium occurs, periodic oral progestin administration has been recommended to prevent endometrial hyperplasia. If dyspareunia continues to be a problem after 5 years of continuous topical estrogens, it may be preferable to counsel patients in the use of inert, water-soluble lubricants prior to intercourse.

3. **Osteoporosis.** Although the optimal duration of therapy to reduce the risk of osteoporosis is not known, estrogen use through age 74 has been demonstrated to protect against hip fractures. Estrogen replacement therapy is rarely indicated after age 75 unless there are clear medical indications to continue treatment (see Chapter 84).

TABLE 82–3. KEY QUESTIONS TO UNCOVER SEXUAL PROBLEMS DURING THE PERIMENOPAUSAL AND POSTMENOPAUSAL PERIODS

1. Are you sexually active?
2. Do you have a partner at the present time?
3. Has there been any change in your interest in or desire for sexual activity?
4. Is intercourse pleasurable?
5. Do you experience any discomfort during intercourse?
6. Have you noticed any change in lubrication when you become aroused?
7. Do you reach orgasm satisfactorily?
8. Does your partner have any problems with your sexual relationship?

Adapted, with permission, from Iddenden DA: Sexuality during the menopause. Med Clin North Am 1987;**71**:87.

4. Cardiovascular protection. There is controversial information coming to light in a few small studies that show that estrogen has a protective effect against cardiovascular disease. In women at high risk for cardiovascular disease, without other contraindications, estrogen replacement therapy may play a beneficial role in cardioprotection and the physician may therefore opt for indefinite low-dose estrogen therapy.

REFERENCES

Clisham PR, et al: Comparison of continuous versus sequential estrogen and progestin therapy in postmenopausal women. Obstet Gynecol 1991;**77**:21.

Delmas PD, et al: Effects of raloxifene on bone mineral density, serum cholesterol concentrations, and uterine endometrium in postmenopausal women. N Engl J Med 1997;**337**(23):1641.

Greendale GA, et al: The menopause: Health implications and clinical management. J Am Geriatr Soc 1993;**41**:426.

Henderson BE, et al: Decreased mortality in users of estrogen replacement therapy. Arch Intern Med 1991;**151**:75.

Iddenden DA: Sexuality during the menopause. Med Clin North Am 1987;**71**(1):87.

Sessions DR, et al: Current concepts in estrogen replacement therapy in the menopause. Fertil Steril 1993;**59**(2):277.

Speroff L, Glass RH, Kase NG: *Clinical Gynecologic Endocrinology and Infertility,* 5th ed. Williams & Wilkins; 1994.

Utian WH: Overview of menopause. Am J Obstet Gynecol 1987;**156**:1280.

Walsh BW, et al: Effects of raloxifene on serum lipids and coagulation factors in healthy postmenopausal women. JAMA 1998;**279**(18):1445.

Whitehead MI: The menopause. Practitioner 1987;**231**:37.

---

83   Obesity

Jack A. Yanovski, MD, PhD, & Susan Zelitch Yanovski, MD

I. **Definition.** *Obesity* is defined as the presence of an abnormally large amount of adipose tissue. Some individuals, such as muscular athletes, are overweight without being obese; however, most people who are overweight also have too much body fat. While most clinicians are familiar with determining overweight through weight-for-height tables, the current preferred method is to use a measure known as the *body mass index* (*BMI*), which is calculated by dividing the weight (in kg) by the height (in meters squared), or the weight (in pounds) × 704.5 divided by the height (in inches squared). A chart converting weight and height into BMI is shown in Table 83–1. BMI provides a more accurate estimate of body fat than relying solely on weight, and is gender and frame-size independent. The Clinical Guidelines on the Identification, Evaluation, and Treatment of Overweight and Obesity in Adults, recently issued by the National Institutes of Health (NIH), define overweight as a BMI of 25–29.9 kg/m², and obesity as a BMI ≥30 kg/m². Obesity itself can further be subdivided into Classes I–III, based on degree of severity (Table 83–2).

II. **Epidemiology**

A. In the United States, 97 million adults, 59% of men and 51% of women, are considered overweight or obese (BMI >25); 20% of men and 25% of women meet criteria for obesity (BMI ≥30). The percentage of adult Americans with a BMI ≥30 kg/m² has almost doubled in the past 30 years, with most of the increase occurring in the past decade.

B. Among women, there is an inverse correlation between socioeconomic status and obesity, although this association is most strong in non-Hispanic whites.

C. Minority populations are disproportionately affected. One-third of Mexican-American and 37% of African American women are obese, and 10% of African American women meet criteria for Class III Obesity (BMI ≥40 kg/m²).

D. Children and adolescents are also becoming heavier. The prevalence of overweight among 6- to 17-year-olds has more than doubled since the 1960s and 1970s. Approximately 1 in 5 children in the United States is now overweight. The Obesity Evaluation and Treatment Expert Committee sponsored by the National Institutes of Health recommends that any child with a BMI for age and sex greater

TABLE 83–1. BODY MASS INDEX: HOW TO MEASURE OBESITY[1]

Body Mass Index

Height (inches)	19	20	21	22	23	24	25	26	27	28	29	30	31	32	33	34	35
									Body Weight (pounds)								
58	91	96	100	105	110	115	119	124	129	134	138	143	148	153	158	162	167
59	94	99	104	109	114	119	124	128	133	138	143	148	153	158	163	168	173
60	97	102	107	112	118	123	128	133	138	143	148	153	158	163	168	174	179
61	100	106	111	116	122	127	132	137	143	148	153	158	164	169	174	180	185
62	104	109	115	120	126	131	136	142	147	153	158	164	169	175	180	186	191
63	107	113	118	124	130	135	141	146	152	158	163	169	175	180	186	191	197
64	110	116	122	128	134	140	145	151	157	163	169	174	180	186	192	197	204
65	114	120	126	132	138	144	150	156	162	168	174	180	186	192	198	204	210
66	118	124	130	136	142	148	155	161	167	173	179	186	192	198	204	210	216
67	121	127	134	140	146	153	159	166	172	178	185	191	198	204	211	217	223
68	125	131	138	144	151	158	164	171	177	184	190	197	203	210	216	223	230
69	128	135	142	149	155	162	169	176	182	189	196	203	209	216	223	230	236
70	132	139	146	153	160	167	174	181	188	195	202	209	216	222	229	236	243
71	136	143	150	157	165	172	179	186	193	200	208	215	222	229	236	243	250
72	140	147	154	162	169	177	184	191	199	206	213	221	228	235	242	250	258
73	144	151	159	166	174	182	189	197	204	212	219	227	235	242	250	257	265
74	148	155	163	171	179	186	194	202	210	218	225	233	241	249	256	264	272
75	152	160	168	176	184	192	200	208	216	224	232	240	248	256	264	272	279
76	156	164	172	180	189	197	205	213	221	230	238	246	254	263	271	279	287

TABLE 83–1. (*continued*)

Height (inches)	Body Mass Index																		
	36	37	38	39	40	41	42	43	44	45	46	47	48	49	50	51	52	53	54
	Body Weight (pounds)																			
58	172	177	181	186	191	196	201	205	210	215	220	224	229	234	239	244	248	253	258
59	178	183	188	193	198	203	208	212	217	222	227	232	237	242	247	252	257	262	267
60	184	189	194	199	204	209	215	220	225	230	235	240	245	250	255	261	266	271	276
61	190	195	201	206	211	217	222	227	232	238	243	248	254	259	264	269	275	280	285
62	196	202	207	213	218	224	229	235	240	246	251	256	262	267	273	278	284	289	295
63	203	208	214	220	225	231	237	242	248	254	259	265	270	278	282	287	293	299	304
64	209	215	221	227	232	238	244	250	256	262	267	273	279	285	291	296	302	308	314
65	216	222	228	234	240	246	252	258	264	270	276	282	288	294	300	306	312	318	324
66	223	229	235	241	247	253	260	266	272	278	284	291	297	303	309	315	322	328	334
67	230	236	242	249	255	261	268	274	280	287	293	299	306	312	319	325	331	338	344
68	236	243	249	256	262	269	276	282	289	295	302	308	315	322	328	335	341	348	354
69	243	250	257	263	270	277	284	291	297	304	311	318	324	331	338	345	351	358	365
70	250	257	264	271	278	285	292	299	306	313	320	327	334	341	348	355	362	369	376
71	257	265	272	279	286	293	301	308	315	322	329	338	343	351	358	365	372	379	386
72	265	272	279	287	294	302	309	316	324	331	338	346	353	361	368	375	383	390	397
73	272	280	288	295	302	310	318	325	333	340	348	355	363	371	378	386	393	401	408
74	280	287	295	303	311	319	326	334	342	350	358	365	373	381	389	396	404	412	420
75	287	295	303	311	319	327	335	343	351	359	367	375	383	391	399	407	415	423	431
76	295	304	312	320	328	336	344	353	361	369	377	385	394	402	410	418	426	435	443

[1] Body mass index (BMI) is usually measured with the Quetelet index as follows: weight divided by height squared (W/H² [kg/m²]).
To use the table, find the appropriate height in the left-hand column. Move across to a given weight. The number at the top of the column is the BMI at that height and weight. Pounds have been rounded off.
Reprinted from Clinical guidelines on the identification, evaluation, and treatment of overweight and obesity in adults—The evidence report. Obes Res 1998;**6**:[suppl 2]:1S2S.

TABLE 83-2. CLASSIFICATION OF OVERWEIGHT AND OBESITY BY BMI, WAIST CIRCUMFERENCE, AND DISEASE RISK

	BMI kg/m²	Obesity Class	Disease Risk[1] Relative to Normal Weight and Waist Circumference	
			Men ≤102 cm (≤40 in) Women ≤88 cm (≤35 in)	>102 cm (>40 in) >88 cm (>35 in)
Underweight	<18.5		—	—
Normal[2]	18.5–24.9		—	—
Overweight	25.0–29.9		Increased	High
Obesity	30.0–34.9	I	High	Very high
	35.0–39.9	II	Very high	Very high
Extreme obesity	≥40	III	Extremely high	Extremely high

[1] Disease risk for type 2 diabetes, hypertension, and CVD.
[2] Increased waist circumference can also be a marker for increased risk even in persons of normal weight.
BMI, Body mass index; CVD, cardiovascular disease.
Reprinted from Clinical guidelines on the identification, evaluation, and treatment of overweight and obesity in adults—The evidence report. Obes Res 1998;6[suppl 2]: p. 62.

than the 95th percentile should undergo an in-depth medical assessment. Revised reference growth curves displaying BMI percentile curves by age and sex will be released soon by the National Center for Health Statistics (NCHS).

III. **Pathophysiology.** People gain weight because of increased caloric intake relative to the body's expenditures. Caloric intake may exceed demand as a result of several factors.

A. **Psychosocial and environmental causes.** The current American environment may be considered a "toxic" one because it facilitates the development of overweight in susceptible individuals. Most Americans are less active than is optimal for health, with up to 40% reporting being totally sedentary. Despite the increasing availability of low-fat foods, Americans consume more calories than they did 10 years ago. More Americans eat out frequently at restaurants, where large portions of high-fat foods contribute to the problem. In addition to environmental and social cues, some people overeat in response to emotional distress. A minority of obese individuals have binge eating disorder (see Chapter 97). These individuals may have more difficulty in completing weight loss treatment or maintaining a weight loss than those without an eating disorder. However, obesity itself is neither a cause nor a result of psychiatric disorders, and the obese population that does not seek treatment shows no more evidence of underlying psychopathology than the nonobese.

B. **Genetic predisposition.** Studies of identical twins and adoptees indicate that obesity has a strong genetic component. Energy expenditure and fat distribution appear to be particularly influenced by heredity. Individuals with a family history of obesity may be viewed as having a vulnerability to obesity, with the environment playing a protective or permissive role in its ultimate development. Patients should be advised that the genetic predisposition to obesity does not necessarily mean that they are destined to be obese. There may, however, be limitations on the amount of weight that an individual can comfortably lose and maintain. This is particularly true of those with more severe degrees of obesity and those who have been obese since childhood.

An explosion of knowledge regarding the genetics and neuroendocrinology of energy regulation has occurred over the past several years, and candidate genes for susceptibility to obesity in humans are being identified at a rapid rate. One example is the newly described hormone leptin, which is secreted by fat cells and supplies the hypothalamus with a measure of the amount of fat stored in adipose tissue. Several case reports of humans with differing genetic mutations leading to severe obesity have been identified; however, the vast majority of patients have not been found to have these mutations. Abnormalities in single genes are probably not the cause of most human obesity. Research advances are likely to lead to improvements in both prevention and treatment of obesity, but translation of these advances to treatments that can be applied to patients is unlikely during the next decade.

C. High "set point." There is some evidence that body weight is regulated by homeostatic mechanisms around a certain weight, or set point, that is defended against change through adjustment of the metabolic rate. There is no evidence that obese individuals have an unusually efficient metabolism compared with those of normal weight. However, recent evidence supports the suggestion that the body tends to defend its weight, increasing its energy expenditure above that predicted when weight is gained, and decreasing energy expenditure below predicted when weight is lost. This is true of individuals who are lean or obese, and appears to be independent of race or sex. It may be that some obese individuals have their weight regulated at a higher level than the nonobese, and the decrease in energy requirements when weight is reduced to a more "normal" level (amounting to 200–300 kcal/day with a 10–20% weight loss) may provide some explanation as to why so many people tend to regain lost weight. The decrease in energy expenditure occurs primarily in nonresting energy expenditure, which includes the energy expended in physical activity. Thus, increasing physical activity may provide a way to offset some of the increase in metabolic efficiency seen with weight loss. Some experts believe that factors such as the amount of fat in the diet or the degree of physical activity may help to modify an individual's set point.

D. "Organic" causes of obesity. Rarely, endocrine or primary neurologic dysfunction causes obesity via a decreased metabolic rate or hyperphagia. Midline hypothalamic tumors such as craniopharyngioma can cause significant obesity. Unusual genetic syndromes such as Prader–Willi syndrome are associated with both obesity and dysmorphisms. Only a few cases of genetic mutations of known obesity genes, such as the leptin or leptin receptor genes, have been reported. Those individuals were severely obese since childhood. Medications such as corticosteroids, tricyclic antidepressants, and phenothiazines may also cause obesity. Severe hypothyroidism may also cause a 5- to 20-lb weight gain.

IV. Diagnosis

A. Symptoms and signs

1. Obese patients often have decreased exercise tolerance as well as symptoms and signs attributable to the many medical conditions that accompany obesity. An important component of assessment of risk status is determination of the presence of concomitant cardiovascular risk factors, glucose intolerance or type 2 diabetes, and other obesity-associated conditions. The physician should inquire about a personal or family history (or both) of hypertension, diabetes, and cardiovascular disease; symptoms of sleep apnea; and presence of gynecologic abnormalities, osteoarthritis, gallstones, and stress incontinence. Tobacco use and the amount of habitual physical activity should be determined. Blood pressure should be measured with an appropriately sized cuff. The physician should be alert to other medical conditions that may contribute to the patient's obesity.

   a. Hypothyroidism is a common disorder, although it is rarely the sole cause of obesity (see Chapter 91).

   b. Cushing's disease is rare and is generally associated with other symptoms and signs, such as striae, muscle weakness, and hypertension. Central obesity is predominant.

   c. The patient with hyperphagia resulting from neurologic dysfunction will generally have other neurologic symptoms and signs that will be detected by a thorough history and physical examination.

   d. The physician should inquire about symptoms of atypical depression, such as hypersomnolence.

2. The normal-weight or mildly obese young woman who requests a weight loss diet should be asked about binge eating and purging behaviors. This is the most common presentation of bulimia nervosa to the primary care physician (see Chapter 97).

3. Significant obesity is usually evident to the practitioner. However, there are several ways to classify obesity that have implications for degree of risk from medical complications, prognosis, and treatment.

   a. **Body weight.** The patient's height and weight are measured and BMI is calculated, as noted above. This method is inexpensive, easily administered, and accurate. The major disadvantages are that the percentage of body fat is not measured directly, and distribution of body fat is also not obtained.

      b. Percentage of body fat. This can be determined by skin fold measurement or by bioelectrical impedance analysis (often called "body fat analyzers"), but both require specialized equipment or training and are not practical for the average primary care physician. Measurement of body fat using bioelectrical impedance analysis is not reliable in the severely obese and is not useful to track short-term changes in body composition such as those seen with diet or exercise. Total body fat of >25% in men or >30% in women is consistent with obesity.

      c. Body fat distribution. Measurement of the waist circumference with a tape measure is inexpensive, accurate, and easily done by the physician or the physician's staff. A waist circumference of >102 cm (40 in) in men or >88 cm (35 in) in women is indicative of central, or android, as opposed to peripheral, or gynoid, obesity, and places the patient at greater relative risk for obesity-associated disease. Waist circumference correlates better with visceral obesity than the waist-to-hip ratio.

      d. Combination of BMI and body fat distribution. These determinations, which are easily and inexpensively obtained by the primary care physician, provide data that can aid in risk assessment and treatment. Table 83–2 shows the classification of overweight and obesity by BMI, waist circumference, and associated disease risk.

B. Laboratory evaluation. Few tests are routinely indicated in the obese patient. Because of the concomitant increases in the rates of non–insulin-dependent diabetes mellitus, hypercholesterolemia, and hypertriglyceridemia in the obese, it is prudent to obtain a fasting blood glucose value and a lipid panel consisting of cholesterol, high-density lipoprotein, and triglycerides (see Chapter 79).

V. Treatment. The physician and the patient should work together to determine realistic goals for weight loss, taking into account the degree of obesity, weight history, family history, patient motivation, and degree of medical risk. A BMI ≥30 kg/m² or ≥25 kg/m² in those with two or more accompanying comorbid conditions or risk factors (such as diabetes or dyslipidemia) should prompt weight loss intervention. In those who are overweight but not obese (BMI 25–29.9) and who have less than two risk factors, the clinician should focus on prevention of further weight gain. The NIH Guidelines treatment algorithm, based on degree of overweight and associated risk factors, is shown in Figure 83–1. The entire text of the guidelines is available on the world wide web at: http://www.nhlbi.nih.gov/nhlbi/cardio/obes/prof/guidelns/ob_home.htm

A. Diet. A nutritionally sound and flexible diet that allows for the food preferences and lifestyle of the patient should be developed. Merely handing the patient a preprinted diet sheet is ineffective. Although a hypocaloric diet that provides less energy than the patient expends is necessary for weight loss, diet must be combined with other modalities to optimize outcome.

    1. A nutritionally adequate, low-fat, reduced-calorie diet should be developed for mildly obese individuals. Caloric intake should not be restricted below 1000 kcal/day, since diets much lower in caloric density are likely to be nutritionally inadequate. Greater minimal caloric intake may be required for growing children.

      a. Merely reducing portion size while maintaining the usual percentage of fat (about 35% of calories in the typical diet in this country) is unlikely to be helpful. Reducing dietary fat to 20–30% of the total calories enhances weight loss, helps to ensure an adequate intake of nutrient-rich foods, and is consistent with health recommendations for the prevention of cardiovascular disease.

      b. Patients should be encouraged to avoid skipping meals and to divide their caloric intake evenly throughout the day.

      c. A caloric deficit of 500–1000 kcal/day will result in the loss of approximately 1–2 lbs/week, which is an appropriate rate of weight loss for most persons.

    2. Very low-calorie diets (VLCDs), under medical supervision, have a limited role in the treatment of individuals with moderate to severe obesity. These diets usually replace meals with supplements of high-quality protein in powder or solid form, along with varying amounts of carbohydrate and small amounts of fat. Most formulations contain the Recommended Dietary Allowance of vitamins and minerals. Daily caloric intake is usually 800 kcal or less.

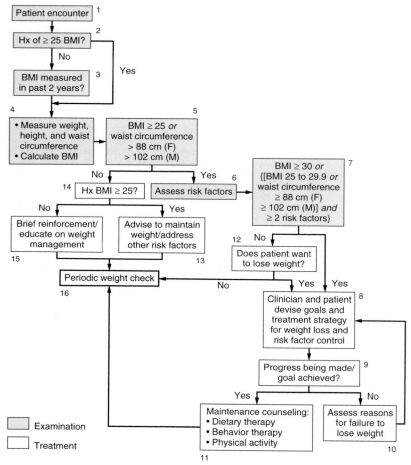

FIGURE 83–1. Treatment algorithm. This algorithm applies only to the assessment for overweight and obesity and subsequent decisions based on that assessment. It does not reflect any initial overall assessment for other conditions and diseases that the physician may wish to do. BMI, Body mass index; F, female; Hx, history; M, male. (Reprinted from Clinical guidelines on the identification, evaluation, and treatment of overweight and obesity in adults—The evidence report. Obes Res 1998;**6** [suppl 2]:66.)

Recent studies have shown that formulations providing <800 kcal do not provide any larger or more rapid weight loss than those providing 800 kcal/day. Therefore, formulations containing <800 kcal are not recommended.

The primary advantage of VLCDs is that larger weight losses are obtained than with conventional diets, which may be advantageous in some patients whose health is compromised by their obesity, such as patients with sleep apnea or Pickwickian syndrome. Weight loss with these diets averages 0.9–2.7 kg (2–6 lbs)/week, and the diets are generally continued for 12–16 weeks, after which foods are gradually reintroduced. Weight losses of >20 kg (44 lbs) are common. While these diets have been shown to be safe when carried out under close medical supervision, patients tend to regain lost weight more quickly than with low-calorie diets (LCDs), so that LCDs are just as effective in producing weight loss after 1 year.

    a. Patients using VLCDs are at increased risk for cholelithiasis. This risk can be ameliorated through the concomitant use of ursodeoxycholic acid (ursodiol) 300 mg twice daily during the period of rapid weight loss.

  3. Nonprescription "formula" diets sold in supermarkets and pharmacies are meant to replace only one or two meals a day. Such diets should not be confused with VLCDs, which should be administered only by physicians. "Formula" diets are very popular with patients because of their low expense and easy availability. Used as directed, these diets have few side effects, although obese patients often tire of these regimens, quickly regaining any lost weight.

  4. Starvation diets are those in which the patient maintains an intake of <200 kcal/day. These diets are potentially dangerous, with complications including hypotension, gout, and cardiac dysrhythmias. Lost weight is generally rapidly regained. Starvation diets have largely been replaced by VLCDs.

  5. "Fad diets," which rely on unusual combinations of foods, restriction of whole classes of foods (ie, proteins or carbohydrates), or which promise to alter the body's metabolism or utilization, have been shown to be unhelpful in long-term weight loss. Some of these diets are potentially dangerous, particularly in adolescents or in individuals with underlying medical problems.

B. Psychological therapies

  1. *Behavioral therapy* for obesity refers to the applications of psychological techniques of learning theory to obesity treatment. It has evolved over the years from the rote application of techniques (eg, eating slowly and putting down one's fork between bites) to a comprehensive treatment system involving dietary modification, nutrition education, promotion of physical activity, and cognitive restructuring. Behavioral therapy is now an accepted modality in most weight management programs.

    The primary advantages of behavioral therapy include the low attrition rate, as compared with other therapies, and the lack of any adverse effects. The major disadvantages are the relatively modest degree of weight loss using behavioral techniques alone, which averages <10 kg (22 lbs) in most studies, and the slow rate of weight loss, usually <0.45 kg (1 lb)/week, which can be discouraging to the patient who requires substantial weight loss. Behavioral therapy may be combined with other modalities, including medication, when appropriate.

    a. Behavioral treatment of obesity consists of a number of components, often provided together in a "package" of services. These include the following.

      (1) Self-monitoring. Patients should keep detailed records of the type and amount of food eaten, the places in which foods are eaten, with whom the foods are eaten, and emotional factors that accompany food intake. This helps patients to identify the antecedents to their eating and the patterns that perpetuate their obesity.

      (2) Stimulus control. Patients learn methods such as restricting the places in which eating is permitted, eating more slowly, and limiting reading or watching television while eating. These techniques enable the patient to separate eating from other activities.

      (3) Self-reward. This includes nonfood incentives, such as buying new clothes, for reaching defined goals.

      (4) Cognitive restructuring, in which self-defeating attitudes, such as "all-or-none" thinking, are examined and challenged, can be helpful in relapse prevention.

      (5) Physical activity is frequently included as a major target for behavioral change, helping patients to develop strategies for increasing energy expenditure by activities that can easily be incorporated into their routine, such as climbing stairs rather than taking an elevator, as well as strategies for increasing more structured forms of exercise.

    b. A long-term maintenance component, which includes continued monitoring, posttreatment contacts with the therapist, and the establishment of social supports, may improve long-term results. Relapse prevention, which helps to "inoculate" the patient against the escalation of inevitable "slips" into full-scale relapse, should also be emphasized. Adjuncts such as assertiveness training, nutrition education, and formal exercise prescriptions are often included in behavior modification programs.

    c. Behavior modification treatment, which typically lasts 12–20 weeks, is usually provided in a group setting. Work-site groups have proven particularly popular. Written materials may also prove useful—either as an adjunct to formal treatment or as a self-help program. A useful resource is the LEARN manual (available by calling 1-800-736-7323), which instructs the patient step by step in designing an individualized behavioral program and which may also be used in conjunction with treatment by the physician. Behavior modification is an essential adjunct in the treatment of more severe obesity by VLCD or surgery.

  2. Commercial weight loss programs and self-help groups span a range of approaches. Some provide prepackaged food, some provide a structured diet, and most offer support, often in a group setting. The abilities of leaders of such groups vary dramatically, and few leaders have formal training in psychology, nutrition, or related fields. Cost can range from negligible, in nonprofit self-help groups, to quite expensive, in programs that require the purchase of food or nutritional supplements. Behavior modification is a component of many of these programs, which vary widely in approach. Patients may need to try more than one to find a group with which they feel comfortable. Self-help groups may be a useful adjunct to other forms of therapy, and many patients benefit from the support that such groups provide. Attrition is a major problem in both commercial weight loss programs and self-help groups, and has been estimated at up to 80% in 1 year. Few data are available on the efficacy of commercial weight loss programs or self-help groups in helping patients to achieve or sustain long-term weight loss.

  3. Insight-oriented or psychoanalytic psychotherapy may be indicated for patients with concomitant psychiatric illness or for those individuals with problems exacerbated by obesity. The common belief in the United States that slimness is necessary for beauty may lead to a poor self-image in individuals who are obese and is also a contributing factor in the development of eating disorders. However, nonbehaviorally oriented psychotherapy alone is usually ineffective in promoting or maintaining weight loss.

    Patients who have difficulties with binge eating may benefit from referral to a therapist experienced in the treatment of eating disorders (see Chapter 97).

  4. The effectiveness of **hypnosis** for long-term weight loss has never been documented in controlled studies.

C. Exercise. When combined with a hypocaloric diet and behavior modification, exercise may contribute to both initial weight loss and its maintenance. Moderate exercise, which does not increase food intake in obese individuals, may help to preserve lean body mass during the period of weight loss. Exercise can aid in improving the patient's sense of well-being and has been shown to be correlated with long-term weight maintenance. It also leads to increased insulin sensitivity, improved glucose tolerance, and a more favorable lipid profile. Exercise is also an important component of obesity prevention, particularly in individuals who are genetically at risk.

  1. Rather than "prescribing" specific exercise for the patient, the physician and the patient can negotiate a plan for increasing physical activity, such as starting with a 10-minute walk after lunch. The Centers for Disease Control and Prevention and the American College of Sports Medicine recommend that moderate-intensity physical activity (eg, brisk walking or gardening) should be carried out for at least 30 minutes on most days. The exercise does not have to be done all at one time in order to confer significant health benefits. Thus, patients may find it more convenient to spread their physical activity throughout the day.

  2. Exercise is most likely to be sustained if it is in a form that is enjoyable for the patient and fits the patient's lifestyle, such as walking or riding a bicycle. Patients should be encouraged to examine everyday activities with a view toward increasing energy expenditure (eg, climbing stairs instead of riding elevators or walking to the store instead of driving). Patients who have underlying medical problems, such as hypertension, cardiovascular disease, or diabetes mellitus, should undergo thorough medical evaluation prior to undertaking any new exercise program.

D. **Pharmacotherapy.** The use of pharmacologic agents to aid patients in the long-term control of this serious and refractory chronic condition is promising. Short-term use of medication makes little sense, as the weight loss attributable to the medication is maintained only for the duration of the drug use. This is not evidence of a lack of efficacy of these medications—other medications, such as antihypertensives or oral hypoglycemics, also fail to work when discontinued! Unfortunately, the ideal pharmacologic agent that curbs appetite, enhances weight loss, and can safely be used over extended periods remains undiscovered. The withdrawal of fenfluramine and dexfenfluramine because of their association with valvular heart disease reinforced the reality that all medical treatments may carry unanticipated risks. At present, no medications have Food and Drug Administration (FDA)-approved indications for the treatment of pediatric obesity and should not be used in children under the age of 16 years outside of the research context. For adults, clinicians should carefully balance the risks of an individual patient's obesity and the potential benefits of additional or more sustained weight against the risks of the proposed treatment.

1. **Prescription-only appetite suppressants,** both adrenergic and serotoninergic, have been shown to significantly increase weight loss relative to placebo; these differences are usually modest, however, averaging 2.5–10 kg (5–22 lbs) more than that lost with behavioral treatment alone. There is great variability in response to weight loss medications, with some patients losing little weight, and others losing 50 lbs or more. In general, twice as many patients will lose 10% or more of initial body weight while taking weight loss medications than placebo. This is often enough to confer significant health benefits.

a. **Amphetamines** and similar compounds act on catecholamine neurotransmitters. Their side effects include increases in heart rate and blood pressure. The significant abuse potential of amphetamines in particular outweighs any benefits these drugs may have as anorectic medications.

b. **Other adrenergic compounds,** such as phentermine and mazindol, have limited abuse potential, compared with amphetamines, although some abuse has been reported. Phentermine hydrochloride is generally given at a dosage of 18.75–37.5 mg once daily in the morning, while an equivalent dose of phentermine resin is 15–30 mg once daily. Mazindol is started at a dosage of 1 mg/day and may be increased to a maximum of 1 mg three times daily. Side effects are those of adrenergic stimulation, including insomnia. These medications should be avoided in patients with symptomatic cardiovascular disease, uncontrolled hypertension, untreated hyperthyroidism, known hypersensitivity or idiosyncratic response to sympathomimetic amides, or concomitant use of monoamine oxidase (MAO) inhibitors. None of these medications are approved by the FDA for long-term use.

c. **Fenfluramine and dexfenfluramine,** which act through both release and reuptake of serotonin, have been associated with both primary pulmonary hypertension and valvular heart disease. They were withdrawn from the market in September 1997 and are no longer available. Patients exposed to either of these medications, either alone or in combination, should be evaluated by their physicians for signs or symptoms of valvular heart disease.

d. **Fluoxetine,** which has been used as an antidepressant for several years, causes significant weight loss in high dosages (eg, 60 mg/day). Unfortunately, after approximately 6 months, slow regain of lost weight is often seen, even while the patient is taking the medication. Fluoxetine and related selective serotonin reuptake inhibitors (SSRIs), however, remain useful choices for obese patients with depression, because weight gain usually does not occur.

e. **Sibutramine** is a serotonin-norepinephrine reuptake inhibitor, which is approved for long-term use in the treatment of obesity. Safety and efficacy have not been demonstrated beyond 1 year of use. Sibutramine has not been associated with valvular heart disease or primary pulmonary hypertension. Weight loss with sibutramine is similar to that found with other weight loss agents. Side effects include insomnia, dry mouth, headache, and constipation, and tend to be self-limited. The adverse effect of most concern is an increase in pulse and blood pressure, which is usually small, but which may be substantial in some patients. Therefore, physicians should routinely monitor pulse and blood pressure in patients undergoing treatment. Sibutramine should not be combined with other serotonergic drugs or with MAO inhibitors, and should not be used in patients with cardiovascular disease, uncontrolled hypertension, or severe hepatic or renal disease. The usual starting dose is 10 mg daily, which may be increased to 15 mg after 4 weeks if response to the 10 mg-dose is inadequate.

   f. Orlistat is a gastrointestinal lipase inhibitor that interferes with absorption of about one-third of dietary fat. Weight loss is similar to that seen with other agents. It is taken three times daily, with meals. Fat-soluble vitamin absorption is also decreased, but this may be ameliorated through supplementation with a daily multivitamin. Side effects are primarily gastrointestinal, including oily spotting, soft stools, and more frequent stools, but this usually improves over time and with adherence to a lower-fat diet. Orlistat is FDA-approved for use in adults, both for weight reduction and for prevention of weight regain, and has been found effective for periods of up to 2 years. The usual dose is 120 mg by mouth three times daily.

   g. Leptin and other drugs, including those with potential to affect both food intake and energy expenditure, are currently in earlier stages of development and are unlikely to be available for the next several years.

   h. Combination pharmacotherapy. With the withdrawal of fenfluramine from the market, the popular fenfluramine/phentermine (fen/phen) combination is no longer available. Others have reported using combinations of SSRIs with an adrenergic agent (such as fluoxetine/phentermine, "fen/pro") or two adrenergic agents (such as phentermine/phendimetrazine). These combination therapies have never been rigorously evaluated for safety or efficacy, and their use is not recommended, except in the context of clinical trials with appropriate oversight by an Institutional Review Board.

2. Hormones such as L-thyroxine or human chorionic gonadotropin (hCG) should never be administered in the absence of recognized medical indications, such as laboratory-proven deficiency states. Several well-controlled studies have shown hCG to be of no benefit. The use of L-thyroxine in the euthyroid person is dangerous; it has been associated with increased protein loss and adverse cardiovascular effects.

3. Nonprescription diet aids and supplements are popular among patients.

   a. One of the most commonly used over-the-counter appetite suppressants is phenylpropanolamine. This compound is similar in both action and effectiveness to the prescription-only appetite suppressants, although its abuse potential is less. Over-the-counter appetite suppressants are contraindicated in patients with hypertension, those with cardiovascular disease, or individuals who are receiving MAO inhibitors.

   b. Increasingly popular weight loss aids are dietary supplements, including so-called "herbal fen-phen" products. Many of these weight loss aids contain Ephedra, which has been linked to stroke and death. Other dietary supplements sold for weight loss include garcinia, chitosan, pyruvate, chromium picolonate, and others. Controlled human trials on the safety and effectiveness of dietary supplements for the treatment of obesity are frequently unavailable, and the remainder either show no effect or inconsistent effects. The use of these products for weight loss is not recommended.

E. Invasive treatment

   1. Gastrointestinal surgery may serve either to decrease the amount of food intake or to interfere with its absorption. This type of surgery is generally limited to patients with severe obesity or to those with lesser degrees of obesity who have serious medical conditions exacerbated by their weight. In these patients, who are notoriously resistant to more conventional therapies, surgery may be the treatment of choice, although more conservative therapies should be attempted first. Although weight losses as a result of surgery are usually dramatic, averaging 40–70 kg (88–154 lbs), most patients do not approach ideal body weight. They can, however, substantially reduce their risk of serious morbidity and attain a more satisfactory quality of life.

  a. Gastric operations work by reducing food intake via a restricted gastric reservoir. Reoperations are frequent, usually because of difficulties with anastomotic connections or inadequate weight loss. Operative mortality is usually <1%. Gastroplasty narrows the connection between the fundus and the antrum via wrapping procedures, vertical banding, or horizontal banding. Vertical banded gastroplasty is currently the most popular procedure. Gastric bypass separates the antrum and the fundus of the stomach via a loop enterostomy or a Roux-en-Y anastomosis. Gastric bypass appears to have a somewhat better success rate in long-term weight loss than does gastroplasty, as well as allowing larger weight loss. However, it is associated with a greater risk of micronutrient deficiencies. A more recent operation, known as biliopancreatic diversion, combines gastric bypass with diversion of bile and pancreatic juices into the distal ileum. It is more effective than gastroplasty or gastric bypass in allowing patients to achieve an "ideal body weight." However, the greater degree of malabsorption with this procedure also corresponds to an increase in morbidity, and experience with its use in the United States is limited.

  2. Liposuction is an operative procedure in which localized fat deposits are removed via a suction probe. It is most useful for removing small, well-defined areas of fatty tissue that do not respond to diet and exercise, such as "saddlebag hips." Serious complications, including infection and death from fat emboli, have been reported. It is not an option for the treatment of generalized obesity.

VI. Management strategies. Few conditions are as frustrating for primary care physicians (or their patients) as obesity. Obesity should be viewed not as a "moral weakness," but as a chronic disease of multifactorial origin which requires an ongoing, flexible, and supportive relationship between the physician and the patient. The physician should consider the following factors.

  A. The **degree of obesity** should influence the management strategy, with conservative approaches being supplemented by more hazardous and high-cost treatments as the degree of medical risk from obesity increases. The presence of central as opposed to peripheral obesity as well as medical conditions exacerbated by obesity should be viewed as independent risk factors. Affected patients who would otherwise be in a lower-risk category should be more aggressively treated. Nonobese high-risk individuals with a strong family history of obesity can best benefit from strategies designed to prevent obesity. Nutritional education as well as institution of an exercise program may be helpful.

  B. The **patient's motivation** should be carefully evaluated prior to beginning any weight loss program. The unmotivated or ambivalent patient is unlikely to adhere to even the most excellent and well-thought-out treatment plan. The psychological effects of potential failure probably outweigh the benefits of any short-term weight loss that might be attained. Such individuals should be encouraged to eat a healthful diet and to increase their physical activity with the goal of improving their health, rather than attaining weight loss. Attainment and long-term maintenance of ideal body weight are likely to be met with only partial success. More limited goals can have positive effects on the patient's health and well-being, however.

  1. Even modest degrees of weight loss (ie, <10% of initial body weight) can decrease blood pressure significantly in the hypertensive patient or improve glycemic control in the patient with type 2 diabetes.

  2. Some degree of weight regain after treatment is usual. Avoid perpetuating the patient's "all-or-none" thinking with regard to weight maintenance. Be supportive of the patient's struggle and encourage continuing involvement in a treatment program.

  3. Prevention of further weight gain in the already obese patient is also a useful strategy in the patient who is unable to lose weight. It is the recommended goal in patients who are overweight but not obese and have no risk factors or one risk factor for obesity-related conditions.

    A. Nutritional education by a dietitian, physician, or other medical personnel or through written materials can help the patient to monitor food intake and choose appropriate foods. An excellent resource for patient-oriented materials on nutrition and obesity is the National Institute of Diabetes and Digestive and Kidney Diseases' Weight Control Information Network. Patients may call 1-800-946-8098, or access materials via the world wide web at: http://www.niddk.nih.gov/health/nutrit/nutrit.htm

    B. Childhood obesity is of special concern, and is increasing dramatically in prevalence. Body weight in the first year of life does not correlate well with adult obesity, but by the age of 6 years, overweight children have more than five times the risk of being overweight as adults than do thinner children.

        1. The physician must pay special attention to the nutritional needs of the growing child or adolescent. The high-fiber, low-fat diet recommended for adults is not appropriate for infants and young children. For some, weight loss will not be required, but merely a slowing of the rate of weight gain so that the child's increasing height will enable him to "grow out" of his obesity. VLCDs can be considered in severely obese children and adolescents, but only in the context of specialized treatment programs.

        2. Involvement of the parents of preadolescents is essential and should include education about nutrition and menu planning, behavioral treatment, and emphasis on physical activity and decreasing sedentary behaviors (eg, watching television). In adolescents, the degree of parental involvement should be individualized.

        3. An algorithm for evaluation of children where obesity is a concern is available on the world wide web at: http://www.pediatrics.org/cgi/content/full/102/3/e29

        4. Behavioral weight loss treatment for children may be more effective than for adults: Improvements in weight centile lasting for more than 10 years are seen in as many as half of all children treated with an intensive program.

VII. Natural history and prognosis. In general, obesity is chronic and refractory to treatment.

    A. Patients with central obesity are at risk for numerous medical complications, such as cardiovascular disease and diabetes mellitus.

    B. Patients with severe or morbid obesity have a greatly increased risk of sudden, premature death compared to individuals of average weight.

    C. Even the most effective weight loss programs, which emphasize long-term changes in lifestyle, including diet and physical activity, show limited success in producing long-term, stable weight maintenance. A pattern of slow regain is most common. However, as most data on weight loss treatment come from research programs in which patients with more refractory obesity are frequently studied, the figures generally cited for successful treatment may be unduly pessimistic.

REFERENCES

Anonymous: Long-term pharmacotherapy in the management of obesity: National Task Force on the Prevention and Treatment of Obesity. JAMA 1996;**276:**1907.

Anonymous: Sibutramine for obesity. Med Lett Drugs Ther 1998;**40:**32.

Barlow SE, Dietz WH: Obesity evaluation and treatment: Expert Committee Recommendations. Pediatrics 1998;**102**(3):1. http://www.pediatrics.org/cgi/content/full/102/3/e29

Blackburn G: Effect of degree of weight loss on health benefits. Obes Res 1995;**3**(suppl 2):211s.

Kellum JM, DeMaria EJ, Sugerman HJ: The surgical treatment of morbid obesity. Curr Probl Surg 1998;**35**(9):791.

National Institutes of Health Technology Assessment Conference: Methods for voluntary weight loss and control. Ann Intern Med 1992;**116:**942.

Pi Sunyer FX, Becker DM, Bouchard C, et al: Executive summary of the clinical guidelines on the identification, evaluation, and treatment of overweight and obesity in adults. Arch Intern Med 1998;**158**(17):1855. Full report available at: http://www.nhlbi.nih.gov/nhlbi/cardio/obes/prof/guidelns/ob_home.htm

Sjostrom L, Rissanen A, Andersen T, et al: Randomized placebo-controlled trial of orlistat for weight loss and prevention of weight regain in obese patients: European Multicentre Orlistat Study Group. Lancet 1998;**352:**167.

Wadden TA: Treatment of obesity by moderate and severe caloric restriction: Results of clinical research trials. Ann Intern Med 1993;**119:**688.

Yanovski SZ: A practical approach to treatment of the obese patient. Arch Fam Med 1993;**2:**309.

84   Osteoporosis

Mark W. Zilkoski, MD

I. **Definition.** Osteoporosis is a generalized metabolic bone disorder characterized by a decreased bone mass but a normal bone mineral-to-matrix ratio, that is, a decreased amount of normal bone. In contrast, osteomalacia, a potentially treatable metabolic bone disorder caused by inadequate intake of vitamin D, is characterized by abnormal bone.

II. **Epidemiology**
   A. Between 15 and 20 million people (mostly women) have osteoporosis in the United States. Sixty-six percent of women who are over 65 years old and 15% of men older than 50 years old have radiologic evidence of osteoporosis.
   B. **Costs** for osteoporosis in 1990 exceeded $10 billion.
   C. **Risk factors** for osteoporosis are shown in Table 84–1.

III. **Pathophysiology.** Bone is constantly remodeling through the process of resorption and formation. This process occurs at age-related rates, ranging from complete renewal of all bones in the first year of life to renewal of 15–30% of the skeleton per year in adults.
   A. Unfortunately at **menopause,** the rate of bone resorption exceeds the rate of bone formation. Bone mass reaches a peak by age 35, with bone loss beginning by age 40 in both sexes. Over her lifetime, a woman loses 35% of her cortical bone and 50% of her trabecular bone. A man loses only two-thirds of the bone that a woman loses, usually only as his muscle mass decreases.
   B. **Primary osteoporosis** is an age-related bone disorder. There are two types of primary osteoporosis.
       1. **Type I.** Postmenopausal osteoporosis usually affects women within 10–20 years after menopause, regardless of whether the menopause is natural or induced by surgery.
           a. Type I osteoporosis primarily affects the trabecular bone that is found largely in vertebrae. Cortical bone loss accelerates to 2–3% per year after menopause. The accelerated phase or trabecular bone loss after menopause is much greater (8–10% per year), although it is of shorter duration, lasting only a few years.
           b. The accelerated phase of trabecular bone loss is caused by an increase in bone resorption, which results in increased parathyroid hormone and calcitonin secretion.

TABLE 84–1. RISK FACTORS FOR OSTEOPOROSIS

Risk Factor	Favors Development of Osteoporosis
Menopause	Physiologic menopause
	Surgically induced menopause
Age	Increasing age
Sex	Female
Family history	Positive
Race	White, Asian
Body build	Lean build, short stature, small bone
Weight	Light, nonobese
Tobacco	Heavy smoking
Diet	High-protein diet, calcium deficiency
Immobility	Sedentary existence or lack of exercise
Malabsorption	Decreased absorption of calcium
Liver or renal disease	Decreased absorption of liver
Endocrine disease	Hyperparathyroidism, thyrotoxicosis
Drugs	Alcohol, steroids, phenytoin, heparin

Adapted from and used with permission from Zilkoski MW, Morrow LB: Osteoporosis. *Am Fam Physician* 1987;**36:**178 (published by the American Academy of Family Physicians).

2. **Type II.** "Senile" osteoporosis affects men and women after the age of 70. The most important age-related factors are decreased osteoblast formation and impaired production of vitamin D, which leads to decreased calcium absorption and secondary hyperparathyroidism.

    a. Type II osteoporosis involves both cortical and trabecular bone loss. Trabecular thinning associated with this slow phase of bone loss leads to gradual and often painless vertebral deformation.

    b. The effects of type I osteoporosis and type II osteoporosis are additive.

C. **Secondary osteoporosis** (Table 84–2). Although secondary factors can cause osteoporosis, it is important to consider them as additive risk factors to primary osteoporosis and as potentially treatable. Each factor causes interference with either adequate bone formation or an increase in bone resorption.

    1. **Premature menopause** leads to increased loss of bone secondary to estrogen deficiency.

    2. **Diet.** Inadequate dietary calcium in bone-forming years may lead to less skeletal bone mass at menopause. A high-protein diet increases urinary excretion of calcium (>120 gm/day leads to calciuria).

    3. **Drugs**

        a. **Alcohol** depresses bone formation.

        b. **Tobacco** use leads to decreased circulation of estrogen.

        c. **Glucocorticoids** cause osteoporosis by impairing calcium and phosphate absorption, inhibiting new bone formation, increasing calcium resorption, and producing hypercalciuria. The incidence of osteoporosis secondary to steroids is highest in growing children and postmenopausal women. Thirty percent to 50% of individuals treated with systemic steroids have osteoporosis.

        d. Use of **heparin, phenytoin,** excess **thyroid** medications, loop **diuretics,** and chronic use of **tetracycline** may induce osteoporosis. Each drug produces osteoporosis through a different mechanism.

    4. **Immobilization** leads to increased bone resorption and to loss of muscle mass.

TABLE 84–2. CAUSES OF SECONDARY OSTEOPOROSIS

Endocrine disorders
Cushing's disease
Thyrotoxicosis
Hypogonadism
Hyperparathyroidism
Hyperprolactinemia
Type I diabetes mellitus

Malignancies
Leukemia
Lymphoma
Multiple myeloma
Ectopic adrenocorticotropic hormone syndrome
Ectopic parathyroid hormone syndrome

Drugs
Alcohol
Glucocorticoids
Heparin
Methotrexate
Anticonvulsants

Genetic abnormalities
Osteogenesis imperfecta
Ehlers–Danlos syndrome
Homocystinuria

Adapted from and used with permission from Zilkoski MW, Morrow LB: Osteoporosis. *Am Fam Physician* 1987;**36:**178 (published by the American Academy of Family Physicians).

IV. Diagnosis

A. Symptoms and signs. By the time symptoms are present, a significant loss of bone has already occurred.

1. **Back pain** may be caused by acute compression fractures or mechanical deformity secondary to multiple old fractures.

2. **Fractures** of vertebra, hip, and forearm produce pain and disability. Fractures may result from such minimal trauma as bending, lifting, or getting out of bed. Some fractures do not produce pain but may lead to other complications, such as restrictive lung disease, early satiety, decreased exercise tolerance, and loss of self-esteem.

3. **Loss of height** is associated with loss of bone, and fractures of the vertebrae and may be accompanied by disfiguring cosmetic changes.

4. **Mechanical deformity** (kyphosis, or dowager's hump) caused by vertebral compression fracture may interfere with both respiration and abdominal processes and may cause early satiety, bloating, and constipation.

B. Laboratory tests (Table 84–3)

1. **X-rays.** By the time osteoporosis is evident on x-ray, 40% of bone is lost. The following changes can be seen on plain x-ray: increased lucency, cortical thinning, increased density of end plate, anterior wedging and biconcavity of vertebrae, and loss of horizontal trabeculae.

2. **Bone mineral densitometry.** The primary goals in performing these tests are to screen certain asymptomatic women for risk of fracture, to measure bone density in patients with osteopenia, and to monitor changes associated with therapy. Although dual energy x-ray absorptiometry (DXA) may be the method of choice for axial osteopenia because of precision, accuracy, low radiation dose, and high patient acceptability, QCT, dual photon absorptiometry (DPA), and bone ultrasound (QUS) are reliable ways of determining bone

TABLE 84–3. SCREENING TESTS FOR OSTEOPOROSIS

Technique	Bones Measured	Examination Time (min)	Possible Accuracy Error (0%)	Effective Radiation Dose (USV)[1]
Dual energy x-ray absorptiometry (DXA) uses a double beam from an x-ray source	Spine, hip, total body	10–20	3–9	7
Dual photon absorptiometry (DPA) uses a double beam from a radioactive energy source	Spine, hip, total body	20–40	4–140	5
Quantitative computed tomography (QCT) uses a conventional CT scanner with specialized software	Spine	10–15	5–20	60[2]
Peripheral QCT (pQCT) is a special version of QCT that measures only the bone density of the wrist	Wrist	10	4–8	3
Ultrasound heel	Heel			0
Single energy x-ray absorptiometry (SXA) uses an x-ray source to measure bone	Wrist, heel	4	5	<1
Single photon absorptiometry (SPA) uses a single beam from an energy source passed through water	Wrist	15	4–6	<1

[1] Effective dose refers to radiation that reaches internal organs. For comparison, one chest x-ray gives a radiation dose of about 50 USV, a lateral spine x-ray 500–1,000 USV, an abdominal CT scan about 4,000 USV, and natural background radiation is about 2000–3000 USV per year.

[2] Radiation doses may be up to 600 USV on older CT scanners.

Adapted from Prescriber's Letter Document No. 141114, fall 1998.

mineral density (BMD). Evidence shows that QUS, which is the least expensive method, may be an excellent way to predict fracture risk.

There is controversy over who should be screened. Most authorities do not support the use of noninvasive measurement of bone mass as a routine screen in perimenopausal women. As a screening tool, noninvasive measurement of bone mass should be reserved for those in whom additional information about fracture risk is needed to enable the physician to decide on prophylactic estrogen therapy or other therapies.

3. **Blood studies** are important for the diagnosis and management of secondary osteoporosis.

   a. **Serum calcium, phosphate, and alkaline phosphate levels** are normal in patients with primary osteoporosis, but results of these tests can be used to rule out secondary causes.

   b. **Levels of parathyroid hormone (PTH) and 1,25-dihydroxycholecalciferol** are normal in osteoporosis but can be abnormal in secondary causes such as osteomalacia. Vitamin D deficiency is likely to occur in elderly patients who have little access to sunlight or vitamin D–fortified milk or who take anticonvulsants such as phenytoin (Dilantin).

   c. If multiple myeloma is suspected, a **complete blood count** and **immunoelectrophoresis** may be helpful.

4. **Studies of bone turnover and resorption** when combined with BMD may be helpful in prognosticating the risk of fracture. Immunoassays for bone formation are osteocalcin, bone alkaline phosphate, and intact I collagen *N*-terminal propeptides. Immunoassays for bone resorption and pyridium cross-links are some type I collagen breakdown products in urine and serum. Bone biopsy, which is the only definite way of diagnosing osteoporosis, is rarely needed, but it can help the physician to rule out osteomalacia or secondary causes of osteoporosis.

V. **Treatment** can be divided into three types of prevention: primary, secondary, and tertiary (after a fracture has occurred). The effect of any treatment regimen is ultimately measured not by increases in bone mass but by a decrease in the incidence of fractures.

   A. **Primary prevention** is the best and most cost-effective approach.

   1. **Calcium.** The recommended amount of calcium varies for each age group (Table 84–4). Calcium therapy is generally safe except in patients with hypercalcemia or nephrolithiasis.

      a. **Estimating calcium intake.** To determine whether supplementation is indicated and how much additional calcium is necessary, a person's calcium intake must be estimated. An estimation of the patient's intake can be made quickly and easily with Repka's rules of 300: the basal diet contains 300 mg of calcium, and each serving of dairy products, such as 8 oz milk, 8 oz yogurt, 11/2 oz cheese, or 2 cups cottage cheese, provides 300 mg of calcium.

      b. **Dosage.** Because calcium absorption is inefficient, chewable tablets with the highest percentage of calcium, or those known to dissolve in the stomach, such as Tums or OsCal, 500-mg tablets, should be recom-

TABLE 84–4. RECOMMENDED DAILY ALLOWANCE FOR CALCIUM FROM THE NATIONAL ACADEMY OF SCIENCE (1984)

Age (yr)	Calcium (mg)
<0.5	400
0.5–1	600
1–10	800
11–24	1200–1500
25–49	1000
Postmenopausal (taking estrogen) <65 yr	1000
Postmenopausal (not taking estrogen) <65 yr	1500
Pregnant or lactating	1200–1500
Men 65 and older	1500

Developed by NIH consensus development on osteoporosis.

mended. Each 500-mg Tums tablet contains 200 mg of elemental calcium. Excellent sources of nondairy calcium include sardines (372 mg in 3 oz) and pink salmon (167 mg in 3 oz).
2. **Exercise** should be weight-bearing and skeletal-stressing, such as walking, jogging, aerobic dance, or cross-country skiing. Swimming is not helpful. Exercising to the point of producing amenorrhea in menstruating women is associated with accelerated bone loss and should be discouraged or treated (see Chapter 5). Some studies in males have also shown that high levels of exercise may lead to bone loss.
3. Factors that can decrease calcium absorption, increase bone resorption, or impair bone formation, such as smoking, excessive alcohol intake, and medications associated with osteoporosis, should be avoided. If a medication such as a glucocorticosteroid cannot be avoided, calcium supplements should be used. Consideration can also be given to the addition of a biphosphonate.
4. **Secondary causes of osteoporosis** should be sought and treated.
5. Since the ultimate goal in the prevention of osteoporosis is to prevent fractures, **other risks for fracture,** such as orthostatic hypotension, especially in the frail, elderly patient, should be sought and reduced. Other factors that have been identified as potential risks for hip fractures in women include lower limb dysfunction, drug use, and visual impairment. A safe home environment should be maintained to prevent accidental falls.
B. **Secondary prevention**
   1. **Calcium intake at menopause** should be continued at 1200–1500 mg per day to prevent negative calcium balance. Although calcium without estrogen has not been shown to be effective in the prevention of early postmenopausal bone loss, postmenopausal women whose calcium intake falls below 400 mg per day did show reduced bone loss with supplementation. New studies are suggesting that calcium administered with estrogen may lower the dose of estrogen necessary to prevent bone loss by 50%.
   2. **Estrogen replacement therapy (ERT).** Since all women should be considered at risk for osteoporosis at menopause, those who have no specific contraindication to estrogen therapy should begin ERT. ERT when taken for at least 7 years decreases the risk of hip, distal forearm, and vertebral fractures by 50%. Although there is yet no conclusive evidence that ERT prevents osteoporosis in patients who have been postmenopausal for more than 20 years, recent studies suggest that ERT may also benefit the elderly with established osteoporosis. No route of administration is superior to another, although vaginal administration of estrogen is erratically absorbed.
      a. **Conjugated estrogens** (Premarin), 0.625 mg orally every day, is the lowest recommended dosage (days 1–25 of the month). Micronized estradiol (Estrace), 1 mg, is equivalent.
      b. **A progestogen** such as Provera, 5–10 mg orally, should be added in a cyclical fashion in women with a uterus, because it has been shown that progestin taken for 13 days of the month (days 13–25) decreases the risk of endometrial cancer and does not reduce estrogen effect.
      c. **Continuous ERT** can be offered. New studies suggest that continuous ERT is safe and efficacious. If continuous therapy is elected, Provera, 2.5 mg orally every day (days 1–25 of the month), should be added to ERT.
      d. **Transdermal estrogen** (Estroderm .05) recently has been shown to be effective in postmenopausal women with established osteoporosis. Although this form of estrogen has less of an effect on raising high-density lipoprotein (HDL) cholesterol than do oral estrogens, it appears to be as cardioprotective.
   3. **Exercise** should be encouraged. Some studies show a retardation in bone loss as a result of exercise.
   4. **Calcitonin** opposes PTH activity, thus inhibiting bone resorption, and may increase bone mass when taken for as long as 2 years. Bone pain also decreases because of the increase in endorphins stimulated by calcitonin.
      a. **Indications.** Calcitonin is indicated in patients who cannot take ERT, in patients who have been postmenopausal for more than 15 years, in patients with significant pain from vertebral fracture, and in patients who are taking long-term corticosteroid therapy.

      b. Dosage. A nasal calcitonin spray (Miacalcin), 200 IU or 1 spray per day, is now available and has replaced calcitonin, which is initially administered 50–100 U subcutaneously three times per week.

      c. Patients should receive 1500 mg of calcium per day, and adequate vitamin D intake (400 U daily or 50,000 U twice weekly) should be supplied.

      d. Side effects. Skin testing prior to the first dose of calcitonin is important because of hypersensitivity reactions. The side effect of nausea can be prevented by the administration of calcitonin at bedtime.

      e. Therapy should be continued for 2 years.

   5. Fluoride (see section V,C)

   6. Vitamin D therapy has no place in the secondary treatment of osteoporosis other than to ensure that the elderly patient is not vitamin D–deficient or to be used in conjunction with calcitonin.

   7. Thiazides in doses of 50 mg per day may be beneficial in treating the high urine calcium of patients with idiopathic hypercalciuria via improving gastrointestinal absorption of calcium. Thiazides should be used only in conjunction with other therapies for osteoporosis.

C. Tertiary prevention. After a patient has had a fracture, prolonged immobilization should be avoided. Patients should be assisted to normal functioning as soon as possible.

   1. Bisphosphonate. Therapy with alendronate sodium (Fosamax) has been shown to significantly increase spinal bone and reduce new vertebral fractures in women. These drugs inhibit osteoclast-mediated bone resorption. Food and Drug Administration approval has been awarded to alendronate sodium, which shows no inhibition of bone mineralization.

      a. Indications. Fosamax is indicated for the prevention and treatment of osteoporosis in women.

      b. Dosage. Alendronate sodium should be taken 10 mg, 1 tablet in the morning with 8 oz water with adequate vitamin D intake indefinitely. Since it is poorly absorbed, it must be given on an empty stomach. A calcium supplement of 500 mg per day is also suggested.

   2. Fluoride therapy is still controversial, and most authorities no longer recommend it for the treatment of osteoporosis. Studies continue to determine whether lower doses are effective and whether sustained-release fluoride is more efficacious than slow-release.

   3. Calcitonin (see section V,B)

   4. Raloxiphene (Evista), a selective estrogen receptor modulator, has been shown to decrease spinal fractures if taken for 2 years. Raloxiphene may be an excellent choice for those who cannot or will not take estrogen.

   5. Intermittent PTH administration is under investigation.

   6. Nonsteroidal anti-inflammatory drugs (NSAIDs) such as sulindac (Clinoril) or ibuprofen (Motrin), may be provided for relief of pain. Although narcotics should generally be avoided, judicial use in elderly patients with contraindications to NSAIDs can be effective.

   7. Back braces and corsets and physical therapy may provide support and pain relief.

D. Patient education

   1. The new National Resource Center on Osteoporosis is a federally funded clearinghouse for the latest risks, prevention, and treatment of and information on osteoporosis. Phone (202) 223-0344. National Osteoporosis Foundation http://www.nof.org

   2. All women should be counseled regarding the benefits of hormone replacement therapy, preventive measures associated with fracture risk, and smoking cessation. Evidence shows that hip packs and anchor rugs in the elderly decrease hip fractures.

VI. Prognosis

A. An estimated 50% of women in the Western world still have a fracture from osteoporosis. Twenty-five percent of women by the age of 70 and 50% of women by the age of 80 have had a vertebral fracture. Colles' fractures are the most common fractures in white women up to age 75.

B. Hip fractures are the 12th leading cause of death in people older than age 65. The mortality rate within 1 year of hip fracture ranges from 12% to 20%.

C. Ten percent of women who fracture their hips become functionally dependent in activities of daily living, whereas almost 50% require nursing home placement. Of these, 15–25% will require long-term care for at least 1 year.

D. Osteoporosis carries an overall mortality rate of 6%. Causes of death include hip fracture, pulmonary embolus, decubitus ulcers, urinary tract infections, and other infections.

REFERENCES

Birkhauser MH, Haemggi W: Benefits of different routes of administration. Int J Fertil 1994; **39**(suppl 1):11.

Ettinger B: An update for the obstetrician-gynecologist on advances in the diagnosis, prevention, and treatment of postmenopausal osteoporosis. Curr Opin Obstet Gynecol 1993;**5**:396.

Filer MD, Filer RB: Transdermal estrogen and prevention of osteoporosis. Am Fam Physician 1994;**49**:1639.

Garneru P, Delmas PD: Diagnostic evaluation update: Osteoporosis. Endocrinol Metab Clin North Am 1997;**26**(4):913.

Kaplan FS: Prevention and management of osteoporosis. Clin Symp 1995;**47**:2.

Lindsay R: Hormone replacement therapy for prevention and treatment of osteoporosis. Am J Med 1993;**95**:5A.

Lufkin EG, et al: Treatment of postmenopausal osteoporosis with transdermal estrogen. Ann Intern Med 1992;**117**:1.

Morley JD, Gundy MC: Epidemiology of bone loss with aging. Clin Geriatr Med 1994;**10**:557.

Smith R: Molecular, cellular, and metabolic mechanisms of osteoporosis. Rev Clin Gerontol 1993;**3**:107.

---

85   Parkinson's Disease

Mark W. Zilkoski, MD

I. Definition. Parkinson's disease (PD) is an idiopathic progressive degenerative central nervous system disorder involving predominantly the substantia nigra. PD is characterized by bradykinesia, resting tremor, gait abnormalities, rigidity, and postural instability.

II. Epidemiology. PD is the third most common neurologic disease seen in the elderly, **affecting 1 million people in the United States.** Its incidence ranges from 100 to 150 cases per 100,000 of the US population. The annual incidence in the United States is 20 per 100,000, which increases with age up to its greatest incidence in the eighth decade.

    A. Men and women are equally affected.

    B. The onset of PD is usually between 50 and 70 years of age. The average age of onset is during the seventh decade, ranging from 61.6 to 66.4 years. Onset in persons under 30 years of age is rare (only 5% of persons affected are less than 40).

III. Pathophysiology

    A. The etiology of PD is unknown and probably multifactorial.

        1. Although 10–15% of PD patients have a first-degree relative with the disease, the role of genetics is presently unclear (possibly autosomal dominant).

        2. Infection may play an etiologic role. Although atypical PD developed in some people who contracted Economo's encephalitis between 1919 and 1926, less than 5% of patients with PD have had documented encephalitis.

        3. Environmental toxins (rural living, well water, pesticides, wood pulp mills) may be involved in the pathogenesis of symptoms similar to those of PD.

            a. Acute parkinsonism developed in a few drug abusers exposed to the synthetic narcotic "designer drug" methyl-4-phenyl-1,2,3,6-tetrahydropyridine (MPTP), which selectively destroys the substantia nigra.

            b. Poisoning with manganese, carbon monoxide, methanol, or cyanide produces clinical abnormalities similar to those of PD.

        4. Repeated head trauma may result in PD; some boxers have developed "pugilistic" PD.

5. Although the incidence of PD increases with age, **aging** may not be a primary cause. Age-associated changes may potentiate the effects of toxic or degenerative causes.

B. The **pathology** of PD consists of degeneration of neurons in the substantia nigra, locus ceruleus, dorsal vagal nucleus, ventral tegmentum, and sympathetic ganglion. The **Lewy body,** an eosinophilic cytoplasmic inclusion in affected neurons, is a histologic marker of PD. Lewy bodies are specific for idiopathic PD and are not found in other conditions that produce parkinsonism, such as MPTP toxicity; poisoning with manganese, carbon monoxide, methanol, or cyanide; multiple basal ganglia infarcts; progressive supranuclear palsy; and the Shy–Drager syndrome.

    1. Progressive depletion of the neurotransmitter dopamine occurs in the substantia nigra concomitant with nigral degeneration. Symptoms develop when 80% of dopaminergic activity is destroyed.

    2. Studies of the neurotoxic effects of MPTP suggest that the enzyme monoamine oxidase B [MAO(B)] and free radicals may be involved in the pathogenesis of neuronal destruction and dopamine depletion.

IV. Diagnosis

A. Signs and symptoms. The onset of symptoms of PD is often insidious, with initial complaints being vague and nonspecific, such as stiffness, weakness, or clumsiness of hands.

    1. Tremor is the most common specific early complaint.

        a. The typical "pill-rolling" tremor of 4–6 cycles per second may begin unilaterally in an upper extremity, but bilateral involvement occurs as the disease progresses.

        b. The tremor is present at rest, increases with anxiety or fatigue, and disappears during sleep. Most prominent in the hands, the tremor may also involve the tongue, jaw, eyelids, and feet.

        c. A **postural tremor** (action tremor occurring during voluntary muscle contraction), which must always be differentiated from the typical resting tremor of PD of 8–10 cycles per second and is most evident in the hand, develops eventually in most PD patients.

    2. Muscle rigidity, which is present during the entire arc of movement of a joint, also occurs. "Cogwheeling," a jerky, ratcheting effect demonstrated on passive motion (usually at the wrist or elbow), is characteristic of PD. Early in the course, cogwheel rigidity may be evident only on passive movement of a joint when the contralateral joint is actively and repetitively moved, that is, when the person draws a circle in the air with the contralateral arm.

    3. Bradykinesia, a general slowness of movement characterized by difficulty initiating motion and inability to perform rapid repetitive movements, is another hallmark of PD. The severity of bradykinesia may fluctuate markedly during the course of the day.

    4. The combination of rigidity and bradykinesia results in such characteristic features of PD as loss of facial expression; decreased frequency of blinking; fixed flexion of the trunk, neck, and extremities; slow hesitant gait with reduced arm swing; postural instability; micrographia; dysarthria; dysphagia; and general poverty of movement.

    5. Other **common clinical features of PD** include constipation, sialorrhea, depression, intellectual impairment, orthostatic hypotension, bladder instability, eczema, sleep disturbance, and abnormal sensations, such as burning and tingling and restless leg syndrome.

    6. Neurologic findings that are not consistent with PD include focal weakness, hemiparesis, cranial nerve palsies, objective sensory deficits, and oculogyric crises. Such signs suggest the presence of a different disorder. PD must be distinguished from drug-induced parkinsonism secondary to reserpine, metoclopramide, and antipsychotic drugs, as well as a group of disorders resembling PD, the Parkinson Plus syndromes, which are not medication-responsive (Table 85–1).

B. Laboratory evaluation contributes little to the clinical diagnosis of PD. The diagnosis is based on the presence of typical signs and symptoms and the exclusion of alternative explanations such as tumors, infarcts, hydrocephalus, and AIDS.

TABLE 85–1. DIAGNOSIS OF PARKINSON DISEASE (PD) BASED ON CLINICOPATHOLOGIC STUDIES

Features characterizing PD
  Progressive onset and slow progression of asymmetric (unilateral) akinesia
  Excellent and sustained levodopa response
  Either classical pill-rolling rest tremor or rigidity
Features suggestive of an alternate diagnosis
  Motor
    Early instability and falls
    Rapid disease progression
    Absent, poor, or waning response to levodopa
    Pyramidal signs
    Cerebellar signs
    Early dysarthria and/or dysphagia
  Oculomotor
    Supranuclear gaze, palsy, slowing of saccades, difficulty initiating saccades
  Cognitive and behavioral
    Early dementia[1]
    Visual hallucinations not treatment induced
    Apraxia
    Sensory or visual neglect, cortical disturbances
  Autonomic
    Early autonomic failure unrelated to treatment (Orthostatic hypotension, impotence, or urinary disturbances)

[1] Dementia occurs in approximately 15% of patients with PD but is not an early feature.
Reprinted from JAMA 1998;**280**(19):1654.

1. **Magnetic resonance imaging (MRI)** may be useful in excluding secondary causes of PD or atypical PD. A recent MRI study shows that 25% of diagnosed PD actually is not PD.
2. **Positron emission tomography (PET)** may help to differentiate atypical PD and to diagnose certain medication-resistant parkinsonian syndrome.

V. **Treatment** of PD, although controversial, is usually begun when the patient begins to experience functional impairment and requires a multidisciplinary approach, such as nonpharmacologic therapy, pharmacologic therapy, physical therapy, occupational therapy, or surgery.

  A. **Pharmacologic therapy** consists of anticholinergic agents, dopamine precursors, dopamine agonists, catechol *O*-methyltransferase inhibitors, and MAO(B) inhibitors (Table 85–2).

    1. **Anticholinergic agents.** In use for more than 40 years, anticholinergic drugs work on the theory that as PD progresses, dopaminergic activity decreases, cholinergic activity becomes predominant, and motor dysfunction results. Anticholinergic agents produce a 25% improvement in the manifestations of PD, with some believing that they work best with tremor. They are a reasonable treatment choice initially in younger patients. Since anticholinergic drugs produce unacceptable side effects, such as confusion and delirium in the elderly, they have a very limited role in that age group.

      a. **Specific anticholinergic regimens** include trihexyphenidyl (Artane), 6–15 mg/day; biperiden (Akineton), 6–30 mg/day; and benztropine mesylate (Cogentin), 2–6 mg/day; each in three divided doses. The antihistamine diphenhydramine (Benadryl), 50–150 mg/day, has been used as an anticholinergic agent with some success in treating early disease. An anticholinergic drug may be used as an adjunct to carbidopa/levodopa (L-dopa) therapy if tremor remains a problem. Trihexyphenidyl is usually started at 0.5–1 mg twice daily (bid) with gradual increases to a maximum of 15 mg/day, if necessary.

      b. **Adverse effects of anticholinergic agents** include dry mouth, acute narrow-angle glaucoma, mental confusion, visual blurring, and urinary hesitancy or retention, particularly in the elderly.

    2. **Dopamine precursors.** The major dopamine precursor L-dopa is the most effective drug in the treatment of PD. L-dopa is transported into the central nervous system and converted to dopamine. Unlike dopamine, L-dopa crosses the blood–brain barrier. When administered as L-dopa, most of it is

TABLE 85–2. PHARMACOLOGIC THERAPY FOR PARKINSON'S DISEASE

Agent	Available	Starting Dose	Dosage Range	Cost ($)[1]
I. Anticholinergic agents				
Trihexyphenidyl (Artane)	2-mg tab 2 mg/5 mL elixir	0.5–1 bid	1–15 mg	4.75
Biperiden (Akineton)	2 mg	2.0 tid	2–8 mg	37.00
Benztropine (Cogentin)	0.5, 1, 2 mg	0.5 bid	0.5–6	6.40
II. Dopamine precursors				
Carbidopa (of L-dopa)	10/100	tid	400–1500	35.00
(Sinemet)	25/100	tid	400–1500	37.00
(Sinemet)	25/250	tid	400–1500	85.00
(Sinemet CR)	50/200	bid	500–800 mg	86.50
	25/100	bid	500–800 mg	76.00
III. Dopamine agonists				
Amantadine (Symmetrel)	100-mg tab 50 mg/5 mL syrup	100 mg po qd	200–400	7.50
Bromocriptine (Parlodel)	2.5, 5-mg tab	1.25 qd	2.5–100	29.50
Pergolide mesylate (Permax)	0.05, 0.25,1-mg tab	0.05 qd	0.5–5 mg	17.50
Pramipexole (Mirapex)	0.125, 0.25 0.5, 1, 1.5	0.125 tid	1.5–4.5	55.00
Ropinirole (Requip)	0.25, 0.5 1, 2, 5	0.25 tid	0.75–24	110.00
IV. COMT inhibitors				
Entacapone (Comtan)	200	200 tid	600–1600	183.00
Tolcapone (Tasmar)	100, 200	100 mg	300–600	185.00
V. Antioxidants				
Selegiline (Eldepryl)	5-mg tab	5 mg po bid	5–10	145.00
Vitamin E	400 IU	400 IU bid	400 IU–1600 IU	2.50

[1] Based on a 1-month supply at starting dose and generic cost when generic is available.
COMT, Catechol o-methyltransferase.

decarboxylated to dopamine peripherally and only a small proportion enters the central nervous system. Consequently, large doses of L-dopa are required to increase dopamine levels in the substantia nigra. Side effects frequently complicate the use of such high doses of L-dopa. The addition of carbidopa, a dopa decarboxylase inhibitor, decreases the peripheral metabolism of L-dopa, allowing more of the precursor to enter the central nervous system.

With the addition of carbidopa, a therapeutic effect can be achieved with smaller doses of L-dopa and fewer adverse effects; thus, L-dopa is rarely used alone.

Because evidence exists that the introduction of L-dopa may actually lead to progression of PD, initial drug therapy with L-dopa is controversial.

   a. Carbidopa/L-dopa combination (Sinemet) is available for oral administration in three dosage forms: 10 mg carbidopa and 100 mg L-dopa (10/100); 25 mg carbidopa and 100 mg L-dopa (25/100); and 25 mg carbidopa and 250 mg L-dopa (25/250); and a controlled-release Sinemet CR (50/200) and (25/100). The usual daily dose of L-dopa (in the form of carbidopa/L-dopa) ranges from 400 to 1500 mg, given in three to four divided doses. In general, at least 75 mg of carbidopa per day is necessary to block the peripheral conversion of L-dopa to dopamine.

   A growing body of evidence suggests that treatment should begin with a long-acting Sinemet (Sinemet CR), which may be associated with a delay in the onset of L-dopa side effects. Start at 50/200 bid and increase to 800 mg per day. When more than 800 mg is needed, the addition of dopamine agonist should be considered.

   b. Although L-dopa improved all the major symptoms of the disease, in 80% of patients rigidity and bradykinesia generally respond better than tremor. Satisfactory initial control of symptoms is usually achieved with 400–800 mg of L-dopa per day. Further increases in dosage are frequently needed in subsequent months or years.

c. The most common side effect of L-dopa is **nausea.** Taking the drug with a light meal frequently relieves this symptom. If nausea persists, the use of domperidone, 10–20 mg, 30 minutes before administration of carbidopa/L-dopa may be effective. If low doses of carbidopa/L-dopa are used, the addition of carbidopa (Lodosyn) 25 mg by mouth three times daily may be helpful.

d. **Heavy meals,** particularly those containing milk, milk products, or meat, may impair absorption owing to protein absorption competition and should be avoided. This is usually not a problem until late PD.

e. Other side effects of L-dopa are orthostatic hypotension, cardiac arrhythmia, leukopenia, mental confusion, and agitation.

f. **Abrupt cessation** of L-dopa therapy may precipitate a neuroleptic malignant syndrome. "Drug holidays" from L-dopa may be dangerous, may have no lasting improvement, and are generally not recommended.

g. Two-thirds of patients after 5 years of therapy develop a number of distressing side effects: dyskinesias (choreiform movements, dystonia), end-of-dose failure, and "on/off" fluctuations in performance and neuropsychiatric symptoms.

(1) The **end of dose** or "wearing-off phenomenon" results from fluctuating plasma level of L-dopa and may be relieved by more frequent dosing. The addition of a controlled-release formulation of Sinemet CR or a catechol *O*-methyltransferase inhibitor may relieve this phenomenon.

(2) The unpredictability of the on/off experience makes it more difficult to manage. Adding a dopamine agonist to the regimen may help resolve this problem. Apomorphine, which is experimental in the United States, has been shown to be useful.

(3) Dyskinesias, which are common in the elderly, are less likely to be improved.

(4) It has been suggested that early combination therapy using dopamine precursors and agonists results in fewer dyskinesias and fluctuations. Unfortunately for the older patients, side effects are not tolerable, particularly postural hypotension, confusion, and dementia.

(5) L-dopa should be avoided in patients with malignant melanoma, since the drug may activate that form of skin cancer.

3. **Dopamine agonists, which directly stimulate dopamine receptors,** used alone or in conjunction with carbidopa/L-dopa, often provide some therapeutic benefit. Data now exist that suggest initiation of treatment with dopamine agonist may be neuroprotective and may prevent or delay development of motor complications seen with Sinemet.

a. **Amantadine** (Symmetrel), an antiviral agent, probably has both anticholinergic and dopaminergic effects. It enhances the release of dopamine from presynaptic terminals. It is less effective with tremor.

(1) In a dose of 100 mg twice a day (or 100 mg once a day in patients over 70), amantadine has a favorable effect in approximately two-thirds of patients with mild disease. The therapeutic response is evident within a few days; if no benefit is seen within 1 week, the drug should be stopped. Unfortunately, the favorable effect of amantadine usually disappears in a few months to a maximum of 1 year as depletion of striatal dopamine progresses.

(2) Side effects of amantadine include livedo reticularis, ankle edema, headaches, and visual hallucinations and dizziness. The drug should be avoided in patients with severe renal insufficiency.

b. **Bromocriptine** (Parlodel) is the drug of choice to start with, according to some neurologists.

(1) The starting dose is 1.25 mg twice a day, to be increased by 2.5 mg a day every 1–2 weeks until a satisfactory response is achieved.

(2) Although not as effective as L-dopa in improving function, bromocriptine may be used alone. A combination of bromocriptine and carbidopa/L-dopa is increasingly used as early therapy for mild PD.

There is some evidence of a synergistic effect in the use of bromocriptine. The most common approach is to add bromocriptine when the daily dose of L-dopa reaches 400–600 mg and to titrate the bromocriptine to a daily dose of 15–30 mg.

    (3) Side effects of bromocriptine are anorexia, nausea, vomiting, headache, orthostatic hypotension, hallucinations, and confusion. Gastrointestinal side effects may be diminished by taking the drug with meals. Dyskinesias, which may occur after several years, are less common with bromocriptine than with L-dopa. The development of erythromelalgia of the lower extremities, a pleural effusion, or pulmonary fibrosis should prompt immediate cessation of bromocriptine. A baseline chest x-ray may be helpful in assessing later pulmonary changes.

  c. Pergolide (Permax) is a dopamine agonist that, in combination with carbidopa/L-dopa, may provide benefit for patients with advanced PD.

    (1) The starting dose is 0.05 mg/day and is gradually advanced to 0.25 mg three times per day within 2–3 weeks. The maximum daily dose is 5 mg administered in divided doses.

    (2) Side effects limit the use of pergolide and include angina pectoris, leukopenia, confusion, and hallucinations. The use of pergolide should be restricted to physicians with extensive experience in the management of PD.

  d. Pramipexole (Mirapex) and Ropinirole (Requip), non-ergot dopamine agonists, avoid ergot-related side effects (pulmonary fibrosis, livedo reticularis) of other dopamine agonists and selectively stimulate D_2 and D_3 receptors.

4. Catechol *O*-methyltransferase (COMT) inhibitors are adjuncts to L-dopa treatment. They block metabolism and enhance absorption of L-dopa. They possibly decrease risk of L-dopa induced motor complications.

  a. Entacopone (Comtan) and tolcopone (Tasmar) enhance antiparkinson effects of L-dopa in patients with fluctuating and nonfluctuating PD.

    (1) Exacerbation of dyskinesia can occur with initiation of treatment, so one must decrease L-dopa within 1–2 days (by 20–30%).

    (2) Side effects include dyskinesia, diarrhea, and liver enzyme abnormality.

5. Neuroprotective drugs constitute another approach to the early treatment of patients with PD.

  a. Selegiline (Eldepryl), 5 mg orally twice daily, an nonreversible inhibitor of MAO(B), is believed by some to delay the onset of disability associated with early untreated PD and should be started as soon as the diagnosis of PD is made. It probably has symptomatic antiparkinsonian effect as well. This drug may be effective as an adjunct to carbidopa/L-dopa therapy in patients who experience fluctuations in response but may also increase dyskinesia and neuropsychiatric side effects in the elderly.

  b. Vitamin E, an antioxidant, is postulated to offer neuroprotection, but studies have not yet substantiated that claim.

6. Surgical treatments are considered for individuals whose condition is unable to be controlled with medical therapy. Three procedures available are pallidotomy, deep brain stimulation, and fetal nigral transplantation. The long-term safety of these treatments is still unknown.

VI. Management strategies. Although no cure for PD exists, available therapy can generally be expected to reduce symptoms and enhance the quality of life. The goal of treatment is to maintain function and independence for as long as possible. Treatment should be individualized and based on the particular needs and expectations of the patient and family, including nonpharmaceutical as well as pharmaceutical treatment.

Therapeutic decisions involve assessing the potential benefits and complications and considering the financial status of the patient.

A. Rehabilitation medicine treatments, which include physical, occupational, and speech therapy, are as important as pharmacologic therapy as PD progresses. Stretching and active exercises may maintain or enhance physical activity, as well as mood. Other helpful approaches include gait training, developing effective turning techniques, providing bathtub and toilet grab bars, using walkers, and using Velcro bands and zippers.

B. **Educational and psychological support** in determining the emotional needs and coping mechanisms of both patient and family are important. The nature of the disease and disabilities and the usual course should be discussed with an emphasis on the ability of current therapy to control symptoms and prolong useful function. PD support groups and the American Parkinson Disease Association (APDA) are invaluable to patients and their families. The APDA can be reached at 1-800-223-2732. The National Parkinson's Foundation can be reached at 1-800-433-7022. "We move" Foundation can now be reached on the Internet (www.wemove.org) It is an excellent source of information for family, patients, and health care providers.

C. **Advanced PD.** The impairment produced by PD gradually progresses despite pharmacologic therapy. In addition, distressing side effects (ie, on/off fluctuations, end-of-dose failure, and dyskinesia) may limit the efficacy of various drugs. The approach to disease progression consists of increasing the dosage of drugs (ie, L-dopa to 1.5–2 g/day; bromocriptine to 75–100 mg/day) and using drug combinations. L-dopa remains the cornerstone of treatment and is included in combination therapy unless its side effects are intolerable. Surgery and electroconvulsive therapy may be helpful in selected patients with advanced PD.

D. **Patient follow-up.** Patients with PD should be seen at regular intervals every 2–6 months to monitor response to therapy and to assess side effects and disease progression. The **UPDRS (Unified Parkinson's Disease Rating Scale)** is helpful to quantitate therapy and progression of disease. It can be downloaded from www.wemove.org

VII. **Natural history and prognosis**

A. The course of PD is highly variable. If left untreated, the disease progresses from minimal dysfunction to severe disability in 3–10 years. Treatment generally retards but does not completely halt the progression of the disease. Current treatment may extend independent functioning and longevity by 5–15 years.

B. In general, the prognosis is better in younger patients with the classic triad of resting tremor, rigidity, and bradykinesia than in older patients with less tremor but more bradykinesia, gait disturbance, postural instability, and cognitive impairment.

C. Death usually results from pneumonia, septic complications of urinary tract infection, or decubitus ulcers.

REFERENCES

Koller WC, et al: An algorithm for the management of Parkinson's disease. Neurology 1994;**44**(suppl 10):51.

Lieberman A: An integrated approach to patient management in Parkinson's disease. Neurol Clin 1992;**10**(2):553.

Mutch WJ: Parkinson's disease. Rev Clin Gerontol 1995;**5**:11.

Olanow CW, et al: An algorithm (decision tree) for the management of Parkinson's disease: Treatment guidelines. Neurology 1998;**50**(3):PS001.

Ward C: Rehabilitation in Parkinson's disease. Rev Clin Gerontol 1992;**2**:254.

---

86   Peptic Ulcer Disease

Jay A. Swedberg, MD

I. **Definition.** Peptic ulcer disease (PUD) is a chronic, relapsing disorder resulting in inflammation and ulceration of areas of the upper gastrointestinal (GI) mucosa due to the action of gastric acid and pepsin.

II. **Epidemiology.** In the United States the overall incidence of PUD for all age groups in 1994 was 17.5 cases per 1000. The incidence increases with age, peaking at 36 cases per 1000 in the 65- to 74-year-old group. The lifetime prevalence of PUD is about 10%.

A. **Risk factors** strongly associated with PUD

1. **Helicobacter pylori.** Persistent presence of *H pylori* in gastric (antral) mucosa is strongly associated with PUD and is almost always present in chronic duodenal ulcer disease. Most peptic ulcers are associated with *H pylori,* and

eradication of this organism enhances ulcer healing and markedly decreases ulcer recurrence.

2. **Use of nonsteroidal anti-inflammatory drugs (NSAIDs).** Use of NSAIDs is associated with erosions and ulceration in the upper GI mucosa. NSAIDs increase the risk of recurrence and of GI complications (bleeding, perforation) two- to sixfold, depending on dose, half-life of agent, frequency of administration, and duration of use.

3. **Zollinger–Ellison syndrome.** This is a rare hypersecretory state that is associated with PUD.

B. The incidence of **recurrence or persistence** of ulcers increases with the following:

1. **Persistence of _H pylori_** in gastric mucosa.
2. **Continued long-term use of NSAIDs.**
3. **Prior history of ulcers or ulcer complications.**
4. **Incomplete ulcer healing** after treatment with H_2 receptor antagonists or proton pump inhibitors for 8 weeks.
5. **Continued smoking** (more than 10 cigarettes per day) increases the rate of ulcer recurrence and complications threefold, especially if _H pylori_ is present in gastric mucosa.

C. Other factors less strongly associated with peptic ulcers include a strong family history of PUD in first-degree relatives, poor coping or adaptation to stress, and fall or spring seasons. Diet does not have a significant impact on PUD or its recurrence.

III. **Pathophysiology.** Peptic ulceration occurs when digestive gastric secretions (gastric acid and pepsin) overcome gastroduodenal mucosal defenses. Mucosal defenses are impaired by _H pylori_ infection or use of NSAIDs.

A. **Aggressive factors**

1. _H pylori_ is associated with nonerosive gastritis and duodenal ulceration in 90–98% of patients. _H pylori_ is a gram-negative, microaerophilic, urease-producing bacterium, which grows beneath the mucus layer of gastric epithelium and is nearly always associated with histologic gastritis. Most peptic ulcers occur in association with _H pylori_ infection of the gastric mucosa. The infectious process requires the presence of acid as an essential factor for ulcer formation. Eradication of _H pylori,_ however, leads to ultimate cure of the ulcer diathesis.

2. NSAIDs and aspirin are frequently associated with hemorrhagic gastritis and gastric ulcers but have less impact on duodenal ulcers. Gastric ulcers occur in 15–20% of patients taking NSAIDs chronically, whereas duodenal ulcers are related to NSAID usage in 5–10% of patients.

3. Gastric acid is associated with upper GI ulcers; ulcers are rarely seen in the absence of acid. Whereas duodenal ulcers are associated with an increased total acid secretion, especially when nocturnal, gastric ulcers usually occur in association with normal or reduced acid secretion.

4. Pepsin (a proteolytic enzyme) requires a strong acid environment to be active.

5. Bile acids, lysolecithin, and pancreatic secretions can induce gastritis.

B. **Defensive factors** regulated by endogenous prostaglandin synthesis include mucus layer (barrier); bicarbonate secretion (buffer); mucosal blood flow; the physical barrier provided by the epithelial cell apical surface; and the response to injury by restitution (movement of cells to cover gaps), cellular regeneration, and repair.

IV. **Diagnosis**

A. **Symptoms and signs**

1. A history of **recurrent epigastric discomfort,** 30 minutes to 1 hour after meals (indigestion) and in the early morning hours, is typical. The discomfort is often relieved with food or antacids, at least temporarily. Nausea is often associated with epigastric discomfort.

2. A history of **recurrent vomiting, hematemesis, or melena** in patients with a history of recurrent epigastric discomfort suggests complications associated with PUD.

3. Symptoms of PUD are not reliable indicators of an ulcer crater. Clinically, 50–60% of patients with symptoms of PUD do not have pathology demonstrated by endoscopy.

4. **Lack of symptoms** does not necessarily indicate the absence of an ulcer. Asymptomatic ulcers are common, especially in the geriatric age group and in patients taking NSAIDs. An estimated 25–40% of peptic ulcer complications occur in asymptomatic patients.

B. **Laboratory tests**

1. **Diagnosis of *H pylori* infection. Serology** for antibody to *H pylori* indicates previous infection but cannot establish whether the infection is current. Positive serology for *H pylori* may be sufficient to treat patients for *H pylori* who have PUD and have not been previously treated for *H pylori*. Serology is not sufficient to diagnose *H pylori* infection when PUD is resistant to treatment or associated with complications (perforation, bleeding, obstruction) or has previously been treated for *H pylori*. A C^{13} or C^{14} **urea breath test** is a non-invasive test that reliably indicates a current *H pylori* infection. A positive breath test is sufficient to diagnosis active *H pylori* infection requiring initial treatment and to identify persistent *H pylori* infection after treatment. **Gastric biopsy** by endoscopy for Clo test (pH color indicator of conversion of urea to ammonia by *H pylori* urease), histology (gastritis with *H pylori* organism evident), or culture is diagnostic of active *H pylori* infection.

2. **Hemoglobin, hematocrit, and red blood cell indices** should be measured, and stool samples should be checked for occult or gross blood in patients with symptoms of PUD to determine the presence of acute or chronic GI bleeding. Nasogastric aspiration may be performed to look for evidence of blood in the stomach when acute bleeding is suspected.

3. **An upper GI x-ray series or esophagogastroduodenoscopy** should be used to confirm the diagnosis in patients with suspected PUD who do not respond to an empirical trial of H_2 receptor antagonists after 2 weeks or in patients with recurrent symptoms or evidence of complications from PUD.

   Endoscopy is the most sensitive method for detection of PUD and for identification of other causes of dyspeptic symptoms through direct visualization, cytology, and biopsy. A biopsy or brushing for cytology is warranted to rule out gastric carcinoma in patients who have gastric ulcers that fail to heal or that recur.

4. **Ultrasonography** of the gallbladder or **computed tomography (CT)** scan of the abdomen to image the pancreas should be considered in selected patients if no evidence of PUD is obtained through endoscopy or upper GI series in order to determine the cause of the patient's symptoms.

5. **A fasting serum gastrin level** should be considered in patients with refractory or recurrent ulcer disease unrelated to *H pylori* to rule out acid secretory failure or gastrinoma (Zollinger–Ellison syndrome).

V. **Treatment.** Goals of treatment include relief of pain and healing of ulceration, minimization of recurrence, prevention of complications, and use of cost-effective therapy (Figure 86–1).

A. **Eliminate *H pylori* infection** if present in gastric mucosa.

1. *H pylori* infection can usually be eradicated with triple therapy (ie, two antibiotics in combination with a proton pump inhibitor (omeprazole, or lansoprazole) or a bismuth compound for 7–14 days.

2. The treatment regimen ideally is simple, well tolerated, and cost-effective and results in a bacterial eradication rate of 90% or better.

B. **Reduction of gastric acid secretion.** If acid secretion is inhibited by at least 60%, healing rates improve significantly.

1. H_2 **receptor antagonists** are effective and well tolerated. These agents heal more than 90% of duodenal ulcers and more than 70% of gastric ulcers. In general, duodenal ulcers may be treated with night-time acid suppression, whereas gastric ulcers and gastroesophageal reflux disease usually require 24-hour acid suppression.

2. **Proton pump inhibitors** (hydrogen/potassium ATPase inhibitors) such as omeprazole (Prilosec) and lansoprazole (Prevacid), cause marked acid suppression, resulting in gastric pH of 2.5 and higher. Omeprazole and lansoprazole are indicated in the following conditions:

   a. **Erosive or ulcerative esophagitis**

   b. **Symptomatic gastroesophageal reflux disease** that has exhibited poor response to previous treatment

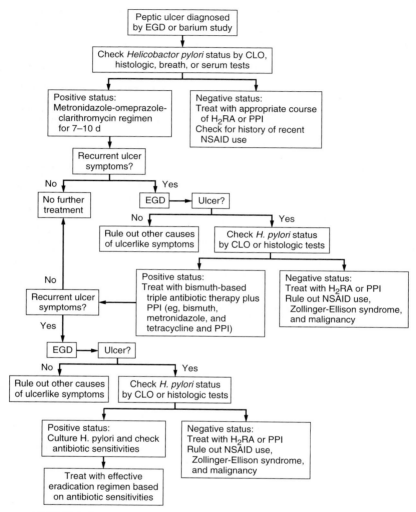

FIGURE 86–1. Recommended algorithm for the eradication of *Helicobacter pylori*. CLO, Campy-lobacter-like organism; EGD, esophagogastroduodenoscopy; H$_2$RA, histamine$_2$-receptor antagonist; NSAID, nonsteroidal anti-inflammatory drug; PPI, proton pump inhibitor. (Reprinted with permission from Salcedo JA, Al-Kawas F: Treatment of *Helicobacter pylori* infections. Arch Intern Med 1998; **158**:848.)

    c. Ulcers that have been unresponsive to 8–12 weeks of full-dose H$_2$ re-ceptor antagonist therapy and have been biopsied to rule out *H pylori* infection and cancer

    d. Pathologic hypersecretory conditions such as those found in Zollinger–Ellison syndrome

    e. Ulcer disease associated with multiple endocrine adenomas or sys-temic mastocytosis

    f. Treatment of *H pylori* when used in combination with two antibiotics and sometimes a bismuth compound for 7–14 days

g. **As a palliative measure** to heal ulcers, suppress ulcer recurrence, and reduce complications in patients who must continue use of NSAIDs or have *H pylori* infection resistant to treatment

3. **Anticholinergic agents.** These agents decrease acid secretion by 30–50% and have been used in combination with other agents such as H_2 receptor antagonists. The usefulness of these agents, however, is limited by their side effects.

   a. **Doxepin** (Sinequan) is an antidepressant that acts as a selective antimuscarinic receptor inhibitor.

   b. **Pirenzepine** is a selective antimuscarinic compound, which has been used in Canada and Europe. It is not yet available in the United States.

C. **Cytoprotective agents.** Mucosal defensive factors should be increased or maintained.

   1. **Sucralfate** (Carafate) and **bismuth compounds** such as bismuth subsalicylate (Pepto-Bismol) or colloidal bismuth subcitrate (De-Nol) achieve healing rates for duodenal ulcers similar to those of the H_2 receptor antagonists.

      a. These medications probably work by decreasing acid back diffusion and stimulating prostaglandin synthesis, which increases mucus secretion. Bismuth compounds reduce recurrence rates after the initial duodenal ulcer has healed, probably by inhibiting *H pylori*.

      b. The use of sucralfate and an H_2 receptor antagonist (combination therapy) is not contraindicated, although the usefulness and cost-effectiveness of this method in patients with routine PUD have not been demonstrated.

   2. **Prostaglandins** such as **misoprostol** (Cytotec) decrease recurrent ulcerations in patients who require NSAIDs.

      a. These agents improve mucosal defenses by increasing mucosal bicarbonate, mucus secretion, cell renewal, and blood flow and by decreasing vascular damage after injury. They also may decrease acid secretion. Prostaglandins, however, have not been shown to increase the rate of ulcer healing.

      b. The usefulness of prostaglandins is limited by side effects such as diarrhea, uterine bleeding, and spontaneous abortion.

D. **Surgery** is reserved for those patients in whom ulcer complications develop or for those who choose a surgical approach rather than daily maintenance therapy.

   1. Ulcer recurrence rates after surgery are 2–3%, compared with 20–30% with medical maintenance therapy. After stopping maintenance therapy, 50–80% of ulcers will recur within 1 year.

   2. Ulcer recurrence is less than 2% when documented *H pylori* infection has been eradicated. Treatment failures for *H pylori* occur in approximately 10–15% of patients.

   3. Surgical procedures include highly selective (proximal) vagotomy, vagotomy with pyloroplasty or antrectomy, and partial gastric resection for failed selective vagotomy.

VI. **Management strategies**

A. **Prevention.** Recent studies have demonstrated feasibility for an immunization strategy in treatment and prevention of *H pylori* infection. Oral administration of vaccine can stimulate an IgA antibody response to *H pylori* in gastric secretions and result in recruitment of T and B lymphocytes in gastric mucosa.

B. **Reduction of risk factors.** This includes cessation of smoking, reduction or discontinuance of NSAIDs, and consideration of **misoprostol** (Cytotec) for those who must continue use of NSAIDs.

C. **Empirical treatment trial.** An empirical treatment trial of full-dose H_2 receptor antagonist or proton pump inhibitor can be done for 4–8 weeks.

   1. **Indications.** An empirical treatment trial is indicated only in patients with typical symptoms of duodenal ulcer and no history or evidence of complications from PUD. PUD is considered complicated if any of the following factors are present.

      a. Bleeding, perforation, obstruction, or significant weight loss

      b. History of refractory or recurrent PUD

      c. Significant comorbid disease

   2. **Failure to symptomatically respond** to empirical therapy after 2 weeks, recurrence of symptoms, or occurrence of complications requires further

evaluation and confirmation of the diagnosis with an upper GI series or esophagogastroduodenoscopy. If PUD is confirmed, testing to identify *H pylori* infection is indicated.

   D. Treatment of *H pylori* is required in patients with PUD if *H pylori* has been identified. Treatment with **triple therapy** consists of use of two antibiotics plus either a bismuth compound or a proton pump inhibitor (Table 86–1).

   E. Maintenance therapy is a palliative measure that heals ulcers, suppresses ulcer recurrence, and reduces complications from PUD. Continuous therapy with a proton pump inhibitor or H_2 receptor antagonist is indicated in the following circumstances:

   1. **Failure to eradicate** *H pylori* infection
   2. **High-risk individuals** with complications of PUD (bleeding, perforation); risk factors such as serious concurrent illness, old age (frailty), continued NSAID use, or recalcitrant disease; or both
   3. **Hypersecretory states (Zollinger–Ellison syndrome)** or ulcer disease associated with multiple endocrine adenoma or systemic mastocytosis

VII. Natural history and prognosis

   A. Treatment for PUD significantly changed after 1977 when cimetidine became available. Elective surgery for PUD decreased fourfold. Although ulcers healed with acid suppression therapy (H_2 receptor antagonists, proton pump inhibitors), recurrence of ulcers remained a major problem. Approximately 75% of peptic ulcers recur within 1 year after acute or maintenance therapy is discontinued, regardless of the duration of maintenance therapy. The natural history of this chronic recurrent disease was not changed until the early 1990s, when *Helicobacter pylori* was shown to cause most cases of PUD, and eradication of *H pylori* infection cured the disease and eliminated recurrence. When the underlying cause of PUD (*H pylori infection,* NSAIDs) is eliminated, then recurrence is not a problem and the natural history of the disease process can be changed.

   B. Complications (bleeding, perforation, obstruction) occur with an annual incidence of 2–5% in patients with PUD.
   1. More aggressive diagnosis and treatment of *H pylori* infection should reduce the prevalence of PUD and decrease its complications.

TABLE 86–1. EFFECTIVE TREATMENT REGIMENS TO ERADICATE *HELICOBACTER PYLORI*

Metronidazole	Amoxicillin	Tetracycline	Clarithromycin	Proton Pump Inhibitor	Bismuth Compound[1]	Duration of Treatment
1 500 mg bid			500 mg bid	Omeprazole 20 mg or Lanzoprazole 30 mg bid		7–10 days
2	1 g bid		500 mg bid	Omeprazole 20 mg or Lanzoprazole 30 mg bid		7–10 days
3		500 mg qid	500 mg tid		Bismuth subsalicylate 302 mg (2 tabs) qid	14 days
4 500 mg tid		500 mg qid		Omeprazole 20 mg or Lanzoprazole 30 mg bid	Bismuth subsalicylate 302 mg (2 tabs) qid	14 days

[1] Bismuth subsalicylate (Pepto-Bismol) 151 mg/tablet; colloidal bismuth subcitrate (De-Nol outside the United States); ranitidine bismuth citrate.
Data from Arch Intern Med 1998;**158:**849.

2. Complications will continue in elderly patients and patients taking H_2 receptor antagonists (prescription or over-the-counter). Complications are especially likely if patients are also taking NSAIDs, since many will have asymptomatic ulcers that will be identified through complications of their PUD rather than through their symptoms.

REFERENCES

Chan FKL, Sung JJY: The medical care of patients with gastrointestinal bleeding after endoscopy. Gastrointest Endosc Clin N Am 1997;**7**(4):671.

Czinn SJ: What is the role for vaccinations in *Helicobacter pylori?* Gastroenterology 1997;**113**:S149.

Howden CW: For what conditions is there evidence-based justification for treatment of *Helicobacter pylori* infection? Gastroenterology 1997;**113**:S107.

Kleanthous H, Lee CK, Monath TP: Vaccine development against infection with *Helicobacter pylori.* Br Med Bull 1998;**54**(No. 1):229.

Neil GA, et al: Do ulcers burn out or burn on? Managing duodenal ulcer diathesis in the *Helicobacter pylori* era. Am J Gastroenterol 1997;**92**(3):387.

NIH Consensus Panel on *Helicobacter pylori* in Peptic Ulcer Disease: *Helicobacter pylori* in peptic ulcer disease. JAMA 1994;**172**:65.

Salcedo JA, Al-Kawas F: Treatment of *Helicobacter pylori* infections. Arch Intern Med 1998;**158**:842.

---

87   Peripheral Vascular Disease

Franklin Hargett, MD

I. **Definition**
   A. **Arteriosclerosis obliterans (ASO)** is a pathologic process that results in decreased blood flow to the limbs secondary to segmental atherosclerotic narrowing or obstruction of the lumen in arteries supplying the limbs.
   B. **Sudden arterial obstruction** is the acute or sudden obstruction of an artery supplying an extremity caused by embolus or in situ thrombus formation.
   C. **Varicose veins** are prominent, abnormally distended, and tortuous superficial veins, usually of the lower extremity.
II. **Epidemiology**
   A. **ASO.** The onset of ASO is usually between ages 50 and 70, although it may occur in younger individuals with hyperlipidemia disorders and diabetes mellitus, especially those who smoke. Men are more commonly affected than women. Symptomatic occlusive peripheral vascular disease occurs in 2% of men and 1% of women over the age of 65. Recent studies of institutional elderly individuals revealed a prevalence rate of 88% for this condition.
   B. The prevalence of **sudden arterial obstruction** is unknown, although it is increasing in frequency due to a growing elderly population, extended survival of patients with cardiac disease, and the increasing use of cardiac prostheses.
   C. **Varicose veins** are common. This disorder occurs in approximately 12% of the population in the United States. It affects approximately 20% of the adult population, and the incidence may reach 50% in age groups over 50. An additional 6–7 million US citizens have chronic, disabling lower extremity venous hypertension; some of these individuals also have leg ulcers. A family history is present in 50% of all cases. Women are five times more likely to develop this condition than men.
III. **Pathophysiology**
   A. The primary lesion in **ASO** is intimal plaque and progressive narrowing with thrombus formation, degeneration, or calcification and, in many cases, complete blockage of the vessel. The final result is atherosclerosis.
   B. **Sudden arterial obstruction** resulting from embolization can generally be regarded as a manifestation of underlying cardiovascular disease. Arterial emboli usually arise from within the heart. Another source of arterial emboli, however, is arteriosclerotic plaques that break off from arterial walls and embolize, usually to the digital artery ("blue toe" syndrome).

    1. Once emboli have been released from the heart, approximately 70% proceed to the lower extremities, 20% to the cerebral circulation, and 10% to the upper extremities or visceral arteries.

    2. The most common cause of an arterial embolus is mural thrombus from a myocardial infarction. Other cardiac sources of emboli are atrial fibrillation, aortic and mitral valvular disease, or, rarely, myxomas of the heart.

C. Varicose veins result from superficial venous insufficiency, which refers to incompetent valves in the greater or lesser saphenous veins or both.

    1. Obstruction secondary to thromboses or pregnancy may elevate venous pressure. Prolonged pressure changes create varicose veins secondary to destruction of valvular competency.

    2. The development of **postphlebitic syndrome** (ie, loss of valvular mechanism in the deep venous system) results in edema, induration, and fibrosis.

    3. Ulcers usually occur above the medial malleolus as a result of prolonged venous insufficiency and secondary atrophic skin changes.

    4. Rupture is an uncommon complication of varicose veins. The skin overlying varices can become thin, and erosion can occur spontaneously or with minor trauma.

IV. Diagnosis

A. Symptoms and signs

    1. ASO. The specific evaluation at the bedside is twofold: (1) The patient's systolic blood pressure perfusion is determined. Raise the patient's leg 60–75°, and check color and temperature. Then have the patient pump his or her foot (heel taps) 20–30 times, and check color and temperature. Coolness and pallor following these maneuvers indicate obstruction. (2) The severity of the obstruction is then determined. Have the patient dangle his or her legs over the side of the bed, and check timing of color return and dorsal vein refilling. Normally, color should return within 10 seconds and venous filling should develop within 15 seconds. In moderate obstruction, color return should take less than 25–30 seconds and venous filling time should be 30 seconds. In severe obstruction, color return and venous filling time take more than 35–40 seconds.

        a. Pain is the cardinal symptom in ASO. Exercise-induced leg pain, or **intermittent claudication,** is a cramping pain in the muscle. The pain is relieved with rest and worsened by increased workload. Calf claudication means that the occlusion is at or proximal to the popliteal artery, whereas hip claudication indicates aortoiliac disease.

        b. Aortoiliac atherosclerosis may produce not only claudication but also **impotence (Leriche's syndrome).**

        c. Diminished, absent, or asymmetrical pulses often pinpoint the exact site of arterial obstruction.

        d. A **bruit** denotes turbulent flow past a stenotic lesion or through an arteriovenous fistula.

        e. Loss of normal skin texture, loss of hair, trophic nail changes, and dependent rubor are signs of ASO.

        f. Atrophy and **ulceration** are common in more advanced disease and in diabetics with neuropathy.

    2. Sudden arterial obstruction. Peripheral arterial emboli appear as abrupt attacks of ischemia.

        a. Pallor, pain, pulselessness, paresthesia, and paralysis are the classic "five Ps" of acute arterial occlusion. Sudden abrupt pain occurs in about 50% of the patients. The remainder experience mild pain or numbness and paresthesia.

        b. Diminished or absent pulses distal to the occlusion and **signs of ischemia** are present.

        c. Paresthesia and **paralysis** are signs of poor salvageability.

    3. Varicose veins. Inspection for varicose veins will be sufficient to diagnose this condition.

        a. The most common reason women bring varicose veins to the attention of the physician is purely **cosmetic,** although **dull, nagging aches** or **discomfort** in the calf and ankle may occur occasionally.

        b. Excessive bleeding may result from spontaneous rupture, minor injury, or puncture of superficially located veins.

    c. **Trendelenburg's test** can identify defective valves and incompetent communicating veins. With the patient recumbent, elevate the leg to empty the veins, and apply a tourniquet over the saphenofemoral junction. Ask the patient to resume the erect position. No filling of the varicosities is seen if the communicating or perforating veins are competent. Rapid filling of the varicosities with the tourniquet in place indicates incompetent perforating veins.

    d. **Perthes' test** can be used to assess deep venous patency. Compress the superficial varicosities by wrapping the extremity with elastic bandages. Severe crampy leg pain with exercise suggests an obstructed deep venous system.

B. Laboratory tests

  1. **ASO.** Vascular laboratory evaluation of the lower extremity includes ultrasonographic Doppler measurement of the ankle and arm systolic blood pressures and examination of directional Doppler velocity and waveforms. Segmental pressures obtained with either the Doppler technique or plethysmography are used to localize the level of disease. The response to standardized exercise completes the noninvasive evaluation of ASO.

    a. The American Heart Association has recommended the **ankle/arm pressure index (AAI)** as the best noninvasive method to detect atherosclerotic peripheral arterial disease in population studies. Normally, the patient has the same systolic blood pressure in the ankle and the arm (ie, AAI = 1).

    b. Indications for **angiography** in the work-up of peripheral vascular disease are rest pain, ulceration or gangrene, presurgery, and evaluation-unexplained leg pain.

  2. **Sudden arterial obstruction.** Routine admission laboratory tests are usually not helpful; however, they may reveal metabolic acidosis, hyperkalemia, and myoglobinuria in delayed presentations with muscle necrosis.

    a. **Electrocardiography** may confirm dysrhythmia, myocardial infarction, or ventricular aneurysm.

    b. **Chest x-rays** may reveal an enlarged heart or prosthetic valve. Complete cardiac evaluation and determination of surgical risk should be done in the majority of patients.

    c. **Doppler ultrasonographic evaluation** of the arterial system can substantiate the clinical findings.

    d. **Angiography** may be performed preoperatively, intraoperatively, or interventionally when coupled with thrombolytic therapy, balloon angioplasty, or laser interventions.

  3. **Varicose veins.** Direct venous pressure by needle and strain gauge provides the most accurate assessment of venous hemodynamics, but the procedure is invasive.

    a. A **directional Doppler test** can be used to determine venous patency and valvular competence. **Duplex scanning** is the most promising new technique. The combination of ultrasonographic duplex scanning using a B-mode imager with a pulsed Doppler instrument provides both imaging and flow patterns.

    b. The **strain gauge plethysmograph** measures venous capacity and outflow, making it more valuable for acute thrombosis than for chronic changes.

V. Treatment

A. ASO. The treatment of intermittent claudication involves lifestyle modification and pharmacologic therapy. Rest pain or chronic ulcer may require surgical intervention.

  1. **Lifestyle modifications** include weight reduction, cessation of tobacco smoking, exercise, control of hypertension, control of diabetes mellitus, management of hyperlipidemia, and foot care.

  2. **Pentoxifylline** (Trental), 400 mg orally three times a day with meals, is efficacious. Blind, controlled, randomized studies have revealed improved treadmill performance in patients with intermittent claudication who take pentoxifylline. Improvement may not be noted for 2–4 weeks, however. The patient may observe as much as a 50% increase in walking distance.

3. **Vasodilators** are no longer approved for use in intermittent claudication or obstructive artery disease. Platelet inhibitors have no proven efficacy in the treatment of these conditions.

4. **Surgical intervention** is chosen based on the location and the extent of the occlusive process. With proper selection of patients and appropriate management of comorbid conditions, the operative mortality is <2% and successful revascularization is obtained in 90–95% of patients.

   a. **Endarterectomy** may be used in selected patients with isolated segmental stenosis or occlusion.

   b. **Aortoiliac or aortofemoral bypass** procedures using prosthetic graft material are utilized most commonly for terminal aortic or iliac occlusive disease. Concomitant femoropopliteal, or tibial, bypass techniques may be necessary in patients with significant distal occlusive disease. Extra-anatomic bypass procedures using axillofemoral or femorofemoral bypass can be performed in selected patients when intra-abdominal procedures are contraindicated.

   c. **Percutaneous transluminal angioplasty (PTA)** has become a safe and effective procedure to improve blood flow in the iliac and femoropopliteal arteries.

   d. **Intra-arterial infusion of thrombolytic agents** is a useful adjunct to surgery and PTA. Streptokinase, urokinase, and tissue plasminogen activators allow lysis of clot in runoff vessels after PTA and lysis of thrombus when bypass grafts have become thrombosed.

   e. New techniques using **laser technology** are being investigated. These devices flatten, vaporize, remove, or remodel atheromatous material.

B. **Sudden arterial obstruction.** Treatment for the source of the embolus (eg, atrial fibrillation, endocarditis, or myocardial infarction) should be instituted. If an entire limb is ischemic, a "golden period" of 6–8 hours during which revascularization can be achieved usually occurs.

   1. **Systematic heparinization** is used to prevent distal propagation of thrombus (see Chapter 23 for a heparinization protocol).

   2. **Surgical embolectomy** is a procedure performed under local anesthesia that uses a balloon embolectomy catheter to extract clots.

   3. A regimen of **intra-arterial streptokinase bolus/infusion,** 25,000–250,000 IU, followed by continuous infusion of 5000–15,000 IU/hr or intra-arterial urokinase bolus/infusion 60,000–120,000 IU followed by 240,000 IU/hr for 2 hours, 120,000 IU for 2 hours, then 60,000 IU/hour, can be used. Trials are under way using tissue plasminogen activator.

   4. **Fasciotomy** must be considered for any limb that is tightly swollen or with prolonged muscle ischemia.

   5. **Aggressive fluid resuscitation** and meticulous electrolyte and acid–base therapy are mandatory.

C. **Varicose veins.** Therapeutic goals are to relieve chronic discomfort, to provide an acceptable cosmetic result, and to prevent long-term sequelae of chronic venous hypertension.

   1. **Graded compression stockings** are the mainstay of medical therapy. The disadvantages of compression stockings are the need for lifelong use and relatively frequent replacement, the difficulty of application in elderly patients, and heat intolerance in a warm climate. Compliance is essential for compression hose to afford protection from chronic venous stasis sequelae and to control symptoms related to varicosities. Stockings to the knee should be prescribed, since thigh and pantyhose garments are less well tolerated.

   2. Mandatory periods of lower extremity **"ankle above atrium" elevation** for 20 minutes four times a day aid in controlling discomfort and edema.

   3. **Operative management** should be considered for those patients with severe primary varicose veins (uncontrollable discomfort and rapid progression) or for those who consider the cosmetic burden intolerable. Ligation and stripping of primary varicosities are the best operation; all of the superficial varicosities are excised. A well-executed operation provides durable protection from local recurrence for at least 10 years.

   4. **Transcutaneous sclerotherapy** using sodium morrhuate or sodium tetradecyl sulfate is best reserved for small primary or recurrent varicosities.

   5. **Local wound care** for ulcers includes the use of an Unna boot or hydro-colloid dressing (Duoderm) for clean ulcers.
   6. Correction of anemia and poor nutrition and correction of blood sugar in patients with diabetes mellitus will improve the patient's chances of healing.

VI. **Management strategies**
   A. **ASO.** Patients with ASO should be informed of the progressive course of the disorder and the systemic nature of the atherosclerotic process. They must be advised that cigarette smoking cessation, regular daily exercise, and weight reduction are essential components of the management of intermittent claudication. Beta blockers should not be used. Surgical intervention is needed for individuals with rest pain and severe ulcers. Amputation is reserved for patients with gangrene, advancing infection, recalcitrant ulceration, and unremitting pain. The frequency of patient follow-up is determined by the severity of the process. Initial visits should be frequent to determine the rate of progression of the disease and the effects of medical management. If the process is stable and the patient is knowledgeable of the planned treatment, follow-up may be planned for twice a year.
   B. **Sudden arterial obstruction.** Both the patient and his or her family should be informed that an acute peripheral embolus is usually a manifestation of underlying cardiac or peripheral vascular disease. They should understand the possibility of limb loss and the inherent risk of cardiac disease. The patient should be educated about the need for and the risks of long-term anticoagulation, if such treatment is deemed necessary. Long-term management of the postembolectomy patient includes correction of any obvious sources of emboli and monitoring of anticoagulants if needed.
   C. **Varicose veins.** Patient education is the most important element in the long-term management of this condition. Extended periodic follow-up is essential for patients managed with medical or surgical treatment. The medically treated patient should be followed up every 3–6 months, and the stable medical or surgically stable patient should be followed up yearly, for signs of recurrent varicosities.

VII. **Natural history and prognosis**
   A. The natural history of **ASO** is dependent on the severity of disease and treatment compliance. In the absence of diabetes mellitus, ASO is a slowly progressive disease. The location of the lesion influences the prognosis. When larger vessels are involved, the probability of successful surgical intervention or percutaneous angioplasty is higher, and the prognosis is better than in patients in whom smaller vessels are involved. Untreated intermittent claudicants seldom require amputation, but patients with rest pain often face a major amputation or early death. Mortality usually results from arteriosclerotic involvement of other vascular beds, such as coronary or cerebral circulation, with death from myocardial infarction or stroke.
   B. In sudden arterial obstruction, the natural clinical course depends on the location of the occlusion, the degree of completeness of luminal blockage, the extent of the thrombosis, and the amount of collateral circulation. If embolectomy is performed during the "golden period," the function of the limb is not compromised. Overall, limb salvage among reported series is approximately 60%. The inhospital mortality rate is approximately 25%.
   C. The natural history and prognosis of **varicose veins** are those of a progressive worsening of venous flow. The development of massive distention of superficial varices may lead to clinical thrombophlebitis, significant hemorrhage from local trauma, or the chronic changes of stasis dermatitis or skin ulceration. With treatment, these complications can be avoided.

REFERENCES

Bradbury A, Evans C, Allan P, et al: What are the symptoms of varicose veins? Edinburgh vein study cross sectional population survey. BMJ 1999;**318**:353.

Gahtan V: The noninvasive vascular laboratory. Surg Clin North Am 1998;**78**:507.

McNamara DB, Champion HC, Kadowitz PJ: Pharmacologic management of peripheral vascular disease. Surg Clin North Am 1998;**78**:447.

Stemmer EA, Aronow W, Wilson S: Peripheral vascular disease in the elderly: Part II. Clin Geriatr 1995;**3**:16.

Working Party on Thrombolysis in the Management of Limb Ischemia: Thrombolysis in the management of lower limb peripheral arterial occlusion: A consensus document. Am J Cardiol 1998;**81**:207.

88   Premenstrual Syndrome

Janice E. Daugherty, MD

I. **Definition.** Premenstrual syndrome (PMS) is the cyclic recurrence in the luteal phase of the menstrual cycle of a combination of distressing physical, psychological, and behavioral changes of severity that results in deterioration of interpersonal relationships or interference with normal activities.

The *Diagnostic and Statistical Manual of Mental Disorders,* 3rd edition, revised 1987, included late luteal phase dysphoric disorder as a proposed diagnostic category needing further study. The subsequent use of these criteria has had considerable impact on standardizing the diagnosis for research in PMS. The designation *premenstrual dysphoric disorder* (PDD) was included in the 4th edition of the manual. Principles of treatment may be applied to patients whose symptoms are similar, but not adequately severe to meet formal diagnostic criteria. Symptoms commonly noted (Table 88–1) include depressed mood or feelings of hopelessness or self-deprecation; anxiety; affective lability; irritability; anger; feelings of difficulty concentrating; decreased energy; change in sleep, appetite, or both (increase or decrease); feelings of being out of control; and physical symptoms of bloating, breast tenderness, muscle or joint aches, and headache. These symptoms must interfere with usual daily activities.

The National Institute of Mental Health has recommended that, for a diagnosis of PMS, there must be a marked change in intensity (at least 30%) of symptoms measured from cycle days 5 to 10 compared to the 6-day interval prior to menses for at least two consecutive cycles.

II. **Epidemiology.** Most women report at least some minor physical and emotional symptoms in the postovulatory phase of the menstrual cycle. Thirty percent to 40% have symptoms of moderate intensity, and it is estimated that 3–5% of women of reproductive age suffer PMS of an intensity that is temporarily disabling.

    A. **Age.** Symptoms of PMS may occur at any age in the reproductive years; incidence of presenting for care peaks in the mid-30s. Some women experience cyclic symptoms even after menopause.

    B. **Social class.** No clinically useful differences have been defined.

TABLE 88–1. RESEARCH CRITERIA FOR PREMENSTRUAL DYSPHORIC DISORDER

In most menstrual cycles during the past year, five (or more) of the following symptoms were present for most of the time during the last week of the luteal phase, began to remit within a few days after the onset of the follicular phase, and were absent in the week postmenses, with at least one of the symptoms being either (1), (2), (3), or (4):

(1) markedly depressed mood, feelings of hopelessness, or self-deprecating thoughts
(2) marked anxiety, tension, or feeling of being "keyed up" or "on edge"
(3) marked affective lability (eg, feeling suddenly sad or tearful or having increased sensitivity to rejection)
(4) persistent and marked anger or irritability or increased interpersonal conflicts
(5) decreased interest in usual activities (eg, work, friends, or hobbies)
(6) subjective sense of difficulty in concentrating
(7) lethargy, easy fatigability, or marked lack of energy
(8) marked change in appetite, overeating, or specific food cravings
(9) hypersomnia or insomnia
(10) a subjective sense of being overwhelmed or out of control
(11) other physical symptoms, such as breast tenderness or swelling, headaches, joint or muscle pain, a sensation of "bloating," or weight gain

The disturbance must seriously interfere with work or usual social activities or relationships, and not be merely an exacerbation of the symptoms of another disorder, such as major depression, panic disorder, dysthymia, or a personality disorder (although it may be superimposed on any of these).
The criteria must be confirmed by prospective, daily self-ratings during at least two cycles.

Adapted with permission from American Psychiatric Association (APA): *Diagnostic and Statistical Manual of Mental Disorders.* 4th ed. APA; 1994.

C. Race. PMS is reported to occur in all ethnic groups. Cultural variation in the prevalence rates and patterns of symptoms occur, but no clinically useful diagnostic or therapeutic differences have yet emerged.

D. Reproductive factors. Women with regular (ovulatory) menstrual cycles, as well as those with longer cycles and heavier menstrual flow, report symptoms of swelling, mood swings, and depression more than other women. PMS may occur in spontaneous anovulatory cycles and following oophorectomy or hysterectomy. More than half of PMS patients have a history of pre-eclampsia or postnatal depression.

III. Pathophysiology. No single theory currently accounts for all the clinical and pathophysiologic features of PMS. The similarity of PMS to depressive illness, as well as its similar response to antidepressant therapy, suggests shared metabolic abnormalities. The interaction of several pathways may result in the development of PMS. Recent research seems to point toward an interaction of hormones, neurotransmitters, nutrients, and behavioral or environmental factors in the development of significant symptoms.

A. Gonadal hormones. Deficiency of progesterone or changes in the progesterone–estrogen ratio or elevated levels of prolactin have all been suspected as causes of PMS, but controlled studies have not yet yielded definitive results. Studies conflict on whether circulating levels of estrogen are elevated or normal. Serum levels of free testosterone were found to be significantly higher throughout the menstrual cycle in women with the diagnosis of PDD. A number of factors complicate the process of clarifying the relationship of hormones to PMS. Significant physiologic fluctuations of sex hormones and gonadotrophins occur throughout the day, rendering single serum levels difficult to interpret. Levels measured in serum include both bound (inactive) and free (active) hormone, and binding globulin levels are influenced by several factors. Other possible measurements (eg, salivary or urinary hormone levels) have not come into standard use.

Studies of hormone supplementation have also been difficult to interpret on a large scale because of supplementation with differing estrogens, or with synthetic progestins that exhibit significantly differing pharmacologic properties. Supplementation with progesterone has shown effectiveness in some studies of PMS, but extensive first-pass hepatic degradation of progesterone administered orally mandates a non-oral route. Intramuscular, transrectal, or transvaginal routes engender obvious compliance issues; transdermal administration has been reported as successful but has not yet been confirmed in large, controlled trials.

B. Other hormones. Various abnormalities of the hypothalamic–pituitary–adrenal axis have been implicated. Some of the clinical symptoms of PMS, such as fatigue, mood swings, and depression, are reminiscent of hypothyroidism. The common complaint of "water retention" has led to speculation that abnormalities of the renin–angiotensin–aldosterone system could cause PMS, but no such abnormalities have yet been found. Recurring elevations of plasma insulin, released in response to hyperglycemia resulting from stress-related epinephrine release, dietary simple sugar intake, or both, are a likely cause for the edema of PMS.

C. Other biochemical abnormalities. Women with PDD have been shown to have premenstrual abnormalities in serotonin, and trials of drugs that influence central nervous system levels of serotonin and other neurotransmitters have shown effectiveness of these drugs over placebo in this disorder. Results incorporating plasma measurements of neurotransmitters have not shown definitive differences, but platelet uptake of serotonin has been found to be abnormal. Women with PDD also have been shown to have altered levels of plasma β-endorphin, lowered plasma adrenocorticotropic hormone levels, differences in the episodic secretion rates of progesterone and luteinizing hormone in the luteal phase, higher nocturnal core body temperatures, and changes in the rhythm of melatonin secretion. The clinical significance of each of these abnormalities is yet to be understood.

D. Vitamin or mineral deficiencies. Deficiency of **vitamin B_6** (pyridoxine), an enzyme cofactor in the formation of serotonin, dopamine, and norepinephrine, has been proposed, but studies have failed to demonstrate vitamin B_6 deficiency in PMS patients, and supplementation has not relieved symptoms in blinded trials. Deficiency of intracellular **magnesium,** but not in serum or erythrocytes, has been shown, and supplementation with magnesium has shown to provide significant relief of symptoms over placebo in several well-designed studies.

Low-calcium diets have been shown in metabolic study to be associated with significant undesirable affect and behavioral changes throughout the menstrual cycle, with poorer mental concentration during the premenstrual phase, as well as increased dysmenorrhea. **Low-manganese diets,** comparable to the typical dietary intake of women in the reproductive years, reproduced the same symptoms, even in the presence of adequate calcium. Daily supplementation of calcium was shown to improve negative premenstrual affect and water retention, as well as dysmenorrhea.

Vitamin E may block the synthesis of excess prostaglandins and may modulate central neurotransmitters. Vitamin E supplementation produced significant improvement in both physical and affective symptoms of PMS in randomized controlled trials.

E. **Other hypotheses.** Abnormalities of specific prostaglandins have not been proven. Disorders of carbohydrate metabolism have been proposed, but insulin clamp studies have shown no abnormalities. It has been postulated that carbohydrate craving is an attempt to increase brain tryptophan and serotonin, but this connection is unclarified. Deficiencies of linoleic acid and its metabolites have been reported in women with PMS, and dietary supplementation with evening primrose oil, a source of gamma-linoleic acid, has been reported effective in relieving symptoms.

IV. **Diagnosis.** For the woman who presents with symptoms of PMS, beginning the diagnostic process with an open-ended inquiry will provide tremendously useful information. In some studies, up to 50% of women presenting to PMS clinics did not meet diagnostic criteria for that disorder, but instead were assigned another diagnosis: most frequently, major depression, followed in frequency by dysthymia, anxiety disorder, menopause, or another gynecologic or medical disorder. "PMS" may be a diagnosis that is more acceptable to the patient than is depression or anxiety. By starting the evaluation in an unstructured manner, the clinician can avoid a premature (and possibly erroneous) diagnosis.

Once an overview of the symptoms has been obtained, the patient's symptoms can be rated to establish a baseline (Table 88–2), and other essential information can be requested, including: Is there a previous diagnosis of PMS? What criteria were used to make the diagnosis? Have the symptoms changed over time? What previous treatments have been successful or unsuccessful? Many patients will self-diagnose PMS from information found in the lay literature. Other important questions include the following.

A. **Is there a history of treatment for an affective disorder?** As many as 10% of women with PMS may report suicidal ideas and death wishes and thoughts.

Are there vegetative symptoms of depression? (See Chapter 96.) Of women with major depression, over half will have exacerbation of symptoms in the premenstrual phase, including increased severity of usual symptoms or the appearance of new symptoms such as increased aggression, suicidal tendencies, or depersonalization.

TABLE 88–2. SHORTENED PREMENSTRUAL ASSESSMENT FORM

The patient is asked to consider the changes currently experienced with regard to her menstrual period:

Pain, tenderness, enlargement, or swelling of breasts
Feeling unable to cope or overwhelmed by ordinary demands
Feeling under stress
Outbursts of "irritability" or bad temper
Feeling sad or blue
Backaches, joint and muscle pain, or stiffness
Weight gain
Relatively steady abdominal heaviness, discomfort, or pain
Edema, swelling, puffiness, or "water retention"
Feeling bloated

Patients may rate each change on this list on a scale from 1 (not present or no change from usual) to 6 (extreme change, perhaps noticeable even to casual acquaintances)

Adapted with permission from Allen SS, McBride CM, Pirie PL: The shortened premenstrual assessment form. J Reprod Med 1991;**36**:769.

B. **Is there seasonal variation of the depressive symptoms?** "Seasonal" PDD has been shown to improve with phototherapy.

C. **Does she consider her general health to be good, or is there chronic disease?** PMS must be differentiated from symptoms arising from other chronic disorders but which are exacerbated during the premenstrual phase of the cycle ("premenstrual magnification"). Some patients experience exacerbation or precipitation of other medical problems, such as asthma, migraine, epilepsy, or manic–depressive illness just prior to menstruation.

D. **Are her menses regular? Has she had pelvic inflammatory disease, surgery, or endometriosis? What contraceptive method does she use?** PMS is associated with ovulatory cycles, which are usually regular. A primary complaint of pain may be related to gynecologic disease. By suppression of ovulation, oral contraceptives may provide relief of PMS, but studies have been inconsistent in this regard. Marked relief of symptoms was noted in the majority of women treated with depot medroxyprogesterone acetate in one study.

E. **Has she been pregnant? What was the outcome? Were her symptoms present during pregnancy? Did she have postpartum depression?** PMS is not present during pregnancy. Current affective symptoms could relate to a pregnancy outcome, such as abortion, other fetal loss, or abnormality. Postpartum depression is frequently found in patients with PDD.

F. **Is the patient taking medications? Is she taking vitamin or mineral supplements, and on whose advice? What alternative therapies has she tried?** Diuretic therapy can result in paradoxical water retention, especially in "idiopathic edema." Large amounts of dairy products may interfere with magnesium absorption, leading to chronic deficiency, which has been noted in PMS. Some women will take large amounts (200 mg or more) of vitamin B_6 in an attempt to relieve PMS symptoms, without understanding the risk of peripheral neuropathy. However, some supplements, in the correct amounts, can be therapeutic for PMS. Women, in the search for PMS treatment, may have encountered clinicians who were less than empathetic toward their complaints. Many seek care from alternative practitioners, who may provide some relief of their symptoms, and this alternative treatment may be continued along with the traditional prescription obtained from the clinician. An understanding of all current treatments is necessary to avoid adverse interactions.

G. **Is there a personal history of alcohol or drug abuse?** Compared with the general population, women seeking treatment for PMS are more likely to have lifetime histories of depression, anxiety disorder, suicide attempts, panic disorder, and substance abuse.

H. **Is there a history of smoking?** Women who smoke are more likely to experience PMS symptoms.

I. **Is there evidence of bulimia? Does she have food cravings? Does she follow any particular diet regimen?** Electrolyte imbalances from frequent vomiting can yield behavioral symptoms, especially fatigue. Ingestion of large amounts of sugar can exacerbate symptoms in at least two ways: refined sugar increases the urinary excretion of magnesium (as do diuretics) and also interferes with renal clearance of sodium and water. In response to a large sugar load, the production of keto acids is suppressed by an insulin surge. The resulting impairment in excretion of sodium and water causes expansion of the extracellular fluid volume with resultant edema, bloating, and breast tenderness. This sodium retention is resistant to aldosterone inhibitors. Table salt enhances the intestinal absorption of glucose, which enhances this insulin response and contributes to the edema. Alcohol may play a role in reactive hypoglycemia of PMS.

J. **Was there early victimization and trauma?** Up to 40% of patients diagnosed with PMS have a history of sexual abuse.

K. **Is there a family history of PMS, affective disorders, substance abuse, or alcoholism?** Familial occurrence is documented.

L. **Symptom clusters.** PMS symptoms may fall into "clusters," which may be helpful in choosing therapy. Some women experience more anxiety, irritability, or mood swings. For some, the primary symptoms are weight gain, swelling, and bloating; for others changes in appetite or cravings, fatigue, and headache are most troublesome. Still others have depression, sleep disturbance, or cognitive difficulties. Some women experience any or all of these, with variations in severity and symptoms from cycle to cycle. Treatment success is not contingent upon identifying a particular symptom cluster.

M. Timing of symptoms. A calendar of symptoms experienced relative to phase of the menstrual cycle (Figure 88–1) can help confirm that they are indeed premenstrual; some women experience erratic symptom patterns and incorrectly attribute them to PMS. Basal temperature measurements can help rule out disorders of ovulation and provide further confirmation of the premenstrual timing of symptoms.

N. Physical examination. General physical and pelvic examinations are indicated to exclude rheumatologic disease, anemia, electrolyte imbalance, neoplasms, endometriosis, or menopause.

O. Laboratory tests. There are no specific laboratory tests for PMS at this time. Other laboratory or physiologic tests may be necessary in individual cases to rule out other potential causes of symptoms.

    1. A complete blood cell count if there is chronic fatigue or menorrhagia.

    2. SMA-18 chemistry profile if there is chronic fatigue or suspicion of electrolyte disorder.

    3. Thyroid-stimulating hormone (unless done within the last 3 months), as the prevalence of thyroid disease is high for women in this age group.

    4. Follicle-stimulating hormone and **luteinizing hormone** for women over 40, with irregular menstrual cycles or hot flashes, or who are posthysterectomy.

    5. Serum prolactin in patients with galactorrhea, an irregular menstrual cycle, history of infertility, decreased libido, or atypical presentations of mastalgia.

    6. Chlamydia and gonorrhea testing if there is high-risk behavior, cervicitis, or pain upon pelvic examination.

V. Treatment

A. Patient education. Patients are exposed to information about PMS from many nonmedical sources and may have strong convictions about the condition and its treatment. Neither the physician nor the patient is helped by the uncertainties in the literature. Empathy and affirmation are particularly useful in dealing with PMS.

    Patient education alone may lead to a dramatic reduction in symptoms during the 3 months when the patient is completing the symptom diary. In addition, such general advice builds patient self-esteem and ability to cope with symptoms. In controlled trials of PMS treatment, the placebo response rate is typically greater than 20% and sometimes as high as 50%. This finding likely reflects the therapeutic value of discussing symptoms with a caring clinician.

B. Symptomatic treatments. Encourage proper diet with adequate composition according to the current U.S. Recommended Daily Allowances and Dietary Guidelines for healthy adults. Following the Food Guide Pyramid (http://www.nal.usda.

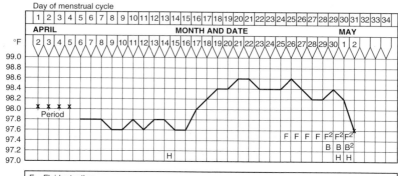

FIGURE 88–1. Premenstrual syndrome symptom diary. A minimum of two symptomatic cycles must be included to establish the diagnosis.

gov/fnic.html) with specific emphasis on avoiding salt and animal fats will often provide symptom relief and potentially confer general health benefits as well.

Supplementation may be necessary to assure adequate amounts of certain nutrients, including calcium (1000 mg of elemental calcium per day), vitamins (vitamin E, 400 IU/day), and trace minerals (magnesium, 400 mg/day; manganese, 6 mg/day). Regular aerobic exercise and elimination or reduction of adverse health habits, such as tobacco and alcohol use, may directly improve PMS through the pathophysiologic mechanisms previously described.

Teaching women to take control of symptoms through reduction of negative emotions by cognitive restructuring, improving problem-solving skills, and developing responsible assertiveness to deal with discomforts has been shown to provide significant relief of both physical and emotional symptoms. If there is suboptimal improvement after 2–3 months of the treatments described above or if symptoms are severe, secondary treatment modalities may be considered.

1. **Anxiety, irritability, and mood swings.** The same drugs used for depressive symptoms have been found to alleviate anxiety symptoms as well in many cases. Also, buspirone, 30 mg/day (10 mg three times a day) for 12 days prior to menses, is effective not only for social dysfunction but also for fatigue, cramps, and general aches and pains. Clonidine, 0.1 mg twice a day, and verapamil, 80 mg three times a day or one 240-mg sustained-release capsule once a day, have also been reported to have beneficial effects on mood.

2. **Weight gain, swelling, and bloating.** Spironolactone, 25 mg orally four times a day, has produced relief of weight gain and abdominal bloating. Metolazone, 1–5 mg/day 1 week prior to and continuing through menses, produced less weight gain and improvement in mood. Diuretic therapy is to be recommended only in addition to restriction of intake of simple sugars and salt.

3. **Breast tenderness.** Vitamin E, 400 IU twice daily, may reduce mastodynia if lower doses are ineffective. Treatment is usually continued for 4–6 months and resumed if symptoms recur.

4. **Changes in appetite, cravings, and fatigue.** Adherence to dietary guidelines, achievement of adequate sleep, and management of the environment to minimize exposure to added stress may offer some mitigation of symptoms.

5. **Depression, sleep disturbance, and cognitive difficulty.** Antidepressant therapy with both tricyclic antidepressants (TCA) and selective serotonin reuptake inhibitors (SSRI) has been shown to be significantly more effective than placebo, with SSRIs preferred because of a lower side effect profile. Several SSRI antidepressants have been found effective for PMS, including fluoxetine (20–40 mg daily), paroxetine (10–20 mg daily) or sertraline (50–100 mg daily). Treatment doses for PMS are the same as for depressive illness, and continuous therapy was found to more effective than medication only during the luteal phase. In studies of depression, hypericin 300 mg three times a day (the principal active component of St. John's wort) was found to be as effective as TCAs, with fewer side effects and at lower cost. At this time there are no published data on efficacy of treatment longer than 6 months, and information about potential adverse interactions of hypericin with other medication is lacking. L-Tryptophan (2 g three times daily with meals, from day 14 through day 3 of the cycle) has been a useful adjunct to antidepressant therapy.

6. **Pain syndromes.** Isolated headaches and general muscular pains are best treated with simple analgesics, such as acetaminophen and aspirin. Migraine headaches occurring as part of PMS may be alleviated by daily treatment beginning approximately 10 days prior to menstruation. Fenoprofen (400 mg four times daily), naproxen sodium (550 mg twice a day), propranolol (40–160 mg twice a day), or ergotamine suppository (1–2 mg at bedtime) are recommended as possible preventive measures. If a migraine attack occurs, conventional treatment should be used (see Chapter 35).

C. **Treatments based on presumed hormonal cause**

1. **Progesterone.** Although progesterone therapy has been widely used, well-controlled clinical trials have failed to prove consistent benefits, possibly because of the dosing and measurement barriers noted above.

2. **Contraceptives.** Reports conflict, but generally an oral contraceptive low in estrogenic activity or a progestin-only pill is recommended. Relief may be found with long-acting progestin contraceptives, but studies are few.

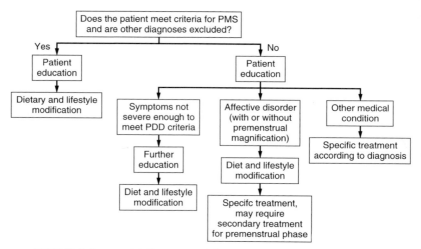

FIGURE 88–2. An approach to the management of premenstrual syndrome (PMS). PDD, Premenstrual dysphoric disorder.

3. **Gonadotropin-releasing hormone analogs.** Leuprolide has been shown to be effective in reducing symptoms of PMS, but side effects are symptoms of menopause, which may be equal to or more troubling than PMS.

VI. **Management strategies.** An approach to PMS management is diagrammed in Figure 88–2.

VII. **Natural history and prognosis.** PMS ceases in the majority of patients at the time of menopause. Many therapies have been found to provide significant relief to a proportion of patients; therefore, the prognosis for improvement of symptoms in PMS is excellent. The medical team must be empathetic, creative, patient, and persistently willing to try different or multiple therapies.

REFERENCES

American Psychiatric Association (APA): *Diagnostic and Statistical Manual of Mental Disorders,* 4th ed. APA; 1994.

Budeiri DJ, Li Wan Po A, Dornan JC: Clinical trials of treatments of premenstrual syndrome: Entry criteria and scales for measuring treatment outcomes. Br J Obstet Gynecol 1994;**101**:689.

Budeiri DJ, Li Wan Po A, Dornan JC: Is evening primrose oil of value in the treatment of premenstrual syndrome? Control Clin Trials 1996;**17**:60.

Daugherty JE: Treatment strategies for premenstrual syndrome. Am Fam Physician 1998;**58**:183.

Johnson WG, Carr-Nangle RE, Bergeron KC: Macronutrient intake, eating habits, and exercise as moderators of menstrual distress in healthy women. Psychosom Med 1995;**57**:324.

Wallin MS, Rissanen AM: Food and mood: Relationship between food, serotonin, and affective disorders. Acta Psychiatr Scand Suppl 1994;**377**:36.

---

89   Seizure Disorders

William L. Toffler, MD, & Scott A. Fields, MD

I. **Definition.** A seizure is a sudden change in consciousness, manifested through motor, sensory, or behavioral changes, brought about by an alteration in cortical electrical activity. Seizures can be further divided into four categories.

A. **Generalized seizures** cause loss of consciousness. This category includes absence (loss of consciousness or posture), myoclonic (repetitive muscle contractions), and tonic-clonic (a sustained contraction followed by rhythmic contractions of all four extremities).

B. Partial (focal) seizures may occur with or without loss of consciousness.

C. Febrile seizures are one or more generalized seizures occurring between 3 months and 5 years of age associated with fever without evidence of any other defined cause.

D. Status epilepticus is a neurologic emergency involving repetitive generalized seizures without return to consciousness between seizures.

II. Epidemiology

A. Four million people in the United States have had at least one seizure, 2 million people have had two or more seizures, and more than 200,000 people have more than one seizure per month despite receiving anticonvulsant therapy. The prevalence of seizures in close relatives of seizure patients is three times that of the overall population. There is no significant difference in prevalence between genders.

B. About 1 in 15 children will have a seizure during their first 7 years of life. The prevalence of seizures in children delivered breech is 3.8% as compared with a prevalence of 2.2% in children delivered vertex.

C. Febrile seizures occur in 3–4% of all children. Fifty percent of febrile seizures occur during the second year of life and almost 90% before the third birthday. Most children with febrile seizures (64%) will have only one episode, but the earlier the age of onset, the more likely the child is to have more febrile seizures. No evidence exists that recurrent febrile seizures increase the risk of epilepsy.

D. The annual incidence of recurrent seizures is 54 in 100,000, excluding febrile convulsions, and 120 in 100,000, if all types of seizures are included. The prevalence of chronic, recurrent epilepsy is 10 in 100,000. The risk of recurrence after a single unprovoked seizure is about 35%.

E. More than 10,000 episodes of status epilepticus occur in the United States each year.

III. Pathophysiology.
A seizure occurs when an inordinate number of neurons depolarize synchronously, resulting in an increase in excitation with a decrease in inhibition. This event may occur in a focal area of the involved cerebral cortex, resulting in a focal seizure, or it may be secondary to an abnormality in a deeper structure such as the thalamus, which leads to a generalized seizure.

A. The possible causes of a seizure can be grouped into the following categories.
1. **Focal brain disease,** including cerebrovascular events (eg, stroke), head trauma, and neoplasm
2. **Infection,** such as meningitis, encephalitis, and abscess
3. **Drug-related causes,** such as cocaine, amphetamines, and alcohol withdrawal
4. **Metabolic derangements,** including uremia, hyponatremia, hypoglycemia, and deficiency states such as phenylketonuria
5. **Subacute conditions,** such as Creutzfeldt–Jakob disease and subacute sclerosing panencephalitis
6. **Toxins,** such as lead poisoning (especially in children) and mercury poisoning in adults
7. **Conditions causing syncope,** including vasovagal episodes, postural hypotension, and arrhythmias
8. **Asphyxia** from hypoxia, carbon monoxide poisoning, or birth injury
9. **Idiopathic seizures,** in which no clear etiology is found

B. Abnormalities leading to seizures may be at the cellular level, such as with tumors, or at the subcellular level, such as with drug or alcohol withdrawal or febrile seizures. The exact mechanism by which a focal lesion creates seizure activity is not known.

C. The age of the patient may help to identify the most likely cause of a seizure (Table 89–1).

IV. Diagnosis

A. Symptoms and signs
1. **Fever** may indicate an infectious cause such as meningitis or encephalitis, or it may directly trigger a febrile seizure.
2. **Focal neurologic findings** may indicate a possible tumor or a localized injury to the brain.

TABLE 89–1. POSSIBLE CAUSES OF RECURRENT SEIZURES BASED ON AGE

Age at Onset (Yrs)	Most Likely Causes
Infancy (0–2)	Perinatal hypoxia Birth injury Congenital abnormality Metabolic 　Hypoglycemia 　Hypocalcemia 　Hypomagnesemia 　Vitamin B_{12} deficiency 　Phenylketonuria Acute infection
Childhood (2–10)	Febrile seizure Idiopathic Acute infection Trauma
Adolescent (10–18)	Idiopathic Trauma Drug and alcohol withdrawal AV malformations
Early adulthood (18–25)	Idiopathic Drug and alcohol withdrawal Tumor
Middle age (25–60)	Drug and alcohol withdrawal Trauma Tumor Vascular disease
Late adulthood (over 60)	Vascular disease Tumor Degenerative disease Metabolic 　Hypoglycemia 　Uremia 　Hepatic failure 　Electrolyte abnormality Drug and alcohol withdrawal

AV, Atrioventricular.

3. **Papilledema** indicates increased intracranial pressure that may be caused by an intracranial hemorrhage or tumor.
4. **Hemorrhagic eye grounds** suggest underlying high blood pressure and may be a cause of seizure associated with hypertensive intercranial bleeding.
5. **Stiff neck (meningismus)** may be present with inflamed meninges (meningitis).
6. **Headache** is a nonspecific complaint compatible with infection or hemorrhage.
B. **Laboratory tests**
　1. The following laboratory tests should be ordered for all patients with a new seizure and for those with recurrent seizures if indicated by the history and physical examination.
　　a. **Serum tests** (glucose, sodium, potassium, calcium, phosphorus, magnesium, blood urea nitrogen, and ammonia levels) should be ordered in any clinical situations associated with dehydration, nausea, vomiting, alteration in consciousness, or drug ingestion.
　　b. **Anticonvulsant levels.** The most common cause of recurrent seizures in children as well as many adults is subtherapeutic anticonvulsant drug levels. Drug levels should be obtained in all individuals already taking anticonvulsant medication who present with recurrence of their underlying seizure disorder.

    c. Drug and toxic screens, including a screen for alcohol, should be ordered, especially if an adequate history cannot be obtained.

    d. A complete blood count assists in the evaluation of a possible underlying infection.

    e. Brain imaging is useful unless the physician can confidently attribute the seizure to a metabolic cause.

        (1) Computed tomography (CT). A head CT scan is indicated in the routine tonic-clonic seizure work-up.

        (2) Magnetic resonance imaging (MRI). A MRI of the head is superior in evaluation of temporal lobe lesions.

  2. The following tests should be ordered only if the results might alter management.

    a. Electroencephalogram (EEG). Unfortunately, any EEG, normal or abnormal, is compatible with the diagnosis of epilepsy. Thus, the diagnosis of epilepsy is not made on the basis of EEG, unless the EEG captures a clinical seizure. The sensitivity, specificity, and predictive value of this test depends on the underlying cause and anatomic location of a seizure focus. An EEG should not be ordered or repeated unless the results will alter management. Specific patterns are described below:

        (1) Delta waves (less than three waveforms per second) are an indication of a disturbance of cerebral function.

        (2) Generalized slowing is related to an acute disturbance such as encephalitis, encephalopathy, anoxia, or a metabolic disturbance. Generalized slowing may occur with hyperventilation, sleep, and drowsiness. Generalized slowing is age-dependent; it is more common in young patients.

        (3) Focal slowing implies acute local disturbance, such as contusion, stroke, local infection, or tumor. Focal slowing may occur as a postictal phenomenon that may last hours or days after a focal seizure. Slowing also varies with age and state of arousal.

        (4) Spikes generally represent an old disturbance seen after brain damage, but they may take years to develop. Spikes are less of an indication for further evaluation than focal slowing. A spike wave, defined as three spikes per second, is noted in absence seizures.

    b. 24-Hour ambulatory EEG may be very helpful in identifying "events" and is useful in separating true seizures from pseudoseizures or other paroxysmal behavior, especially when the two coexist. The cost of this test with interpretation is often near $1000.

    c. Video monitoring may be coupled with a continuous EEG. It may be useful in localizing seizures such as a frontal seizure or a temporal seizure, when the physician is considering surgical correction. This method may also be useful in evaluating suspected pseudoseizures and other paroxysmal behaviors. The evaluation is generally performed with the patient as an inpatient. Video monitoring can cost up to $1700.

    d. Skull x-rays are not usually helpful except in the evaluation of severe head trauma.

    e. Lumbar puncture is not routinely indicated in a child older than 12 months with a first febrile seizure. In infants younger than 12 months, it should be strongly considered because clinical seizures and symptoms of meningitis may be subtle.

V. Treatment

  A. Acute treatment

    1. The patient's airway must be protected.

    2. No medication is usually necessary.

    3. If seizure activity persists longer than 5 minutes, intravenous medication may be given (Table 89–2).

  B. Drug therapy

    1. Only one drug should be prescribed. Drugs can be chosen from Table 89–3, where they are listed in order of effectiveness. A specific side effect (such as decreased cognitive function) might lead the physician to select a certain drug (such as phenobarbital over phenytoin) in certain circumstances.

    2. Dosage should be increased as tolerated to achieve a therapeutic blood level. Clinical response is more reliable than blood levels, however.

TABLE 89–2. DRUGS USED IN THE TREATMENT OF SEIZURE DISORDERS

Drug of Choice for Particular Type of Seizure	Adult Dose (mg/day)	Pediatric Dose (mg/kg/day)	Adult Starting Dose	Side Effects	Therapeutic range (µg/mL)
Generalized—tonic-clonic					
Phenytoin (Dilantin)	300–400	4–7	100 mg bid–tid	Decrease in cognitive function, sedation, ataxia, diplopia, gingival hyperplasia	10–20
Phenobarbital	120–250	4–6	30–60 mg bid	Respiratory depression, hyperactivity, sedation	15–40
Carbamazepine (Tegretol)	600–1200	20–30	200 mg bid–qid	Sedation, diplopia, ataxia, aplastic anemia, hypo-osmolality	6–12
Valproic acid (Depakene)	1000–3000	10–60	250 mg tid	Sedation, nausea, vomiting, weight gain, hair loss, GI hematologic toxicity	50–100
Primidone (Mysoline)	750–1500	10–25	250 mg tid–qid	Sedation, vertigo, nausea, ataxia, change in behavior	6–12
Generalized—absence					
Ethosuximide (Zarontin)	250–1000	20–40	250 mg bid	Nausea, vomiting, lethargy, hiccups, headache blood dyscrasias	40–100
Valproic acid (Depakene)	1000–3000	10–60	250 mg tid	Sedation, nausea, vomiting, weight gain, hair loss, GI hematologic toxicity	50–100
Clonazepam	1.5–20	0.01–0.3	0.5 mg tid	Drowsiness, ataxia, change in behavior	0.013–0.072
Generalized—myoclonic					
Valproic acid (Depakene)	1000–3000	10–60	250 mg tid	Sedation, nausea, vomiting, weight gain, hair loss, GI hematologic toxicity	50–100
Clonazepam	1.5–20	0.01–0.3	0.5 mg tid	Drowsiness, ataxia, change in behavior	0.013–0.072
Phenytoin (Dilantin)	300–400	4–7	100 mg bid–tid	Decrease in cognitive function, sedation, ataxia, diplopia, gingival hyperplasia	10–20
Partial					
Carbamazepine (Tegretol)	600–1200	20–30	200 mg bid–qid	Sedation, diplopia, ataxia, aplastic anemia, hypo-osmolality	6–12
Phenobarbital	120–250	4–6	30–60 mg bid	Respiratory depression, hyperactivity, sedation	15–40
Valproic acid (Depakene)	1000–3000	10–60	250 mg tid	Sedation, nausea, vomiting, weight gain, hair loss, GI hematologic toxicity	50–100
Primidone (Mysoline)	750–1500	10–25	250 mg tid–qid	Sedation, vertigo, nausea, ataxia, change in behavior	6–12
Status epilepticus					
Lorazepam (Ativan)	0.05 mg/kg IV	0.05 mg/kg IV	2–4 mg q20–30 min	Respiratory depression, sedation	
Diazepam (Valium)	0.25–0.5 mg/kg IV	0.25–0.5 mg/kg IV	5–10 mg q20–30 min	Respiratory depression, sedation	—
Phenytoin (Dilantin)	15–20 mg/kg IV drip at 30–50 mg/min	15–20 mg/kg IV drip at 0.5–1.6 mg/min	—	Decrease in cognitive function, sedation, ataxia, diplopia, gingival hyperplasia	10–20
Phenobarbital	300–800 mg IV drip at 25–50 mg/min	20 mg/kg IV drip at 25–50 mg/min	—	Respiratory depression, sedation	15–40

GI, Gastrointestinal.

TABLE 89-3. STATUS EPILEPTICUS TREATMENT

1. Ensure airway—assist ventilation if necessary
2. IV with normal saline
3. Dextrostix, or give 50 mL of 50% dextrose solution
4. Diazepam IV, 0.25–0.4 mg/kg (up to 10 mg) at a maximum rate of 1 mg/min; may need to repeat in 20–30 min
5. If seizures continue, phenobarbital IV, 10–15 mg/kg; 20% of total dose every 5–10 min at a rate of less than 50 mg/min; preferred over phenytoin especially in very young children
6. Phenytoin, loading dose of 15 mg/kg, undiluted, at a rate of 0.5–1.5 mg/kg/min; an additional 5 mg/kg can be given after 12 hr
7. General anesthesia can be considered and given

   3. Another drug can be substituted if therapy is ineffective. Only after failure of each single agent should combination therapy be considered.
   4. Several newer agents—felbamate (Felbatol), gabapentin (Neurontin), and lamotrigine (Lamictal)—have been approved primarily for partial seizures. Gabapentin has a relatively short half-life, necessitating multiple doses. Dosage adjustments are necessary with lamotrigine and felbamate when used with other anticonvulsants. Felbamate has been associated with aplastic anemia. Patients taking this medication should probably have it discontinued unless benefits clearly outweigh this potential complication.

C. **Treatment during pregnancy**
   1. Drug metabolism may be drastically altered during pregnancy.
   2. There is about a twofold risk of congenital malformation (predominantly facial cleft and neural tube defects) in mothers who take anticonvulsants to control seizures. Malformations are most strongly associated with trimethadione and valproic acid.

D. **Converting from polytherapy to monotherapy**
   1. The single agent most likely to be successful should be chosen. The dosage of the agent should be slowly increased while the undesirable drug is slowly withdrawn. Long-acting drugs should be discontinued slowly over 1–3 months by halving the dose once per week.
   2. The plan, including the alternatives and the risks, should be fully discussed with the patient. It should be modified if control of seizures is diminished.

E. **Febrile seizures**
   1. In general, anticonvulsants are not indicated for a patient with febrile seizures. Anticonvulsant prophylaxis for febrile seizure should be considered, however, if the neurologic examination is abnormal, if the seizure activity lasts for more than 15 minutes, if a transient or permanent neurologic defect is present, or if there is a family history of nonfebrile seizures.
   2. Phenobarbital or other anticonvulsant therapy is effective in preventing recurrence of febrile seizures. Treatment does not affect the percentage of individuals who will develop epilepsy in the future, however.

VI. **Natural history and prognosis.** Follow-up and prognosis are dependent on the type of seizure the patient has experienced.
   A. Seizures beginning early in life may be caused by developmental defects, perfusion defects of the brain, intrauterine hypoxemia, or fetal infection. Assisting the patient with developmental problems such as learning deficits is as important as controlling the seizures.
   B. In 80% of childhood seizures, no clear cause is found despite an exhaustive workup. If the seizures are controlled, normally no impairment in development occurs. If seizures are poorly controlled, difficulties with scholastic, emotional, and social development may arise.
   C. New onset of seizures in adolescence generally has no adverse effect on the patient's development as long as the seizures are controlled. Compliance with treatment is a significant problem in this age group.
   D. New onset of seizures in adults may indicate serious disease, including alcoholism or drug abuse. Patients in early adulthood or middle age must be screened carefully regarding the use of alcohol and "recreational" drugs, as well as the appropriate use of prescription drugs. Identification and intervention may prevent an extensive work-up.

E. Onset of seizures late in life indicates possible cerebral vascular disease or tumor. If the cause of the seizures is not investigated, a potentially correctable problem may be missed and control of the seizures may be difficult to achieve.

F. With time, seizure activity may become quiescent. Withdrawal of therapy should be considered after the patient has been seizure-free for 2 years. The relapse rate of patients who have been medication-free for 3 years is about 33%. Relapse is related to seizure type. Patients with complex partial seizures with generalization have the worst prognosis, and those with partial seizures without generalization have the best prognosis.

REFERENCES

American Academy of Pediatrics Provisional Committee on Quality Improvement, Subcommittee on Febrile Seizures: Practice parameter: The neurodiagnostic evaluation of the child with a first simple febrile seizure. Pediatrics 1996;**97**(5):769.

Cascino GD: Epilepsy: Contemporary perspectives on evaluation and treatment. Mayo Clin Proc 1994;**69**:1199.

Hauser WA, Rich SS, Lee JRJ, et al: Risk of recurrent seizures after two unprovoked seizures. N Engl J Med 1998;**338**(7):429.

Marson AG, Kadir ZA, Hutton JL, et al: The new antiepileptic drugs: A systematic review of their efficacy and tolerability. Epilepsia 1997;**38**(8):859.

Parles BR, Dostiow UG, Noble SL: Drug therapy for epilepsy. Am Fam Physician 1994;**50**:639.

Sadot B: Epilepsy: A progressive disease? Still no answer to the controversy over whether seizures beget more seizures. BMJ 1997;**314**(7078):391.

Schoenenburger RA, Heim SM: Indication for computed tomography of the brain in patients with first uncomplicated seizure. BMJ 1994;**309**:986.

---

90   Stroke

Ellen R. Evans, MD

I. Definition. Stroke is a clinical syndrome consisting of the sudden or rapid onset of a constellation of neurologic deficits that persist for more than 24 hours secondary to a vascular event. "Brain attack" is a term used to alert health care providers, patients, and their families and friends of the emergency condition that threatens the life and function of irreplaceable brain tissue.

II. Epidemiology. The most frequent disabling (and lethal) neurologic disease of adults, stroke accounts for half of all hospitalizations for acute neurologic disorders. Six hundred thousand Americans have new or recurrent stroke each year. Although the incidence and mortality of stroke in the United States have been declining since the 1940s, still nearly one-third of stroke victims die each year, keeping stroke the third leading cause of death in this country. With about one-third of the approximately 4 million Americans who have survived a stroke requiring help to care for themselves, stroke is the leading cause of chronic disability or long-term institutionalization in this country.

Childhood stroke is complicated by delayed diagnosis, in part because this type of stroke is rare (an annual incidence rate of about 2.5/100,000/year in one large study).

A. Well-documented risk factors for adult stroke are classified as treatable and untreatable by the American Heart Association (AHA). AHA untreatable (in relation to stroke) risk factors are age (risk doubles each decade beyond 55 years of age), family history of stroke, male gender, race (African American), diabetes mellitus (an independent risk factor that may be related to an abnormality of fibrinolysis), and prior stroke. The approximate risk of recurrent stroke within the first year after an ischemic stroke is 12% and within 5 years is 50%. AHA treatable risk factors are hypertension, cardiac disease, cigarette smoking ("dose-related"), transient ischemic attack (TIA has a 10-fold increase in stroke risk), and polycythemia. Heavy alcohol use predisposes one to stroke. Use of oral contraceptives with cigarette smoking increases stroke risk as well. Nonvalvular atrial fibrillation, which leads to almost 50% of cardiogenic brain embolizations, carries an annual risk of embolus of about 5% if left untreated. While elevated cholesterol is a more significant risk factor for coronary artery disease than for occlusive cerebrovascular disease, high plasma homocysteine and Lp(a) lipoprotein levels may be equally important to both. Atherosclerotic vascular occlusive disease in other areas of the body (ie, coronary artery disease and peripheral arterial disease) may herald coexistent cerebrovascular disease. Childhood stroke is believed to have similar risk factors, but its diverse and numerous causes coupled with its relative rarity preclude precise risk factor analysis. Leukemia and sickle cell disease are noted risks.

B. The **differential diagnosis for stroke** includes mass lesions (eg, subdural hematoma or neoplasm), metabolic abnormalities (eg, hypoglycemia, hyponatremia, or hypernatremia), infectious processes (eg, meningitis or cerebral abscess), inflammatory processes (eg, temporal arteritis), and idiopathic processes (eg, epilepsy). Clinical history and physical examination identify nonischemic events, suggested by slow onset of gradually progressive symptoms affecting multiple vascular territories. Symptoms of coronary ischemia, cardiac arrhythmias, congestive heart failure, and valvular disease implicate cardiac causes.

C. Types of stroke. In adults, 80% of strokes are **ischemic: atheroembolic/ atherothrombotic stroke** (60–70% of strokes), **cerebral embolic,** and **lacunar (small vessel occlusive).** The rest of adult strokes are **hemorrhagic strokes.** Childhood strokes are more often hemorrhagic than ischemic.

D. Prognosis. Third nerve palsy (signaling uncal herniation), increased age of the patient, and hemorrhagic events are associated with grave immediate prognoses. In hemorrhagic events, the prognosis for total unilateral motor deficit and coma is poor. Brain stem infarctions such as pontine hemorrhages have an extremely poor prognosis. Lacunar infarctions involve subcortical small vessels and have the lowest mortality rate of all strokes.

III. Pathophysiology

A. Atherothrombotic/atheroembolic stroke results from progressive arterial stenosis with eventual occlusion resulting from platelet-mediated thrombus formation involving adhesion, activation, and aggregation. First, an atherosclerotic plaque becomes unstable. Its rupture exposes adhesive proteins to which circulating platelets adhere. Through a cascade of steps the adherent platelets are activated: Different agonists (eg, collagen, thrombin, serotonin, epinephrine) bind to specific platelet receptors and work in concert to trigger the release of aggregating agents such as adenosine diphosphate and thromboxane A_2. These agents bind to specific receptor sites on the platelets and activate the GpIIb/IIIa receptor complex, which undergoes a conformational change allowing fibrinogen to bind. Fibrinogen, then, links platelets together, forming platelet aggregates. This growing thrombus is stabilized by activation of the coagulation cascade (secondary hemostasis) and thereby expands and eventually occludes the affected vessel. Deficiencies of endogenous fibrinolysis have been shown to be associated with increased risk of cerebrovascular occlusion. This may be the mechanism of diabetic risk as well as the increased risk seen with those having deficiency of free fraction of protein S (in young patients) and decreased tissue plasminogen activator (tPA) antigen.

The resultant thrombus occlusion causes ischemia. Within hours of the onset of ischemia, polymorphonuclear leukocytes (PMNs) accumulate and obstruct the microvasculature by interacting with the microvascular endothelium (via rolling, adhesion, and transmigration into the parenchyma). This process is influenced by inflammatory mediators such as cytokines. Monocyte and macrophage cells follow the PMNs. Under conditions of ischemia and reperfusion, PMNs and the endothelium are activated. The free radicals and proteases, which are thereby generated, contribute to microvascular and parenchymal tissue injury. Extensive recent and ongoing research reveals amazing insight into the vast complexity of mechanisms through which ischemic brain tissue is injured: for example, complement activation, free radical–mediated injury, and other mechanisms, such as extracellular calcium ion influx. These findings offer many new sites for targeted clinical intervention to achieve cessation or reversal of the ischemic process: for example, antiplatelet therapy, free radical scavenging, or antioxidant therapy. Immune and neuropharmacologic protection (including calcium channel–voltage sensitive antagonists, glutamine release inhibitors, GABA agonists ([γ-aminobutyric acid], adenosine, naloxone, and gangliosides) as well as nitric oxide (NO) inhibition (blockade) and other interventions are under investigation (including even phase III efficacy trials). (Regarding NO inhibition, while the vasodilatory action of NO might increase cerebral blood flow [CBF], the mediation of glutamate action at *N*-methyl-D-aspartate receptors by NO promotes ischemic damage with the formation of highly injurious peroxynitrite radicals.)

B. Embolic stroke occurs from sudden mobilization into the bloodstream of material that lodges in any conceivable trunk or branch of a cerebral vessel: fragments of bland mural thrombus (eg, the heart or the great vessels), thrombus–bacteria complexes, cholesterol fragments, microscopic tumor aggregates, gas bubbles, fat, or foreign bodies. The resulting ischemia is subject to the mechanisms reviewed above (see section III,A.)

C. About 75% of **lacunar infarctions** occur in patients with hypertension. The perforating cerebral arteries are occluded by lipohyalinosis, segmental arterial hypertensive degeneration, or microatheroma (small perforating arteries).

D. Hemorrhagic strokes are classified by location.

    1. Intracerebral hemorrhage (ICH) is usually related to hypertension. Other causes of ICH include arteriovenous malformations, tumors, and blood dyscrasias (eg, anticoagulation). Cerebral amyloid angiopathy is a recognized cause of spontaneous lobar ICH in elderly normotensive patients. Spontaneous midbrain hemorrhage is a rare but unique brain stem vascular lesion, which usually results in alteration of consciousness and headache with associated neuro-ophthalmologic abnormalities and less frequent hemiparesis, hemisensory loss, and ataxia.

    2. Subarachnoid hemorrhage (SAH), unlike other types of stroke, represents a common cause of stroke in young persons and occurs rarely in elderly individuals. The cause is usually a ruptured congenital berry aneurysm located in the circle of Willis, internal carotid, anterior communicating, or middle cerebral arteries. SAH produces direct injury to cerebral tissue and delayed vasospasm contributing to ischemic injury.

IV. Diagnosis. Three obvious clinical presentations of cerebrovascular disease are encountered acutely: completed stroke (static neurologic deficits), stroke in progress (progressively worsening deficits, most common with large vessel thrombosis, but also with lacunes and emboli), and TIA (quickly resolving neurologic deficit that may be the forerunner of subsequent stroke). With the cascade of discoveries about both cellular-level pathophysiology and near-microscopic diagnostic evaluation of acute stroke, the clinical presentation is fast approaching a continuum of diagnostic and therapeutic considerations. Even apparently completed stroke is viewed as being potentially amenable to therapeutic interventions (eg, neurotransmitter therapy to enhance recovery and improve function)!

Early presentation coupled with rapid imaging and prompt treatment are key goals for health care providers and the communities they serve. The placid acceptance of the inevitable course of stroke of the past must become the vigorous battleground of active intervention to affect positively and dramatically the "brain attack" of today. This goal applies regardless of the age of the patient.

A. Symptoms and **signs** of stroke reflect the cerebrovascular territory affected by the stroke process. The vessels most often involved and common clinical presentations are listed in Table 90–1.

B. Laboratory tests (see also Chapter 81)

    1. A **complete blood cell count** identifies anemia or polycythemia. The **coagulation profile** (ie, prothrombin time, activated thromboplastin time, and platelet count) provides baseline information for anticoagulation and thrombolysis. The International Normalized Ratio (INR) provides accurate monitoring of warfarin anticoagulation therapy. Evaluation of additional specific coaguation factors (eg, levels of coagulation factors such as proteins C and S and antithrombin III) identifies prothrombotic states. In young patients with progressive intracranial occlusion, such evaluation for prothrombotic states is warranted. Recent studies have shown tPA antigen levels and homocysteine levels to be elevated in patients at risk for stroke. Other measures of metabolic abnormalities identify potential aggravators of cerebral ischemia: **blood glucose, serum electrolytes, blood urea nitrogen,** and **creatinine.** Because a significant number of patients with carotid artery disease have concomitant asymptomatic coronary artery disease, cholesterol and lipid status is evaluated for treatment in the post-stroke patient.

TABLE 90–1. CLINICAL PRESENTATION OF STROKE

Stroke Type/ Artery or Site Involved	Clinical Presentation	Special Considerations
Atherothrombotic stroke Internal carotid artery (mostly extracranial) Vertebral artery (mostly intracranial) Basilar artery	Stuttering onset, can occur upon waking; cerebellar infarction causes severe edema/brain stem compression	Preceded by TIA in 50% of cases
Embolic stroke Middle cerebral artery Anterior cerebral artery Posterior cerebral artery	Sudden onset of maximal deficit	
Lacunar infarction (penetrating arteries) Middle cerebral perforator– lenticulostriate Posterior cerebral perforator Basilar artery perforating branches	Develops suddenly or over several hours; headache, loss of consciousness, and emesis do not occur	Lacunar syndromes: pure motor hemiparesis, pure sensory loss, crural paresis, and ataxia/dysarthria (clumsy hand syndrome)
Intracerebral hemorrhage Deep cerebral hemisphere (putamen) Subcortical white matter (lobar intracranial hemorrhage) Cerebellar Thalamic Midbrain	Smooth onset, although can be sudden; emesis and loss of consciousness do occur	Selective surgical clot evacuation; unpredictable course in cerebellar ICH; most midbrain ICHs improve with supportive care
Subarachnoid hemorrhage (ruptured aneurysm) Circle of Willis Internal carotid artery Anterior communicating artery Middle cerebral artery	Sudden onset ("brutal" headache, emesis, loss of consciousness then awakening with headache and stiff neck); **note:** aneurysms are rarely symptomatic before rupture	Complications: rerupture, obstruction of spinal fluid flow (communicating hydrocephalus), vasospasm 3–14 days postevent

ICH, Intracerebral hemorrhage; TIA, transient ischemic attack.

2. Initial **brain imaging** detects the presence of hemorrhage and excludes other causes (eg, tumor, abscess, or subdural hematoma). Advances in brain imaging promise early distinction of the core area of ischemic tissue with severely compromised CBF from the "penumbra," that is, the surrounding rim of moderately ischemic brain tissue with impaired electrical activity but preserved cellular metabolism and viability. Coupled with upcoming breakthroughs in therapy, this advanced brain imaging may offer clear diagnostic indications for specific therapeutic interventions directed at relieving the stunned penumbra and salvaging the ischemic core. Accurate prediction of the eventual outcome is another expectation.

   a. **Computed tomography (CT)** gives reliable differentiation of hemorrhagic from ischemic stroke with scanning obtained during the first 72 hours of the stroke. CT will show a subarachnoid hemorrhage with 95% sensitivity if performed within 5 days of the event. Normal CT scans are frequently obtained in lacunar or brain stem infarctions when the lesions are small. Early in the course of an ischemic infarction, plain CT scans are usually negative unless edematous changes are present; however, various quantitative CBF imaging techniques with high sensitivity and good spatial resolution have been demonstrated: xenon-enhanced

CT as well as radiolabeled microsphere, 133Xe and iodoantipyrine CBF techniques. Although the diagnostic yield of plain CT scanning in ischemia is greatest 7 days after the event, most current tPA-administration protocols call for a pretreatment CT scan within 3 hours of the onset of symptoms. Initial noncontrast CT scans are readily available and provide quick and accurate diagnosis of hemorrhagic events for which thrombolysis is contraindicated. Used mostly in research, single photon emission computed tomography (SPECT) defines CBF and function. Spiral computed tomographic angiography is another research tool that defines vascular lesions.

b. **Magnetic resonance imaging (MRI)** is more sensitive than CT in detecting ischemic stroke. New MRI techniques for assessing acute cerebral infarction provide more functional information about the status of the brain on presentation of stroke symptoms: fluid-attenuating inversion recovery imaging, diffusion-weighted imaging (DWI), perfusion-weighted imaging (PWI), functional MRI, and magnetic resonance spectroscopy. These techniques promise ever increasing delineation of infarcted (irreversibly damaged) tissue from "stunned" (at-risk, potentially reversibly ischemic) tissue. Abnormalities often appear within hours of stroke onset.

c. **Positron emission tomography (PET),** which demonstrates regional blood flow and localized cerebral metabolism, has a high yield in lesion localization and has provided wonderful information about the ischemic brain; however, its expense and limited availability coupled with the marked advances in CT and MRI techniques have relegated PET to the research and investigational realm.

3. **Imaging of the extracranial and intracranial vessels** is indicated by the case presentation. The initial evaluation of patients with symptoms of acute cerebrovascular ischemia includes **carotid noninvasive testing** (carotid duplex ultrasonography and color Doppler flow imaging), looking for significant lesions of the carotid arteries. **Transcranial Doppler ultrasonography (TCD)** detects middle cerebral and distal (intracranial) internal carotid artery stenosis with a sensitivity of 92% and a specificity of 100%. However, this technique is insufficient to detect stenosis or occlusion in the posterior circulation, and the middle cerebral artery cannot be seen in up to a fourth of patients. TCD is capable of detecting microembolic material of both gaseous and solid states within intracranial cerebral arteries. **Spiral computed tomographic angiography** provides definition of vascular lesions; however, the preferred technique for screening patients for extracranial carotid and intracranial artery disease (including the posterior circulation) is **magnetic resonance angiography (MRA). Cerebral angiography,** the "gold standard" of vascular imaging, is performed on a case-specific basis, primarily when surgical intervention is considered or when angiographic confirmation of stenosis detected by other techniques is required. **Digital subtraction angiography** is another technique. **Oculoplethysmography** offers an indirect measure of carotid arterial blockage by measuring arterial pulsations in the retinal artery.

4. **Echocardiography** (transthoracic or transesophageal) and **24-hour Holter monitoring** are performed when an embolic process is suspected, when surgical intervention is planned, or when the stroke patient has significant risk factors for emboli (eg, atrial fibrillation, suspected infective endocarditis, prosthetic heart valve, dilated cardiomyopathy, or recent anterior myocardial infarction).

5. A **lumbar puncture** is useful when brain imaging is normal and subarachnoid hemorrhage or meningitis is suspected. While cerebrospinal fluid is usually bloody in ventricular extension of a hypertensive hemorrhage, vascular malformation, and ruptured aneurysm, a clear tap does not guarantee absence of hemorrhage. Leukocytosis in the cerebrospinal fluid suggests infection.

6. **Electroencephalography** may show slow waves in strokes involving the cortex and is performed when seizure activity has occurred or is suspected.

V. **Treatment.** Brain attack is a medical emergency. The first step is patient education directed at encouraging patients to seek medical care as soon as symptoms develop. Initiation of diagnosis and treatment within the first few hours of onset enhances the very real chances to minimize irreversible ischemic damage and thus improve outcomes. Care in specialized stroke units has been shown to improve outcomes. Attention to rehabilitation goals begins as soon as possible after the acute event. Childhood stroke is believed to be amenable to treatment modalities similar to those discussed below based on research and experience in adults. (Pediatric neurologic or neurosurgical consultation would be expected.)

A. **Stabilization of the patient** involves blood pressure (BP) control, arrhythmia detection and treatment, airway protection, and, if needed, ventilatory assistance and supplementary oxygenation. Proper positioning to avoid pressure sores, diligent correction of metabolic disturbances, and skilled monitoring of stroke progression via repeated neurologic examinations are important. Continuous cardiac monitoring during the first 24 hours is advised because of the high risk of cardiac arrhythmias.

The prevention of neurologic and cardiovascular compromise caused by the extremes of BP poses a unique clinical challenge in the stroke patient. Poststroke BP elevation usually declines spontaneously by about 10% in the first 24 hours. In fact, elevated BP can be a physiologic response to acute brain ischemia. Normalization of BP often occurs when specific effects of stroke are controlled: pain, nausea, agitation, bladder distention, increased intracranial pressure, stress of stroke, and underlying hypertension. Data supporting specific BP guidelines for treatment of poststroke hypertension are lacking, however. Furthermore, exaggerated responses to antihypertensive drugs can cause sudden drops in BP that compromise cerebral perfusion and thus worsen neurologic status. Thus, the National Stroke Association recommends pharmacologic therapy for hypertension associated with **ischemic stroke** only for specific indications (eg, myocardial infarction or arterial dissection) or for systolic BP >219 mm Hg or diastolic BP >119 mm Hg on repeated measurements over a 30- to 60-minute period. Oral therapy is preferred. In patients with extremely elevated BP (>130 mm Hg *mean* or >200 mm Hg systolic), cautious administration of parenteral agents is recommended by the American Heart Association's Stroke Council. The approach to blood pressure control must take into account whether the pre-event blood pressure was known to be normotensive or not. Additionally, patients with **hemorrhagic stroke,** after **thrombolysis** and in the **postoperative period** (eg, carotid endarterectomy or hematoma removal) require more aggressive treatment of hypertension.

B. **Limitation of ischemia**
  1. **Reperfusion** therapy aimed at recanalization of the affected vessel(s) in the acute stroke is a very recent advancement. Pharmacologic, angioplastic, and surgical recanalization are the current options.
     a. **Pharmacologic agents** are infused during the initial 3 hours after onset of stroke symptoms. Streptokinase has serious adverse side effects with questionable efficacy in stroke. It has not been studied in the 3-hour window. Urokinase is primarily used in angioplasty. Recombinant tissue-type plasminogen activator (tPA) is approved by the Food and Drug Administration (FDA) for treatment of CT-proved nonhemorrhagic stroke within the first 3 hours of onset of symptoms. More recent studies and experience have extended the window of infusion to 6 or 7 hours with variable results. Still, much of the debate returns to the axiom that "brain attack" is an emergency that is best treated within minutes to a couple of hours after onset of symptoms. Furthermore, studies show the sooner the intervention, the greater the chance of a good outcome. While the guidelines for choice of optimal agent, dose, rate, and delivery mechanism are evolving, the advantages of reperfusion in selected patients are a well proved reality. Intra-arterial administration of tPA is recommended for patients with occlusions of the internal carotid, main stem middle cerebral, and basilar arteries. Intravenous tPA is best for patients with intracranial circumferential branch artery occlusions. The greatest risk of thrombolysis in acute stroke is ICH. Intensive care unit monitoring after thrombolysis includes attention to signs of ICH: decreased consciousness, headache, nausea, vomiting, and increased neurologic focal deficits. The risk of ICH is decreased by close blood pressure control (treat for systolic >185 and diastolic >110). Neither aspirin nor anticoagulation is given for the initial 24 hours after thrombolysis, and neither is initiated after that

until a repeat CT scan shows no hemorrhage. Expect specific selection criteria and protocols for thrombolysis to evolve as the data are collected and the evidence is studied.

b. Angioplasty of extracranial and intracranial vessels is an emerging treatment modality. Increasing numbers of reports of successful angioplastic intervention in acute stroke are published. The advances in imaging and increased experience with angioplasty in acute stroke are expected to allow selection of appropriate angioplasty candidates based on evaluation of tissue reversibility and related risk factors. Randomized and controlled trials are desirable.

c. Carotid endarterectomy (CEA) for ipsilateral severe (70–99%) carotid artery stenosis in symptomatic patients with recent nondisabling carotid artery ischemic events (TIA or stroke) is clearly beneficial. Based on preliminary data, it appears that delay of CEA in such patients beyond 3 days after an event merely increases their risk of recurrent stroke. CEA, which is one of the most common surgical procedures performed, is not beneficial for symptomatic patients with less than 30% stenosis. The potential benefit of CEA for symptomatic patients with carotid artery stenosis of 30–69% is under investigation: NASCET (North American Symptomatic Carotid Endarterectomy Trial).

Recommendation for prophylactic CEA in **asymptomatic** patients based on the AHA Guidelines for CEA is related to surgical risk. The surgeon's specific morbidity and mortality statistics are a significant factor in estimating this risk. Patient selection and postoperative management of modifiable risk factors apply as well. For asymptomatic patients with a life expectancy of at least 5 years and a surgical risk less than 3% ipsilateral, CEA is considered a proven benefit when stenosis is greater than 59%, regardless of plaque characteristics (eg, ulceration), contralateral carotid status, or antiplatelet therapy. Unilateral CEA is acceptable at the time of indicated coronary artery bypass grafting in asymptomatic patients whose ipsilateral carotid artery stenosis is greater than 59%. Those whose surgical risk is greater than 3% have no proven indication.

Aspirin therapy (30–1300 mg daily) beginning before CEA is recommended for all patients unless contraindicated (eg, allergy). The perioperative risks of CEA include stroke, myocardial infarction, and death. Postoperative complications include cranial nerve palsy, wound hematoma, seizure, recurrent stenosis, hypertension (highly correlated with the presence of preoperative hypertension, although nearly a fourth of normotensive patients develop this), hypotension, intracerebral hemorrhage, and hyperperfusion syndrome. Cerebral hyperperfusion syndrome is characterized by unilateral headache, seizures, and occasional altered mental status or focal neurologic deficits. Poor control of BP after CEA is the greatest risk factor. TCD, which shows increased MCA blood velocity, may play a role in monitoring this condition.

2. The use of **heparin** in the acute phases of TIA and nonhemorrhagic stroke is based mainly on the historic stroke observation that evolving stroke has a poor outcome. Preliminary studies from the International Stroke Trial indicate that excess major bleeding complications may negate any benefits. The use of heparin remains a matter of preference of the treating physician. Even for patients with recent cardioembolic stroke, the data regarding the safety and efficacy of heparin are inconclusive. Within the first few hours after TIA, selected patient scenarios are considered to have a high risk for recurrence: high stenosis in the affected vascular territory, current antiplatelet therapy (ie, failed antiplatelet therapy), cardioembolic cause, or crescendo TIA (ie, attacks occurring with increasing frequency). Small, stable brain ischemia with arterial or cardiac cause and a high risk of worsening because of recurrent embolization or thrombus extension is treated with anticoagulation. Although no firm data exist to support its predictable efficacy, common practice in any of these situations is to initiate anticoagulation therapy with heparin followed by warfarin (see Chapter 23). The risk of central nervous system hemorrhage is 1–4% in anticoagulated patients having TIA or acute or progressive stroke. Obvious contraindications are increased risk of worsening because of intra-

parenchymal bleeding, active bleeding elsewhere, and uncontrolled hypertension. Strokes with increased bleeding risk are large; they may be embolic and may reveal the hypodensity of hemorrhagic transformation on early CT. **Note that the heparin bolus is NOT given in patients with acute cardioembolic stroke because of the increased risk of hemorrhagic transformation. Furthermore, after initiation of heparin therapy for stroke/TIA, avoid additional boluses of heparin; instead, adjust the rate of infusion according to the goal of partial thromboplastin time of 50–60.**

Low-molecular weight heparin used within 48 hours of onset of stroke has been shown to decrease death and dependency during the first 6 months.

3. **Cerebral edema** is a leading cause of death in the first week of stroke. Treat or avoid conditions that tend to increase intracranial pressure (ICP): fever, pain, hypoxia, agitation, fluid overload, hypercarbia, and drugs that dilate intracranial vessels. Corticosteroids are ineffective in managing brain edema secondary to stroke. The two medical modalities used to treat cerebral edema are **osmotherapy** (eg, mannitol and glycerol) and **hyperventilation therapy** in patients with markedly increased ICP. Surgical intervention (eg, decompression hemicraniectomy) is sometimes necessary to control increasing ICP.

4. **Nimodipine** is a dihydropyridine calcium channel blocker that affects mainly the central nervous system vasculature. Approved for treating cerebral ischemia associated with subarachnoid hemorrhage, nimodipine is recommended at a dosage of 60 mg orally every 4 hours for 21 days (the period of time during which neurologic deficit from vasospasm is most likely).

5. **Therapies under investigation** are numerous. (See section III regarding pathophysiology and proposed mechanisms.)
   a. Other **calcium channel blockers** and ***N*-methyl-D**-aspartate receptor blockers may succeed in limiting cerebral ischemia.
   b. **Agents to improve anticoagulant therapy**, such as other low-molecular weight heparinoids and ancrod, a thrombin-like enzyme derived from pit viper venom, are being evaluated.
   c. **"Super-aspirins"** are platelet IIb–IIIa receptor blockers that keep platelets from clumping and forming blood clots that can trigger myocardial infarction and stroke. Intravenous infusion (generic: Eptifibatide, tirofiban, and abciximab) has been studied.
   d. **Gangliosides** are glycosphingolipids found in highest concentration in the mammalian brain. **Ganglioside GM$_1$** is the simplest of four major brain gangliosides shown to have neurotogenic and neuronotrophic activity and to facilitate repair of neuronal tissue. Initial research has shown beneficial effects of ganglioside GM$_1$ in the treatment of stroke and spinal cord injuries, particularly within the first few hours of the acute event.
   e. **Hyperbaric oxygen therapy** has been used in hypertensive intracerebral hemorrhage.
   f. Although some approaches are still experimental, tremendous advances have been achieved in the treatment of the patient with intracranial aneurysm. The evolution of **minimally invasive surgical techniques,** using such innovative occlusion devices as detachable latex and silicon balloons, liquid polymers, and intravascular lasers and stents, may increase treatment options. Silicon microballoon angioplasty has been used in treating vasospasm following subarachnoid hemorrhage.

C. **Prevention of stroke recurrence** is key to continued reduction of morbidity and mortality of stroke.
   1. **Risk factor modification.** BP control (mean arterial BP goal of <100 mm Hg), smoking cessation, and cardiac disease treatment are essential. Most stroke and TIA patients succumb to cardiac disease.
   2. The role of **CEA** has been discussed (see section V,B,1).
   3. **Long-term anticoagulation therapy** with **coumadin** (warfarin sodium) is recommended on a case-specific basis. Warfarin therapy has been shown to decrease the risk of stroke in those with atrial fibrillation associated with rheumatic valvular disease, prosthetic valve disease, and, more recently, nonvalvular atrial fibrillation. High-risk subgroups of patients with atrial fibrillation include those with hypertension, previous embolic events, structural heart disease, and older age. Younger patients with lone atrial fibrillation

have low embolic rates not warranting anticoagulation, although aspirin therapy is recommended.

Anticoagulation also results in stroke reduction in those who have had a myocardial infarction. A smaller risk reduction is seen in those who are not candidates for long-term anticoagulation therapy and who take aspirin instead. Aspirin plus low-dose warfarin therapy and very low-intensity anticoagulation are under investigation. The American College of Chest Physicians has recommended long-term warfarin therapy with an INR of 2.0–3.0 for selected patients (ie, those with atrial fibrillation with associated cardiovascular disease, thyrotoxicosis, or age over 59 years).

Survivors of stroke who have a definite cardiac–embolic cause and those TIA patients who have surgically inaccessible lesions and remain symptomatic when taking aspirin are considered candidates as well. Anticoagulation therapy is contraindicated when cerebral embolism is associated with subacute bacterial endocarditis, in which rapid treatment of the infection is indicated instead. Therapy should generally continue at least 6–12 months or even for the patient's lifetime.

4. **Antiplatelet therapy**
    a. **Aspirin** is currently recommended for stroke and TIA patients whether or not CEA has been performed. Aspirin decreases production of prostaglandins, which are hormone-like substances that cause platelet activation and aggregation. Although the optimum dosage has not been established, daily dosage ranges of 50–1300 mg have been studied. Randomized, prospective studies comparing four dosages are under way at the NASCET centers. Recent data raised doubt about the effectiveness of low-dose aspirin. For now, 325 mg daily is the favored dosage. Those patients at high risk for cerebral hemorrhage would be excluded. The effect of intravenous acetylsalicylic acid (aspirin) on microemboli has been evaluated by TCD.
    b. **Dipyridamole** (Persantine) has been studied in a capsule form combined with aspirin: 400 mg dipyridamole with 50 mg aspirin. In the European Stroke Prevention Study, the combined capsule was studied compared with aspirin alone and with dipyridamole alone for second stroke prevention in patients with recent completed ischemic stroke or TIA. The capsule showed an additive effect for marked reduction in re-stroke (37% decreased risk versus aspirin (18%) or dipyridamole (16%). FDA approval is expected for this combination capsule. Dipyridamole prevents clot formation by inhibition of platelet activation and aggregation.
    c. **Ticlopidine hydrochloride** (Ticlid), 250 mg orally twice a day, is currently indicated for use in patients who are intolerant of aspirin. It inhibits platelet aggregation by interfering with fibrinogen–platelet binding and subsequent platelet interaction. Side effects include diarrhea and skin eruptions. Reversible, absolute neutropenia is an uncommon but serious side effect of ticlopidine. Weekly monitoring of white blood cell counts is necessary within the first few months of starting ticlopidine. Ticlopidine offered a 21% relative risk reduction for recurrent stroke compared with aspirin at the end of 3 years in the Ticlopidine/Aspirin Stroke Study.
    d. **Clopidogrel bisulfate** (Plavix) is a potent, noncompetitive inhibitor of adenosine diphosphate–induced platelet aggregation. Its irreversible effect lasts the duration of platelet life (7–10 days). It inhibits activation of the GpIIa/IIIa receptor binding site for fibrinogen, thus blocking fibrinogen-linked platelet aggregation. The Clopidogrel versus Aspirin in Patients at Risk of Ischemic Events showed clopidogrel to be marginally more effective than aspirin at reducing secondary stroke. A dosage of 75 mg daily is recommended. Side effects include: skin eruption, diarrhea, and thrombotic thrombocytopenic purpura (TTP), which can be fatal.
5. Two cholesterol-lowering medications have been approved by the FDA for prevention of first stroke or TIA in coronary artery disease. Pravastatin (Pravachol) is approved for patients with average cholesterol (<240) and a personal history of heart disease. Simvastatin (Zocor) is approved in patients with high cholesterol and coronary artery disease. (See Chapter 79.)
6. **Antioxidant therapy** is under investigation for prevention and treatment of stroke (see discussion above).

VI. Management strategies. Stroke indicates generalized vascular disease; it is one event in a prolonged and ongoing process. Management strategies center on prevention of further manifestations of the disease and maximization of poststroke function during the three stages of stroke.

    A. Stage I. The **acute stage** of stroke spans the first week. Attention to evaluation, maintenance, and return of function includes passive range of motion of extremities, proper positioning, frequent turning, and maintenance of good hygiene.

    B. Stage II. The **subacute stage** of stroke usually lasts 3 months. Return of neurologic function is greatest during this interval. **Rehabilitation** involves interdisciplinary assessment and treatment by a team of nurses, physical therapists, occupational therapists, speech therapists, a dietitian, and the physician to maximize functional return and independence. Selection of the site of rehabilitation (eg, a formal rehabilitation unit, a skilled nursing home, the patient's home with home health care agency coordination, or outpatient facilities) depends on the patient's medical condition, the family situation (supports and weaknesses), financial considerations, and available resources. To benefit from any kind of rehabilitation, the patient must be able to communicate (verbally or nonverbally), follow a two- to three-step command, and remember what is learned. Rehabilitation units require that a patient's cardiopulmonary endurance allows 2–3 hours of intense therapy daily. Patients with marked dementia, severe chronic obstructive pulmonary disease, marked limitation of cardiovascular reserve, or severely debilitating multiple joint disease are not likely to benefit from acute inpatient rehabilitation, although such patients may receive benefit from skilled or subacute care in the immediate posthospitalization period.

    C. Stage III. The **chronic stage** of stroke recovery begins after 3 months. Neurologic return may continue for as long as 1 year after an event and functional recovery can occur for as long as 2 years. Maintenance of the functional gains achieved in the subacute stage is important.

        1. Involvement of the family or caregiver in the acute and intermediate phases of stroke care enhances their knowledge and expectations regarding the patient's condition. The format for an adult chronic illness family conference is listed in Table 90–2. Careful coordination of patient and family involvement with discharge planning involves family or caregiver teaching sessions with the patient and with each of the patient's regular therapists and team nurse.

TABLE 90–2. FORMAT FOR FAMILY CONFERENCE IN ADULT CHRONIC ILLNESS

       1. Introduction (family members and health care professionals)

       2. Presentation of case summary
          a. Patient's current medical history
          b. Pertinent clinical findings
          c. Short-term concerns, prognosis, and plans
          d. Long-term concerns, prognosis, and plans

       3. Review of family genogram
          a. Psychosocial factors
          b. Environmental factors
          c. Family dynamics

       4. Listening to family and patient responses
          a. Feelings
          b. Health questions
          c. Future plans

       5. Summary
          a. Formalizing a plan
          b. Gaining a consensus
          c. Identifying and recognizing resources
          d. Assigning specific tasks

Modified with permission from Evans ER, Green-Walsh MA, Department of Family Practice, Creighton University School of Medicine, Omaha, Nebraska.

TABLE 90-3. BARTHEL INDEX

A score above 60 usually means that less than 2 hours of personal care assistance is required each day. A score of 60 or less indicates that 4 or more hours of personal care assistance is needed daily. A score of 0 is given when a criterion cannot be met.

Functional activity	Dependent	Independent
1. Feeding	5	10
2. Transfer from bed to wheelchair, back to bed (includes sitting up in bed)	15 5 = assisted out of bed only 10 = some help/cueing	
3. Grooming (wash face, comb hair, shave, including preparing razor, clean teeth, and apply own make-up if worn)	0	5
4. Toileting (transfer on/off toilet, handling clothing, wiping, and flushing)	5	10
5. Bathing (tub, shower, or complete sponge bath)	0	5
6. Ambulation, 50 yards, level surface		
a. Walking (assistive device allowed)	10	15
or		
b. Unable to walk (eg, wheeled walker or wheelchair required)	(0)	(5)
7. Ascending/descending stairs (mechanical assistive devices allowed)	5	10
8. Dressing (includes tying shoes and donning assistive devices; excludes nonprescribed girdles or bras)	5	10
9. Bowel continence (suppository, enema allowed)	5	10
10. Urinary continence	5	10

Modified with permission from Mahoney FI, Barthel DW: Functional evaluation: The Barthel index. Md Med J 1965;**14**:61.

2. **Home health care agency involvement** allows for smooth transition and capable problem solving as the patient returns home.
3. **Monitoring of the patient by the physician** at regular intervals is important to assess and promote risk management strategies, identify and treat complicating illness (eg, depression), evaluate recurrence of symptoms, assess functional status (Barthel index [Table 90–3]), negotiate potential blocks to maintenance of function, and facilitate the patient's acceptance of disability.

VII. **Natural history and prognosis.** Overall, the vast majority of initially alert patients survive the acute phase of stroke. Acute phase deaths are generally due to cerebral causes related to irreversible failure of vital function of the brain stem. Pulmonary embolism and cardiac events contribute to early mortality in stroke patients. Systemic causes (eg, pneumonia, pulmonary embolism, ischemic heart disease, or recurrent stroke) are the usual causes of death in the subacute and chronic phases. The risk of recurrence of stroke is substantial. The major complications of stroke are aspiration, infection (eg, urinary tract infection or pneumonia), pressure sores, corneal abrasion, and depression.

REFERENCES

Biller J, et al: Guidelines for carotid endarterectomy: A statement for health care professionals from a special writing group of The Stroke Council, American Heart Association. Stroke 1998;**29**:554.

Caplan LR: New therapies for stroke. Arch Neurol 1997;**54**:1222.

del Zoppo GJ, Wagner S, Tagaya M: Trends and future developments in the pharmacological treatment of acute ischaemic stroke. Drugs 1997;**54**(1):9.

Goertler M, et al: Rapid decline of cerebral microemboli of arterial origin after intravenous acetylsalicylic acid. Stroke 1999;**30**:66.

Macko RF, et al: Elevated tissue plasminogen activator antigen and stroke risk: The stroke prevention in young women study. Stroke 1999;**30**:7.

Sacco I, et al: Risk factors. Stroke 1997;**28**:1506.

Schafer AI: Antiplatelet therapy. Am J Med 1996;**101**:199.

Ueda T, et al: Angioplasty after intra-arterial thrombolysis for acute occlusion of intracranial arteries. Stroke 1998;**29**:2568.

ELECTRONIC RESOURCES

www.amhrt.org is the website for the American Heart Association. Three times a year, STROKE, a publication of AHA, publishes a synopsis of the current ongoing multicenter trials related to stroke. American Heart Association. 1998 Heart and stroke statistical update provided statistics. www.ninds.nih.gov is the National Institute of Neurologic Disorders and Stroke (NIH) website. www.stroke.org is the website for the National Stroke Association.

---

91   Thyroid Disease

Stephen F. Wheeler, MEng, MD

I. Evaluation of thyroid function

  A. Physiology. Thyrotropin-releasing hormone, secreted by the hypothalamus, stimulates the anterior pituitary to produce thyroid-stimulating hormone (TSH). The major hormone released by the thyroid gland in response to TSH is thyroxine (T_4), which is converted peripherally to triiodothyronine (T_3), a more potent hormone. T_4 and T_3 are both highly but reversibly bound to plasma thyroid-binding globulin (TBG) and, to a lesser extent, to albumin and prealbumin. Only the minute unbound (free) fractions are metabolically active. The most sensitive indicator of thyroid status is the level of TSH, which is controlled in classic negative-feedback fashion by the concentration of unbound thyroid hormones.

  B. Laboratory tests. Diagnosis of thyroid disease depends on symptoms, clinical signs, and laboratory tests. Since thyroid function tests cannot be accurately interpreted without appropriate clinical data, their inclusion on multiphasic profiles for patients at low risk of having thyroid disease is discouraged.

    1. Sensitive TSH (sTSH). The inverse log/linear relationship between sTSH and unbound T_4 (free T_4) estimates means that sTSH will always be more sensitive than free T_4 estimates at indicating thyroid function. Thus, a normal sTSH, except in rare instances, excludes both hypothyroidism and hyperthyroidism.

      a. In addition to hyperthyroidism, sTSH may be **suppressed** by severe nonthyroidal illness, by use of dopamine, and by glucocorticoid therapy. Also, sTSH may be suppressed in some euthyroid elderly patients.

      b. sTSH may be mildly **elevated** during recovery from severe nonthyroidal illness, by various drugs, including lithium and amphetamines, and in some euthyroid elderly patients.

    2. Serum total T_4 (T_4) and total T_3 (T_3). These tests measure both protein-bound and free hormone by radioimmunoassay and are affected by changes in the concentration of thyroid-binding proteins.

    3. T_3 resin uptake (T_3 RU). A laboratory assessment of the protein binding of both T_4 and T_3. T_3 RU is **not** a measure of circulating T_3 levels. Rather, it is inversely proportional to the unsaturated hormone binding sites on TBG and is most useful in helping to interpret a given level of T_4.

    4. Free thyroxine index (FTI) is the product of T_4 and T_3 RU and provides an estimate of free T_4 by adjusting for variations in total hormone concentration secondary to altered protein binding.

    5. Free T_4 can be measured directly and reliably. Severe or chronic nonthyroidal illness, which affects other types of free T_4 assays, has been the major indication for this test, although its use is being increasingly recommended for the routine diagnostic evaluation of thyroid disease.

  C. Diagnostic evaluation versus screening

    1. Table 91–1 lists the most common symptoms and signs of hypothyroidism according to frequency.

TABLE 91–1. SYMPTOMS AND SIGNS OF HYPOTHYROIDISM

Symptom or Sign	Percent of Cases
Weakness	99
Dry skin	97
Coarse skin	97
Lethargy	91
Slow speech	91
Edema of eyelids	90
Sensation of cold	89
Decreased sweating	89
Cold skin	83
Thick tongue	82
Edema of face	79
Coarseness of hair	76
Cardiac enlargement (x-ray)	68
Pallor of skin	67
Memory impairment	66
Constipation	61
Gain in weight	59
Loss of hair	57
Pallor of lips	57
Dyspnea	55
Peripheral edema	55
Hoarseness	52
Anorexia	45
Nervousness	35
Menorrhagia	32[1]
Palpitation	31
Deafness	30
Poor heart sounds	30
Precordial pain	25
Poor vision	24
Fundus oculi changes	20
Dysmenorrhea	18[1]
Loss of weight	13
Atrophic tongue	12
Emotional instability	11
Choking sensation	9
Fineness of hair	9
Cyanosis	7
Dysphagia	3

[1] In 41 premenopausal women.
Adapted from DeGroot LJ: *The Thyroid and Its Diseases.* John Wiley & Sons; 1984.

2. Table 91–2 lists the most common clinical findings of hyperthyroidism according to frequency.
3. Patients with many **other health problems** can present with these symptoms and signs. One study found that the probability of thyroid metabolic disorders was related to the number of symptoms and signs exhibited by the patient. Seventy-eight percent of patients with five or more findings had proven thyroid disease, compared with 2.9% of patients with three or four findings and only 0.45% of those with one or two findings.
4. **Diagnostic evaluation** of patients with signs and symptoms suggestive of thyroid dysfunction often requires multiple specific tests, beginning with sTSH and FTI or free T_4. Further work-up depends on the clinical situation and the initial laboratory results.
5. **Screening** patients at low risk of having thyroid disease is not recommended. However, certain populations are at higher risk of having overt but unrecognized illness. **Suspect populations** include newborns; postpartum women 4–8 weeks after delivery; persons with a family history of thyroid disease; patients with dyslipidemias; women older than 50 years; and patients with immunologically mediated diseases such as Addison's disease, insulin-

TABLE 91–2. SYMPTOMS AND SIGNS OF HYPERTHYROIDISM

Symptom or Sign	Percent of Cases
Goiter	87
Dyspnea on exertion	81
Tiredness	80
Hot hands	76
Palpitation	75
Preference for cold	73
Hands sweating	72
Excessive sweating	68
Regular pulse rate: over 90 bpm	68
Finger tremor	66
Lid lag	62
Nervousness	59
Weight loss	52
Goiter, diffuse enlargement of thyroid gland	49
Hyperkinesis	39
Exophthalmos	34
Goiter, nodular	32
Increased appetite	32
Auricular fibrillation	19
Scant menses	18
Constipation	15
Diminished appetite	13
Diarrhea	8
Weight gain	4
Goiter, single adenoma	4
Excessive menses	3

Adapted from Wayne EJ: The diagnosis of thyrotoxicosis. Br Med J 1954;**1**:411.

dependent diabetes mellitus, and rheumatoid arthritis. The initial screening test of choice is sTSH, with follow-up of abnormal values using FTI or free T_4 and other tests as indicated.

II. Hypothyroidism

A. Definition. Hypothyroidism results from insufficient production of thyroid hormones.

B. Epidemiology. Overt hypothyroidism is found in 1–3% of the general population. It is at least twice as common in females as in males and prevalence increases progressively with age.

C. Pathophysiology

1. **Primary hypothyroidism,** most commonly from chronic autoimmune (Hashimoto's) thyroiditis, radioactive iodine therapy, or surgery, accounts for the overwhelming majority of hypothyroidism cases.

2. **Secondary hypothyroidism** results from decreased pituitary secretion of TSH. This condition is usually accompanied by other manifestations of pituitary hyposecretion. Causes include postpartum pituitary necrosis (Sheehan's syndrome) and pituitary tumors.

D. Diagnosis

1. In a patient with suggestive signs and symptoms, a high sTSH (>15 µU/mL) and a low FTI or free T_4 are diagnostic of primary hypothyroidism. When autoimmune thyroiditis is the presumptive cause, confirmation with a serum antithyroperoxidase level (formerly called antimicrosomal antibody) is helpful.

2. In the setting of overt hypothyroidism, a sTSH that is normal or only mildly elevated suggests secondary hypothyroidism. Concurrent amenorrhea, galactorrhea, postural hypotension, loss of axillary and pubic hair, and visual field deficits may be present.

E. Treatment

1. **Levothyroxine** is preferred for routine replacement therapy. Recent interchangeability studies of levothyroxine products have not shown significant fluctuations in hormone levels when switching among name brand or generic preparations.

   2. Adults require approximately 1.7 µg/kg/day for full replacement, with an average maintenance dose of 125 µg/day. Older patients may need <1 µg/kg/day. Therapy is usually initiated with the full replacement dose in patients under 50 years of age. In patients older than 50 years, or in younger patients with known or suspected cardiac disease, a lower initial dose of 12.5–50 µg/day is indicated.
   3. Clinical and biochemical **re-evaluation** at 6- to 8-week intervals is necessary until the levothyroxine dose has been titrated to produce a normalized sTSH. Subsequently, an interim history and physical examination pertinent to thyroid status and a sTSH should be performed at least annually.
   4. **Drugs** such as cholestyramine, ferrous sulfate, sucralfate, and antacids containing aluminum hydroxide may interfere with levothyroxine absorption. Other drugs, such as phenytoin, carbamazepine, and rifampin, may accelerate levothyroxine metabolism, necessitating higher replacement doses.

III. **Subclinical hypothyroidism**
   A. **Definition.** Subclinical hypothyroidism is distinguished by an elevated sTSH, a normal FTI or free T_4, and few, if any, hypothyroid symptoms.
   B. **Epidemiology.** As many as 15% of geriatric patients, as well as many younger adults, meet these criteria. Generally, women show a higher prevalence than men.
   C. **Clinical course.** Subclinical hypothyroidism does not always progress to overt hypothyroidism. Risk factors for progression include the presence of thyroid autoantibodies, age greater than 65 years, female gender, and a higher sTSH level ($\geq$10 µU/mL). Patients who do not progress are considered to be euthyroid with a reset thyrostat, probably because of a subtle insult to the thyroid gland.
   D. **Treatment** must be individualized, based on risk factors for progression and the presence of subtle symptoms and signs, including elevated lipids. In some patients, levothyroxine may ameliorate vague symptoms or those attributed to other sources. Patients **not treated** should be monitored clinically and biochemically at yearly intervals for evidence of progressive thyroid dysfunction.

IV. **Hyperthyroidism**
   A. **Definition.** Hyperthyroidism results from elevated levels of thyroid hormones.
   B. **Epidemiology.** Hyperthyroidism is less common than hypothyroidism in the general population. Community-based studies have found prevalences of 1.9% in women and 0.16% in men. Approximately 15% of cases occur in persons over 60 years of age. Graves' disease, which accounts for about 90% of hyperthyroidism in those younger than 40 years, demonstrates a familial predisposition.
   C. **Pathophysiology.** Hyperthyroidism encompasses a heterogeneous group of disorders.
      1. **Graves' disease** is an autoimmune disease that results from the action of thyroid-stimulating immunoglobulin G antibody (TS Ab) on thyroid gland TSH receptors.
      2. **Toxic multinodular goiter (Plummer's disease),** the most common cause of hyperthyroidism in those older than 40 years, occurs when a patient with nontoxic multinodular goiter develops one or more autonomous hyperfunctioning nodules.
      3. **Toxic adenoma,** the least common cause of hyperthyroidism, is produced by one or more hyperfunctioning thyroid adenomas capable of functioning independently of TSH or other thyroid stimulators.
      4. **Thyroiditis** may produce transient hyperthyroidism as hormone leaks from an inflamed gland. Transient hypothyroidism often follows as the intrathyroidal stores of hormone are depleted.
   D. **Diagnosis**
      1. In a patient with suggestive signs and symptoms, a suppressed sTSH and an elevated FTI or free T_4 level are diagnostic of hyperthyroidism. In a clinically hyperthyroid patient with a suppressed sTSH and a normal FTI or free T_4 level, T_3 should be measured to evaluate for possible T_3 thyrotoxicosis.
      2. The **history** and the **physical examination** are critical to distinguish among the causes of hyperthyroidism (Table 91–3).
      3. **Radioactive iodine (^{123}I) uptake** can help clarify hyperthyroidism of uncertain origin. Diffuse increase in ^{123}I uptake is consistent with Graves' disease, whereas nodular concentration indicates toxic adenoma or multinodular goi-

TABLE 91–3. DIAGNOSIS OF HYPERTHYROIDISM

Gland Size	Nodule	Tender	Other Findings	Suggested Diagnosis
I	0	NT	Proptosis; pretibial myxedema; thyroid bruit in 50%	Graves' disease
I	0	T	Recent viral illness in many	Subacute thyroiditis
Modest I	0	NT	Some postpartum	Silent thyroiditis (consider Hashimoto's thyroiditis)
I	Multiple	NT		Toxic multinodular goiter (consider Hashimoto's thyroiditis)
D	0	NT		Consider extrathyroid source
D	Single	NT		Toxic adenoma

D, Decreased; I, increased; NT, nontender; T, tender.

ter. If ^{123}I uptake is decreased, a serum **thyroglobulin** measurement can distinguish between exogenous (factitious) hyperthyroxinemia (thyroglobulin decreased) and thyroiditis, iodine-induced thyrotoxicosis, or struma ovarii (thyroglobulin increased).

E. Therapeutic modalities
  1. The **antithyroid drugs (ATDs)** methimazole and propylthiouracil (PTU) inhibit thyroid hormone synthesis. PTU also inhibits peripheral conversion of T_4 to T_3. ATDs suppress thyroid autoantibodies, decrease TS Ab, and lead to remission in some patients with Graves' disease.
     a. The usual starting doses are 10–30 mg/day for methimazole and 100–150 mg three times daily for PTU. If there is no decrease in FTI in 4–8 weeks, the dose should be increased. Doses as high as 60–90 mg/day of methimazole and 300 mg three or four times daily of PTU may be required to normalize thyroid function. TSH may remain suppressed for several months after thyroid hormone levels normalize.
     b. Once euthyroidism is achieved (usually within 6–8 weeks), the dose can be titrated down to maintain euthyroidism. Typical maintenance doses are 100–200 mg PTU or 10–20 mg methimazole daily.
     c. Most clinicians treat patients for 12–24 months before attempting to withdraw antithyroid therapy. ATDs induce long-lasting remissions in only about 50% of patients who have been treated for periods of 18–20 months and 33–50% of those who respond will relapse.
     d. Adverse reactions, which are encountered in 1–5% of patients taking ATDs, include rash, itching, fever, arthralgias, and hepatic abnormalities. The most serious reaction to ATDs is agranulocytosis, which occurs in about 0.3% of patients. Onset is usually within 2 months and rarely after 4 months. Patients developing fever, chills, jaundice, sore throat, or bleeding gums should stop taking the drug immediately and contact their physician for appropriate evaluation, including a complete blood count with differential.
  2. **Radioactive iodine (RAI, ^{131}I),** usually administered orally, concentrates in the thyroid gland, where it destroys follicular cells.
     a. A single dose permanently controls hyperthyroidism in about 90% of patients. If symptomatic hyperthyroidism persists 3–6 months after therapy, a second ^{131}I treatment is given.
     b. RAI exerts its full effect over a 2- to 3-month period. Follow-up at 4- to 6-week intervals to measure FTI or free T_4 and assess clinical response is appropriate until thyroid function stabilizes within the normal range or hypothyroidism ensues.
     c. The most common complication of therapy is the early or late development of hypothyroidism. Thyroid replacement therapy should be initiated as the FTI and sTSH pass from normal into the hypothyroid range. The end point of replacement is a normal sTSH.

    d. RAI is contraindicated during pregnancy, and it is usually advised that pregnancy be postponed 6 months following therapy. Treatment with ^{131}I does not cause cancer or infertility and has not been shown to produce ill effects in subsequent children of those so treated.

  3. Surgery for hyperthyroidism has declined in popularity because of the effectiveness of ATDs and ^{131}I.

    a. Specific indications include patients unwilling or unable to take ATDs or to be treated with ^{131}I as well as those with neck obstruction, very large goiters that may be relatively resistant to ^{131}I, or cosmetic concerns.

    b. Any patient undergoing surgery for hyperthyroidism should be pretreated with methimazole until euthyroid status is attained. Alternative regimens using various combinations of methimazole, potassium iodide, and a β-adrenergic antagonist are also effective at reducing postoperative thyrotoxic crisis.

    c. Complications of surgery depend on the skill and experience of the surgical and anesthesiology teams. Potential complications are transient hypocalcemia, transient hypothyroidism, thyroid crisis, permanent hypoparathyroidism, recurrent laryngeal nerve damage, and postoperative hemorrhage. The mortality rate for elective surgery is close to 0%, and the rate of complications is reported to be less than 4%.

    d. Recurrent hyperthyroidism occurs in at least 10% of patients who are treated surgically. Permanent hypothyroidism occurs in 5% of patients within the first year, and subsequently in 1–2% of patients per year. Up to 50% of patients are hypothyroid 25 years after surgery.

  4. Adjunctive medical therapies are useful for relieving symptoms in patients undergoing definitive therapy with other agents or in those with transient forms of hyperthyroidism.

    a. β-Adrenergic antagonists provide prompt symptomatic relief of the hyperadrenergic manifestations of hyperthyroidism. Propranolol is the most widely used beta blocker for this purpose. Initial doses of 20–40 mg four times daily are adjusted to control tachycardia and symptoms.

    b. Calcium channel blockers such as diltiazem or verapamil may be used in patients who cannot tolerate, or have contraindications to, beta blockers.

F. Choice of therapy

  1. Graves' disease

    a. RAI is the treatment of choice for most elderly patients.

    b. For children and adolescents, ATDs have commonly been recommended for initial therapy, with surgery or RAI reserved for patients who either fail ATD therapy or experience complications. However, the high failure rate of ATDs and the efficacy and apparent safety of RAI have prompted increasing use of RAI in this age group.

    c. The treatment of young adults is also controversial. Specific patient characteristics, along with the risks and benefits of each treatment, should be considered. In young women with this condition who are anticipating pregnancy, RAI is often preferred to obviate future concern about ATDs causing fetal goiter or hypothyroidism.

    d. RAI therapy may exacerbate **ophthalmopathy** in Graves' disease. This exacerbation is often transient and can be prevented by moderate doses of prednisone. Although it is controversial, some physicians substitute ATDs for RAI in patients with active eye disease, until pertinent signs and symptoms stabilize. Avoidance of clinical hypothyroidism after therapy may also be important in minimizing subsequent eye abnormalities. Aggressive treatment with high-dose glucocorticoids can also be considered for progressive and severe ophthalmopathy.

  2. Toxic multinodular goiter. There are no spontaneous remissions of hyperthyroidism resulting from nodular thyroid disease. RAI is usually the treatment of choice. Surgery may be appropriate for very large goiters, if there is concern about thyroid cancer, or in children, adolescents, or young adults. ATDs are valuable as pretreatment before thyroid surgery and before or after RAI in elderly patients and those with concurrent health problems.

  3. Toxic adenoma. RAI is usually the treatment of choice. Surgical removal may be appropriate in young patients.

    4. Thyroiditis produces only transient hyperthyroidism, so treatment focuses on symptom control with adjunctive medical therapies. Inflammatory symptoms and pain can usually be controlled with salicylates. Aspirin, started at 650 mg four times daily, is titrated as symptom response and early manifestations of toxicity, such as tinnitus and mild deafness, allow. Severe symptoms respond to prednisone, 20–60 mg/day. Transient hypothyroidism may follow the initial hyperthyroid phase and may be symptomatic enough to warrant levothyroxine therapy.

V. Subclinical hyperthyroidism

A. Definition. Subclinical hyperthyroidism is distinguished by a low or undetectable sTSH and normal T_3 and FTI or free T_4 in an asymptomatic person.

B. Epidemiology

1. Subclinical hyperthyroidism is more common than overt hyperthyroidism among the elderly. Various studies have shown a prevalence of 4–12%. Excluding patients receiving thyroid hormone therapy, 0.9–1.9% of older persons meet these criteria.
2. Excessive thyroid hormone replacement is the most common cause. Other important causes include nodular thyroid disease, subclinical Graves' disease, and thyroiditis.
3. Factors that can suppress sTSH levels, such as severe illness, high-dose glucocorticoids, dopamine, and pituitary dysfunction, should be excluded.
4. Laboratory findings consistent with subclinical hyperthyroidism can be a normal variant in the elderly.

C. Clinical course. Subclinical hyperthyroidism often disappears, and progression to overt hyperthyroidism is uncommon. However, it does increase the risk for atrial fibrillation and may increase the risk for other atrial arrhythmias, left ventricular hypertrophy, muscle weakness, neuropsychological dysfunction, and accelerated bone loss.

D. Treatment

1. If excessive hormone replacement is the cause, the dose should be reduced.
2. If subclinical hyperthyroidism is associated with nodular thyroid disease, subclinical Graves' disease, arrhythmias, other cardiac disorders, or accelerated bone loss, antithyroid treatment should be seriously considered.
3. In patients not meeting the above criteria, careful follow-up is acceptable.

VI. Thyroid nodules

A. Epidemiology

1. Palpable nodules are present in 4–7% of adults. However, physical examination is relatively insensitive, and up to 50% of patients demonstrate thyroid nodules by ultrasonography or at autopsy. Prevalence is four to nine times greater in women than in men. Approximately 5% of all solitary nodules are carcinomas.
2. Prior radiation exposure increases the rate of development of both benign and malignant new nodules to about 2% per year. Peak incidence is 15–25 years after exposure.
3. Up to 35% of glands examined at surgery or autopsy contain tiny, clinically unimportant papillary carcinomas.
4. Since similar frequencies of cancer have been found in patients who have solitary or multiple nodules on palpation, dominant nodules in multinodular glands should also be considered for diagnostic evaluation.

B. Thyroid cancer risk factors

1. **Family history** of familial goiter, medullary or papillary cancer, or familial polyposis.
2. **Personal history** of prior head and neck radiation exposure. Childhood exposures increase thyroid cancer risk 10-fold.
3. **Physical findings** suggestive of cancer are nodule size greater than 4 cm, recurrence of cystic nodules after aspiration, progressive or rapid growth, firmness, fixation to surrounding structures, local lymphadenopathy, and hoarseness.
4. **Other risk factors** include age less than 20 or greater than 60 years and male gender.

C. Diagnostic and management strategies

1. A thorough **history** and **physical examination** should focus on thyroid cancer risk factors.

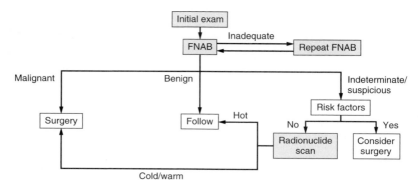

FIGURE 91–1. Treatment of a solitary or dominant thyroid nodule. FNAB, Fine-needle aspiration biopsy.

2. Serum **sTSH** identifies patients with unsuspected thyroid dysfunction. Other tests may be beneficial in specific settings: FTI or free T_4 if sTSH is abnormal; serum antithyroperoxidase if sTSH is elevated; basal serum calcitonin if there is a family history of medullary thyroid cancer or multiple endocrine neoplasia, type II.

3. **Fine-needle aspiration biopsy (FNAB)** should be the initial test in most patients. It is safe and inexpensive and more effectively selects patients for surgery than any other test. FNAB has reduced the number of patients undergoing thyroid surgery by 25–50%, increased the yield of carcinoma in those who do have surgery from 15% to 30–40%, and decreased the cost of care by 25%.

4. An algorithm for the evaluation and management of nodular thyroid disease is displayed in Figure 91–1. Follow-up of thyroid nodules not surgically explored should include clinical examination with palpation and consideration of repeat FNAB. Thyroid ultrasonography and sTSH may also be helpful in following selected patients.

5. **Thyroid hormone suppression** has been used routinely in the past in both the diagnosis and treatment of thyroid nodules. Recent controlled trials have not shown it to be efficacious for these purposes. If suppressive therapy is considered, the risks associated with subclinical hyperthyroidism must be included in the risk–benefit analysis.

REFERENCES

American Association of Clinical Endocrinologists (AACE) Thyroid Guidelines Task Force: *AACE Clinical Practice Guidelines for the Evaluation and Treatment of Hyperthyroidism and Hypothyroidism.* Endocr Pract 1995;**1:**54.

Franklyn JA: The management of hyperthyroidism. N Engl J Med 1994;**330:**1731.

Hefland M, Redfern CC: Screening for thyroid disease: An update. Ann Intern Med 1998;**129:**144.

Singer PA, et al: Treatment guidelines for patients with hyperthyroidism and hypothyroidism. JAMA 1995;**273:**808.

Singer PA, et al: Treatment guidelines for patients with thyroid nodules and well-differentiated thyroid cancer. Arch Intern Med 1996;**156:**2165.

SECTION III. Psychiatric Disorders

92   Alcohol & Drug Abuse

Richard L. Brown, MD, MPH

I. **Definition.** There is increasing evidence that the difficulty in controlling substance use by substance-dependent individuals results from alterations in the neurophysiology of the mesolimbic system. Genetics probably accounts for much of the differential susceptibility to these alterations. The body of biomedical evidence for the disease model of substance dependence continues to grow. Substance abuse, which, by definition, is under voluntary control, cannot be characterized as a disease. The most important practical point, however, is that when physicians treat alcohol and drug problems as intently and empathically as they do other medical problems, they are more likely to attain positive results.

   A. **Substance abuse** is present when patients continue to use a psychoactive substance despite repeated adverse consequences of such use. Repeated substance use in physically hazardous situations also qualifies individuals for a *Diagnostic and Statistical Manual of Mental Health Disorders,* 4th edition (DSM-IV), diagnosis of substance abuse.

   B. **Physical (or pharmacologic) dependence** is a physiologic phenomenon consisting of either tolerance or withdrawal. Tolerance occurs when a drug used repeatedly elicits less effect, which can lead to escalation in use. Withdrawal is the phenomenon in which abrupt diminution or cessation of drug use results in stereotypical symptoms. Some patients, such as those who take opioids continuously for chronic pain or those who take benzodiazepines continuously for anxiety disorders, have physical dependence without substance abuse or substance dependence.

   C. **Substance dependence** is the repeated use of substances that results in negative consequences plus frequent loss of control over use, preoccupation with obtaining substances, and cravings to take the substances. There may or may not be physical dependence. Synonyms include alcoholism and addiction.

   D. **At-risk substance use** occurs when individuals use amounts associated with a risk of negative consequences. For men, consumption of more than four drinks (one standard drink is 1–1.5 oz of hard liquor, 5–6 oz of wine, or 12 oz of beer) per occasion or more than 14 drinks per week confers risk. For women, consuming more than three drinks per occasion or more than 11 drinks per week confers risk. Although most users of illicit drugs do not satisfy the criteria for substance abuse or dependence, use of such drugs carries more risk of abuse or dependence than does alcohol. Therefore, any illicit drug use is considered at-risk substance use.

II. **Epidemiology.** Estimates of the prevalence of substance-related disorders among American adults range from 10% to 20%. Affected individuals account for at least 10% of all ambulatory visits, 40% or more of all emergency room visits, and at least 25% of general hospital inpatients. Although alcohol continues to be the most widely abused drug, abuse of alcohol in combination with other drugs is becoming more common, especially among individuals under age 40. While cocaine use has decreased among the general population, cocaine abuse and dependence continue to be prevalent, especially among certain disadvantaged groups. There is concern about the use of marijuana among young people, since marijuana use is often a gateway to the use of "hard" drugs. Risk factors for current or future substance abuse include a family history of substance abuse; antisocial personality disorder; alcoholic blackouts (loss of memory of events during a period of intoxication); frequent substance use to the point of intoxication; use in social isolation; and use for pharmacologic effect, including relieving psychological symptoms, controlling sleep, and alleviating social anxiety. Fewer than 5% of substance abusers are stereotypical vagrants. Differences in prevalence among ethnic and gender groups are eroding with acculturation and evolution of gender roles. Abuse of alcohol and prescription drugs is being increasingly recognized as a problem in the elderly.

III. **Pathophysiology**

   A. **Genetics and family.** Research has demonstrated the importance of genetic transmission of substance abuse disorders. Individuals with an alcoholic parent are at three to four times the baseline risk for alcohol dependence. Monozygotic twins of proband alcoholics have a higher incidence of alcoholism than dizygotic twins. However, penetrance is incomplete and may be influenced by environmental factors. For example, families that preserve rituals, such as holiday celebrations and vacations, despite an alcohol-abusing parent, transmit alcohol problems less frequently to their children than do families whose rituals are lost.

B. **Molecular biology.** In animal models, regular use of cocaine and other commonly abused substances leads to persistent translation of different DNA sequences in reward centers of the brain, even months after cocaine is discontinued.

C. **Psychiatric disorders and stress.** Some substance-related disorders are secondary to self-medication of psychiatric disorders, including anxiety, depression, and schizophrenia. Although self-medication can alleviate symptoms acutely, it can also exacerbate the underlying condition, leading to more substance abuse and dependence. Physicians should take care, however, not to attribute substance abuse automatically to life stresses, as is often the tendency of patients in denial. Stress is often an *effect* of the adverse consequences of substance abuse, not the cause of the substance use.

D. **Iatrogenic physical dependence** on drugs appropriately prescribed and used as directed should not necessarily be viewed as a problem. For selected patients with certain conditions, such as end-stage cancer, acute pain, severe anxiety, or chronic noncancer pain, the advantages of maintenance medications may outweigh the disadvantages of physical dependence. This can hold true even for some patients with a history of substance dependence, although such patients should be monitored very closely. For all patients, though, it is best to try nonpharmacologic and nonaddictive treatments before instituting long-term therapy with potentially addictive medications.

IV. **Diagnosis**

A. **Early diagnosis** of substance abuse should be the goal of all physicians. The benefits of early diagnosis seem to include avoidance of additional reversible or irreversible biomedical and psychosocial consequences, a need for less intensive treatment, and a greater likelihood of acceptance and success of treatment.

B. **Symptoms and signs**

1. **Frequency, quantity, and pattern** (eg, when, where, and with whom a drug is used) can suggest a problem but are minimized by some patients. Direct or implied challenges to responses make patients more defensive and less willing to reveal sensitive information. To facilitate accurate responses, delay asking about substance use until rapport is established through a brief social history, and link the questions to a clinical issue. For example, "I see that you're under a lot of stress. How do you cope? Does alcohol ever help you relax or be social? How much do you drink? On how many days a week? Have you ever experimented with any drugs, such as marijuana or cocaine?"

2. A **detailed social history** taken in a nonjudgmental, supportive manner is crucial for making an early diagnosis of substance abuse, since most early symptoms are psychosocial. Subsequent questions investigating links between potential adverse consequences and substance use, such as "Do you think your spouse/boss/friends would be happier with you if you stopped drinking?," can be helpful. The history should aim to uncover the negative consequences of substance use (see section VII).

3. The **four CAGE questions** are recommended to screen male adults for alcohol abuse. For primary care populations, one positive response to the CAGE questions warrants further assessment. Follow-up of positive responses helps elicit adverse consequences of substance use. The four CAGE questions are shown below.

—Have you ever felt you ought to **c**ut down on your drinking? (Follow-up: What made you feel that way?)

—Have people **a**nnoyed you by criticizing your drinking? (Follow-up: Who? What do they criticize you about?)

—Have you ever felt bad or **g**uilty about your drinking? (Follow-up: Can you give me an example of when you felt guilty?)

—Have you ever had a drink first thing in the morning to steady your nerves or get rid of a hangover (**e**ye-opener)?

One positive response suggests a need for further assessment.
4. The **TWEAK** is recommended as an alcohol screening device for women.
   —How many drinks does it take before you begin to feel the first effects of alcohol? (This item assesses for **T**olerance. Three drinks or more is considered a positive response and scores two points.)
   —Have your friends or relatives **W**orried or complained about your drinking in the past year? (A positive response scores two points.)
   —Do you sometimes take a drink in the morning (**E**ye-opener) when you first get up? (Positive responses to this and the remaining items each score one point.)
   —Are there times when you drink and afterwards you can't remember what you said or did (**A**mnesia or blackouts)?
   —Do you sometimes feel the need to cut down on your drinking? (The **K** sound of the "c" of "Cut" completes the mnemonic.)
   A score of two or more for pregnant women and a score of three or more for other women suggests a need for further assessment.
5. The **Two-Item Conjoint Screen (TICS)** has nearly 80% sensitivity and specificity for an alcohol or drug disorder:
   —In the past year, have you ever drank or used drugs more than you meant to?
   —Have you ever felt you ought to cut down on your drinking or drug use?
   One positive response suggests a need for further assessment.
6. The **physical examination** commonly reveals clues to protracted substance abuse but is usually negative for early abusers. The odor of alcohol on a patient seeking nonurgent care is virtually diagnostic but not sensitive. Track marks and signs of injury to the nasal mucosa can suggest drug problems.
C. **Laboratory studies** sometimes provide clues to substance abuse.
   1. **Elevations in γ-glutamyltransferase (GGT)** levels can indicate alcohol abuse. Sensitivity ranges from 35% to 54%. Specificity is approximately 85%. False-positive results are due to obstructive liver disease and medications that induce microsomal enzymes. GGT diminishes within days of abstention.
   2. **Elevations in mean corpuscular volume** can indicate alcohol abuse. Macrocytosis can take months to resolve after cessation of drinking, and occurs in early alcohol abusers without vitamin B_{12} or folate deficiency.
   3. **Elevations in serum aspartate aminotransferase (AST)** levels (often double the serum alanine aminotransferase [ALT] level), **uric acid,** and **triglycerides** are common but nonspecific laboratory signs of excessive alcohol use.
   4. **Surreptitious urine drug testing** usually destroys the patient–physician relationship and confirms only recent drug use, not abuse. Parental worries about adolescent substance use can stem from a variety of individual and family problems. When a parent asks for a urine drug screen on an adolescent, seek permission from all adults and adolescents to perform or arrange a thorough family assessment along with the drug screen.
D. **Written questionnaires,** such as the Michigan Alcoholism Screening Test (MAST) and the Drug Abuse Screening Test (DAST), are quite insensitive to early substance abuse. The AUDIT (Alcohol Use Disorders Identification Test) is sensitive to early alcohol abuse, but many physicians consider this 10-item questionnaire too lengthy for routine use as a screening tool.
E. **Further assessment** is warranted when suspicions of substance abuse cannot be verified. Possible strategies include a family interview; referral to a substance abuse treatment expert for evaluation; and a 1-month trial of no substance use, or of specified, limited substance use, to assess the patient's ability to control substance use and the effect on potential adverse consequences. If the patient refuses these options, expressions of concern and watchful waiting for additional consequences are appropriate.
V. **Treatment**
   A. **Overview**
      1. The **ultimate goals** for the individual are to ameliorate the current effects of substance use and to prevent future negative consequences.
         a. For **substance-dependent patients,** these goals are usually best met by abstinence and strategies aimed at minimizing the frequency, duration,

and intensity of relapses. Traditional treatment objectives include full acceptance of the diagnosis and attenuation of potential triggers for relapse, including guilt and shame from previous substance use and its consequences, environmental cues such as peer pressure, family dysfunction, and coexisting psychiatric disorders.

    b. For many **at-risk users** and **substance abusers,** these goals can be met by reducing consumption and modifying circumstances of substance use.

  2. Research comparing the efficacy of treatment modalities has been hampered by the difficulty in identifying or creating comparable groups entering treatment. Studies suggest, however, that all forms of treatment have some efficacy. Twenty-five percent to 30% of abusers exhibit spontaneous improvement in 1 year. Thirty percent of the most chronic dependents have an improved quality of life 1 year posttreatment. This rate increases to 60–70% for individuals with intact jobs and families, and to 90% for practicing physicians. Optimal treatment plans take into account patients' individual characteristics, such as cultural background, sexual preference, and need for child care or special hours that would allow retention of employment.

B. Treatment options

  1. Physician-administered brief interventions may suffice for early abusers and at-risk users (see section VI,D).

  2. Self-help programs such as Alcoholics Anonymous should be a mainstay of treatment for substance-dependent patients who will embrace them.

  3. Professionally administered outpatient treatment, including individual, group, and family therapies, appears to enhance the efficacy of self-help programs and may succeed without them.

  4. Inpatient programs are recommended primarily for patients who cannot remain abstinent in outpatient programs.

  5. Halfway houses and day programs are recommended for patients who have the most chronic, resistant problems and require a structured environment to prevent relapse.

  6. Family treatment. Al-Anon and Al-A-Teen may be extremely helpful for family members, whether or not the abuser chooses treatment. These programs help family members face *their* problems and their limitations in controlling others' substance use. For some individuals, family therapy is an important component of treatment; sometimes it succeeds as the sole treatment. Some adult children of alcoholics (ACOAs) may have difficulties forming stable relationships and may benefit from ACOA meetings, psychotherapy, or both.

C. Assessment and treatment for withdrawal. Before advising patients to abstain or decrease consumption, assess the potential for withdrawal. For patients without unstable medical conditions, detoxification from opioids, cocaine, other stimulants, and hallucinogens is not life-threatening. Withdrawal from alcohol and other sedative–hypnotic drugs can be fatal. Patients with prior severe reactions to sedative withdrawal, complicating medical conditions, inability to abstain, or poor social support should be detoxified under supervision.

  1. Alcohol withdrawal

    a. Diazepam, chlordiazepoxide, and phenobarbital are the drugs most commonly used to treat alcohol withdrawal. Minor withdrawal (eg, agitation, tachycardia, hypertension, tremor, agitation, nausea, and sleep disturbance) can be treated with diazepam, 10–20 mg orally or intravenously (or equivalent), every 2 hours until mild sedation occurs. For major withdrawal (hallucinations plus exacerbation of the above symptoms), this dose should be repeated every 30 minutes until mild sedation is achieved. Often, a total dose of 60–200 mg is required. Once the patient is mildly sedated, additional doses should be given only as needed. Infrequent reevaluation of the patient is the most common cause of poor outcomes, such as aspiration or delirium tremens, which is severe major withdrawal plus disorientation. Most withdrawal seizures are self-limited. If prolonged seizures do not respond to benzodiazepines, carbamazepine is preferred over phenytoin, and intracranial injury should be considered.

    b. Shorter-acting medications such as **lorazepam** are indicated only for patients with severe hepatic dysfunction. The patient may be given 5 mg orally or intramuscularly every 30–120 minutes until mild sedation occurs and then 2–4 mg every 4 hours for 24 hours. The dose should be decreased by one-third on each succeeding day.

   c. **Vitamins and minerals** should be given to patients at risk for or experiencing alcohol withdrawal. Thiamine, 100 mg orally or intramuscularly every day for 3 days; folate, 1 mg orally every day; and multivitamins are indicated. To prevent seizures, hypomagnesemic patients should receive 2 mL of 50% magnesium sulfate intramuscularly every 4–8 hours until normal levels are restored.

   d. **β-Adrenergic blockers** such as **propranolol,** 20 mg every 6 hours, or **atenolol,** 50–100 mg every day for 2–3 days, may ameliorate some symptoms but mask autonomic signs that may warn of more severe alcohol withdrawal.

   e. **Haloperidol,** 1–2 mg orally or intramuscularly every 4 hours, may be used to control hallucinations that do not respond to sedatives. Other antipsychotics are more likely to precipitate seizures.

  2. **Benzodiazepine detoxification** is best accomplished with a long-acting benzodiazepine or phenobarbital, which should be tapered over 8–12 weeks. The taper must be particularly gradual as very low doses are reached. Alternatively, benzodiazepines may be reduced by one-third the starting dose for each of 3 days with initiation of carbamazepine, 200 mg three times a day, adjusted after 1 week to a serum level of 7–12 mg/mL, maintained for an additional 2 weeks, and then tapered over several days.

  3. **Withdrawal from other sedative–hypnotics** should be treated with an initial daily dose of 30 mg of phenobarbital for each 50 mg of butabarbital; 100 mg of amobarbital, pentobarbital, or secobarbital; 250 mg of chloral hydrate or glutethimide; or 400 mg of meprobamate. This daily dose should be divided every 6 hours and tapered over 1–2 weeks.

  4. **Opioid withdrawal**

   a. **Daily methadone,** tapered over 1–2 weeks, provides the most comfortable withdrawal from opiates. The starting daily dose is 10–40 mg and can be determined by the patient's response to as many as four 10-mg test doses during the first 24 hours. Pregnant women who are dependent on narcotics should be maintained on 10–20 mg of methadone, since opiate withdrawal may cause fetal demise, especially in the first trimester.

   b. **Clonidine** (a 0.1-mg test dose followed by up to 0.3 mg orally every 4 hours or the equivalent transdermal preparation) can control autonomic symptoms. Anticholinergic medications, nonsteroidal anti-inflammatory drugs, and hypnotics may be used at their usual doses for relief of other symptoms.

 D. **Adjunctive pharmacologic treatment**

  1. **Naltrexone,** 50 mg, reduces the cravings for alcohol by alcohol-dependent patients and increases retention and success in treatment.

  2. **Desipramine,** 75–200 mg orally every day, may reduce the cravings of cocaine addicts, but is, at best, an adjunct to other treatment.

  3. **Disulfiram,** 125–500 mg orally every day, and **naltrexone,** 50 mg orally every day after an initial 0.8-mg test dose of naloxone IV, can be helpful adjuncts for the treatment of alcohol and opioid dependence, respectively.

  4. **Methadone maintenance** sustains physical dependence on opioids, while ameliorating most of the negative consequences of opioid dependence. Many studies have demonstrated its effectiveness.

VI. **Management strategies**

 A. **Eliciting the patient's acceptance** of the need for and commitment to behavioral change is the first, most crucial, and often most difficult step. Prochaska's stages of readiness for behavioral change and Miller's motivational interviewing techniques provide a useful framework for promoting change. The stages of behavioral change are listed below.

  1. **Precontemplation.** Patients in this stage are not even considering whether to decrease their substance use. Aim questions and information to help patients determine whether continued substance use will allow them to attain their goals for themselves and other individuals important to them. For patients who have learned helplessness from previous relapses, reframe failures to helpful learning experiences.

2. **Contemplation.** Patients in this stage are ambivalent about decreasing their substance use. Questions and information should help them weigh the pros and cons of continuing their substance use relative to their goals. Other ways of attaining the advantages of continued substance use should be explored.
3. **Preparation.** Patients in this stage have decided to decrease their substance use soon, often within 1 month. Questions and information should help them identify the behavioral strategies that will work best for them. Positive reinforcement of their decision is helpful.
4. **Action.** Patients in this stage have begun to change their behaviors. Provide positive feedback, encouragement, emotional support, and assistance in identifying and managing new cues and impulses to resume their previous behaviors.
5. **Maintenance.** Patients in this stage have learned their new behaviors well but remain susceptible to relapse. Patients should be monitored for adherence to their behavioral strategies. Possible indications of impending or current relapse are nonadherence to treatment plans, cessation of pharmacologic therapy, failure to keep appointments, and any potential adverse consequence of substance use.
6. **Termination.** In this stage, maintenance of the behavior change is well learned and almost automatic. Many substance-dependent patients in recovery never reach this stage.

B. The **process of behavioral change** is dynamic and difficult to predict. Patients may move forward and backward through the above stages. Effective clinicians understand and accept where patients are in their process of change and aim their counseling accordingly.

C. **Patient education** can help patients accept their need to change. Clinicians must discuss honestly and supportively with patients how their substance use hurts or jeopardizes their lives. Blamelessness for having these problems, their commonness, their lack of association with undesirable character traits such as weakness, and their amenability to assistance can help patients accept their condition. For most patients with severe disorders, eventual acceptance and understanding of their diagnosis are helpful. For patients with less severe disorders, and initially for most patients, diagnostic labeling can impede acceptance of the need for behavioral change.

D. **Brief interventions** consist of feedback to patients on their substance use, education about their risk or consequences, a suggestion to quit or cut down, a negotiation around future substance use, concrete and specific goal setting, and follow-up. In several randomized controlled trials for alcohol abuse or at-risk drinking, brief interventions have resulted in decreased alcohol use, fewer hospitalizations, and improved work attendance.

E. **Behavioral contracts** can be useful. For patients willing to accept the need for change but not treatment, contracts to accept treatment in the event of further consumption or negative consequences should be attempted. For patients who are ambivalent about the need for change, 1-month trials of abstinence or decreased substance use can help patients determine whether their substance use was harmful and whether it is under their control. For those able to reduce consumption, negotiate long-term plans for safer substance use. For those who are not, recommend abstinence and treatment.

F. **Johnson's "intervention"** is a risky but usually effective tool for engaging in treatment the most chronic, resistant substance-dependent patients. At a meeting arranged as a surprise to the substance-dependent individual, caring associates (eg, family members, friends, coworkers, clergy, and physicians) cite firsthand evidence of the problem and insist on immediate acceptance of treatment. Intervention should be coordinated by a trained professional.

G. **Family dynamics** can be important in the maintenance, if not the initiation, of substance-related disorders. Family members are to be held as blameless as the individual who is abusing substances. Family members often need help to avoid enabling (ie, allowing the abuser to continue abusing without facing the natural consequences of the abuse) and allowing a recovering individual to resume normal family roles and responsibilities. Engage family members in treatment by emphasizing that the family needs help to recover whether or not the substance abuse continues.

H. Clinicians' beliefs about substance abuse can interfere with their effectiveness. Challenge pessimism and judgmental views toward substance abusers by witnessing recovery at self-help group meetings and treatment programs.

I. Prevention for youth
1. **Later onset of substance use** is associated with fewer substance-related problems.
2. **Closer parental supervision and moderate consumption of alcohol by parents** are associated with less substance use by offspring.
3. **Imparting knowledge** alone does not alter substance-related behaviors.
4. **School-based programs** can be effective. Factors linked to effectiveness include a focus on refusal skills, booster sessions, peer trainers, involvement of parents and teachers, and links with local media.

VII. Natural history and prognosis. Substance abuse and dependence follow variably relapsing and remitting courses, much like rheumatoid arthritis. Most individuals in remission have never received treatment or professional advice. Some individuals with substance-related problems respond to advice and do not have further adverse consequences. Many have unpredictable, intermittent flares of uncontrolled substance use that may remit spontaneously. Others have a progressive course despite treatment and strong motivation, especially males with a young age at onset and a strong family history. Adverse consequences of substance abuse may occur in all facets of patients' lives and comprise the symptoms of substance abuse.

A. Biomedical consequences. Alcohol abuse contributes to many major causes of mortality, including cardiovascular diseases, selected cancers, cirrhosis, suicide, and trauma, including motor vehicle accidents.
1. Early consequences of alcohol abuse include dyspepsia, gastritis, nonhealing peptic ulcers, acute or subclinical pancreatitis, chronic diarrhea, labile or unresponsive hypertension, weight gain, and injuries from accidents and altercations. Common consequences of protracted, excessive alcohol consumption include hepatitis, cirrhosis, chronic pancreatitis, cardiomyopathy, bone marrow suppression, dementia, neuropathy, malnutrition, and several types of cancer.
2. Episodes of intoxication may result in aspiration pneumonia, trauma, and blackouts, which are losses of memory for events while intoxicated.
3. Loss of interest in food and sex often accompanies cocaine abuse. Acutely, cocaine can cause arrhythmias and coronary or other arterial vasospasm. Chronic cocaine snorting can lead to vasoconstrictive injury to the nasal mucosa.
4. Individuals who barter sex for drugs may present frequently with sexually transmitted diseases.
5. Intravenous drug abuse, commonly of heroin, cocaine, or amphetamines, causes local skin and soft tissue infection, endocarditis, viral hepatitis, and human immunodeficiency virus (HIV). As homosexual males have increasingly practiced safe sex, intravenous drug abuse and other substance abuse, through its association with risky sexual behavior, have become more important causes of HIV transmission.
6. Overuse of narcotics, stimulants, or phencyclidine (PCP) and withdrawal from sedatives can produce seizures.
7. Complaints regarding sleep and sexual performance are common among abusers of alcohol and many other drugs.
8. Maternal alcohol use in the first trimester may cause full-blown fetal alcohol syndrome or partial fetal alcohol effect.
9. Ongoing controlled studies will determine whether maternal cocaine use or related environmental factors cause behavior and learning problems in offspring.

B. Psychological consequences
1. The most common psychological effects of substance abuse are situational anxiety and depressive symptoms emanating from the consequences of abuse. Patients may present with somatic symptoms, such as headache, back pain, and abdominal discomfort.
2. Use of even small quantities of alcohol or other drugs can precipitate anxiety disorders, major depression, or psychosis in susceptible individuals.
3. Withdrawal from benzodiazepines and other sedatives produces agitation. Cessation of cocaine use can induce a depressive state.

        4. Amphetamines can cause episodes of psychosis that mimic schizophrenia.
- **C. Family dysfunction.** Substance abuse may be a manifestation or source of family dysfunction.
    1. Child and spouse abuse and violence are obvious consequences of substance abuse (see Chapter 95).
    2. Marital problems; behavioral problems in children (eg, discipline problems or a decline in school performance); and anxiety, depression, and somatic symptoms in family members of substance abusers are common. Family dissolution may occur, but denial and embarrassment of family members often lead to chronic, stable family dysfunction, with rigid roles and stunted growth and maturation.
    3. ACOAs and adult children of other drug abusers may be at risk for difficulties with self-esteem, close relationships, perfectionism, and expression of feelings.
- **D. Social problems.** Substance abusers often alienate nonabusing friends and gravitate toward individuals with similar lifestyles. Much of crime is linked to substance abuse.
- **E. Work or school difficulties.** Performance at work and school often drops, although in highly motivated students or professionals, including those in health care, it may be preserved. Other signs of work or school difficulties are frequent changes of job or selection of employment that allows intoxication, absences, especially on Mondays, and requests for notes from physicians.
- **F. Legal and financial problems**
    1. Most people arrested for driving while intoxicated have a substance-related disorder. Fights and other disruptive behaviors also can lead to arrest.
    2. Substance abuse is expensive and may result in theft and drug dealing, even among middle-class individuals. Selling of personal and family items is common among cocaine abusers.

REFERENCES

American Psychiatric Association (APA): *Diagnostic and Statistical Manual of Mental Health Disorders,* 4th edition (DSM-IV). APA; 1994.

Botvin GJ, et al: Long-term follow-up results of a randomized drug abuse prevention trial in a white middle-class population. JAMA 1995;**273:**1106.

Department of Health and Human Services (DHHS): *Drug Abuse and Drug Research: The Third Triennial Report to Congress* (ADM 91-1704). DHHS; 1991.

Department of Health and Human Services (DHHS): *Eighth Special Report to the U.S. Congress on Alcohol and Health* (NIH Publication No. 94-3699). DHHS; 1994.

Fleming MF, Barry KL: *Addictive Disorders.* Mosby–Year Book; 1992.

Institute of Medicine: *Broadening the Base for Treatment for Alcohol Problems.* National Academy Press; 1990.

Institute of Medicine: *Treating Drug Problems,* vol 1. National Academy Press; 1990.

Miller WR, Rollnick S: *Motivational Interviewing: Preparing People to Change Addictive Behavior.* Guilford; 1991.

Prochaska JO, DiClemente CC, Norcross JC: In search of how people change: Applications to addictive behaviors. Am Psychologist 1992;**47:**1102.

Volpicelli JR, Alterman AI, Hayashida M, et al: Naltrexone in the treatment of alcohol dependence. Arch Gen Psychiatry 1992;**49:**876.

---

93   Anxiety

John C. Rogers, MD, MPH

- **I. Definition.**
    - **A. Generalized anxiety disorder** is a syndrome of excessive or unrealistic anxiety or worry about two or more life circumstances for 6 months or longer.
    - **B. Panic disorder** is the recurrence of episodic periods of intense fear or apprehension accompanied by at least four somatic symptoms, such as diaphoresis, dyspnea, faintness, paresthesias, or flushing.

C. A **phobia** is a persistent fear of an object, activity, or situation that is out of proportion to the objective danger.

D. **Post-traumatic stress disorder** develops after an individual experiences emotionally or physically distressing events that are outside the range of usual human experience and would be extremely traumatic for virtually any person. Examples include combat experience, natural catastrophes, assault, rape, serious threat or harm to one's family members, or sudden destruction of one's home or community.

II. Diagnoses

A. **Generalized anxiety disorder.** Diagnostic criteria are specified in Table 93–1. Diagnoses that must be ruled out include medical disorders and diagnosable mental disorders.

1. **Biomedical disorders** may include thyrotoxicosis, paroxysmal atrial tachycardia, mitral valve prolapse, hyperventilation, caffeine intoxication, stimulant abuse, alcohol withdrawal, and sedative or hypnotic withdrawal.

2. **Mental disorders** may include panic disorder, phobias, obsessive–compulsive disorder, adjustment disorder with anxious mood, depression, dysthymia, somatization disorder, and schizophrenia.

B. **Panic disorder.** Diagnostic criteria are displayed in Table 93–2. **Panic attacks,** which are spontaneous, unexpected episodes that occur in the absence of any apparent precipitant, generally last no more than 20–30 minutes, with attacks of 1 hour being rare. Fear without any apparent source and an impending sense of death and doom are characteristic. Such mental thoughts are associated with somatic symptoms, typically tachycardia, palpitations, dyspnea, and sweating. As many as 20% of patients may experience syncope during panic attacks.

C. **Phobia.** Diagnostic criteria are listed in Table 93–3.

1. The most common **biomedical disorders** are intoxication with hallucinogens, sympathomimetics, and other drugs of abuse; small cerebral tumor; and cerebrovascular accidents.

2. The most common **mental disorders** in the differential diagnoses are depression, schizophrenia, obsessive–compulsive disorder, and personality disorders (schizoid, avoidance, or paranoid).

D. **Post-traumatic stress disorder.** Diagnostic criteria are specified in Table 93–4.

1. **Biomedical conditions** to be ruled out include head injury and alcohol and drug abuse.

TABLE 93–1. DIAGNOSTIC CRITERIA FOR GENERALIZED ANXIETY DISORDER

A. Excessive anxiety and worry (apprehensive expectation), occurring more days than not for at least 6 months, about a number of events or activities (eg, work or school performance)

B. The person finds it difficult to control the worry

C. The anxiety and worry are associated with three or more of the following six symptoms (with at least some symptoms present for more days than not for the past 6 months). **Note:** Only one item is required in children
  (1) Restlessness or feeling keyed up or on edge
  (2) Being easily fatigued
  (3) Difficulty concentrating or mind going blank
  (4) Irritability
  (5) Muscle tension
  (6) Sleep disturbance (difficulty falling or staying asleep, or restless unsatisfying sleep)

D. The focus of the anxiety and worry is not confined to features of an axis I disorder; for example, the anxiety or worry is not about having a panic attack (as in panic disorder), being embarrassed in public (as in social phobia), being contaminated (as in obsessive–compulsive disorder), being away from home or close relatives (as in separation anxiety disorder), gaining weight (as in anorexia nervosa), having multiple physical complaints (as in somatization disorder), or having a serious illness (as in hypochondriasis), and the anxiety and worry do not occur exclusively during post-traumatic stress disorder

E. The anxiety, worry, or physical symptoms cause clinically significant distress or impairment in social, occupational, or other important areas of functioning

F. The disturbance is not due to the direct physiologic effects of a substance (eg, a drug of abuse or a medication) or a general medical condition (eg, hyperthyroidism) and does not occur exclusively during a mood disorder, psychotic disorder, or pervasive developmental disorder

---

Adapted with permission from American Psychiatric Association (APA): *Diagnostic and Statistical Manual of Mental Disorders,* 4th ed. APA; 1994.

TABLE 93–2. DIAGNOSTIC CRITERIA FOR PANIC DISORDER WITHOUT AGORAPHOBIA

A. Both (1) and (2):
   (1) Recurrent, unexpected panic attacks (see below)
   (2) At least one of the attacks has been followed by 1 month (or more) of one or more of the following:
       (a) Persistent concern about having additional attacks
       (b) Worry about the implications of the attack or its consequences (eg, losing control, having a heart attack, or "going crazy")
       (c) A significant change in behavior related to the attacks
B. Absence of agoraphobia
C. The panic attacks are not caused by the direct physiologic effects of a substance (eg, a drug of abuse or a medication) or a general medical condition (eg, hyperthyroidism)
D. The panic attacks are not better accounted for by another mental disorder, such as social phobia (eg, occurring upon exposure to feared social situations), specific phobia (eg, on exposure to a specific phobic situation), obsessive–compulsive disorder (eg, upon exposure to dirt in someone with an obsession about contamination), post-traumatic stress disorder (eg, in response to stimuli associated with a severe stressor), or separation anxiety disorder (eg, in response to being away from home or close relatives)
E. Criteria for panic attack: A discrete period of intense fear or discomfort, in which four or more of the following symptoms developed abruptly and reached a peak within 10 minutes
       (1) Palpitations, pounding heart, or accelerated heart rate
       (2) Sweating
       (3) Trembling or shaking
       (4) Sensations of shortness of breath or smothering
       (5) Feeling of choking
       (6) Chest pain or discomfort
       (7) Nausea or abdominal distress
       (8) Feeling dizzy, unsteady, lightheaded, or faint
       (9) Derealization (feelings of unreality) or depersonalization (being detached from oneself)
       (10) Fear of losing control or going crazy
       (11) Fear of dying
       (12) Paresthesia (numbness or tingling sensations)
       (13) Chills or hot flushes

Adapted with permission from American Psychiatric Association (APA): *Diagnostic and Statistical Manual of Mental Disorders,* 4th ed. APA; 1994.

TABLE 93–3. DIAGNOSTIC CRITERIA FOR SPECIFIC PHOBIA

A. Marked and persistent fear that is excessive or unreasonable, cued by the presence or anticipation of a specific object or situation (eg, flying, heights, animals, receiving an injection, or seeing blood).
B. Exposure to the phobic stimulus almost invariably provokes an immediate anxiety response, which may take the form of a situationally bound or situationally predisposed panic attack. **Note:** In children, the anxiety may be expressed by crying, tantrums, freezing, or clinging.
C. The person recognizes that the fear is excessive or unreasonable. **Note:** In children, this feature may be absent.
D. The phobic situation(s) is avoided or else is endured with intense anxiety or distress.
E. The avoidance, anxious anticipation, or distress in the feared situation(s) interferes significantly with the person's normal routine, occupational (or academic) functioning, or social activities or relationships, or there is marked distress about having the phobia.
F. In individuals under age 18 years, the duration is at least 6 months.
G. The anxiety panic attacks, or phobic avoidance associated with the specific object or situation, are not better accounted for by another mental disorder, such as obsessive–compulsive disorder (eg, fear of dirt in someone with an obsession about contamination), post-traumatic stress disorder (eg, avoidance of stimuli associated with a severe stressor), separation anxiety disorder (eg, avoidance of school), social phobia (eg, avoidance of social situations because of fear of embarrassment), panic disorder with agoraphobia, or agoraphobia without history of panic disorder. Specify type.

       (1) Animal type
       (2) Natural environment type (eg, heights, storms, or water)
       (3) Blood–injection–injury type
       (4) Situational type (eg, airplanes, elevators, or enclosed places)
       (5) Other type (eg, phobic avoidance of situations that may lead to choking, vomiting, or contracting an illness; in children, avoidance of loud sounds or costumed characters).

Adapted with permission from American Psychiatric Association (APA): *Diagnostic and Statistical Manual of Mental Disorders,* 4th ed. APA; 1994.

TABLE 93–4. DIAGNOSTIC CRITERIA FOR POST-TRAUMATIC STRESS DISORDER

A. The person has been exposed to a traumatic event in which both of the following were present:
  (1) The person experienced, witnessed, or was confronted with an event or events that involved actual or threatened death or serious injury, or a threat to the physical integrity of self or others
  (2) The person's response involved intense fear, helplessness or horror. **Note:** In children, this may be expressed instead by disorganized or agitated behavior
B. The traumatic event is persistently re-experienced in one or more of the following ways:
  (1) Recurrent and intrusive distressing recollections of the event, including images, thoughts, or perceptions. **Note:** In young children, repetitive play may occur in which themes or aspects of the trauma are expressed
  (2) Recurrent distressing dreams of the event. **Note:** In children, there may be frightening dreams without recognizable content
  (3) Acting or feeling as if the traumatic event were recurring (includes a sense of reliving the experience, illusions, hallucinations, and dissociative flashback episodes, including those that occur upon awakening or when intoxicated). **Note:** In young children, trauma-specific re-enactment may occur
  (4) Intense psychological distress at exposure to internal or external cues that symbolize or resemble an aspect of the traumatic event
  (5) Physiologic reactivity upon exposure to internal or external cues that symbolize or resemble an aspect of the traumatic event
C. Persistent avoidance of stimuli associated with the trauma and numbing of general responsiveness (not present before the trauma), as indicated by at least three or more of the following:
  (1) Efforts to avoid thoughts, feelings, or conversations associated with the trauma
  (2) Efforts to avoid activities, places, or people that arouse recollections of the trauma
  (3) Inability to recall an important aspect of the trauma
  (4) Markedly diminished interest or participation in significant activities
  (5) Feeling of detachment or estrangement from others
  (6) Restricted range of affect (eg, unable to have loving feelings)
  (7) Sense of a foreshortened future (eg, does not expect to have a career, marriage, children, or normal life span)
D. Persistent symptoms of increased arousal (not present before the trauma), as indicated by two or more of the following:
  (1) Difficulty falling or staying asleep
  (2) Irritability or outbursts of anger
  (3) Difficulty concentrating
  (4) Hypervigilance
  (5) Exaggerated startle response
E. Duration of the disturbance (symptoms in B, C, and D) is more than 1 month.
F. The disturbance causes clinically significant distress or impairment in social, occupational, or other important areas of functioning. Specify if:

  Acute: if duration of symptoms is less than 3 months
  Chronic: if duration of symptoms is 3 months or more

  Specify if:
  With delayed onset: if onset of symptoms is at least 6 months after the stressor

Adapted with permission from American Psychiatric Association (APA): *Diagnostic and Statistical Manual of Mental Disorders,* 4th ed. APA; 1994.

    2. Psychiatric conditions include generalized anxiety disorder, panic disorder, depression, adjustment reaction, factitious disorder, malingering, borderline personality disorder, and schizophrenia.

III. Epidemiology
    A. Generalized anxiety disorder is the fourth most common mental disorder, following substance abuse, major depressive disorder, and phobias. Two percent to 5% of the US population exhibits this disorder in any given year.

      1. The mean age at onset of symptoms is in the mid-20s, with most cases developing between the ages of 16 and 40. The mean duration of symptoms before treatment is about 5 years.

      2. In the general medical care setting, the female–male ratio is 2–3:1, but among psychiatric patients, the sex ratio is 1:1. First- and second-degree relatives of a person affected by generalized anxiety disorder have at least a threefold increased risk of being affected.

      3. Comorbidity with depression is frequent (just over 50% of depressed patients have concurrent generalized anxiety disorder).

   B. Panic disorder occurs in 1.4% of the US population.
   1. The mean age at presentation is 25 years, with onset generally between 17 and 30 years of age.
   2. The female–male ratio is 2.5–3 : 1. This disorder has a familial tendency, with first-degree relatives having a twofold increased risk of being affected compared to control subjects.
   3. Comorbidity with depression occurs (nearly 10% of depressed patients have panic disorder) and leads to more frequent and severe symptoms.
   C. Phobia is the most common anxiety disorder. Fifteen percent to 20% of the population may be affected by phobias.
   1. Social phobia usually begins during the early to late teens. Simple phobias can begin at any age, however, depending on typical exposure to the object or situation. The most common objects of simple phobia are, in descending order and frequency, animals, storms, heights, illness, and death.
   2. Social phobia is reportedly more frequent in males than in females, whereas simple phobias are more frequent in females than in males.
   3. Comorbidity with depression is common (over 20% of depressed patients have concurrent phobia).
   D. Post-traumatic stress disorder affects 0.5% of men and 1.2% of women in the general population. Onset may be at any age, but because of the types of precipitating situations that are most common, this disorder is most common in young adults. The initiating trauma for men is usually combat experience. The initiating trauma for women is most often assault or rape.
IV. Pathophysiology
   A. Generalized anxiety disorder
   1. Psychosocial theories about the genesis of the anxiety include stress, psychoanalytic, behavioral, and existential theories. Stress is the imbalance between perceived threats or pressures and a person's resources and coping responses. Chronic stress produces the psychological and biologic characteristics of anxiety. Patients with this disorder tend to have increased sympathetic tone and to overrespond autonomically to stimuli.
   2. Noradrenergic and serotoninergic systems in the frontal and limbic lobes of the brain, along with increased γ-aminobutyric acid (GABA) activity, are believed to be involved in this disorder.
   B. Panic disorder
   1. A general cognitive model of anxiety proposes that all persons scan the environment for threats and cognitively appraise stimuli for potential danger. Pathologic anxiety arises from errors in cognitive appraisal, such as overestimating the likelihood and severity of a feared event and underestimating coping resources and social support factors.
   2. The autonomic nervous systems of patients with panic disorder tend to exhibit increased sympathetic tone, adapt more slowly to repeated stimuli, and respond excessively to moderate stimuli. Abnormalities in the hippocampus, locus ceruleus, and GABA–benzodiazepine receptors have been associated with this disorder.
   C. Phobias
   1. Psychoanalytic theory suggests that a fundamental anxiety (eg, separation) is displaced onto a symbol that can then be avoided to escape underlying anxiety.
   2. Behavioral theory proposes a traditional stimulus–response model of conditioned reflex in which the object of the phobia is a neutral stimulus that was contiguous with an active stimulus. Operant conditioning then occurs when avoidance of the now active stimulus is reinforced by diminished anxiety.
   D. Post-traumatic stress disorder. The cause of this disorder is related to the severity of stressor, the social environment of the victim and availability of social supports, the personality traits of the victim, and the victim's premorbid biologic vulnerability.
   1. Biologic theories propose that individuals affected by this disorder are prone to excessive autonomic reactions to stress and that symptoms may result from an endogenous opiate withdrawal syndrome.
   2. Psychoanalytic theories propose that the trauma reactivates incautious, unresolved conflicts from early childhood. Secondary gain from the patient's

environment may also be involved, such as increased attention or monetary gain.

V. Treatment

A. Generalized anxiety disorder treatment is directed toward reduction in symptoms so that patients can function in relationships and work. To achieve this goal, the physician must provide patience, realistic reassurance, education about the condition, and encouragement to socialize and assume work and family responsibilities.

1. **Elimination of caffeine and other stimulants** and **regular exercise** may help reduce symptoms.

2. **Pharmacologic therapy**

   a. **Benzodiazepines** have been the mainstay of pharmacologic treatment of this disorder. The pharmacologic properties of common benzodiazepines are displayed in Table 93–5. Patients respond best to anxiolytic agents with short half-lives. Use of rapid-acting benzodiazepine as needed may be superior to routine dosing. The problems with the use of these drugs are that 20–30% of patients fail to respond to these agents, tolerance and dependence may occur, and impaired alertness and increased risk of accidents are possible.

   b. **Antidepressants** such as **imipramine** are being used more frequently to treat this disorder. Imipramine starts at 50–75 mg/day and is increased every 2 weeks, depending on response, to a maximum of 150 mg/day in divided doses. The efficacy of monoamine oxidase (MAO) inhibitors is unknown. Selective serotonin reuptake inhibitors (SSRIs) have shown comparable efficacy to benzodiazepines in acute treatment of generalized anxiety disorder and are appropriate for patients with concurrent depression.

   c. **Beta blockers** are used to treat peripheral somatic symptoms such as tremor or palpitation. **Propranolol** can be started at 60–80 mg/day in divided doses and gradually increased to optimum response or a maximum dose of 240 mg/day. Combination of a beta blocker and a benzodiazepine is more effective than a benzodiazepine alone.

   d. **Azapirones** act on the serotoninergic system and may become the drug of choice for this disorder. These drugs do not act through the GABA–benzodiazepine receptor complex, so problems of tolerance, dependence, and impaired alertness are avoided. The available azapirone buspirone, should be started at 5 mg three times a day for 3–7 days and then increased to 10 mg twice or three times daily, the usual maintenance dose. The dose should not exceed 60 mg/day.

B. Panic disorder treatment is directed toward control of symptoms so that the patient may be as functional as possible.

1. **Selective serotonin reuptake inhibitors** are being considered as the first-line pharmacologic treatment: they are as effective as benzodiazepines in improving anxiety, have fewer side effects than the alternatives, have no interference with cognitive behavioral therapy, and provide treatment of concurrent depression. Fluoxetine, 5–40 mg/day, is recommended as a single morning dose. The starting dose is 5 mg (2 mg if there is significant insomnia or agitation) with increases each week. The dose for sertraline is 25 mg/day to start with a maximum of 200 mg/day. The starting dose for paroxetine is 10 mg/day with 50 mg/day maximum. Fluvoxamine starts at 25 mg twice a day, with a maximum of 150 mg twice a day. Full response occurs after at least 4 weeks, and perhaps 8–12 weeks. Treatment should continue for 12–24 months with slow discontinuation over 4–6 months.

2. **Tricyclic antidepressants. Imipramine** and **desipramine** are effective agents. Imipramine, 150–300 mg/day, is recommended as a single bedtime dose. The starting dose is 50–100 mg/day, which can be increased every 2 weeks until an optimum response or maximum dose is reached. Desipramine is sometimes better tolerated by patients than is imipramine.

3. **MAO inhibitors. Phenelzine,** 45–90 mg/day, and iproniazid, up to 150 mg/day, are effective in controlling symptoms. Administration of MAO inhibitors may be either divided equally three times a day or given according to whether an activating or sedating effect occurs in the patient, in which case a morning dose (activating effect) or an evening dose (sedating effect) is prescribed

TABLE 93–5. DRUG TREATMENT OF ANXIETY DISORDERS

Drug	Starting Dosage (mg)	Usual Daily Dosage (mg)	Maximum Daily Dosage (mg)	Rate of Onset	Half-life (hr)	Common Side Effects
Benzodiazepines						
Alprazolam (Xanax)	0.25 tid	0.5–4	10	Intermediate	12–15	Transient drowsiness, alexia, confusion, depression
Chlordiazepoxide (Librium, Lipoxide, Mitran, etc)	5 tid or qid	15–80	100	Intermediate	5–30	Withdrawal symptoms upon abrupt discontinuation
Clorazepate (Tranxene)	7.5 qd or bid	15–30	60	Rapid	30–100	
Diazepam (Valium, Vazepam)	2 bid–qid	4–40	40	Very rapid	20–80	
Halazepam (Paxipam)	20 tid or qid	60–160	160	Intermediate to slow	14	
Lorazepam (Alzapam, Ativan)	1 bid or tid	2–4	10	Intermediate	10–20	
Oxazepam (Serax)	10–15 tid or qid	30–90	120	Intermediate to slow	5–20	
Prazepam (Centrax)	20 hs	20–40	60	Slow	30–100	
Azepirone						
Buspirone (BuSpar)	5 tid	20–30	60	Delayed	2–3	Dizziness, nervousness, nausea, headache
Tricyclic antidepressants						
Imipramine (Tofranil, Janimine)	75 qd or hs	50–150	200	Delayed	11–25	Sedation, anticholinergic effects, orthostatic hypertension
Desipramine (Norpramin, Pertofrane)	50 qd	100–200	300	Delayed	12–24	
Monoamine oxidase inhibitor						
Phenelzine (Nardil)	15 tid	45–60	90	Delayed	NA	Orthostatic hypotension, dizziness, jitteriness, overstimulation
Beta blockers						
Propranolol (Inderal)	40 bid	80–120	320	Rapid	3–5	Bradycardia, dizziness, fatigue, depression, impotence
Selective Serotonin Reuptake Inhibitors						
Fluoxetine (Prozac)	5 mg qd	10–20	40	Delayed	Days	Insomnia, agitation, anorgasmia
Sertraline (Zoloft)	25 mg qd	50–100	200	Delayed	26	Insomnia, nausea, sexual dysfunction
Paroxetine (Paxil)	10 mg qd	20–40	50	Delayed	21	Drowsiness, fatigue, delayed ejaculation
Fluvoxamine (Luvox)	25 mg bid	100–150	300	Delayed	15	Drowsiness, nausea, anorgasmia

to blend with the patient's sleep routines. The possibility of a serious reaction such as a hypertensive crisis or intracranial bleeding must be kept in mind, and patients must be warned to avoid certain foods and beverages.

4. **Benzodiazepines. Alprazolam** is as effective as imipramine and phenelzine in treating this disorder. Clonazepam and lorazepam also appear to be effective. High-dose diazepam (mean of 30 mg/day) can also markedly decrease panic attacks. The disadvantages of using benzodiazepines are that nearly half of patients with panic disorder have concurrent major depression that is not helped by benzodiazepines, abuse can be a potential problem, and benzodiazepines are more difficult to taper than are tricyclic antidepressants or MAO inhibitors.

C. Treatment of **phobia** requires commitment on the part of the patient and clear identification of the phobic object or situation.

1. **Behavioral treatment** techniques are the most effective, with systematic desensitization being used more frequently. A cognitive strategy of suggesting new ways of thinking about the phobic object or situation may be used in addition to muscle relaxation techniques.

2. **Pharmacologic therapy**

   a. **Beta blockers** such as propranolol may be useful just prior to direct challenge by the phobic situation. Propranolol, 10–20 mg 1 hour before exposure to the phobic object, or up to 40 mg, should be effective.

   b. **Tricyclic antidepressants, MAO inhibitors, and SSRIs** (fluvoxamine and sertraline) may be of use, particularly in patients with social phobia.

D. **Post-traumatic stress disorder** treatment consists primarily of psychotherapy. Pharmacotherapy is used most often when the patient has symptoms of depression or a paniclike disorder.

1. **Time-limited psychotherapy** uses cognitive and supportive approaches to minimize the risk of dependency and chronicity. The patient is encouraged to garner support from friends and relatives; to review emotional feelings associated with the event; to consciously re-enact the event through imagination, words, or actions; and to plan for future recovery. Group and family therapies have been particularly effective.

2. **Drug therapy** may include tricyclic antidepressants (amitriptyline and imipramine), MAO inhibitors (phenelzine), benzodiazepines, propranolol, lithium, anticonvulsants, or antipsychotic medications, such as chlorpromazine, trifluoperazine, or mesoridazine.

VI. **Management strategies**

A. **Generalized anxiety disorder.** Physician time and involvement need not be extensive. Education of the patient about the disorder and the scheduling of frequent, short office visits are the physician's primary responsibilities. Listening carefully to the patient's account of problems is very beneficial. Specific management techniques include being supportive of patient choices, expanding coping strategies, normalizing symptoms through reassurance, encouraging confrontation of anxiety-provoking situations, and being available for brief clinical encounters.

B. **Panic disorder.** Patients with panic disorder should be reassured that they have a treatable condition. The patient's somatic symptoms should be discussed in such a way as to avoid the attachment of any stigma to the patient. Eliciting the patient's explanation of the symptoms and goals for treatment is crucial. Behavioral treatment dealing with fear-provoking circumstances and psychotherapy for specific psychosocial problems are integral parts of the treatment plan.

C. **Phobias.** The goal of therapy is for the affected person to discover that the feared situation is not as much of a threat as previously thought. Avoidance should be discouraged, and behavioral techniques should be used until the phobic object or situation has been fully confronted. Hypnosis may be used as an adjunct method of relaxation and as a method of offering alternative cognitive appraisals of the phobic object. Family therapy may be particularly useful in this condition.

D. **Post-traumatic stress disorder.** Physicians caring for patients with this disorder must deal effectively with suspicion, paranoia, and mistrust on the part of the patient. Gentle confrontation is necessary to overcome the patient's denial of the traumatic event and to encourage the individual to remain in the treatment program of therapy and medications. Groups of individuals suffering similar events, such as assault self-help groups, may also be useful. Hospitalization may be necessary if the patient is suicidal or a danger to others.

VII. Natural history and prognosis

A. Generalized anxiety disorder is a chronic condition with a typical duration of illness just over 10 years. Affected individuals usually respond to treatment, but relapse after withdrawal of treatment may occur in as many as 80% of patients, nearly 25% of whom may go on to develop panic disorder.

B. Panic disorder is a chronic, remitting, and relapsing condition that is often precipitated by stressful life events. In one study, at 5-year follow-up, 30% of affected patients were moderately to severely impaired and 50% were mildly impaired; at 20-year follow-up, 15% had moderate to severe symptoms, and 70% had mild symptoms with no disability. Between 30% and 70% of patients experience a major depressive disorder subsequent to the onset of the panic attacks. These individuals are at increased risk for suicide, alcohol and drug dependence, and obsessive–compulsive disorder. Once an effective drug dose is achieved, the medication should be continued unchanged for 6–12 months. At that time, the medication is slowly tapered. Drug treatment should be reinstituted if symptoms return. Patients with good function prior to development of symptoms of brief duration tend to have a better prognosis.

C. Phobias beginning in childhood may resolve without treatment, but others may become chronic. Those that are chronic in nature seem to increase after middle age. Most affected individuals experience little disability, since the phobic object or situation can usually be easily avoided.

D. Post-traumatic stress disorder. The full syndrome usually develops sometime after the traumatic event, and delay can be from 1 week to as long as 30 years. Symptoms fluctuate with exacerbations during periods of stress. Individuals with a good prognosis usually have rapid onset of symptoms, symptoms of less than 6 months' duration, good functioning before the onset of the syndrome, strong social support, and the absence of any other medical or emotional disorders. Over time, 10% of affected patients remain unchanged or become worse, 20% have moderate symptoms, 40% have mild symptoms, and 30% recover.

REFERENCES

American Psychiatric Association (APA): *Diagnostic and Statistical Manual of Mental Disorders,* 4th ed. APA; 1994.

Peebles-Kleiger MJ, Zerbe KJ: Office management of posttraumatic stress disorder. A clinician's guide to a pervasive problem. Postgrad Med 1998;**103:**181, 187, 194.

Roy-Byrne P, Stein M, Bystrisky A, et al: Pharmacotherapy of panic disorder: Proposed guidelines for the family physician. J Am Board Fam Pract 1998;**11:**282.

Saeed AS, Bruce TJ: Panic disorder: Effective treatment options. Am Fam Physician 1998;**57:** 2405, 2419.

Sherbourne CD, Jackson CA, Meredith LS, et al: Prevalence of comorbid anxiety disorders in primary care outpatients. Arch Fam Med 1996;**5:**27.

---

94   Attention-Deficit/Hyperactivity Disorder

Thomas M. Johnson, PhD

I. Definition. Attention-deficit/hyperactivity disorder (ADHD), formerly termed "attention deficit disorder" or "ADD," is a neurologically based behavioral disorder characterized by symptoms of hyperactivity (excessive motor restlessness), impulsivity, inability to sustain attention, or all three. In order to meet criteria for ADHD, symptoms must be present prior to age 7, be maladaptive and inconsistent with developmental level, cause social impairment at least two settings, and not be associated with another psychiatric disorder. The *Diagnostic and Statistical Manual of Mental Disorders,* 4th edition (DSM-IV) describes three subtypes of ADHD:

A. A predominantly hyperactive–impulsive subtype (typically with more overt motor symptoms like fidgetiness)

B. A predominantly inattentive subtype (manifested by more subtle symptoms such as easy distractibility)

C. A mixed subtype (with features of both) ADHD also is recognized to persist into adulthood, although usually not with the same array of signs and symptoms. In such cases, the terms "residual type" or "in partial remission" are used.

II. Epidemiology. Prevalence estimates in the United States vary from 2% to 20% depending on the diagnostic criteria used. Clinical practice among school-age children suggests a true prevalence of 6–8%, making ADHD the most common chronic behavioral disorder in this age group. More children are being diagnosed and treated now than in the past, but it is unclear whether the true prevalence is increasing or if the increase in rates is a result of better surveillance. An estimated 60% of children with ADHD will have at least one residual symptom persisting into adulthood.

A. Although DSM criteria stipulate that symptoms occur prior to age 7, most children with ADHD exhibit symptoms before age 3.

B. ADHD formerly was thought to occur in a male to female ratio of from 4 : 1 to 9 : 1, but more recent data suggest that only the predominantly hyperactive forms of ADHD appears more often in boys than girls. The sex ratio may be as low as 2 : 1 when the inattentive type is included.

C. Attention problems occur among all social classes and in other cultures, but different diagnostic traditions and rates of recognition result in differences in apparent prevalence.

D. ADHD is more common in first-degree relatives, suggesting a genetic basis for the disorder.

III. Etiology. The cause (or causes) of ADHD remains unknown. It is likely that ADHD is a syndrome with most cases resulting from inherited abnormalities in regional central nervous system neurotransmitter/receptor function and only a very small percentage of cases caused by acquired neurologic insults or metabolic processes. In cases in which presumed ADHD is associated with nongenetic factors, the overall symptom picture usually is atypical.

A. Genetic influences are apparent, and inheritance probably accounts for most cases.

  1. Twin studies demonstrate a higher concordance for ADHD symptoms in monozygotic than dizygotic twins.

  2. Siblings of children with ADHD are at greater risk for ADHD; this risk increases if one or both parents have an ADHD history.

  3. Adopted children with biological parents who had psychiatric problems are more likely to have ADHD than adopted children without parents with such problems.

B. Many acquired factors have been implicated, but research data indicate that *none* of the following are significant contributors to ADHD:

  1. Perinatal problems: intrapartum hypoxia or maternal substance abuse.

  2. Infectious processes: bacterial meningitis or encephalitis.

  3. Toxins: drug ingestion by the child; heavy metal poisoning.

  4. Foods: artificial dyes, additives, or sugar.

  5. Sequelae of metabolic disorders.

  6. Head trauma.

  7. Medical disorders and treatments: thyroid dysfunction, theophylline, phenytoin, or phenobarbital therapy for seizures.

IV. Pathophysiology. Central nervous system abnormalities appear to cause ADHD, although no single, specific pathophysiologic pathway has been identified. Presently, searches for a single, primary cause of ADHD have been supplanted by belief that multiple interacting genetic and environmental factors cause ADHD. Scientific evidence for a presumptive central nervous system pathophysiology of ADHD currently is based on emerging neuroimaging technologies and inferences from psychopharmacotherapy of ADHD.

A. People with ADHD may have *hypo*activity of the alerting centers in the reticular activating system, which normally stimulate the cerebral cortex and result in more effective cognitive control over behavior and emotions.

B. There may be central catecholaminergic problems, with deficits of norepinephrine production and distribution; problems with α_2-adrenergic receptor number or sensitivity in the locus ceruleus; or both. These hypothetical defects combine to create a lowered threshold for incoming sensory stimuli, leading to a state of hypervigilance.

    C. Frontal lobe metabolic dysfunction has been suggested by positron emission tomography hypoprofusion of white matter in people with ADHD. Methylphenidate administration results in increased metabolism in the premotor and superior prefrontal cortex, and decreased activity in the motor and primary sensory areas of the cortex.

    D. There may be inadequate activity in the prefrontal cortex, since stimulant medications appear to increase dopamine output from the basal ganglia,

    E. Single photon emission computed tomography imaging studies, combined with clinical experience, suggest that there may be at least five clinically significant subtypes of ADHD, with distinctive patterns of neurologic dysfunction correlated with specific symptom clusters.

V. Diagnosis. Diagnostic challenges result from the multitude of symptoms that define the syndrome of ADHD, the absence of any specific biological markers indicating the presence of ADHD, and the need for multiple sources of diagnostic data. In addition, the presenting symptoms differ with gender and change with age. Some parents and professionals defer diagnosis in all children younger than school age, for fear of harmfully labeling them. Others disagree, arguing that such children typically are "labeled" variously as "bad" anyway and that very early treatment is important in minimizing morbidity.

    A. Symptoms and signs. For ADHD to be diagnosed, some signs and symptoms must have been present prior to age 7. Symptoms also must have: (1) been maladaptive and inconsistent with developmental level; (2) caused impairment in two or more settings; (3) resulted in clinically significant impairments in social and academic/occupational functioning; (4) not been the result of another psychiatric disorder.

        1. DSM criteria. DSM-IV describes both hyperactive–impulsive and inattentive symptoms. In order to make the diagnosis of ADHD, a child must exhibit six or more of the symptoms in (a), (b), or both, below:

            a. A child with hyperactive–impulsive signs and symptoms *often:*
                (1) Fidgets with hands or feet, or squirms in his or her seat.
                (2) Leaves his or her seat in the classroom or in other situations in which remaining in one's seat is expected.
                (3) Runs about or climbs excessively in inappropriate situations.
                (4) Has difficulty playing quietly.
                (5) Is often "on the go" or acts as if "driven by a motor."
                (6) Talks excessively.
                (7) Blurts out answers before questions have been completed.
                (8) Has difficulty waiting for his or her turn.
                (9) Interrupts or intrudes on others.

            b. A child with inattentive signs and symptoms *often:*
                (1) Fails to give close attention to details or makes careless mistakes.
                (2) Has difficulty sustaining attention in tasks or play.
                (3) Does not seem to listen when spoken to directly.
                (4) Does not follow through on instructions and fails to finish schoolwork, chores, or tasks.
                (5) Has difficulty organizing tasks or activities.
                (6) Avoids, dislikes, or is reluctant to engage in tasks requiring sustained mental effort.
                (7) Loses things necessary for tasks or activities.
                (8) Is easily distracted by extraneous stimuli.
                (9) Is forgetful in daily activities.

        2. Problems with DSM criteria. A major problem with DSM-IV is that the criteria for ADHD refer, and apply most easily, to children between the ages of 7 to early teens. Residual symptoms of ADHD that persist into adulthood are different from those in children (see section 3, below). In the absence of the more overt hyperactive–impulsive signs and symptoms, inattentive symptoms alone are subtle and easily overlooked. Finally, ADHD clearly is framed by DSM as a diagnosis of exclusion, only being diagnosed if symptoms are not better accounted for by pervasive developmental disorder (autism), schizophrenia or other psychotic disorder, mood disorder, anxiety disorder, or dissociative disorder.

3. **Age-specific features**
   a. **Infancy to 5 years of age.** Although ADHD often is not diagnosed until school age, many children with ADHD exhibit what appear to be prodromal symptoms from birth, such as colic, fussy eating, irritability, sensitivity to touch and noise, sleep problems, and toilet-training delays. 3- to 5-year-old children with ADHD often exhibit extreme hyperactivity, disregard of danger, talkativeness, and disrespect for parental limit-setting.
   b. **Adolescence.** Longitudinal studies of children with ADHD demonstrate that as many as 70–80% continue to have problems with impulsivity and inattention into adolescence. Overt hyperactivity typically is replaced by subtler but pervasive feelings of restlessness. When compared with normal controls, adolescents with ADHD have more academic problems, lower self-esteem, more oppositional or antisocial behavior (school suspensions or juvenile arrests), relationship problems, and greater cognitive immaturity, all independent of socioeconomic status or of prior treatment with stimulants during childhood. Nonspecific electroencephalogram abnormalities in children with ADHD tend to normalize in adolescence, but this is not predictive of outcome.
   c. **Adulthood.** Core symptoms of inattention, impulsivity, and hyperactivity of childhood ADHD tend to be obscured in adults because they may affect fewer areas of functioning, be more situational, and be less constant. Adults with ADHD typically have learned to accommodate to their neurologic dysfunction, yet those with untreated, residual ADHD commonly present with concerns that include:
      (1) Distractibility often manifested as difficulty listening or focusing.
      (2) Short attention span or forgetfulness—"loses things."
      (3) Daydreaming.
      (4) Procrastination and chronic lateness.
      (5) Chronic anxiety; low frustration tolerance.
      (6) Low self-esteem.
      (7) Employment problems such as frequent job changes.
      (8) Substance abuse or addiction.
      (9) Disorganization or inefficiency in work, resulting in inability to complete tasks.
      (10) Chronic boredom or restlessness.
      (11) Frequent and unpredictable mood swings.
      (12) Relationship problems—often avoiding group activities or having frequent marital problems.
         In short, adults with ADHD tend to exhibit symptoms that result from both ongoing neurologic dysregulation and lifelong problems in adapting to occupational and interpersonal demands.
B. **Differential diagnosis.** The following are several conditions that can lead to behavior that mimics ADHD, but it also is common for any of these other conditions to be comorbid with ADHD, considerably complicating diagnosis. In fact, the triad of **ADHD/Tourette's syndrome/obsessive–compulsive disorder** is recognized as such a common comorbidity that if a child has one of the three, careful screening for the remaining two is indicated. Of children with ADHD, 30% will have **major depression,** 30% (boys) to 40% (girls) will have **anxiety disorders,** 10–25% will have childhood **mania. Specific learning disabilities** also co-occur with ADHD in about 30% of cases.
   1. **Normal development.** Some children are naturally more hyperactive but exhibit none of the other symptoms of ADHD. Parents also typically have difficulty assessing their own preschool children, because they may have accommodated to high levels of hyperactivity over time. In milder cases, the possibility of ADHD may only be raised later by teachers.
   2. **Parent–child relational problem** can be an appropriate diagnosis when inadequate or ineffective discipline worsens the behavior of children who would not otherwise meet criteria for ADHD. Disruptive behaviors in this scenario tend to be person- or situation-specific, manipulative, and attention-seeking.
   3. **Adjustment disorder with disturbance of conduct** is diagnosed in circumstances in which family disruptions and social upheavals (such as a move, divorce, abuse, birth of a sibling, etc) result in behavioral dyscontrol, but such

problems will not have been present prior to the stressor, and onset typically will be sudden.

4. **Oppositional–defiant disorder (ODD) and conduct disorder (CD)** are more ominous conditions with some symptoms resembling ADHD. Confusingly, these disorders often emerge progressively, as younger children with untreated ADHD mature. In older children, ADHD, ODD, and CD may be comorbid conditions. Unlike the generalized behavioral disruptions of ADHD, these disorders involve specific, patterned behaviors of excessive defiance toward authority figures and persistent violation of age-specific social norms, the rights of others, or both. In adolescents, substance abuse is common. There is some evidence that the progression from ODD to CD continues on to become antisocial personality disorder with age.

5. **Bipolar disorder** formerly was thought to appear only in the late teens to early twenties, but symptoms now are recognized to occur even in very young children. Mania in young children may mimic hyperactivity of ADHD, but is more intense. The characteristics of bipolar disorder in children that best differentiate it from ADHD are:
   a. Significant, often cyclical, sleep disorder.
   b. Angry, hostile tantrums lasting from 30 minutes to 3 hours.
   c. Grandiosity manifested as inappropriate sarcasm or hostile irritability toward adults.
   d. Threatening or hostile behavior toward adults.
   e. Pressured speech that is difficult to interrupt.
      Table 94–1 distinguishes mania from ADHD in greater detail. Mania in adults also can be difficult to differentiate from ADHD, but symptoms typically become progressively more florid with age; in contrast, symptoms of ADHD become more subtle with age. A family history of mood disorder, and in particular bipolar disorder, coupled with symptoms that look like ADHD, is highly suggestive.

6. **Depression** in children and adolescents commonly is manifested behaviorally by irritability and anger, which may appear to be the impulsivity and hyperactivity of ADHD. But ADHD is a chronic behavioral pattern that clearly dates from before age 7, often with normal affect. Depression tends to be episodic, often is unrecognized prior to age 7, and usually includes more dysphoria.

7. **Separation anxiety disorder, simple phobia, social phobia, generalized anxiety disorder, post-traumatic stress disorder, and obsessive–compulsive disorder** all are characterized by anxiety that can impair concentration and also can cause jumpiness, restlessness, agitation, or fidgeting that may resemble the inattentiveness, impulsivity, and hyperactivity of ADHD. Anxious children, however, usually are able to describe the specific traumatic event or circumstances causing their worry or fear, whereas children with ADHD have little or no awareness of, and even less insight into, their symptoms. Anxiety levels fluctuate from one situation to another, whereas symptoms of ADHD are manifested in multiple settings. Distinguishing ADHD from anxiety disorders is critical, since at least 25% of people with ADHD have comorbid anxiety disorders, with anxiety often made worse by the stimulant medications commonly used to treat ADHD. Obsessive–compulsive disorder is a particularly common ADHD comorbidity (see section V,B, above) and must be distinguished because it responds to a completely different class of medications.

8. Far less common conditions—**temporal lobe seizures and intermittent explosive disorder**—also can cause impulsive behavior. Poor behavior control also is a feature of **pervasive developmental disorder** and **mental retardation,** but their overall symptom pictures—including language and cognitive delays—make these conditions easily distinguishable from ADHD.

9. Adults with ADHD often have chronic interpersonal and occupational problems suggesting **Axis II (personality) disorders.** This suggestion is buttressed by the fact that many adults with ADHD have accommodated to their neurologic dysfunction to the extent that personal qualities that vex and exasperate others are ego-syntonic and not identified as problems by the sufferers. Less resourceful children with more severe ADHD often progress on to conduct disorder as adolescents, and then to **antisocial personality disorder** as adults.

TABLE 94–1. DIFFERENTIATING MANIA FROM ADHD IN CHILDREN

	Mania	Attention-Deficit/ Hyperactivity Disorder
Behavior		
Hyperactivity:	Multiple, shifting goals	Random, not goal-directed
Impulsivity:	Targeted; purposeful	Nonspecific
Thrill or risk-seeking:	Intentional	Thoughtless
Grandiose behavior:	Yes	No
Belief in grandiose ideas:	Yes	No
Talkativeness:	Acutely variable	Regularly a little overtalkative
Interrupt when speaking?	Difficult or nearly impossible	Stops–then restarts
Agitation:	Yes	No–just hyperactivity
Destructiveness:	When angry	Inadvertent–non-angry
Use of physical force:	Controlled (unless severe)	Poorly regulated–sloppy
Tantrums/rage:	Extreme	Less severe and frequent
Duration of tantrums:	45 minutes to 4 hours	0–30 minutes
Enjoys power struggles:	Usually	Rarely
Fights:	Seeks them out	Inadvertent
Accidents:	Thrill-seeking	Careless
Hitting walls:	Intentional	Random, accidental
Cognition		
Inattention:	Over-scanning, too many ideas	Forgetful or mixed up
Cognitive looseness:	Tangential, jumps	Illogical leaps
Watching TV:	Stays tuned	In and out of attention/room
Punning and joking:	Precocious (age 2–3 years)	Age-appropriate
Sexual interest:	Precocious	Age-appropriate
Obliviousness:	To limits/limitations	To physical objects
Sleep, appetite, energy		
Hours of sleep:	None or low (4–6 hours)	Normal
Pre-bedtime:	Agitated; 1–4 hours	Minor difficulties to settle
Dreams:	Intense; gory; mutilation; blood	Normal
Hyper when asleep:	Episodic	Persistent
Morning arousal:	Slow	Fast
Mood on arousal:	Irritable; snippy; mute	Like rest of day
Appetite/thirst:	Acute increase	No changes
General energy:	Acute increase	Variable; chronically high
Sexual energy:	High	Normal
Emotions/affect		
Intensity:	Theatrical	Variable; less intense
Feelings "too strong":	Often	Sometime
Irritability:	Most individuals	Minority of individuals
Emotional lability:	Marked	Linked to changes in attention
Behavior in office		
Waiting room:	Loud or isolative	Hyperactive
Walking in hall:	Intentionally hits walls/jokes	Accidentally scrapes walls
First minute:	Dysphoric, rejecting, hostile	Overly vigilant and exploratory
Minutes 2–5:	Dysphoric, rejecting, hostile	Habituates toward normal
Interview tolerance:	Disruptive, insulting	Becomes bored, frustrated
Toward interviewer:	Directly challenging	Normal variability

Adapted from Popper C, 1997; personal communication.

     10. Although uncommon, other conditions with features of ADHD include hearing loss or visual disturbances, side effects of medications, thyroid disorders, and exposure to certain toxins.
  C. Diagnostic strategies. Diagnosis of ADHD in children and adults involves assessing the presence of key symptoms, documenting their presence in multiple settings, and establishing their presence prior to age 7.
    1. Clinical observation. ADHD cannot be diagnosed on the basis of behavior in the office alone, particularly in cases of predominantly inattentive symptoms. Indeed, as few as 20% of children with ADHD demonstrate their hyperactivity

and impulsivity in the initial office visit. Nonetheless, careful assessment in the office can increase or decrease the index of suspicion for ADHD and guide effective use of behavioral checklists and neurologic tests.

   a. Listen for parents to volunteer key complaints:

     (1) "He just can't sit still."

     (2) "She's constantly fidgeting."

     (3) "He is always interrupting and bothering other kids."

     (4) "She only can get homework done when there are no distractions."

     (5) "She sits and works but never gets anything done."

   b. Observe behavior in the office to determine whether or not the child's hyperactivity and impulsivity are volitional:

     (1) Inform parents that you will be watching the child carefully while you are listening to them and asking them questions.

     (2) Watch to see if the child is involved with others or "off in a world of his own." Children with ADHD quickly become uninvolved with others in the room and move randomly from one activity to another, seldom staying interested in one task for more than a few minutes. If a child repeatedly looks back at his or her parent(s), as if checking for reactions or trying to get attention, that is not a sign of ADHD.

     (3) Observe patterns of discipline in the interaction of children and parents. Are parents unwittingly reinforcing unwanted behavior by constantly paying attention to it and reacting with extreme emotionality? Or do parents consistently and unemotionally intervene despite ongoing hyperactivity and impulsivity?

     (4) A child with normal hearing whose name has to be called repeatedly before responding, or a child who sits quietly but does not follow conversations (persistently responding with a puzzled look or responding "what?") suggests the possibility of the predominantly inattentive type of ADHD.

2. Interviews

   a. Employ key questioning of parents:

     (1) Are there any situations at home in which the child is able to remain still and focused? Some activities, such as playing video games or watching cartoons, are so fast-paced that they uniquely captivate the attention of children with ADHD.

     (2) What environmental variables (eg, types of settings, numbers and types of people, times of day, etc) tend to be associated with behavioral control or lack of control?

     (3) What do people in other settings (day care, school, church, youth groups, etc) say about the child's behavior?

     (4) Is the child able to complete tasks, games, chores, and projects, or is there a constant trail of half-finished activities around the house?

     (5) Are there any dietary relationships with hyperactivity? Some parents report that caffeinated beverages actually calm children and make it easier for them to fall asleep. Some adolescents and adults initially present with gastritis resulting from unrecognized self-medication with caffeine. Many parents report that sugar or food dyes cause their children to become more hyperactive; while well-intentioned, such popular theories never have been substantiated scientifically.

   b. Gather developmental data from parents. There must be evidence of symptoms prior to age 7. The following often are associated with ADHD:

     (1) Excessive hyperactivity in utero.

     (2) Great difficulty in quieting.

     (3) Fidgeting even when asleep.

     (4) Early walking.

     (5) Mixed dominance for handedness.

     (6) Feeding problems.

     (7) Accident proneness; frequent falls and scrapes.

     (8) Obliviousness to danger (eg, climbing cabinets or running away from parents in stores).

   c. Assess family disruptions, such as recent moves, birth of a sibling, parental discord or divorce, change of schools, and so on, that may be resulting in behavioral problems.

      d. Evaluate the family history for evidence of ADHD in relatives:
- **(1)** Does the child resemble anyone else in the family?
- **(2)** Is that person a chronic underachiever despite normal intelligence?
- **(3)** Has anyone else in the family ever been diagnosed or treated for ADHD?
- **(4)** Is there substance abuse in relatives?

3. Physical examination. The routine physical examinations of most children with ADHD are completely normal.

    a. "Soft" neurologic signs and minor congenital anomalies should be noted, but not considered of any diagnostic significance.

    b. Vision and hearing should be checked in any child with attention problems.

    c. Multiple scars on knees, shins, elbows, and foreheads are common.

4. Checklists and questionnaires. Because of the need to document the presence of symptoms in multiple settings and over time, standardized behavioral checklists should be used. These permit systematic data gathering from different people, as well as the collection of retrospective data to help in the assessment of adults.

    a. Conners Parent and Teacher Rating Scales

    b. Achenbach Child Behavior Checklist

    c. ADD-H Comprehensive Teacher Rating Scales

    d. Child Behavior Checklist

    e. ACTers

    f. Wender-Utah Rating Scale (retrospective self-report for adults)

    g. Attention-Deficit Scale for Adults (retrospective self-report for adults)

5. Performance tests. A number of computerized continuous performance tests have been designed and standardized. They can differentiate children with ADHD from normal controls with modest reliability. They also are useful in discriminating ADHD of the predominantly inattentive subtype in children, as well as residual symptoms in adults—both of which are more difficult to discern because of the absence of overt hyperactivity. They also can be useful in documenting medication response.

    a. Test of Variables of Attention (TOVA)

    b. Conner's Continuous Performance Test

VI. Treatment. The initial step in treatment is to assess parents' attitudes. What beliefs do the parents have about ADHD? Is there fear and uncertainty about using medications, or are there positive expectations? What are the bases for either positive or negative expectations? What types of behavioral approaches and disciplinary strategies have been tried in the home? Optimal treatment plans almost always combine pharmacotherapy and behavioral interventions. Medication trials only should be initiated when there is a presumptive diagnosis of ADHD based on data collected (above). Response to medication should never be the sole criterion for diagnosing ADHD. Lack of response to a given medication does not rule out ADHD. When using medication, mechanisms for monitoring desired responses and adverse effects should be established. Duration of therapeutic effects for any specific drug shows great interindividual variability.

A. Medications used to treat ADHD

    1. Stimulants. Psychostimulants are the preferred initial choice for medication trials. Seventy percent to 80% of children with ADHD respond to stimulant medication. Choice of specific stimulant can be based on prior experience by family members, attitudes of parents, or both. Although dosing on a mg/kg basis often is advocated (typically 0.3–0.8 mg/kg/dose of methylphenidate or equivalent), such guidelines are less helpful clinically because of great interindividual variability in response.

      a. Methylphenidate (Ritalin)
- **(1)** Supplied as 5-, 10-, and 20-mg scored tablets.
- **(2)** Usual starting dose: 5 mg at 7 AM and noon, titrating up every 4–7 days based on response. A three times daily initial dosing is used in older children, so that parents can evaluate response in the home.
- **(3)** Effects usually begin 30–45 minutes after dose. Duration of action varies from 2–6 hours, with 3–4 hours being the most common effective range.
- **(4)** Adverse effects: nausea, anorexia, headache, dizziness, and insomnia. Minimize adverse effects by giving with food. Food increases blood levels.

    (5) Advantages/disadvantages: rapid response; predictable and safe because of great experience with use. Very short duration of action; end-of-dosing-cycle irritability/dysphoria is common.

b. Methylphenidate–Sustained Release (Ritalin–SR)

    (1) Supplied as 20-mg tablets, *but which deliver only the equivalent of 7.5–10 mg of regular methylphenidate.* Parents may be alarmed when switching their children from 5 mg of regular methylphenidate to the SR formulation because of the "20-mg" designation, making parent education/reassurance important. To avoid potentially dangerous confusion, "SR" and "regular" designation always should be stated explicitly in medical charts when referring to any 20-mg methylphenidate prescription.

    (2) Sustained-release preparations seldom are used for initial treatment in younger children, but a normal starting dose would be one 20-mg SR tablet every morning and at 2:00–3:00 PM.

    (3) Advantages/disadvantages: Slower initial rise and more gradual end-of-dosing-cycle fall in blood levels can reduce incidence of side effects, but also may reduce effectiveness.

    (4) Effective duration of action ranges from 5–9 hours, with 6–7 hours being most common.

    (5) In children, SR and regular preparations can be combined effectively both to increase absolute dose and to decrease end-of-dosing-cycle adverse effects. SR preparations are used more often in adults and adolescents, for whom taking fewer doses each day increases adherence.

c. Dextroamphetamine (Dexedrine)

    (1) How supplied: 5-mg tablets; 10-, 15-, and 20-mg "spansules" (sustained release); elixir. Unlike methylphenidate, regular and sustained-release preparations are equivalent strength, and differ only in duration of action.

    (2) Advantages/disadvantages: predictable and safe because of great experience with use and rapid onset of action.

    (3) Dextroamphetamine is about 2 times as potent as methylphenidate on a mg/kg basis. Usual starting dose in younger children is 2.5–5.0 mg, given two or three times daily at intervals of every 3–4 hours.

    (4) Effective duration of action is 3–4 hours for regular, and 8–10 hours for sustained-release preparations.

    (5) Side effects are similar to those for methylphenidate.

d. Adderall (compound of dextroamphetamine sulfate, amphetamine sulfate, dextroamphetamine saccharate, and amphetamine aspartate)

    (1) How supplied: 5-, 10-, 20-, and 30-mg scored tablets.

    (2) Advantages/disadvantages: long duration of action, flexible dosing.

    (3) Effective duration of action is 8–12 hours. Most children and adults require only one or two doses per day. If more than one dose is required, the dosing interval should be approximately every 6 hours.

    (4) Initial starting dose is 5–10 mg every morning or twice daily in children over 6, and 2.5 mg in the same schedule for children under 6. Dosage can be increased in 2.5- to 5.0-mg increments weekly. Patients seldom require >40 mg/day, although 60 mg/day is necessary in some circumstances.

    (5) Side effects are similar to those for methylphenidate.

e. Pemoline (Cylert)

    (1) How supplied: 18.75-, 37.5-, and 75-mg tablets; 37.5-mg chewable tablets.

    (2) Pemoline is inherently long-acting, with behavioral effects of each dose lasting 12–24 hours. Onset of action is very long: clinical response may not occur for 2–4 weeks.

    (3) Advantages/disadvantages: is given in a single AM dose; possibly fewer side effects than other stimulants; relatively high incidence of liver toxicity, especially in children. Although elevations in liver enzymes usually are reversible upon withdrawal of the drug, evidence that the risk of liver failure has been underreported has led the manufacturer to market Cylert as *not* an appropriate first- or second-line treatment for ADHD in children. Baseline and periodic liver function tests must be done.

    (4) Starting dose is 18.75 mg every morning. Dosing can be increased by 18.75 mg every morning weekly.

2. **Antidepressants.** Several antidepressants have been effective in the treatment of ADHD, but purely serotonergic antidepressants, such as fluoxetine (Prozac), sertraline (Zoloft), and paroxetine (Paxil), are of no benefit. Only antidepressants with noradrenergic—and perhaps dopaminergic—properties are effective, but the effects of antidepressants on hyperactivity and impulsivity in children are not as robust as are the stimulant medications. Recent data suggest that adults' responses to noradrenergic antidepressants and stimulants are equivalent.

    a. Tricyclic antidepressants (TCAs). TCAs—especially **imipramine** (Norpramin) and **desipramine** (Tofranil)—often are used when the side effects of stimulants are debilitating (such as when anorexiant effects lead to significant weight loss or failure to maintain growth within an acceptable range). TCAs also are more effective when insomnia, irritability, and anger outbursts are part of the clinical picture (either from comorbid depression or as part of ADHD). Positive effects of TCAs on ADHD usually occur at lower doses than those needed for treating depression. TCAs can be combined with stimulants, but may increase concentrations of dextroamphetamine in the brain dramatically. Although TCAs have been used extensively in children—such as imipramine for nocturnal enuresis—they theoretically can cause cardiac conduction problems. Isolated case reports tell of sudden death in eight children taking TCAs, but the contribution of TCAs to the deaths remains unclear. Cautious use of TCAs in children < age 14 (particularly desipramine) and baseline electrocardiograms are recommended by specialists. This is not necessarily the standard of care in the ambulatory treatment of patients with no history of cardiac problems, particularly at lower doses. Initial dosing is 10–25 mg imipramine or desipramine at bedtime, titrating up to a maximum daily dose of 300 mg (in divided doses if >100 mg every day).

    b. Bupropion (Wellbutrin). This atypical antidepressant frequently is used in lieu of stimulant medications. It is available in both regular and extended-release preparations. Although jitteriness or nervousness is a common side effect, and although less effective than stimulants in treating hyperactivity and impulsivity in children, bupropion appears to be effective in adults with predominantly inattentive ADHD. Use of extended-release preparation is associated with fewer side effects. Starting dose in children is 75 mg of extended-release bupropion every morning.

    c. Venlafaxine (Effexor), which possesses both serotonergic and noradrenergic activity, has been shown to be beneficial in some children and adults with ADHD. Starting and maximum daily doses are 18.75 and 150 mg, respectively.

3. **Antihypertensive medications.** Central α-noradrenergic receptor agonists have proven useful in themselves and also to augment stimulant medication. They have been particularly effective in facilitating calming, reducing frustration tolerance and aggression, and reducing sleep disturbance associated with stimulant medications. Although there is a theoretical danger of rebound hypertension with abrupt discontinuation, there are few such events reported in clinical practice with children. Parents should be cautioned not to discontinue medication in their children without tapering it, however, and blood pressure should be monitored at each visit. Start at the lowest possible dose. These medications cause sedation—both initially and with each increase in dose—that usually is alarming to parents and teachers because of the dramatic changes in activity level, so careful explanation of this effect prior to initiating treatment is essential. Sedation usually subsides after 3–4 days on a given dose.

    a. Clonidine hydrochloride (Catapres) is supplied as 0.1-, 0.2-, and 0.3-mg tablets (which have an effective duration of action of 3–6 hours) or equivalent transdermal patches (which last 5 days). Usual oral dosing is 0.05 mg at bedtime and titrating upward by additional 0.05 doses every 3–7 days until four times daily dosing is achieved. The maximum daily dose is supposed to be 0.3 mg per day, but 0.4–0.5 mg sometimes is used. Side effects include sleepiness (which typically subsides several days after initiating treatment), headache, dizziness, and nausea. Transdermal patches can be cut to permit precise dosing, but they can cause local skin reactions and often are not effective in children because they tend to remove them.

   b. Guanfacine (Tenex) is similar to clonidine in its actions, but is preferred by some physicians because of its longer half-life, decreased sedative side effects, and more selective binding profile.

B. General principles of pharmacotherapy for ADHD

1. Dosing

   a. Although common advice is to use the smallest effective dose of any medication, incomplete treatment is inappropriate. If a child is exposed to any medication, use whatever amount is necessary to control symptoms.

   b. Stimulants typically have bimodal effects: lower doses can treat inattention, but higher doses often are required to control hyperactivity. If hyperactivity persists after maximal or tolerable dosing of two different stimulants, consider augmentation.

2. Medication choice

   a. First-line medications for ADHD in most children are stimulants (other than pemoline).

   b. There is no consensus whether dextroamphetamine or methylphenidate is preferable.

   c. Specific algorithms for treating individual patients can be based on unique symptom clusters (see section V,C below).

3. Generic versus brand-name medication:
Currently, no controlled studies have demonstrated that generic forms of medications for ADHD are any less effective than brand-name, although some parents insist that generics are inferior.

4. Growth

   a. Stimulants frequently cause loss of appetite and a flattening of growth curves in children, although there is no evidence that there are long-term deleterious effects. In fact, some very hyperactive children eat better when they take stimulants.

   b. Growth charts should be in the medical records of every child being treated for ADHD. As a general rule, a loss of 20 percentile points in weight or height should prompt reconsideration of treatment strategy.

5. When to start medication.
In the past, pharmacotherapy was not initiated until children reached school age. Current practice is not as restrictive, and medicine is used as early as age 2. Dextroamphetamine elixir is available, although many young children can swallow the small methylphenidate or dextroamphetamine pills if they are given with food like chunky applesauce or tapioca pudding. Children younger than age 5 do not respond to stimulant medications (only about a 50% stimulant response rate) as frequently as older children, and failure to respond before age 5 should not be interpreted as misdiagnosis or an indication that stimulants will not work in the future.

6. When to give medications.
Side effects like nausea, headache, and jitteriness often remit after several days, or can be mitigated by administering medicines with food. For very young children, parents should be encouraged to give medication with food or juice immediately upon arising to minimize side effects and increase absorption, although acidic juices can lower absorption of amphetamines.

7. Relative cost of stimulant medications.
The relative cost of different stimulant medications is presented in Table 94–2. Prices are based on actual costs to pharmacists based on average wholesale prices. Cost to the patient will be higher.

8. "Drug holidays."
Although medications used to be withheld on weekends, current thinking is that more harm than good is done by the frustration that this strategy causes for patients and families. Children should be taken off

TABLE 94–2. COST PER PILL FOR TYPICAL STARTING DOSE OF STIMULANT AND ANTIDEPRESSANT MEDICATIONS COMMONLY USED TO TREAT ADHD[1]

Medication	Generic	Brand
Methylphenidate 5 mg	$0.33	$0.38
Methylphenidate—SR 20 mg[3]	$1.06	$1.23
Dexedrine 5 mg	$0.18	$0.24
Dexedrine Spansule 5 mg[3]	NA[2]	$0.52
Pemoline 18.75 mg[3]	NA	$0.65
Adderail 5 mg[3]	NA	$0.33
Wellbutrin 100 mg	NA	$1.05
Wellbutrin-SR 150 mg[3]	NA	$1.39
Effexor-XR 37.5 mg[3]	NA	$2.00
Imipramine 25 mg[3]	$0.47	$0.54
Desipramine 25 mg[3]	$0.28	$0.72

[1] Average wholesale prices taken from *Drug Topics Red Book Annual Edition*—1999, 103rd ed: Medical Economics Data. Cost to patients likely will be higher. Note that the starting dose is not likely to be the ultimate therapeutic dose and that shorter-acting medications typically require multiple doses each day.
[2] NA = Generic form not available.
[3] Extended-release or inherently long-acting preparation.

medication at least once each year to assess for continuing presence of symptoms. Summer frequently is chosen, although the first two weeks of the new year (week 1 out of school and week 2 in school) are a more realistic trial off medication, permitting assessments by multiple raters in different settings.

9. **In school.** Care should be taken to dispense medications or remind children discreetly. Children with ADHD already may feel "different" and further embarrassment will reduce adherence.

10. **As children grow.** Children with ADHD generally require increasing amounts of medication until they reach puberty, when requirements typically decrease. Young children taking stimulants usually require only morning and noon doses; as children progress in school and have to do homework in the evening, a third dose may be added in the late afternoon.

11. **Tic disorders.** Although formerly thought to induce tics, stimulant medications now are felt only to exacerbate tics in individuals already at risk.

C. **Specific pharmacotherapy algorithms for children.** Although all children with ADHD should have a core of symptoms in common, experts recognize that there are several subtypes of ADHD with specific behavioral manifestations, and which seem to be associated with abnormal function in different areas of the brain. These specific symptoms may appear prior to treatment, or after initial treatment with stimulants, and commonly require special medication regimens (see sections C,3–C,6, below).

1. Initial treatment for **all ADHD:**
   a. Initiate treatment (any **ONE** of the following):
      (1) 5 mg regular methylphenidate every morning and noon
      (2) 2.5–5.0 mg regular dextroamphetamine every morning and noon
      (3) 5 mg Adderall every morning or twice daily (AM + 2 PM)
   b. Monitor response:
      (1) *How effective is the symptom control?*
         (a) Symptoms **ARE** controlled:
            (i) Prescribe that dose on a schedule based on the effective duration of action.
            (ii) Although 0.3–0.8 mg/kg/dose of methylphenidate equivalent is a general guideline for dosing, 60 mg/day is an accepted upper limit.
         (b) Symptoms **ARE NOT** controlled:
            (i) Increase each dose by the initial starting dose and continue increasing by that amount every 4–5 days.
            (ii) Switch to a different stimulant.
            (iii) Switch to an antidepressant: imipramine 10–300 mg every day or bupropion 75–400 mg every day.

(2) *How long do the effects of a single dose last?*
  (a) Symptoms **DO NOT** recur between doses:
    (i) Prescribe enough doses daily to prevent symptom break-through during waking hours.
    (ii) Reevaluate periodically.
  (b) Symptoms **DO** recur between doses:
    (i) Shorten dosing interval.
    (ii) Switch to a sustained-release or longer-acting medications.
(3) *Are there persistent side effects?*
  (a) Discontinue and start another medication (see section C,1,(a).
  (b) Add a medication (see sections C,2–C,6 below) to counteract side effects.

2. Special algorithm when ADHD involves primarily **inattention** (short attention span, distractibility, disorganization, low motivation, going off-task):
  a. Follow section C,1 above.
  b. Typically requires relatively lower levels of stimulant medication.

3. Special algorithm when **hyperactivity–impulsivity symptoms** (restlessness, excessive talking, interrupting, poor judgment, sleep problems) predominate:
  a. Follow section C,1 above.
  b. If hyperactivity is decreased by stimulants but symptoms persist:
    (1) Add a TCA—typically imipramine at 25 mg at bedtime (10 mg if weight <50 lbs) **OR**
    (2) Add guanfacine (Tenex) 1–2 mg every morning, or clonidine (Catapres) 0.05–0.2 mg every day—twice daily.

4. Special algorithm when **temporal lobe symptoms** (irritability, aggressivity, anger outbursts, low frustration tolerance, anxiety, visual/auditory illusions, frequent déjà vu, head or abdominal pain, history of head injury, family history of rages, dark thoughts) predominate:
  a. Initiate treatment with an anticonvulsant:
    (1) First-line choices: divalproate (Depakote) 125–2100 mg every day or twice daily, gabapentin (Neurontin) 100–1800 mg every day or twice daily, or carbamazepine (Tegretol) 100–600 mg twice daily.
    (2) Second-line choices: phenytoin (Dilantin) 30–150 mg twice daily, or lamotrigine (Lamictal) 25–500 mg every day.
  b. Add a stimulant medication as in section C,1 above.

5. Special algorithm when **depressive/limbic system symptoms** (negativity, moodiness, irritability, low energy, lack of motivation, low self-esteem, social isolation, anhedonia, guilt, helplessness) predominate:
  a. Initiate treatment with an antidepressant:
    (1) First-line choices: imipramine 10–30 mg every day, bupropion 75–400 mg every day divided, or desipramine 10–300 mg (age >14).
    (2) Second-line choices: venlafaxine 18.75–150 mg every day to three times daily or nortriptyline (Pamelor) 10–150 mg every day.
  b. Add a stimulant medication as in section C,1 above.

6. Special algorithm when **overfocus symptoms** (having cognitive inflexibility, being bound by perfectionism, having trouble shifting attention, being stuck on negative thoughts or behaviors, worrying, holding grudges, being oppositional, having difficulty with change, needing ritual or routine) predominate:
  a. Initiate treatment with an antidepressant:
    (1) First-line choices: venlafaxine 18.75–175 mg every day to twice daily, fluoxetine 10–80 mg every day, sertraline 25–200 mg every day, or paroxetine 10–50 mg every day.
    (2) Second-line choices: fluvoxamine 50–300 mg every day, clomipramine (Anafranil) 10–250 mg every day, or nefazodone (Serzone) 20–600 mg every day.
  b. Add a stimulant medication as in section C,1 above.

7. Always combine pharmacotherapy with behavioral interventions.

D. **Behavioral interventions.** Rather than list specific behavioral interventions for ADHD, below are some general principles for nonpharmacologic treatment.
  1. Focus on positive reinforcement of desired behaviors. Ignore or "robot" undesired behavior.

2. Try to make the environment as simple as possible—permit only one friend at a time. In school, avoid "open" classrooms and position the child at or near the front of the room.
3. Establish routines in the home and at school, trying to make study time, bedtime, and mealtime as consistent as possible.
4. Assign one task at a time, speaking quietly and slowly. In the classroom, give assignments one at a time and break them down into manageable steps. Check frequently on child and reward task completion.
5. Avoid repetition of words like "No!" or "Stop it!"
6. Use visual cues to augment verbal commands.
7. Use "stickers and stars" on calendars or charts to monitor/reward accomplishments.
8. Avoid crowded places like amusement parks or malls, which have many visual and auditory stimuli.
9. Establish a quiet study area, placing a full-size mirror in front of the child so that the child can self-monitor distractibility.
10. Reward self-monitoring and self-control of specific behaviors (such as behavioral contracting that provides rewards for completing chores or homework); do not emphasize getting better grades, since there are many factors beyond the control of a child that affect grades.
11. Provide opportunities for exercise to discharge energy, but also avoid extreme fatigue.
12. Avoid constant linking of medications with behavior (avoid saying, for example, "You're being so good today. You must have taken your medication!" or "Why are you being so squirmy? Did you forget to take your medication?").

E. Parent/patient education
1. Have handouts available in the office. An excellent source of educational materials—as well as both national and local support groups—is ChADD (Children and Adults with Attention Deficit Disorders).
2. Develop a brief talk to help parents understand what a person with ADHD experiences, and how medications work: *"Most people's brains work very hard to screen out distracting stimuli—sounds, movements, and even sensations in the body like itching or hunger. This active filtering by the brain occurs unconsciously, and permits people who don't have ADHD to concentrate, plan, sit still, have patience, and so on. Filtering occurs because certain areas of the brain are working very hard 'in the background'; in people with ADHD these areas of the brain do not work hard enough, so the world seems chaotic. Instead of 'turning down' the brain, ADHD medications work by stimulating those areas of the brain that filter and focus."*
3. Emphasize to parents that children and adults with ADHD are not "bad" and that ADHD and intelligence are unrelated.
4. Because of controversial media reporting, parents often have reservations about using medication. Common fears are that their children will become "like zombies" or will become "addicted," or that ADHD treatment is like "experimenting on a child."
   a. Parents need reassurance that medications often make children appear overly quiet and sluggish, but that this may be magnified because the parents have become accustomed to high levels of hyperactivity.
   b. Some medications *do* have sedating side effects that disappear over time; some children are more sensitive to medications and will require unexpectedly smaller doses than usual. Close cooperation and frequent communication between parents/patients and their physicians is imperative.
   c. Parents should be told **prior to initiating treatment** that medication type, dose, and timing of doses typically will change as many as 4–6 times over the first 6 months to minimize misperceptions of "experimenting" on their children.
   d. Confirm that there are children and adults who abuse stimulant medications to get "high," but that people with ADHD do not get "high" when taking them. It is important, however, to keep medications in a safe place and to teach responsible use.

F. Family therapy/counseling. It is common for parents to disagree strongly about the approach to a child with ADHD. This is true in intact families as well as after divorce. In addition, normal sibling rivalry frequently is complicated when the attention received by one child with ADHD results in unafflicted siblings feeling comparatively neglected. In such situations, the treatment of a child with ADHD becomes more complicated, and unaffected siblings can begin to exhibit acting-out behavior. Family therapy is particularly helpful for newly diagnosed adults with ADHD, whose family members may have had very dysfunctional, long-term adaptations to problems associated with untreated ADHD in a parent.

1. In families that have a child with ADHD, it is imperative that there be a strong parental coalition: Disagreements about diagnosis and treatment should be resolved or at least not discussed in front of children. This is true of divorced parents sharing custody, whose mixed messages typically only serve to confuse children, sabotage treatment, and result in other behavioral problems not related to ADHD itself.

2. One technique for minimizing sibling rivalry is to give vitamin pills or small cinnamon candies to unaffected children who become jealous of siblings' morning medication rituals.

3. Older siblings often are left in charge of younger children with ADHD. This sibling "parenting" can cause major problems in families, which can be addressed in family therapy.

G. **Controversial treatments.** Over the past two decades, there has been increased public interest in ADHD and its treatment. Several controversial treatments have captured the attention of the public. Since many parents will have heard of them and may question their physicians, it is important that practitioners understand both the theories and the evidence for each.

1. **Dietary interventions.** Suggestions that ADHD symptoms might occur in children sensitive to aspirin have led to diets eliminating artificial flavorings, colorings, and preservatives. All well-controlled studies to date have failed to demonstrate the efficacy of such elimination diets. Any behavioral benefits from elimination diets in case reports may be due to the effects of the rigorous attention by parents that such diets entail. In naturalistic studies of the effects of sugar on hyperactivity, there were no differences in the actual behavior of the children; only in the vigilance of parents toward their children's behavior, with parents who believed their children were ingesting sugar consistently noticing and commenting about disruptive behaviors more frequently than if they were told their children were not receiving sugar.

2. **Megavitamin and mineral supplementation.** There is a complete lack of scientific evidence to support use of supplementation in ADHD, and megavitamin therapy has potential hepatotoxicity.

3. **Anti-motion sickness medications.** Based on the theory that children with ADHD have problems in the inner ear causing balance and coordination problems, proponents claim a success rate greater than 90%. Their results are unpublished.

4. *Candida albicans* elimination. Based on the idea that toxins produced by *Candida albicans* overgrowth in the body weakens the immune system and increases susceptibility to ADHD and other psychiatric conditions, antifungal medicines and low-sugar diets have been used. Only testimonials have been offered as proof; and the theory of *Candida albicans*/immune dysregulation is not consistent with compelling theories about the cause and pathophysiology of ADHD.

5. **Biofeedback.** Using electroencephalogram monitoring and feedback training, children can "learn" to increase frontal lobe activity associated with attention and to decrease activity associated with inattention. Theoretically, such children will be able to control hyperactivity, impulsivity, and inattention better. A few studies have demonstrated impressive results, but the studies are flawed in many ways. Although promising, the approach is expensive and time-consuming. Parents should be cautious and consider biofeedback as an adjunctive therapy, if at all.

VII. **Natural history and prognosis.** Without treatment, children with ADHD are at much greater risk for academic failure, oppositional–defiant behavior, truancy, substance abuse, motor vehicle accidents, anxiety, depression, and low self-esteem. Treatment can mitigate these risks, especially if initiated early. Unfortunately, even with treatment, children with ADHD have higher rates of social and psychological maladjustment as adults. Historically, ADHD was not thought to persist into adulthood. Prospective, long-term proband studies now suggest that symptoms of ADHD persist into adulthood in 20–60% of people who had ADHD as children. Neuroimaging studies confirm that childhood abnormalities in brain functioning associated with ADHD can persist into adulthood. Adult "core" symptoms of ADHD tend to be similar to children, but hyperactivity/impulsivity tends to be less pronounced, making the presentation in adults more subtle. Many adults with ADHD—perhaps because of chronic underachievement, disorganized interpersonal relationships, and low self-esteem—exhibit symptoms mimicking Axis II (personality) disorders. Lifelong treatment may be helpful to many adults with residual symptoms of ADHD.

REFERENCES

Amen DG, Goldman B: Attention-deficit disorder: A guide for primary care physicians. Primary Psychiatry 1998;**5**(7):76.

American Psychiatric Association (APA): *Diagnostic and Statistical Manual of Mental Disorders,* 4th ed. APA; 1994.

Baran M: Attention-deficit/hyperactivity disorder. Patient Care, December 1995;56.

ChADD (Children and Adults with Attention Deficit Disorders) 499 NW 70th Avenue, Suite 101. Plantation, FL. www.chadd.org (305)587-3700.

Council on Scientific Affairs, American Medical Association (Goldman LS, Genel M, Bezman RJ, Stanetz PJ). Diagnosis and treatment of attention-deficit/hyperactivity disorder. JAMA 1998; **270:**1100.

Fargason RE, Ford CV: Attention deficit hyperactivity disorder in adults: Diagnosis, treatment, and prognosis. South Med J 1994;**87**(3):302.

Lin-Dyken DC, Wolraich ML: Attention-deficit hyperactivity disorder. In: Greydanus DE, Wolraich ML, eds. *Behavioral Pediatrics.* Springer-Verlag, 1992; 167.

Taylor MA: Evaluation and management of attention-deficit hyperactivity disorder. Am Fam Physician 1997;**55:**887.

Wender PH: *The Hyperactive Child, Adolescent, and Adult: Attention Deficit Disorder Through the Lifespan.* Oxford Univ Press; 1987.

Wilens TE, Biederman J, Spencer TJ, et al: . Psychotherapy of adult attention deficit/hyperactivity disorder: A review. J Clin Psychopharmacol 1995;**15**(4):270.

Zametkin AJ, Ernst M: Problems in the management of attention-deficit hyperactivity disorder. N Engl J Med 1999;**340**(1):40.

---

95   Child, Elder, & Family Violence

F. David Schneider, MD, MSPH, Linda M. Ivy, MD,
& Melissa A. Talamantes, MS

I. **Introduction.** Family violence has become an increasingly important problem in the United States. Many barriers exist to the detection of violence by physicians, including lack of training and confidence to treat the problem adequately. This chapter focuses on three aspects of family violence: (1) child abuse and neglect, (2) partner abuse, and (3) elder abuse and neglect.

II. **Child abuse and neglect**
   A. **Definition.** *Child physical abuse* is defined as "inflicted injury to a child." These injuries include bruises, welts, burns, lacerations, abrasions, fractures, and abdominal or intracranial injuries such as subdural hematomas. *Sexual abuse* is the exposure of an adolescent or child to sexual materials or sexual contact with an adult. Another form of abuse is *emotional abuse,* "coercive, demeaning, or overly distant behavior by a parent or other caretaker that interferes with a child's normal social development." *Child neglect* is a deprivation of the basic needs of the child: "inadequate nutrition, clothing, shelter, emotional support, love and nurturing, education, safety, and medical and dental care."

   B. **Epidemiology.** There are 2 million reported cases of child abuse and neglect in the United States annually; 250,000 of these cases involve sexual abuse, 160,000 involve serious or life-threatening injuries, and 2000–4000 result in death. Eighty percent of children who die from child abuse and neglect are under the age of 5, with 40% of such deaths occurring during the first year of life.

C. Diagnosis. Physicians often lack the proper training to recognize potential cases of abuse or neglect, and as a result do not intervene. Since abuse is not unique to any specific socioeconomic group, the physician must always be sensitive to its existence. When taking a history, patients should be screened for abuse by asking all newly enrolled families about violence: "Have you ever been in a relationship where children or adults were hit or hurt by another member of the household?" and "When you were a child, did anything ever happen that you considered to be physically or sexually abusive?" If there are injuries or behaviors that seem odd or uncomfortable, then the physician's suspicion of the possibility of family violence should be heightened.

If one suspects abuse, then extra time must be spent to investigate suspicions. Children rarely make false disclosures of abuse. A thorough history and extensive physical examination must be performed. The physical signs of abuse are listed in Table 95–1. The clinician should keep the following points in mind.

   1. Remain calm and act professionally. Both children and parents are more likely to continue to remain trusting if you remain objective. Remain empathetic; however, your questions concerning the abuse should be direct and specific. Use objective, open-ended questions, and do not lead the patient.

   2. Be sure to obtain the entire past medical history, especially episodes of injury that required medical treatment.

TABLE 95–1. SIGNS AND SYMPTOMS THAT SHOULD AROUSE CONCERN ABOUT CHILD ABUSE OR NEGLECT

Subnormal growth
Weight, height, or both <5th percentile for age
Weight <5th percentile for height
Decreased velocity of growth

Head injuries
Torn frenulum of the upper or lower lip
Unexplained dental injury
Bilateral black eyes with history of a single blow or fall
Traumatic hair loss
Retinal hemorrhage
Diffuse or severe central nervous system injury with history of a minor to moderate fall (<3 m)

Skin injuries
Bruise or burn in the shape of an object
Bite marks
Burn resembling a glove or stocking or with some other distribution suggestive of an immersion injury
Bruises of various colors (ie, in various stages of healing)
Injury to soft tissue areas that are normally protected (eg, thighs, stomach, or upper arms)

Injuries of the gastrointestinal or genitourinary tract
Bilious vomiting
Recurrent vomiting or diarrhea witnessed only by a parent
Chronic abdominal or perineal pain with no identifiable cause
History of genital or rectal pain
Injury to the genitals or the rectum
Sexually transmitted disease

Bone injuries
Rib fracture in the absence of major trauma such as a motor vehicle accident
Complex skull fracture after a short fall (<1.2 m)
Metaphyseal long-bone fracture in an infant
Femur fracture (any configuration) in a child <1 year old
Multiple fracture in various stages of healing

Laboratory studies
Implausible or physiologically inconsistent laboratory results (polymicrobial contamination of body
   fluids, sepsis with unusual organisms, electrolyte disturbances inconsistent with the child's clinical
   state or underlying illness, wide and erratic variations in test results)
Positive toxicologic tests in the absence of a known ingestion or medication
Bloody cerebrospinal fluid (with xanthochromic supernatant) in an infant with altered mental status and
   no history of trauma

Reprinted with permission from Wissow LS: Child abuse and neglect. N Engl J Med 1995;**332**:1425.

3. The physical examination should be performed separately from the history, after the child has developed a level of trust with the provider.

4. If possible, question the child alone or without the caregiver present.

5. Make sure the history explains the medical evidence appropriately.

6. Determine the level of ongoing risk to the child and siblings.

7. Documentation is extremely important. These medical records are often the only objective evidence of the abuse. Word-for-word documentation of statements made by the child are helpful. Tape the interview if possible. A detailed description of any injuries, including the size, location, number, and degree of healing. Photographs and laboratory data, including imaging studies, should be included. Drawings are very helpful in the event that a case of abuse ends up in court. All documentation should be objective. The physician's opinions do not belong in the documentation of the history or physical examination; these should be included only in the assessment portion of the progress note. Here, an opinion as to whether the injuries were adequately explained by the history is appropriate. If the case goes to court, the physician should be able to testify that the record was completed at the time of the examination and was "made in accordance with routinely followed procedures," and he or she will need to discuss the care and access to the medical record.

8. Deprivational syndromes are marked by poor weight gain (or "falling off the growth curve"), poor hygiene, developmental delay, delay in obtaining treatment for medical problems, inadequate well-child care, or failure to obtain necessary immunizations.

9. Physical examination in victims of suspected child abuse should include cultures for sexually transmitted diseases, a pregnancy test in postmenarcheal girls, and blood tests for syphilis and human immunodeficiency virus (HIV) infection.

D. **Management strategies.** Presenting suspicions of abuse or neglect to the family or the patient can be anxiety provoking for the physician. The physician's job is to make sure that the victim of abuse is safe and that appropriate referrals are made (see section II,E). Although the majority of abuse stops once it has been identified, it continues in approximately one-third of cases. Remain objective when presenting this to the family. Do not investigate the offense or confront the abuser. If possible, the therapeutic relationship with the family can be continued. The trauma of the investigation, often taking months, can be psychologically damaging.

   The physician should never try to manage a case of child abuse or neglect on his or her own. Besides being legally obligated to report the abuse, it is more appropriate to take a multidisciplinary approach to management. Become aware of the resources available. Local Child Protective Services (CPS), the local health department, or the local hospital social work department can acquaint physicians with these community resources.

   In cases of sexual abuse, the patient often feels that he or she has been visibly altered. In order to lessen this perception by the victim, explain that there is "a small scratch that only a doctor can see." Patients who have been sexually abused often need referral for long-term counseling, whether the abuse event(s) was recent or in the distant past.

E. **Legal responsibilities.** Physicians are obligated to report child abuse or neglect to the local CPS in all states. Even if the physician has never seen the child but has learned about abuse from an adult, physicians are mandated to report the incident. Initial reports may be made by telephone to the local agency. Some states require a written report within a few days of the initial report. In most states, failure to report a suspected case of child abuse or neglect is a criminal offense.

F. **Prognosis.** Abused children often (1) are more aggressive toward peers, (2) show avoidance or withdrawal toward their peers, (3) have learning disorders, and (4) demonstrate criminal behavior.

   As adults, these people are more likely to be substance abusers; have affective, anxiety, or eating disorders, borderline personality, and sexual dysfunction; and abuse their own children.

III. **Partner abuse**

A. **Definition.** *Wife abuse* is often used interchangeably with *domestic violence* or **partner abuse. Abuse** is a broad term that can include verbal harassment or threats, sexual assault, isolation of the victim, denial of personal freedom, and physical attacks. The battering syndrome, which includes all of these forms of abusive behavior, is used to gain control of the victim's behavior. Examples of these forms of abuse include the following.

1. **Verbal abuse,** which ranges from repeated insults or insinuations up to threats to hurt or kill the victim or loved ones.
2. **Sexual assault,** which includes any form of nonconsensual sexual activity, occurs in about 35–40% of battered women.
3. **Isolation** of the victim from family and friends serves to give the abuser complete control over the victim's environment as well as to conceal any physical abuse.
4. **Physical abuse,** in its extreme, includes punching, kicking, choking, and use of a knife or a gun.

B. **Epidemiology.** A minimum of 2–4 million women are abused by male partners. More than 1.8 million women are seriously assaulted annually. The abuse can become lethal; domestic violence causes 30–40% of female murders in the United States. Ninety percent of these cases are the result of males' violently assaulting their female partners. Although mutual battering exists, studies have shown that men are more likely than women to perform more severe acts of violence. Men who admit to acts of violence often cite a desire to control or alter their victim's behavior. On the other hand, women who admit to violence indicate that they are responding to a perceived threat.

C. **Cyclic pattern of violence.** Within an abusive relationship, there is usually a typical pattern of tension building, violence, and reconciliation. Over the duration of an abusive relationship, this cycle recurs many times, often with the violence increasing in severity.

1. Tension building is characterized by frequent hostile verbal attacks, heightened surveillance of the victim, and escalating demands. This part of the cycle is actually the most destructive to the woman's ego and self-esteem.
2. Violence occurs after a build-up of days or months of increasing tension. This can be precipitated by a particular event or can come without warning. Some women have been awakened by beatings.
3. The reconciliation phase quickly follows. The attacker is often remorseful and promises never to be physically abusive again.

D. **Diagnosis**

1. **Awareness.** The key to identification by the primary care physician is the realization that anyone could be a battered woman. Stereotypes regarding poor, uneducated, minority women or the woman who somehow "provokes" her partner to attack her must be dispelled. A heightened awareness is necessary to consider battering when evaluating women. Victims of abuse commonly present with multiple somatic complaints, including headache, abdominal pain, muscle aches, joint pain, fatigue, vaginal or pelvic complaints, anxiety disorders, or depression. Battered women often go from doctor to doctor and are frequently identified as "difficult patients." Feelings of guilt, shame, and low self-esteem are the primary reasons that many battered women are hesitant to discuss the abuse.
2. **Screening** for abuse should be done routinely as part of any history and physical examination. By asking about abuse, the physician lets the patient know that he or she is approachable and willing to help. Battered women who do not reveal abuse at an initial visit may discuss it later if they feel that their doctor is receptive. A nonjudgmental statement such as "I often see depression in women who have been hurt by someone close to them. Has this ever happened to you?" is a good screening question for partner abuse. This statement lets the patient know that her physician is willing and able to help.

E. **Treatment.** Often physicians are reluctant to elicit a history of abuse because they are unsure about how to proceed if abuse is reported. Consider the following in offering treatment to victims of domestic violence.

1. The therapeutic process has already begun when the patient can talk to the physician about the abuse. The physician needs to convey that there are many women who have had similar experiences and that the patient is not crazy. It is normal to feel overwhelmed and in need of support. It is also important that the patient understands that her symptoms are a reaction to the abuse. Reassurance helps decrease the sense of isolation and helplessness.

2. The level of continuing danger must be assessed. If there is imminent danger of serious harm or death, arrangements for a shelter should be made before the patient leaves the office. If children are involved in the abuse, by law this must be reported.

3. The patient needs to know what resources are available, even if she is not yet ready to leave an abusive relationship. Group sessions with women who have had similar experiences are especially helpful. The patient should be given the telephone number of a women's shelter before she leaves the office.

4. Documentation including as many details as possible in the history and physical examination is very helpful. Drawing figures or diagrams, depicting exact areas of ecchymoses, swelling, lacerations, and so on, further documents the abuse.

5. The physician may feel frustrated because the patient cannot or will not leave an abusive relationship. The physician cannot make this decision for the patient. The role of physician is that of facilitator, helping the woman work through the process of recovery.

F. **Prognosis.** Effects on the victim vary, but certain emotional and behavioral sequelae are commonly seen in an abused partner.

1. Depression is one of the most common manifestations suffered by battered women. Depression can come from anger at the abuser turned inward, and feelings of guilt or self-blame for "allowing the abuse to happen." Suicide is not uncommon. Depression can persist after the victim has left the abusive relationship.

2. Living in an abusive relationship produces high levels of anxiety, and, even after the relationship has terminated, many women will still have environmental triggers that can provoke anxiety attacks. Both anxiety and depression are common ways battered women will present to the primary care physician.

3. Self-destructive behavior is common and can manifest itself as substance abuse, smoking, or failure to use safety items such as seat belts.

IV. **Elder abuse.** Abuse is a symptom of underlying family dysfunction. Treatment must include the family unit as well as the victim of abuse. The physician cannot treat elder abuse alone; a team approach, using social workers, mental health professionals, and lawyers, is more likely to be successful.

A. **Definitions.** The term *elder abuse* is used interchangeably with *elder mistreatment* and includes many types of abuse against older adults. The National Aging Resource Center on Elder Abuse (NARCEA) has developed working definitions for elder abuse and neglect. The types of elder abuse include physical, psychological, and sexual abuse; psychological and physical neglect; violation of rights; and financial or material abuse. Neglect and physical and psychological abuse may also be self-inflicted.

1. **Physical abuse** is the act of causing physical pain or injury resulting in bruising, fractures, dislocations, abrasions, burns, welts, lacerations, and other multiple injuries. Physical abuse can be intentional or unintentional and includes at least one act of violence including beating, slapping, burning, cutting, inappropriate use of physical restraints, and intentional overmedicating.

2. **Physical neglect** is the failure by a caregiver to meet care obligations such as providing goods and services such as food, clothing, shelter, and medical and personal care. Indicators of neglect may include malnutrition, dehydration, decubitus ulcers, poor hygiene, and lack of caregiver compliance with medical regimens.

3. **Psychological neglect** is the failure to provide a dependent elder with meaningful social contact or stimulation. Examples of this type of neglect include isolating or ignoring the elder for long periods. This commonly results in depression, extreme withdrawal, or agitation.

4. **Psychological abuse** includes the infliction of mental anguish through intimidation, threats, verbal assaults, berating, deprivation, infantilization (treating the older adult like an infant), humiliation, or the provocation of internal fear. The end result of this type of abuse is similar to that of psychological abuse in which the elder is depressed, withdrawn, or fearful, and can present with symptoms of "failure to thrive."

5. **Sexual abuse** is defined as molestation or forced sexual activity. Although this type of abuse is the most underreported, it may occur more often than previously suspected.

6. **Violation of personal rights** includes preventing elders from making their own decisions regarding housing arrangements, financial matters, and personal decisions such as marriage, divorce, and medical treatment. Physicians can observe for signs of violation of personal rights through observation of the caregiver–elder interaction. Does the caregiver insist on being present for the examination? Does the caregiver interrupt the elder's conversation, never allowing the elder to respond to the physician's questions? Does the caregiver deny the elder the right to make health care decisions?

7. **Material or financial abuse** refers to the illegal exploitation of monetary or material assets. This type of abuse includes control of the elder's income and assets by the caregiver; coercion in signing contracts or making changes in a will or durable power of attorney; or the theft of money or property. Specific indicators include a caregiver's refusal to release funds to purchase needed care or patient complaints that they have inadequate funds to buy medication.

B. **Epidemiology**
   1. **Prevalence and incidence.** The NARCEA estimates that between 1.5 and 2 million older adults in the United States suffer from physical abuse or neglect annually. Elder abuse occurs in all communities, regardless of gender, ethnicity or race, socioeconomic status, or religious affiliation. Because of the variation in state reporting requirements, it is difficult to determine the actual rate of elder abuse; however, the majority of state adult protective and regulatory agencies responsible for the identification, investigation, and prevention of elder abuse report an increase in reported cases over the last decade. In Boston, 3.2% of elders reported experiencing some form of physical or psychological abuse or neglect. A longitudinal study in Connecticut found that mistreated older adults reported to Adult Protective Services were more likely to die within the 13-year follow-up study period than older adults who experienced self-neglect or those who were not reported to Adult Protective Services (Lachs et al, 1998).
   2. **Identity and background of the perpetrators.** Physical abuse is perpetrated most often by spouses with acute or chronic health problems or responsibilities for providing companionship, financial resources, or property maintenance for their dependent spouse. Adult children tend to psychologically abuse and neglect their parents as well as financially exploit them. These children are often financially dependent on the parent and have a history of mental illness or substance abuse. Pillemer and Suitor (1992) found that 64% of abusers were financially dependent on their victims and 55% were dependent on them for housing needs.
   3. **Risk factors for abuse.** Increased life expectancy, dependency, learned helplessness, poor physical health, and stress and burnout experienced by the caregiver are primary risk factors for abuse. Other risk factors include living arrangements, caregivers with mental illness or substance abuse, or a family history of violence. Lachs et al (1997) found that mistreated elders were likely to live with someone and have fewer social networks. Potential predictors of elder mistreatment include poverty, race, and cognitive impairment.

C. **Diagnosis.** A comprehensive biopsychosocial assessment of the elderly patient is important to determine whether there are clinical findings to support abuse or neglect. Table 95–2 outlines the clinical procedures for detecting abuse.

D. **Management strategies.** The American Medical Association (AMA) recommends that all physicians ask their patients about family violence regardless of whether there is clinical evidence or suspicion of abuse or neglect. If the elderly patient is not cognitively impaired, a thorough interview, separate from the caregiver, should occur to assess whether the patient is safe. Nonthreatening questions should be asked, such as (1) "Do you feel safe in your home?," (2) "Who helps you with your personal care, such as bathing, taking your medications, preparing your meals?," (3) "What happens if your family member becomes tired or cannot help you?," (4) "What happens if you have a disagreement?," and (5) "Who helps you pay your bills?" If the patient has cognitive impairment, history and screening questions must be obtained from the caregiver or family member if available.

If the elder does not feel safe and accepts physician intervention, hospitalization should be considered. If hospitalization is not an option, the physician should discuss other placement options with Adult Protective Services (APS). APS has

TABLE 95–2. CLINICAL PROCEDURES FOR THE DETECTION OF ABUSE OF AN ELDERLY PATIENT

Focus	Procedure or Item To Be Noted
History	Interview the patient and the suspected abuser separately and alone. Make direct inquiries about physical violence, restraints, or neglect. Request precise details about the nature, frequency, and severity of events. Assess the patient's functional status (independence, activities of daily living). Inquire of the designated caregiver whether impairment of activities of daily living is present. Assess recent psychological factors (eg, bereavement, financial stress). Elicit the caregiver's understanding of the patient's illness (care needs, prognosis, etc).
Behavioral observation	Withdrawal
	Infantilizing of the patient by the caregiver
	Caregiver insists on providing the history
General appearance	Hygiene
	Cleanliness and appropriateness of dress
Skin and mucous membranes	Skin turgor, other signs of dehydration
	Multiple skin lesions in various stages of evolution
	Bruises, decubitus ulcers
	Evaluate how skin lesions have been cared for
Head and neck	Traumatic alopecia (distinguishable from male pattern alopecia on the basis of distribution)
	Scalp hematomas
	Lacerations, abrasions
Trunk	Bruises, welts. The shape may suggest an implement (eg, iron or belt)
Genitourinary tract	Rectal bleeding
	Vaginal bleeding
	Decubitus ulcers, infestations
Extremities	Wrist or ankle lesions suggesting the use of restraints, or immersion burn (stocking–glove distribution)
Musculoskeletal system	Examine for occult fracture, pain. Observe gait
Neurologic–psychiatric status	Conduct a thorough evaluation to assess focality
	Depressive symptoms, anxiety
	Other psychiatric symptoms, including delusions and hallucinations
	Formal mental status testing (eg, Mini-Mental State Examination or Mental Status Questionnaire)
	Cognitive impairment suggesting that delirium or dementia has a role in assessing decision-making capacity
Imaging and laboratory tests	As indicated from the clinical evaluation
	Albumin, blood urea nitrogen, and creatinine levels; toxicologic screening (assess the caregiver's compliance with the medical regimen)
Social and financial sources	Inquire about other members of the social network available to assist the elderly person and about financial resources
	This information is crucial in considering interventions that include alternative living arrangements and home services

Reprinted with permission from Lachs MS, Pillemer K: Abuse and neglect of elderly persons. N Engl J Med 1995;**332**:437.

several emergency, court-ordered options available and can facilitate this process. The following approach with the caregiver facilitates the interview process and reduces some of the tension that may exist: "It must be very difficult to care for your mother with this type of illness. Do you find yourself feeling tired, frustrated, and unable to deal with the situation?" Advising the family member that you will be making a report to APS in order to help reduce some of the stress that the caregiver may be experiencing may be less threatening to the caregiver. The caregiver should be informed of available resources such as adult day care, respite care, home health care, senior companion programs, and caregiver support groups.

E. Ethical and legal obligations. Physicians play a critical role in the assessment of elder abuse and neglect, as well as in the intervention process. In long-term physician-patient relationships in which trust has been established, the process is facilitated.

Physicians have a legal responsibility to report suspected cases of abuse or neglect. Mandatory reporting laws exist in most states. Designated state agencies are responsible for conducting investigations and interventions. APS is the agency assigned to investigate and intervene with elder abuse cases. Persons who are licensed, registered, or certified to provide health care, education, and social, mental health, and other human services are required to report abuse. Anonymous reports can be made. Physicians usually are granted immunity from civil suits in reporting cases of suspected abuse or neglect. Failure to report suspected abuse can result in civil liability and fines for any subsequent damages that may occur. Failure to follow state guidelines for reporting abuse may result in criminal prosecution, professional delicensure, or other penalties.

REFERENCES

American Medical Association (AMA): *Diagnostic and Treatment Guidelines on Abuse and Neglect.* AMA; 1992.
Brown A: Violence against women by male partners: Prevalence, outcomes, and policy implications. Am Psychol 1993;**48**:1077.
Campbell JC, Lewandowski LA: Mental and physical health effects of intimate partner violence on women and children. Psychiatr Clin North Am 1997;**20**:353.
Ferris LE, Norton PG, Dunn EV, et al: Guidelines for managing domestic abuse when male and female partners are patients of the same physician. JAMA 1997;**278**:851.
Hamberger LK, Burge SK, Graham AV, et al: *Violence Issues for Health Care Educators and Providers.* Haworth Maltreatment and Trauma Press; 1997.
Hendricks-Matthews MK: Survivors of abuse: Health care issues. Prim Care 1993;**20**:391.
Kini N, Lazortiz S: Evaluation for possible physical or sexual abuse. Pediatr Clin North Am 1998;**45**:205.
Lachs MS, Pillemer K: Abuse and neglect of elderly persons. N Engl J Med 1995;**332**:437.
Lachs MS, Williams CS, O'Brian S, Pillemer KA, Charlson ME: The mortality of elder mistreatment. JAMA 1998;**280**:5.
Lachs MS, Williams C, O'Brian S, et al: Risk factors for reported elder abuse and neglect: A nine year observational cohort study. Gerontologist 1997;**37**:4.
Melvin SY, Rhyne MC: Domestic violence. Adv Intern Med 1998;**43**:1.
Nimkin K, Kleinman PK: Imaging of child abuse. Pediatr Clin North Am 1997;**44**:615.
Pillemer K, Suitor JJ: Violence and violent feelings: What causes them among family caregivers? J Gerontol 1992;**47**:165.
Wissow LS: Child abuse and neglect. N Engl J Med 1995;**332**:1425.

---

96   Depression

Michael L. Parchman, MD

I. **Definition.** Major depressive disorder (MDD) is a mood disorder characterized by at least 2 weeks of depressed mood or a loss of interest or pleasure in daily activities associated with other findings, such as sleep disturbance and appetite changes.
II. **Other diagnoses with depressive features**
   A. **Uncomplicated bereavement** (formerly known as "adjustment disorder with depressed mood"). This type of mood disorder is readily attributable to a recent psychosocial stressor such as a loss of a loved one or employment and should resolve as the stressor decreases. It is distinguished from an MDD by its milder severity and shorter time course. Some bereaved patients manifest primarily psychological symptoms and seek counseling, while others develop somatic symptoms and seek medical attention. Unfortunately, many individuals with MDD have stressors that may be identified as the cause of their depression, and thus their illness may be overlooked.
   B. **Dysthymia.** Formerly known as neurotic depression, dysthymia is a chronic mood disorder in adults that lasts for at least 2 years. Patients with dysthymia may be thought of as having a depressive personality or character style. Although depressive symptoms in dysthymia are not as severe as those of major affective disorder, they are too prolonged to be thought of as adjustment responses.
   C. **Organic mood disorder.** This condition is diagnosed when a prominent mood disturbance can be attributed to a specific organic factor, such as an endocrine impairment; acquired immunodeficiency syndrome (AIDS) encephalopathy; a tumor

involving the limbic area; stroke; or the side effects of drugs and medications such as beta blockers, levodopa, steroids, reserpine, and oral contraceptives.

D. Anxiety. Distinguishing between anxiety and depression may be very difficult. Patients with MDD may present with such a predominance of anxiety symptoms that subtler symptoms of depression, such as loss of appetite, fatigue, or loss of pleasure, may be overlooked.

E. Other psychiatric disorders. Depressive symptoms may also be present in other psychiatric disorders, although they are not predominant. Therefore, the evaluation of depressive symptoms should include a psychiatric history and a brief review of systems, looking for psychotic features, phobias, panic attacks, somatization, and personality disorders.

III. Epidemiology. The point prevalence of MDD in Western industrialized nations is 2.3–3.2% for men and 4.5–9.3% for women. The risk of developing MDD over one's lifetime is 7–12% for men and 20–25% for women. The point prevalence of MDD in primary care patients is 4.8–8.6%; 14.6% of adult medical inpatients meet criteria for MDD. Depression is the seventh most common outpatient diagnosis.

A. A depressive disorder may begin at any age, but the average age at onset is the late 20s. Psychosocial events or stressors may play a significant role in precipitating the first or second episode of MDD, but may play little or no role in subsequent episodes.

B. Multiple studies support the finding that major depression is more common in women than in men. This gender difference is found in community samples and is not the result of higher rates of help-seeking behavior by women. Recent studies have disproved the belief that the incidence of depression in women increases during the climacteric.

C. Some studies suggest that the age of onset has decreased, and the lifetime risk of MDD has increased over each of the past several generations since 1940. Prevalence rates for MDD are unrelated to race, education, or income.

D. Certain individuals are at increased risk for depression, including alcohol and drug abusers, hypochondriacs, patients with a life-threatening disease such as a stroke or myocardial infarction, individuals recovering from major surgery, women in the postpartum state, and patients with a family history of depression.

IV. Pathophysiology

A. Multiple lines of research point to a genetic or inherited predisposition for MDD that is activated or precipitated by psychosocial or physiologic stressors. The general understanding of how these stressors interact with a genetic predisposition to produce clinical depression is limited.

   1. Potential mediating stressors include life-threatening illnesses; unresolved losses, either current or during childhood; current stressful life events; impact of life events on lifestyles; symbolic meaning of life events; inadequate social support; deficient social skills; and personality traits.

   2. The interaction among these environmental and inherited factors is postulated to culminate in the final common pathway of limbic–hypothalamic dysfunction, which is clinically manifested as a depressive illness.

B. It was originally believed that a depletion of neurotransmitters, including norepinephrine, serotonin, and γ-aminobutyric acid, in hypothalamic centers of the brain contributed to the symptom complex of depression. More recent studies suggest a dysregulation hypothesis rather than depletion of a single neurotransmitter. Such an imbalance is the physiologic explanation for symptomatology, but does not explain symptom development.

V. Diagnosis. Recent studies have documented improvements in the recognition and treatment of MDD in primary care settings, with two-thirds of patients recognized and nearly half prescribed antidepressants.

A. Symptoms and signs

   1. The clinical diagnosis of depression depends on recognition of an identifiable cluster of signs and symptoms suggesting the disorder. See Table 96–1 for a list of criteria for diagnosing MDD according to the *Diagnostic and Statistical Manual of Mental Disorders,* 4th edition (DSM-IV). Any of the symptoms listed may represent the leading edge of a cluster of depressive symptoms. For example, a recent study found that 80% of patients with the chief complaint of fatigue go on to be diagnosed with an affective disorder. The DSM-IV requires that five or more symptoms be present during the same 2-week pe-

TABLE 96–1. DSM-IV CRITERIA FOR MAJOR DEPRESSIVE EPISODE

Five (or more) of the following symptoms have been present during the same 2-week period and represent a change from previous functioning; at least one of the symptoms is either (1) depressed mood or (2) loss of interest or pleasure.

Note: Do not include symptoms that clearly result from a general medical condition or mood-incongruent delusions or hallucinations.

(1) Depressed mood most of the day, nearly every day, as indicated by either subjective report (eg, feels sad or empty) or observation made by others (eg, appears tearful). **Note:** In children and adolescents, can be irritable mood
(2) Markedly diminished interest or pleasure in all, or almost all, activities most of the day, nearly every day (as indicated by either subjective account or observation made by others)
(3) Significant weight loss when not dieting or weight gain (eg, a change of >5% of body weight in a month) or decrease or increase in appetite nearly every day. **Note:** In children, consider failure to make expected weight gains
(4) Insomnia or hypersomnia nearly every day
(5) Psychomotor agitation or retardation nearly every day (observable by others, not merely subjective feelings of restlessness or being slowed down)
(6) Fatigue or loss of energy nearly every day
(7) Feelings of worthlessness or excessive or inappropriate guilt (which may be delusional) nearly every day (not merely self-reproach or guilt about being sick)
(8) Diminished ability to think or concentrate, or indecisiveness, nearly every day (either by subjective account or as observed by others)
(9) Recurrent thoughts of death (not just fear of flying), recurrent suicidal ideation without a specific plan, or a suicide attempt or a specific plan for committing suicide

Reprinted with permission from American Psychiatric Association (APA): *Diagnostic and Statistical Manual of Mental Disorders,* 4th ed (DSM-IV). APA; 1994.

riod and that at least one be either a depressed mood or loss of interest or pleasure. It is important to note that the DSM-IV includes a loss of interest in all, or almost all, activities as an alternative to depressed mood as the primary symptom. Often, a patient may deny feelings of sadness but may admit to "not caring anymore."

2. Although the DSM-IV is useful in evaluating the possibility of depression in a patient, it was designed primarily by and for psychiatric researchers and was validated on a psychiatric population. DSM-IV criteria may not be as applicable to a primary care population.

3. The wide application of the term *depression* often leads to confusion about its diagnosis. The following guidelines are suggested to distinguish bereavement or dysphoric symptoms from clinical depression.
    a. Patients with established clinical depression do not respond to positive changes in the psychosocial environment.
    b. A clinical disorder is usually incapacitating and interferes with work performance and relationships.
    c. Diurnal variation of symptoms, which become worse in the morning, is more common with clinical depression.
    d. Psychomotor retardation, which may be associated with depression, is almost never observed with bereavement.
    e. Recurrence is especially characteristic of a mood disorder. A prior history of a similar episode is strong evidence for clinical depression.
    f. Finally, a positive family history of a similar disorder is characteristic of a primary mood disorder.

4. **Age-specific features** in the diagnosis of depression
    a. Elderly patients with psychomotor retardation, slow thinking, and indecisiveness may be misdiagnosed as having dementia (see Chapter 77).
    b. Prepubertal children often present with somatic complaints, irritable mood, or a psychomotor agitation that may manifest itself as a marked drop in school performance.
    c. In adolescents, similar findings may occur. Antisocial behavior, restlessness, agitation, aggression, withdrawal from social activities, and increased emotional sensitivity are also common. Children and adoles-

cents are often unable to recognize these changes or to associate them with depression.

B. Laboratory tests

1. The clinical interview remains the most effective method for detecting depression. No reliable biochemical markers for depression exist. Only a limited number of laboratory tests should be conducted to detect potential general medical causes of depressive symptoms. No standard "screening" work-up can be used to rule out potential underlying organic causes for depressive symptoms. The evaluation should be directed by demographic and historical clues. For example, hypothyroidism should be considered in an older patient who presents with depressive symptomatology. Medications known to be associated with depressive symptoms should be stopped, especially if recently prescribed.

2. Several **self-administered questionnaires** have been designed to help identify patients with depressive symptomatology. These tests, which are more useful as case-finding instruments than as screening tests, possess sensitivities in the 70% range and specificities in the 80% range. They are easily administered and well accepted by patients. Widely used tests include the following.

   a. Beck Depression Inventory, including the short-form version with 13 items.

   b. The National Institute of Mental Health (NIMH) Center for Epidemiologic Studies Depression Scale (CES-D), which has 20 items.

   c. The Zung Self-Rating Depression Scale (SDS), which also has 20 items.

VI. Treatment. The treatment of MDD is well within the domain of the primary care physician. The objectives of treatment are (1) to resolve all signs and symptoms of the depressive syndrome, (2) to restore occupational and psychosocial functioning to baseline, and (3) to reduce the likelihood of relapse and recurrence. Treatment may be divided into three phases: acute, continuation, and maintenance.

A. Acute phase treatment. In primary care, the most common acute treatment modalities are medication, psychotherapy or counseling, or a combination of medication and psychotherapy.

1. **Medication**

   a. Medications have been shown to be effective in all forms of MDD and should be considered first-line therapy in moderate to severe MDD.

   b. Medication selection should be based on side effect profiles; history of prior response; and patient symptoms, concurrent medical conditions, and concurrently prescribed medications (Table 96–2). No one antidepressant medication is clearly more effective than another. No single medication results in remission for all patients.

   c. In order to be proficient in the treatment of depression, the primary care physician should learn how to use at least three or four antidepressants well and become familiar with dosages, side effects, and serum levels. The chosen medications should have varying side effect profiles and be applicable to different types of presenting symptomatologies.

   d. Suggested guidelines for selection include the following.

      (1) If the patient has insomnia and early morning awakening, a more sedating medication should be chosen.

      (2) If the patient's symptoms are characterized by an excessive need for sleep, then a more stimulating and less sedating medication should be selected.

      (3) If anxiety is a major component of the symptom complex, then a medication with fewer insomnia or agitation side effects is recommended.

   e. Elderly patients are especially sensitive to the orthostatic and anticholinergic side effects of some antidepressants. As a result, the selective serotonin reuptake inhibitors (SSRIs) have replaced tricyclic antidepressants as first-line therapy in the elderly. Careful observation of cardiac function, vital signs, cognitive functioning, and physical complaints will often help identify potential problems early.

   f. If the medication is relatively sedating, compliance can be improved by having the patient take the entire dosage either at bedtime or a few hours before.

TABLE 96–2. ANTIDEPRESSANTS

Drug	Starting Dose	Therapeutic Daily Dose	Cost	Adverse Effects				
				Sedation	Anticholinergic	Orthostatic Hypotension	Cardiac Conduction	Insomnia
Tricyclics								
Amitriptyline (Elavil)	50 mg qhs[1]	75–300 mg	$	High	High	High	High	Very low
Doxepin (Sinequan)	50 mg qhs[1]	75–300 mg	$	High	Moderate	Moderate	Moderate	Low
Imipramine (Tofranil)	50 mg qd[1]	75–300 mg	$	Moderate	Moderate	High	High	Very low
Nortryptiline (Pamelor)	25 mg qd[1,2]	40–200 mg	$$	Low	Low	Low	Moderate	Low
Heterocyclics								
Trazodone (Desyrel)	150 mg qhs[1]	75–300 mg	$$	High	Very low	Moderate	Very low	Very low
Bupropion (Wellbutrin)	100 mg bid[3]	200–450 mg	$$	Low	Very low	Very low	Very low	Moderate
Selective serotonin reuptake inhibitors								
Fluoxetine (Prozac)	10–20 mg qam	10–80 mg	$$$	Very low	Very low	Very low	Very low	High
Paroxetine (Paxil)	10–20 mg qd	10–60 mg	$$$	Low	Low	Very low	Very low	Low
Sertraline (Zoloft)	50 mg qd	50–200 mg	$$$	Very low	Low	Very low	Very low	Low
Serotonin/norepinephrine reuptake inhibitor								
Venlafaxine (Effexor)	37.5 mg bid	75–300 mg	$$	Low	Low	Very low	Low	Low

[1] May be better tolerated if given in divided doses.
[2] Begin at lower dose in the elderly, titrate to serum level of 50–150 ng/mL.
[3] Not to exceed 150 mg/dose to minimize seizure risk.
$, least expensive; $$, moderately expensive; $$$, most expensive.

2. Psychotherapy

   a. Brief counseling or psychotherapy are well within the domain of the primary care physician.

   b. Depression rarely occurs independent of psychosocial issues. It is vital that the patient begin to address these issues if true recovery is to occur. If relationships within the family, such as a poor marital relationship, prove to be a precipitating factor, then involvement of other family members in counseling may be important.

   c. Psychotherapy alone may be preferable in patients with milder forms of MDD who do not desire medication, who have unacceptable side effects to medication, and who have medical conditions limiting medication options. There appear to be few differences in the 1-year outcome between patients with milder forms of MDD who are treated with cognitive therapy alone and those who receive pharmacotherapy alone.

   d. A complete discussion of all available psychotherapeutic techniques is beyond the scope of this chapter.

      (1) Often, the patient needs only a sympathetic listener to be able to work through the conflicts he or she is experiencing.

      (2) Encounters need not be lengthy. Ten or 15 minutes is enough time to allow the patient to explore problems in a therapeutic way, with the physician facilitating this process by asking open-ended questions.

      (3) It is not important that the physician produce a final answer to all of the patient's questions, doubts, or problems.

   e. Many physicians establish a good working relationship with a local psychiatrist, psychologist, or family therapist to whom they can refer patients for counseling or psychotherapy.

3. Patient education

   a. A key element in acute phase treatment is the provision of adequate information to both the patient and his or her family about the condition. In addition, the provision of support, advice, reassurance, and hope is critical for depressed patients who are experiencing fatigue, low mood, and poor concentration. Several studies have found that patient education improves adherence to treatment in depressed outpatients.

   b. An important point to make with many patients is that antidepressant medication is not habit-forming or addictive. Many patients are fearful of "nerve pills" because of friends or relatives who may have developed a drug dependence.

   c. Side effects such as dry mouth, constipation, and sedation should be discussed, and patients should be reassured that most will resolve with time.

   d. Patients should be told not to expect overnight results. It often takes 4–6 weeks for noticeable improvement to occur. It is often helpful to remind patients that their symptoms developed over a similar, if not longer, time interval.

B. Continuation and maintenance treatment

   1. The goal of continuation treatment is to decrease the likelihood of relapse (a return of the current episode of depression).

   a. Patients who respond well to acute treatment should be continued on the same dosage for at least 6–12 months after they have resolved their depressive symptoms. There is very strong evidence that continuation of treatment for this time interval is effective at preventing relapse and recurrence.

   b. **Common mistakes** in continuation treatment

      (1) Too little. A subtherapeutic dosage is often used by primary care physicians because many of the somatic symptoms will improve on this lower dose. Unfortunately, the depression does not completely resolve and often has a higher relapse rate if the dosage is not increased to the recommended therapeutic range.

      (2) Too short. The second criticism of primary care physicians is that treatment is discontinued much too soon. As previously mentioned, once the maintenance dosage is attained and symptoms resolve, treatment should continue for 6–12 months.

2. The goal of maintenance therapy is to prevent the recurrence of a subsequent depressive episode once the current episode has resolved.
   a. Patients who have had three or more lifetime episodes of MDD are candidates for long-term antidepressant medication.
   b. Patients who have a recurrence shortly after discontinuation of medication after an adequate initial treatment period of 6–12 months may require long-term medication, similar to diabetic or hypertensive patients.
   c. Maintenance medications should be prescribed at the same type and dosage found effective in previous acute phase treatment.

VII. Management strategies

A. Overcoming patient resistance

1. **Depression** is often difficult for the primary care physician to treat because the diagnosis itself is often socially unacceptable and culturally invalid for many patients. A recent survey of 350 family practice physicians revealed that the major obstacle to treatment of depressed patients was patient resistance to the diagnosis.
2. Many physicians find it useful to approach an explanation of the illness in terms that are better understood by the patient.
   a. Such an explanation often begins by explaining how the human body responds to stress and then defining the illness as an imbalance of chemical messengers in the nervous system.
   b. Patients are often more accepting of the diagnosis of depression and more willing to address the psychosocial precipitants, as well as use medication properly, when such an explanation is given.
3. It is often useful, if not crucial, to involve the family in such an explanation, since their support is vital to a successful outcome.

B. Suicide. Suicide potential and prevention must always be considered when the diagnosis of depression is made.

1. Many physicians are leery of asking about suicide out of fear that it may precipitate a suicide attempt. Such fears are unfounded. The evidence to date suggests that patients appreciate the concern demonstrated by such questioning. Many physicians find it useful to ask a patient who has considered suicide to form a suicide pact or agreement. The patient agrees to call the physician or another health provider before taking any action. No studies exist to support the efficacy of this arrangement, however.
2. Those individuals at highest risk for suicide attempt are young females. These attempts are usually gestures and are often not successful. Medication overdose is a common method of suicide in females. If suicide is judged to be a risk, it is prudent to limit the amount of medication prescribed to <1500 mg of a tricyclic antidepressant at any one time.
3. Those persons at highest risk for successful suicide are middle-aged to older men.

C. Referral or hospitalization. Even though most depressed patients who present to primary care settings can be managed as outpatients, some will need hospitalization in an inpatient psychiatric unit or referral to a psychiatrist. General recommendations are given below.

1. The patient who presents with suicide ideation and specific suicide plans is at serious risk, and hospitalization should be strongly considered.
2. The patient whose depression is severe enough to interfere with activities of daily living, such as dressing and feeding, should probably be hospitalized.
3. Referral should be considered if the patient has a strong history suggestive of bipolar disorder.
4. Referral should be sought if evidence of a thought disorder or psychotic features of the depression itself, such as fixed delusions, are present.
5. If the patient fails to respond to treatment after 3 months, referral to a psychiatrist should be considered.

D. Frequency of office visits

1. Follow-up should be scheduled at 2 weeks after the initial diagnosis for most mild to moderate depression. Patients with more severe forms of MDD should be seen weekly for the first 4–6 weeks of treatment. Subsequent visits may be scheduled at 4- to 12-week intervals, depending on the degree of response and the need for office counseling.

    2. Therapeutic blood levels of antidepressant drugs have been established. Nortriptyline, imipramine, and amitriptyline have well-established minimal therapeutic blood levels. Drug levels should be obtained in the following instances.

      a. When an adequate response is not achieved on full therapeutic doses. Nonresponsiveness to a medication cannot be established unless the steady-state serum level is within the therapeutic range for 2–4 weeks.

      b. When serious side effects occur at normal doses. Similarities exist between depressive and toxic symptoms in patients who are clinically deteriorating.

      c. When symptom breakthrough occurs after an initial full response.

      d. When an overdose has occurred.

VIII. Natural history and prognosis

  A. Prognosis without treatment

    1. An untreated episode of depression typically lasts 6 months or more. A remission of symptoms then occurs, and functioning often returns to the premorbid level.

    2. Of those patients with recurrent episodes, 5% will have a manic attack at a later date, resulting in a change in their diagnosis to a bipolar mood disorder.

    3. The toll in lives lost is high; half of all suicide victims are thought to have had a major depression. Suicide occurs in 1% of patients with an acute episode of depression and in 25% of patients with a chronic depression.

  B. Prognosis with treatment

    1. Treatment with tricyclic antidepressants usually results in resolution of all symptoms in 65–70% of patients.

    2. Treatment of the initial episode of MDD with an adequate course of tricyclics (eg, over a period of 4–9 months) has been shown to decrease the incidence of recurrent episodes of depression by at least half.

REFERENCES

American Psychiatric Association (APA): *Diagnostic and Statistical Manual of Mental Disorders,* 4th ed. APA; 1994.

Depression Guideline Panel: *Depression in Primary Care,* vol 1 (*Detection and Diagnosis*), Clinical Practice Guideline No. 5. Agency for Health Care Policy and Research (AHCPR); 1993. AHCPR Publication No. 93–0550.

Depression Guideline Panel: *Depression in Primary Care,* vol 2 (*Treatment of Major Depression*), Clinical Practice Guideline No. 5. Agency for Health Care Policy and Research (AHCPR); 1993. AHCPR Publication No. 93–0551.

---

97   Eating Disorders

Aliza Acker-Bernstein, MD

  I. Definition. Eating disorders are psychophysiologic disorders characterized by serious disturbances in eating behavior (Table 97–1).

    A. Anorexia nervosa (AN) is characterized by refusal to maintain a normal body weight, accompanied by a fear of gaining weight. Low weight in anorexia nervosa may be maintained solely by restriction (restrictive subtype) or by compensatory behaviors, such as vomiting or laxative abuse, with or without binge eating (binge eating/purging type).

    B. Bulimia nervosa (BN) is characterized by frequent episodes of binge eating accompanied by emotional distress plus the presence of frequent compensatory behaviors. In the purging subtype, the most frequent compensatory behaviors include vomiting (80–90%) and laxative abuse (33%). Less common behaviors include abuse of diuretics or diet pills, use of thyroid hormones, and enemas. Diabetic patients may omit or reduce insulin as a form of purging behavior. Rarely, ipecac may be used to induce vomiting. In the nonpurging subtype, compensatory behaviors include fasting, strict dieting, and excessive exercise in response to binge eating.

TABLE 97–1. DIAGNOSTIC CRITERIA FOR EATING DISORDERS

Anorexia nervosa
A. Refusal to maintain body weight at or above a minimally normal weight for age and height
B. Intense fear of gaining weight or becoming fat, even though underweight
C. Disturbance in the way in which one's body or shape is perceived
D. In postmenarchal females, amenorrhea
E. Type
    1. Restricting type
    2. Binge eating/purging type

Bulimia nervosa
A. Recurrent episodes of binge eating
B. Recurrent inappropriate compensatory behaviors in order to prevent weight gain
C. Binge eating and inappropriate compensatory behaviors both occur, on average, at least twice a week for 3 months
D. Self-evaluation is unduly influenced by body weight and shape
E. Type
    1. Purging type
    2. Nonpurging type

Binge eating disorder
A. Recurrent episodes of binge eating
B. Binge eating episodes are associated with at least three behavioral indicators of loss of control
C. Marked distress regarding binge eating
D. Binge eating occurs, on average, at least twice a week for 6 months
E. Binge eating is not associated with the regular use of inappropriate compensatory behaviors and does not occur exclusively during the course of anorexia nervosa or bulimia nervosa

Summary of the American Psychiatric Association's *Diagnostic and Statistical Manual of Mental Disorders,* 4th ed, criteria.

    C. Binge eating disorder (BED) is listed in an appendix to the 4th edition of the *Diagnostic and Statistical Manual of Mental Disorders* (DSM-IV) as an example of an eating disorder, not otherwise specified. It is characterized by frequent episodes of binge eating accompanied by emotional distress, but without evidence of frequent compensatory behaviors.
  II. Epidemiology. The prevalence of eating disorders appears to be rising.
    A. Anorexia nervosa
        1. AN primarily affects adolescent and young adult women, although onset has been reported in prepubertal girls and (rarely) in postmenopausal women.
        2. From 90% to 95% of individuals with anorexia nervosa are female.
        3. AN is most prevalent in industrialized societies. While more common in those with higher socioeconomic status and among whites, it is becoming increasingly recognized in other racial and ethnic groups and in lower socioeconomic groups.
        4. The prevalence of **AN** among adolescent and young adult women is estimated to be 0.5–1%, although a larger number exhibit impairment resulting from symptoms not severe enough to meet diagnostic criteria for the disorder.
    B. Bulimia nervosa
        1. BN affects primarily adolescent and young adult women. The age at onset is generally older than for **AN,** in late adolescence or young adulthood.
        2. Approximately 50–60% of individuals with **BN** have a past history of **AN.**
        3. As with **AN, BN** affects individuals in most racial and ethnic groups and is observed throughout the socioeconomic spectrum.
        4. From 1% to 4% of adolescent and young adult women meet diagnostic criteria for **BN,** but a much larger percentage have significant impairment caused by disordered eating, which is subthreshold for a diagnosis.
        5. Female athletes are at increased risk for BN. Female college gymnasts are at the highest risk.
        6. Approximately 90% of individuals with **BN** are female. Among males, **BN** is found with increased frequency in the homosexual population and among athletes (eg, wrestlers and gymnasts) who must achieve a certain body weight for competition.

C. **Binge eating disorder**
   1. **BED** affects 2–5% of the general population.
   2. It is more common among those who are obese. Among the mildly obese not seeking treatment, the prevalence of BED is approximately 5%, increasing to 10–15% among those enrolled in commercial weight loss programs, and 30% in those attending university-based weight management programs.
   3. Approximately 60% of individuals with BED are female.
   4. Age at onset is often in the young adult period, but many patients present at an older age (eg, mid- to late 30s) when seeking weight loss treatment.
   5. BED is associated with considerable psychiatric comorbidity.

III. **Pathophysiology.** Eating disorders are multifactorial disorders, which probably result from a number of individual, familial, biological, and cultural predisposing factors.
   A. **Sociocultural influences.** Common to all of the eating disorders is the national preoccupation with weight and shape, and the idealization of thinness as a standard of feminine beauty. Dissatisfaction with body weight and shape may lead to restrictive dieting, which may precipitate eating disorders in vulnerable individuals.
   B. **Familial characteristics**
      1. **Twin studies.** Twin studies of AN suggest a genetic predisposition to the disorder.
      2. **Family history of comorbid psychopathology. AN, BN,** and **BED** have all been associated with an increased relative risk of mood disorders in first-degree relatives. Substance abuse disorders have also been reported to be more prevalent in relatives of patients with BN and BED.
      3. **Family history of obesity.** Some evidence shows that individuals with **BN** have an increased prevalence of obesity in first-degree relatives compared with those without the disorder. Those with **BN** are also more likely than their peers to have been overweight prior to the development of their eating disorder. Obese individuals with BED frequently report a family history of obesity similar to that of obese individuals without the disorder.
   C. **Psychiatric comorbidity**
      1. **Affective disorders**
         a. Many individuals with **AN** show evidence of clinical depression while underweight, but some of this symptomatology may improve when weight is restored.
         b. Both **BN** and **BED** are associated with an increased lifetime prevalence of major depression and dysthymic disorder—often reported as over 50%. It is not known whether this depression is primary, secondary to the eating disorder, or the result of some unspecified third factor. Symptoms often improve with treatment of the eating disorder.
      2. **Personality disorders,** especially those with a primary component of impulse control, such as borderline personality disorder, are seen in one- to two-thirds of eating disorders accompanied by binge eating, purging, or both, including the binge eating/purging subtype of **AN, BN,** and **BED.**
      3. **Substance abuse disorders**
         a. In **AN,** substance abuse is most frequently seen in patients with the binge eating/purging subtype.
         b. Both **BN** and **BED** have been associated with an increased prevalence of drug or alcohol abuse or both.
      4. **Obsessive–compulsive disorders.** An increased prevalence of obsessive–compulsive disorder has been reported in both **AN** and **BN.** Most often, obsessions are seen in areas related to the eating disorder. In order to make a diagnosis of obsessive–compulsive disorder, obsessions or compulsions must be present that do not relate to food, body shape, or weight.
      5. **Anxiety disorders,** including panic disorder and social phobia, are seen with increased frequency in patients with **AN, BN,** and **BED.**
   D. A **history of sexual abuse,** particularly in childhood, is frequently cited as being extremely prevalent in patients with eating disorders, with a cited prevalence of 20–50%. However, some experts have suggested that the rate of sexual abuse among patients with eating disorders is no higher than that found among patients with other psychiatric disorders, or even that within the general population.
   E. **Neurobiological alterations.** Many endogenous neurotransmitters and related neurochemicals involved in regulating processes of eating have been studied.

These include hunger signals (norepinephrine, norpeptide y and yy), satiety signals (serotonin and cholecystokinin), food reward signals (dopamine and endorphins), and metabolic signals (leptin). Some differences in these signals have persisted in people with eating disorders, despite attaining normal weight and eating habits. This finding suggests future studies that may result in better pharmacologic treatment for these disorders.

IV. Diagnosis
A. Presentation to the physician
1. **Anorexia nervosa.** Approximately 50% of the time, a family member brings the patient to the physician because of concern about weight loss or low body weight. Those patients rarely complain of weight loss or loss of appetite. They will usually present with nonspecific complaints such as fainting, fatigue, low energy (despite high physical activity), dry skin, cold intolerance, blue hands and feet, constipation, bloating, amenorrhea, nerve compression symptoms (from loss of fat padding), hair loss, easy bruising (from K+ abnormalities), frequent fractures, sexual disinterest, and sexual dysfunction.
2. Patients with **BN** often present to physicians requesting a weight loss diet, or with nonspecific symptoms (mostly related to purging), such as fainting, weakness, oligomenorrhea, amenorrhea, easy bruising, muscle cramps, nonspecific chest pain, heartburn, abdominal pain, severe constipation, and dental caries. Most will not reveal binge eating/purging spontaneously, but will admit to these behaviors if asked in a sympathetic manner.
3. Most patients with **BED** present requesting treatment of obesity, or for other medical complaints. Most will not admit to difficulties with binge eating unless asked in a sympathetic manner.

B. Physical examination and laboratory evaluation.
Suggested evaluation of patients with eating disorders is listed in Table 97–2. All patients with eating disorders should receive a thorough physical examination, with special attention to the cardiovascular and gastrointestinal systems. Anthropometric evaluation (eg, skin

TABLE 97–2. SUGGESTED MEDICAL EVALUATION OF PATIENTS WITH EATING DISORDERS

Evaluation	Anorexia Nervosa — Restricting Type	Anorexia Nervosa — Binge/Purge Type	Bulimia Nervosa — Purging Type	Bulimia Nervosa — Nonpurging Type	Binge Eating Disorder
Weight for height	X	X	X	X	X
Temperature, pulse, blood pressure	X	X	X	X	X
Physical examination	X	X	X	X	X
Dental examination		X	X		
Electrocardiogram	X	X	X		
Complete blood cell count	X	X	X	X	X
Urinalysis	X	X	X	X	X
Blood urea nitrogen/creatinine	X	X	X	X[1]	
Amylase		X[1]	X[1]	X[1]	
Sodium/potassium/chloride/bicarbonate	X	X	X	X[1]	
Magnesium	X	X	X[1]		
Calcium	X	X	X[1]		
Phosphate	X	X	X[1]		
Albumin	X	X	X[1]		
Bone mineral densitometry[2]	X[1]	X[1]	X[1]	X[1]	
Luteinizing hormone/follicle-stimulating hormone/estradiol[2]	X[1]	X[1]	X[1]	X[1]	
Liver enzymes	X	X	X		
Thyroid-stimulating hormone, T₄	X	X	X	X	X
Cholesterol	X	X	X	X	X
Glucose	X	X	X	X	X
Blood or urine screen for drugs/alcohol/laxatives/diuretics	X[1]	X[1]	X[1]	X[1]	X[1]

[1] May be indicated, depending on the patient's clinical circumstances.
[2] In patients with long-standing amenorrhea.

fold thickness, bioelectrical impedance analysis, or dual energy x-ray absorptiometry) carried out by a nutritionist can be helpful in malnourished patients.

1. **Anorexia nervosa**
   a. By DSM-IV criteria, on physical examination, there must be at least low weight for age and height, though subterfuge about it is common, with patients wearing heavy clothes, carrying heavy objects while being weighed, or drinking a lot of water prior to being weighed. Other findings may include acrocyanosis, lanugo, pitting edema of extremities, hypotension or orthostatic hypotension, sinus bradycardia, cardiac murmur (due to mitral valve prolapse, reversible with weight gain), slow relaxation of tendon reflexes, and skin changes (coarse, dry, yellow/orange tinged, loose and flabby).

      In females, there may be breast atrophy and atrophic vaginitis. In males, there may be hypotropic hypogonadism.
   b. Laboratory abnormalities may include leukopenia (though no increased risk for infection), thrombocytopenia, normocytic normochromic anemia or elevated hemoglobin (may be falsely elevated secondary to dehydration), erythrocyte sedimentation rate normal or low, low blood urea nitrogen (poor protein intake) or high low blood urea nitrogen (dehydration), or cholesterol falsely elevated (starvation reaction).
   c. Endocrine abnormalities may include thyroid abnormalities (euthyroid sick syndrome (low T_4, normal thyroid-stimulating hormone), growth hormone abnormalities (often increased with abnormal response to stimulation tests), and plasma cortisol abnormalities (mildly elevated and decreased response to insulin induced hypoglycemia).
   d. In the presence of purging behaviors, a variety of electrolyte abnormalities may be seen, including hypochloremic metabolic alkalosis (resulting from vomiting), metabolic acidosis (caused by laxative abuse), and hypokalemia.
   e. X-ray and bone density studies may show signs of osteopenia or osteoporosis.

2. Patients with **BN** frequently have no abnormalities upon physical examination. Occasionally they may present with specific abnormalities on physical examination such as the following:
   a. Swollen cheeks, secondary to painless parotid inflammation, may be secondary to chronic vomiting and salivary stimulation. This generally resolves within a few weeks after cessation of vomiting.
   b. Erosions of the lingual surfaces of the teeth and multiple dental caries are frequent, secondary to vomiting. Dental evaluation is recommended in all patients who purge by vomiting.
   c. Patients may have scarring or calluses on the dorsum of the hand from self-induction of vomiting (Russell's sign).
   d. Laboratory abnormalities are similar to those seen in the purging subtype of **AN.**
   e. Elevated serum amylase, primarily the salivary isoenzyme, is present in about 30% of patients who purge by vomiting. If elevated, this may be useful in confirming the presence of vomiting when patient denial is suspected.
   f. Additional useful laboratory testing, which should be guided by the history and the physical examination, includes serum or urine testing for drugs of abuse, alcohol, laxatives, and/or diuretics.

3. Patients with **BED** frequently have no physical abnormalities upon physical examination attributable to their eating disorder, other than obesity. No specific laboratory abnormalities are seen. Because they are frequently obese, testing for the medical complications of obesity may be useful (see Chapter 83).

V. **Medical complications of eating disorders**
   A. **Anorexia nervosa.** The most dangerous complications of **AN** are secondary to starvation, purging, or both.
      1. **Cardiomyopathy,** secondary to low weight or ipecac abuse, and **cardiac arrhythmias,** secondary to electrolyte abnormalities, may lead to sudden death. Electrocardiographic (ECG) abnormalities may include sinus bradycardia, ST-segment depression, and U waves if hypokalemia or hypomagnesemia

is present. Monitoring of pulse, blood pressure, and ECG during treatment is recommended.

2. **Gastrointestinal complications** include delayed gastric emptying, duodenal dilatation, and constipation.

3. **Amenorrhea** is a diagnostic feature of **AN** and may persist for some time after restoration of normal body weight.

4. **Renal abnormalities,** seen in up to 70% of these patients, include decreased glomerular filtration rate, increased blood urea nitrogen, and pitting edema. Monitoring of renal function during treatment is strongly recommended.

5. **Osteoporosis** may be severe. Bone densitometry should be considered in patients with chronic amenorrhea.

6. **Suicide** is a major cause of death in **AN** (see section VI).

7. **Aggressive refeeding** can lead to edema and severe electrolyte and cardiac abnormalities (see section VI,B).

8. **Multiple dental caries** may be seen. Patients who have been vomiting for 4 years or more demonstrate enamel erosions.

B. **Bulimia nervosa.** Medical complications of purging **BN** are similar to those seen in purging **AN**, including electrolyte abnormalities and cardiac arrhythmias.

1. Laxative abuse can lead to "cathartic colon" with severe and refractory constipation. This can be managed with increased fluids, lactulose, and bulk laxatives and may take up to 6 months to resolve.

2. Rare but serious complications of binge eating include gastric or esophageal rupture and megacolon secondary to chronic laxative abuse.

C. **Binge eating disorder.** The primary complications of **BED** are secondary to the obesity that may be caused or worsened by binge eating, including type II diabetes mellitus, hypertension, and dyslipidemias.

VI. **Treatment.** The initial treatment goal for **AN** and **BN** is nutritional rehabilitation, with an aim of weight restoration, establishment of normal healthy eating patterns, and correction of physiologic and psychological dysfunction that may be secondary to malnutrition. Longer-term goals are aimed at preventing relapse.

A. **Indications for hospitalization.** While eating disorders are now primarily treated in the outpatient setting, patients with severe or refractory eating disorders—particularly those with **AN**—may require inpatient hospitalization. Indications for hospitalization include severe malnutrition (<70%–75% of ideal body weight for height, arrested growth and development), physiologic instability (syncope, dehydration, hypotension, orthostatic changes, hypothermia, symptomatic bradycardia), electrolyte imbalance (hypokalemia, hypophosphatemia), ECG abnormalities (bradycardia <50 beats per minute, prolonged corrected QT, arrhythmias), psychiatric instability (suicidality, severe concomitant psychiatric disorders), social considerations (lack of local availability of suitable outpatient treatment program), and lack of progress in outpatient treatment. In less severe situations day hospitalization may be considered.

B. **Nutritional rehabilitation.** Rapid refeeding may lead to edema, cardiac decompensation, and gastrointestinal symptoms.

1. The usual starting intake is 30–40 kcal/kg/day (1000–1600 kcal/day), with increases up to 70–100 kcal/day necessary during refeeding for some patients. Replacement of abnormal electrolytes, vitamins, and trace elements is particularly important in the initial phase of refeeding.

2. Reasonable targets for weight gain are 1–3 lbs/week in the inpatient setting and 0.5–2 lbs/week in the outpatient setting. Checking weight 2–3 times a week is sufficient; no advantage has been found for more frequent checks.

3. Solid food is preferred; however, some programs initiate treatment with a liquid diet.

4. Oral feeding is preferred, although much encouragement by staff may be necessary. Nutritional supplements may be helpful in some patients. Nasogastric feeding and parenteral nutrition generally should be used only in life-threatening situations.

5. The target weight should be one at which reproductive function normalizes, and will vary with the individual patient. Many patients can be discharged from inpatient treatment at a weight below their target weight and followed up carefully as outpatients.

C. **Psychotherapy.** Most individuals with eating disorders will benefit from referral to a mental health professional with specialized expertise in the treatment of these disorders. Many university-based hospitals and college campuses offer specialized treatment for eating disorders. The American Anorexia/Bulimia Association (418 E 76th Street, New York, NY 10021) also provides referral to qualified professionals.

1. **Anorexia nervosa**

   a. Behavioral programs in which privileges such as time out of bed or permission to exercise are tied to weight gain are frequently used in the initial treatment of AN. Patients who purge after eating may require supervision when using the bathroom after meals or may have to wait an hour before being given permission to use the bathroom.

   b. For adolescents under age 18, whose duration of illness has been less than 3 years, the addition of family therapy has been found to be particularly beneficial.

   c. Older patients benefit more from an emphasis on interpersonal, cognitive–behavioral, and psychodynamic therapies.

   d. Traditional inpatient therapy, individual plus family therapy, and outpatient group plus group family psychoeducational therapy are equally efficacious.

2. **Bulimia nervosa**

   a. **Cognitive–behavioral psychotherapy (CBT)** is the major psychological treatment for **BN** and has been shown to be effective in reducing the severity of binge eating and purging behaviors.

      (1) CBT focuses on altering the patient's faulty cognitions and attitudes regarding food, body image, and weight. Behavioral principles are then applied to enable patients to change their behaviors regarding food and weight (ie, eating regular meals, enhancing problem-solving skills, and receiving relapse prevention training). CBT may be provided in an individual or group setting. Treatments are usually 3–6 months in duration and typically involve 10–20 treatment sessions.

      (2) Reduction of binge eating by completion of treatment is often dramatic, generally ranging from about 50% to 95%. Rates of complete abstinence by the end of treatment are much lower, with most studies reporting about 20–50% of patients completely abstinent from binge eating, purging, or both at the end of treatment.

      (3) While follow-up data are limited, over half of patients generally report >50% reductions in binge eating at follow-up, averaging several months posttreatment. A smaller percentage (generally 20–50%) report total abstinence.

      (4) Maintenance of change appears better at 1 year with CBT than with antidepressant medications alone.

   b. **Interpersonal psychotherapy (IPT)** focuses on helping patients to identify interpersonal triggers to binge eating and to improve their relationships with others. As with CBT, treatment may be provided in a group or individual format and is usually time limited. This form of therapy has been found to be as effective as CBT in the long term, thought it does have a delayed onset of effect.

   c. **Addiction model for treatment.** The efficacy of programs treating eating disorders as addictions themselves has not been proven.

   d. **Self-help groups.** Some patients report being helped by self-help groups (eg, Overeaters Anonymous) that use a 12-step approach to the management of eating disorders. These programs can be quite variable from chapter to chapter. It is recommended that clinicians carefully monitor their patients' response to such programs.

   e. **Treatment of concomitant substance abuse disorders.** In general, unless malnutrition is severe, substance abuse disorders should be addressed prior to treatment of the eating disorder, unless program staff is competent to treat both disorders concurrently.

3. **Binge eating disorder.** Both CBT and IPT have been shown to be efficacious in reducing the frequency of binge eating in BED. Unfortunately, there

is little or no weight change in programs that do not also target changes in eating habits and exercise. Binge eating actually decreased in patients with BED who underwent weight loss programs, including very low-calorie diet programs and behavioral weight control programs, although a subset of patients appear to be at risk for attrition from treatment, early regain of lost weight, or both. Some obese patients may need to receive treatment targeted to their eating disorder before they can successfully lose weight and maintain weight loss.

D. Medication

  1. Anorexia nervosa. There have been few controlled studies using pharmacologic therapy for the treatment of **AN**, although several classes of agents have been used empirically.

  a. Antipsychotic medications. There is no evidence of the efficacy of antipsychotic medications in the treatment of **AN**, and these low-weight patients are at untoward risk for adverse effects. Therefore, the use of these agents is not recommended.

  b. Antidepressant medications. Controlled trials of tricyclic antidepressant agents have not demonstrated efficacy in the treatment of **AN**, although a few open-label trials of fluoxetine in a small number of patients did appear to show some benefit, especially in preventing relapse in weight-recovered patients. Concerns about the cardiotoxicity of antidepressant agents, as well as the frequent amelioration of depressive symptoms with weight restoration, limit the use of antidepressants in the treatment of AN. In the patient with persistent depression, use of these agents should be considered, with careful consideration of any underlying medical contraindications to their use.

  c. Cyproheptadine is a serotonin antagonist known to promote increased appetite and weight gain. Controlled trials at doses up to 32 mg/day have shown little efficacy compared with placebo, although there is some evidence that more severely ill patients derive some benefit. In particular, anorectic patients in the restricting (nonbulimic) subgroup may be more likely to benefit from treatment with this agent.

  d. There is insufficient evidence to recommend the use of other agents, such as lithium carbonate or anticonvulsants, for the treatment of **AN**.

  e. Metoclopramide. A recent double-blind controlled study suggests that this medication may be beneficial in assisting with weight gain by alleviating symptoms of both vomiting and slow gastric emptying.

  f. Hormone replacement therapy is suggested by some authorities when there has been long-standing amenorrhea, though a recent study suggests that hormone replacement may not ameliorate the osteoporosis in AN.

  g. Vitamin D and calcium may at this time be the only treatment available for osteoporosis when caused by AN.

  2. Bulimia nervosa. Numerous studies have shown the efficacy of antidepressant medications in the treatment of **BN**.

  a. Antidepressant medications generally cause a marked reduction (50–66%) in the frequency of binge eating and purging.

  b. Total "abstinence" from binge eating/purging behaviors is much lower—approximately 25% over the short term (ie, <1-year follow-up).

  c. Fluoxetine is frequently used in the treatment of **BN**. The required dosages are often higher than those used in the treatment of depression—generally 60 mg/day.

  d. Other tricyclic and tetracyclic antidepressant agents and serotoninergic agents are frequently used in the treatment of **BN**, including imipramine, desipramine, trazodone, paroxetine, and sertraline. Selective serotonin reuptake inhibitors (SSRIs), including fluoxetine, paroxetine, and sertraline, have the advantage of not causing weight gain. Bupropion has been associated with an increased incidence of seizures in patients with eating disorders, and its use is not recommended in this population. Monoamine oxidase inhibitors, such as phenelzine and isocarboxazid, may be useful in some patients who have been unresponsive to the tricyclic antidepressants or SSRIs, but they have the disadvantages of dietary restrictions and interaction with various medications. For most antidepressant medications, the dosages are similar to those used to treat depression (see Chapter 96).

    e. Even patients without significant depressive symptomatology may respond well to antidepressant treatment of bulimia. The onset of effects, as in the treatment of depression, is gradual.

    f. Patients who do not respond to one class of antidepressant medication may respond favorably to an agent from a different class.

    g. Studies have found that intensive CBT may be more effective than antidepressant treatment alone.

    h. Integrating antidepressant medicine and psychotherapy seems to offer the best available treatment at this time. A stepwise approach has been suggested. Combining different approaches, the steps could be as follows:

        (1) Start with CBT only. If there is a good response, continue with maintenance therapy. If there is inadequate clinical response, continue to step 2.

        (2) Give CBT and an SSRI. If there is a good response, continue with maintenance therapy. If there is inadequate clinical response, continue to step 3.

        (3) Change to another antidepressant, or change the psychotherapy to IPT.

        In a patient with BN and without depression, start with step 1. In the bulimic patient with evidence of depression, start with step 2. It may be necessary to try up to three antidepressants before there is a good response. In order for a particular antidepressant to be considered as failed, at least 4 weeks of adequate doses of the antidepressant are recommended. In bulimic patients taking medication who appear to be responding poorly, consideration should be given to the possibility that continued purging makes it unlikely that adequate medicine levels are maintained.

    i. Maintenance therapy. There do not appear to be long-term studies published that prove how long maintenance therapy should continue or what form this therapy should take. There does, however, seem to be an understanding that therapy should continue for at least 12 months.

  3. Binge eating disorder.

    a. Antidepressant medications appear to have similar efficacies in **BED** and in **BN,** although fewer studies have been conducted in BED. SSRIs, such as fluoxetine, 60–80 mg/day, appear to have advantages over tricyclics in the prevention of weight gain.

    b. A combined medicine and physiotherapy treatment plan, such as is used in BN, seems to be beneficial. Sometimes, however, early treatment with SSRIs is recommended, to help with short-term weight loss.

  4. Eating disorders and complementary medicine. Currently no published trials are available on use of complementary medicine in the treatment of eating disorders. Much anecdotal evidence is, however, available about various modalities, including acupuncture, mind–body techniques, Chinese medicine, herbs, and so on. Since St. John's wort has SSRI-like pharmacologic effects, it might be as beneficial as other SSRI medication in the treatment of eating disorders.

VII. Natural history and prognosis

  A. Anorexia nervosa

    1. The course of **AN** is quite variable. Some patients have a single episode, others have an intermittent course characterized by relapses and remissions, while others have a chronic and unrelenting course.

      a. In a follow-up of hospitalized patients and patients from a referral center at least 4 years after treatment, slightly fewer than half showed good outcome, with near-normal weight restoration and regular menses, while 24% had poor outcome, with continued low weight and menstrual dysfunction.

      b. Mortality is extremely high—estimated to be 10–20% at 20 years. Death primarily results from inanition, electrolyte imbalance, and suicide.

      c. About two-thirds of patients continue to have food preoccupation, up to 40% show continued bulimic symptoms, and frequent comorbid psychopathology persists.

      d. Onset in early adolescence, early referral for treatment, and absence of binge eating/purging are favorable prognostic indicators.

B. Bulimia nervosa
1. **BN** tends to be characterized by remissions and relapses.
   a. While some symptoms often persist, those treated as outpatients frequently manifest long-term improvement.
   b. Over a 1- to 2-year period, untreated bulimic patients report modest improvement, with reductions in binge eating and purging of about 24%.
2. Good prognostic indicators for **BN** include more mild symptoms at presentation, the presence of at least a few close friendships, a lack of concomitant personality disorders, and absence of laxative abuse. The presence of depression does not significantly affect prognosis.

C. Binge eating disorder. Not enough is known about long-term outcomes of BED, with and without treatment. Weight is often regained within 12 months. Short-term treatment appears to be as successful as with BN. More studies are needed to assess long-term management and the influence of the comorbid factors.

REFERENCES

American Psychiatric Association (APA): *Diagnostic and Statistical Manual of Mental Disorders,* 4th ed. (DSM-IV). APA; 1994.

Crow SJ, et al: Integrating cognitive therapy and medications in treating bulimia nervosa. Psychiatr Clin North Am 1996;**19**(4):755.

Grinspoon S, et al: Mechanisms and treatment options for bone loss in anorexia nervosa. Psychopharmacol Bull 1997;**33**(3):399.

Hudson JI, et al: Antidepressant treatment of binge-eating Disorder: Research findings and clinical guidelines. J Clin Psychol 1996;**57**(8):73.

Jimerson DC, et al: Medications in the treatment of eating disorders. Psychiatr Clin North Am 1996;**19**(4):739.

Massimo C, Mauri et al: Neurobiological and psychopharmacological basis in the therapy of bulimia and anorexia. Prog Neuropsychopharmacol Biol Psychiatry 1996;**20**:207.

Schwitzer AM, et al: Eating disorders among college women: Prevention, education, and treatment responses. J Am Coll Heath 1998;**46**:199.

Wiseman CV, et al: Eating disorders. Med Clin North Am 1998;**82**:(1);145.

---

98   Personality Disorders

Brian Hertz, MD

I. **Definition.** Personality disorders are a heterogeneous group of diagnoses that typically present as difficult patient encounters. These difficulties may arise in managing or diagnosing general medical conditions, or with patients who mobilize intense feelings toward their provider, such as anger, impotence, or hatred. However, in defining personality disorders, the traits that produce these difficulties must be a part of the patient's underlying personality and not arise from a general medical condition or another psychiatric disorder or be secondary to medication or substance abuse.

    Personality disorders manifest as enduring patterns of inner experience or behavior, both inflexible and maladaptive. This enduring pattern must cause functional impairment or personal distress, and must pervade a broad range of personal and social situations.

    The 4th edition of *the Diagnostic and Statistical Manual of Mental Disorders* (DSM-IV) outlines 10 specific personality disorders, divided into three clusters:

A. Cluster A (odd, eccentric) disorders:
1. **Paranoid disorder.** Patients may expect exploitation or harm, question loyalty and fidelity, or bear grudges. They expect to be taken advantage of and challenge other's intentions toward them. Wariness and jealousy are common.
2. **Schizoid disorder.** Patients appear aloof and indifferent to praise or criticism. Patients are typically loners with a constricted affect.
3. **Schizotypal disorder.** Patients appear like schizophrenics without psychotic symptoms. They relate poorly to others, often with magical beliefs, non-

delusional ideas of references, or inappropriate silliness, excessive anxiety, constricted affect, or odd dress.

B. Cluster B (dramatic, erratic) disorders:

1. **Antisocial disorder.** Patients exhibit cruelty, problems with authority, unlawful behavior, dishonesty, and irresponsibility, frequently exploiting others. Antisocial patients often have a childhood history of delinquent behavior, such as arson, cruelty to animals, truancy, or fighting.

2. **Borderline disorder.** Patients' moods may shift rapidly and to extremes. These patients have unstable work and are characterized by unstable lives. Patients quickly shift from idealizing others to totally devaluing them, and their relationships tend to be intense and unstable.

3. **Histrionic disorder.** Patients show exaggerated emotions and need to be in the limelight. They tend to overstate physical complaints. Although seductive behavior is common in individuals with histrionic personality disorder, patients usually do not wish to engage in actual sexual contact with their physician. Their descriptions are generalized and vague; in other words, they see the forest but never the trees. Patients are usually overly concerned about their appearance.

4. **Narcissistic disorder.** Patients are self-centered and vain. They feel special and superior and react with anger, depression, or shame if criticized. They believe they deserve special attention. They lack empathy for others.

C. Cluster C (anxious) disorders:

1. **Avoidant disorder.** Affected patients are shy and fearful. They want relationships with others but are often too fearful to seek them. Criticism wounds them deeply. Men with avoidant behavior are usually unmarried.

2. **Dependent disorder.** Patients with this disorder want other individuals to run their lives for them. Often clinging and demanding of their physician's time, they welcome "doctor's orders" and are usually compliant. Dependent disorder patients often become depressed when they feel uncared for and try to avoid being alone.

3. **Obsessive–compulsive disorder.** Patients are perfectionists who demand neatness and orderliness. Unlike histrionic disorder patients, these individuals tend to see the trees and miss the forest. Many patients with obsessive–compulsive disorder are workaholics. Their emotions are restricted, and they rarely show their feelings, except for anger. In addition, they are often stingy.

4. **Passive–aggressive disorder.** Affected patients feel put upon by social and job demands. They respond to these demands by passive resistance, such as forgetting to do things, being late, obstructing others, or working slowly. Passive–aggressive patients complain frequently and respond poorly to criticism.

II. Epidemiology. The community prevalence rates of personality disorders vary widely, averaging 11% in adults. As a group, patients tend to have less education, greater problems with alcohol abuse, more marital difficulties, and more unemployment than individuals in the general population.

A. Cluster A disorders are uncommon and are seen more often in males. Schizotypal disorder is more common in first-degree relatives of patients with schizophrenia.

B. Cluster B disorders. Antisocial behavior, which is more common in the lower socioeconomic classes, more often affects males than females. Borderline disorder is common and is found much more often in females. Patients with borderline personality disorder have an increased incidence of attention-deficit/hyperactivity disorder. Mood disorders commonly coexist with personality disorders. Some authorities believe that mood disorders may predispose individuals to borderline personality disorder. Women are more often diagnosed with histrionic disorder, but the actual prevalence between both sexes may be the same. Narcissistic disorder affects both sexes equally.

C. Cluster C disorders. Avoidant, passive–aggressive, and dependent disorders have a nearly equal male–female ratio. Men have a greater prevalence of obsessive–compulsive disorder.

III. Psychopathology. The formation of personality disorders is not completely understood. These disorders probably develop from an interaction between inherited temperaments and life experiences, particularly early life experiences.

A. **The social learning model** considers personality to be the sum total of complex patterns of learned behavior. Rewards and punishments for behaviors throughout life shape the individual's personality.

B. **The psychoanalytic model** considers personality to be formed developmentally. Failure to negotiate a developmental step may result in long-standing difficulties. For example, the patient with a borderline personality disorder is believed to be "stuck" in the separation–individuation phase of development as a result of some type of emotional trauma. Patients with personality disorders are thought to use primitive defenses (eg, splitting, in which the world is viewed in "all-or-none" terms) or make maladaptive use of defenses (eg, inappropriate isolation of affect in which ideas or thoughts are separated from their associated feelings).

C. Some authorities view personality disorders as representing an extreme end of a **continuum of personality traits.** Others assert that such disorders are not part of a spectrum from normal to abnormal, but are **discontinuous pathologic conditions.**

D. **A major genetic role** is postulated for schizotypal personality disorder and antisocial personality disorder. Antisocial personality disorder is genetically linked to somatization disorder, which is seen mainly in women. The early life history of patients with this disorder is often characterized by emotional deprivation or physical abuse, although some cases of antisocial personality disorder result from organic brain disease, such as a head injury or encephalitis.

IV. **Diagnosis.** Symptoms, signs, and feelings of patients define specific disorders, based on criteria described in the introductory section.

A. **Laboratory tests.** There are currently no clinically available biologic markers helpful in diagnosing personality disorders, even those with a strong genetic contribution. However, several structured interviews or psychological tests can assist in the diagnosis of personality disorders. The administration and interpretation of all the tests described below require special training, although screening inventory techniques for primary care are being studied. Referral to a psychologist may be needed if testing is desired.

1. Structured interviews commonly used to identify personality disorders include the **Structured Interview for the DSM-III Personality Disorders (SIPD)** and the **Personality Diagnostic Questionnaire (PDQ).**

2. The **Minnesota Multiphasic Personality Inventory (MMPI)** is a classic test measuring various dimensions of personality, but it does not define DSM-IV categories directly.

3. The **Millon Clinical Multiaxial Inventory (MCMI)** is a written test that provides scales that can be directly translated into DSM-IV diagnostic categories. Shorter versions of the Millon test, such as the brief personality inventories described by Clark et al (1998), may provide useful screening tools in primary care.

4. Projective testing provides more subjective data on personality dynamics. Common examples include the **Thematic Apperception Test** and the **Rorschach Inkblot Test.**

V. **Treatment.** Most approaches to the treatment of personality disorders combine psychotherapy, medication, and directed behavioral therapy. The goals of therapy are to alleviate symptoms and minimize dysfunctional behaviors.

A. **Psychotherapy** may be either individual or group. Theoretical approaches include psychoanalytic, psychodynamic, cognitive, behavioral, strategic, supportive, and experiential psychotherapies. None has been shown to be superior to the others. Many therapists use an eclectic approach, which is a mixture of a variety of theoretical schools.

Treatments for some specific personality disorders are described below.

1. **Antisocial disorders.** Antisocial disorder patients are best treated in special groups within institutional settings where external controls are available. Antisocial criminals have participated in special 2- to 4-week wilderness programs, which have decreased the incidence of criminal recidivism.

2. **Avoidant and dependent** disorder patients often benefit from assertiveness training. Passive–aggressive disorder patients may also benefit by learning to substitute assertive techniques for their passive–aggressive behavior.

3. **Obsessive–compulsive** disorder patients have been successfully treated with the serotonin reuptake inhibitors, such as paroxetine HCL (10–40 mg

daily), and the tricyclic compound, clomipramine (starting at 25 mg twice daily and increasing to 100 mg twice daily over the first 2 weeks, with a maximum daily dose of 250 mg).

B. Several associated symptoms and comorbid conditions may benefit from psycho-pharmacologic agents.

    1. Depression occurs commonly with personality disorders. If depressive symptoms are typical, a tricyclic antidepressant or selective serotonin reuptake inhibitor can be used (see Chapter 96). If symptoms are atypical (eg, increased appetite, increased sleep, or rejection sensitive), a monoamine oxidase inhibitor should be considered. Phenelzine, 15 mg three times a day, may be used.

    2. Borderline disorder patients may have brief **psychoses, paranoia, or dissociative symptoms,** which can be treated with low doses of antipsychotics, such as risperidone. Risperidone is typically started at a dose of 0.5–1 mg twice daily and increased as needed by no more than 2 mg at a time each week, up to no more than 6 mg daily.

    Borderline disorder patients with episodic dyscontrol (episodes of angry outbursts often associated with violent ideation directed at either themselves or others) can be administered carbamazepine, 200 mg twice daily initially, increasing up to 1000 mg/day as necessary. A sleep-deprived electroencephalogram should be obtained beforehand to assess temporal lobe epilepsy.

    Avoid prescribing benzodiazepines in borderline disorder patients, as these agents are potentially addictive and may cause disinhibition with uncontrolled rage or dysphoria.

VI. Management strategies

A. Cluster A disorders

    1. Paranoid disorder patients should be treated with a courteous, professional attitude without trying to be too close. Physicians should not argue with these patients about their beliefs, nor should they reinforce them.

    2. Schizoid and schizotypal disorder patients are uncomfortable with closeness. Their desire to be left alone should be accepted. Physicians should show reasonable interest in these patients without necessarily expecting them to reciprocate.

B. Cluster B disorders

    1. Antisocial disorder patients are best managed by "sticking to the rules" in a nonjudgmental but matter-of-fact way. The physician should not tolerate dangerous behavior and should avoid prescribing addictive medications.

    2. Borderline disorder patients represent a major challenge to the physician. They often stir up angry feelings in clinicians, who must struggle to maintain a calm, reasoned approach. Since patients with borderline disorders fear both closeness and rejection, it is best to stay in the "middle ground." The clinician should not be drawn into trying to fill excessive demands (eg, more time, more tests, or special care). Appropriate limits should be set in a nonpunitive manner. Sometimes a written treatment contract is helpful. At times, medication may be needed (see section V,B,2). Avoid prescribing addictive drugs. Observe patients carefully for drug abuse. Co-manage the patient with the help of a mental health professional. Splitting care among health care providers should be minimized; ensure frequent communication among those involved. Patients often play one provider against another.

    3. Histrionic disorder patients should be given "bottom lines," since they often forget details. These patients should be allowed to express their fears. The physician should not let the seductiveness of this type of patient evolve into a nonprofessional relationship.

    4. Narcissistic disorder patients will often challenge the physician's authority. The physician should not become defensive but should express himself or herself as a competent clinician. Acknowledging the patient's accomplishments, intelligence, and abilities, insofar as they truly exist, may establish the patient as an ally.

C. Cluster C disorders

    1. Avoidant disorder patients should be approached in an open, caring way. Their need for privacy should be respected when possible. Outright criticism should be avoided. Once these patients come to know and trust their physician, they are quite loyal and appreciative.

2. **Dependent** disorder patients feel best if the physician expresses willingness to care for the patient. These patients respond well to reassurance. Sometimes their needs are so great they become too demanding, however. In this case, set limits in a nonpunitive way.

3. **Obsessive–compulsive** disorder patients fear a loss of self-control. Everything should be explained to them in great detail, and patients should be given choices whenever possible. They are reassured by a physician who is organized, on time, and thorough.

4. **Passive–aggressive** disorder patients are most cooperative when they are approached with requests rather than demands. Noncompliance may be a clue that the patient is responding in a passive–aggressive way.

VII. **Natural history and prognosis.** Personality disorders are primarily formed, and are identifiable, by adolescence or young adulthood.

A. Persons affected by cluster A (odd, eccentric) disorders tend to remain much the same throughout adult life. Individuals with cluster B (dramatic, erratic) and cluster C (anxious) disorders tend toward spontaneous improvement throughout adult life until old age, when some experience an exacerbation.

B. Personality disorders increase vulnerability to major psychiatric syndromes such as mood disorders, anxiety disorders, somatoform disorders, substance abuse disorders, and psychoses.

C. The prognosis with treatment is usually only fair. Successful treatment usually requires a well-motivated patient who is capable of psychological insight. Most treatments are lengthy; the treatment of patients with antisocial and borderline disorders may require an institutional setting where external controls are available.

REFERENCES

American Psychiatric Association (APA): *Diagnostic and Statistical Manual of Mental Disorders,* 4th ed. APA; 1994.

Carpenter LL, et al: A risk-benefit assessment of drugs used in the management of obsessive-compulsive disorder. Drug Saf 1996;**15:**116.

Clark JW, et al: Initial evidence for reliability and validity of a brief screening inventory for personality disorders. Psychol Rep 1998;**82:**1115.

Emerson J, Paukratz L, Joos S, et al: Personality disorders in problematic medical patients. Psychosomatics 1994;**35:**469.

Oldham JM: Personality disorders: Current perspectives. JAMA 1994;**272:**1770.

Rey JM, et al: Continuities between psychiatric disorders in adolescents and personality disorders in young adults. Am J Psychiatry 1995;**152:**895.

Sanislow C, et al: Treatment outcomes of personality disorders. Can J Psychiatry 1998;**43:**237.

---

99   Schizophrenia

James T. Flannick, PsyD

I. **Definition.** Schizophrenia is a recurrent mental disorder marked by characteristic psychotic symptoms and by deterioration in social and occupational functioning and in self-care. Type I schizophrenia is characterized by the predominance of positive symptoms such as hallucinations, delusions, and disorganized thinking, whereas in type II schizophrenia negative symptoms such as apparent lack of emotional responsiveness, withdrawal, apathy, and poor grooming are more prominent.

II. **Epidemiology.** Schizophrenia, which affects more persons than any other functional psychosis, occurs with remarkably similar frequency throughout the world. The lifetime prevalence of schizophrenia among people living in the United States, using US definitional criteria, is 1.5%; the 6-month prevalence is 0.9%.

A. Schizophrenia occurs in both sexes with equal frequency. The first symptoms usually occur in late adolescence or the early 20s. Males often experience an earlier onset and a more severe course than females.

   B. Risk factors of the disease include a history of schizophrenia among biologic relatives, especially first-degree relatives; environmental stress; and premorbid behavior characterized by suspiciousness, eccentricity, withdrawal, or impulsivity.

III. **Pathophysiology.** No single cause or pathophysiologic process has been established for schizophrenia. The disease probably represents a heterogeneous group of disorders with similar symptoms.

   A. Genetic factors. At least some (and probably all) persons with schizophrenia have an inherited genetic vulnerability. The likelihood of developing schizophrenia increases with genetic closeness to, and severity of illness in, the proband. Concordance in identical twins is about 40%; in fraternal twins, it is about 12%. When one parent has schizophrenia, offspring have about an 8% chance of developing the disorder; with two parents with schizophrenia, the odds increase to about 40%.

   B. Brain structure and function. Postmortem and structural and functional brain imaging studies (computed tomography [CT], magnetic resonance imaging [MRI], brain electric activity map [BEAM], single photon emission computed tomography [SPECT], and positron emission tomography [PET]) have revealed differences between the brains of persons with schizophrenia and the brains of controls without the disease. In most persons with schizophrenia, typical findings include enlarged ventricles, atrophy in and around limbic structures, a smaller thalamus, and reduced prefrontal cortical activity. A hyperdopaminergic state as the final common pathway is the most widely accepted pathophysiologic explanation for schizophrenia. Consistent with this etiologic model, the potency per milligram of neuroleptic drugs has been found to correlate moderately with their ability to block postsynaptic dopamine type 2 receptors, and the dopamine agonists amphetamine and cocaine are capable of producing symptoms that mimic schizophrenia.

IV. **Diagnosis**

   A. Symptoms and signs. No characteristic psychotic symptom or sign is present in all persons with schizophrenia. Furthermore, all schizophrenic signs and symptoms have been observed in persons without schizophrenia secondary to central nervous system lesions or other physical disorders. A diagnosis of schizophrenia is therefore a clinical judgment based in part on current signs and symptoms, the patient's past psychiatric history, and exclusion of any known organic cause, including acute substance intoxication or withdrawal. The onset of psychotic symptoms in schizophrenia is often preceded by a prodromal phase, during which a deterioration from previous functioning occurs. Besides this functional decline, the prodrome may include social withdrawal; peculiar ideation, perceptions, or behavior; disturbed communication; lack of initiative or interests; and blunted or inappropriate affect. The length of the prodromal phase is extremely variable.

   1. Characteristic psychotic symptoms and signs. Except as otherwise noted, at least two of the following five symptoms and signs should be present before a diagnosis of schizophrenia is made.

   a. Delusions, which are false beliefs that persist in the face of overwhelming evidence to the contrary. In the case of bizarre delusions such as thought broadcasting, no other psychotic symptom need be present to make the diagnosis.

   b. Prominent hallucinations, which are sensory perceptions without external stimulation of the relevant sensory organ. Auditory hallucinations are especially characteristic. Hallucinations in other sensory modalities in the absence of auditory hallucinations suggest a diagnosis other than schizophrenia. No other psychotic symptom is necessary to diagnose schizophrenia if the content of the auditory hallucinations is unrelated to elation or depression, if the hallucinations are of a voice that keeps up a running commentary on the patient's behavior or thoughts, or if the hallucinations are of two or more voices conversing.

   c. Disorganized thinking, so that contiguous ideas are either unrelated or only obscurely related to each other. The greater the disorganization, the less coherent is the patient's speech.

   d. Marked motor disturbance, such as excited, purposeless motor activity; resistance to instruction or attempts to be moved; assumption of an inappropriate or bizarre posture for a long period of time; stereotyped movements, prominent mannerisms, or prominent grimacing; echolalia; echopraxia; stupor; mutism; and waxy flexibility, or maintaining the position in which limbs are placed.

   e. Negative symptoms such as flat affect, poverty of thought, or loss of motivation.

2. **Role performance.** Persons with schizophrenia invariably experience a substantial reduction in performance at work, in social relations, or in self-care. Reduced role performance may be the only discernible symptom of schizophrenia, especially in an ambulatory setting. When deterioration in role performance occurs, a question about auditory hallucinations ("Do you sometimes hear people talking to you when no one is there?") may yield an unexpected positive response.

3. **Duration.** To make a diagnosis of schizophrenia, some signs of the illness should be present for at least 6 months, and, during that period, the characteristic psychotic symptoms and signs previously noted should be present for at least 1 month, less if treated.

B. Differential diagnosis

1. Symptoms and signs of a mood disorder must be brief relative to the duration of the symptoms and signs of schizophrenia. Otherwise, a diagnosis of schizoaffective disorder, or mood disorder with psychotic features, is more appropriate.

2. Any known or presumed organic cause, such as central nervous system tumors, chronic alcohol abuse, acute amphetamine intoxication, Alzheimer's disease, or hypoglycemia, rules out the diagnosis of schizophrenia. If disorientation or memory impairment is present and persists or if hallucinations in modalities other than auditory are prominent, an organic cause should be actively investigated (see Chapter 14).

C. Laboratory tests. No consistent abnormality in laboratory tests has been discovered in schizophrenia. Structural and functional brain imaging is not sufficiently specific to be clinically useful in diagnosis.

V. Treatment

A. Pharmacotherapy

1. **Neuroleptic drugs.** Consideration of a trial of neuroleptic agents is always in order, since about 65% of persons with schizophrenia achieve substantial benefit from them during the acute stage of the illness and some of the remaining 35% experience benefits, although not as marked. However, the risk of tardive dyskinesia (4% in younger individuals, 28% in older individuals after 1 year of exposure) must be weighed in the balance and discussed with the patient and family before a final decision is made about prescribing neuroleptics. Contraindications to their use include central nervous system depression, comatose or greatly obtunded states, severe heart disease, liver damage, suspected or established subcortical brain damage (perphenazine and fluphenazine), Parkinson's disease (haloperidol), blood dyscrasias, presence of signs and symptoms of Reye's syndrome, bone marrow depression, and use of highly anticholinergic neuroleptics (eg, chlorpromazine, thioridazine, molindone) in patients with prostatic hypertrophy or angle closure glaucoma. Patients with a history of neuroleptic malignant syndrome or tardive dyskinesia, or pregnant or nursing women, should be offered psychosocial treatment alone or referred to a psychiatrist for a careful analysis of the risk–benefit ratio of neuroleptic medication.

   a. Initial choice of drug. Although the milligram potency between drugs varies, group data reveal all neuroleptic drugs to be equally effective, with the exception of the superior efficacy of clozapine (superiority most apparent in treatment-resistant patients), the possible superiority of risperidone in nontreatment-resistant patients, and the superiority of olanzapine and quetiapine in reducing negative symptoms. Olanzapine and quetiapine have the added benefit of a much lower incidence of extrapyramidal side effects (EPS).

   The high rate of potentially life-threatening agranulocytosis associated with clozapine (1.3% in 1 year), the requirement of weekly blood monitoring, and its much higher cost relegate it to use as a second-line medication; its use can be justified only after a patient has failed at least two adequate trials with two different neuroleptic agents. Besides the more effective or potentially more effective olanzapine, quetiapine, and risperidone, other medications to consider initially are those neuroleptics to which the patient has had a positive response in the past, since group outcome data obscure the fact that individual patients differentially respond to different agents. Additional considerations in choosing a neuroleptic drug are described in the text that follows.

   (1) **Side effect profile.** High-potency neuroleptics often produce more EPS, whereas low-potency agents usually have more anticholinergic and sedative side effects and are associated with a higher incidence of postural hypotension. The new, atypical neuroleptics olanzapine and quetiapine have minimal EPS and less frequent hyperprolactinemia, but are sedating and cause postural hypotension. EPS can be ameliorated with antiparkinsonian agents, but the sedation and postural hypotension of low-potency and atypical medications cannot be countered. Sedation is a particularly troubling problem for patients who are employed, but may be desirable if a substantial sleep disturbance is present. Weight gain is another relevant consideration. Because molindone is the only neuroleptic that does not cause weight gain, it should be considered seriously for obese patients and women: Obese patients should not be exposed to the increased health risks of additional weight gain, and women are more likely to discontinue a treatment regimen that causes weight gain. Each neuroleptic drug has other side effects peculiar to itself, which also should be considered in the context of the patient's medical status.

   (2) **Subjective response.** A dysphoric response to a given neuroleptic agent within 48 hours of treatment initiation is associated not only with poor treatment response, but with noncompliance. Suicide can even result from the induced dysphoria. Neuroleptic-induced dysphoria is suggested when the patient reports that the medication makes him or her feel "weird" or like a "zombie," tired or sluggish, anxious or agitated, controlled, or coerced into taking the medication.

   (3) **Cost.** Excluding clozapine from the analysis, a 10-fold difference exists between the least and most expensive neuroleptic agents. After clozapine, olanzapine is one of the most expensive, if not the most expensive, neuroleptic.

   (4) **Compliance.** The likelihood of patient compliance must also be determined. If compliance is doubtful, the depot neuroleptic drug haloperidol decanoate should definitely be considered.

   b. **Patient response.** When the patient responds poorly to a 2- to 3-week trial of the initial agent or if significant dysphoria results within the first few days, the medication should be discontinued, and a neuroleptic from a different class should be initiated (Table 99–1). In the case of a 2- to 3-week trial, blood levels should first be obtained to ensure that dosing and compliance have been adequate. The use of two neuroleptics simultaneously is not recommended. If a patient fails two or more adequate trials of a neuroleptic, referral for psychiatric consultation should be entertained.

   c. **Dosage and administration.** In general, after a dosage increase 1–2 days after commencement, levels can continue to be titrated upward at semiweekly intervals until symptoms remit. After remission of acute symptoms for 2 weeks, the dosage should be reduced to the lowest amount possible. Once or twice daily dosing is possible, given the long half-life of neuroleptic drugs. Taking the medication at bedtime reduces problems with side effects, but increases the likelihood of nightmares.

2. **Antidepressant drugs.** When tricyclic antidepressants or monoamine oxidase inhibitors (MAOIs) are used alone or in combination with neuroleptic agents, exacerbation of symptoms of schizophrenia has been observed in some cases. In other cases, particularly when depression is persistent and positive symptoms are absent, the addition of imipramine to a neuroleptic regimen has been associated with a reduced rate of relapse.

B. **Psychosocial interventions.** By reducing environmental stressors or enhancing coping skills or social support, psychosocial interventions have a very favorable impact on relapse rate and quality of life. Psychosocial interventions that have

TABLE 99–1. NEUROLEPTIC AGENTS

Drug	Trade Name	Usual Starting Dose (mg)	Maximum Daily Dose (mg)
Phenothiazines			
Aliphatic			
Chlorpromazine	Thorazine	25 bid or tid	1000
Piperidine			
Thioridazine	Generic Only	50–100 tid	800
Mesoridazine	Serentil	50 tid	400
Piperazine			
Prochlorperazine	Compazine	5–10 tid or qid	150
Perphenazine	Trilafon	4–8 tid	64
Trifluoperazine	Stelazine	2–5 bid	40
Fluphenazine	Generic Only	2.5 qd–qid	40
Thioxanthenes			
Thiothixene	Navane	2–5 bid	60
Butyrophenones			
Haloperidol	Haldol	0.5–5 bid or tid	100
Indoles			
Molindone	Moban	25 bid or tid	225
Dibenzoxazepines			
Loxapine	Loxitane	10–25 bid	250
Benzisoxazole			
Risperidone	Risperdal	1 bid	6
Thienobenzodiazepine			
Olanzapine	Zyprexa	5–10 qd	20
Dibenzothiazepine			
Quetiapine	Seroquel	25 bid	750

Important note: Before prescribing any medication, physicians should consult product information and the current edition of the *Physician's Desk Reference* to check for changes in recommended dosages or scheduling of doses and to avoid the possibility of patient injury or death resulting from inadvertent errors in this table.
bid, twice daily; qd, daily; qid, four times daily; tid, three times daily.

an educational component or that focus on specific behaviors have been shown to be superior to those interventions that primarily provide support or focus on increased self-awareness. The greatest benefits of psychosocial treatment are achieved when the acute stage of the illness has passed.

1. **Family-centered intervention** should not seek to encourage exploration or expression of feelings, or enhance awareness of semiconscious impulses or motivations. The following are goals of such intervention.
   a. Education of the patient and family about the nature of schizophrenia and about the importance of medical and psychosocial treatments in preventing relapse.
   b. Reduction or elimination of family guilt over development of the illness. Portraying schizophrenia as a brain disorder is helpful in this regard.
   c. Enhancement of family tolerance for nonharmful dysfunctional behaviors. Family criticism has been strongly associated with relapse.
   d. Reduced parental involvement in the patient's emotional life. This can be accomplished in part by encouraging the parents to invest the time necessary to strengthen their own marital relationship. Like family criticism, parental overinvolvement is predictive of relapse.
   e. Identification of problematic behaviors in the patient and family members, and concrete guidance for both patient and family members concerning appropriate, psychologically innocuous ways of requesting change in those problematic behaviors.
2. **Individual-centered psychotherapy,** psychodynamic- or insight-oriented, has not been shown to be beneficial for persons with schizophrenia and may be actually harmful to some. Individual therapy is beneficial if it provides information and education about schizophrenia and the usefulness of both medical and psychosocial treatments; if it focuses on stress management,

problem-solving, or the enhancement of specific social skills; and if it occurs in the context of a therapeutic relationship characterized by empathy, non-possessive warmth, genuineness, and positive, realistic expectations for improvement. Empathic understanding of the patient's confusion, strong fears, and demoralization are particularly important.

VI. **Management strategies.** The goal of maintenance treatment is prevention of the reappearance of psychotic symptoms while minimizing side effects. Without treatment, 70% of persons with schizophrenia in remission have a relapse within 1 year. Therefore, indefinite pharmacotherapy or psychosocial treatment is warranted in most instances.

A. **Continuous treatment.** Indefinite prophylactic administration of neuroleptic drugs is indicated in persons prone to relapse when medication is discontinued. The likelihood of such relapse may be predicted by a previous history of return of symptoms following discontinuation. The lowest effective drug dosage should be used, since side effects and subsequent noncompliance are dose-related and since tardive dyskinesia is directly related to cumulative neuroleptic exposure. The optimal frequency and longitudinal course of contacts for psychosocial treatment have not been empirically established, but initial weekly sessions are a good place to start. Contacts need to be even more frequent during crises or acute exacerbations. Gradual spacing of visits to once every 4–8 weeks after stabilization may be possible. As is the case for medication, indefinite psychosocial treatment will likely be desirable.

B. **Intermittent treatment.** Persons who are at less risk for relapse upon discontinuation of medication should be considered for intermittent neuroleptic treatment, especially because the lifetime risk of tardive dyskinesia is thereby lowered. Medication can be weaned and eventually discontinued during remission, then reinstated during the early stages of relapse. This approach requires the patient and members of the support system to be educated about the early symptoms of exacerbation peculiar to that individual patient. Routine monthly or bimonthly psychosocial treatment sessions should be arranged even when no medication is being prescribed. Unfortunately, recent evidence indicates that intermittent treatment with neuroleptic drugs results in significantly elevated relapse rates compared with continuous treatment. However, since this evidence is culled from group data, the practitioner should still consider intermittent neuroleptic treatment for every patient with schizophrenia until experience proves this to be nonviable.

VII. **Natural history and prognosis**

A. **A residual phase** often follows remission of fully developed psychotic symptoms, especially during the initial years of the disorder. The symptoms and signs during this phase are similar to those of the prodrome; mild psychotic symptoms persist in about 50% of patients. Complete recovery lasting at least 3 years occurs in 10% of patients, whereas significant improvement occurs in up to two-thirds of cases. Many persons with schizophrenia experience intermittent exacerbations, especially in response to stressful environmental circumstances. Males have been observed to experience a more severe course of the disorder. Ten percent of those with schizophrenia die by suicide.

B. **Good prognosis** has been associated with absence of prodromal behavioral disturbance, a clear environmental precipitant, abrupt onset, onset in midlife, the presence of confusion, a family history of mood disorder, and a support system that is noncritical and not overly intrusive in the patient's life. Type I schizophrenia does not necessarily have a better prognosis than type II.

REFERENCES

American Psychiatric Association (APA): *Diagnostic and Statistical Manual of Mental Disorders* (DSM-IV), 4th ed. APA; 1994.

Awad AG, Hogan TP: Subjective response to neuroleptics and the quality of life: Implications for treatment outcome. Acta Psychiatr Scand 1994;**89**(suppl 380):27.

Moller H-J: Review: Treatment of schizophrenia—State of the art. Eur Arch Psychiatry Clin Neurosci 1996;**246**:229.

Schooler NR, Keith SJ, Severe JB, et al: Maintenance treatment of schizophrenia: A review of dose reduction and family treatment strategies. Psychiatr Q 1995;**66**:279.

Sheitman BB, Lee H, Strauss R, et al: The valuation and treatment of first-episode psychosis. Schizophr Bull 1997;**23**:653.

100   Somatization

John L. Coulehan, MD, MPH

I. **Definition.** Somatization is a process by which persons experience and express emotional discomfort or psychosocial stress using physical symptoms.
II. **Epidemiology**
   A. **Prevalence**
      1. Between 60% and 80% of healthy persons experience somatic symptoms in any given week.
      2. About one-third of all primary care patients have ill-defined symptoms not attributable to physical disease, and 70% of those with emotional disorders present a somatic complaint as the reason for their office visit. The prevalence of **somatization disorder,** as defined in the *Diagnostic and Statistical Manual of Mental Disorders,* 4th edition (DSM-IV), is less than 1% in community-based studies, 5% among primary care outpatients, and 9% among hospitalized medical and surgical patients. The great majority of these patients are female. Clinical somatization is more common than these percentages suggest. Patients who report multiple unexplained symptoms (eg, between four and 12), although fewer than the number required by DSM-IV diagnostic criteria, have utilization patterns, clinical features, and outcomes similar to those with somatization disorder.
      3. The prevalence of **psychogenic pain disorder** is unknown, but the disorder appears to be quite common in medical settings.
      4. In primary care practice, the prevalence of **hypochondriasis,** a preoccupation with the fear or belief that one has serious illness, may be as high as 10%. Full-blown somatization disorder is quite rare in men, but hypochondriasis appears in both sexes with equal frequency.
      5. **Conversion symptoms** (eg, sudden blindness or paralysis), while apparently common several decades ago, are now infrequent.
   B. **Personal characteristics** associated with somatization include female gender, older age, currently unmarried state, lower level of education, lower socioeconomic class, and urban residence.
   C. **Cultural factors.** Somatization occurs throughout the world, but is more prevalent in cultures in which emotional distress is generally couched in nonpsychological terms. In the United States, somatization appears to be particularly frequent among Hispanic and Asian populations.
III. **Pathophysiology**
   A. Multiple theories have been proposed to explain somatization (Table 100–1). These are not mutually exclusive, and it is likely that somatization is a complex phenomenon with multiple "risk factors" playing a role in its causation. In a given patient, one might distinguish the following sets or clusters of factors.
      1. **Predisposing factors** include the patient's biologic, developmental, personality, and sociocultural characteristics. Some studies have shown an association in women between sexual abuse and somatization and chronic pelvic pain. One theory is that a predilection for somatization results from abnormal central nervous system regulation of incoming sensory information (**corticofugal inhibition**).
      2. **Precipitating factors** include stressful life events, such as illness, and interpersonal conflict. Somatization may be precipitated by positive life events (eg, job promotion) as well as negative ones (eg, death in family).

TABLE 100–1. THEORIES OF SOMATIZATION ETIOLOGY

1. **Neurobiologic.** Abnormal central nervous system regulation of incoming sensory information leads to an impairment in attentional processing.
2. **Psychodynamic.** Somatization is a defense mechanism.
3. **Behavioral.** Somatization is a learned behavior in which environmental reinforcers maintain abnormal illness behavior.
4. **Sociocultural.** "Correct" ways of dealing with emotions and feelings are culturally determined.

3. **Maintaining factors** include interactions among patient, family, physician, and social system. Financial rewards and other forms of secondary gain reinforce somatization, as do iatrogenic factors such as unnecessary testing, side effects of medication, and complications of invasive studies.

B. **Origin of symptoms.** The process of somatization may lead to symptoms in several ways. A given patient may present with symptoms in all three categories. This is particularly true in somatization disorder.

   1. Patients may **amplify symptoms** of acute or chronic organic diseases, or preferentially report somatic symptoms (while de-emphasizing emotional symptoms) of psychiatric conditions such as major depression or panic disorder.
   2. Patients may report **psychophysiologic disturbances** (eg, headaches, irritable bowel, or palpitations) mediated through autonomic or other known mechanisms.
   3. Patients may experience **conversion symptoms** that serve a symbolic function and may not correspond with known physiologic mechanisms. Such symptoms constitute a language in which emotion or conflict is represented by perceived physical dysfunction, rather than being experienced in the affective realm.

IV. **Diagnosis.** Somatization is a complex, multifactorial process. Rather than considering its variants as separate entities, it is perhaps best to think of somatization as a spectrum that ranges from occasional functional somatic symptoms to full-blown DSM-IV somatoform disorders.

   A. **Differential diagnosis**
      1. **Occult physical disease** in which somatization might play a role or which might be confused with somatization include **fibromyalgia** or **fibromyositis** (see Chapter 48), **chronic fatigue syndrome** (see Chapter 28), **hypothyroidism** or **hyperthyroidism** (see Chapter 91), and **mitral valve prolapse syndrome,** which is the coexistence of mitral valve prolapse with a constellation of common symptoms (eg, atypical chest pain, palpitations, lightheadedness, fatigue, or anxiety attacks). Since both the functional symptoms and the anatomic finding are quite prevalent in the population, their conjunction in this so-called syndrome may have little significance.

         Other disorders with vague, multiple, and confusing symptoms (eg, multiple sclerosis, porphyria, systemic lupus erythematosus, or musculoskeletal and neuropsychiatric manifestations of Lyme disease) must also be considered, although their prevalence in the primary care setting is quite low.
      2. **Amplified symptoms** of underlying organic disease may also be involved in somatization.
      3. **Psychiatric disorders** in which somatization is not the primary process may be "masked" by an array of somatic complaints. These disorders include **major depression** (see Chapter 96), **alcohol and substance abuse** (see Chapter 92), and **generalized anxiety** and **panic disorders** (see Chapter 93). Physician recognition of psychiatric distress is decreased when patients present with high levels of somatization. Among somatizers in one primary care study, 24% had major depression, 17% had dysthymia, and 22% had generalized anxiety disorder.
      4. **Somatoform disorders**
         a. **Somatization disorder** (Table 100–2).
         b. **Conversion reaction** (Table 100–3).
         c. **Hypochondriasis** (Table 100–4).
         d. **Psychogenic pain disorder** (Table 100–5).
      5. **Factitious disease** is the conscious reporting of false symptoms for secondary gain. Patients with "disability neurosis" may have factitious symptoms, but more likely suffer from true somatization to which secondary gain serves as a maintaining factor. Less than 5% of patients referred to psychiatrists for evaluation of unexplained somatic symptoms have factitious disease. Patients who persistently report factitious disease have **Munchausen syndrome.** Diagnostic tests and medical interventions often lead to additional symptoms (eg, drug side effects), findings (eg, surgical scars), and dysfunction (eg, intestinal adhesions) in these patients.

   B. **Symptoms and signs**
      1. Symptoms favoring somatization are presented in Table 100–6. The presence of several of these characteristics strongly suggests somatization, even though evidence of organic disease may also be present.

TABLE 100–2. DIAGNOSTIC CRITERIA FOR SOMATIZATION DISORDER

A. A history of many physical complaints beginning before the age of 30, occurring over a period of several years and resulting in treatment being sought or significant impairment in social or occupational functioning
B. Each of the following criteria must have been met at some time during the course of the disorder. To count a symptom as significant, it must not be fully explained by a known general medical condition, or the resulting complaints or impairment is in excess of what would be expected from the history, physical examination, or laboratory findings
  1. Four pain symptoms: a history of pain related to at least four different sites or functions (eg, head, abdomen, back, joints, extremities, chest, rectum, during sexual intercourse, during menstruation, or during urination)
  2. Two gastrointestinal symptoms: a history of at least two gastrointestinal symptoms other than pain (eg, nausea, diarrhea, bloating, vomiting other than during pregnancy, or intolerance of several different foods)
  3. One sexual symptom: a history of at least one sexual or reproductive symptom other than pain (eg, sexual indifference, erectile or ejaculatory dysfunction, irregular menses, excessive menstrual bleeding, or vomiting throughout pregnancy)
  4. One pseudoneurologic symptom: a history of at least one symptom or deficit suggesting a neurologic disorder not limited to pain (conversion symptoms such as blindness, double vision, deafness, loss of touch or pain sensation, hallucinations, aphonia, impaired coordination or balance, paralysis or localized weakness, difficulty swallowing, difficulty breathing, urinary retention, or seizures; dissociative symptoms such as amnesia or loss of consciousness other than fainting)

TABLE 100–3. DIAGNOSTIC CRITERIA FOR CONVERSION DISORDER

A. One or more symptoms or deficits affect voluntary motor or sensory function, suggesting a neurologic or general medical condition
B. Psychological factors are judged to be associated with the symptom or deficit because the initiation or exacerbation of the symptom or deficit is preceded by conflicts or other stressors
C. The symptom or deficit is not intentionally produced or feigned (as in factitious disorder or malingering)
D. The symptom or deficit cannot, after appropriate investigation, be fully explained by a neurologic or general medical condition and is not a culturally sanctioned behavior or experience
E. The symptom or deficit causes clinically significant distress or impairment in social, occupational, or other important areas of functioning or warrants medical evaluation
F. The symptom or deficit is not limited to pain or sexual dysfunction, does not occur exclusively during the course of somatization disorder, and is not better accounted for by another mental disorder

TABLE 100–4. DIAGNOSTIC CRITERIA FOR HYPOCHONDRIASIS

A. Preoccupation with fears of having, or the idea that one has, a serious disease based on the person's misinterpretation of bodily symptoms
B. The preoccupation persists despite appropriate medical evaluation and reassurance
C. The belief in A is not of delusional intensity (as in delusional disorder, somatic type) and is not restricted to a circumscribed concern about appearance (as in body dysmorphic disorder)
D. The preoccupation causes clinically significant distress or impairment in social, occupational, or other important areas of functioning
E. The duration of the disturbance is at least 6 months
F. The preoccupation does not occur exclusively during the course of generalized anxiety disorder, obsessive–compulsive disorder, panic disorder, a major depressive episode, separation anxiety, or another somatoform disorder

TABLE 100–5. DIAGNOSTIC CRITERIA FOR PSYCHOGENIC DISORDER

A. Pain in one or more anatomic sites is the predominant focus of the clinical presentation and is of sufficient severity to warrant clinical attention
B. The pain causes clinically significant distress or impairment in social, occupational, or other important areas of functioning
C. Psychological factors are judged to have an important role in the onset, severity, exacerbation, or maintenance of the pain
D. The pain is not better accounted for by a mood, anxiety, or psychotic disorder and does not meet criteria for dyspareunia

TABLE 100-6. POSITIVE CRITERIA FOR DIAGNOSIS OF PSYCHOGENIC SYMPTOMS

1. The patient's descriptions of symptoms are vague, inconsistent, or bizarre
2. Symptoms persist despite apparently adequate medical therapy
3. The illness began in the context of a psychologically meaningful setting (eg, death of relative, conflict with spouse, or job promotion)
4. The patient denies that any emotional distress or psychological factors play a role in symptom development
5. The patient has visited several physicians or has had several operations
6. There is evidence of an associated psychiatric disorder
7. The patient has features suggesting a hysterical personality style
8. Discussion reveals that the patient attributes an idiosyncratic meaning to symptoms
9. Alexithymia (ie, difficulty describing emotions or inner processes in words) is present

Adapted and abridged with permission from Kaplan C, Lipkin M, Gordon GH: Somatization in primary care: Patients with unexplained and vexing medical complaints. J Gen Intern Med 1988;**3**:177.

2. **Pain** is the most frequent single complaint, present in over 80% of patients with somatization.
3. **Three frequent symptom clusters suggestive of somatization secondary to depression, anxiety, or panic disorder are described below.**
   a. **Atypical chest pain, palpitations, tachycardia, and/or difficulty catching one's breath** (sighing, not true dyspnea).
   b. **Headache, dizziness, lightheadedness, presyncope, or paresthesias.**
   c. **Dyspepsia, heartburn, "gas," flatulence, and/or other gastrointestinal symptoms.**
4. **Globus hystericus,** the sensation of a lump in the throat that interferes with swallowing, is a frequent symptom of anxiety or conversion.
C. **Laboratory tests.** Laboratory and radiographic studies serve only to rule out organic disease, although evidence of a disease entity does not exclude the diagnosis of somatization. Moreover, abnormalities unrelated to the patient's symptoms may be discovered with sophisticated diagnostic technology. For example, the presence of minimal mitral valve prolapse on echocardiography cannot explain an array of somatic symptoms.
V. **Treatment.** Appropriate treatment for the underlying problem is the first priority. Additionally, treatment is not likely to be effective unless maintaining factors are addressed and minimized.
A. **Basic treatment principles**
   1. The patient's problem should be considered as deserving of attention. This requires attentive listening, empathic responses, and avoidance of statements that the patient might construe to mean "There's nothing wrong with you" or "It's all in your head."
   2. Clear explanations of symptoms should be presented in functional or physiologic terms. The physician should describe the problem in terms the patient can understand, and in a way that fits in with his or her belief system about health and illness. Disease labels should be avoided as much as possible. When you do not understand and cannot explain a symptom, tell the patient in unambiguous terms.
   3. A well-defined treatment program should be initiated. Even if treatment consists only of explanation, reassurance, observation, and symptomatic measures, the physician should provide relatively definite information about how to proceed, how long the symptoms might last, and what to do next. Ambiguity increases anxiety.
   4. It is important to engage the patient's active participation in treatment by behavioral means, such as by keeping a diary to identify factors that influence symptoms, which may serve to make the problem appear less unpredictable and out of control. General behavior change techniques also may be initiated. For example, an exercise program to enhance "muscle tone" or a diet for weight reduction, if successful, generally enhances the patient's sense of control and self-mastery.
B. **Multifaceted treatment approach required by primary chronic somatization**
   1. **Pharmacotherapy.** There are no adequate clinical trials of drug treatment for primary somatization per se. However, drugs may be effective in the following situations.

    a. Specific intractable symptoms such as headaches, myalgias, and other forms of chronic pain may be ameliorated by **tricyclic antidepressants** or **selective serotonin reuptake inhibitors** (see Chapter 96).

    b. Even when DSM-IV criteria for depression are not present, patients who demonstrate somatic symptoms of depression often benefit from adequate doses of antidepressants. Likewise, anxious patients may experience relief of somatic symptoms in response to **benzodiazepine therapy,** even though they do not fulfill DSM-IV criteria for panic or anxiety disorders (see Chapter 93).

    c. Because patients who somatize often have a low tolerance for the side effects of medications, symptomatic medications (eg, analgesics or antispasmodics) should be used sparingly and in the minimal effective doses.

    d. There is rarely, if ever, a place for narcotic analgesics in treating somatization symptoms.

  2. **Psychiatric consultation** has been shown over the short term (ie, 1 year) to be effective in reducing hospitalizations and overall medical costs of patients with somatization disorder. In one study, a single consultation report to the primary physician was associated with a 12% reduction in costs. The physician should refer the patient to a consultation–liaison service or to a psychiatrist comfortable with patients with this condition. Such a consultation may lead to short-term psychotherapy, in addition to the recommended management strategies for the primary care physician. There are no adequate controlled studies of specific psychotherapy in hypochondriasis or somatization. Most patients with somatization disorder do not respond well to open-ended referral for psychiatric care.

  3. Patients with severe chronic somatization may benefit from comprehensive inpatient treatment programs that include individual, group, and family therapy; educational programs; physical and occupational therapy; biofeedback; and vocational rehabilitation.

VI. Management strategies. Optimal management of somatizing patients requires relief of symptoms, treatment of underlying medical or psychiatric disorders, and avoidance of the pathologic cycle of intervention (medical treatment, temporary improvement, renewal of symptoms, disappointment, patient and physician anger).

  A. The **therapeutic contract** should be emphasized and its parameters defined. While recognizing the reality of the patient's symptoms, one should attempt to develop a broader framework for physician–patient interaction by following the guidelines described below.

    1. Tolerate symptoms and scale down the goals of therapy. Speak in terms of reduction, lessening, and coping, rather than complete symptom alleviation. Evaluate new symptoms as they occur, but do so conservatively in a stepwise fashion. Openly discuss the risks of medication side effects and the possibility of complications with invasive procedures.

    2. Discuss psychiatric or psychosocial issues not as direct causes of symptoms, but rather as possible aggravating factors or as unfortunate results of physical symptoms.

    3. Promote stability in the physician–patient relationship by scheduling office visits at regular intervals (usually ranging from 1 to 4 weeks, depending on patient and physician tolerance), thereby diminishing the patient's need for a "ticket of admission." Increase the length of office visits to allow relatively unrushed attention. Schedule them at times when interruptions will be minimal, not on particularly "emergency-prone" days such as Mondays or Fridays.

    4. Explicitly discourage dependent behaviors, such as unscheduled phone calls or drop-in visits. Prearranged follow-up phone calls may allow a reduction in the frequency of office visits. Ask the patient not to "doctor shop" or to seek specialist care without consulting the primary care physician.

  B. Somatization may be a sign of **family dysfunction** in which the identified patient's symptoms may serve to stabilize a pathologic family situation. It may be necessary to enlist family members in behavioral strategies to "wean" the patient from secondary gain (eg, using somatization to avoid household tasks, to require special meals, or to excuse irritability and angry outbursts).

  C. While remaining supportive of the symptomatic person, the physician should attempt to avoid certifying the person as **permanently and totally disabled.** The label of *disability* can be viewed as another "medical intervention" with adverse consequences as well as benefits. The physician should realize that severe and chronic somatization is a disabling condition, however. Chronic pain syndrome, for example, may qualify under Medicare as a cause of total disability. While not desirable in terms of "curing" the somatization, disability may, in certain cases, for economic and social reasons be the best palliative option.

D. Physicians develop a great deal of **anger** and **frustration** when treating patients who somatize. To maintain equanimity, the physician may use the following strategies.

    1. Make the diagnosis of somatization and modify treatment objectives accordingly, rather than wallowing in frustration over the absence of objective findings of disease.

    2. Set up firm and explicit guidelines as described above, and review them frequently with the patient. Arrange office appointments so that somatizers are not clustered together.

    3. Develop an informal relationship with a psychiatrist or a psychologist to whom feelings about these patients can be ventilated and with whom treatment problems can be discussed. More structured group experiences (eg, Balint groups) for providers are also quite effective.

VII. Natural history and prognosis

A. A large proportion of patients with functional somatic symptoms recover without specific intervention. Favorable prognostic factors include acute onset and short duration of symptoms, younger age, higher socioeconomic class, absence of organic disease, and absence of personality disorder.

B. The long-term prognosis for patients with somatization disorder is guarded, and usually lifelong supportive treatment is required. If somatization is a mask for another psychiatric disorder, its prognosis depends on that of the primary problem. In one study of patients with emotional disorders presenting with a recent onset of physical symptoms, 40% subsequently developed chronic somatoform disorders.

C. If hypochondriasis is conceptualized as an "amplifying somatic style," patients who exhibit this condition are likely to have recurrent physical complaints and require frequent medical intervention. Appropriate treatment for somatization should minimize these complaints by providing education and reassurance, by reducing anxiety, and by enhancing the patient's coping skills.

D. Discrete conversion symptoms have a better prognosis. They may resolve spontaneously when no longer "required" or may respond to specific psychotherapy.

REFERENCES

Baughman OL: Rapid diagnosis and treatment of anxiety and depression in primary care: The somatizing patient. J Fam Pract 1994;**39**:378.

Blackwell B, DeMorgann NP: The primary care of patients who have bodily concerns. Arch Fam Med 1996;**5**:457.

Coulehan JL, Block MR: Seal up the mouth of outrage: Interactive problems in interviewing. In: *The Medical Interview: Mastering Skills for Clinical Practice.* Davis, 1997; 183.

Kathol RG: Reassurance therapy: What to say to symptomatic patients with benign or non-existent disease. Int J Psychiatry Med 1997;**27**:173.

McWhinney IR, Epstein RM, Freeman TR: Rethinking somatization. Ann Intern Med 1997;**126**: 747.

SECTION IV. **Reproductive Health**

101   Contraception

Laura B. Frankenstein, MD

The demand for birth control is great; an estimated 41 million women in the United States are sexually active. Three million women in this country between the ages of 15 and 44 do not use contraception, however. Forty percent of these women are not using any birth control methods because they are afraid of either real or imagined side effects. Most unintended pregnancies occur either because contraceptives are not used or because they are used sporadically or incorrectly. Other nonusers who are at risk for unintended pregnancy are those women who have no prior sexual experience, those who have lost partners to separation or death, and those who believe they are protected because they are postpartum or nursing. Age, socioeconomic class, and level of education are inversely correlated with the failure rate of contraceptives. In the United States, 92% of pregnancies in adolescents aged 15–19 years are unintentional.

  I. **Choosing a birth control method.** There are no perfect methods of birth control except abstinence. Correct use of any contraceptive device does not guarantee protection; 20% of women who experienced unintended pregnancy used their selected methods consistently and properly. Consideration of the following factors will help patients and physicians make the best possible choices.

   A. **Theoretical efficacy rates** are defined as the number of unintended pregnancies per 100 women that occur during the first year of use of a given contraceptive method (if the method is used correctly). **Actual efficacy rates** reflect the percentage of women who become pregnant during the first year of contraceptive use. The efficacy of a given contraceptive method is influenced by the fertility, individual motivation, and risk-taking attitude of each partner; the frequency of intercourse; the ability of the patient to master the method; and the theoretical efficacy rate of the method. Using two forms of contraception at once significantly lowers the risk of accidental pregnancy.

   Patient education and physician understanding promote increased efficacy of a birth control method by minimizing discontinuation of a particular method or switching to another form of contraception. Too often, women quit using a method in frustration and then conceive. For example, 50% of users of oral contraceptives stopped taking the pills after less than 1 year. When discussing the possible side effects of a particular method of birth control with patients, the physician should explain how problems can be minimized and point out the benefits and risks. When a patient reports breakthrough bleeding while taking the pill, use this as a chance to see if she is able or willing to take the pill daily, since spotting may reflect missed pills. For complete information for patients concerning each form of contraception, see the appropriate chapter in *Contraceptive Technology* (Hatcher et al, 1998).

   B. **Safety concerns** include risks of morbidity and mortality as well as noncontraceptive safety benefits such as protection from sexually transmitted diseases (STDs) or the resolution of menstrual problems.

   C. **Acceptability** of a method depends on the following factors.
    1. **Financial cost** of the product, as well as the cost of time and money in physician visits and necessary medical tests.
    2. **Individual preferences and experiences.** The effect of a birth control method on subsequent fertility should be considered if future pregnancy is desired. See Table 101–1 for questions women should ask themselves before selecting a contraceptive method.

 II. **Hormonal contraception** works by suppressing ovulation and changing cervical mucus so that sperm are less effective. When hormonal contraception is used as postcoital emergency contraception, inhibition or delay of ovulation and alteration of the transport of sperm or ova prevents pregnancy. If a woman is already pregnant, there will be no impact.

   A. **Oral contraceptives.** This birth control method, used by 18 million women, is the most popular reversible form of contraception in the United States. Except for the

TABLE 101–1. QUESTIONS A WOMAN SHOULD ASK BEFORE SELECTING A BIRTH CONTROL METHOD

1. Am I afraid of using this method?
2. Would I rather not use this method?
3. Will I have trouble remembering to use this method?
4. What are my chances of becoming pregnant using this method?
5. Will I have trouble using this method carefully?
6. Do I have unanswered questions about this method?
7. Does this method cost more than I can afford?
8. Could this method ever cause me serious health problems?
9. Do I object to this method because of religious beliefs?
10. What problems can I expect?
11. Is my partner opposed to this method?
12. Am I using this method without my partner's knowledge?
13. Will using this method embarrass me or my partner?
14. Will I enjoy intercourse less because of this method?
15. Will this method interrupt my lovemaking?

Modified from Hatcher RA, et al: *Contraceptive Technology 1994–1995.* 16th ed. Irvington; 1994.

progestin-only pills, all oral contraceptive pills have different doses of two types of estrogen and nine types of progestin. Biphasic and triphasic oral contraceptives contain different amounts of hormone throughout the menstrual cycle in an attempt to more closely mimic natural hormone production. Choosing among the many oral contraceptives can be done on the basis of characteristics of both the patient and the contraceptive. Low-dose pills (30–35 µg of estrogen) may be used initially, and the dosage may be altered as needed (see Table 101–2 for suggestions).

1. The **failure rate** for the ideal user is 0.1% for combined pills and 0.5% for progestin-only pills. Actual failure rates are 5% for both types of contraceptives.
2. **Contraindications**
   a. **Women over age 35 who smoke.** Healthy women who do not smoke can safely use oral contraceptives until menopause if they desire.
   b. **Women with cardiovascular problems,** such as a history of thromboembolic disease, cerebrovascular disease, and ischemic heart disease. Other conditions, such as breast cancer, liver tumor, or undiagnosed vaginal bleeding, preclude oral contraceptive use.
   c. Use of pills with **third-generation progestins** (gestodene and desogestrel) are controversial, as these progestins can increase a woman's risk of thromboembolic disease, but they may also reduce the risk of myocardial infarctions. More studies of this issue are in progress.
   d. **Lactating women** less than 6 weeks postpartum because of the theoretical risk to infants and because oral contraceptives can diminish breast milk production.
   e. **Relative contraindications** include diabetes mellitus, migraine or vascular headaches, systolic blood pressure >140 mm Hg or diastolic blood pressure >90 mm Hg, sickle cell disease, or active gallbladder disease.
3. **Side effects** are much less of a problem than they were in the past because the amounts of estrogen and progestin in oral contraceptives have decreased. In the United States, it is safer for women to use oral contraceptives than to deliver a baby. Many of the side effects are temporary. If the woman can tolerate spotting, acne, breast tenderness, and nausea, these conditions often improve after 3 months. Continued spotting may be a symptom indicating that a woman is not taking her pills every day.
   a. **Breast cancer.** Results of studies conflict, but the Food and Drug Administration (FDA) currently considers evidence suggesting that long-term use of oral contraceptives increases the risk of breast cancer to be insufficient.
   b. **Cervical neoplasia** rates are higher in women who use oral contraceptives, but studies have not determined whether oral contraceptives or other factors are responsible.

TABLE 101–2. CHOOSING AMONG THE MANY TYPES OF ORAL CONTRACEPTIVES (OCPs)

Characteristic	Oral Contraceptive	Comment
Nursing women	Ovrette Micronor Nor-QD	Progestin-only pills will not interrupt the milk supply
Nausea or breast tenderness when taking OCPs	Ovrette Micronor Nor-QD	Progestin-only pills
No previous use of oral contraceptives	Ovcon-35 Ortho-Novum 1/35 Triphasil Tri-Levlen Ortho-Novum 777	Low-dose oral contraceptive pills minimize side effects
Acne, hirsutism, or obesity	Ovcon-35 Modicon Brevicon Triphasil	Least androgenic oral contraceptive pills
Hypertension Hyperlipidemia Diabetes mellitus	Desogen Ortho-Cept Ortho Cyclen Ortho Tricyclen Ovcon-35 Modicon Brevicon	All produce a favorable high-density lipoprotein and low-density lipoprotein cholesterol pattern
Scanty or absent withdrawal bleeding on low-dose pill	Pills with increased estrogen or progestin content	Build up endometrium
Spotting, if persists more than 3 months	Pills with increased progestin or estrogen content	Build up endometrium
	Estrostep Low Ovral Ortho-Cyclen Ortho-Cept Desogen	
Minimize risk of thrombosis or nausea	Loestrin 1/20 Alesse	Less estrogen
Use of Rifampin or Dilantin, which increases breakthrough bleeding	Use estrogen 50 mcq OCPs	Increase estrogen
Hirsutism, chronic anovulation due to increased testosterone	New progestin OCPs Ovcon-35	Decrease free testosterone level

c. **Lactation** can be interrupted because estrogen inhibits milk production. Nursing mothers who want to use oral contraceptives should use progestin-only pills.

d. **Gallbladder disease** symptoms may be precipitated by oral contraceptives that contain estrogen, although the incidence of gallbladder disease is not itself increased.

e. **Normal menses and fertility** may be slightly delayed, but most women have no trouble conceiving within the first year after oral contraceptives are discontinued. Ninety-nine percent of women resume regular menses within the first 6 months after they stop taking contraceptive pills.

f. **Estrogen-related effects** such as nausea, breast tenderness, cyclic weight gain, headaches, and growth of fibroids may occur. Progestin-related effects include increased appetite, weight gain, depression, fatigue, decreased libido, acne, decreased glucose tolerance, headaches, and increased levels of low-density lipoprotein (LDL) cholesterol and decreased levels of high-density lipoprotein (HDL) cholesterol.

g. **Mild mood swings and depression** have been described by women using oral contraceptives. Contraceptive pills deplete vitamin B_6 (pyridoxine) levels. Symptomatic women should receive supplements. Pyridoxine, 50–100 mg/day, is the usual dose.

h. **Low-dose oral contraceptive pills** do not impact glucose metabolism adversely. Some progestins do decrease HDL cholesterol and increase LDL cholesterol (see Table 101–2 to choose wisely).

4. **Noncontraceptive benefits** of low-dose estrogen oral contraceptives ($\geq$50 μg)

   a. **Protection from endometrial cancer** after 1 year of use.

   b. **Reduction in the risk of ovarian cancer** after 6 months of use.

   c. **More regular and** *less painful* menstrual periods with less bleeding and iron deficiency anemia. Premenstrual syndrome is less common and less severe in women using oral contraceptives, as are benign breast disease and benign ovarian cysts, endometriosis, acne, hirsutism, and anovulatory bleeding. Pelvic inflammatory disease (PID) caused by *Chlamydia* occurs less often because of the effects oral contraceptives have on the menses, cervix, and mucus.

5. **Acceptability** of oral contraceptives may be limited if remembering a pill daily is difficult. The cost is $100 to $130 per year for generic pills and $200 to $300 per year for nongeneric pills.

6. **Evaluation and follow-up.** Monitoring includes yearly Pap smears and blood pressure monitoring.

B. **Injectable hormones.** Depo-Provera (depo-medroxyprogesterone acetate) has been used safely by over 10 million women worldwide. It has been approved in over 90 countries, including the United States. It is given as a deep intramuscular injection of 150 mg every 12 weeks.

1. The **failure rate** is very low—only 0.3% failure in ideal and actual cases. Low body weight decreases the efficacy.

2. **Contraindications.** This method should not be used in women who are at significant risk for breast cancer or who have been treated for this type of cancer.

3. **Side effects**

   a. **Breast cancer** is most feared because of data from animal studies, but recent studies have not supported this association in humans, nor has the large experience worldwide.

   b. **Menstrual irregularities** occur, with more time elapsing between menses the longer Depo-Provera is used. After 6 months (two injections), one-half of the women are amenorrheic, and most women are without menses after 1 year of therapy. Normal menses and fertility will not return immediately upon stopping the drug and may take more than 1 year to normalize. The average time to conception after the last injection is 8–9 months. If menses do not resume within 1 year of discontinuation, a work-up for amenorrhea is necessary.

   c. **Headache** is experienced by 1–3% of women. Weight gain, resulting from an increase in appetite, averages 5 lbs in the first year and up to 14 lbs by year four of treatment.

4. **Noncontraceptive benefits**

   a. **Amenorrhea** is a consequence that many women enjoy. Baseline luteinizing hormone and follicle-stimulating hormone levels do not change, so these women have no symptoms of estrogen deficiency.

   b. **Lactation** is not adversely affected if the hormone is given immediately postpartum; trace amounts are detectable in breast milk without adverse outcome to infants.

   c. **Women with epilepsy** have fewer seizures.

5. **Acceptability** is high for women who need or want very effective birth control that is not coitally dependent, and who prefer or do not mind amenorrhea.

6. **Administration.** Give Depo-Provera, 150 mg intramuscularly, every 3 months. The first injection should be given immediately postpartum or within the first 5 days of a woman's menses.

C. **Norplant** is a fully reversible method of contraception, approved by the FDA in 1990. Norplant consists of six flexible silicone rubber rods, each of which is 1.3 inches long and contain 36 mg of levonorgestrel. Inserted subdermally at the inside of the upper arm, the rods continuously release a low dose of this progestin, which inhibits ovulation and causes thickening of the cervical mucus, preventing conception for up to 5 years.

1. The **failure rate** is less than 1% per year. It is less effective in women weighing more than 150 lbs.

2. **Contraindications** include active thrombophlebitis or thromboembolic disorders, undiagnosed abnormal vaginal bleeding, known or suspected pregnancy, acute liver disease, benign or malignant liver tumors, or known or suspected carcinoma of the breast.

3. **Side effects**
   a. Irregular bleeding usually subsides within 3–6 months, but the change in frequency or duration or the increase in blood flow or amenorrhea can be bothersome. Women who are told that these changes may occur handle them better.
   b. The rods can be felt by touching the arm but usually are not seen. Complications from insertion are negligible.
   c. Occasional acne and weight loss or gain have been reported.
   d. Removal of the device can be more difficult and take longer than insertion.

4. **Noncontraceptive benefits** are not yet well described, except that if a woman wants to conceive, fertility rates reach preinsertion levels within days of removal of the Norplant.

5. **Acceptability** is enhanced if a women prefers a method that is not coitally related. Counseling is especially important when this method is considered; the 7–10% discontinuation rate the first year is largely the result of the frequency of irregular menses. Headaches, weight gain, and depression are other common reasons for early removal. If women understand the possibility of this inconvenience, they are more likely to tolerate it. This method can be used by nursing mothers 6 weeks postpartum; studies have not been done for the immediate postpartum period.

D. **Emergency contraception (ecp)** using oral contraceptive pills containing ethinyl estradiol and norgestrel or levonorgestrel reduces the risk of pregnancy after unprotected intercourse; it will not interrupt an existing pregnancy. Therefore, it is wise to check a pregnancy test before supplying ecp. It is also important to discuss future contraception plans and whether the woman is at high risk for STDs (see Chapters 106, 108, and 110), and to counsel her about risk reduction activities.

1. When used within 72 hours of unprotected intercourse, ecp prevents at least 3 of 4 pregnancies that would have occurred.

2. Pregnancy is the only contraindication, not because ecp harms the pregnancy, only because ecp does not terminate a pregnancy. There are no medical contraindications.

3. Side effects include nausea in 30–50% of women and vomiting in 15–25%, as well as fatigue, breast tenderness, abdominal pain, headache, and dizziness for a day or two. Supplying the patient with antiemetic medication to be taken 1 hour before the first dose of ecp helps.

4. Noncontraceptive benefits for society include the cost-effectiveness of this method for preventing unintentional pregnancies. This method is an essential part of treatment for victims of sexual assault.

5. Acceptability is limited because many women and their health care providers are unaware of ecp. The FDA, in 1996, approved of ecp, and the American College of Obstetrics and Gynecology only recently developed guidelines on its use. ecp is not recommended for routine use because it is less effective than other forms of contraception.

6. **Administration.** Nordette (4 light orange pills/dose), Levlen (4 light orange pills/dose), Lo/Ovral (4 white pills/dose), Triphasil (4 yellow pills/dose), Tri-Levlen (4 yellow pills/dose), Ovral (2 white pills/dose), and Alesse (5 pink pills/dose) all work. Give one dose within 72 hours of unprotected intercourse and a second dose 12 hours later. Women using ecp can then use the rest of the pills in the pack as their birth control method; otherwise, women should begin a new pack of their regular pills. Progestin-only forms of ecp cause less nausea and vomiting, but the first dose must be taken within 48 hours. Women should expect their menses within 3 weeks of taking ecp; otherwise, they need a pregnancy test.

III. **Barrier methods** prevent contraception by providing a mechanical barrier to sperm. If such methods are used with a spermicide, sperm inactivation results. Avoid using oil-based lubricants and medications (Femstat, Monistat, estrogen, and Vagisil creams), because they cause the latex in condoms to deteriorate.

   A. **Condoms** are made of latex, the cecum of lambs ("skins"), or polyurethane (for latex-sensitive individuals). Most condoms have a shelf life of 5 years if stored properly in a cool place. Condoms for women offer increased coverage of the external genitalia and line the vagina entirely. They can be inserted 8 hours before intercourse. Acceptance has been limited because of the condom's bulkiness. Female and male condoms should not be used together because they can adhere, causing one or both to slip out of position.

   1. **Failure rates** for the ideal user are 3%. For the actual user, they are 14%. Latex condoms with spermicide are the most effective.

   2. **Contraindications.** Condoms should not be used if one or both partners are allergic to them.

   3. **Side effects** are limited to allergy to latex or spermicide.

   4. **Noncontraceptive benefits** include protection from STDs, including HIV, for latex and polyurethane condoms; skin condoms are too porous. Protection from infertility and from cervical intraepithelial neoplasia also occurs. Seventy-five percent of men agree that using condoms "shows you are a caring person," while 32% agree that using a condom "makes sex last longer."

   5. **Acceptability** is limited if a couple finds using condoms distracting or embarrassing. Expense is minimal, although specialty items are more costly. Condoms are available over the counter. No office visit is required. Patient instructions are given by the manufacturer. At least 25% of men are still embarrassed to buy condoms and may not know how to negotiate condom use with partners.

   B. **Diaphragms** are dome-shaped, rubber cups with arching or coiled rims. They must be left in place for at least 6 hours and not more than 24 hours after intercourse. Additional spermicide must be inserted before each coital act.

   1. The **failure rate** is 3% ideally and 18% actually. Efficacy improves as patient age and duration of use increase.

   2. **Contraindications.** If a woman has a cystocele, is allergic to latex or spermicide, has a history of toxic shock syndrome (TSS), is less than 12 weeks postpartum, or is too squeamish to use a diaphragm properly, another birth control method should be chosen.

   3. **Side effects**

   a. **Spermicide sensitivity** is the most common problem. Allergic reactions to latex may also occur.

   b. **Cystitis** is more common in women using this birth control method than in women not using a diaphragm. This is often because of improper fit and resolves when a smaller diaphragm is used.

   c. **TSS** occurs in no more than 10 per 100,000 users.

   4. **Noncontraceptive benefits** are similar to those of condoms (see section III,A). Cervical neoplasia rates are markedly less than those for other non-barrier forms of contraception.

   5. **Acceptability** is limited if a couple dislikes having to plan ahead before each coital act. The diaphragm, as well as contraceptive jelly or cream, must be purchased, and the diaphragm must be fitted by a physician.

   6. **Fitting the diaphragm.** The diaphragm is available in 11 sizes. The posterior rim of the diaphragm should fit in the posterior fornix, and the anterior rim should lie snugly behind the pubic bone.

   a. Use the largest rim size that is comfortable for the patient. Since much depends on muscle tone, recheck the position of the diaphragm after self-insertion when the patient is more relaxed.

   b. Always allow the patient to practice insertion, and then recheck diaphragm placement. Make sure the patient feels comfortable removing it.

   C. **Cervical caps** are thimble-shaped, rubber cups that fit over the cervix with an airtight seal dependent on suction. They can be left in place up to 48 hours. The cap has been used extensively in Europe, where it has been more popular than the diaphragm. The style available in the United States, the Prentif cap, received FDA approval in 1988.

1. The **failure rate** is 5% ideally and 18% in reality.
2. **Contraindications**
    a. Herpes papillomavirus (HPV) infection, atypia on smear, acute PID or cervicitis, undiagnosed vaginitis, and cervical biopsy or surgery within the past 12 weeks are absolute contraindications.
    b. A woman who has an abnormal Pap smear or an infection should not be fitted for a cervical cap. A normal Pap smear within the last 3 months is required.
    c. Anatomic abnormalities that preclude a good fit, including a vaginal septum or an extremely long or shallow cervix, preclude the use of this device.
    d. Allergy to latex or spermicide is also a contraindication.
    e. History of TSS is a contraindication.
3. **Side effects**
    a. Cervical atypia is accelerated in 0.9% of cap-wearing women, a percentage that is comparable to the rest of the population. However, this problem is of concern, because if women are selected improperly, the incidence of this condition is higher. Women should return for a Pap smear 3 months after beginning to use the cap and yearly thereafter.
    b. Allergic reaction to the latex or spermicide can occur.
    c. Vaginal discharge may occur if the cap is worn more than 48 hours at a time.
    d. Cervical or vaginal trauma caused by a poor-fitting cap or by prolonged wear (ie, more than 5 days continuously) is infrequent.
    e. TSS has not been reported, although it is a theoretical possibility.
4. **Acceptability** is similar to that of the diaphragm, except that inserting the cervical cap is more difficult to master. The availability of the cap is limited, because only health care providers who receive training by personnel recognized by the manufacturer can purchase and distribute the cap; pharmacies do not sell them.
D. **Vaginal sponges** are disposable, cylindrical pieces of polyurethane that are impregnated with nonoxynol 9. Each sponge is effective for 24 hours and is left in place if intercourse occurs more than once. It should not be removed for at least 6 hours after intercourse. Unfortunately, the vaginal sponge has not been manufactured since January 1995. The sponge remains safe to use, if it can be found. A new sponge is undergoing clinical trials in Europe.
    1. **Failure rates** range from 5% to 8% in ideal situations. In actual cases, the failure rate is 18–28%. Parous women have the highest rates of failure.
    2. **Contraindications.** If a woman has a history of TSS, if she has anatomic abnormalities such as prolapse or a vaginal septum, and if either partner has an allergy to polyurethane or nonoxynol 9, vaginal sponges should not be used.
    3. **Side effects**
        a. TSS occurs once per every 2 million sponges used. The risk is greatest if the sponge is used either during the menstrual or postpartum period or when the sponge is left in place for more than 24 hours.
        b. Allergic symptoms affect 2% of users.
        c. Vaginal infections (both monilial and bacterial vaginosis) occur more frequently in some women.
        d. Occasionally, women present for medical help because they cannot remove a sponge themselves.
    4. **Noncontraceptive benefits.** Nonoxynol 9 and octoxynol 9 destroy chlamydiae, herpes, gonococci, trichomonas, and human immunodeficiency virus (HIV). Women who use spermicides are one-third as likely to have cervical cancer as are other sexually active women.
    5. **Acceptability** is high for those who prefer a nonprescription method.
IV. **Chemical methods** inactivate the sperm by interfering with motility. Spermicides are available in the form of gels, creams, foams, suppositories, and film. The two most widely used are nonoxynol 9 and octoxynol 9. Douching is not a reliable contraceptive even when women put spermicide in the solution, because it is too late to inactivate the sperm. Women who routinely douche have an increased risk of PID and ectopic pregnancy.
    A. The **failure rate** is 3% ideally and 21% actually. Using a barrier method with a chemical method together increases efficacy.

    B. Contraindications. Spermicides should not be used if either partner has an allergy to the spermicidal agents.

    C. Side effects are limited to allergy. There is no increased risk of congenital malformation if conception occurs while using spermicides.

    D. Noncontraceptive benefits (see section III,D,4).

    E. Acceptability is high for those individuals or couples who like nonprescription, fairly inexpensive protection but low for people who find this method to be messy.

V. Intrauterine devices (IUDs) immobilize sperm, prevent implantation of the fertilized ovum, and dislodge the blastocyst from the endometrium. Both IUDs that are available are T-shaped; the ParaGard T380A has copper wound around the base, and the Progestasert is impregnated with progesterone. Both have fine, nylon tails that hang through the cervix, which allows women to check for the presence of the IUD.

    A. The **failure rates** are 0.5% for the first year and 1.9% after 4 years of use.

    B. Contraindications

        1. Women who are not in mutually monogamous relationships, who are at risk of acquiring STDs for other reasons, or who have acute pelvic infections should not use IUDs.

        2. It is not wise to insert an IUD in a nulliparous woman because of the concern about infertility.

        3. Pregnancy is a contraindication.

        4. Pre-existing severe dysmenorrhea will become worse with the copper IUD.

        5. To women with valvular heart disease, some physicians give prophylactic antibiotics before IUD insertion. Some practitioners will not use IUDs in such cases.

        6. Copper allergy or Wilson's disease precludes the use of the T380A IUD.

    C. Side effects

        1. Salpingitis with subsequent infertility and ectopic pregnancy are the most feared problems. If PID occurs, the IUD should be removed and another form of birth control can be used. The patient should wait 3 months before having the IUD replaced.

        2. Perforation of the uterus at insertion or at a later time occurs with 1 in 2500 users.

        3. Menometrorrhagia and dysmenorrhea are problems for some women with the copper IUD. Iron deficiency anemia may also result.

        4. If pregnancy occurs with an IUD in place, spontaneous abortions are more likely. If left in place, 50% of intrauterine pregnancies will spontaneously abort. If the IUD is removed, the rate is only 25%.

        5. Spotting may occur.

        6. Expulsion of the IUD, which often goes undetected, occurs in 5–8% of users the first year. This rate is highest for women who are parous.

    D. Noncontraceptive benefits. The Progestasert decreases the volume of menstrual blood and dysmenorrhea in symptomatic women.

    E. Acceptability is high for women who want a reversible, safe method of contraception when they are fairly sure their family is complete. Expense and availability can be a problem, since not all health insurance policies cover costs. An IUD costs at least $150. Some women are very uncomfortable with the idea of the IUD inside them, and other women dislike the idea that conception is not prevented. Yearly replacement of the device, which is required for the Progestasert IUD, is not accepted by some women.

    F. Insertion and removal. Always read the manufacturer's instructions for the specific kind of IUD to be used. The insertion and removal of an IUD are office procedures. A consent form must be signed. Both types of IUDs come with lengthy forms that take considerable time for women to complete.

        1. One size of both IUDs discussed above fits all women.

        2. One dose of a nonsteroidal anti-inflammatory drug (NSAID) such as Anaprox or Motrin is helpful if taken 1 hour prior to insertion or removal.

        3. Insertion is easiest during menses because the cervix is slightly dilated, although the incidence of expulsion and infection is slightly higher if the IUD is inserted at this time. Any time during the cycle is acceptable for insertion. The preferred time for removal is at the menses both for comfort and to insure that recent exposure will not result in pregnancy.

4. Leave a tail of at least 4 cm to allow the patient to check for expulsion of her IUD and to allow for easy removal. Let her feel the remnant of string so that she knows what to feel for monthly after her menses.

5. The Lippes Loop, which was available from 1974 to 1986, is the only IUD that can stay in place until menopause. All other IUDs may stay in place for a maximum of 4 years. The Progestasert must be replaced yearly.

VI. Fertility Awareness Method or Natural Family Planning

A. **Periodic abstinence** depends on avoidance of coitus during fertile days, which are determined by length of past menstrual cycles (rhythm or calendar method), or the changes in cervical mucus and basal body temperature that predict ovulation. Abstinence is required for about 17 days of each cycle. Some couples use barriers or withdrawal during the fertile time.

1. The **theoretical failure rate** is 2–10%, with an actual rate of 20% if mucus and temperature changes are monitored. For the calendar rhythm alone, actual failure rates are 14–47%. Natural family planning used with barrier methods reduces the failure rate to 10%.

2. **Contraindications.** Periodic abstinence should not be used in women who are nursing or nearing menopause or in women who have irregular cycles.

3. **Side effects.** A small chance that offspring will have more frequent malformations exist. Subsequent spontaneous abortions and birth defects may occur because overripe eggs are fertilized. Research studies conflict and are not conclusive.

4. **Noncontraceptive benefits** include self-knowledge of a woman's cycles, which can be helpful when pregnancy is desired. This information may also enhance both partners' awareness and involvement in family planning and can be helpful to couples trying to conceive.

5. **Acceptability** is most limited by the fairly extensive period of abstinence required, the work involved to keep track of changes in temperature and mucus consistency, and the high failure rate. This method, along with barrier contraception, works well for some couples, particularly because of the lack of side effects, the affordability, and acceptance by most religions. Many couples engage in noncoital sexual activities to make this method work for them.

6. **Patient instructions** are complex and should not be undertaken unless the health care provider is very secure that he or she can teach the techniques thoroughly. A lengthy teaching time is necessary. Handing a woman a chart to record changes without detailed instructions will most likely result in pregnancy. Workbooks are available to guide patients thoroughly.

B. **Coitus interruptus,** also known as the withdrawal method, depends on withdrawal of the penis from the vagina before ejaculation occurs.

1. The **failure rate** is estimated at 4% if used ideally and is actually 19%. This is, in part, because of the presence of pre-ejaculatory fluid, which contains up to millions of sperm per drop, particularly if ejaculation has recently occurred.

2. **Contraindications.** This birth control method should not be used if either partner will not be able to exercise enough control to prevent semen from reaching the vagina.

3. **Side effects.** Interruption of the sexual cycle can diminish pleasure.

4. **Noncontraceptive benefits** do not include protection from STDs, since mixing of secretions occurs even before ejaculation. Women have become infected with HIV while their partners consistently practiced this method.

5. **Acceptability** is enhanced because the method is free and involves no chemicals or devices, but for many couples the sacrifice and lack of spontaneity are too large a price to pay.

6. **Patient instructions.** Emphasize that any fluid on the tip of the penis must be wiped off before intercourse. Intercourse should not be repeated.

VII. Sterilization is a permanent form of birth control resulting from obstruction of the vas deferens in males (vasectomy) or the fallopian tubes in females (tubal ligation). It is the most widely relied-on form of birth control in the United States. It is used by about one-third of women to prevent pregnancy.

A. The **theoretical failure rate** is 0.15%, and the actual rate is less than 3% for a vasectomy.

B. **Contraindications.** Sterilization is contraindicated if any doubt about wanting permanent sterilization exists, since reversal of either a vasectomy or a tubal ligation is not always successful.

C. Side effects

1. Vasectomy

   a. Swelling, bruising, and pain are common. Hematomas occur in less than 2% of cases, and infections, including epididymitis, result less than 3% of the time.

   b. The risk of cardiovascular problems does not increase, as was once believed.

   c. The mortality rate in the United States is essentially 0%.

2. Tubal ligation

   a. Women often report a change in their menses, including menorrhagia and dysmenorrhea, although studies do not clearly support this. Some women may notice a change after discontinuing oral contraceptives prior to the ligation.

   b. Infection and hemorrhage are infrequent.

   c. Mortality is low, with 3 deaths per 100,000 cases in the United States. It is even lower if general anesthesia is not used.

   d. Ectopic pregnancy must be ruled out if signs of pregnancy occur after tubal occlusion.

D. Noncontraceptive benefits are limited to a diminished rate of PID in women who have had tubal ligations.

E. Acceptability is high for individuals who desire a permanent, effective birth control method. Cost is high initially if it is not covered by insurance, particularly for tubal ligations, but the expense is reasonable if five or more potential childbearing years remain. Vasectomy is an office procedure that takes about 20 minutes to perform. These patients return to work in a few days, depending on the nature of their job. Tubal ligation requires at least outpatient surgery and has a longer recovery period, depending on the method used and the surgeon.

F. Patient instructions

1. Informed consent is critical for either procedure and must describe the methods as irreversible, yet acknowledge a small risk of failure and pregnancy (possibly ectopic for the tubal ligation).

2. It is important for patients to think carefully about whether any change such as death or separation from a partner or from a child would make them regret the choice.

REFERENCES

American College of Obstetrics and Gynecology (ACOG). *Emergency Oral Contraception.* ACOG; 1996.

Dickey RP: *Managing Contraceptive Pill Patients,* 8th ed. Essential Medical Information Systems; 1994.

Earl DT, David DJ: Depo-Provera: An injectable contraceptive. Am Fam Physician 1994;**49:**891.

Hatcher RA, Trussell J, Stewart F, et al: *Contraceptive Technology,* 17th ed. Ardent Media; 1998.

Sivin I: Contraception with Norplant implants. Hum Reprod 1994;**9:**1818.

---

102   Infertility

Keith A. Frey, MD, MBA

I. Definition. *Infertility* is defined as 1 year of unprotected intercourse in which a pregnancy has not been achieved. Fifteen percent of couples in the United States are infertile.

II. Common diagnoses. The causes of infertility include abnormalities of any portion of the male or female reproductive system. Although infertility results from a single cause in the majority of couples, more than one factor contributes to infertility in as many as 40% of couples. "Unexplained" infertility, in which no specific cause is identified, occurs in approximately 10% of infertile couples. The following causes of infertility have been identified.

A. Male factors (35% of infertile couples).

B. Ovulatory dysfunction (15% of infertile couples).

    C. Tubal and pelvic pathology (35% of infertile couples).

    D. Unusual problems (5% of infertile couples).

III. Pathophysiology

  A. Male factors. The most commonly encountered cause of male infertility is a varicocele. Other causes include oligospermia or azoospermia, disorders of sperm function or motility (asthenospermia), and abnormalities of sperm morphology (teratospermia). Male infertility associated with antisperm antibodies is quite rare.

  B. Ovulatory dysfunction. The possible causes of anovulation may be grouped into four major categories.

    1. Hypothalamic anovulation (psychogenic trauma, anorexia nervosa, pseudocyesis, pharmacologic agents, anatomic defects, or congenital defects).

    2. Pituitary anovulation (pituitary tumors or ischemia).

    3. Ovarian anovulation (ovarian dysgenesis, premature ovarian failure, pseudoovulation, or ovarian tumors).

    4. Integrative anovulation (polycystic ovarian syndrome or nonpsychogenic weight disturbances).

  C. Tubal and pelvic pathology. Infertility may be associated with tubal damage or adnexal adhesions. Tubal obstruction may result from acute salpingitis, although many cases of tubal occlusion are encountered in which no episodes of salpingitis are recalled. Anatomic distortion of adnexal structures may also be caused by endometriosis (see section III,D). The chronic inflammation associated with endometriosis may disrupt normal conception by causing tubal damage or by interfering with ovum capture and gamete and embryo transport.

  D. Unusual problems. Cervical mucus abnormalities occur if at the time of ovulation the mucus is either insufficient in quantity or poor in quality. Factors contributing to the formation of such "hostile" (unreceptive) cervical mucus include cervical infections, previous surgery or cautery, and clomiphene therapy.

IV. Diagnosis. The physician should arrange a meeting with the couple early in the diagnostic work-up. This provides an important opportunity to review reproductive biology and the rationale for subsequent laboratory test results.

  A. Signs and symptoms. Since infertility may arise from one or more areas of the reproductive system, it requires a comprehensive diagnostic evaluation. The initial assessment of both the male and the female partner consists of a thorough history and physical examination. Specific areas requiring extra attention are noted in Table 102–1.

  B. Laboratory tests (Tables 102–2 and 102–3). In addition to a comprehensive history and physical examination, each couple must be evaluated by a series of routine laboratory tests and appropriately timed studies to evaluate each major reproductive factor that may be the cause of infertility. This comprehensive diagnostic survey can and should be completed for most couples in 6–12 months.

TABLE 102–1. THE INFERTILITY WORK-UP IN OUTLINE: HISTORY (MALE, FEMALE, OR BOTH)

Marriage	Occupation and habits	Review of systems
Duration of infertility	Exposure to radiation, chemicals,	Focus on endocrine conditions
Fertility in previous relationships	excessive heat (saunas, hot	(diabetes, thyroid disorders)
Frequency of intercourse	tubs, etc)	
Sexual potency and techniques		**Gynecology**
Use of coital lubricants	**Childhood illness**	Coital frequency and techniques
	Cryptorchidism	Contraceptive use
Adult illnesses	Timing of puberty	Diethylstilbestrol use by mother
Acute viral or febrile illness in past		Douche and lubricant use
3 months	**Surgery**	Exposure to radiation and
Mumps orchitis	Herniorrhaphy	chemicals
Renal disease	Retroperitoneal surgery	Fertility in previous relationships
Radiation therapy	Vasectomy	Menarche
Sexually transmitted disease		Menses (regularity and flow)
Stress and fatigue	**Drug use**	Mittelschmerz
Tuberculosis	Alcohol, tobacco, and drugs	
	Alkylating agents	
	Anabolic steroids	
	Nitrofurantoin	
	Sulfasalazine	
	Cimetidine	

TABLE 102–2. THE INFERTILITY WORK-UP IN OUTLINE: PHYSICAL EXAM/ROUTINE LABORATORY TESTS (MALE AND FEMALE)

Male		Female	
Physical Examination	**Routine Laboratory Tests**	**Physical Examination**	**Routine Laboratory Tests**
Hair pattern	**CBC**	**Breast formation**	**CBC**
Genitalia	**Semen analysis**	**Distribution of body fat**	**Pap smear**
Meatus size and location	Abstinence of 2 days	**Galactorrhea**	**Urinalysis and urine culture if indicated**
Prostate and seminal vesicles	Masturbation into sterile vessel	**Hair pattern (virilization)**	**VDRL test**
Scrotum	To laboratory (warm) within 2 hours	**Height and weight**	**At-home test**
Testicular size (≥4 cm in long axis)	Results	**Neurology**	**Basal body temperature**
Varicocele (standing and Valsalva's	Volume: 2–5 mL	Anosmia	Measure temperature for 5–10 minutes orally before
maneuver)	Liquefaction: complete within 30 minutes	Visual fields	arising
Neurology	Sperm count: 60–150 million/mL	**Pelvis**	Measure temperatures throughout evaluation and
Anosmia	Sperm motility: >60%	External genitalia	treatment
Visual fields	Morphology: >60% normal forms	Retrovaginal area (endometriosis)	Bring chart on each visit
	2–3 tests as necessary	Uterus and adnexa	
	Urinalysis and urine culture if indicated	Vagina and cervix	
	VDRL test		

CBC, complete blood cell count; VDRL, Venereal Disease Research Laboratory.

TABLE 102–3. THE INFERTILITY WORK-UP IN OUTLINE: FURTHER DIAGNOSTIC TESTS

Postcoital (Sims–Huhner) test
Determines the number and condition of sperm and their ability to penetrate cervical mucus
Performed around the time of ovulation

Hysterosalpingography
Preferred test of tubal patency
Performed 2–6 days after cessation of menstrual flow
May enhance fertility temporarily

Laparoscopy
Performed if hysterosalpingography is unproductive
Permits examination of pelvic contents

Endometrial biopsy
Determines whether luteal phase defect exists
Performed 2–3 days before expected menses
Informed consent required
Requires histologic dating

Serum progesterone
May be an alternative to endometrial biopsy
Sample drawn 5–7 days after supposed ovulation
Serum level >3 ng/mL is compatible with ovulation

Each couple's evaluation must be individualized based on the findings of the history and the physical examination. However, an initial survey of each major reproductive factor is necessary in *all* couples and can be coordinated by the primary care physician.

    1. Male factors. Evidence of oligospermia after two or more semen analyses will require further diagnostic evaluation, including blood levels for luteinizing hormone (LH), follicle-stimulating hormone (FSH), and testosterone. Testicular biopsy may be required, particularly if aspermia is discovered.

    2. Tubal factors. The female partner must undergo an evaluation for tubal patency. If the history or the physical examination shows no clear evidence of tubal damage, proceed with a hysterosalpingogram; otherwise, refer the patient for laparoscopy.

    3. Ovulatory dysfunction. Anovulation or inconsistent ovulation may be diagnosed by the history (irregular menses), a nonbiphasic basal body temperature pattern, abnormally low serum progesterone levels, or endometrial biopsy.

    4. Cervical mucus factors. When a significant number of white blood cells is noted on cervical mucus samples at the time of expected ovulation (ie, during the postcoital test), a specific bacteriologic diagnosis should be sought. See Chapter 55 for specific recommendations.

V. Treatment. Generally, treatment should not be initiated until the diagnostic evaluation is completed. The male and female partners should be treated as a couple whenever possible. Therapy should proceed at a rate that the couple finds comfortable.

    A. Male factors. Specific antibiotics are used to treat infections such as prostatitis and epididymitis (see Chapters 3 and 64). Consultation with a urologist will generally be required to complete the evaluation and coordinate treatment.

    B. Ovulatory dysfunction. If anovulation is diagnosed, consider treatment with clomiphene.

        1. Clomiphene treatment. Amenorrheic and oligomenorrheic women attempting to conceive are among the patients best suited for clomiphene. Patients with other causes of anovulation generally respond best to specific therapy, such as surgery for a pituitary tumor. The usual starting dose is 50 mg/day orally on days 5–9 of the menstrual cycle. The dose may be increased by 50 mg/day in the second and third cycles. A careful evaluation for galactorrhea and a prolactin level should precede treatment.

            Common side effects include vasomotor flushes (10%), abdominal or pelvic discomfort (5.5%), nausea (2.2%), and breast tenderness (2%).

        2. Expected results. Ovulation should be expected 5–10 days after the treatment ends; this should be confirmed by biphasic basal body temperature

(BBT) and an elevated level of serum progesterone on day 21. If ovulation does not occur despite clomiphene therapy, consultation with a reproductive endocrinologist is recommended.

C. Tubal and pelvic pathology. Tubal blockage or deformity may necessitate surgical correction. The management of endometriosis in a woman desiring to achieve pregnancy depends on the degree and location of endometrial deposits. Conservative surgical treatment may enhance fertility potential by destroying endometrial implants and endometriomas. Laparoscopic conservative surgical treatment should be considered as a treatment option for mild endometriosis-associated infertility. For patients with more severe tubal and pelvic pathology, referral for assisted reproductive technologies is warranted.

D. Unusual problems. For cervical mucus abnormalities, antibiotics should be used to treat the specific bacterial cause of the problem. Low-dose estrogens are often the best treatment for poor cervical mucus that does not result from infectious causes. Conjugated estrogens, 0.625 mg/day for 9 days preceding the expected time of ovulation, may be used.

VI. Management strategies. The work-up, diagnosis, and treatment of infertility can precipitate intense emotional reactions. The sensitive physician should discuss such emotions as anger, guilt, self-doubt, depression, and grief with the couple. The actions described below may also prove beneficial.

    A. Help the couple understand their motives for parenting, which may include desires (1) to parent, (2) to experience a pregnancy, (3) to meet the expectations of others, and (4) to promote genetic continuity.

    B. Assist the couple in the development of mutual support and an adaptive "couple-coping" style. Discuss sexual issues, and encourage the couple to nurture their intimacy; they will need its strength to deal with the problems associated with infertility. Periodic meetings with the couple to review diagnostic progress provide further opportunity to reinforce coping skills.

    C. Help the couple broaden their support systems, including self-help groups, such as Resolve, Inc.

VII. Prognosis. The exact prognosis of infertility is difficult to define because of the multiple potential causes. For most of these, conception will not be achieved without specific treatment. However, with specific therapy, subsequent pregnancy rates have been studied and the results are favorable. "Unexplained" infertility is the persistent inability to conceive after a comprehensive diagnostic assessment of the couple fails to establish a specific diagnosis. If a comprehensive diagnostic work-up fails to identify a cause, or if the appropriate treatment is unsuccessful, the physician should discuss adoption options with the couple.

REFERENCES

Howard SS: Treatment of male infertility. N Engl J Med 1995;**332**:312.
Petrie K, Frey KA: *Preconception Care/Infertility.* Monograph, Edition No. 234, Home Study Self-Assessment program. American Academy of Family Physicians; November 1998.
Speroff L, Glass RH, Kase NG: *Clinical Gynecologic Endocrinology and Infertility,* 5th ed. Williams & Wilkins; 1994.

ELECTRONIC RESOURCES

Assisted Reproductive Technology Success Rates: National Summary and Fertility Clinic Reports 1995.
http://www.cdc.gov/nccdphp/drh/arts/index.htm
RESOLVE National Home Page. http://www.resolve.org

---

103   Prenatal Care

Megeen Parker, MD

I. Goals

    A. Antenatal care refers to a comprehensive approach to medical care and psychosocial support of the family that ideally begins prior to conception and ends with the onset of labor.

B. **Preconception care** is the physical and mental preparation of both parents for pregnancy and childbearing prior to conception in order to improve pregnancy outcomes.

C. **Prenatal care** formally begins with the initial diagnosis of pregnancy and includes ongoing risk assessment, education, and counseling to promote health as well as identification and management of problems.

II. **Preconception care**

A. **Medical history.** All women of childbearing age are potential candidates for preconception evaluation. Identifying conditions and risks that could adversely affect a future pregnancy, followed by appropriate interventions and counseling to improve the outcome of pregnancy, are the primary tasks of the preconception evaluation.

1. **Chronic medical conditions** should be evaluated both for potential effects on pregnancy and for effects that pregnancy may have on the medical condition. Significant chronic illnesses include diabetes mellitus, hypertension, thyroid disorders, anemias, coagulopathies, seizure disorders, asthma, and cardiovascular diseases. A history of infectious diseases such as HIV/AIDS, hepatitis B and C, toxoplasmosis, rubella, and varicella is also of critical importance in identifying risks that may be lowered prior to conception with appropriate immunizations and counseling. Also notable are a past history of recurrent urinary tract infections and phlebitis.

2. Note **previous surgeries,** particularly abdominal and pelvic procedures.

3. A thorough review of **prescription and over-the-counter medications** currently being taken is helpful to anticipate and minimize adverse effects, particularly during the period of organogenesis from the fourth to the tenth weeks of gestation. The Food and Drug Administration's Pregnancy Categories and other reviews such as the Teris classifications are useful in determining risk versus benefit and teratogenic risk. Drugs clearly proven to have significant teratogenic risk in humans include alcohol, chemotherapeutic agents, anticonvulsants, androgens, warfarin, lithium, and isotretinoin.

4. Note **allergies and sensitivities** to medications and anesthetics.

5. **Current methods of contraception.** Ideally, some methods should be discontinued several menstrual cycles prior to conception to assist with accurate dating (see Chapter 101).

6. **Genetic risk assessment** performed in the preconception period as opposed to the prenatal period allows women and their partners to consider a greater number of options in family planning. The background incidence of congenital malformations is approximately 3%. Genetic causes account for about 20% of anomalies. Genetic counseling and further testing may be of benefit when the following conditions are identified: advanced maternal (over 35 years) or paternal (over 55 years) age; family history of or previous child with neural tube defect (NTD), congenital heart disease, hemophilia, thalassemia, sickle cell disease, Tay–Sachs disease, cystic fibrosis, Huntington's chorea, muscular dystrophy, mental retardation, Down syndrome, or other inherited disorders; maternal metabolic disorders; recurrent pregnancy loss (three or more); use of alcohol, recreational drugs, and medications; and environmental or occupational exposures.

7. **Obstetric and menstrual history.** Review the number, date, length, and outcome of prior pregnancies. Record any history of significant pregnancy-related health concerns, such as gestational diabetes, intrauterine growth retardation, preterm labor, or hemorrhage. Make note of any complications during labor and delivery. A detailed menstrual history is helpful, paying particular attention to irregular menses and infertility.

B. **Psychosocial history.** This is a critical area of the history, since significant risks may be identified that may be addressed prior to pregnancy. A potential pregnancy may also serve as an incentive to the patient to alter certain unhealthy habits. High-risk behaviors include tobacco use, alcohol consumption, illicit drug use, and poor nutrition. Psychosocial risks include a past history of mental illness, inadequate personal supports and coping skills, high stress, exposure to domestic violence or abuse, single marital status, inadequate housing, low income, and less than high school education.

C. **Immunization history.** Rubella, varicella, and hepatitis B immunity are best addressed prior to conception.

D. Physical examination
   1. Height and weight. Patients who weigh more than 200 lbs or less than 90 lbs may be at greater risk for problems in pregnancy.
   2. Blood pressure
   3. Breast examination
   4. Pelvic examination, including clinical pelvimetry (although pelvimetry is unlikely to affect the outcome of the pregnancy).
E. Laboratory tests
   1. Recommended laboratory tests include hemoglobin or hematocrit, rubella titer, urine dipstick for protein and glucose, Pap smear, gonococcal culture, hepatitis B surface antigen, and syphilis serology. Counseling regarding HIV testing should occur with all patients.
   2. Additional screening may be appropriate for women with the following, who are identified to be at greater risk: *Chlamydia,* tuberculosis, toxoplasmosis, cytomegalovirus, herpes simplex, varicella, and hemoglobinopathies.
F. Health promotion
   1. Optimize management of pre-existing medical conditions such as diabetes and hypertension.
   2. Administer appropriate immunizations (see Chapter 107).
   3. The US Public Health Service recommends that all women of childbearing age should consume 0.4 mg of folic acid per day to reduce the risk of NTDs.
   4. Provide counsel and educate regarding the following topics.
      a. Pregnancy planning. Accurate recording of menstrual cycles is helpful. Oral contraceptives should be discontinued and a barrier method should be used to establish normal cycles prior to attempting pregnancy.
      b. Nutrition and weight correction, if necessary.
      c. Smoking cessation and avoidance of alcohol and illicit drugs.
      d. Genetic risks, if any.
      e. Avoidance of teratogens, including prescription and nonprescription medications, and occupational and environmental exposures.
      f. Preparation of the family for pregnancy and enhancement of social support.
      g. Proper exercise.
III. Prenatal care
  A. Initial diagnosis of pregnancy
   1. Symptoms include cessation of menses, breast tenderness and enlargement, nausea, fatigue, and frequent urination.
   2. Signs such as uterine enlargement and a dark bluish coloring of the cervix and vaginal mucosa (Chadwick's sign) are present.
   3. Urinary tests for elevated levels of β-human chorionic gonadotropin (β-hCG) are generally positive at about the time of the first missed menses and have a sensitivity of 98% and a specificity of 99%.
  B. The **first prenatal visit** should occur before 8 weeks' gestation, as it is critical for determining an accurate delivery date, evaluating risk status, and providing essential patient education. The visit may be abbreviated if a recent preconceptual visit has occurred.
   1. Patient history (see section II). A detailed menstrual history as well as the last contraceptive method used is important for establishing dates. The estimated date of delivery (EDD) should be established before 20 weeks' gestation, when techniques for dating are most accurate. The date of the start of the last menstrual period is the most accurate predictor for EDD. A first-trimester ultrasound can confirm gestational age within ±4 days, although routine use for dating is controversial. In addition, a history of illnesses, medications, and exposures since the last menstrual period (LMP) should be obtained. A patient's questions concerning common symptoms in early pregnancy can be answered at this time.
   2. Complete physical examination. This should include evaluation of fetal heart tones and pelvic examination that documents uterine size and evaluates the bony pelvis (the conjugate diameter, evaluation of the ischial spines, the shape of the sacrum, the distance between the ischial tuberosities, and the angle of the pubic arch).

3. **Routine laboratory work.** In addition to testing recommended during the preconception visit (see section II,E), blood and Rh type, antibody screen, microscopic urinalysis, and urine culture should be performed.

4. **Patient education** early in pregnancy is critical. Important issues to be addressed are described below.

   a. **High-risk behaviors**

   (1) **Smoking** has been associated with intrauterine growth retardation (IUGR), prematurity, placenta previa, placental abruption, and preterm rupture of membranes.

   (2) **Alcohol use** is linked to fetal alcohol syndrome (craniofacial abnormalities, limb and cardiovascular defects, growth and mental retardation).

   (3) **Cocaine** is associated with increases in spontaneous abortions, placental abruption, preterm labor and delivery, low birth weight, neonatal withdrawal syndromes, and central nervous system damage.

   (4) **Opiates** may cause IUGR, preterm delivery, and an increased rate of intrauterine hypoxemia and fetal distress.

   (5) Daily consumption of more than 300 mg of **caffeine** (about three cups of coffee) has been associated with an increased risk of IUGR and low birth weight.

   b. **Nutrition and weight gain.** Total weight gain of 25–35 lbs is recommended for women at an appropriate weight at the time of conception. Women at less than 90% or greater than 120% of ideal body weight (IBW) should gain 30–35 pounds or 18–20 pounds to minimize risks. A weight gain of less than 10 lbs at 20 weeks' gestation is associated with increased complications.

   (1) The average pregnant woman needs approximately 1900–2750 kcal/day (300 kcal more than nonpregnant patients). The best clue to adequate caloric intake is maternal weight gain.

   (2) The diet should include increased amounts of calcium (1200 mg daily, equivalent to 3–4 milk servings), iron (30 mg essential iron), vitamins C and D, and folic acid (0.4–0.8 mg daily) and consist of 50–60% complex carbohydrate, up to 20% protein, and no more than 30% fat. A prenatal multivitamin and mineral supplement is recommended when dietary intake is inadequate. Vegetarians require additional iron, vitamin B_{12}, and zinc. Excessive doses of vitamins, particularly vitamins A, C, and D, can be harmful to the fetus.

   c. **Patient expectations,** the benefits of childbirth education classes, and family issues should be discussed.

   d. **Sexual intercourse** during pregnancy is contraindicated only for patients with placenta previa and for those at risk for abortions or premature labor.

   e. **Physical activity** should not be significantly increased during pregnancy; however, regular, low-intensity exercise (walking, swimming, bicycling) should be encouraged. Contact sports, activities requiring repeated Valsalva maneuvers or rapid changes in direction, or those involving unpredictable risk should be discouraged.

   f. **Symptoms for which patients need to promptly contact their physician** should be clearly outlined. These include any vaginal bleeding or escape of fluids from the vagina, swelling of the face and fingers, severe continuous headache, dimness or blurring of vision, abdominal pain, persistent vomiting, chills or fever, dysuria, and change in frequency or intensity of fetal movements.

C. **Common symptoms**

   1. **Nausea and vomiting,** which usually begin at about 6 weeks and disappear by 14–16 weeks, are commonly worse in the morning and occur in up to 70% of pregnant women. Nonpharmacologic therapies include having frequent, small meals; avoiding greasy, spicy foods; having a protein snack at bedtime; eating dry crackers before getting out of bed in the morning; and avoiding drinking liquids on an empty stomach. Purposeful stimulation of the P6 (Neiguan) acupuncture point located three fingerbreadths proximal to the distal wrist crease and between the two central flexor tendons of the forearm, via pressing firmly with the fingers for 5 minutes every 4 hours while

awake or via use of Seabands, can be quite helpful. Pharmacologic measures include antiemetics such as meclizine or metoclopramide, pyridoxine (vitamin B_6) 25 mg two or three times daily or in combination with 10 mg of doxylamine found in Unisom. Sipping red raspberry, German chamomile, or peppermint tea can also be helpful. Reassurance that symptoms may be related to higher levels of maternal estrogens and an associated improved pregnancy outcome may also be useful.

2. **Headache** is common before 20 weeks' gestation and is usually benign, although in most cases no specific cause can be found. This symptom may be safely treated with acetaminophen. Relaxation and use of warm compresses may help. The pattern of migraine may change during pregnancy. The physician must consider pre-eclampsia, particularly later in pregnancy.

3. **Gastrointestinal symptoms common during pregnancy**
    a. Heartburn occurs in about one-half of pregnant women at some time. This condition has been attributed to a number of factors, including decreased tone in the lower esophageal sphincter, displacement and compression of the stomach by the uterus, and decreased gastric motility. Treatment consists of having frequent small meals and avoiding bending over or lying flat soon after eating. Low-sodium liquid antacids are helpful and safe; however, those agents that contain magnesium or aluminum hydroxides impair absorption of iron.
    b. Constipation is common in pregnancy because of steroid-induced changes in bowel transit time. Dietary measures are the mainstay of treatment and include high-fiber foods, liberal consumption of water and other liquids, and regular, low-intensity exercise. Mild laxatives, such as milk of magnesia, stool softeners, and bulk laxatives, are safe and effective.
    c. Abdominal pain may occur in pregnancy and warrants evaluation. The physician should consider the same causes for abdominal pain that occur in the nonpregnant state. However, these conditions may present differently in pregnant patients. Types of abdominal pain specific to pregnancy are described below.
        (1) Ectopic pregnancy should be ruled out in women with lower abdominal or pelvic pain early in pregnancy (see Chapter 55).
        (2) Pre-eclampsia may be associated with upper abdominal pains in the epigastrium or the right upper quadrant.
        (3) Placental abruption should be considered when pain is associated with bleeding, particularly in the third trimester.
        (4) Urinary tract infections (see Chapter 24).
        (5) Other, less significant causes include round ligament or broad ligament discomfort, which results from increased tension on these structures as the uterus enlarges.

4. **Urinary complaints,** such as increasing frequency and stress incontinence, are often noted, especially during the first and third trimesters, because of uterine pressure on the bladder. Decreasing night-time fluid intake (without any overall restrictions) and Kegel's exercises can be helpful. Infection, however, is common and should be considered when frequency is associated with dysuria.

5. Increased **vaginal discharge (leukorrhea)** is common, often with no pathologic cause. This physiologic discharge is related to increased estrogen. Infectious causes should be ruled out (see Chapter 67) in the presence of associated symptoms of itching, burning, foul odor, or labial swelling.

6. **Vaginal bleeding** may occur at any time during pregnancy and should always be considered significant enough to warrant further evaluation.
    a. Bleeding in the first trimester is a relatively frequent occurrence. Causes range from physiologic bleeding as a result of implantation to life-threatening conditions. Extrauterine pregnancy should be considered when bleeding occurs during this time, even in the absence of pain. Any bleeding occurring in the first half of pregnancy, particularly with cramping, may be associated with spontaneous abortion.
    b. Bleeding in the later half of pregnancy occurs less frequently and may be associated with cervical trauma during coitus. Painless bleeding may suggest placenta or vasa previa, whereas painful bleeding is classically associated with placental abruption.

7. **Edema in the feet and the ankles** is common, particularly during the third trimester. This edema is secondary to sodium and water retention combined with increased lower extremity venous pressure. Edema should raise concerns of pre-eclampsia when it is accompanied by hypertension and proteinuria. Benign edema normally responds to leg elevation, avoidance of long periods of sitting or standing, and use of support stockings.

8. **Backache** is relatively common during pregnancy and is partially related to increased joint laxity as well as compensatory postural changes that occur as the uterus enlarges. Avoiding excessive weight gain, wearing flat or low-heeled shoes, and improving posture may provide some relief. Chiropractic care may be effective and is safe during pregnancy.

9. **Varicose veins** are aggravated by pregnancy, prolonged standing, and advancing age. This condition usually worsens as pregnancy advances, because of increased femoral pressure. Treatment is limited to periodic rest with leg elevation and elastic stockings; more definitive treatment is delayed until after pregnancy.

10. **Hemorrhoids** are the result of increased pressure on hemorrhoidal veins by the uterus and by the tendency toward constipation during pregnancy. Effective treatments include sitz baths with warm water for 20 minutes and followed by local application of witch hazel, topically applied anesthetics, and stool softeners (see Chapter 57).

D. **Additional prenatal care.** Traditionally, prenatal visits should occur every 4 weeks through the 28th week of pregnancy, every 2 weeks through the 36th week, and then weekly until delivery. The frequency of visits may be altered based on the risk status of the patient. Measurement of weight, blood pressure, and fundal height; assessment of edema; check of a urine dipstick for protein and glucose, and documentation of fetal heart rate should occur at every visit. Other tests and interventions may be needed at specific times during pregnancy, as noted below.

1. **Care prior to 14 weeks (first trimester).** Initial care during the first trimester can prepare both clinician and patient for a healthy pregnancy.

   a. Review initial laboratory work and define maternal risk status more precisely.

   b. Counsel patients regarding the initial troubling symptoms of pregnancy, such as nausea, fatigue, and emotional changes. Encourage good nutrition. Review signs of miscarriage. Inquire about the partner's adjustment.

   c. Offer early prenatal diagnostic studies to all patients with genetic risk factors (see section II,A,6). Chorionic villus sampling (CVS) is performed between 9 and 12 weeks' gestation, which allows for earlier termination of pregnancy with less maternal morbidity. Amniocentesis is usually performed after 15 weeks, but can be done as early as 13 weeks' gestation. Unlike amniocentesis, CVS cannot be used for prenatal diagnosis of NTDs and may be associated with limb reduction defects. Amniocentesis carries a 0.5–1% risk of fetal loss. The risk from CVS is slightly higher. A detailed ultrasound scan performed in the second trimester can also assist in the evaluation of fetal anomalies but is not recommended as a screening test.

   d. Fetal heart tones are first heard with Doppler ultrasound between 10 and 12 weeks' gestation and sometimes as early as 8 weeks in multigravidas.

2. **Care between 14 and 28 weeks' gestation (second trimester).** An obviously pregnant body and the first sensations of fetal movement often lead to an increased appreciation of being pregnant. The second trimester is an excellent time to schedule a joint visit with the patient and her partner to discuss expectations about parenting.

   a. **Confirmation of the estimated date of delivery.** At approximately 20 weeks' gestation, the uterine fundus is at the level of the umbilicus, and fetal heart tones can usually be heard with a fetoscope. The sensation of fetal movement (quickening), which may first be a fluttering sensation, is usually felt at 16–20 weeks.

   b. **Routine prenatal screening for neural tube defects and chromosomal abnormalities** such as Down syndrome (trisomy 21) are offered during this time. NTDs occur in 4 per 10,000 live births. Screening involves measuring the **maternal serum α-fetoprotein (MSAFP)** between 16 and

18 weeks' gestation. Approximately 50 of 1000 women will have an elevated (>2.5 multiples of the median) MSAFP, indicating the possibility of an NTD. Most will be falsely positive, resulting from inaccurate dating, multiple gestation, or other anomalies. A targeted anatomic ultrasound to confirm dates can detect 90–95% of NTDs. An amniocentesis is more accurate in detecting NTD but carries a small but discrete risk of fetal loss (0.5–1%). Reduced levels of MSAFP (<0.7 multiples of the median) indicate an increased risk of Down syndrome. An association with reduced levels of estradiol and elevated levels of hCG (the "triple screen") lowers the false-positive rate from 20% to 5% and will identify approximately 60% of cases. Amniocentesis offers the only definitive diagnosis, once dating is confirmed by ultrasound. Parents should be carefully advised of the benefits and risks of these screening tests with documentation of the discussion and their decision recorded in the chart.

   c. Despite growing controversy that **screening for gestational diabetes** does not meet criteria for a screening test, universal screening between 24 and 28 weeks is widely recommended and practiced. Measurement of plasma blood glucose 1 hour after ingesting a 50-g oral glucose load is most commonly done, and fasting is not required. Levels over 140 mg/dL require further evaluation with a 3-hour oral glucose tolerance test. Women with borderline levels between 130 and 140 may benefit from repeated testing in several weeks. Some physicians advocate earlier screening (prior to 24 weeks), when conditions increasing risk for gestational diabetics are present. Such conditions include a past history of gestational diabetes or a macrosomic infant (>4000 g), family history of type II diabetes, or a maternal weight over 200 lbs.

   d. The hemoglobin or hematocrit can be repeated at the same time as screening for diabetes, along with antibody screening for D (Rh)-negative women.

   e. **D (Rh)-negative** women should be given D (Rh) immune globulin at 28 weeks' gestation, if the antibody screening is negative. D (Rh) immune globulin should be given earlier if an event has occurred exposing the patient to fetal blood (eg, CVS, amniocentesis, or significant trauma). A repeat dose given within 72 hours after delivery is also necessary.

3. Care beyond 28 weeks of gestation (third trimester). This is often a period of increasing discomfort for the patient, with sleep disturbances, dyspnea, urinary frequency, and fatigue being common. The incidence of complications such as pre-eclampsia, maternal hypertension, and malposition of the fetus lead to a need for more frequent and intensive monitoring. Allow time to discuss expectations and wishes regarding labor and delivery, and review indications for calling the office.

   a. **Blood pressure** should be carefully monitored. Systolic blood pressures >140 mm Hg or a rise >30 mm Hg or diastolic blood pressures >90 mm Hg or a rise of >15 mm Hg is diagnostic of transient hypertension and warrants further evaluation for pre-eclampsia, particularly when associated with proteinuria or edema.

   b. **Fetal position** should be regularly assessed. Most babies are vertex by the final month of pregnancy. For other presentations, external version is often successful and increases the chances of a vaginal delivery.

   c. Testing for **sexually transmitted diseases** in high-risk women, if appropriate, should be repeated at 36–38 weeks' gestation. Testing allows for treatment prior to delivery.

   d. **Screening for group B streptococcal (GBS) infection** remains controversial. GBS sepsis occurs in approximately 1.8 per 1000 live births and is related to intrapartum exposure when the mother is colonized. One of two equally acceptable strategies for lowering the risk of neonatal GBS sepsis involves universal screening with rectovaginal swab for culture at 35–37 weeks' gestation in the absence of risk factors (previous infant with invasive GBS disease, GBS bacteriuria, or preterm labor). Intrapartum antibiotic prophylaxis is then given to all women who test positive or have other intrapartum risk factors (intrapartum fever or prolonged rupture of membranes). Antepartum prophylaxis is not recommended. The alternative strategy does not involve any antenatal screening cultures but instead focuses on intrapartum risk assessment with subsequent intrapartum antibiotic prophylaxis of women with one or more risk factors.

E. Medications in pregnancy. Most drugs should be used only when benefits clearly outweigh risks, particularly in the first trimester. Patients need to understand that taking any medication during pregnancy involves some small degree of risk.

1. **Antihistamines** are generally acceptable when used in normal therapeutic doses, with the possible exception of brompheniramine.
2. **Antiemetics** may be used safely if other conservative measures are not effective.
3. **Decongestants.** Phenylephrine and phenylpropanolamine should be avoided, but pseudoephedrine is relatively safe to use. Use it in the lowest dosages possible, since large doses may influence uterine perfusion. Decongestants are contraindicated when uteroplacental insufficiency is suspected. Try recommending the substitution of saline nose spray or irrigation or judicious use of topical decongestants.
4. **Oral analgesics and anti-inflammatory agents**
   a. Acetaminophen is the drug of choice for mild analgesia and antipyresis. Continuous high doses may cause maternal anemia and fatal kidney disease in the newborn.
   b. Low-dose aspirin has been used to lower the risk of pre-eclampsia in high-risk women. Although there is no clear consensus regarding the benefits related to pre-eclampsia, aspirin has proven to be a relatively safe drug. There does seem to be an increased risk of placental abruption. Caution should be used in the second half of pregnancy.
   c. Nonsteroidal anti-inflammatory drugs, such as ibuprofen and naproxen, have a theoretical risk of prenatal closure of the ductus arteriosus when used near term. Indomethacin, if used after 34 weeks' gestation, may lead to persistent pulmonary hypertension of the newborn, inhibition of labor, and prolongation of pregnancy. There is no evidence of adverse effects in the first half of pregnancy.
   d. Codeine is not absolutely contraindicated, although association with malformations has been reported. Neonatal withdrawal has been documented. Hydrocodone–acetaminophen combinations (Vicodin) may be safer in pregnancy than codeine.
5. **Antibiotics**
   a. Penicillins (with or without clavulanate) and cephalosporins are among the most effective and least toxic of available antibiotics and can be used at any time during pregnancy.
   b. Erythromycin has not been reported to be of harm to the fetus, except as the estolate salt, which is contraindicated in pregnancy.
   c. Tetracyclines and quinolones are contraindicated in pregnancy because of adverse effects on developing teeth and bones.
   d. Sulfonamides may be used in the first two trimesters. Use near term and during nursing should be avoided, since sulfonamides may cause significant jaundice or hemolytic anemia in the newborn.
   e. Oral metronidazole is contraindicated in the first trimester, since it may result in fetal malformations. Topical metronidazole is safe throughout pregnancy.
   f. Nitrofurantoin should be used with care in late pregnancy since it has the ability to induce hemolysis in neonatal red blood cells.
6. **Antidepressants and benzodiazepines**
   a. Tricyclic antidepressants should be used with caution, as no extensive studies of their use in the first trimester are available.
   b. Selective serotonin reuptake inhibitors, particularly fluoxetine, have generally been proven to be relatively safe during pregnancy. Several recent studies found no increased teratogenesis, pregnancy loss, or childhood developmental abnormalities. Use in the third trimester may require caution, however, as there is some evidence of increased rate of preterm births.
   c. Lithium is contraindicated during pregnancy.
   d. Benzodiazepines should be used cautiously, if at all, as there is some evidence of an increased risk of cleft palate or cleft lip.

IV. Preterm labor (PTL) is defined as regular uterine contractions accompanied by descent of the presenting part and progressive dilatation and effacement of the cervix occurring before 37 weeks from the first day of the last menstrual period. PTL complicates only 8–10% of pregnancies but is responsible for over 60% of all perinatal morbidity and mortality. Risk factors include occult maternal genitourinary tract infections, maternal smoking, high levels of stress, low socioeconomic status, maternal age less than 18 or greater than 35, cervical dilatation >1 cm or cervical effacement >30% between 26 and 34 weeks' gestation, and uterine anomalies. Risk factors most likely are synergistic.

A. Diagnosis. Early diagnosis is crucial, as tocolysis is most effective before 3 cm of cervical dilatation or 50% effacement. Symptoms suggestive of regular uterine contractions should be evaluated with serial examinations for cervical change and by external monitoring of uterine activity.

B. Treatment. The risks of preterm delivery must outweigh the risks to mother and fetus of tocolysis. Advancing gestational age clearly improves the preterm infant's prognosis until approximately 35 weeks, when delaying delivery has less effect overall. Survival increases to 90% at 29 weeks; mortality then decreases about 1% per week. The acuteness and severity of preterm labor suggest the type of treatment.

   1. Uterine irritability without significant cervical change may benefit from rest at home, intake of fluids, and treatment of causative factors, such as urinary tract infection, if present.

   2. Tocolytic therapy is indicated in preterm labor if no contraindications, such as severe pre-eclampsia or chorioamnionitis, exist. All tocolytics have potentially severe side effects for both mother and fetus. Choices include β-sympathomimetics, magnesium sulfate, nifedipine, and Indocin.

   3. Evaluation for possible triggers, particularly occult urinary tract infection, is indicated. Randomized controlled trials have found no clear benefit to the use of antibiotics in PTL with intact membranes on prolonging gestation or improving neonatal morbidity or mortality. Treatment with antenatal corticosteroids given between 34 weeks' gestation and greater than 24 hours but less than 7 days prior to delivery has been shown to be of benefit in reducing the incidence and severity of respiratory distress syndrome and improves neonatal survival rates.

V. Fetal assessment and postdates pregnancy

A. Fetal assessment. Several methods have been developed to assess the wellbeing of the fetus when risk factors exist. Fetal assessment begins between 34 and 36 weeks' gestation or whenever the risk develops. Major indications for antenatal testing include diabetes mellitus, hypertensive disorders, maternal substance abuse, third-trimester bleeding, IUGR, previously unexplained stillbirth, D (Rh) sensitization, oligohydramnios, multiple gestation, and decreased fetal movement as perceived by the mother. Fetal assessment techniques also are routinely applied when a pregnancy becomes postdates (42 weeks from the LMP).

   1. Fetal movement counts. A quantitative method of counting fetal movements has been developed as a means of fetal assessment near term. The patient is asked to count fetal movements during a 2-hour period each day and report less than 10 movements during that period. A positive test (fewer than 10 movements) is an indication for additional fetal assessment. The advantages of this test are its low cost and maternal involvement.

   2. Fetal heart rate testing

      a. The nonstress test (NST) is a noninvasive method based on the premise that in a healthy fetus, acceleration of the heart rate occurs during fetal movement. An external monitor is used to record the fetal heart rate while the mother reports fetal movement. A reactive or normal test has two or more accelerations of more than 15 beats per minute, each lasting for 15 seconds, in a 20-minute period and in the absence of decelerations. If fetal movement does not occur in 20 minutes, abdominal palpation or vibro-acoustic stimulation may be applied to awaken a sleeping fetus. A reactive NST accurately identifies a healthy fetus 98% of the time.

      Evaluation of a nonreactive NST should include extending the testing period to 60–90 minutes when possible. Nonreactive NSTs and variable decelerations on reactive NSTs must be followed by a contraction stress test.

    b. The contraction stress test (CST) is a test of the fetal heart rate in response to uterine contractions. The uterus may be stimulated to contract through intermittent stimulation of one breast nipple or through intravenous infusion of low-dose oxytocin. A satisfactory test requires at least three contractions in 10 minutes. The test is interpreted as negative, or normal, if there are no decelerations and positive, or abnormal, if late decelerations follow 50% or more of contractions. A nonreactive, positive CST is highly suggestive of fetal distress and must be treated immediately with oxygen, positional changes, labor induction, or cesarean section. Equivocal results occur with occasional late decelerations and should be repeated in 24 hours.

    3. An **amniotic fluid index** is used to complement fetal heart rate testing. Ultrasonography is used for estimating amniotic fluid volume, which is an indirect measure of placental function. The largest anteroposterior fluid depths in each of four quadrants of the uterus is measured. The sum should exceed 5 cm.

    4. The **biophysical profile** is a quantitative score that combines the NST with ultrasonic observation of the fetus for up to 30 minutes and measurement of the amniotic fluid index. A score of 2 is given **for each normal result** (fetal breathing movements, gross body movements, tone, amniotic fluid index, and NST) and 0 for an abnormal condition. A total score of 8–10 is reassuring, 6 is equivocal, and 4 or less is worrisome. A combination of NST and amniotic fluid evaluation is considered comparable to the biophysical profile in assessing fetal well-being.

B. Postdates pregnancy. Defined as lasting longer than 42 weeks from the beginning of the LMP, approximately 3.5–12% of pregnancies are postdates. Prolonged pregnancy is one lasting longer than 41 weeks. Accurate dating is essential to avoid mislabeling a pregnancy as postdates.

    1. Chronic uteroplacental insufficiency leading to fetal compromise occurs in up to 20% of postdates pregnancies. Additional complications include oligohydramnios, meconium passage, and macrosomia, which may contribute to a higher cesarean section rate.

    2. Evaluation. Fetal assessment testing should be performed in all postdates pregnancies, and some nonrandomized studies suggest that beginning noninvasive fetal assessment at 41 weeks with a biweekly NST may lower the rate of stillbirths and intrapartum fetal distress.

    3. Management. International randomized controlled clinical trials have shown a clear benefit to induction of labor at 41–42 weeks' gestation. The fetal mortality rate of 2 per 1000 at this gestational age is lowered to virtually zero, and cesarean rates are lowered. Elective induction with pitocin, using prostaglandins for cervical ripening, is relatively safe and effective.

VI. Normal labor and delivery. Signs of labor include passage of the mucus plug, bloody show (small amount of blood-tinged mucoid vaginal discharge), regular uterine contractions, and spontaneous rupture of membranes. In the general population, about 90% of women should be able to have a healthy birth outcome without medical intervention. Family-centered birthing focuses on safety for the mother and child and fostering a positive experience for the woman, her partner, and family. Since most labor occurs in the hospital, a full discussion of labor and its complications is beyond the scope of this chapter.

REFERENCES

American Academy of Pediatrics and The American College of Obstetricians and Gynecologists: *Guidelines for Perinatal Care,* 4th ed. American Academy of Pediatrics; 1997.

Briggs GG, Freeman RK, Yaffe SJ: *Drugs in Pregnancy and Lactation: A Reference Guide to Fetal and Neonatal Risk,* 5th ed. Williams & Wilkins; 1998.

Cochrane Database of Systematic Reviews (available in the Cochrane Library). The Cochrane Collaboration, Issue 1. Update Software; 1997. Available from BMJ Publishing Group.

Ratcliffe SD, Byrd JE, Sakornbut EL (eds): *Handbook of Pregnancy and Perinatal Care in Family Practice: Science and Practice.* Hanley and Belfus; 1996.

US Preventive Services Task Force: *Guide to Clinical Preventive Services: Report of the US Preventive Services Task Force,* 2nd ed. Williams & Wilkins; 1996.

104   Postpartum Care

Jeannette E. South-Paul, MD

I. **Definition.** The postpartum period, or puerperium, is that period of time that begins with the delivery of the placenta and ends with the resumption of ovulatory menstrual cycles, which, in nonlactating women, usually occurs 6–8 weeks after delivery.

II. **Normal physiologic changes during the postpartum period**

    A. **Uterus.** The uterus decreases in size dramatically following delivery (involution); it weighs only about 500 g at the end of the first week and lies again in the true pelvis. This change is accompanied by a high level of uterine activity (contractions, afterpains) that diminishes smoothly and progressively after the first 2 hours postpartum. The placental implantation site sheds organized thrombi and obliterated arteries in order to prevent scar formation and preserve normal endometrial tissue.

    B. **Cervix.** The cervical os admits two fingers for the first 4–6 days postpartum, but constricts thereafter and admits only a small banjo curette by the end of the second week.

    C. **Vagina.** Large and smooth-walled following delivery, the vagina begins to develop rugae by the end of the fourth week. It regains its nonpregnant size by the end of the sixth to eighth week.

    D. **Lochia.** The uterine discharge, which is bright red at delivery, changes within a few days to the reddish-brown lochia rubra, composed of blood and decidual and trophoblastic debris. Lochia serosa, a more serous combination of old blood, serum, leukocytes, and tissue debris, appear 1 week postpartum and last for a few days. Lochia alba, a whitish-yellow discharge that contains serum leukocytes, decidua, epithelial cells, mucus, and bacteria, then begins and continues until approximately 2–4 weeks postpartum. Lochia rubra that lasts more than 4 weeks suggests the presence of retained secundines or the formation of placental polyps, organized placental fragments.

    E. **Urinary tract.** Passage of the infant through the pelvis traumatizes the bladder, and its wall may be edematous. Trauma or conduction analgesia may also cause the bladder to be insensitive to changes in intravesicular pressure, resulting in an impaired urge to urinate. Symptoms of urinary incontinence increase with parity. Practice of pelvic muscle exercise by primiparas has resulted in fewer urinary incontinence symptoms during late pregnancy and the puerperium. The glomerular filtration rate remains elevated during the first postpartum week. Urinary output, which often reaches 3 L in a 24-hour period, exceeds fluid intake. This output, combined with insensible losses, accounts for the approximately 12-lb weight loss seen during this period. The pregnancy-induced dilation of the ureters and renal pelves subsides to normal within 6 weeks.

    F. **Abdominal wall.** The abdominal wall begins to resume a nonparous condition in about 6–7 weeks. The skin remains lax, but the muscles regain substantial tone with proper exercise.

    G. **Cardiovascular changes.** Cardiac output decreases to nonpregnant levels within 2–3 weeks postpartum. Lower-extremity varicosities and pelvic varices regress during this period. Plasma volume decreases more rapidly than do cellular components initially, so that the hematocrit increases slightly during the first 72 hours postpartum.

    H. **Weight change.** Weight gain during the first 20 weeks of pregnancy predicts postpartum retained weight. The influence of lactation on weight loss postpartum is unclear. Women lose approximately half of the average weight gain of pregnancy (25 lbs) in the first 2 weeks after delivery. The remainder is lost during the following weeks. Women should return to their nonparous weight in approximately 8 weeks.

    I. **Breasts.** Milk production and engorgement begin within 3 days postpartum, following the decrease in estrogen and the increase in prolactin produced by suckling. Suckling is the single most important stimulus for the maintenance of milk production. A mother wishing to stop breast feeding need only discontinue suckling. The accumulation of milk in the alveoli and major ducts leads to increased intra-alveolar and intraductal pressure, resulting in the cessation of milk formation. The historical practice of breast binding is thought to work by the same mechanism.

J. **Hypothalamic–pituitary–ovarian function.** Forty percent of nonlactating women will resume menstruation within 6 weeks following delivery, 65% within 12 weeks, and 90% within 24 weeks. Approximately 50% of the first cycles are ovulatory. In nursing mothers, menstruation is resumed within 6 weeks in only 15% and within 12 weeks in only 45%. In 80% of these women, the first ovulatory cycle is preceded by one or more anovulatory cycles. Rapid decreases in blood levels of estrogen, progesterone, human placental lactogen, and insulin occur following delivery.

III. Abnormalities of the puerperium

A. **Puerperal infections.** *Puerperal infection* is defined as infection of the genital tract that sometimes extends to other organ systems. Onset is insidious and may occur 2–5 days postpartum. Nonspecific symptoms are malaise, anorexia, and fever. In many cases, a temperature of 38 °C (100.4 °F) or higher on any 2 of the first 10 days postpartum, exclusive of the first 24 hours, indicates a puerperal infection. Extragenital infections and noninfectious causes of fever must be excluded. The differential diagnosis includes urinary tract infections (UTIs), mastitis, and thrombophlebitis, as well as other causes of fever unrelated to the postpartum state. Onset of fever after the tenth postpartum day is usually of a nonobstetric nature. Puerperal infections that are usually polymicrobial in origin are caused predominantly by anaerobes and sometimes by aerobes. *Escherichia coli* and group B streptococci are very common. Multiple bacteria of low virulence, common in the genitourinary tract, may become pathogenic as a result of hematomas and devitalized tissue. Cultures are of limited usefulness, since the same organisms are identified in patients with or without infections.

1. **Predisposing factors**
   a. **Antepartum.** Premature or prolonged rupture of membranes, malnourishment, and anemia increase the likelihood of puerperal infections.
   b. **Intrapartum.** Soft tissue trauma, residual devitalized tissue, prolonged labor, and hemorrhage are also risk factors.
   c. **Late-onset indolent metritis** has been attributed to antepartum *Chlamydia trachomatis* cervical infection, but this organism has not been isolated at the time these infections developed postpartum.

2. **Specific puerperal infections**
   a. **Endometritis.** This term describes inflammatory involvement, especially leukocytic infiltration, of the superficial layers of the endometrium or decidual layer. When severe, endometritis may be accompanied by chills, extreme lethargy, lower abdominal pain, and fever. Temperature spikes to 40 °C (104 °F) usually indicate associated sepsis. It is not necessarily associated with significant uterine tenderness by abdominal or vaginal palpation. The prevalence of this type of infection, which is relatively uncommon following uncomplicated vaginal delivery, has decreased from 2.5% to 1.3% in the last 15 years. This prevalence approaches 6%, however, in high-risk women: those with protracted labor and prolonged rupture of membranes, prior history of gynecologic infections, hematomas or devitalized tissue, postpartum anemia, maternal age <17 years, and where there is manual removal of the placenta. Prior to the common use of perioperative antimicrobials for women undergoing cesarean section, these women had an extraordinarily high risk of developing endometritis. The reported overall prevalence of postoperative uterine infection was 13–50%, depending on the socioeconomic group of the parturient.

   The polymicrobial cause of endometritis necessitates broad-spectrum therapy. A combination of clindamycin and gentamicin has been used traditionally. Clindamycin is administered intravenously in a dose of 2.4–2.7 g/day in three or four divided doses. Gentamicin is given in a loading dose of 2 mg/kg and then 1.5 mg/kg every 8 hours thereafter. Other treatment regimens have been evaluated recently, but the number of subjects studied has been small. Regimens reported to be as effective as clindamycin plus gentamicin include cefoxitin, moxalactam, cefoperazone, cefotaxime, piperacillin, cefotetan, and clindamycin plus aztreonam.

Evidence now suggests that ampicillin (2 g) and sulbactam (1 g) intravenously every 6 hours is equally as effective as the clindamycin/ gentamicin regimen for clinical cure, bacterial eradication, and incidence of adverse experiences. In all cases, intravenous therapy should be continued until the patient has been free of symptoms for approximately 48 hours.

    b. Parametritis. This infection involves the broad ligament adjacent to the uterus. Parametritis is usually associated with endometritis. In its most isolated mild form, it may follow cesarean section. Treatment is the same as for endometritis.

    c. Perineal infection. Such an infection is more likely in the presence of a small, unnoticed hematoma. Examination of the perineum reveals an edematous, erythematous lesion with purulent drainage. Sutures must be removed to enhance drainage.

    d. Mastitis (see Chapter 10).

B. Nonpuerperal complications

  1. Urinary tract infections. The high incidence of UTIs during the postpartum period is usually attributed to trauma-induced hypotonicity of the bladder and frequent catheterization. Most patients with cystitis have had a negative initial screening culture and no urologic abnormalities. A 10- to 14-day course of antibiotics (amoxicillin, 500 mg orally three times daily for 10–14 days) is begun before cultures are ready (see Chapter 24). For a penicillin-allergic patient, refer to the alternative medications noted in Chapter 24, Table 24–1. Cystitis usually results in local symptoms without fever. In contrast, the symptoms of pyelonephritis are more severe: flank pain, shaking chills, and fever to 40 °C (104 °F) are frequent accompaniments.

  2. Thrombophlebitis and **thromboembolic disease.** These conditions occur in fewer than 1% of all parturients, but occur significantly more often in the parturient than in the nonpregnant woman.

    a. Disorders of the deep veins in the postpartum period have been attributed to sluggish circulation, trauma to pelvic veins secondary to pressure from the fetal head, estrogen-induced hypercoagulability, and pelvic infection. Deep vein thrombophlebitis is characterized by fever, deep vein tenderness, Homans' sign, and extremity swelling secondary to venous obstruction. A useful, reliable diagnostic procedure is venography. The accuracy of Doppler ultrasonography depends on the skill of the technician (see Chapter 44).

    b. Superficial thrombophlebitis usually involves the saphenous system and is palpable on physical examination. Tenderness and increased skin warmth are also evident. Treatment methods include **elastic support stockings, walking, elevation of the legs at rest, a combination of analgesic drugs,** and **application of moist local heat** to the area. To prevent this form of thrombophlebitis, women should remain active and refrain from taking estrogens to suppress lactation or oral contraceptives, since these agents increase the risk of hypercoagulation. They should also avoid anti-inflammatory agents during pregnancy and lactation because of risk of premature closure of the fetal ductus arteriosus.

    c. *Right ovarian vein syndrome,* or **pelvic thrombophlebitis,** is the term used to describe thrombophlebitis occurring in the ovarian veins and other pelvic vessels. The patient often complains of abdominal pain and fever. If no evidence of pelvic abscess exists, and appropriate antibiotic therapy has resulted in no improvement in 72 hours in a patient with suspected endometritis, the diagnosis of ovarian vein syndrome should be considered. A sausage-shaped, tender mass may be palpated in the right midabdomen. Dramatic improvement usually results once **anticoagulation with heparin** is initiated, but defervescence may only occur after 4–5 days of heparin therapy, in doses similar to those used for the treatment of pulmonary embolism (see Chapter 23). Currently available imaging studies (computed tomography scan and ultrasound) are poor in diagnosing this entity, so clinical suspicion is important.

    d. Massive pulmonary embolism is characterized by the sudden onset of pleuritic chest pain, cough (with or without hemoptysis), fever, apprehension, and tachycardia. Friction rub, signs of pleural effusion and atelectasis, hypotension, diaphoresis, electrocardiographic signs of right heart strain, and increasing central venous pressure may all be present in severe cases (see Chapter 23).

3. **Parametrial phlegmon.** A phlegmon, a three-dimensional mass that is palpable adjacent to the uterus on pelvic examination, develops most frequently when appropriate antimicrobial therapy has been delayed following evaluation of a postcesarean fever. A parametrial phlegmon is an intense area of induration within the leaves of the broad ligament occurring when endometritis and accompanying parametrial cellulitis follow cesarean delivery. The infection can be localized in the retroperitoneal area and presents with symptoms of peritonitis, such as an adynamic ileus. Treatment includes **bed rest, hydration with intravenous fluids, decompression of the bowel,** and **maintenance of electrolyte balance.** Clinical response occurs following intravenous antimicrobial therapy (the same antibiotics as are used for endometritis), although not usually until 5–7 days after initiation of treatment.

4. **Toxic shock syndrome (TSS).** Toxic shock syndrome toxin-1, an exotoxin produced by *Staphylococcus aureus,* causes TSS by provoking severe endothelial injury. Nearly 10% of pregnant women have been found to be colonized vaginally by *S aureus,* and TSS has been reported in parturients. The syndrome most commonly occurs in young menstruating women who are using tampons. This severe, multisystem, acute febrile illness is characterized by a fever of 38.9 °C (102 °F) or higher; a macular erythematous rash, especially on the palms and the soles, that desquamates 1–2 weeks after onset of illness; hypotension, <90 mm Hg systolic, or orthostatic syncope; and involvement of three or more of the following organ systems: gastrointestinal, muscular, mucous membrane, renal, hepatic, hematologic, or central nervous.

   Initial management includes hospitalization, fluid and electrolyte resuscitation (up to 12 L/day), and administration of packed red blood cells and coagulation factors as necessary. In addition to baseline laboratory studies, blood and vaginal cultures of *S aureus* should be obtained promptly. Treatment with a β-lactamase–resistant antibiotic, such as nafcillin, oxacillin, or methicillin, is indicated; the dosage is 1 g intravenously every 4 hours. Vancomycin, 100 mg every 6 hours, is effective if the patient is allergic to penicillin.

5. **Necrotizing fasciitis.** This deep, soft tissue infection that involves muscle and fascia may develop adjacent to myofascial edges, including surgical incisions and other wounds. Such infections rarely develop during the postpartum period in healthy women, but are seen in diabetic and immunocompromised women. Symptoms most commonly occur 3–5 days following delivery. The microbes implicated in these perineal infections are similar to those causing other pelvic infections, but anaerobes predominate. A high index of suspicion is necessary with rapid surgical exploration if the diagnosis is probable. Therapy consists of **broad-spectrum antibiotics** (eg, clindamycin, 2.4 g/kg in four divided doses) plus gentamicin (1.5 mg/kg every 8 hours), or others as noted above, as well as vigorous surgical **debridement.**

C. **Postpartum hemorrhage**

1. **Uterine atony.** This condition, which is the most common cause of postpartum hemorrhage, can result from excessive uterine stretching secondary to hydramnios, multiple gestation, multiparity, prolonged labor, and certain general anesthetic agents. Initial management includes **fundal massage, removal of any remaining placental fragments,** and **oxytocin** (10 U intramuscularly every 4 hours, or 10–40 U intravenously diluted in 1000 mL of 0.5 normal saline titrated intravenously) to control atony. Methylergonovine maleate (0.2 mg intramuscularly every 4 hours for 48 hours) may be used instead of oxytocin.

2. **Lacerations.** Routine inspection of the cervix, vagina, and perineum immediately following delivery affords the opportunity for timely repair of extensions to the episiotomy or lacerations.

3. **Hematomas.** Perineal pain and noticeable mass suggest hematomas, which usually occur at the sites of lacerations or episiotomy repair. If managed within the first 24 hours after delivery with incision, drainage, and ligation of bleeding vessels, the cavity can be closed with a figure-of-eight suture.

    4. Less common causes of postpartum hemorrhage are placenta accreta, inverted uterus, coagulation defects (eg, associated with amniotic fluid embolism or pre-eclampsia–eclampsia), retained placental fragments, or uterine rupture. Digital examination of the uterus and lower uterine segment upon delivery is necessary to detect uterine rupture, especially after a vaginal delivery following prior cesarean section.

D. Postpartum emotional disorders

    1. "Baby blues," or "postpartum blues." This transient depression, which is encountered in 70–80% of women during the first week postpartum, usually on the second or third day following delivery, can be accompanied by tearfulness. This self-limited disorder usually resolves within 3–7 days. Twelve percent of women will present with clinically relevant depressive disorders within 6 weeks postpartum, but 90% of these cases are associated with a situational or longstanding problem. Postpartum depression, occurring between 2 weeks and 12 months postpartum, is related to employment factors in the working parturient, such as work hours and duration of maternity leave, maternal fatigue, and quality of prenatal social support. If the symptoms are severe enough to interfere with the new mother's ability to cope with ordinary daily tasks and activities, counseling and pharmacotherapy are advisable (see Chapter 96).

    2. Psychiatric disorders. If the patient exhibits excessive or no tearfulness, lack of interest in the baby, or excessive concern with the problems that will be encountered upon returning home that persist more than 24 hours while still in the hospital, or does not respond to counseling about problems developing subsequently, psychiatric evaluation is needed. Not only can major affective disorders appear during this time, but the stress of gestation and parturition are nonspecific factors that may contribute to the development of various psychotic disorders.

IV. Management strategies

    A. Immunizations

        1. Nonisoimmunized D-negative women who deliver a D-positive infant should be given 300 mg of anti-D immune globulin (Rhogam) shortly after delivery.

        2. The postpartum hospitalization period is also an appropriate time for vaccination of women not already immune to rubella. Some hospitals also give a tetanus toxoid booster injection prior to discharge unless it is contraindicated.

    B. Discharge instructions

        1. Periods of rest during the day are advisable for the **first month postpartum.** All parturients, especially those who have been sedentary during pregnancy, become detrained during the third trimester and the postpartum period and should begin exercising at a baseline level. If vaginal bleeding increases upon resumption of exercise, parturients should stop for 2–3 days to allow further uterine involution and then resume activity. The parturient may gradually increase her activity and exercise level as soon as 2 weeks following an uncomplicated delivery. Only half of women seem to regain their usual level of energy by 6 weeks postpartum, however.

        2. Sitz baths, basins designed to fit over the toilet seat and be filled with warm water and 1 oz of Betadine solution, or tub baths for 30 minutes two to three times daily, are helpful for painful episiotomies or lacerations.

        3. Sexual intercourse

            a. For some time, **abstinence** has been recommended in the 6 weeks following delivery. The most common complaint is concern about dyspareunia during this period, which can be minimized by careful episiotomy. This period of discomfort can be shortened safely if no episiotomy is needed or if episiotomy repair is done meticulously so that healing occurs rapidly and comfortably. If tender areas in the episiotomy scar or in the vaginal wall persist after healing, a 1:1 steroid–lidocaine (1–2 mL of 1% Xylocaine without epinephrine and 1–2 mL of triamcinolone acetonide, 10-mg per milliliter) injection to the painful area can be used for relief.

            b. Otherwise, **sexual intercourse** can be resumed between the second and third postpartum weeks. The parturient can be encouraged to resume sexual activity when bleeding slows and when acceptable contraception has been provided. Contraception should be discussed and a method should be selected prior to discharge from the hospital (see Chapter 101). Intrauterine devices, diaphragms, sponges, and foams are not advised until after the puerperium.

4. Breast feeding

a. Components of milk

(1) Colostrum. This liquid is secreted by the breasts for the first 5 days of parturition. It contains more protein, mostly globulin, and minerals and less sugar and fat than the more mature milk that is ultimately secreted. Host resistance factors, such as complement components, macrophages, lymphocytes, lactoferrin, lactoperoxidase, and lysozyme, as well as immunoglobulin, are present in colostrum and milk.

(2) Milk. The major components are proteins (α-lactalbumin, β-lactoglobin, and casein), lactose, water, and fat. All vitamins except vitamin K are present in human milk in variable amounts. Iron is present in low concentrations, and iron levels in breast milk do not seem to be influenced by maternal iron stores. The predominant antibody present is secretory immunoglobulin A. These antibodies are thought to act locally within the infant's gastrointestinal tract.

b. Nursing

(1) Advantages

(a) Accelerates involution of the uterus via oxytocin release.

(b) Gives ideal nourishment. Breast milk meets the nutritional needs of the infant.

(c) Provides immunologic advantage. In addition, breast-fed babies are less prone to respiratory and enteric infections than are bottle-fed babies.

(d) Contributes to bonding. Nursing is generally well tolerated by infants.

(e) Delays ovulation.

(2) Disadvantages

(a) Privacy is needed for frequent feedings.

(b) Contraindications include concurrent usage of certain drugs (eg, chloramphenicol, streptomycin, metronidazole, sulfa drugs, antithyroid drugs, some anticancer agents, certain anticonvulsants, some diuretics, and radioactive agents). Women with certain maternal illnesses (eg, active hepatitis A or B or tuberculosis) should not engage in breast feeding.

(c) Nursing can be an additional stressor in an already stressed mother.

c. Breast care. Cleanliness and attention to fissures on the nipples are important. Water and mild soap can be used to cleanse the areolae before and after nursing. Lanolin-containing cream is recommended for nipple protection during the initial weeks of breast feeding to deter chapping and cracking of the nipples. Should severe irritation of the nipples occur, a nipple shield can be used for 24 hours or more.

5. Suppression of lactation. Women who do not wish to breast feed should avoid all breast stimulation, suckling, manipulation, and showers, and should utilize breast support, binding, and analgesia for 1 week. Minor symptoms of tenderness and a sense of fullness are common. Otherwise, there are no risks or side effects. Neither parenteral Deladumone nor oral bromocriptine is currently recommended. Following the use of Deladumone, rebound symptoms are common; in 25% of cases, there is an associated risk of thromboembolism, and use of the medication rarely results in substantial decrease in lactation. Rebound symptoms affect approximately 25% of women using bromocriptine as well. Furthermore, additional risks include hypotension, nausea, headache, dizziness, strokes, and early ovulation.

6. Postpartum examination. The postpartum visit is usually scheduled for 6–8 weeks after delivery, since most of the systemic signs of pregnancy have resolved by this time. Recent research evaluating optimal timing of the postpartum examination demonstrates that scheduling the Pap smear at least 8 weeks following delivery, rather than at 4–6 weeks, results in an approximately 30% decrease in the number of abnormal smears requiring follow-up or colposcopic examination. Following normal labor and puerperium, the postpartum evaluation should consist of blood pressure and weight determinations, palpation of the thyroid gland, a breast examination, a pelvic examination with cytologic examination of the cervix, evaluation of rectal sphincter tone, examination of abdominal wall tone, and urinalysis. Routine postpartum hematocrits are unnecessary in clinically stable patients with an estimated blood loss of less than 500 cc.

REFERENCES

Collins NL, et al: Social support in pregnancy: Psychosocial correlates of birth outcomes and postpartum depression. J Pers Soc Psychol 1993;**65:**1243.

Ely JW, et al: The association between manual removal of the placenta and postpartum endometritis following vaginal delivery. Obstet Gynecol 1995;**86:**1002.

Ely JW, et al: Benign fever following vaginal delivery. J Fam Pract 1996;**43:**146.

Gall S, Koukol DH: Ampicillin/sulbactam vs clindamycin/gentamicin in the treatment of postpartum endometritis. J Reprod Med 1996;**41:**575.

Gibbs RS: Chorioamnionitis and bacterial vaginosis. Am J Obstet Gynecol 1993;**169:**460.

Gjerdingen DK, Chaloner KM: The relationship of women's postpartum mental health to employment, childbirth, and social support. J Fam Pract 1994;**38:**465.

Gray RH, et al: Risk of ovulation during lactation. Lancet 1990;**335:**25.

Howie PW, et al: Protective effect of breast feeding against infection. BMJ 1990;**300:**11.

Janney CA, Zhang D, Sowers M: Lactation and weight retention. Am J Clin Nutr 1997;**66:**1116.

Muscati SK, Gray-Donald K, Koski KG: Timing of weight gain during pregnancy: Promoting fetal growth and minimizing maternal weight retention. Int J Obes Relat Metab Disord 1996;**20:**526.

Nicol B, Croughan-Minihane M, Kilpatrick SJ: Lack of value of routine postpartum hematocrit determination after vaginal delivery. Obstet Gynecol 1997;**90:**514.

Rarick TL, Tchabo JG: Timing of the postpartum Papanicolaou smear. Obstet Gynecol 1994;**83:**761.

Resnik E, et al: Early postpartum endometritis: Randomized comparison of ampicillin/sulbactam vs ampicillin, gentamicin and clindamycin. J Reprod Med 1994;**39:**467.

Sampselle CM, Miller JM, Mims BL, et al: Effect of pelvic muscle exercise on transient incontinence during pregnancy and after birth. Obstet Gynecol 1998;**91:**406.

South-Paul JE, Deuster PA: Physical activity during pregnancy. Clin Consult Obstet Gynecol 1993;**5:**245.

Wang IY, Fraser IS: Reproductive function and contraception in the postpartum period. Obstet Gynecol Surv 1994;**49:**56.

Witlin AG, Sibai BM: Postpartum ovarian vein thrombosis after vaginal delivery: A report of 11 cases. Obstet Gynecol 1995;**85**(5 Pt 1):775.

Witlin AG, et al: Septic pelvic thrombophlebitis or refractory postpartum fever of undetermined etiology. J Matern Fetal Med 1996;**5:**355.

---

105   Sexual Dysfunction

John G. Halvorsen, MD, MS

I. **Definition.** The sexual dysfunctions represent disturbances in sexual desire and in the psychophysiologic changes that characterize the sexual response cycle.

II. **Common diagnoses.** The *Diagnostic and Statistical Manual of Mental Disorders,* 4th edition (DSM-IV), classifies the dysfunctions according to the following system. All must be "persistent or recurrent," "cause marked distress or interpersonal difficulty," and not be "better accounted for by another Axis I disorder" or "due exclusively to the direct psychophysiologic effects of a substance (eg, a drug of abuse, a medication) or a general medical condition." Subtypes are also provided for all disorders to indicate the onset (lifelong type or acquired type), the context (generalized type or situational type), and the causative factors (caused by psychological factors or by combined factors) associated with each dysfunction.

   A. **Sexual desire disorders (SDDs)**
      1. **Hypoactive sexual desire disorder:** deficient (or absent) sexual fantasies and desire for sexual activity.

2. **Sexual aversion disorder:** extreme aversion to, and avoidance of, genital contact with a sexual partner.

B. **Sexual arousal disorders**

1. **Female sexual arousal disorder:** inability to attain or maintain an adequate lubrication–swelling response of sexual excitement until sexual activity is completed.

2. **Male erectile disorder (ED):** inability to attain or maintain an adequate erection until sexual activity is completed.

C. **Orgasmic disorders**

1. **Female orgasmic disorder:** delayed or absent orgasm following normal sexual excitement.

2. **Male orgasmic disorder:** delayed or absent orgasm following normal sexual excitement.

3. **Premature ejaculation (PE):** ejaculation with minimal stimulation before it is wanted, either before, on, or shortly after penetration.

D. **Sexual pain disorders**

1. **Dyspareunia:** genital pain in either men or women associated with sexual intercourse.

2. **Vaginismus:** involuntary vaginal muscular spasm that interferes with sexual intercourse.

E. **Sexual dysfunction due to a general medical condition:** sexual dysfunction that is fully explained by the direct physiologic effects of a defined medical condition.

F. **Substance-induced sexual dysfunction:** sexual dysfunction that develops during or within 1 month of substance intoxication or when medication use is causally related.

III. **Epidemiology.** Research indicates that sexual problems occur in almost half of all marriages and in at least 75% of couples who seek marital therapy. In one study from a family medicine center, 56% of patients reported one or more sexual problems when asked.

A. **SDDs.** Couples with relational problems (eg, anger, resentment, hostility, fear, disappointment, or loss of trust) are at highest risk for SDD. Libido is also influenced by organic factors such as chronic illness, pregnancy, drugs, and endocrine alterations. Over half of all couples who seek marital counseling experience SDD. In the National Health and Social Life Survey (NHSLS), a large, randomly chosen, representative national sample, 15% of men and 33% of women indicated lack of interest in sex for at least 1 of the past 12 months.

B. **Sexual arousal disorders.** Research estimates indicate that over 10 million men in the United States experience **ED,** and that 4–9% of all men and 25% of men over 65 have organic impotence. In a large cross-sectional, random sample survey of men aged 40–70, the prevalence of minimal ED was 17%; of moderate ED, 25%; and of complete ED, 10%. Multiple organic and psychogenic risk factors are associated (Table 105–1).

Estimates of arousal disorders in women range from 20% to 48%. Causative factors in women are less well known, but are presumed to include many of the same factors as in **ED.**

C. **Orgasm disorders**

1. **Female orgasmic disorder.** Surveys suggest that 5–25% of women are anorgasmic and 20–48% report problems lubricating or reaching orgasm. Underlying psychogenic factors include fears of pregnancy, vaginal damage, or rejection by a sexual partner; hostility toward men; and guilt feelings associated with sexual impulses. Some women equate orgasm with losing control or with aggressive, destructive, or violent behavior. These women may express their associated fear through inhibited arousal or orgasm. Cultural expectations and societal restrictions on women may also contribute. Organic factors include chronic illness and the effects of medications and drugs of abuse.

2. **Male orgasmic disorder.** Recent studies indicate a prevalence of 4–10%. Many men with this disorder were raised in rigid, puritanical families that considered sex sinful and the genitalia dirty. These men also experience problems with closeness in relationships. Underlying organic factors include genitourinary surgery, neurologic disease that affects the lumbar or sacral spinal cord, and some medications.

TABLE 105–1. COMMON ORGANIC AND PSYCHOGENIC FACTORS ASSOCIATED WITH SEXUAL DYSFUNCTION

Organic Factors

1. Chronic illness
   a. Congenital illness or malformation
   b. Endocrine disease (eg, diabetes mellitus; gonadal dysfunction; pituitary, adrenal, or thyroid disorders)
   c. Neurologic disorders (eg, multiple sclerosis, spinal cord injury)
   d. Vaginal or pelvic pathology (eg, vaginal atrophy, infections, endometriosis, childbirth injury)
   e. Genital trauma
   f. Cardiovascular and peripheral vascular disease
   g. Postsurgical complications (eg, after prostatectomy, abdominal vascular surgery, sympathectomy, gynecologic procedures)
2. Pregnancy (especially in the first and last trimesters)
3. Pharmacologic agents

	Primary Affects			
	Desire	Arousal	Orgasm	Hormones
a. Anticholinergics		+		
b. Antidepressants	+	+	+	
c. Antihistamines	+	+		
d. Antihypertensives	+	+	+	+
e. Antipsychotics	+	+	+	+
f. Anxiolytics	+		+	
g. Narcotics	+	+	+	+
h. Sedative–hypnotics	+	+	+	
i. Other drugs				
Cimetidine	+	+		+
Clofibrate	+	+		
Digitalis	+	+		
Ethinyl estradiol		+		+
Levodopa			+	
Lithium		+		
Ketoconazole	+	+		
Niacin	+			
Norethindrone	+	+		+
Phenytoin	+	+		
Primidone	+	+		
4. Drugs of abuse				
a. Alcohol	+	+	+	+
b. Amphetamines	+	+	+	
c. Cocaine		+	+	
d. Heroin	+	+	+	
e. Marijuana	+			
f. MDMA	+	+	+	
f. Methadone	+	+	+	
g. Phencyclidine (PCP)	+		+	
h. Tobacco		+		

Psychogenic Factors

1. General psychogenic factors
   a. Personal problems (eg, depression, anxiety, diminished self-esteem, intrapsychic conflict)
   b. Relationship problems (eg, poor communication, unrealistic marital expectations, unresolved conflict, lost trust, poor relationship models, family system distress, sex role conflicts, divergent sexual values)
   c. Psychosexual factors (eg, prior sexual failure, chronic performance inconsistency, negative learning and attitudes about sex, prior sexual trauma, sexual performance anxiety, gender identity conflict, paraphilias)
2. Remote versus immediate factors
   a. Remote factors have historical origins (eg, negative sexual learning in childhood, dysthymic depression, prior relationship failures)
   b. Immediate factors occur during sexual activity (eg, sexual anxiety, denial of erotic feelings, ineffective sexual behaviors, failure to communicate desires and feelings)

Sexual Enactment Factors

Skill and knowledge deficits (eg, inadequate penile stimulation, inadequate stimulation for vaginal lubrication, unfavorable pelvic position for intercourse)

MDMA, 5-methoxy-3, 4-methylenedioxy amphetamine.

3. **PE.** PE is more common in college-educated men and may relate to excessive concern for their partner's satisfaction. It has also been related to anxiety about the sex act, societal conditioning about men's sex roles, and stressful marriage relationships. Thirty-five percent to 40% of men treated for sexual dysfunction experience PE. The community prevalence rate in one recent study was 36–38%. In the NHSLS, 28% of men reported climaxing too early.

D. **Sexual pain disorders**

1. **Dyspareunia.** As many as 30% of surgical procedures on a woman's genital tract result in temporary dyspareunia, and 30–40% of the women seen in sex therapy clinics for dyspareunia have identified pelvic disease. In the NHSLS, 5% of men and 15% of women experienced dyspareunia in the past 12 months.

2. **Vaginismus.** Vaginismus most often occurs in highly educated women from higher socioeconomic groups. Sexual trauma (eg, rape or incest) and a strict religious background that associates sex with sin are also risk factors. Incidence estimates for vaginismus arising from sexual dysfunction clinics range widely, from 7.8% to 42%.

IV. **Pathophysiology.** Because organic and psychosocial factors affect sexual functioning, the physician who evaluates patients with sexual dysfunction should consider those factors listed in Table 105–1 during the diagnostic evaluation. Causes for the particular dysfunctions include the following.

A. **SDDs.** Problems in a couple's relationship are the most common cause of SDD. Hate and love are mutually exclusive; as one increases, the other decreases. Voluntarily blocking sexual arousal is a passive–aggressive way to manage a power imbalance or to maintain emotional distance, and it can be a powerful tool for maintaining equilibrium within the relationship. Negative past experiences also affect desire. These include strict religiosity (particularly if the partners do not share common religious beliefs), mixed societal messages that teach one to appear sexually attractive but then chastise one for behaving that way, incest or sexual assault, and experiencing or fearing a sexually transmitted disease.

Family of origin issues are also important. Parental attitudes and modeling are latent predisposing factors that influence sexual interest later in life. Other hypothesized family factors include an incestuously eroticized relationship with the opposite-sex parent, exposure to a distressed relationship between parents, and failure to introject the sex role of the same-sex parent.

Common organic problems associated with SDDs include chronic illness, thyroid disorders, disfiguring trauma, congenital disfigurement, pituitary disorders, and the first and last trimesters of pregnancy.

B. **Sexual arousal disorders.** Numerous psychological, social, cultural, environmental, and experiential factors are causally important in ED. Developmental and family of origin factors include unopposed maternal or paternal dominance in a two-parent home, permanent absence of one parent, overt mother–son sexual encounters, conflicting parent–child relationships, negative family attitudes toward sexuality, repressive religiosity regarding sexual expression, traumatic childhood sexual experiences, traumatic first coital experiences, and teenage homosexual experiences. Emotional and affective factors include performance anxiety, spectating during sexual encounters, guilt, poor self-esteem, fears about the consequences of sex or about continued erectile difficulty following an erectile failure, depression, mania, and anxiety or guilt created by "forbidden" intrusive thoughts and fantasies. Interpersonal and relationship factors include inadequate sexual cues from a partner; anger, hostility, and distrust toward the partner; diminished physical attraction to the partner; poor communication; sex role conflicts; divergent sexual preferences; and overanxious concern for the partner's pleasure. Knowledge and perception factors involve negative attitudes and misconceptions about sex and ignorance concerning sexual anatomy, physiology, and techniques.

Cognitive interference is a broad concept that some contemporary theorists suggest explains how anxiety, depression, anger, and stress interact to cause erectile dysfunction. Men with ED develop a negative-feedback loop. The sexual invitation or demand is followed sequentially by negative expectations, underestimated arousal, perceived lack of erectile control, attentional focus on the consequences of erectile failure, and subsequent avoidance of future sexual activities.

Occasionally, another sexual disorder underlies the ED. Men with paraphilias (eg, transvestitism, voyeurism, or pedophilia) may attempt to manage these disorders by suppressing arousal. ED may also represent a conscious attempt to inhibit arousal to resolve a more severe problem with PE. ED is associated with over 100 distinct organic origins, including genetic, cardiovascular, endocrine, hematologic, hepatic, infectious, neurologic, nutritional, poisoning, pulmonary, renal, urologic, surgical, and traumatic problems.

Most research on the causes of arousal disorders has examined problems in men. Many clinicians assume that the organic and psychogenic findings apply to women as well. Further research on arousal disorders in women will establish whether this assumption is warranted.

C. **Orgasm disorders**

1. **Female orgasmic disorder.** Anxiety as a cause for orgasm disorders in women is supported by little evidence other than the effectiveness of psychosexual treatment. Recent investigations suggest that excessive anxiety alone is an insufficient causative explanation. Depression, however, may inhibit both arousal and orgasm. Relationship problems are important. Infidelity, real or imagined, can break trust in the relationship and manifest itself as anorgasmia. Many women need to sense mutual commitment in order to experience orgasm. Other relationship factors that may underlie a woman's orgasmic disorder are listed in Table 105–1. Family of origin issues, especially negative attitudes toward sexuality, oedipal problems, and unresolved interpersonal conflicts, also inhibit sexual arousal and orgasm. To date, no common organic causes have been identified for women's orgasmic disorders other than some of the same pharmacologic agents that cause arousal problems in men.

2. **Male orgasmic disorder.** Orgasmic disorders are more common in men with obsessive–compulsive personality disorders and in those with unexpressed hostility toward women. Cognitive interference theories focus on a number of factors that interfere with a man's ability to receive erotic stimuli. These factors include worries about possible pregnancy, ambivalence about commitment to the relationship, performance anxiety focused on not achieving orgasm, loss of sexual attraction to the partner, and partner demands for a greater relationship commitment. In some cases, men have established an excitability threshold that is too high for the ejaculatory reflex. As is the case with women, to date no common organic causes other than pharmacologic agents have been identified as causes for men's orgasmic disorders.

3. **PE.** The developmental background and psychodynamics of PE and ED appear similar. Definitive data on the causes of PE are only hypothesized, with some studies suggesting that groups of men with and without PE do not differ significantly in rates of arousal, absolute amount of arousal, or number of sexual situations to which they respond. Men with PE, however, ejaculate at lower sexual arousal levels and have longer periods of abstinence from intercourse and ejaculation. Some research also suggests that penile sensory thresholds are lowered by infrequent sexual activity. Organic problems only rarely cause PE. Surgical trauma to the sympathetic nervous system, pelvic fracture, localized infections, and drug withdrawal from narcotics or trifluoperazine have been associated with PE.

D. **Sexual pain disorders.** Dyspareunia is associated with many medical conditions in women (eg, inadequate vaginal lubrication, pelvic or urinary tract infections, vaginal or hymenal scar tissue, endometriosis, estrogen deprivation, allergic reactions, and gastrointestinal conditions). Most vaginismus is psychogenic. Dyspareunia in men may relate to structural abnormalities in the penis, Peyronie's disease, priapism, urethral stricture, prior genital surgery, or genital infections. Psychogenic theories of dyspareunia and vaginismus are similar. The analytic literature suggests that these disorders result from phobic reactions, major anxiety conflicts, specific unconscious intrapsychic conflicts, hostility toward specific partners or the opposite sex in general, aversion to sexuality, or conversion hysteria. The learning theory postulates that, through ignorance or faulty learning, a woman enters early sexual encounters with a set of negative expectations. These may become so strongly entrenched that they distort the actual experience or inhibit natural responses enough so that intercourse is uncomfortable. These early unpleasant experiences thereby reinforce the learned dysfunction. The operant conditioning model explains that random negative concrete experiences can create a preconditioned "negative set" that may then distort reality or alter physiologic responses so that further sexual encounters become uncomfortable.

V. Diagnosis

A. Symptoms. Physicians should include a brief query about sexual relationships during routine clinical encounters. A general question such as "Are you having any problems sexually?" gives patients "permission" to discuss this area with the physician if they wish. Specific questions that inquire into problems with various phases of the sexual response cycle are appropriate. These include queries such as "Do you and your partner have different levels of sexual interest?," "Do you or your partner have any problems becoming sexually aroused?," "During sex, do you have any problems with erections?," "Is intercourse painful for you or your partner?," and "Do you or your partner have any problems sexually satisfying each other?" If the patient responds affirmatively to probing questions about sexual dysfunction, the physician can collect more historical detail.

1. **Present history.** Define the sexual problem better by collecting the following data: date and mode of onset; problem duration; situational context; current sexual interactions of the couple, including frequency of intercourse or sex play, frequency that the patient and his or her partner would prefer, time of day for lovemaking, presence of fatigue during lovemaking, difficulties with privacy, verbal and nonverbal communication of desires, type and pleasurability of sex play that precedes intercourse, arousal level during intercourse, orgasm frequency, thoughts, visualizations, and fantasies during sex, pain felt during intercourse (this symptom itself must be pursued in more detail), and any exacerbations or remissions of the problem; effects of any attempted treatment; and the presence of any associated symptoms in other body systems.

2. **Sexual history.** Explore early experiences, emotional reactions, attitudes toward sexuality, sexual knowledge, frequency and types of past sexual practices, acceptance of cultural myths, current sexual relationship development, masturbation practices and fantasies, homosexual experiences, and any past negative sexual experiences (eg, incest or sexual assault).

3. **Developmental and family history.** Discuss family attitudes toward sexuality, parental modeling, religious influences, relationships with parents and siblings, family violence, and level of family function in the couple's families of origin.

4. **Nature of the current relationship.** Focus on the development and stability of the current relationship, changes in feeling toward the partner, the presence of unresolved conflict, loss of trust or fidelity, and communication problems (eg, failures to listen and understand, hidden agendas, or using sex for power in the relationship).

5. **Current stressors.** Inquire about stresses that are both intrafamilial (eg, death, illness, or problems with children) and extrafamilial (eg, financial, occupational, or legal). Focus both on stresses and strains that normally occur as the individual and family progress through their life cycle stages and on stresses and strains that occur unexpectedly.

6. **Past medical history.** Identify any acute or chronic disease, injury, or surgery that could affect sexual functioning. Inquire specifically about those organic factors included in Table 105–1.

   Many commonly used drugs may contribute to sexual dysfunction (Table 105–1). Drug effects vary by individual, depending on age, absorption, body weight, dosage, duration of use, rates of metabolism and excretion, presence of other drugs, underlying disorders, patient compliance, and suggestibility.

7. **Habits.** See Table 105–1 for the types of sexual dysfunctions associated with the common drugs of abuse.

8. **Questionnaires.** The **International Index of Erectile Function (IIEF)** is a 15-item inventory designed to assess erectile function, orgasmic function, sexual desire, intercourse satisfaction, and overall sexual satisfaction. A shortened 5-item version, the **IIEF-5**, is useful as a screening instrument. These tools can help the busy physician focus the history-taking process. Modified versions of the IIEF are now also being used to study sexual disorders in women.

B. Signs. A comprehensive physical examination will help identify any concurrent acute or chronic illness and any associated physical conditions that could affect sexual functioning or treatment.

1. **Focus special attention on the following.**
   a. **General:** obesity, cachexia, and vital signs.
   b. **Cardiovascular:** bruits (especially femoral), peripheral pulses, evidence of venous stasis, arterial insufficiency (especially in the lower extremities), and pulsatile epigastric mass.
   c. **Abdominal:** pain, tenderness, mass, guarding, tympany, and bowel activity.
   d. **Neurologic:** gait, coordination, deep tendon reflexes, pathologic reflexes, sensation, motor strength, integrity of the sacral reflex arc (S-2–S-4) with perineal sensation, anal sphincter tone, and bulbocavernosus reflex.

2. Observe the **male genitalia** for testicular size and consistency, penile size, malformations, and lesions. Obtaining **penile blood pressure** measurements on any man with ED can help to diagnose arterial insufficiency. Place and inflate a 3-cm pediatric blood pressure cuff around the base of the penis and auscultate the central artery of the corpora cavernosa with a 9.5–MHz Doppler stethoscope as the cuff is deflated. The penile systolic pressure is the pressure at which the arterial pulse is first heard. The ratio between the penile systolic pressure and the brachial systolic pressure should exceed 0.75. If it is below 0.60, significant penile vascular insufficiency likely exists.

3. **Female pelvic examination.** Focus on the following:
   a. **External genitalia:** dermatitis, vulvar inflammation, episiotomy or other scars, clitoral inflammation, and adhesions.
   b. **Introitus:** hymenal rigidity, tags, or fibrosis; urethral carbuncle; and Bartholin's gland inflammation.
   c. **Vagina:** spasm of the vaginal sphincter and adduction of the thighs with attempted vaginal examination, atrophy, discharge, inflammation, stenosis, relaxation of supporting ligaments, and tenderness along the vaginal urethra or posterior bladder wall.
   d. **Bimanual examination:** cul-de-sac masses or tenderness; adnexal mass or tenderness; and position, size, mobility, and tenderness of the uterus.
   e. **Rectovaginal examination:** hemorrhoids, fissures, constipation, and tenderness.

C. Laboratory tests

1. **Evaluation for systemic disease. Baseline studies** include a complete blood cell count, fasting blood sugar level, urinalysis, tests for sexually transmitted diseases, lipid profiles, and tests of thyroid, liver, and renal function.

2. **Evaluation for specific disorders**
   a. **SDDs.** Obtain a morning **serum testosterone** level in men with SDDs. If levels are low or borderline, or if the low desire is associated with little or no masturbation history, obtain a **serum prolactin** level. Correlation between **sexual desire** and **levels of follicle-stimulating hormone (FSH), androstenedione, luteinizing hormone (LH),** and **estradiol is presently inconclusive.**
   b. **Female sexual arousal disorder.** Experimental techniques for measuring nocturnal vaginal blood flow using a specially designed vaginal probe demonstrate that vaginal engorgement cycles occur in women during rapid eye movement (REM) sleep with the same frequency that erectile cycles occur in men. Several companies now make devices that measure blood flow in the clitoris as well as the vagina. Some can be used at home while the woman sleeps. They may help to determine whether arterial factors cause arousal problems in women, and they may also help to differentiate psychogenic from organic causes.
   c. **Male erectile disorder**
      (1) **Serum tests.** Obtain a morning **serum testosterone** level to screen for hypogonadism. If the level is low, obtain **FSH, LH,** and **prolactin** levels. If FHS and LH are low and prolactin is normal, then the diagnosis is pituitary or hypothalamic failure. If FSH and LH are high and prolactin is normal, then the diagnosis is testicular failure. If FSH and LH are low, but prolactin is high, then there is a 25–40%

chance of a pituitary adenoma. In this case request a **computed tomographic (CT) scan** or **magnetic resonance imaging (MRI)** scan of the sella turcica.

(2) **Nocturnal penile tumescence (NPT) evaluation.** Because sleep eliminates the psychological factors that inhibit arousal, NPT evaluation helps to differentiate psychological from organic ED. Normally, three or four erections occur each night during REM sleep. Organic interference persists during sleep, disturbing erections. Psychogenic interference should not persist and erections will occur. Several techniques evaluate and quantify NPT.

The **snap gauge** is a ring of opposing Velcro straps that are connected by three plastic strips. The ring is wrapped around the penis before sleep. During a normal rigid nocturnal erection, all bands break. By noting whether no, one, two, or three bands break, one can estimate the maximum erectile response during sleep. This is a useful screening tool, since it is inexpensive, is simple, and can be performed at home. False-negative results occur if it is not applied tightly enough. False positives occur if bands break while turning during sleep. This method only detects the maximal erectile event during sleep and does not measure erection duration, maximum number, or actual rigidity. Furthermore, one cannot correlate erections with REM sleep cycles.

The **Rigiscan** is a small computer with two cords leading to rings that encircle the base and tip of the penis. Inside each ring is a cable that the central unit can loosen or tighten during monitoring. The cables detect tumescence by expanding passively and rigidity by contracting actively, detecting resistance. The Rigiscan records all erectile events; measures erection duration, tumescence, and rigidity; and can be performed at home. It cannot correlate erections with REM sleep cycles, and the dynamic nature of bands actively contracting may induce or augment erections during the test.

NPT monitoring is performed in a sleep laboratory, where electroencephalographic tracings can detect sleep cycles. Mercury strain gauges are placed around the base and tip of the penis to detect tumescence. Rigidity is assessed either visually or by applying a handheld tonometer to the penis to detect the force required to "buckle" it. This approach records all erectile events; measures duration, tumescence, and rigidity (but not as well as the Rigiscan); and correlates erections with REM sleep. However, it is expensive, is time- and labor-intensive, and must occur in an unnatural sleep environment.

(3) **Duplex ultrasonographic scanning** provides high-resolution real-time ultrasonographic imaging and pulse Doppler analysis of the actual blood flow in the cavernous arteries before and after injection of a vasodilator. Normal vessels should double in size with an initial peak systolic flow velocity of .30 cm/sec.

(4) **Intracavernous injection of vasoactive drugs** helps screen for a vascular cause. Injecting 30–60 mg of papaverine or 40 μg of PGE_1 should cause within 10 minutes an erection that lasts at least 30 minutes. An erection delay of 15–20 minutes suggests arterial insufficiency. A prompt, rigid erection that is lost quickly suggests a cavernous leak.

(5) **Pudendal angiography.** Selective internal pudendal angiograms can determine whether an arterial block exists that could be corrected by penile revascularization. This technique is used most commonly in younger patients with clinical and noninvasive findings that suggest an arterial cause for their ED and who are candidates for reconstructive surgery.

(6) **Cavernosometry and cavernosography** evaluate the venoocclusive mechanisms of the corpus cavernosum. Through a butterfly needle inserted into the corpus cavernosum, the procedural physician first infuses a vasoactive agent (20 μg of PGE_1), then hepa-

rinized saline and finally radiographic contrast. X-rays are taken to identify leaks in specific veins and to evaluate for glans or spongeosal leaks. These procedures are performed less frequently now since surgical procedures designed to correct venous leaks are less successful than anticipated.

(7) **Bulbocavernosus reflex latency tests** measure the integrity of the sacral reflex arc (S-2–S-4). When the glans penis is stimulated with a pinch or a squeeze, electromyographic needles in the bulbocavernosus muscle record muscle contraction. The time delay from stimulation to contraction is calculated. Longer times suggest a neurologic cause for ED.

(8) **Somatosensory evoked potentials** record waveforms over the sacrum and the cerebral cortex in response to dorsal penile nerve stimulation, and can therefore help localize neurologic lesions to peripheral, sacral, or suprasacral locations.

(9) **Summary of evaluation for ED.** After conducting a comprehensive history, physical examination, and laboratory screening, one must form a "most probable" hypothesis for the man's ED. Is it psychological or organic? If it is organic, is the cause likely neurologic, vascular, endocrine, or a combination of these factors?

If one cannot separate psychological from organic factors, consider an **NPT evaluation.** If the hypothesis is "organic: neurologic or vascular," consider a therapeutic trial of one of the noninvasive agents used to treat ED. If the trial succeeds, continue therapy. If it fails, then consider further specific procedural evaluation for neurologic or vascular causes.

If the hypothesis is "organic: endocrine," then obtain a **serum testosterone** level. If this is low, then obtain **FSH, LH,** and **prolactin** serum levels. If the serum testosterone is normal, revise the hypothesis and consider a therapeutic trial.

d. **Sexual pain disorders.** Laboratory evaluation, guided by the clinical evaluation, helps to detect associated organic factors.

(1) **Office laboratory procedures** include saline and potassium hydroxide wet mounts of vaginal secretions to diagnose vaginitis or vaginosis; urinalysis, urine culture, and examination of prostatic secretions to diagnose associate genitourinary infections; and tests to diagnose chlamydial, herpes simplex, and gonococcal infections (see Chapters 24, 55, 64, and 67).

(2) **Colposcopy** may be useful in diagnosing specific vaginal or cervical disease such as human papillomavirus infections.

(3) **Pelvic ultrasonography** can help diagnose adnexal, uterine, or cul-de-sac problems.

(4) **Laparoscopy** can help diagnose, and in some cases treat, adnexal or intraperitoneal disease.

(5) **Anoscopy or sigmoidoscopy** is used to identify associated colorectal problems (see Chapter 57).

VI. **Treatment**

A. **Therapeutic strategies.** Physicians can relate to patients with a sexual problem at one of five levels.

1. **Level 1: Case finding.** Ask the initial sexual history question, but then refer to another professional for evaluation and treatment.

2. **Level 2: Evaluate the chief complaint.** Collect the basic sexual history during routine visits and provide basic education about normal anatomy, physiology, and sexual functioning. When there are sexual concerns, obtain a "history of present illness" with appropriate symptom pursuit and perform a focused physical examination. Refer to another professional if treatment involves more than reassurance or basic education.

3. **Level 3: Comprehensive evaluation.** Obtain a detailed sexual history that includes both the psychosocial and medical history. Perform a comprehensive physical examination and evaluate for organic causes with appropriate laboratory tests and diagnostic procedures.

4. **Level 4: Manage organic problems and refer for psychosexual therapy.** Treat any organic problems or coordinate care with another physician if a special procedure such as a penile implant is required. Continue to provide psychological support, but refer psychosexual therapy to a sexual therapist.

5. **Level 5: Manage both organic and psychosexual therapy.**

Before primary physicians determine which role to play, they must ascertain their own interest in sexual concerns and the care they wish to provide. They must also build a professional referral network to provide care that is beyond their own competence or interest. Membership in or certification by one or more of the following organizations is one indication of a sexual therapist's competence: Society for Sex Therapy and Research (SSTAR); American Association for Sex Education, Counseling and Therapy (AASECT); and Society for Scientific Study of Sex (SSSS).

B. **Medical management**

1. **Testosterone** does not benefit men with normal serum levels. In fact, it can compound the problem in men with ED who have normal levels by increasing sexual desire without concomitantly increasing arousal. In hypogonadal men with testosterone values <100 ng/dL, intramuscular testosterone enanthate (200 mg every 2–3 weeks) is the preferred treatment. Transdermal systems are also available and effective methods for replacing testosterone (Androderm 2.5–7.5 mg daily or Testoderm 4–6 mg daily). Oral agents are less effective and may cause hepatic disorders (eg, cholestatic jaundice).

A 2% testosterone vaginal cream has also been used to enhance desire in women. Convincing evidence to support its use, however, is lacking.

2. **Bromocriptine mesylate** (Parlodel) treats hyperprolactinemia. Doses begin at 1.25 mg/day and increase by 1.25 mg every 3–7 days until the serum prolactin level is normal. The usual treatment dose is 2.5 mg twice daily.

3. **Yohimbine** is an α_2-adrenoceptor antagonist that theoretically enhances penile erections by restricting penile venous outflow and increasing libido through a central nervous system effect. Dosage is 6 mg orally three times daily. To date, few double-blind, placebo-controlled studies have been performed to document its efficacy. The American Urological Association now states that it "should not be recommended as a treatment for the standard patient" based on lack of proven effectiveness.

4. **Sildenafil** is an orally active inhibitor of the type-V cyclic guanosine monophosphate-specific phosphodiesterase (the predominant isoenzyme in the human corpus cavernosum). It increases levels of nitrous oxide (NO), which relaxes the endothelial muscles, increasing blood flow into the corpora cavernosa. It is effective in ED of organic, psychogenic, and mixed etiology. It enhances the erectile mechanism with sexual stimulation, and does not work without stimulation. A man takes a single oral dose of 50–100 mg about an hour before intercourse. Sildenafil's activity begins in 30 minutes and lasts up to 4 hours. The most common adverse effects are headache (16%), flushing (10%), dyspepsia (7%), nasal congestion (4%), urinary tract infection (3%), visual effects (3%), and diarrhea (3%). Drug levels are increased by other drugs that are metabolized by or that inhibit the cytochrome P450 system. Sildenafil also potentiates the hypotensive effects of nitrates and is **absolutely contraindicated** in patients using organic nitrates in any form.

Studies to evaluate sildenafil's effectiveness in treating women with arousal disorders are now in process.

5. **Phentolamine mesylate** is an oral adrenergic receptor antagonist that causes erections by relaxing smooth muscle tissue and dilating arteries. It has been studied in men with minimal ED of broad-spectrum etiology. A man takes 20–80 mg about 15 minutes prior to intercourse. Side effects include headache, facial flushing, and nasal congestion. The drug appears safe and effective for treatment of mild ED.

6. **Apomorphine** is believed to cause erections through its effect as a dopaminergic agonist. It has also been studied on men with minimal or insignificant organic disease. It is taken as a transbuccal tablet in dosage strengths of 2 mg, 4 mg, or 6 mg. The main adverse effect is nausea. Other observed adverse effects include persistent yawning, vomiting, and hypotension.

7. **Nitroglycerin** has a local effect on penile smooth muscle, causing relaxation and subsequent engorgement. Although controlled studies that support its effectiveness are sparse, men with mild vascular, neurologic, or mixed arousal dysfunction may benefit from a therapeutic trial with nitroglycerin before starting more invasive therapies. Men apply 0.5–1 inch of 2% ointment to the penile shaft just prior to intercourse, using a condom during intercourse to avoid vaginal absorption of the nitroglycerin and adverse systemic effects in their partners. A transdermal nitroglycerin patch applied 1–2 hours prior to intercourse also reportedly improves erections.

   Several studies indicate that men can also apply topical 2% **minoxidil** solution to the glans to produce erections, and that it may be even more effective than nitroglycerin. Several companies are now testing PGE_1 compounded with an agent that enhances absorption through the skin. This may result in more effective topical agents in the future. These agents may benefit women as well as men.

   When using these vasodilators, prophylactic analgesics help manage any associated headache.

8. **Intracavernous injection of vasoactive drugs.** Patients may inject either **papaverine** or PGE_1 into a corpus cavernosum with a 27-gauge needle to induce an erection. This technique is quite successful in men with neurogenic disorders, mild vascular problems, or combined neurogenic and vascular disorder, and in selected men with psychogenic causes for whom psychosexual treatment has failed. Therapy begins with a low dose of either drug, gradually titrating the dose to provide an adequate erection that lasts 1–2 hours. This usually requires 10–30 mg of papaverine or 10–20 µg of PGE_1. Injections are limited to three times per week and 10 times per month. Complications include priapism (0.33%), cavernous tissue fibrosis (2.8%), hematoma, cavernositis, pain, and changes in blood pressure (usually orthostatic hypotension). Erections that last more than 4 hours should be reversed by irrigating the corpora cavernosum with diluted phenylephrine.

   VIP 0.025 mg mixed with phentolamine 2.0 mg is a new investigational agent. It comes as a prefilled, ready-to-use autoinjector that demonstrates a reported overall efficacy of 80% and a 70% efficacy in men who failed other intracavernosal therapy. The most common adverse reaction is transient facial flushing (53%). The incidence of priapism, fibrosis, and pain occurs less frequently than with other injection therapies.

   Intracavernosal injections may be used to treat PE as well as ED. In the case of PE they may allow sexual activity to continue despite the man's premature climax.

9. **Intraurethral PGE_1** therapy requires a man to insert a medicated pellet into his urethra with an applicator following urination. When absorbed through the mucosa, the PGE_1 relaxes smooth muscles and dilates arteries. Following insertion, the man must manually stimulate the penis for 10 seconds and then walk around for another 10 minutes to promote erection. The maximal response occurs in 20–25 minutes. Pellets are available in 125-, 250-, 500-, and 1000-mcg dosage strengths. Adverse effects include penile pain (32%), urethral burning (12%), minor urethral bleeding (5%), testicular pain (5%), hypotension (3%), and dizziness (2%).

10. **Tricyclic antidepressants** may help treat PE because they inhibit the cholinergic component of ejaculation. Men take a low initial dose (eg, 25 mg of amitriptyline) 3–5 hours prior to sexual activity, increasing subsequent doses until they experience ejaculatory control, have side effects, or reach the maximal recommended dose.

11. **Thioridazine,** at standard antidepressant doses, may also benefit men with PE. It is the most potent anticholinergic and α-adrenergic blocking agent in its class and presumably delays ejaculation through these effects.

12. **Phenoxybenzamine (PBZ)** is an α-adrenergic blocker indicated for treating hypertension. Used by men with PE in daily doses of 20–30 mg, PBZ benefits ejaculation and erection with minimal side effects. It is best used by men who do not wish to procreate, since PBZ inhibits seminal emission.

13. **Clomipramine** may benefit PE by increasing the sensory threshold for stimuli from the genital area. A man takes doses of 25–50 mg 3–5 hours prior to sexual activity. The most common side effect is dry mouth.

14. **Sertraline** may also delay ejaculation through its serotonergic effects. The usual dose is 50–100 mg taken 3–5 hours prior to sexual activity. The most common side effect is drowsiness.
15. **Fluoxetine** has also been used to treat PE at doses of 20–60 mg.
16. A new **lidocaine–prilocaine cream** has also been used to prevent PE. In pilot studies men applied 2.5 g to the glans 30 minutes before sexual contact, and then covered the penis with a condom.
17. For information on **managing endocrine disorders,** see Chapters 78 and 91.

C. **Surgical management**
   1. **Arterial revascularization.** Successful surgery for proximal artery occlusion (eg, endarterectomy, transluminal balloon angioplasty, or graft placement) reportedly improves blood flow through the hypogastric vessels. Success depends on whether the distal vessels are disease free and can accept the increased flow and whether surgery damages the autonomic nerves that course over the vessels. Many surgical techniques can revascularize the corpora when distal vessels (internal pudendal and penile arteries) are occluded (eg, end-to-side anastomosis of artery to corpora, direct anastomosis to the dorsal or deep cavernous artery, and anastomosis of the epigastric artery to the dorsal vein with ligation of the vein's distal end, thus forming a direct retrograde connection to the corporal spaces). Best long-term results occur when the arterial lesion is localized and the bypass is placed into normal vessels. Procedures are most often performed on younger men.
   2. **Venous surgery.** Surgical procedures vary, depending on where venous incompetence occurs. If a shunt is found from the corpus to the deep dorsal vein, the surgeon ligates the vein, any accessory veins, and all the circumflex and emissary veins that join the dorsal vein, thus providing added resistance to venous outflow. These procedures are now performed much less frequently, since their long-term success rates have not reached expectations.
   3. **Penile prosthesis.** The penile prosthesis is the most reliable surgical option in the United States, with the inflatable prosthesis implanted most frequently. Manufacturers now provide reliable protheses consisting of cylinders that expand in both girth and length, a single scrotal pump, and an abdominal reservoir. To decrease the chance of mechanical failure in multicomponent devices and to mimic natural erection, self-contained inflatable devices have also been designed that include an inflation chamber, reservoir, and pump mechanism in a self-contained cylinder. Prosthesis implantation is relatively uncomplicated, but most devices require replacement after 48–60 months. Potential complications include mechanical failure (0–3.2%), infection (1.9–8.3%), erosion, penile gangrene, improper sizing, and silicone shedding.

D. **Mechanical management.** Penile vacuum pumps can also aid erections. The man places a lubricated cylinder over his penis, and using an attached handheld pump to withdraw air, he creates a vacuum that draws blood into the corpora cavernosum. When his penis is erect, he maintains engorgement by applying an elastic band around the penile base and removes the cylinder. Potential complications include penile edema, decreased penile sensation, impaired ejaculation, subcutaneous bleeding, and penile necrosis. These devices no longer require a physician's prescription.

E. **Psychosexual therapy**
   1. **Standard principles.** Several basic principles undergird current psychosexual therapy.
      a. People are responsible for their own sexuality.
      b. Growth in sexual attitudes, performance, and feelings results from behavioral change.
      c. Every person deserves sexual health.
      d. Physiologic relaxation is the foundation for sexual excitement.
      e. Boundaries must be established with the nonsexual aspects of sexual dysfunction (eg, career stress or marital problems).
   2. **Cognitive–behavioral therapy** that incorporates behavioral therapy into other treatments is the treatment of choice for managing most sexual dysfunctions. Behavior therapists assume that sexual dysfunction is learned maladaptive behavior that causes patients to fear sexual interaction. During treatment, the therapist establishes a hierarchy of anxiety-provoking situations for

the patient and then helps him or her master the anxiety through systematic desensitization. This process inhibits the learned anxious response by encouraging antianxiety behaviors. The therapist may also prescribe sexual exercise homework assignments that are also based on a hierarchy, starting with those activities that have proved most pleasurable and successful in the past. Assignments often enlist a cooperative partner's support and participation.

3. **Masters and Johnson dual-sex therapy** requires a man–woman cotherapy team to work with couples. It acknowledges that men and women differ in sexual experiences and roles and establishes the therapeutic importance of gender fairness and balance. Few centers currently use dual-gender treatment teams, since other models are successful and dual-gender teams carry financial and logistical limitations.

4. **Sensate focus.** The original behavioral tasks developed by Masters and Johnson are termed "sensate focus" exercises, since they heighten sensory awareness to touch, sight, sound, and smell. As patients focus on their own sensations, they often relax, overcoming those barriers that impede natural physiologic responses. Partners first learn to enjoy touching, stroking, exploring, massaging, and fondling all the contours of each other's bodies except for their genitals. When both partners are adept and comfortable exchanging nongenital caresses, they add genital stroking exercises. Erogenous stroking progresses to vaginal penile containment, first without genital thrusting and then to full intercourse with orgasm. Couples learn to use fantasies to distract them from obsessive performance concerns and to communicate mutual needs verbally and nonverbally.

5. **Hypnotherapy** begins with a series of nonhypnotic sessions to build a secure doctor–patient relationship and to establish treatment goals. Therapy focuses on removing symptoms and altering attitudes. Patients are taught to use relaxation techniques before a sexual encounter, and they also learn alternative ways to deal with anxiety-provoking sexual situations.

6. **Group therapy** methods can also examine patients' intrapsychic and interpersonal problems. Groups provide a strong support system and can counteract sexual myths, correct misconceptions, and provide accurate information about sexual anatomy, physiology, and varieties of behavior. Groups composed of sexually dysfunctional married couples are particularly effective in consensually validating individual preferences and enhancing self-esteem and self-acceptance.

7. **Traditional marital therapy** is also important, since marital or relationship problems that generate stress, fatigue, and dysphoria commonly underlie the sexual dysfunctions. Therapy helps the couple develop communication skills, establish realistic marital expectations, resolve conflict, and build trust.

F. **Specific sexual therapy techniques**

1. **Directed masturbation** is the most effective treatment program to date for primary orgasmic dysfunction in women. Beginning with basic education in sexual anatomy and physiology, women progress through the stages of tactile and visual self-exploration, manual stimulation to areas of pleasurable sensation, sexual fantasy and image development, sensate focus exercises alone and then with a partner, and finally sharing effective masturbation techniques with a partner.

2. The **stop–start or squeeze technique.** The stop–start technique of Semans and the squeeze technique modification of Masters and Johnson are used to treat PE. The technique begins as the couple embrace and caress one another until the man's penis is erect. He then lies on his back, his partner begins stimulating his penis, and he concentrates on his arousal sensations. Just before he reaches the point of imminent ejaculation, he tells his partner to stop stimulation. At this point, Masters and Johnson direct the woman to squeeze the penis firmly between her thumb and forefinger, under the corona of the glans. Most current therapists now suggest that the man apply the squeeze himself. When the woman applies the squeeze, it paradoxically suggests that control over erections is hers rather than the man's. With or without the squeeze, the couple wait for several minutes until arousal sensations dissipate. This process of stimulation and stopping repeats several times before ejaculation is permitted.

After four or five successful stimulation–stopping sessions, the couple tries the stop–start process with the penis in the vagina. The woman assumes the woman-superior position and the man glides her slowly up and down the shaft of his penis. As he again almost reaches the point of ejaculation, he ceases moving his partner until the need subsides. This process is also repeated several times before he ejaculates.

When the man can control ejaculation with this level of stimulation, his partner begins to stimulate the penis with vaginal thrusting until the man begins to feel the need to ejaculate. At this point, he tells her to stop stimulation until arousal wanes. This sequence is also repeated several times before he ejaculates.

The couple completes a start–stop sequence at least weekly until they learn to use it automatically during intercourse. Eventually, they use the method with other sexual positions. Most men, however, experience the greatest difficulty controlling ejaculation in the man-superior position. The couple-on-their-side often becomes the favored position for intercourse.

3. **Sexologic examination.** The vaginal sexologic examination helps treat women with arousal and orgasmic disorders by assisting them and their partners to identify specific erotically sensitive vaginal areas. The examination is performed with the sexual partner present and with the woman's signed consent.

After performing a complete pelvic examination, the physician systematically explores the vagina with lubricated, gloved fingers, starting with the posterior vaginal wall and slowly proceeding toward the lateral and anterior aspects of the vaginal canal. Light pressure is applied to all vaginal surfaces as the woman concentrates on her sensations, verbalizing her sensory feelings during stimulation. Once an erotically sensitive area is located, stimulation continues long enough to reach early arousal.

When the physician's examination is complete, the woman's partner takes the physician's place and under the woman's instruction he proceeds with similar examination and stimulation so that he can also identify her erotically sensitive areas and achieve success with helping her become aroused.

4. **Systematic desensitization** is a technique used to treat both dyspareunia and vaginismus. The pelvic examination is the first step in the treatment process and must be conducted with care, reassurance, and proper education. The examination confirms the absence of pelvic disease, demonstrates that vaginal comfort is possible, confirms that vaginal events are under the woman's control, allows the woman to see the psychophysiologic components of the dysfunction (eg, involuntary introital contractions can be seen with a mirror, allowing the woman to visualize the relationship between psychological conditioning and a physical event), and allows the physician to reassure the woman about her normality and to teach her specific techniques to help her overcome the disorder. During the examination, the physician also educates the partner in anatomy and psychosomatic physiology. It is important that he observes the process of successful vaginal containment.

The first desensitization step after examination is to assure the woman that she is in complete control. When she says "Stop!," the examination stops. It may take several sessions to demonstrate painless vaginal insertion. The woman is given a handheld mirror to use throughout the examination so that the physician can teach vulvar and vaginal anatomy and so that she can visualize her own muscle contractions. She is taught to contract and relax her abdominal, medial thigh, and vaginal introital muscles sequentially. By identifying and contracting these muscles, she will have an easier time relaxing them.

The woman is then taught to "bear down and pull in" while contracting her introital muscles (Kegel exercises). When she can do this easily, the physician (with the patient's permission) places the tip of his or her index finger at the introitus and asks the woman to bear down and push the finger away. When this process is repeated several times, the fingertip will enter the vagina spontaneously. The woman often feels that instead of penetrating the vagina, the finger is "captured" by it. She learns that she can actively control what enters her vagina and that it can be painless.

When the woman comfortably contains the physician's fingertip, she repeats the same process first using her own fingertip and then her partner's. As she contracts and relaxes her vaginal muscles around his finger, she learns that she can control penetration and experience painless vaginal containment.

After the woman is comfortable with these exercises, she progresses through small steps to initiate intercourse. She inserts her partner's penis into her vagina after she is sufficiently aroused. Both partners must understand that the woman always controls the amount of contraction, relaxation, and penetration that occurs during intercourse and that she will not experience vaginal pain.

VII. Natural history and prognosis

A. **SDDs.** The few published studies indicate that SDDs for both men and women resist sustained behavioral change. Following therapy, one study noted initial improvement that was sustained at 3 months, but that had regressed to below pretherapy levels by 3 years. Prognosis is better if the problem is secondary, the symptoms are present less than 1 year, the marital relationship is stable, the partners are emotionally calm, both partners view each other as loving and attractive, both partners find pleasure in sexual behavior, and the couple complies with homework assignments during therapy.

B. **ED.** The natural history and prognosis of ED depend on many variables, particularly the underlying problem. Most data on psychosexual treatment success were obtained before recent diagnostic advances permitted better differentiation between organic and psychogenic causes. Reported success rates range from 50% to 90%. Treatment success for surgical implants is 85–95%. Success with intracavernosal injections is also 85–95%, and satisfaction with the vacuum-constriction device is 68–92%. Reported success rates with intraurethral PGE_1 range from 43–65%. Oral agents also vary in success. From 70–85% of men using sildenafil achieve erections firm enough for intercourse. In men with mild ED, phentolamine has a response rate of 37% at the 40-mg dose and 45% at the 80-mg level. Reported success with apomorphine in mild ED is 46% with 2 mg, 52% with 4 mg, and 60% with 6 mg.

C. **Female orgasmic disorder.** The natural history of untreated disorders is unknown. Women whose orgasmic disorder is primary respond rapidly to treatment with a high success rate when therapy is focused specifically on sexual matters. Women with secondary orgasmic disorders do better when traditional marital therapy is combined with sexual therapy. Masters and Johnson report success rates of 83% for primary disorders and 77% for secondary disorders using dual-gender therapy. Directed masturbation training to treat primary disorders is successful in 80–100% of patients. New pharmacologic management may become integrated into treatment in the near future.

D. **Male orgasmic disorder.** Outcome studies on the treatment of this disorder are limited by its relative rarity. Reported success rates range from 46% to 82%.

E. **PE.** Masters and Johnson report success rates of 95%. Others report more modest rates around 60%. Long-term success rates, however, are disappointing. In one study, men treated for PE showed immediate posttreatment gains in foreplay length, sexual relationship satisfaction, male acceptance, and intercourse duration. By 3 years posttreatment, however, frequency and desire for sexual contact, intercourse duration, and marital satisfaction all regressed, with marital satisfaction and intercourse duration dropping to pretreatment levels.

The best data on pharmacologic management are available for clomipramine, sertraline, and fluoxetine. Sexual satisfaction rates are reported at 53% for clomipramine along with a statistically significant increase in ejaculation latency time. For sertraline, sexual satisfaction rates range from 42–87%, with significantly increased ejaculation latency. The data on fluoxetine's success is variable. Some studies indicate a significant increase in ejaculation latency, but others suggest that it is no better than placebo. In the pilot sample used to study topical lidocaine–prilocaine, 80% graded the result as "excellent" or "better."

F. **Dyspareunia.** The prognosis depends on the nature of any associated organic problems and the success with which they are treated. Women with a pure psychogenic basis for their problem report success rates around 95%.

G. **Vaginismus** is very amenable to treatment. In one group of patients followed up for 4 years, 95% achieved and maintained sexual functioning. A desire for childbearing, a husband-initiated consultation, and a couple's perception that the problem was psychogenic predicted successful outcomes. Unsuccessful outcomes were associated with a perception that the problem was organic, experience with a previous anatomic problem, abundant sexual misinformation, a negative attitude toward genitalia, fear of sexually transmitted disease, and negative parental attitudes toward sex.

REFERENCES

Alexander B: Disorders of sexual desire: Diagnosis and treatment of decreased libido. Am Fam Physician 1993;**47:**832.

American Psychiatric Association (APA): *Diagnostic and Statistical Manual of Mental Disorders,* 4th ed. APA; 1994.

American Urological Association issues treatment guidelines for erectile dysfunction (special medical report). Am Fam Physician 1997;**55:**1967.

Finger WW, Lund M, Slagle MA: Medications that may contribute to sexual disorders: A guide to assessment and treatment in family practice. J Fam Pract 1997;**44:**33.

Goldstein I, Lue TF, Padma-Nathan H, et al: Oral sidenafil in the treatment of erectile dysfunction. N Engl J Med 1998;**338:**1379.

Halvorsen JG: Sexual dysfunction: Classification, incidence and prevalence, aetiology, and initial patient evaluation. Baillieres Clin Psychiat 1997;**3:**43.

Halvorsen JG: Sexual and gender identity disorders. In: Conn RB, Borer WZ, Snyder JW, eds. *Current Diagnosis.* Saunders; 1997.

Lechtenberg R, Ohl DA: *Sexual Dysfunction: Neurologic, Urologic, and Gynecologic Aspects.* Lea & Febiger; 1994.

Rosen RC, Riley A, Vagner G, et al: The international index of erectile function (IIEF): A multidimensional scale for assessment of erectile function. Urology 1997;**49:**822.

Spector IP, Carey MP: Incidence and prevalence of the sexual dysfunctions: A critical review of the empirical literature. Arch Sex Behav 1990;**4:**389.

SECTION V. **Preventive Medicine**

106   Counseling

Angela D. Mickalide, PhD, CHES

Patient education and counseling is one of the most effective prevention strategies available to primary care providers. Efforts by clinicians to influence such behaviors as tobacco use, exercise, nutrition, and alcohol and other drug abuse are more likely to decrease illness and premature death than are many other types of clinical preventive interventions. Forty percent to 70% of the 12 million years of productive life lost annually in the United States is preventable by adopting healthier lifestyles. Unfortunately, physicians, in general, counsel too little. Sparse financial remuneration, lack of behavioral education skills, and organizational constraints are among the factors accounting for low rates of physician counseling.

I. **Behavioral risk factors amenable to counseling**
  A. **Tobacco use.** The effectiveness of clinician counseling in prevention of tobacco use is well documented, particularly when multiple intervention strategies are used, including face-to-face counseling, scheduled reinforcement, behavioral contracts, self-help materials, referral to community programs, and drug therapy (Table 106–1).
    1. Cigarette, cigar, pipe, and smokeless tobacco cessation counseling should be offered to patients who use such products and to nonusers at risk for beginning this habit, for example, adolescents, who should be advised not to start.
    2. The detrimental effects of tobacco use and secondhand smoke on unborn and young children should be discussed with all pregnant women and parents.
  B. **Nutrition.** Clinicians have several roles in nutritional counseling: taking a complete and accurate dietary history, working with patients to identify the obstacles to changing dietary patterns, and providing advice on food selection and preparation. Physicians who lack the time or skills to assist patients with their nutritional knowledge and behaviors should involve registered dietitians, nutritionists, and other trained staff.
    1. Dietary intake of calories, fat (especially saturated fat), cholesterol, complex carbohydrates, fiber, and sodium is among the nutritional topics that clinicians should discuss routinely with patients. Caloric intake should be balanced with energy expenditures through a well-balanced diet and regular exercise.
    2. An ideal diet consists of the Food Guide Pyramid's five major food groups, which together meet nutritional requirements. These are (1) breads, cereals, and grains; (2) fruits; (3) vegetables; (4) milk, yogurt, and cheese; and (5) meats and proteins. Patients should consume fats, oils, and sweets sparingly. An individual's age, gender, and physical activity can help determine the number of servings needed to maintain a well-balanced diet.
    3. Adolescent and adult females should be alerted to the importance of dietary calcium and iron intake.
    4. Pregnant women should be advised of their special nutritional needs, and parents should be counseled about the dietary requirements of infants and young children.
  C. **Exercise.** Clinicians should advise all patients, especially women, ethnic minorities, adults with lower educational attainment, and older adults, to engage in regular moderate-intensity physical activity. Recommendations for regular physical activity should be tailored to the health status and lifestyle of each patient.
    1. Every American adult should accumulate 30 minutes or more of moderate-intensity physical activity over the course of most days of the week. Activities that can contribute to the 30-minute total include walking, gardening, dancing, or washing windows or floors, as well as planned exercise such as jogging, swimming, and bicycling (Table 106–2).
    2. Patients should be given instructions on the safe performance of exercise, and those at increased risk of injury or medical complications should be

TABLE 106–1. SYNOPSIS FOR PRIMARY CARE PROVIDERS: HOW TO HELP YOUR PATIENTS STOP USING TOBACCO

1. Ask about tobacco use at every opportunity
2. Advise all tobacco users to stop
3. Assist the patient in stopping
   a. Help set a quit date
   b. Provide self-help materials
   c. Recommend nicotine gum or prescription drugs for tobacco cessation, especially for highly addicted patients (those who smoke one pack a day or more; those who smoke their first cigarette within 30 minutes of waking; or those who use other tobacco products several times daily)
   d. Consider signing a stop-tobacco contract with the patient
4. Arrange follow-up visits

Modified with permission from Glynn TJ, Manley MW: *How to Help Your Patients Stop Smoking: A National Cancer Institute Manual for Physicians.* National Cancer Institute; April 1990. Publication No. DHHS (PHS) 90-3064.

advised about appropriate physical activity. Clinicians who lack the skills or time to design effective exercise programs for patients should rely on the expertise of accredited fitness centers and exercise specialists.

D. Intentional injuries
    1. Suicide
        a. Clinicians should be alert to suicidal ideation among patients at high risk as a result of recent divorce, separation, unemployment, depression, alcohol and other drug abuse, major medical illnesses, living alone, and recent bereavement. Adolescents are at particular risk for suicide; risk factors include declines in school performance or attendance, isolation or changes in peer relations, and excessive anger or fighting behavior. Older adults are also at excess suicide risk.

TABLE 106–2. EXAMPLES OF MODERATE AMOUNTS OF PHYSICAL ACTIVITY

Activity[1,2]	Relationship of Time Spent and Intensity of Effort
	Less Vigorous, More Time
Washing and waxing a car for 45–60 minutes	
Washing windows or floors for 45–60 minutes	
Playing volleyball for 45 minutes	
Playing touch football for 30–45 minutes	
Gardening for 30–45 minutes	
Wheeling self in wheelchair for 30–40 minutes	
Walking 1¾ miles in 35 minutes (20 min/mile)	
Basketball (shooting baskets) for 30 minutes	
Bicycling 5 miles in 30 minutes	
Dancing fast (social) for 30 minutes	
Pushing a stroller 1½ miles in 30 minutes	
Raking leaves for 30 minutes	
Walking 2 miles in 30 minutes (15 min/mile)	
Water aerobics for 30 minutes	
Swimming laps for 20 minutes	
Wheelchair basketball for 20 minutes	
Basketball (playing a game) for 15–20 minutes	
Bicycling 4 miles in 15 minutes	
Jumping rope for 15 minutes	
Running 1½ miles in 15 minutes (10 min/mile)	
Shoveling snow for 15 minutes	
Stairwalking for 15 minutes	
	More Vigorous, Less Time

[1] A moderate amount of physical activity is roughly equivalent to physical activity that uses approximately 150 Calories (kcal) of energy per day, or 1,000 Calories per week.
[2] Some activities can be performed at various intensities; the suggested durations correspond to expected intensity of effort.
From Centers for Disease Control and Prevention, National Center for Chronic Disease Prevention and Health Promotion, Division of Nutrition and Physical Activity; 1996.

     b. Patients with suicidal ideations should be questioned about the extent of their plans (eg, distribution of possessions, obtaining a weapon, writing a suicide note). If suicidal intent is serious, clinicians should make immediate referrals to mental health professionals and consider possible hospitalization. Persons with suicidal thoughts should also be alerted to community resources such as local mental health agencies and crisis intervention centers.

  2. Violence

     a. Both the history (discussion of previous violent experiences and current risk factors, such as weapons in the home and discord in the peer group and community) and the physical examination (detection of burns, bruises, and other traumatic injuries) can be used to identify victims of abuse or neglect. Clinicians who suspect violence among patients should refer both the victims and the perpetrators to mental health professionals and other community resources to prevent future episodes.

     b. Certain physical, behavioral, and medical signs indicate child neglect and abuse (see Chapter 95). Physicians must report probable cases of such abuse to local child protective service agencies. In addition, clinicians should be alert to risk signs for adolescent violence such as fighting, bullying, chronic victimization, weapon-carrying, history of domestic violence, and changes in peer relations.

E. Unintentional injuries

  1. Motor vehicle-related injuries. Physicians should urge all patients to use federally approved occupant restraints (eg, safety belts and child safety seats), to wear safety helmets when riding motorcycles and bicycles, and to avoid driving while under the influence of alcohol or other psychoactive drugs. Clinician counseling is particularly urged for individuals at increased risk of motor vehicle injury, such as adolescents and young adults, alcohol and other drug users, and patients with certain medical conditions that affect safety. These individuals should be encouraged to discuss with their families transportation alternatives for social activities in which any drugs are being used.

  2. Environmental and household injuries. Although passive interventions (eg, child-resistant containers to prevent poisoning) are the most effective measures to control injuries, clinician counseling may help patients reduce their risks of household and environmental injuries (eg, falls, drowning, fire, poisoning, suffocation, and firearm mishaps).

     a. Patients should be advised to abstain from alcohol or other psychoactive drug use when participating in potentially dangerous activities (eg, swimming, boating, bicycling, driving, or handling firearms).

     b. Smokers should be advised against smoking near upholstery or in bed.

     c. Patients should be urged to install, and check monthly, smoke detectors in their homes and to set hot water heaters at 48.4 °C (120 °F).

     d. Patients with **children in the home** should be counseled to lock all medications, toxic substances, matches, and firearms out of the reach of children; to have a 1-oz bottle of syrup of ipecac available; and to display emergency numbers prominently near telephones (eg, the police department, the fire department, 911, and the local Poison Control Center).

       To prevent falls, adults should be advised to place collapsible gates or other barriers at stairway entrances, to install four-sided fencing with self-latching and self-closing gates around swimming pools and spas, and to install window guards on all windows not designated as emergency fire exits.

       Bicyclists and parents of children who ride bicycles should be made aware of the importance of wearing safety helmets and avoiding riding in motor vehicle traffic.

     e. To prevent falls among **older patients,** clinicians should suggest modifications to their home environments, for example, tacking down carpets and arranging furniture so that pathways are not cluttered; testing their visual acuity periodically; and closely monitoring their use of drugs that can increase the risk of falls. Older patients should receive instructions on appropriate physical exercises to maintain and improve flexibility and mobility. Patients with medical conditions affecting mobility should receive special counseling on measures to prevent falls.

F. Sexual behavior
1. Sexually transmitted diseases (STDs)
   a. Clinicians should take a complete sexual and drug use history of all adolescent and adult patients and offer STD screening according to recommended guidelines (see Chapter 108). Clinicians should discuss sexual behavior with respect, compassion, and confidentiality.
   b. Sexually active patients should be counseled that the most effective strategy to prevent infection with human immunodeficiency virus (HIV) or other STDs is to abstain from sex or maintain a mutually monogamous sexual relationship with a partner known to be uninfected. Patients should be counseled to engage in routine screening since many STDs are asymptomatic. Sexual activity with persons of uncertain infection status should be discouraged. Clinicians should counsel women of childbearing age on the dangers of HIV and STD infection during pregnancy.
   c. Patients should be alerted that a nonreactive HIV test does not rule out infection if the sexual partner has engaged in sexual intercourse during the 6 months prior to testing. Safe (or "safer") sexual practices (eg, massage, hugging, or dry kissing [Table 106–3]) should be encouraged. Reducing the number of sexual partners and consistent and proper use of condoms should be discussed with patients who have multiple sexual partners (see Chapter 101).
   d. Intravenous drug users should be urged to participate in drug treatment programs, warned against sharing and using unsterilized drug para-

---

TABLE 106–3. "SAFER SEX" PRACTICES SUGGESTED FOR REDUCING THE RISK OF SEXUALLY TRANSMITTED DISEASES

The most effective strategies are sexual abstinence or the maintenance of a mutually monogamous sexual relationship. In other cases, the following practices should be observed

_____ Always use a latex condom during sexual intercourse. The application of spermicides and the use of diaphragms by women may also decrease risk

_____ Avoid multiple partners, anonymous partners, prostitutes, persons with multiple partners, persons who use intravenous drugs, and those not known to be seronegative for human immunodeficiency virus (HIV)

_____ Avoid sexual contact with persons who have a genital discharge, genital warts, genital herpes lesions, or evidence of hepatitis B surface antigen

_____ Do not practice anal intercourse. Avoid all sexual activities that could cause cuts or tears in the lining of the rectum, vagina, or penis

_____ Avoid oral–anal sex to prevent enteric lesions

_____ Avoid genital contact with oral herpetic lesions

_____ Persons at increased risk should be especially careful to avoid mouth contact with the penis, vagina, or rectum

_____ Persons who use intravenous drugs should receive treatment and should never use unsterilized or shared injection equipment

_____ Persons at increased risk should have a periodic examination for sexually transmitted diseases

Safe sexual activities
Massage
Hugging
Body rubbing (dry)
Kissing (dry)
Masturbation (on healthy skin)
Hand-to-genital touching or mutual masturbation

Possibly safe sexual activities (these activities are completely safe if both partners are known to be uninfected)
Kissing (wet)
Oral sex on men wearing latex condoms
Oral sex on women (who are not menstruating or experiencing a vaginal infection with discharge)

Data from Novello A: *Surgeon General's Report on Acquired Immune Deficiency Syndrome.* Office of the Surgeon General, US Department of Health and Human Services, Public Health Service; 1993.
Additional data adapted from Sexually transmitted diseases treatment guidelines, September 1993. MMWR 1993;**42:**RR-14.

phernalia, and directed to community programs making uncontaminated equipment available.

2. **Unintended pregnancy.** Clinicians should discuss the efficacy, limitations, and proper use of available contraceptive techniques (see Chapter 101). Clinicians should review the menstrual cycle with patients, as appropriate, so that they better understand their contraceptive options and their own fecundity.

G. Dental disease

1. Clinicians should counsel patients to visit a dentist regularly, to brush their teeth daily with a fluoride-containing toothpaste, and to use dental floss daily to clean between teeth. Young children should have their first dental visit by age 2. Children, particularly those under age 6, should be taught to spit out rather than swallow toothpaste containing fluoride, to prevent dental fluorosis. Patients with dental abnormalities found through visual examination (eg, nursing bottle tooth decay, crowding or malalignment of teeth, dental caries, or periodontal infections) should be referred to their dentist for further evaluation.

2. Patients should be advised to limit their intake of foods containing refined sugar, particularly between-meal snacks. To reduce the risk of early childhood caries, infants should not be put to bed with a bottle. If a bedtime bottle is necessary, only those filled with water should be used.

3. Children living in areas with inadequate fluoride in their drinking water should be prescribed daily fluoride drops or tablets according to recommended guidelines (Table 106–4). Clinicians prescribing fluoride supplements for children must know the concentration of fluoride in the child's drinking water.

4. Clinicians should urge patients to reduce their risk of oral cancer by eliminating tobacco use and limiting alcoholic beverage consumption. All patients who smoke cigarettes, pipes, or cigars or who use spit tobacco should be counseled to stop, and those who do not use tobacco, especially adolescents and young adults, should be encouraged to resist pressure to start.

H. Alcohol and other drugs

1. The routine history for all adolescents and adults should include questions about the quantity, frequency, and other patterns of use of wine, beer, liquor, or other drugs. Questionnaires are available for more systematic detection of problem drinking, but there are limitations in either their accuracy or their suitability for routine use in busy practices.

2. Clinicians should provide substance-abusing patients with information about chemical dependence, the effects of the drug, and its effect on health. Intravenous drug users should be referred for treatment and warned against the use of contaminated or shared needles, which can transmit HIV, hepatitis B virus, and other organisms. Treatment plans should be tailored to the drug of abuse and the individual needs of the patient and his or her family (see Chapter 92).

I. Self-examination. Although widely practiced, self-examination of the breast, testes, skin, and other sites has not been conclusively proven to be an effective maneuver for reducing cancer mortality. The teaching of self-examination is neither specifically recommended nor discouraged.

TABLE 106–4. DIETARY FLUORIDE SUPPLEMENT DOSAGE SCHEDULE

	Fluoride Ion Level in Drinking Water (ppm)[1]		
Age of Child	<0.3 ppm	0.3–0.6 ppm	>0.6 ppm
Birth–6 mo	None	None	None
6 mo–3 yr	0.25 mg/day[2]	None	None
3–6 yr	0.50 mg/day	0.25 mg/day	None
6–16 yr	1 mg/day	0.50 mg/day	None

[1] 1 ppm = 1 mg/L.
[2] 2.2 mg of sodium fluoride contains 1 mg of fluoride ion.
From American Dental Association: Council on Scientific Affairs, association report on dietary fluoride supplements. JADA 1995;**126**:19-S.

J. **Exposure to ultraviolet light**
 1. To prevent skin cancer, clinicians should advise all patients of effective techniques to reduce outdoor exposure to ultraviolet (UV) light. Patients with increased occupational or recreational exposure to sunlight as well as those who live in tropical climates should be counseled to regularly apply broad-spectrum sunscreen with UVA/UVB protection. They should also be advised to wear protective clothing, such as wide-brimmed hats and long-sleeved shirts and slacks and to try to reduce outdoor activity between 10 AM and 3 PM.
 2. Parents should also be reminded to limit their children's exposure to ultraviolet light through similar measures.

II. **Techniques for counseling.** Once the clinician has identified personal health behaviors that require attention, it is important to engage in effective counseling and patient education to initiate and maintain change. Empirical research and clinical experience have yielded certain useful principles that clinicians can use to encourage behavior change among patients.

A. **Develop a therapeutic alliance** in which the clinician is viewed as an expert consultant who is available to help patients remain in control of their own health choices. This perspective facilitates development of a provider–patient partnership.

B. **Respond to the educational needs of all patients** in ways appropriate to their age, race, sex, socioeconomic status, and interpersonal skills. Most patients are eager for health information and guidance and generally want more than clinicians provide. Clinicians tend to talk more with patients who pose more questions. Yet those patients who are quieter are often in greater need of counseling.

C. **Ensure that patients understand the relationship between behavior and health.** Inquire about what patients already know or believe about the relationship between risk factors and health status. Do not assume that they understand the health effects of smoking, lack of exercise, poor nutrition, and other lifestyle factors. Explain in simple terms the idea that certain factors can increase the risk of disease and that combinations of factors can sometimes work together to increase risk beyond the sum of their individual contributions.

D. **Work with patients to assess barriers to behavior change**
 1. Anticipate obstacles to behavior modification. Patients often do not follow the clinician's advice concerning medication use or lifestyle changes. According to one well-studied model, three areas of beliefs influence the adoption and maintenance of behavior change.
    a. Susceptibility to continuing problems if the advice is not followed.
    b. Severity of problems associated with not following the advice.
    c. Benefits of adopting the advice weighed against the potential risks, costs, side effects, and barriers.
 2. Assess those areas and address those beliefs that are not conducive to healthful behaviors. In addition, try to determine other obstacles to change, including lack of skills, motivation, resources, and social support. Help patients determine ways to overcome them.

E. **Gain commitment from patients to change.** Patients typically come into a clinician's office expecting to be treated for a condition. If they do not agree that their behaviors are significantly related to their health outcomes, attempts at counseling may be irrelevant.

F. **Have patients choose one risk factor to change at a time.** Do not overwhelm patients by asking them to try to change all their unhealthful behaviors at the same time. Let patient need, patient preference, and your own assessment of the relative importance to the patient's health dictate your recommendation of which risk factor to tackle first.

G. **Use a combination of strategies**
 1. Educational efforts that integrate individual counseling, group classes, audiovisual aids, written materials, and community resources are far more effective than those strategies using only a single technique. Tailor programs to individual needs and preferences.
 2. Ensure that printed materials are accurate, consistent with the clinician's views, and at a reading level appropriate to the patient population.

H. **Design a behavior modification plan**
 1. Ask patients if they have ever tried to change a specific behavior before and discuss the methods used, the barriers encountered, and the degree of suc-

cess. Agree on a specific, time-limited goal to be achieved, and record the goal in the medical record.

   2. Assist patients in writing action plans, review relevant instructional materials, and stress provider willingness to be of continued assistance.

I. **Monitor progress through follow-up contact**
   1. Schedule a follow-up appointment or telephone call with the patient to evaluate progress in achieving the goal. Reinforce successes through positive verbal feedback.
   2. If patients have not followed the plan, work with them to identify and overcome obstacles. Modify the plan if necessary to facilitate successful risk factor reduction. When necessary, refer patients to community agencies or self-help groups and elicit support for the prescribed regimen from family members or significant individuals in their social networks.

J. **Involve office staff.** Use the team approach to patient education. Share responsibility for patients with nurses, health educators, dietitians, and other allied health professionals, as appropriate.

REFERENCES

Casamassimo P: *Bright Futures in Practice: Oral Health.* National Center for Education in Maternal and Child Health; 1996.

The Food Guide Pyramid. Your Personal Guide to Healthful Eating (brochure). International Food Information Council; 1996.

Healthy People 2010 Objectives (draft for public comment). US Department of Health and Human Services, Office of Public Health and Science; Sept 15, 1998.

Jones DA, Ainsworth BE, Croft JB, et al: Moderate leisure-time physical activity: Who is meeting the public health recommendations? A national cross-sectional study. Arch Fam Med May/June 1998;**7**:285.

McGinnis JM, Foege WH: Actual causes of death in the United States. JAMA 1993;**270**:2207.

O'Donnell GO, Mickalide AD: *SAFE KIDS at Home, At Play & On the Way: A Report to the Nation on Unintentional Childhood Injury.* National SAFE KIDS Campaign; April 1998.

Osofsky JD (ed): *Children in a Violent Society.* Guilford Press; 1997.

US Centers for Disease Control and Prevention: HIV prevention through early detection and treatment of other sexually transmitted diseases: United States. MMWR July 1998; vol 47.

US Preventive Services Task Force: *Guide to Clinical Preventive Services,* 2nd ed. Williams & Wilkins; 1996.

---

107 Immunizations

Cynthia Haq, MD, & David V. Power, MD, MPH

I. **Introduction.** Immunizations have dramatically reduced the rates of childhood and adult infectious diseases and are among the most cost-effective preventive health interventions. Yet many children and adults do not receive recommended vaccines. While immunization coverage has improved in recent years, in the United States in 1997, 24% of 3-year-old children were not fully immunized. Also, in adults over age 65, 35% had not received influenza vaccines and 55% had not received pneumococcal vaccines. Family physicians have the opportunity to work with communities and public health agencies to increase awareness and improve immunization rates across the life span.

II. **Childhood immunizations.** A consensus statement on recommendations for routine childhood immunizations in the United States was first published in 1995 jointly by the American Academy of Pediatrics (AAP), the American Academy of Family Physicians (AAFP), the Advisory Committee on Immunization Practices (ACIP) of the Centers for Disease Control and Prevention, and other bodies. These recommendations are revised and published semiannually. It is important to remain updated on changes in recommendations (http://www.cdc.gov/nip).

   A delay in the recommended immunization schedule does not require restarting the primary series or adding extra doses. A delay does not reduce final antibody concentrations, and the schedule should be continued as directed. However, vaccines should not be given at a shorter interval than recommended. Intramuscular vaccinations are usually given in the anterolateral aspect of the thigh in infants less than 12 months of age, while the deltoid is often preferred in children older than 18 months. Most widely used vaccines are considered safe and effective when administered simultaneously.

Contraindications to all vaccines include previous severe allergic or anaphylactic reactions to prior vaccines or constituents. Precautions for vaccine administration include moderate to severe acute illnesses. In these cases, the vaccine usually should be delayed until the condition has resolved. **In general, prematurity, mild acute illness with low-grade fever, concurrent antibiotic therapy, and minor local reactions to a previous immunization are not considered contraindications to immunizations.** Live vaccines may pose some risk for immunosuppressed family members, and in this context, an inactivated vaccine may be preferred.

A. Routinely recommended vaccines. A standardized immunization schedule is recommended during well-child visits (Table 107–1).

   1. Diphtheria–tetanus–acellular pertussis (DTaP) vaccine

      a. A total of 5 doses is recommended by the time of school entry. Vaccine efficacy is estimated at 70–90%. Immunogenicity wanes, with little protection 5–10 years after the last dose. In 1996, the acellular pertussis vaccine (DTaP) was favored over whole-cell pertussis (DTP) in the primary series because of reduced local inflammation, systemic reactions, and evidence of improved vaccine efficiency. Whole-cell vaccine (DTP) is an acceptable alternative if DTaP is not available.

      b. Serious adverse events include a temperature over 40.5 °C (105 °F), collapse or shock within 48 hours, persistent inconsolable crying over 3 hours, or convulsions within 3 days. These events have been less frequent with use of the DTaP vaccine.

      c. Following serious adverse events, diphtheria and tetanus toxoids (DT) is recommended. Precaution is advised in infants with moderate or severe acute illness or a new or evolving neurologic disorder. In these circumstances, the vaccine should be withheld until the child is stabilized. Stable neurologic conditions and a family history of seizures or minor illnesses are **not** contraindications to pertussis immunization.

      d. DTaP and DTP are administered by deep intramuscular injection. The fourth dose may be administered as early as 12 months of age, provided that at least 6 months have elapsed since the third dose. Acetaminophen or ibuprofen may be given at the time of vaccination and for 24 hours afterward to reduce the possibility of postimmunization fever and systemic reactions.

   2. Poliovirus vaccine

      a. Two types of polio vaccine are available, a live oral poliovirus vaccine (OPV), and an inactivated poliovirus vaccine (IPV) for subcutaneous or intramuscular use. The OPV is easier to administer and less expensive than IPV, but carries a minute risk of vaccine-associated paralytic polio (VAPP) in recipients and their contacts. While protected against infection, persons immunized with OPV can transmit the wild virus to unimmunized contacts. IPV is highly effective and carries no personal risk of VAPP.

      b. Beginning in January 2000, the recommended schedule is four doses of IPV at 2 and 4 months of age, between 6 and 18 months, and between 4 and 6 years. OPV and IPV may be used interchangeably, and if a child has begun the series with OPV, there is little benefit in switching to IPV.

      c. Contraindications to OPV include immunocompromised recipients or children with family members with immunodeficiency disorders, in which case IPV should be given instead.

   3. *Haemophilus influenzae* **type b (Hib) vaccine**

      a. Three types of conjugate vaccines are currently licensed for intramuscular use in the United States; each is 95–100% effective in preventing invasive Hib disease.

         (1) Oligosaccharide–diphtheria conjugate: HbOC (HibTITER).

         (2) Polyribosylribitol phosphate–tetanus toxoid conjugate: PRP-T (ACTHib and OMNIHib).

         (3) Meningococcal protein conjugate: PRP-OMP (PedvaxHib).

      b. Hib vaccines should not be given to infants younger than 6 weeks. The recommended schedule is a dose of Hib at 2, 4, and 6 months and a

TABLE 107–1. RECOMMENDED CHILDHOOD IMMUNIZATION SCHEDULE UNITED STATES, JANUARY–DECEMBER 2000

Vaccines[1] are listed under routinely recommended ages. ☐ Bars indicate range of recommended ages for immunization. Any dose not given at the recommended age should be given as a "catch-up" immunization at any subsequent visit when indicated and feasible. ◯ Ovals indicate vaccines to be given if previously recommended doses were missed or given earlier than the recommended minimum age.

Age ▶ Vaccine ▼	Birth	1 mo	2 mos	4 mos	6 mos	12 mos	15 mos	18 mos	24 mos	4–6 yrs	11–12 yrs	14–16 yrs
Hepatitis B[2]	Hep B		Hep B		Hep B						Hep B	
Diphtheria, Tetanus, Pertussis[3]			DTaP	DTaP	DTaP		DTaP[3]			DTaP	Td	
H. influenzae type b[4]			Hib	Hib	Hib	Hib						
Polio[5]			IPV	IPV		IPV[5]				IPV[5]		
Measles, Mumps, Rubella[6]						MMR				MMR[6]	MMR[6]	
Varicella[7]							Var				Var[7]	
Hepatitis A[8]									Hep A[8]—in selected areas			

Approved by the Advisory Committee on Immunization Practices (ACIP), the American Academy of Pediatrics (AAP), and the American Academy of Family Physicians (AAFP).

On October 22, 1999, the Advisory Committee on Immunization Practices (ACIP) recommended that Rotashield (RRV-TV), the only US-licensed rotavirus vaccine, no longer be used in the United States (MMWR Morb Mortal Wkly Rep. Nov 5, 1999;48(43):1007). Parents should be reassured that their children who received rotavirus vaccine before July are not at increased risk for intussusception now.

[1] This schedule indicates the recommended ages for routine administration of currently licensed childhood vaccines as of 11/1/99. Additional vaccines may be licensed and recommended during the year. Licensed combination vaccines may be used whenever any components of the combination are indicated and its other components are not contraindicated. Providers should consult the manufacturers' package inserts for detailed recommendations.

[2] **Infants born to HBsAg-negative mothers** should receive the 1st dose of hepatitis B (Hep B) vaccine by age 2 months. The 2nd dose should be at least 1 month after the 1st dose. The 3rd dose should be administered at least 4 months after the 1st dose and at least 2 months after the 2nd dose, but not before 6 months of age for infants.

TABLE 107–1. (*continued*)

Infants born to HBsAg-positive mothers should receive hepatitis B vaccine and 0.5 mL hepatitis B immune globulin (HBIG) within 12 hours of birth at separate sites. The 2nd dose is recommended at 1 month of age and the 3rd dose at 6 months of age.

Infants born to mothers whose HBsAg status is unknown should receive hepatitis B vaccine within 12 hours of birth. Maternal blood should be drawn at the time of delivery to determine the mother's HBsAg status; if the HBsAG test is positive, the infant should receive HBIG as soon as possible (no later than 1 week of age).

All children and adolescents (through 18 years of age) who have not been immunized against hepatitis B may begin the series during any visit. Special efforts should be made to immunize children who were born in or whose parents were born in areas of the world with moderate or high endemicity of hepatitis B virus infection.

[3] The 4th dose of DTaP (diphtheria and tetanus toxoids and acellular pertussis vaccine) may be administered as early as 12 months of age, provided 6 months have elapsed since the 3rd dose and the child is unlikely to return at age 15 to 18 months. Td (tetanus and diphtheria toxoids) is recommended at 11 to 12 years of age if at least 5 years have elapsed since the last dose of DTP, DTaP, or DT. Subsequent routine Td boosters are recommended every 10 years.

[4] Three *Haemophilus influenzae* type b (Hib) conjugate vaccines are licensed for infant use. If PRP-OMP (PedvaxHIB or ComVax [Merck]) is administered at 2 and 4 months of age, a dose at 6 months of age is not required. Because clinical studies in infants have demonstrated that using some combination products may induce a lower immune response to the Hib vaccine component. DTaP/Hib combination products should not be used for primary immunization in infants at 2, 4, or 6 months of age unless FDA-approved for these ages.

[5] To eliminate the risk of vaccine-associated paralytic polio (VAPP), an all-IPV schedule is now recommended for routine childhood polio vaccination in the United States. All children should receive four doses of IPV at 2 months, 4 months, 6 to 18 months, and 4 to 6 years. OPV (if available) may be used only for the following special circumstances:

1. Mass vaccination campaigns to control outbreaks of paralytic polio.
2. Unvaccinated children who will be traveling in <4 weeks to areas where polio is endemic or epidemic.
3. Children of parents who do not accept the recommended number of vaccine injections. These children may receive OPV only for the third or fourth dose or both; in this situation, health care professionals should administer OPV only after discussing the risk for VAPP with parents or caregivers.
4. During the transition to an all-IPV schedule, recommendations for the use of remaining OPV supplies in physicians' offices and clinics have been issued by the American Academy of Pediatrics (see *Pediatrics*, December 1999).

[6] The 2nd dose of measles, mumps, and rubella (MMR) vaccine is recommended routinely at 4 to 6 years of age but may be administered during any visit, provided at least 4 weeks have elapsed since receipt of the 1st dose and that both doses are administered beginning at or after 12 months of age. Those who have not previously received the second dose should complete the schedule by the 11- to 12-year-old visit.

[7] Varicella (Var) vaccine is recommended at any visit on or after the first birthday for susceptible children, ie, those who lack a reliable history of chickenpox (as judged by a health care professional) and who have not been immunized. Susceptible persons 13 years of age or older should receive 2 doses, given at least 4 weeks apart.

[8] Hepatitis A (Hep A) is shaded to indicate its recommended use in selected states and/or regions; consult your local public health authority. (Also see *MMWR Morb Mortal Wkly Rep*. Oct 01, 1999;48(RR-12); 1–37).

booster at 12–15 months. Children who have received PRP-OMP at 2 and 4 months do not require a dose at 6 months. The number of doses needed to complete an interrupted series depends on the vaccine type and the child's age.

  c. When possible, the Hib vaccine used at the first vaccination should be used for the entire primary series. After the primary series, any licensed Hib conjugate vaccine may be administered as a booster dose at age 12–15 months.

  d. Combination vaccines containing Hib include the following:
    (1) DTP and Hib (TETRAMUNE and ActHIB)
    (2) DTaP and Hib (TriHIBit)
    (3) Hepatitis B and Hib
      Combinations may be used when the two vaccines are to be administered simultaneously, but separate injections are preferred for the primary series because of possible reduced effectiveness of the combined acellular pertussis vaccine in infancy. The DTaP-Hib combination is only recommended at 12–18 months. Combination vaccines, including DTaP/Hib/HBV and DTaP/Hib/HBV/IPV, are in development.

4. Pneumococcal conjugate vaccine

  a. *Streptococcus pneumoniae* is among the leading causes of death from infection in the world and is a common cause of meningitis, pneumonia, and otitis media in children. Patients with sickle cell anemia, asplenia, an immunocompromised condition, or a chronic illness, children who are attending a day care center, and those who are African American, Native American, or Alaskan Native are at greatest risk.

  b. Early in 2000, the ACIP recommended routine vaccination of children under 2 years of age with a newly developed conjugate heptavalent pneumococcal vaccine. The unconjugated vaccine available for adults is not effective in children under 2 years of age.

  c. The vaccine should be administered in 0.5 mL doses at 2, 4, and 6 months of age, with a fourth dose between 12 and 15 months. The first dose can be given as early as 6 weeks of age, with intervals between the first three doses of 4–8 weeks. The fourth dose should be given at least 2 months after the third. Unvaccinated children between 7 and 11 months of age should receive three doses at least 4 weeks apart with the third dose after 12 months, separated from the second dose by at least 2 months. Unvaccinated children 12–23 months and older children at high risk should receive two doses at least 2 months apart.

  d. Common, self-limited side effects include erythema, swelling, tenderness at the injection site, and low-grade fever. There are no reports of serious adverse reactions to the vaccine.

5. Measles–mumps–rubella (MMR) vaccine

  a. The first dose of MMR vaccine is recommended subcutaneously at 12–15 months of age. The second dose of MMR can be administered at either 4–6 years or 11–12 years of age, in keeping with state school immunization requirements.

  b. The components of MMR are live, and this vaccine is contraindicated in persons with severe allergy to gelatin or neomycin or who have had a severe prior reaction. Egg allergy is not a contraindication to MMR. In persons with moderate or severe illness, receiving high-dose steroids or with recent thrombocytopenia, immunization should be delayed until the condition is resolved. Persons with asymptomatic HIV infection should receive MMR. MMR should be withheld from persons with HIV infection with immunodeficiency (low age-specific CD4 counts).

6. Hepatitis B virus (HBV) vaccine

  a. All infants born to mothers who test negative for hepatitis B surface antigen (HBsAg) should receive 2.5 μg of Recombivax HB or 10 μg of Engerix-B intramuscularly at birth or up to 2 months of age. The second dose should be given between 1 and 4 months of age, as long as 1 month has elapsed since administration of the first dose. The third dose is recommended between the ages of 6 and 18 months. HBV vaccine is more than 90% protective. Larger or additional doses may be required in immunocompromised persons. Immunity lasts at least 13 years. Booster doses and routine serologic testing to assess immune status are not currently recommended.

  b. Infants born to HBsAg-positive mothers should receive immunoprophylaxis with 0.5 mL of hepatitis B immune globulin (HBIG) within 12 hours of birth, as well as either 5 μg of Recombivax HB or 10 μg of Engerix-B, at a separate site. In these infants, the second dose of HBV vaccine is recommended at 1 month of age and a third dose should be given at 6 months of age. Testing for HBsAg positivity (active HBV infection) and HBsAb (immunity) is recommended at 9–15 months of age.

  c. A combination hepatitis B–Hib vaccine (COMVAX) is available for use at 2, 4, 6, and 12–15 months of age. It is not recommended in children under 6 weeks or those born to HBsAg-positive mothers.

7. Varicella-zoster virus (VZV) vaccine

  a. This live vaccine was approved for subcutaneous administration in 1995. ACIP guidelines recommend that susceptible children (no history of chickenpox) without a contraindication should be routinely vaccinated with a single 0.5–mL dose of VZV subcutaneously between 12 and 18 months of age. The vaccine is highly protective (97%) and appears to confer long-lasting immunity; however, about 1% of vaccinees per year develop mild, breakthrough infection that does not appear to be contagious. Studies on the duration of immunogenicity are ongoing.

  b. Serologic testing of children between 12 months and 12 years of age without a reliable history of chickenpox infection is not warranted prior to vaccination because most of these children are susceptible and because the vaccine is well tolerated by seropositive individuals.

  c. Contraindications include prior serious allergic reaction, pregnancy, or immunosuppression. Precautions include acute moderate or severe illness. Adverse reactions include rash. Transient zoster in recipients and transmission to susceptible contacts of vaccinees has been reported.

  d. Varicella-zoster immune globulin (VZIG) is indicated in susceptible individuals following significant exposure and in newborns of mothers with varicella that occurred in the interval from 5 days prior to 2 days following delivery.

8. Rotavirus vaccine. In 1998, the ACIP recommended the use of the live, oral tetravalent rotavirus vaccine (Rotashield) for all healthy infants at 2, 4, and 6 months of age. In 1999, Rotashield recommendations were withdrawn, because of concerns about possible associated intussusception.

B. Other vaccines

1. Influenza vaccine

  a. The ACIP currently recommends influenza immunization for any person of at least 6 months of age who is considered to be at high risk for the complications of influenza (Table 107–2). Influenza vaccine is given by intramuscular injection and may be given at the same time as other routine vaccines.

  b. Two influenza vaccine doses at least 1 month apart are advised for children less than 9 years of age who are receiving the influenza vaccine for the first time. Dosages differ according to the child's age. Only split vaccine is recommended for children younger than 12 years old.

  c. Children with severe immunosuppression often do not respond to the vaccine. Children with anaphylaxis to chicken or egg protein should not receive the vaccine. Chemoprophylaxis with amantadine or other agents during epidemics is an alternative for these children.

2. Hepatitis A virus (HAV) vaccine

  a. HAV was approved for use in the United States in 1995. The two inactivated vaccines available (Havrix and VAQTA) are highly effective (over 90%). ACIP guidelines recommend that HAV be given to eligible children 2–18 years of age in communities with high rates of hepatitis A infection (more than 20 cases/100,000 persons/year) and periodic outbreaks. Additionally, HAV may be provided to eligible children during community-wide outbreaks, at the discretion of local heath authorities, and is rec-

TABLE 107–2. PATIENTS AT INCREASED RISK FOR INFLUENZA-RELATED COMPLICATIONS

Persons aged 65 or over
Residents (any age) of nursing homes or chronic care facilities
Adults and children > 6 mos with:
Chronic disorders of the pulmonary or cardiovascular system (including children with asthma)
Chronic metabolic conditions (including diabetes mellitus)
Renal disease
Hemoglobinopathies
Immunosuppression (including HIV infection)
Children (less than 18 years old) on long-term aspirin therapy
Chronic aspirin therapy (children)
Pregnant women > 14 wks' gestation
Household contacts of high-risk individuals (including children)
Health care providers
Employees of chronic care facilities

HIV, Human immunodeficiency virus.
Adapted from Centers for Disease Control and Prevention: Recommendations of the Advisory Committee on Immunization Practices (ACIP); 1998.

ommended for travelers to regions of the United States or countries with high hepatitis A endemicity. Departments of public health can provide local incidence rates. International travelers less than 2 years of age should be given immune globulin instead.

    b. The dosage of the Havrix HAV vaccine for children 2–18 years of age is two 0.5-mL (360 ELU) doses intramuscularly, administered at least 1 month apart, followed by a booster dose 6–12 months after the first dose or in two doses of 720 ELU 6–12 months apart. The VAQTA HAV vaccine is given as two doses of 25 U, 6–18 months apart.

  3. Bacille Calmette–Guérin (BCG) vaccine

    a. This is a vaccine of an attenuated strain of live *Mycobacterium bovis* that is infrequently given in the United States but used routinely in developing countries where tuberculosis is endemic.

    b. BCG vaccination is recommended for children who are tuberculin negative and will have prolonged and intimate exposure to persons with untreated active tuberculosis (ie, a parent); for those who have repeated exposure to patients with multidrug-resistant tuberculosis (tuberculosis resistant to isoniazid and rifampin); and persons belonging to groups with a high rate of new infection, for whom chemotherapy may not be available.

    c. BCG offers limited protection against pulmonary tuberculosis (50%), but is 80% effective against meningeal and miliary tuberculosis in children.

    d. Contraindications to BCG include children with major burns, skin infections, or significant cellular immunosuppression.

    e. Persons who have received BCG vaccine usually show a positive Mantoux (PPD) skin test from the vaccine and require radiographic testing and cultures to evaluate their tuberculosis status if active disease is suspected.

III. Adolescent immunizations. The 1995 consensus statement calls for a routine preadolescent care visit at 11–12 years of age, at which time the immunization status may be reviewed and missed vaccines can be administered. Vaccinations that should be reviewed at this time include:

  A. HBV vaccine. Recommended for adolescents who have not previously received three doses of vaccine. The second dose should be administered at least 1 month after the first dose, and the third dose should be administered at least 4 months after the first dose.

  B. VZV vaccine. Varicella infection is more severe and associated with a higher rate of pneumonia and other complications in adults. Children over 12 who do not have a history of chickenpox and have not been immunized require two 0.5-mL, subcutaneous doses of the vaccine at least 4 weeks apart. Susceptible family contacts of immunocompromised individuals should receive VZV.

  C. Tetanus–diphtheria toxoid, adsorbed, for adult use (Td). For persons whose last dose of DTP, DTaP, or DT was administered more than 5 years previously, a booster dose of Td should be administered at 11–12 years of age. Administration of Td at 14–16 years of age remains an acceptable alternative.

D. MMR vaccine. Children who did not receive the second dose of MMR at 4–6 years of age should receive their second dose at 11–12 years.

IV. Adult immunizations. Adults are less likely than children to have had recommended immunizations. Health maintenance visits provide the best opportunity to assess adult immunization status. Unfortunately, many adults do not present for regular health maintenance. Urgent care and injury visits offer alternative opportunities to assess the need for immunizations. Age, comorbidity, occupation, and time of last immunization impact guidelines for adults. Guidelines are issued regularly by the American College of Physicians (ACP) and the ACIP. The ACIP recommends that all healthy adults at 50 years of age should be evaluated for their need for primary or booster Td immunization. The presence of risk factors identifies adults who need the pneumococcal vaccine or the commencement of annual influenza immunization.

A. Routinely recommended vaccines

1. Influenza vaccine

a. Influenza vaccine should be administered (0.5 mL intramuscularly) annually to anyone who wishes to reduce their chances of infection, to all persons aged 65 or over, and to those at increased risk for severe influenza (Table 107–2). The ideal time for vaccination is mid-October through November, though the vaccine can be given at any time during the flu season. Influenza vaccine is 90% effective in preventing infection in young healthy adults, but only 30–40% effective in frail elderly or compromised adults. Persons who contract influenza following immunization usually have a milder course and are less likely to have complications.

b. The ACIP recommends immunization of pregnant women after the 13th week of pregnancy or during the early puerperium before the influenza season. Pregnant women with any risk factor listed in Table 107–2 should be immunized before the influenza season, regardless of their stage of pregnancy.

c. Adverse events following influenza immunization (most commonly redness or swelling at the injection site) occur in less than 20% of recipients. Less than 1% of recipients develop fever, malaise, or myalgia. Persons with anaphylactic egg allergy may be at increased risk of hypersensitivity reactions. Since 1976, there has been no association between influenza immunization and Guillain-Barré syndrome.

d. A live attenuated influenza vaccine, administered intranasally, should become available within the next 2 years.

2. Pneumococcal vaccine

a. The unconjugated pneumococcal vaccine should be administered (0.5 mL subcutaneously or intramuscularly) to all persons aged 65 and older and to persons with medical conditions that increase the risk of life-threatening infection (Table 107–3).

TABLE 107–3. PATIENTS AT INCREASED RISK FOR PNEUMOCOCCAL DISEASE

Persons aged 65 or older
Adults and children with
  Chronic cardiopulmonary disorders
  Diabetes mellitus
  Absent or dysfunctional spleen
  Sickle cell disease
  Immunosuppression (including HIV infection)
  Nephrotic syndrome
  Cirrhosis
  Cerebrospinal fluid leakage
  Alcoholism

HIV, Human immunodeficiency virus.
Adapted from Recommendations of the Advisory Committee on Immunization Practices (ACIP): Update on adult immunization; 1998.

    b. The ACIP recommends that persons who have received pneumococcal vaccination before age 65 should be reimmunized at age 65, provided that at least 6 years has passed since they received the first dose.

    c. Because immunity wanes in the elderly, a booster dose of Pneumovax is indicated every 5–7 years.

3. MMR vaccine

    a. All persons born after 1956 who lack evidence of immunity to measles, mumps, or rubella or do not have documentation of having received MMR on or after their first birthday should receive a 0.5-mL subcutaneous dose of MMR. Persons born before 1957 are generally assumed to be immune. MMR or other live-virus vaccines are generally not given during pregnancy.

    b. Any woman who is not pregnant and who has no history of vaccination or evidence of immunity should be immunized with MMR or rubella vaccine (0.5 mL subcutaneously) and agree to avoid pregnancy for 3 months. Susceptible pregnant women should be immunized in the immediate postpartum period, with the same instructions.

4. Td booster

    a. The ACIP recommends Td boosters every 10 years. Alternatively, a single booster can be given at age 50 for people who have completed the primary series.

    b. Patients who have never received a primary series should be given a complete three-dose program of Td. The second dose should be given 4 weeks after the first dose, and the third dose should be given 6–12 months later.

    c. During routine wound management, Td administration is not required unless more than 10 years has elapsed since the last dose for clean, minor wounds. For contaminated or deep wounds, a booster is recommended if it has been longer than 5 years since the last dose or the immunization history is unclear. Tetanus immune globulin (250 IU intramuscularly) is also indicated for contaminated wounds in those with uncertain histories or with less than three primary Td doses.

5. Hepatitis B (HBV) vaccine

    a. HBV should be offered to all young adults, persons with occupational risk (health care workers and public service workers), persons with lifestyle risk (homosexual or bisexual men, heterosexual persons with multiple partners or with any sexually transmitted disease, and injectable drug users), hepatitis C, hemophiliacs and hemodialysis patients, and those with environmental risk factors (including household or sexual contacts of hepatitis B carriers, prison inmates, and immigrants from hepatitis B endemic areas). All pregnant women should be screened prenatally for active HBV infection (HBsAg positive).

    b. HBV vaccine is administered as 1 mL intramuscularly (10 µg of Recombivax HB or 20 µg of Engerix-B), with a second dose given 1 month later and the third dose given at 6 months.

    c. Booster doses of HBV vaccine are not recommended after completion of the primary series in immunocompetent persons. Pre- and postimmunization serologic testing may be considered, based on the patient's risk factors. Immunity has been shown to persist, even with low antibody levels.

    d. Postexposure prophylaxis using 0.06 mL/kg intramuscularly of HBIG, in addition to the HBV vaccine series, should be offered to persons with percutaneous or mucous-membrane exposure to blood or secretions known to be HBsAg positive, as soon as possible after exposure (within 72 hours).

6. Varicella-zoster virus (VZV) vaccine

    a. The ACIP recommends that all persons 13 years of age or older, in addition to high-risk groups, without a reliable history of chickenpox should be offered the VZV vaccine at any routine health care visit. VZV is given in two 0.5-mL doses subcutaneously, spaced 4–8 weeks apart.

    b. Those with a reliable history of chickenpox infection may be assumed to be immune. Those with an unreliable history of infection can be considered as susceptible without serologic testing, although testing may be performed to confirm their immune status.

B. Other vaccines
1. HAV vaccine

   a. The adult dose of this vaccine is 1.0 mL (1440 ELU or 50 U), given intramuscularly, followed by a booster dose 6–12 months later. It is recommended for high-risk individuals (homosexual men, intravenous drug users, persons with chronic liver disease) and travelers to endemic areas. The vaccine is more than 90% effective in immunocompetent individuals, and immunity following a booster dose can be expected for at least 10 years. Studies of the persistence of immunity and need for further booster doses are ongoing.

   b. Immediate protection against hepatitis A can be achieved with immune serum globulin (ISG, 0.02–0.06 mL/kg, intramuscularly). ISG should be given within 2 weeks of exposure to close household and sexual contacts of persons with hepatitis A and to health care workers and patients in centers with active cases of hepatitis A. ISG affords protection against hepatitis A for 3–6 months, depending on the dose given.

   c. The protective effect of HAV immunization takes 4 weeks to develop. For international travelers, it may be necessary to administer ISG at a different site, in addition to the vaccine, if travel is anticipated before 4 weeks has elapsed.

2. Rabies immunization

   a. Rabies vaccine is recommended for persons at increased risk of exposure to rabies virus, such as veterinarians, animal handlers, cave explorers, and hunters. Seemingly insignificant contact with bats has resulted in clinical rabies even in the absence of a bite.

   b. Rabies vaccine is administered as two doses, intramuscularly, 1 week apart, followed by a third dose, 2–3 weeks after the second dose. If exposure continues, booster doses are indicated every 2 years or if antibody titers are found to be inadequate.

   c. Postexposure prophylaxis includes thorough wound washing and human rabies immune globulin (HRIG) 20 IU/kg, with half administered at the bite site and the rest administered intramuscularly. Rabies immunization should be initiated without delay following contact of an unvaccinated person with a potentially rabid animal. Postexposure immunization includes five intramuscular doses on days 0, 3, 7, 14, and 28 following exposure.

3. Lyme disease vaccine. An inactivated vaccine for Lyme disease (LYMErixü) became available in 1999. The vaccine is 60–80% protective. The ACIP recommends consideration of the vaccine for persons aged 15–70 years who reside, work, or recreate in areas of high or moderate risk and whose exposure to tick-infested habitat is frequent or prolonged, based on their risk of exposure. The vaccine should also be considered for persons with a previous history of Lyme disease who are at continued risk of exposure, but not yet for those with treatment-resistant Lyme arthritis or neurologic illness. The vaccine is not recommended for those who travel or work in areas of low risk. The vaccine is not yet recommended for children under age 15, pregnant women, or persons with immunodeficiency.

   The vaccine is administered in three doses by intramuscular injection. The initial dose is followed by a second dose 1 month later, followed by a third dose 12 months after the first dose. Second (year 1) and third (year 2) doses should ideally be administered several weeks before the beginning of the disease-transmission season (usually April). Existing data suggest that boosters might be needed, but additional data are required to make recommendations regarding booster schedules (see the CDC reference under Electronic Resources).

4. Vaccines for international travel

   a. Many additional vaccines are available and recommended for international travelers. Review of these is beyond the scope of this publication. Current information is available from the US Department of Health and Human Services, Centers for Disease Control and Prevention, on the World Wide Web at http://www.cdc.gov, or can be found in the CDC's Health Information for International Travel.

REFERENCES

American Academy of Pediatrics (AAP): *1997 Red Book: Report of the Committee on Infectious Diseases,* 24th ed. AAP; 1997.

American College of Physicians (ACP): *Guide for Adult Immunization/ACP Task Force on Adult Immunization and Infectious Diseases Society of America,* 3rd ed. ACP; 1994.

Atkinson WL: Rotavirus. Needle Tips & the Hepatitis B Coalition News. Fall/Winter 1998–99; **8**(2):16.

Centers for Disease Control and Prevention: *Epidemiology and Prevention of Vaccine-Preventable Diseases: The Pink Book,* 4th ed. Department of Health and Human Services; Feb 1998.

Centers for Disease Control and Prevention: MMWR 1998;**47**(38):707.

Centers for Disease Control and Prevention: MMWR 1998;**47**(44);956.

Centers for Disease Control and Prevention: Recommendations of the Advisory Committee on Immunization Practices (ACIP).

Department of Health and Human Services, Public Health Service; 1995.

US Public Health Service: *Put Prevention into Practice: The Clinician's Handbook of Preventive Services,* 2nd ed. International Medical Publishers; 1998.

ELECTRONIC RESOURCES

http://www.cdc.gov

http://www.cdc.gov/ncidod/dvbid/lymevaccine.htm

Centers for Disease Control, Lyme Disease Vaccine Recommendations, June 1999.

---

108   Screening Tests

Larry L. Dickey, MD, MSW, MPH

I. **General principles**
   A. **Characteristics of screening tests**
   1. **Sensitivity** is the ability of a screening test to correctly detect persons who have a disorder (true-positives). Example: A test with 80% sensitivity will detect 80% of persons with a disorder, but not the remaining 20% (false-negatives).
   2. **Specificity** is the ability of a screening test to correctly identify persons who do not have a disorder (true-negatives). Example: A screening test with a specificity of 80% will correctly identify 80% of unaffected persons as not having a disorder, but incorrectly identify the remaining 20% as positive (false-positives).
   3. **Positive predictive value** is the percentage of persons identified by screening as having a disorder who actually have the disorder. This increases directly with the specificity of the test and the prevalence of the disorder in the population.
   B. Major authorities issuing recommendations for screening
   1. **Governmental organizations**
      a. **National Institutes of Health (NIH).** Several institutes issue recommendations for specific diseases and conditions, such as the National Heart, Lung, and Blood Institute (NHLBI) and the National Cancer Institute (NCI). Recommendations are formulated by convening consensus conferences of experts in the subject area.
      b. **Centers for Disease Control and Prevention (CDC),** particularly for infectious diseases, such as tuberculosis and sexually transmitted diseases (STDs).
      c. **US Preventive Services Task Force (USPSTF)** is a group of academic experts convened by the Agency for Health Care Policy and Research, US Public Health Service.
   2. **Primary care professional organizations**
      a. American Academy of Family Physicians (AAFP)
      b. American Academy of Pediatrics (AAP)
      c. American College of Physicians (ACP)
      d. American College of Obstetricians and Gynecologists (ACOG)

3. **Specialty professional organizations.** Examples are:
   a. American Urological Association (AUA)
   b. American Thyroid Association (ATA)
   c. American Society of Colon and Rectal Surgeons (ASCRS)
   d. American Thoracic Society (ATS)
   e. American Gastroenterological Association (AGA)
4. **Voluntary organizations.** Examples are:
   a. American Cancer Society (ACS)
   b. American Heart Association (AHA)
   c. American Diabetes Association (ADA)
   d. Skin Cancer Foundation (SCF)
   e. American Speech-Language-Hearing Association (ASHA)

C. Reasons for differing screening recommendations between authorities
1. **Differing methods of assessing scientific evidence.** Some authorities, such as the USPSTF, require evidence from well-designed studies, preferably randomized controlled trials, before recommending screening. Others, such as the ACS, may issue recommendations based on less conclusive evidence, including expert opinion.
2. **Differing criteria for defining benefit.** Some authorities, such as the USPSTF, require evidence of improved health outcomes, whereas others consider improved disease detection or health service delivery to be adequate benefits to justify screening. All authorities seek to access cost-benefit to some extent, but the methodology for this is not well standardized or uniformly implemented.
3. **Differing populations.** Screening of populations at high risk for disease leads to increased positive predictive values for screening. Thus, groups that treat patients at high risk are more likely to recommend routine screening than those who treat normal-risk persons.
4. **Economic or professional interests.** Some authorities may represent groups that benefit financially or professionally from screening and the resultant work-up or treatment of patients with positive results.
5. **Patient advocacy.** Some groups, such as some voluntary organizations, may give greater weight to the desire of patients and the public for increased access to screening.

II. **Body measurement screening**
A. **Head circumference.** The AAP has recommended measurement of head circumference at every visit until a child is 2 years of age. Other authorities have not made recommendations for or against this.
B. **Height and weight.** All major authorities have recommended regular measurement of height and weight at all ages. For children, these can be plotted using standard growth curve charts. For adolescents and adults, height and weight charts can be used (Table 108–1). Several authorities recommend calculation of body mass index [BMI = weight (kg)/height^2 (m)] as more reflective of total body fat. According to the US Department of Agriculture, BMI of ≥25 constitutes overweight, the point at which negative health consequences begin.
C. **Waist/hip ratio.** Some authorities, such as the US Department of Agriculture and the US Department of Health and Human Services, have recommended measurement of waist and hip circumferences and calculation of waist/hip ratio (WHR) for adults. By some reports, this may be a more accurate predictor of negative health consequences than height/weight or BMI values. Upper limits of healthy WHR values are usually cited as 0.8 for women and 1.0 for men.
D. **Blood pressure.** All major authorities recommend regular measurement of blood pressure for all persons beginning at 3 years of age. For children, values above the 95th percentile are considered elevated, (Table 108–2), whereas for adults systolic pressures ≥140 mm Hg and diastolic pressures ≥90 mm Hg are considered elevated. Elevated values should be confirmed on at least one or two additional visits before hypertension is diagnosed. The NHLBI has issued recommendations for follow-up of initial blood pressure measurements in adults (Table 108–3).
E. **Bone density.** No major authority recommends the routine screening of women with bone densitometry for the detection of osteoporosis. The USPSTF found insufficient evidence to recommend for or against routine screening of post-

TABLE 108–1. WEIGHT CHART FOR ADULT MEN AND WOMEN

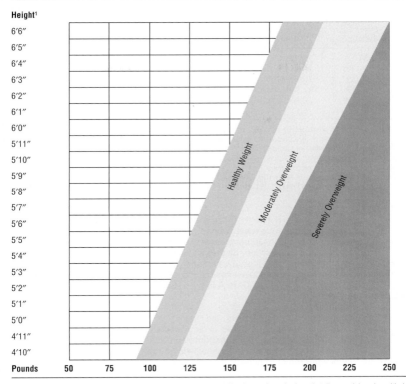

Height[1]

Pounds

¹ The use of shading reflects the lack of consensus about exact cutoff points and emphasizes that disease risk varies with degree of overweight.

Note: To use this chart, find your height in feet and inches (without shoes) along the left side of the graph. Trace the line corresponding to your height across the figure until it intersects with the vertical line corresponding to your weight in pounds (without clothes). The point of intersection lies within a band that indicates whether your weight is healthy or is moderately or severely overweight. The higher weights apply mainly to men, who have more muscle and bone.

Reprinted from US Department of Agriculture, US Department of Health and Human Services: *Nutrition and Your Health: Dietary Guidelines for Americans.* US Government Printing Office; 1995. Home and Garden Bulletin 232.

TABLE 108–2. 95TH PERCENTILE OF BLOOD PRESSURE BY SELECTED AGES IN GIRLS AND BOYS, BY THE 50TH AND 75TH HEIGHT PERCENTILES

Age (Years)	Girls' SBP/DPB		Boys' SBP/DBP	
	50th Percentile for Height	75th Percentile for Height	50th Percentile for Height	75th Percentile for Height
1	104/58	105/59	102/57	104/58
6	111/73	112/73	114/74	115/75
12	123/80	124/81	123/81	125/82
17	129/84	130/85	136/87	138/88

DBP, diastolic blood pressure; SBP, systolic blood pressure.

Reprinted from National Institutes of Health: *The Sixth Report of the Joint National Committee on Prevention, Detection, Evaluation, and Treatment of High Blood Pressure.* US Department of Health and Human Services; 1997. NIH Publication No. 98-4080.

TABLE 108-3. RECOMMENDATIONS FOR FOLLOW-UP BASED ON INITIAL
BLOOD PRESSURE MEASUREMENTS FOR ADULTS

Initial Blood Pressure (mm Hg)[1]		
Systolic	Diastolic	Follow-Up Recommended[2]
<130	<85	Recheck in 2 years
130–139	85–89	Recheck in 1 year[3]
140–159	90–99	Confirm within 2 months[3]
160–179	100–109	Evaluate or refer to source of care within 1 month
≥180	≥110	Evaluate or refer to source of care immediately or within 1 week depending on clinical situation

[1] If systolic and diastolic categories are different, follow recommendations for shorter time follow-up (eg, 160/86 mm Hg should be evaluated or referred to source of care within 1 month).
[2] Modify the scheduling of follow-up according to reliable information about past blood pressure measurements, other cardiovascular risk factors, or target-organ disease.
[3] Provide advice about lifestyle modifications.
Reprinted from National Institutes of Health: *The Sixth Report of the Joint National Committee on Prevention, Detection, Evaluation, and Treatment of High Blood Pressure.* US Department of Health and Human Services; 1997. NIH Publication No. 98-4080.

menopausal women. The AAFP and ACP have recommended against routine screening of postmenopausal women. Since July 1998 Medicare has provided coverage for bone densitometry screening of estrogen-deficient women, including postmenopausal women, as well as for persons at high risk due to receiving long-term glucocorticoid therapy, persons with primary hyperparathyroidism, and persons being monitored to assess the response to an osteoporosis drug therapy approved by the Food and Drug Administration.

III. **Blood test screening**
  A. **Cholesterol**
    1. **Children and adolescents.** No major authority recommends routine cholesterol screening of children or adolescents. Several authorities, including the AAP, AMA, and NHLBI, recommend total cholesterol screening of children >2 years old and adolescents who have a parent with a total cholesterol level ≥240 mg/dL. These authorities also recommend lipoprotein analysis of children >2 years old and adolescents who have a family history of premature cardiovascular disease (before age 55) in a parent or grandparent. The National Cholesterol Education Program (NCEP) recommends screening for at-risk children and adolescents every 5 years. The AMA states that during adolescence screening is needed only once if values are normal. The NCEP has classified cholesterol levels in children and adolescents as follows: acceptable (total <170 mg/dL, low-density lipoprotein [LDL] <110 mg/dL); borderline (total 170–199 mg/dL, LDL 110–129 mg/dL); and high (total = 200 mg/dL, LDL = 130 mg/dL).
    2. **Adults.** Recommendations vary regarding screening of adults. The most aggressive recommendations are those of the NCEP, which recommends screening all adults at least once every 5 years for total cholesterol and at the same time, if accurate results are available, high-density lipoprotein (HDL) cholesterol. The USPSTF recommends screening for total cholesterol in men 35–65 years of age and women 45–65 years. The ACP states that screening of men and women in these same age ranges is appropriate but not mandatory. The ACP and the USPSTF do not recommend screening younger men and women unless they are at high risk. Both ACP and USPSTF state that there is insufficient evidence to recommend for or against screening above 65 years of age. The ACP recommends screening only once, unless the result is near a treatment threshold. The USPSTF states that the appropriate interval for screening is unknown. The NCEP has classified cholesterol level in adults without coronary artery disease as follows: desirable (total <200 mg/dL, LDL <130 mg/dL); borderline (total 200–239 mg/dL, LDL 130–159 mg/dL); and high (total ≥**240 mg/dL, LDL ≥ 160 mg/dL). The NCEP considers HDL levels** <35 mg/dL and ≥60 mg/dL to be positive and negative risk factors, respectively, for coronary artery disease.

B. Hemoglobin/hematocrit

1. Children and adolescents. The AAP recommends screening all children for anemia once between 1 and 9 months of age and once during adolescence for menstruating teenagers. The USPSTF recommends screening infants at high risk for iron deficiency between 6 and 12 months of age. The USPSTF defines high-risk factors as poverty; race—blacks, Native Americans, and Alaskan Natives; immigrants from developing countries; preterm and low-birth-weight infants; and infants whose principal intake is unfortified cow's milk. According to the CDC, the cutoff points for defining anemia in children 6 months to 2 years of age are hemoglobin ≤ **11.0 g/dL and hematocrit ≤ 33.0%.**

2. Adults. No major authority recommends routine screening of asymptomatic, nonpregnant adults for anemia, except ACOG, which recommends screening women with a history of excessive menstrual flow. In nonpregnant women and adolescent girls over 15 years of age, the cutpoints for anemia are hemoglobin ≤12 g/dL and hematocrit ≤36%.

C. Lead.

In 1997 the CDC recommended that state health officials develop plans for targeted blood lead level (BLL) screening of children based on assessments of the lead exposure and screening capacity in specific regions of the state. For targeted screening, the CDC recommends screening of children who reside in a zip code in which >27% of housing was built before 1950; receive services from public assistance programs for the poor, such as Medicaid or the Supplemental Food Program for Women, Infants, and Children (WIC); or whose parents answer "yes" or "don't know" to any of three question of a personal-risk questionnaire (see Table 108–4).

In areas where exposure to lead from older housing is unlikely, the CDC states that the personal-risk questionnaire could contain questions about other risk factors, such as parental occupation or use of lead-containing ceramic ware or traditional remedies.

In the absence of a targeted screening plan or other formal guidance from state health officials, the CDC recommends universal screening of all children at 1 and 2 years of age and of children 36–72 months of age not previously screened.

Diagnostic testing of venous blood should be performed for all patients with elevated blood lead levels >10 μg/dL at a follow-up interval based on degree of elevation of BLL (see Table 108–5).

The AAP has endorsed the 1997 CDC recommendations. The USPSTF recommends screening children at increased risk for lead exposure. The USPSTF

TABLE 108–4. BASIC LEAD PERSONAL RISK PROFILE

1. Does your child live in or regularly visit a house that was built before 1950? This question could apply to a facility such as a home day-care center or the home of a babysitter or relative.
2. Does your child live in or regularly visit a house built before 1978 with recent or ongoing renovations or remodeling (within the last 6 months)?
3. Does your child have a sibling or playmate who has or did have lead poisoning?

Reprinted from Centers for Disease Control and Prevention: *Screening Young Children for Lead Poisoning: Guidance for State and Local Public Health Officials.* US Department of Health and Human Services; 1997.

TABLE 108–5. SCHEDULE FOR DIAGNOSTIC TESTING OF A CHILD WITH AN ELEVATED BLOOD LEAD LEVEL ON A SCREENING TEST

If result of screening test (μg/dL) is:	Perform diagnostic test on venous blood within:
10–19	3 months
20–44	1 month–1 week[1]
45–59	48 hours
60–69	24 hours
≥70	Immediately as an emergency lab test

[1] The higher the screening blood lead level, the more urgent the need for a diagnostic test.

Reprinted from Centers for Disease Control and Prevention: *Screening Young Children for Lead Poisoning: Guidance for State and Local Public Health Officials,* US Department of Health and Human Services; 1997.

states that this screening should occur at about 12 months of age and that the optimal frequency for screening or repeat testing of children with elevated BLLs is left to clinical discretion.

D. **Newborn screening.** The AAP and other authorities have recommended that newborn screening be performed according to each state's regulations. National authorities have made recommendations for the following specific conditions:

1. **Hypothyroidism.** The AAP, ATA, and USPSTF have recommended that all neonates be screened for congenital hypothyroidism between 2 and 6 days of life. Care should be taken to ensure that infants born at home, ill at birth, or transferred between hospitals in the first week of life are screened before 7 days of life.

2. **Phenylketonuria (PKU).** The AAFP and USPSTF have recommended that all infants be screened for PKU prior to discharge from the nursery. Premature infants and those with illnesses should be tested at or near 7 days of age. Infants tested before 24 hours of age should receive a repeat screening. According to the USPSTF, this should occur by the time the infant is 2 weeks of age.

3. **Hemoglobinopathies.** The Sickle Cell Disease Guideline Panel of the Agency for Health Care Policy and Research, US Public Health Service, has recommended universal screening of newborns for sickle cell disease. This recommendation has been endorsed by the AAP, American Nurses Association, and AMA. The USPSTF has also recommended neonatal screening for sickle hemoglobinopathies, but has stated that whether screening should be universal or targeted to high-risk groups should depend on the proportion of high-risk persons in the screening area. All screening must be accompanied by comprehensive counseling and treatment services

E. **Thyroid function.** No authorities recommend screening of asymptomatic adults for thyroid dysfunctions, except for older women. The ACOG recommends measurement of thyroid-stimulating hormone (TSH) levels every 3–5 years in all women over 65 years of age. In 1998, ACP stated, "It is reasonable to screen women older than 50 years of age for unsuspected but symptomatic thyroid disease. The preferred screening method is a sensitive TSH test." This recommendation is based on the estimate that 1 of 71 women over 50 years of age will have unsuspected but symptomatic overt hypothyroidism or overt hyperthyroidism that will respond to treatment. Treatment of subclinical hyperthyroidism or hypothyroidism is of uncertain benefit. Other organizations, such as the USPSTF, have found insufficient evidence for screening of this population, recommending instead that clinicians remain alert for subtle or nonspecific symptoms of thyroid dysfunction when examining older women, postpartum women, and persons with Down syndrome.

IV. **Sensory screening**

A. **Hearing**

1. **Children.** The Joint Committee on Infant Hearing (composed of the AAP, American Speech-Language-Hearing Association, American Academy of Otolaryngology—Head and Neck Surgery, and American Academy of Audiology) has endorsed the goal of universal screening of all neonates. Until this is feasible, these authorities recommend screening neonates with risk factors for hearing impairment prior to hospital discharge, but not later than 3 months of age. Table 108–6 shows a list of neonatal risk factors. The USPSTF has found insufficient evidence to recommend for or against universal screening of neonates. The AAP has recommended routine screening of asymptomatic children with pure-tone audiometry at 3, 4, 5, 10, 12, 15, and 18 years of age. The USPSTF has recommended against routine screening of asymptomatic children. The Joint Committee on Infant Hearing has identified recurrent or persistent otitis media with effusion for at least 3 months to be a risk factor requiring screening.

2. **Adults.** All major authorities recommend screening older adults for hearing impairment. However, the modality for screening remains poorly defined. The American Speech-Language-Hearing Association recommends using a hearing handicap questionnaire or pure-tone audiometry. The USPSTF recommends first questioning patients about hearing impairment and performing audiometry on those reporting abnormalities. Patients found to

TABLE 108–6. NEONATAL RISK FACTORS FOR HEARING IMPAIRMENT

- Family history of hereditary sensorineural hearing loss
- In utero infection, such as cytomegalovirus, rubella, syphilis, herpes, or toxoplasmosis
- Craniofacial anomalies, including those with morphologic abnormalities of the pinna and ear canal
- Birth weight less than 1500 g (3.3 lbs)
- Hyperbilirubinemia at a serum level requiring exchange transfusion
- Ototoxic medications, including but not limited to aminoglycosides, used in multiple courses or in combination with loop diuretics
- Bacterial meningitis
- Apgar scores of 0–4 at 1 minute or 0–6 at 5 minutes
- Mechanical ventilation lasting 5 days or longer
- Stigmata or other findings associated with a syndrome known to include a sensorineural or conductive hearing loss

Adapted from Joint Committee on Infant Hearing: Joint Committee on Infant Hearing 1994 position statement. Pediatrics 1995;**95:**152.

have evidence of hearing loss by screening should be considered for referral to a specialist for comprehensive audiologic evaluation, especially if they feel handicapped by the hearing loss. Because about 10% of persons with hearing loss are amenable to medical or surgical treatment and because some patients are incorrectly identified as having hearing loss by screening, patients should not be referred directly to a hearing aid dealer. The primary care clinician should make sure that appropriate follow-up management is provided to all patients referred for audiologic evaluation. Patients may need considerable support and training to use their hearing aids effectively.

B. Vision

1. Children. Recommendations regarding vision screening for children vary among authorities. The AAP has recommended questioning of parents regarding a child's vision at well-child visits, with the first objective test of visual acuity at 3 years of age. If the child is uncooperative, this should be rescheduled 6 months later. Subsequent objective testing is recommended at 4, 5, 10, 12, 15, and 18 years of age. The USPSTF recommends that clinicians be alert for signs of ocular misalignment in examining all newborns, infants, and children. The USPSTF recommends testing for amblyopia and strabismus once before the child enters school, preferably at 3 to 4 years of age, and states that stereotesting is more effective for this purpose than visual acuity testing. Physical examination procedures for detecting amblyopia and strabismus include the corneal light reflex, fixation, differential occlusion, and cover/uncover tests. The USPSTF has found insufficient evidence to recommend for or against routine visual acuity testing of school children, because refractive errors of consequence present symptomatically and are easily treated with corrective lenses.

2. Adults. Recommendations for vision screening of adults vary considerably among authorities.

a. Visual acuity. All major authorities recommend routine visual acuity screening for normal-risk adults beginning at 65 years of age.

b. Eye examination. No major authority recommends routine examination by primary care physicians, including the use of tonometry to detect glaucoma. Most authorities recommend referral to an ophthalmologist for patients at risk for glaucoma, especially African Americans over 40 years of age. The American Academy of Ophthalmology recommends comprehensive eye examinations by an ophthalmologist every 2–4 years from ages 40–64 and every 1–2 years beginning at 65 years of age. The National Eye Institute recommends comprehensive eye examinations every 2 years starting at 60 years of age. All authorities recommend frequent, yearly, comprehensive eye examinations by eye care specialists for patients with diabetes mellitus.

V. Infectious disease

A. Hepatitis C. In recognition of the heavy burden of disease caused by hepatitis C (1.8% of the US population infected, >$600 million in medical and work-loss expenses annually), the CDC has recommended screening of high-risk populations (Table 108–7).

B. Human immunodeficiency virus (HIV). All major authorities recommend that HIV screening be offered to patients at risk: those with another STD, homosexual and bisexual men, past or present injection drug users, persons with a history of prostitution or multiple sexual partners, persons whose past (or present) sexual partners are HIV-infected or injection drug users or both, patients with a history of blood transfusion between 1978 and 1985, and persons born in, or with long-term residence in, a community in which HIV is prevalent. The AMA also recommends offering testing and counseling to high-risk persons receiving family planning services or undergoing surgery. The CDC recommends that health facilities with an HIV seroprevalence rate of at least 1% or an AIDS diagnosis rate of 1 or more per 1000 discharges should consider a policy of routine counseling and voluntary HIV testing for patients 15–54 years of age.

C. Other sexually transmitted diseases

1. Chlamydia and gonorrhea. The AAP and AMA have advocated screening all sexually active adolescents. For adolescent males, this can be done with dipstick leukocyte esterase test, whereas screening of females requires culture or rapid antigen tests. The USPSTF recommends screening sexually active adolescent females and high-risk adult women. For chlamydia, risk factors are a history of prior STDs, a new partner or multiple sex partners, age under 25, inconsistent barrier contraceptive use, cervical ectopy, and being unmarried. In areas of high prevalence, screening of all women for chlamydia is justified. For gonorrhea, women at risk are commercial sex workers, those with repeated episodes of gonorrhea, and women under 25 years of age with two or more sex partners in the last year.

The USPSTF has stated that in settings in which prevalence is high, such as urban adolescent clinics, broader screening, including screening of males, may be justified. Although dipstick leukocyte testing is convenient and inexpensive, its positive predictive value has been found to be as low as 11% for chlamydia and 30% for gonorrhea. Thus, confirmation with more specific tests is required for all positive results.

Screening of urine for chlamydia with new ligase chain reaction tests has increased specificity to 99% and sensitivity to >90%. However, as of this update, major authorities, including the CDC, have yet to issue revised recommendations for screening based on this new technology.

2. Syphilis. All major authorities recommend that screening be performed for persons at high risk for infection. These persons may include sexual partners

---

TABLE 108–7. PERSONS WHO SHOULD BE TESTED ROUTINELY FOR HEPATITIS C VIRUS (HCV) INFECTION

Persons who should be tested routinely for hepatitis C virus (HCV) infection based on their risk for infection
- Persons who ever injected illegal drugs, including those who injected once or a few times many years ago and do not consider themselves as drug users.
- Persons with selected medical conditions, including
  —Persons who received clotting factor concentrates produced before 1987;
  —Persons who were ever on chronic (long-term) hemodialysis; and
  —Persons with persistently abnormal alanine aminotransferase levels.
- Prior recipients of transfusions or organ transplants, including
  —Persons who were notified that they received blood from a donor who later tested positive for HCV infection;
  —Persons who received a transfusion of blood or blood components before July 1992; and
  —Persons who received an organ transplant before July 1992.

Persons who should be tested routinely for HCV-infection based on a recognized exposure
- Healthcare, emergency medical, and public safety workers after needle sticks, sharps, or mucosal exposures to HCV-positive blood.
- Children born to HCV-positive women.

Reprinted from Centers for Disease Control and Prevention: Recommendations for prevention and control of Hepatitis C Virus (HCV) infection and HCV-related chronic disease. MMWR 1998;**47**(RR-19):1.

of known syphilis cases, those with multiple sexual partners—especially in high-prevalence areas—prostitutes or those who trade sex for drugs, and males who engage in sex with other males. Routine screening of sexually active adolescents has not been advocated.

Because the causative agent of syphilis cannot be cultured, screening relies on serology. A nontreponemal test, either the VDRL or RPR, is recommended for initial screening. Because the specificity of these tests is limited, follow-up testing with a treponemal test, such as the FTA (fluorescent treponemal antibody), is required for positive results. Because the sensitivity of nontreponemal tests may be as low as 75% in primary syphilis, patients who have had recent contact with a person with a documented case of syphilis should be treated, even if serologic tests are negative.

D. Tuberculosis (TB). All major authorities recommend screening of persons at high risk for TB. Recently, the AAP and other pediatric authorities have decided against routine screening of normal-risk children. In general, authorities have not specified how often high-risk persons should be screened, although the AAP has recommended annual screening for children at risk. Populations at risk include (1) medically underserved, low-income populations, including those of African American, Hispanic, Asian, Native American, and Alaskan Native heritage; (2) foreign-born persons from high-prevalence countries (eg, Asia, Africa, and Latin America); (3) persons in close contact with infectious TB cases (sharing accommodations as well as playing or working in the same enclosed area); (4) alcoholics and injection drug users; (5) residents of high-risk environments, including long-term care facilities, correctional institutions, and mental institutions; and (6) persons with medical conditions known to substantially increase the risk of TB, such as HIV infection, diabetes mellitus, and chronic renal failure.

The appropriate criterion for defining a positive skin test reaction depends on the likelihood of TB exposure and the risk of TB if exposure has occurred. For persons with HIV infection, close contacts of infectious cases, and those with fibrotic lesions on chest radiograph, a reaction of ≥5 mm is considered positive. For other at-risk persons, including all infants and children younger than 4 years of age, a reaction of ≥10 mm is considered positive. Persons who are not likely to be infected with *Mycobacterium tuberculosis* should generally not be skin-tested because the predictive value of a positive skin test in low-risk populations is poor. If a skin test is performed on a person who is not in a high-risk category or who is not exposed in a high-risk environment, a cutoff point of ≥15 mm is considered positive, although prophylaxis with isoniazid is not necessarily recommended for these persons.

VI. Cancer screening
A. Breast cancer
1. Clinical breast examination (CBE). All major authorities recommend annual breast examinations for women 50 years of age and older. Recommendations for CBEs for women under 50 vary: AAFP—every 1–3 years for women 30–39 years of age and annually thereafter; ACS—every 3 years for women 20–39 years of age and annually thereafter; ACOG—annually beginning at 18 years of age; and ACP—annually beginning at 40 years of age. The USPSTF does not recommend CBEs for normal-risk women before 50 years of age. It is interesting that CBE may be almost as accurate as mammography in detecting cancer. In one large trial of combined mammography and CBE, two-thirds of the effectiveness of the trial may have been due to the CBE alone. In performing the CBE, the examiner should be systematic, palpating every portion of the breast with the patient in both an upright and supine position. One of the best indicators of examiner accuracy is thought to be the amount of time spent.

2. Mammography. All major authorities recommend regular mammography for women 50 years of age and older. ACS, ACOG, and NCI recommend annual screening. The USPSTF recommends mammography every 1–2 years, and the ACP recommends screening every 2 years. The USPSTF recommends screening up to 69 years of age, and the ACP recommends cessation of screening at 75 years of age. Recommendations for screening of women less than 50 years of age continues to be an area of controversy. The ACS recommends annual screening beginning at 40 years of age. The NCI recommends screening every 1–2 years for women 40–49 years of age. The USPSTF states that there is insufficient evidence to recommend for or against mammography before 50 years of age, whereas the ACP and the Canadian Task Force on the Periodic Health Examination recommend that women under 50 years of age not be screened with mammography. ACOG recommends mammography beginning at 35 for those at high risk, whereas ACP states that women at high risk should follow the same schedule as that of average-risk women.

The controversy regarding mammography screening of women less than 50 years of age hinges on the failure of major trials to detect significantly improved mortality. Breast cancer occurring or treated before 50 years of age may be more aggressive and less responsive to treatment than that occurring after 50 years of age. Some authorities maintain that studies of screening mammography in women less than 50 years of age have been flawed.

The clinician should keep in mind that the sensitivity of a mammogram is limited—about 90%. Thus, symptoms and positive physical findings should not be dismissed strictly on the basis of a negative mammogram. The specificity is similarly limited; thus, women should be counseled against alarm based strictly on a positive mammogram.

B. Cervical cancer. All major authorities recommend routine Papanicolaou (Pap) smears for sexually active adolescent and adult women. The recommended frequency varies among authorities. The ACS and ACOG recommend annual Pap smears, stipulating that after three normal annual tests, Pap smears can be performed less frequently at the discretion of the patient and clinician. After two or three normal annual Pap smears, the ACP recommends screening every 3 years for normal-risk and every 2 years for increased-risk women. The USPSTF recommends screening at least every 3 years, with the interval to be determined by the physician based on risk factors. Important risk factors include early initiation of sexual intercourse, history of multiple sexual partners, and low socioeconomic status. Women with HIV infection are particularly at risk for cervical cancer. The ACP has recommended discontinuing screening of women at 66 years of age if women have been screened within the preceding 10 years. If not, screening should continue until 75 years of age. The USPSTF has found insufficient evidence to recommend an upper age limit for screening.

The use of an endocervical brush and wooden spatula provides the best yield of adequate samples, defined as containing endocervical cells. Although the presence of endocervical cells has not been demonstrated to result in improved clinical outcomes, it remains the accepted standard for adequacy of Pap smears. Women exposed to diethylstilbestrol (DES) in utero should have sampling performed from the upper third of the vagina.

C. Colorectal cancer

    1. Digital rectal examination. Digital rectal examination is no longer recommended by major authorities as a modality for screening for colorectal cancer because of its poor sensitivity (<10%).

    2. Fecal occult blood testing. All major authorities now recommend annual fecal occult blood testing for normal-risk persons beginning at 50 years of age. Some authorities, such as the ACP and USPSTF, state that its use may be optional if sigmoidoscopy or colonoscopy are performed regularly. Some authorities (AAFP, ACS, and AGA) recommend beginning screening at 40 years of age for high-risk patients, such as those with a family history of colon cancer. The ACP has recommended stopping screening at "70 or 80" years of age. The sensitivity and specificity of fecal occult blood testing are limited, resulting in many false-negative and false-positive results. The positive predictive value may be <10%. Those undergoing annual screening have a lifetime risk of about 40% of experiencing a false-positive result. The improved mortality attributed to screening may actually be due to the high rate of sigmoidoscopy and colonoscopy used to evaluate incidental false-positive fecal occult blood tests. Rehydration of samples with a few drops of water before development improves sensitivity but significantly decreases specificity. For this reason, most authorities recommend against rehydration. Clinicians should keep in mind that, because of limited sensitivity and the intermittent nature of colorectal cancer bleeding, cancer cannot be ruled out by repeated fecal occult blood testing after a positive result.

3. **Sigmoidoscopy.** All major authorities now recommend sigmoidoscopy screening for persons beginning at 50 years of age. Some authorities, such as the ACP and USPSTF, state that sigmoidoscopy may be optional for persons undergoing annual fecal occult blood testing. The ACS and AGA recommend sigmoidoscopy every 5 years. Some authorities (AAFP, ACS, and AGA) recommend beginning screening at 40 years of age for high-risk patients, such as those with a family history of colon cancer. The ACP recommends stopping screening at 70 years of age. The sensitivity of sigmoidoscopy is limited by the length of the scope, with about 40% of malignancies being beyond the reach of a 60-cm flexible scope. For this reason, some authorities recommend offering procedures that are able to examine the entire colon, such as colonoscopy and barium enema.

4. **Colonoscopy.** Several authorities (AAFP, ACP, ACS, and AGA) have recommended colonoscopy every 10 years—beginning at 50 years of age for normal-risk and at 40 years of age for high-risk patients—as an alternative to fecal occult blood and sigmoidoscopy screening. The USPSTF found the evidence insufficient to recommend colonoscopy for routine screening.

5. **Barium enema.** Several authorities (AAFP, ACS, and AGA) have recommended a barium enema every 5 years—beginning at 50 years of age for normal-risk and at 40 years of age for high-risk patients—as an alternative to other screening modalities. The USPSTF found the evidence insufficient to recommend barium enema for use in routine screening.

D. **Oral cancer.** The ACS recommends oral cavity examinations every 3 years until 40 years of age and yearly thereafter. The ACOG recommends yearly examinations starting at 40 years. The USPSTF states that there is insufficient evidence to recommend for or against screening examinations, but suggests that clinicians may wish to provide such examinations to persons at risk because of a history of chewing or smoking tobacco or regular alcohol use.

E. **Ovarian cancer**

1. **Bimanual pelvic exam.** All major authorities except the USPSTF recommend screening for ovarian cancer with bimanual pelvic examination at the time of performing a Pap smear. The USPSTF has stated that there is evidence to recommend against screening for ovarian cancer by pelvic examination. The main limitation of pelvic examination for screening is its limited sensitivity, with many tumors becoming large in size before becoming detectable by examination.

2. **Tumor markers.** No major authorities have recommended screening normal-risk women using tumor markers, such as CA-125. An NIH consensus conference has recommended using annual CA-125 measurements and transvaginal ultrasonography to screen women at particularly high risk because of hereditary cancer syndrome. Because of limited specificity and low prevalence of the disease, the use of tumor makers for screening in normal-risk populations results in large numbers of false-positives.

3. **Ultrasonography.** No major authority currently recommends the use of ultrasonography to screen normal-risk women, largely because of its poor positive predictive value. As previously described, some authorities have recommended its use in combination with tumor marker measurement to screen high-risk women.

F. **Prostate cancer**

1. **Digital rectal examination (DRE).** The ACS recommends annual DRE for men beginning at 40 years of age, whereas the AUA recommends annual DRE beginning at 50 years of age for normal-risk men. The USPSTF recommends against DRE in screening for prostate cancer. The DRE has limited sensitivity (33–69%) and positive predictive value (6–33%) for detecting prostate cancer in asymptomatic men.

2. **Prostate-specific antigen (PSA) testing.** The ACS and AUA recommend annual PSA testing for normal-risk men 50 years of age and older, whereas the USPSTF has recommended against such screening. The positive predictive value of PSA testing is estimated to be 10–35%, thus leading to many

unnecessary biopsies. Efforts to refine PSA testing using age, prostate size based on ultrasound findings, and rates of change in PSA over time may lead to improvements in sensitivity and specificity. Because prostate cancer tends to be slow growing, it is unclear to what extent early detection decreases mortality.

   3. Ultrasonography. No major authority currently recommends using transrectal ultrasonography (TRUS) to screen for prostate cancer. Because TRUS cannot distinguish between benign and malignant nodules, its positive predictive value is lower than that of PSA testing.

G. Skin cancer. The American Academy of Dermatology recommends annual skin examinations for all adults. The ACS recommends skin examinations every 3 years from 20–40 years of age and yearly thereafter. The USPSTF has found insufficient evidence to recommend for or against routine skin examinations by primary care clinicians, while recommending that they remain alert for skin lesions with malignant features, particularly in patients at risk. Risk factors include melanocytic precursor or marker lesions (eg, atypical moles); large numbers of common moles; immunosuppression; a family or personal history of skin cancer; substantial cumulative lifetime sun exposure; intermittent intense sun exposure or severe sunburns in childhood; freckles; poor tanning ability; and light skin, hair, and eye color. The USPSTF has recommended that primary care clinicians consider referring patients with melanocytic precursor or marker lesions to skin care specialists.

   Major characteristics that make a lesion suspicious for malignant melanoma may be remembered by the ABCDs: A, asymmetry; B, irregular borders; C, variation in color; and D, diameter greater than 6 mm.

H. Testicular cancer. The AUA recommends annual testicular examinations beginning at 15 years of age. The ACS recommends examinations every 3 years starting from 20–40 years of age and annual examinations thereafter. The USPSTF has found insufficient evidence to recommend for or against routine screening, while stating that patients at increased risk because of history of cryptorchidism or testicular atrophy should be counseled about the risk of cancer and offered the options of physician examinations or self-examinations. A major factor against screening is the excellent prognosis of testicular cancer, regardless of how it is detected.

I. Thyroid cancer. The ACS recommends thyroid palpation every 3 years until 40 years of age and yearly thereafter. The USPSTF has found inadequate evidence to recommend for or against routine screening by thyroid palpation, while stating that screening of persons at high risk because of a history of external upper body radiation in infancy and childhood may be justified on other grounds, such as patient preference or anxiety.

REFERENCES

American Academy of Family Physicians, Commission on Public Health and Scientific Affairs: *Age Charts for Periodic Health Examination.* American Academy of Family Physicians; 1994.

American Academy of Pediatrics, Committee on Infectious Disease: *1998 Red Book.* American Academy of Pediatrics; 1998.

American Academy of Pediatrics, Committee on Practice and Ambulatory Medicine: Recommendations for pediatric preventive health care. Pediatrics 1995;**96**:373.

American Cancer Society: *Summary of American Cancer Society Recommendations for the Early Detection of Cancer in Asymptomatic People.* American Cancer Society; 1992.

American College of Obstetricians and Gynecologists: *The Obstetrician-Gynecologist and Primary-Preventive Health Care.* American College of Obstetricians and Gynecologists; 1993.

American College of Physicians. *Guidelines.* In: Eddy DM, ed. *Common Screening Tests.* American College of Physicians, 1991; 396.

American Medical Association: *Guidelines for Adolescent Preventive Services (GAPS).* Williams & Wilkins; 1994.

US Department of Agriculture, US Dept of Health and Human Services: *Nutrition and Your Health: Dietary Guidelines for Americans.* US Government Printing Office; 1995. Home and Garden Bulletin 232.

US Department of Health and Human Services: *Clinician's Handbook of Preventive Services,* 2nd ed. US Government Printing Office; 1998.

US Preventive Services Task Force: *Guide to Clinical Preventive Services,* 2nd ed. Williams & Wilkins; 1996.

109   Chemoprophylaxis, Travel Medicine, & Alternative Medicine

Gregory H. Blake, MD, MPH

I. **Definition.** Prophylaxis is derived from the Greek (*pro phulax*), which means "to put up a guard before it is necessary." Chemoprophylaxis is the use of a chemical or medication to prevent a disease. Its usage runs from travel medicine to preventing infectious diseases to treating chronic disease states.

II. **Bacterial meningitis**

  A. **Pathogens**

   1. *Haemophilus influenzae*

     a. The mortality rate is about 5%, with 20–30% of survivors having neurologic sequelae.

     b. Eighty-five percent of invasive *Haemophilus* disease occurs in children under 5 years of age.

     c. In the United States, the incidence is greatest in Native Americans, blacks, those in lower socioeconomic groups, and those with complement or immunoglobulin deficiencies.

   2. *Neisseria meningitidis*

     a. The mortality rate is about 10%, with children below 1 year of age having the greatest incidence.

     b. Twelve serogroups of meningococcus have been identified based on capsular polysaccharide. Serogroups B and C account for 50% and 20% of the mortality, respectively.

     c. Meningococci are carried by 15% of contacts in their throats, but only 3–4% will carry a pathogenic strain.

   3. *Streptococcus pneumoniae*

     a. The mortality rate is about 26%, with the greatest mortality in patients over 60 years of age.

     b. Most cases occur during the first 2 years of life, but a second peak occurs in the elderly.

     c. Eighty-eight percent of organisms causing bacteremic disease in the United States are represented in the 23-valent pneumococcal vaccine.

     d. In the United States, the incidence is greatest in patients who are asplenic or alcoholic and those with sickle cell disease, human immunodeficiency virus (HIV) infection, and deficiencies of immunoglobulins and complement.

  B. **Prophylaxis**

   1. Prophylaxis should be considered in invasive disease resulting from *H influenza* type b and *N meningitidis.* Prophylaxis for *S pneumoniae* is recommended only in circumstances of overcrowding.

   2. *H influenza* type b meningitis

     a. Criteria for prophylaxis

       (1) **Members of the same household,** if a contact is younger than 48 months and has not received a complete course of the *H influenza* conjugated vaccine series.

       (2) **Children younger than 2 years of age** in day care with contact of 25 hr/week or greater.

       (3) **Personnel of day care centers,** when two or more cases occur within 60 days.

       (4) **Not needed when all children in day care are older than 2 years of age.**

     b. **Regimen.** Rifampin, administered orally at 20 mg/kg/day in one dose for 4 days (maximum dose, 600 mg/day).

   3. *N meningitidis* meningitis

     a. Criteria for prophylaxis

       (1) **Household, day care, and nursery school contacts.**

       (2) **Personnel, including those involved in health care,** who have had contact with oral secretions of the index case.

b. Regimen
  (1) Rifampin, administered orally every 12 hours at 5 mg/kg per dose in children below 1 year, 10 mg/kg per dose in children aged 1–12, and 600 mg in adults and children aged over 12 years for a total of four doses (maximum 600 mg/day).
  (2) Ceftriaxone, administered as a single intramuscular dose of 125 mg for children younger than 12 years and a dose of 250 mg for adults, may eliminate meningococcal carriage of serogroup A strains.
  (3) Ciprofloxacin, administered as a single oral 500-mg dose in adults.
  (4) Outbreaks of serogroup A strains need antibiotic prophylaxis for all persons 3 months or older and the meningococcal vaccine.

III. Atherosclerosis
A. Coronary heart disease
  1. Low-dose aspirin is indicated for patients with unstable angina and prior myocardial infarction. Data support use in patients with atrial fibrillation, chronic stable angina, valvular heart disease, or prior peripheral or coronary revascularization.
  2. Aspirin irreversibly blocks cyclo-oxygenase, which inhibits platelet aggregability for the life of the platelet. Aspirin (325 mg) provides nearly complete inhibition for 2 days, with return to pretreatment levels in about 8 days. Although the optimal dose of aspirin is unknown, 80 mg of aspirin daily or 325 mg of enteric-coated aspirin daily provides the lowest gastric toxicity and most favorable prostacyclin–thromboxane ratio.
  3. The US Preventive Services Task Force does not recommend routine aspirin prophylaxis for the primary prevention of myocardial infarction for men aged 40 or over because of insufficient evidence. Men with risk factors for coronary heart disease and no contraindications to aspirin use may benefit from prophylaxis. Aspirin prophylaxis is contraindicated in patients with a history of uncontrolled hypertension, liver or kidney disease, peptic ulcer disease, a history of gastrointestinal or other bleeding problems, or other risk factors for bleeding or cerebral hemorrhage.
  4. Although inconsistent findings in women regarding aspirin prophylaxis preclude a formal recommendation for prophylaxis, women taking an average of one to six aspirin tablets per week had an age-adjusted relative risk of 0.68 (95% CI 0.52–0.89) for a first myocardial infarction compared with women receiving placebo.

B. Cerebrovascular disease
  1. Aspirin reduces the risk of stroke in patients with transient ischemic attacks and minor stroke. All aspirin doses are similarly effective. Clopidogrel (75 mg orally each day) and ticlopidine (250 mg twice a day) are effective agents in preventing recurrent ischemia.
  2. Warfarin is the drug of choice for patients with nonvalvular atrial fibrillation. Patients younger than 60 years without specific clinical or echocardiographic risk factors do not need warfarin. Patients at risk or those sustaining focal cerebral ischemia from cardioembolism should receive warfarin, and the International Normalized Ratio (INR) should be maintained at 2.0–3.0. Patients with severe dilated cardiomyopathy, mitral stenosis, or prosthetic valves should receive warfarin with the INR maintained at 2.0–4.5.
  3. In patients with nonrheumatic atrial fibrillation, 325 mg of aspirin per day reduces the occurrence of noncardioembolic strokes.

C. Future direction. Atherosclerosis is a degenerative process in arteries involving endothelial cell injury, accumulation of lipid, proliferation of smooth muscle cells, and thickening of the intimal and medial layers.
  1. Research suggests that free radicals and oxidized lipids influence this process.
    a. Low-density lipoprotein (LDL) particles contain polyunsaturated fatty acids and cholesterol, which can be oxidized by free radicals in the presence of iron and copper catalysts.
    b. Oxidatively modified LDL particles are ingested by subendothelial macrophages (foam cells) and recruit monocytes to the subendothelium, inhibit release of endothelium-dependent vasodilatory nitric oxide, and are cytotoxic to endothelial cells.

    c. Homocysteine activates clotting factors V and XII, increases thromboxane formation, binds lipoprotein to fibrin, causes desquamation of endothelial cells, and is involved in the modification of LDL.

  2. Epidemiologic studies suggest that physiologic antioxidants such as vitamin E, ascorbic acid, flavonoids, and free radical scavenging enzyme systems can inhibit these processes. Folate also blocks the effects of homocysteine.

  3. Prospective randomized controlled trials are in progress testing whether supplemental antioxidants are beneficial in preventing coronary heart disease. However, as of now no recommendation can be made.

IV. Bacterial endocarditis

A. Pathophysiology

  1. Infective endocarditis is a localized infection consisting of fibrin, platelets, and microorganisms that adhere to the cardiac valves.

  2. Without appropriate treatment, the mortality rate approaches 100%.

  3. Clinical manifestations include fever, cardiac murmurs, anemia, splenomegaly, petechiae, pyuria, and peripheral emboli.

  4. The causative organisms for native valves are *Streptococcus viridans* and other streptococci (60%), *Staphylococcus aureus* (25%), enterococci (10%), and other gram-negative organisms (5%). For prosthetic valves beyond 2 months of placement, *Streptococcus viridans* and other streptococci account for 30% of cases; coagulase-negative staphylococci, 20%; *S aureus,* 15%; and enterococci and gram-negative organisms, 10%.

  5. Diagnosis is made by using clinical, microbiologic, and echocardiographic data (Table 109–1).

TABLE 109–1. DIAGNOSTIC CRITERIA FOR INFECTIVE ENDOCARDITIS (IE)[1]

Definite IE
Pathological criteria
Micro-organisms: demonstrated by culture or histology in a vegetation, or in a vegetation that has embolised, or in an intracardiac abscess *or*
Pathological lesions: vegetation or intracardiac abscess present, confirmed by histology showing active endocarditis
Clinical criteria, using specific definitions for these terms as listed below
2 major[2] criteria, or 1 major[2] criterion and 3 minor[3] criteria, or 5 minor[3] criteria

Possible IE
Findings consistent with IE that fall short of[1] Definite,[1] but not[1] Rejected[1]

Rejected
Firm alternate diagnosis for manifestations of IE *or*
Resolution of manifestations of IE, with antibiotic therapy for 4 days or less *or*
No pathological evidence of IE at surgery or autopsy, after antibiotic therapy for 4 days or less

---

[1] Definitions and terminology used in Duke's criteria.

[2] Major criteria: positive blood culture for IE; typical micro-organisms for IE from 2 separate blood cultures; viridans streptococci (including nutritional variants strains), *Streptococcus bovis,* HACEK group or community-acquired *Staphylococcus aureus* or enterococci, in the absence of a primary focus or persistently positive blood culture. A persistently positive blood culture is defined as the recovery of a micro-organism consistent with IE from blood cultures drawn more than 12 hours apart or all of 3 or a majority of 4 or more separate blood cultures, with first and last drawn at least 1 hour apart. Evidence of endocardial involvement includes positive echocardiogram for IE; oscillating intracardiac mass on valve or supporting structures, or in the path of regurgitant jets, or on implanted material, in the absence of an alternative anatomical explanation, or abscess, or new partial dehiscence of prosthetic valve, or new valvular regurgitation (increased or change in pre-existent murmur not sufficient).

[3] Minor criteria: predisposition (predisposing heart condition or intravenous drug use); fever $\geq 38.0\,°C$ (100.4°F); vascular phenomena (major arterial emboli, septic pulmonary infarcts, mycotic aneurysm, intracranial haemorrhage, conjunctival haemorrhages, Janeway lesions); immunological phenomena (glomerulonephritis, Osler's nodes, Roth spots, rheumatoid factor); microbiological evidence [positive blood culture but not meeting major criterion as noted previously (excluding single positive cultures for coagulase-negative staphylococci and organisms that do not cause endocarditis)] or serological evidence of active infection with organism consistent with IE; and echocardiogram (consistent with IE but not meeting major criteria as noted above).

HACEK, *Haemophilus* spp., *Actinobacillus actinomycetemcomitans, Cardiobacterium hominis, Eikenella* spp. and *Kingella kingae.*

Reprinted from Stamboulian and Carbone: Management of endocarditis. Drugs 1997;**54**(5):733.

B. Prophylaxis

1. Although only proved to prevent endocarditis in experimental animals, chemoprophylaxis is recommended for invasive procedures that cause bacteremia in humans having cardiac lesions highly associated with endocarditis. Individuals at highest risk are those with prosthetic heart valves, a previous history of bacterial endocarditis, cyanotic congenital heart disease (single ventricle, transposition of great vessels, and tetralogy of Fallot), or surgically constructed systemic pulmonary shunts or conduits. Individuals at moderate risk are those with uncorrected congenital heart conditions (patent ductus arteriosus, ventricular septal defect, primary atrial septal defect, coarctation of the aorta, and bicuspid aortic valve), acquired valvular dysfunction (rheumatic heart or collagen vascular disease), and hypertrophic cardiomyopathy.

2. Patients with mitral valve prolapse who have prolapsing and leaking valves, evidenced by audible clicks and murmurs of mitral regurgitation or by Doppler-demonstrated mitral insufficiency, should receive prophylactic antibiotics. Men older than 45 years with mitral valve prolapse, without a consistent systolic murmur, may warrant prophylaxis. Patients with thickened mitral valve leaflets on echocardiogram need antibiotic prophylaxis.

3. Patients at negligible risk and not needing antibiotic prophylaxis include those with isolated secundum atrial septal defect, surgically repaired congenital heart lesions (atrial septal defect, ventricular septal defect, or patent ductus arteriosus without residua beyond 6 months), previous coronary artery bypass graft surgery, mitral valve prolapse without valvular regurgitation, previous Kawasaki disease without valvular dysfunction, and previous rheumatic fever without valvular dysfunction.

4. Additional strategies to prevent infective endocarditis include brushing teeth, using oral antiseptics, providing atraumatic care for acneiform pustules, avoiding nail biting, and paying close attention to gum and tooth care.

5. The specific antibiotic prophylaxis guidelines in Tables 109–2 and 109–3 were designed to improve practitioner and patient compliance, reduce cost and potential gastrointestinal adverse effects, and lessen risk of increasing bacterial resistance.

V. Neural tube defects

A. Studies reveal that 20% of women whose pregnancies ended in miscarriages and up to 30% of women with recurrent miscarriages had an inadequate folate level. Several studies suggest that consumption of folic acid decreases the incidence

TABLE 109–2. PROPHYLACTIC REGIMENS FOR DENTAL, ORAL, RESPIRATORY TRACT, OR ESOPHAGEAL PROCEDURES

Situation	Agent	Regimen[1]
Standard general prophylaxis	Amoxicillin	Adults: 2.0 g; children: 50 mg/kg orally 1 h before procedure
Unable to take oral medications	Ampicillin	Adults: 2.0 g IM or IV; children: 50 mg/kg IM or IV within 30 min before procedure
Allergic to penicillin	Clindamycin *or*	Adults: 600 mg; children: 20 mg/kg orally 1 h before procedure
	Cephalexin[2] or cefadroxil[2] *or*	Adults: 2.0 g; children: 50 mg/kg orally 1 h before procedure
	Azithromycin or clarithomycin	Adults: 500 mg; children: 15 mg/kg orally 1 h before procedure
	Clindamycin *or*	Adults: 600 mg; children: 20 mg/kg IV within 30 min before procedure
Allergic to penicillin and unable to take oral medications	Cephazolin[2]	Adults: 1.0 g; children: 25 mg/kg IM or IV within 30 min before procedure

[1] Total children's dose should not exceed adult dose.

[2] Cephalosporins should not be used in individuals with immediate-type hypersensitivity reaction (urticaria, angioedema, or anaphylaxis) to penicillins.

IM, Intramuscular; IV, intravenous.

Reprinted from Dajani et al: Prevention of bacterial endocarditis. CID 1997;**25**:1454.

TABLE 109-3. PROPHYLACTIC REGIMENS FOR GENITOURINARY OR GASTROINTESTINAL (EXCLUDING ESOPHAGEAL) PROCEDURES

Situation	Agents[1]	Regimen[2]
High-risk patients	Ampicillin plus gentamicin	Adults: ampicillin 2.0 g IM or IV plus gentamicin 1.5 mg/kg (not to exceed 120 mg) within 30 min of starting the procedure; 6 h later, ampicillin 1 g IM/IV or amoxicillin 1 g orally Children: ampicillin 50 mg/kg IM or IV (not to exceed 2.0 g) plus gentamicin 1.5 mg/kg within 30 min of starting the procedure; 6 h later, ampicillin 25 mg/kg IM/IV or amoxicillin 25 mg/kg orally
High-risk patients allergic to ampicillin/amoxicillin	Vancomycin plus gentamicin	Adults: vancomycin 1.0 g IV over 1–2 h plus gentamicin 1.5 mg/kg IV/IM (not to exceed 120 mg); complete injection/infusion within 30 min of starting the procedure Children: vancomycin 20 mg/kg IV over 1–2 h plus gentamicin 1.5 mg/kg IV/IM; complete injection/infusion within 30 min of starting the procedure
Moderate-risk patients	Amoxicillin or ampicillin	Adults: amoxicillin 2.0 g orally 1 h before procedure; or ampicillin 2.0 g IM/IV within 30 min of starting the procedure Children: amoxicillin 50 mg/kg orally 1 h before procedure, or ampicillin 50 mg/kg IM/IV within 30 min of starting the procedure
Moderate-risk patients allergic to ampicillin/amoxicillin	Vancomycin	Adults: vancomycin 1.0 g IV over 1–2 h; complete infusion within 30 min of starting the procedure Children: vancomycin 20 mg/kg IV over 1–2 h; complete infusion within 30 min of starting the procedure

[1] Total children's dose should not exceed adult dose.
[2] No second dose of vancomycin or gentamicin is recommended.
Reprinted from Dajani et al: Prevention of bacterial endocarditis. CID 1997;**25**:1455.

of neural tube defects in the fetuses of pregnant women. These studies include trials of folate supplementation, dietary consumption of folate, and folate concentrations in serum and red blood cells.

B. Folic acid supplementation can prevent approximately 70% of neural tube defects by correcting abnormal homocysteine metabolism. Research interest is centered on enzymes of folate metabolism that are involved in the production or degradation of homocysteine.

C. The Food and Nutrition Board of the Institute of Medicine recommends that all women of childbearing age capable of becoming pregnant consume 0.4 mg of folic acid per day. All women should consume 0.6 mg of folate per day during pregnancy and 0.5 mg of folate per day during lactation. Women who have delivered a child with a neural tube defect should consume 4 mg of folate 1 month prior to conception and for the first 3 months of pregnancy. The minimal effective folate dose is unknown.

D. The Food and Drug Administration decided in 1993 to fortify staple foods by adding 1.4 mg folic acid/kg of cereal grain. Folic acid consumption may mask the hematologic manifestations of pernicious anemia in the elderly. Folate doses should be kept under 1 mg/day in those with low vitamin B_{12} levels, particularly those with achlorhydria and gastric atrophy lacking intrinsic factor.

E. Moderate increases in folate supply should also lower serum homocysteine in patients heterozygous for the gene for homocystinuria. Elevated homocysteine levels appear to be a strong independent risk factor for coronary vascular disease.

VI. Rheumatic fever

A. Rheumatic fever is a complication of group A β-hemolytic streptococcal infection of the upper respiratory tract that is most frequently observed in children 5–13 years of age.

B. Diagnosis is based on meeting the Jones criteria: two major criteria or one major and two minor criteria plus evidence of a preceding streptococcal infection (Table 109–4).

C. Prophylaxis

    1. Antibiotic regimens used to prevent recurrences of acute rheumatic fever are inadequate for prevention of bacterial endocarditis.

    2. Continuous antimicrobial prophylaxis provides effective protection from rheumatic fever recurrences.

        a. Patients who have had rheumatic fever with carditis and residual heart disease need prophylaxis for at least 10 years beyond the last episode and until age 40 years or perhaps for life.

        b. Patients who have had rheumatic fever with carditis but without residual heart disease need prophylaxis for at least 10 years since the last episode or well into adulthood, whichever is longer.

        c. Patients who have had rheumatic fever without carditis need prophylaxis for at least 5 years since the last episode or until age 21, whichever is longer.

D. In patients with a previous attack of acute rheumatic fever, secondary prophylaxis is recommended to prevent a recurrence.

    1. The following schedules are effective in preventing colonization or infection of the upper respiratory tract.

        a. Benzathine penicillin G (1,200,000 U intramuscularly every 3–4 weeks).

        b. Penicillin V (250 mg by mouth twice daily).

        c. Sulfadiazine (500 mg/day orally if <60 lbs; 1 g/day orally if >60 lbs).

        d. Erythromycin (250 mg by mouth twice daily).

    2. Although the duration is controversial, secondary prophylaxis should continue for at least 5 years after the most recent attack or until the patient is 18. Others recommend that prophylaxis be extended longer or for life for medical professionals, schoolteachers, those living in overcrowded conditions, and those with significant heart disease.

VII. Travel medicine

A. Definition. Each year, 3–5 million North Americans travel to developing countries, placing themselves at risk for diseases endemic to the areas visited. Travel medicine studies the changing disease patterns and international health requirements for the traveler's protection. It encompasses general preventive anticipatory guidance, immunization updates, chemoprophylaxis consideration, and the diagnosis and treatment of problems developed during travel and upon return to the United States.

B. General considerations

    1. Health requirements are determined from a detailed travel itinerary of the areas to be visited, duration of stay, and medical history. Asymptomatic individuals should be screened at least 6 weeks upon return so that illnesses such as schistosomiasis can be excluded. Routine testing may include stool microscopy, dipstick urinalysis, and complete blood cell count.

    2. Vaccinations required for entry into a country and those recommended because a disease is endemic to the country of destination should be obtained (Table 109–5).

TABLE 109–4. RHEUMATIC FEVER: DIAGNOSTIC CRITERIA

Major	Minor
Carditis	Prolonged PR interval on electrocardiography
Migratory polyarthritis	Arthralgia
Chorea	Fever
Erythema marginatum	Previous rheumatic fever
Subcutaneous nodules	Elevated acute phase reactants (erythrocyte sedimentation rate of C-reactive protein)

TABLE 109–5. IMMUNIZATIONS FOR FOREIGN TRAVEL

Vaccine	Schedule	Precautions/Indications	Contraindications
Toxoids			
Tetanus–diphtheria	Primary: two doses (0.5 mL) IM 4–8 weeks apart; third dose 6–12 mo later; booster every 10 yrs	All adults	First-trimester pregnancy Hypersensitivity or neurologic reaction to previous doses Severe local reaction
Inactivated bacterial vaccines			
Haemophilus influenzae type b (HbOC)	Primary: three doses (0.5 mL) IM at 2-mo intervals Booster: one dose at 2-mo interval	Children 2 mo of age	Hypersensitivity to vaccine components
Haemophilus influenzae type b (PRP-OMP)	Primary: two doses at 2-mo intervals Booster: one dose 12 mo	Children 2 mo of age	Hypersensitivity to vaccine components
Haemophilus influenzae type b (PRP-D)	Primary: one dose (0.5 mL) IM Booster: none	Children 15 mo to 5 yrs	Hypersensitivity to vaccine components
Streptococcus pneumoniae (23 serotypes)	Primary: one dose (0.5 mL) SC or IM Booster: only for high-risk patients	Those 2 yrs or older at risk and those healthy over 65 yrs Asplenia	Safety in pregnancy unknown Prior vaccination
Neisseria meningitidis (A,C,Y,W-135 serotypes)	Primary: one dose (0.5 mL) SC Booster: not recommended		Safety in pregnancy unknown
Typhoid (heat-phenol-inactivated)	Primary: two doses (0.5 mL) SC given 4 or more weeks apart Booster: 0.5 ml SC or 0.1 mL ID every 3 yrs	Travel to epidemic areas Travel to high-risk areas Exposure to contaminated food/water in high-risk areas	Severe local reaction lasting 1–2 d Acetone-killed vaccines not given Avoid pregnancy
Oral live-attenuated Ty21a	Primary: one capsule every other day for 4 doses Booster: every 5 years	Exposure to contaminated food/water in high-risk areas	Not recommended for children <6 Immunocompromised host Avoid in pregnancy Avoid antibiotics
Live-attenuated oral typhoid	Single capsule without food every other day for 4 doses before departure		Avoid antibiotics
Purified Capsular Polysaccharide Typhoid (ViCPS)	Primary: one dose (0.5 mL) IM 2 weeks before departure in adults and children Booster: every 2 yrs	Exposure to contaminated food/water in high-risk areas Not in those >2 yrs	May cause paralytic poliomyelitis in unimmunized adults Avoid in pregnancy
Attenuated live virus vaccines			
Measles	Primary: one dose (0.5 mL) SC unless already immune Booster: none	Born after 1956 and has not received two doses of vaccine or had documented measles	Pregnancy Immunocompromised host Anaphylaxis to eggs or neomycin Do not administer with immune globulin
Mumps	Primary: one dose (0.5 mL) SC Booster: none	Born after 1956 and has not had *documented* mumps	Same as for measles

(continued)

703

TABLE 109–5. (Continued)

Vaccine	Schedule	Precautions/Indications	Contraindications
Poliomyelitis (OPV)	Primary: three oral doses, first two given at 6- to 8-week intervals; third 8–2 mos later Booster: one oral dose	Patients <18 yrs. Boost only if previously immunized	Immunocompromised host or in contact with same
(IPV)	Primary: in unimmunized adults two doses (0.5 mL) SQ 4–8 weeks apart, then a third dose preferably 6–12 mos Booster: one OPV or IPV dose		
Rubella	Primary: one dose (0.5 mL) SC Booster: none	All persons	Pregnancy Immunocompromised host Anaphylaxis to neomycin Do not administer with immune globulin
Yellow fever	Primary: one dose (0.5 mL) SC, 10 days prior to travel Booster: every 10 yrs	Required by country	Avoid in pregnancy Prudent to avoid vaccinating infant <9 mos Immunocompromised host Hypersensitivity to eggs Do not administer with cholera vaccine
Inactivated virus vaccines			
Hepatitis B	Primary: three doses (1.0 mL) IM in deltoid at 0, 1, 6, 6–8 mos Booster: not recommended	Health care workers In high-risk area for >6 mo Blood or body fluid contact	
Influenza	Annually	Patients ≥6 mo old at increased risk of complications of disease Healthy adults ≥65 yrs Medical care workers	First-trimester pregnancy Anaphylaxis to eggs
Japanese B encephalitis	Primary: one dose (1.0 mL) SQ on 5 days 0, 7, and 30 in 3 yrs old and over Booster: 1.0 mL SQ 3 yrs later	Areas of risk with rural exposure	Pregnancy Allergy to mice or rodents Immunocompromised host
Rabies	Pre-exposure: 1 mL IM in deltoid or 0.1 mL ID on days 0, 7, and 21 or 28 Booster: 1.0 mL IM or 0.1 mL ID, depending on risk category and serologic testing	Risk area for >1 mo	Allergy to components Complete ID route ≥30 days before travel Do not use ID route with chloroquine or mefloquine administration Effective antibody levels persist 5–10 yrs
Hepatitis A Havrix	Primary: in adults 1.0 mL IM, in children 2–18 yrs 0.5 mL IM Booster at 6–12 mos	Travel to high-risk area	Antibody response may be delayed 4 weeks Hypersensitivity to vaccine component
VAQTA	Primary: in adults, 1 mL IM, in children 2–17 yrs 0.5 mL Booster: at 6–18 mos		
Passive prophylaxis			
Immune globulin	Travel <3 mo duration; 0.02 mL/kg Travel >3 mo: 0.06 mL/kg every 4–6 mo	Prevention of hepatitis A	

3. Anticipatory guidance should cover protection against mosquitoes and other arthropod vectors, risks from food and drink, and environmental effects.

4. Patients taking prescription medications should carry an adequate supply in their original containers to avoid customs delays.

5. Patients with severe allergies to insect stings should take along an epinephrine injection kit.

6. Individuals with medical problems should take along a physician's letter providing a medical summary, a copy of their electrocardiogram, and the phone number of their primary care physician.

7. Reliable sources for travel information include the Centers for Disease Control and Prevention (CDC) (www.cdc.gov/travel) and the World Health Organization (www.who.ch/programmes/ctd).

C. General anticipatory guidance

1. Mosquitoes and other arthropod vectors
   a. Wear long-sleeved, light-colored shirts and trousers.
   b. Apply insect repellents containing no more than 30% *N*,N-diethyl-*m*-toluamide (DEET) to exposed skin and sleeve and trouser cuffs during the mosquito-biting period. Spray aerosolized insecticides in living and sleeping quarters at dusk. Sleep in a screened or air-conditioned room. If outdoors, use small mesh bed netting without defects, impregnated with permethrin. Use of mosquito nets reduced the mosquito attack rate to 97% compared to 77% for patients using chemoprophylaxis alone.
   c. Tick or mite bites are avoided by tucking pants into socks and wearing boots. Permethrin-based insecticides add protection.

2. **Food and drink precautions**
   a. Travelers should avoid nonchlorinated tap water, even for brushing teeth. Since ice is made frequently from contaminated water or chipped from a large exposed block, its use should be avoided. Alcoholic beverages will not purify contaminated ice. Unpasteurized milk and dairy products should be considered contaminated.
   b. Travelers can drink beer, wine, canned or bottled water, and carbonated beverages if the seal is unbroken. The tops of cans and bottles should be dried before opening. Beverages such as powdered drinks and coffee or tea should be made with boiled water.
   c. Travelers should avoid raw fruits and vegetables unless they peel them themselves. Lettuce and other leafy vegetables, cut-up fruit salad, raw or rare meat and fish, and meat or shellfish not served hot may be contaminated. Foods not cooked to a temperature of 70.4 °C (160 °F) and those purchased from street vendors are not safe. Exercise caution regarding airline food prepared in underdeveloped countries.
   d. Dry items such as bread and hyperosmolar items such as jellies and highly acidic citrus fruits are probably safe.
   e. Avoidance of sexual contact with indigenous people and the use of barrier contraceptive measures will protect patients from hepatitis and sexually transmitted diseases.

3. **Environmental precautions**
   a. Travelers must dress appropriately for the weather and avoid excessive sunlight. Lighter-skinned patients or those traveling at high altitudes need to use topical skin protection.
   b. Travelers should take an extra pair of reading glasses and should wear sunglasses when necessary.

4. **Wear seat belts**

D. Vaccinations

1. For unavoidable exposure to poor sanitary conditions of more than 2–3 weeks, vaccines can be administered (Table 109–5).

2. Most vaccines are contraindicated in pregnant women and the immunocompromised host. Pneumococcal and meningococcal vaccines may be given to the high-risk pregnant woman, but their safety has not been documented. Vaccinations during the first trimester are best avoided. Many countries require HIV testing for long-term travelers prior to entry, and many diseases prevalent in the developing world may manifest severe or prolonged clinical courses in HIV-positive patients. Determination of the CD4 lymphocyte count prior to vaccine administration may predict vaccine risk and therapeutic benefit.

3. Physicians can obtain current information concerning immunization requirements and disease prevalence by contacting the state health department or the CDC. Up-to-date automated information is available from the CDC at 1-888-232-3228 or on the Internet (www.cdc.gov). Another excellent source of information on disease prevalence is calling physicians or health care resources in the country to be visited.

E. Travelers' diarrhea

1. *Travelers' diarrhea* refers to disease acquired when a person goes from an industrialized country to an undeveloped area. The disease consists of passing three or more stools in a 24-hour period, accompanied by at least one of the following symptoms: nausea, vomiting, cramps, fever, fecal urgency, tenesmus, or the passage of bloody, mucoid stools. Travelers' diarrhea generally lasts 3–5 days.

2. Bacterial enteropathogens, in order of frequency, include *Escherichia coli, Shigella* spp, *Clostridium jejuni, Aeromonas* spp, *Plesiomonas shigelloides, Salmonella* spp, and noncholera vibrios. Rotavirus and Norwalk virus may account for up to 10% of cases acquired in Mexico. Uncommon causes include *Giardia* spp, *Cryptosporidium* spp, and *Entamoeba histolytica*. Noninfectious causes include tropical sprue, celiac disease, inflammatory bowel disease, transient lactose intolerance, irritable bowel syndrome, and the chronic use of medications such as magnesium-containing antacids. Alcohol consumption, stress, menstruation, and dietary change account for a portion of the mild cases.

3. Dietary precautions are the first choice in prevention of traveler's diarrhea. If the physician and the patient decide on chemoprophylaxis, the following regimens are available.

a. *Lactobacillus* preparation, which metabolizes carbohydrate in the gut, reduces intraluminal pH and inhibits the growth of enteropathogen by producing lactic and organic acids. Protective efficacy ranges from 0% to 14%.

b. Bismuth subsalicylate, taken as two tablets with meals and at bedtime, has a protection efficacy of 62–65%. Bismuth subsalicylate should not be taken by pregnant patients or those taking aspirin or anticoagulant therapy.

c. Although several antibiotics can prevent traveler's diarrhea, many consultants prescribe medication and instruct the patient to begin treatment promptly when symptoms occur. Immunocompromised patients, those with medical illnesses in whom an episode of diarrhea may cause decompensation, and those with decreased gastric acid should be considered for prophylactic antibiotics. In prescribing medications, physicians should consider the range of antibiotic side effects, and that antibiotic use may enhance antibiotic resistance among likely pathogens, facilitate the onset of *Clostridium difficile* colitis by disturbing normal flora, or promote the acquisition and virulence of *salmonella* or *Campylobacter* organisms. Effective agents include ciprofloxacin (500 mg once daily), levofloxacin (500 mg once daily), ofloxacin (300 mg once daily), or norfloxacin (400 mg once daily) for a maximum of 3 weeks.

4. Travelers' diarrhea can be treated by oral loperamide (4-mg loading dose, then 2 mg after each loose stool up to a maximum of 10 mg/day for adults) and an oral antibiotic. A single dose of ciprofloxacin (750 mg), levofloxacin (500 mg), or ofloxacin (400 mg) usually relieves diarrheal symptoms in less than 24 hours. In the case of severe diarrhea, high fever, or bloody stools, use ciprofloxacin (500 mg twice daily) or ofloxacin (300 mg twice daily) for 3 days in adults.

5. Oral rehydration solutions containing 2.5% glucose and salt are optimal as fluid replacement for dehydration caused by travelers' diarrhea. In these solutions, glucose facilitates water absorption and sodium couples with glucose absorption. The cereal-based preparations provide four times more calories and may decrease stool volume and diarrhea duration. Travelers may prepare their own solutions (Table 109–6).

F. Malaria chemoprophylaxis

1. Malaria is transmitted by infected female mosquitoes of the *Anopheles* genus. *Plasmodium falciparum* may cause kidney failure, coma, and death. *P vivax, P ovale,* and *P malaria* produce a milder illness consisting of fever and flu-

TABLE 109–6. HOW TO USE ORAL REHYDRATION SOLUTIONS

If you have more than 3–4 episodes of diarrhea per day, you may be in danger of becoming dehydrated. In this situation, you should seek medical attention, or take the medication your physician has already provided to stop the diarrhea. In addition, you should replenish your body fluids by drinking an oral rehydration solution, which you can buy ready-made or prepare yourself.

Cereal-Based Recipe (preferred)	Glucose-Based Recipe (use if rice cereal is not available)
1–2 cups rice cereal for infants (eg, Gerber) 4 cups clean water (boiled or chemically purified) ½ teaspoon table salt Mix salt and water in a clean container. Gradually stir in rice cereal.	4½ cups clean water (boiled or chemically purified) ¼ teaspoon salt substitute that contains potassium ½ teaspoon baking soda ½ teaspoon table salt (increase to 1 teaspoon if the salt substitute and baking soda are not available) 2–3 tablespoons glucose (table sugar, honey, or corn syrup) Mix all the ingredients together in a clean container.

With either recipe, you may need to drink up to 3–6 quarts over 2–4 hours to counteract dehydration. Be sure to drink 8–12 ounces after each watery stool. If you are nauseated, begin with 1-ounce sips every 5–10 minutes, and increase the amount as tolerated.
Reprinted from Clev Clin J Med 1997;**64**(9):485.

like symptoms, which may occur at intervals. *P vivax* and *P ovale* may remain dormant in the liver and cause relapses weeks, months, or even years after the initial infection.

2. The risk of malaria varies by season and region of the country visited. Malarial risk is greatest from dusk to dawn in rural areas. The risk is high for travelers to sub-Saharan Africa, Papua New Guinea, the Solomon Islands and Vanuatu; intermediate on the Indian subcontinent and in Haiti; and low in Southeast Asia and Latin America. Most capital cities of the Far East and South America and frequently visited tourist attractions are malaria free.

3. Chloroquine-resistant *P falciparum* malaria is present in most malaria-endemic countries except Haiti, the Dominican Republic, Central America west of the Panama Canal, Iran, Yemen, Oman, and Saudi Arabia. Chloroquine-resistant *P vivax* is present in Indonesia, Papua New Guinea, the Solomon Islands, and Myanmar.

4. No chemoprophylaxis regimen is completely effective because of drug resistance. Malaria chemoprophylaxis preferably begins 1–2 weeks before traveling to malarious areas and continues during travel in the malarious area and for 4 weeks after leaving the region. Daily doxycycline therapy begins 2 days before traveling and continues for 4 weeks after return. For chloroquine-resistant *P falciparum* areas, mefloquine alone is recommended. Chloroquine, once weekly, is recommended in chloroquine-sensitive *P falciparum* areas. Travelers with prolonged exposure to *P vivax* or *P ovale* malaria areas should take primaquine during their last 2 weeks of prophylaxis. However, caution should be exercised in glucose-6-phosphate dehydrogenase–deficient individuals. Table 109–7 outlines chemoprophylaxis regimens.

5. Current information on malaria prevalence and chemoprophylaxis can be obtained by calling the Malaria Branch of the CDC at (770) 488-7788.

VIII. **Complementary or alternative medicine**
   A. **General**
      1. Complementary or alternative medicine (CAM) is defined as those healing techniques that typically fall outside the Western biomedical model of disease, diagnosis, and treatment. The Office of Alternative Medicine of the National Institutes of Health classifies alternative therapies into the following broad categories: (1) mind–body interventions, (2) bioelectromagnetic therapies, (3) alternative systems of medical practice, (4) manual healing methods, (5) pharmacologic and biologic treatments, (6) herbal medicine, and (7) diet and nutrition.

   In 1993 one-third of Americans sought treatment for medical problems outside of conventional medicine. Patients with cancer (54%), HIV (44%), back

TABLE 109–7. CHEMOPROPHYLAXIS REGIMENS AGAINST MALARIA

Drug	Dosage		Efficacy (%)[1]
	Adult	Child	
Mefloquine	228 mg base (250 mg of salt)	15–19 kg: ¼ tablet per week 20–30 kg: ½ tablet per week 31–45 kg: ¾ tablet per week >45 kg: 1 tablet per week	90–100
Doxycycline	100 mg	>8 yr: 2 mg/kg up to 100 mg/day	64–97
Chloroquine phosphate	300 mg base (500 mg of salt)	5 mg/kg base (8.3 mg/kg salt) up to 300 mg base	10
Proquanil	200 mg combined with chloroquine	>2 yr: 50 mg/day 2–6 yr: 100 mg/day 7–10 yr: 150 mg/day >10 yr: 200 mg/day	54–72
Primaquine	15 mg base (26.3 mg of salt) daily for 14 days	0.3 mg/kg base (0.5 mg/kg salt)	

[1] Percentage reduction in risk in users compared with that in nonusers.

pain (36%), and those afflicted with rheumatologic disease frequently seek alternative medicine therapies. Each year $14 billion is spent on alternative medicines. Patients in the United States seek medical advice more frequently from alternative health care providers than their primary care physicians.

B. Manipulative treatment may be classified as soft tissue techniques, articulatory techniques, or direct and indirect methods of joint mobilization.

  1. General

    a. Soft tissue procedures that apply force directly to a specific tissue of the musculoskeletal system are massage, effleurage, kneading, stretching, and friction rub. Indirect soft tissue techniques use reflex mechanisms (Chapman's reflexes, Travell's trigger points, etc) to stimulate the peripheral tissues of the musculoskeletal system.

    b. Articulatory procedures put elements of the musculoskeletal system (particularly articulations) through ranges of motion in a graded fashion to enhance the quantity and quality of motion.

    c. Specific joint mobilization procedures incorporate the method with an intrinsic or extrinsic force. The direct method applies force to move the restricted joint articulation closer to its normal physiologic soft tissue limits. The exaggerated method applies the force against the normal soft tissue limiting barrier in the direction opposite the motion loss. This force is usually a high-velocity, low-amplitude thrust. The indirect method moves the musculoskeletal segment away from the restrictive barrier and holds it there for up to 90 seconds to relax the tissues around the articulation to enhance mobility. Extrinsic forces are operator effort, gravity, and adjuncts such as straps or traction. Intrinsic forces are physiologic mechanisms arising from the patient such as respirations, muscle energy, and reflex activity.

    d. Although most of these methods lack controlled studies establishing their therapeutic value, their usage results in predictable physiologic responses and patient perception of benefit. Since spinal manipulation is used frequently, its efficacy and contraindications will be discussed more fully.

  2. Spinal manipulation

    a. Definition

      (1) Spinal manipulation is the use of a short- or long-lever high-velocity thrust directed to one or more joints beyond its restricted range of motion.

      (2) Spinal mobilization involves low-velocity, passive movements within or at the limit of joint range.

b. Efficacy

    (1) Randomized clinical trials have not demonstrated the efficacy of spinal manipulation for patients with acute or chronic low back pain. However, spinal manipulation had similar effects and costs to those of the McKenzie method of physical therapy for patients with acute low back pain. Both methods only had marginally better outcomes than in those receiving an educational booklet.

    (2) Randomized controlled trials reveal short-term benefit for cervical mobilization for acute neck pain.

    (3) Spinal manipulation for patients with subacute or chronic neck pain showed improvement at 3 weeks in randomized controlled trials compared with muscle relaxants or usual care.

    (4) Spinal manipulation in a randomized controlled trial provided short-term relief for patients with tension-type headache.

c. Contraindications for spinal manipulation

    (1) Absolute contraindications for spinal manipulation include acute arthropathies, acute fractures and dislocations, signs of ligamentous rupture or instability, bone malignancies and metastases, infections of bone and joints, acute myelopathy, and cauda equina syndrome.

    (2) Relative contraindications for spinal manipulation include spondylolisthesis with progressive slippage, articular hypermobility, post-surgical joints, acute soft tissue injuries, osteoporosis, benign bone tumors, clinical manifestations of vertebrobasilar insufficiency, aneurysm, anticoagulant therapy, and blood dyscrasias.

    (3) Contraindications are probable in patients whose age is greater than 50 and in patients with history of significant trauma, fever greater than 100 °F, prolonged use of corticosteroids, unexplained weight loss, history of cancer, adenopathy, history of serious systemic inflammatory arthritides or vasculitides, endocrinopathies affecting calcium metabolism, and presence of a neurologic deficit.

d. Complications of spinal manipulation are not well documented in the literature. Major complications in order of frequency are vertebrobasilar vascular accidents, disk herniation or progression to cauda equina syndrome, and other cerebral complications.

C. Acupuncture

    1. Acupuncture is part of traditional Chinese medicine in which the patient is viewed holistically without separation of mind and body. When the human body is in balance, the flow of vital energy (Qi) necessary for maintenance and nourishment of the organs and associated tissues is unobstructed. The energy flows through several sets of imaginary lines (meridians) that run longitudinally in and around the body. The set of lines is related functionally to a yin and corresponding yang organ.

    a. Types

        (1) Traditional Chinese medicine describes over 1000 acupuncture points, most of which are located along 12 paired and 2 unpaired meridians, or channels. Over 50% of these points are located directly above major nerve trunks. Traditional acupuncture attempts to maintain a balanced energy state and uses classical needle points. Similar diagnoses in two different patients may require using different classical points based on the unique constitution of the patient. The patient's pulse, color, and nature of the tongue and complexion are evaluated prior to selection of needle points to be used at each visit.

        (2) Formula acupuncture places needles at a predefined set of classic points according to a defined pathologic diagnosis.

        (3) Needles may be inserted along or around symptomatic areas. Classical needle points are not used.

        (4) In 1950 auriculotherapy was developed from observations that areas of tenderness or increased electrical activity in the ear may correspond to areas of body dysfunction. Auriculotherapy may be combined with body acupuncture.

        (5) Acupuncture combines the use of acupuncture needles with low-intensity electric current (electroneedling).

      (6) The available studies on traditional acupuncture and electro-needling therapies reveal positive effects on increasing peripheral hemodynamic functions.

  2. It is believed that acupuncture excites nerve fibers or receptors in the stimulated tissue, which are physiologically activated by strong muscle contraction, whose effects on organ function are similar to those obtained with protracted exercise. Experimental and clinical evidence suggests that acupuncture may affect the sympathetic nervous system at the hypothalamic and brain stem level. The stimulated hypothalamic β-endorphinergic systems may inhibit the vasomotor center. Post-stimulatory sympathetic inhibition is maximized within a few hours and can be sustained for as long as 12 hours.

  3. Controlled studies of patients with nociceptive low back pain, sore throat, tension headache, dental postoperative pain, rheumatoid arthritis, osteoarthritis, and neck pain reveal a 50–80% therapeutic response ranging from 2 weeks to 4 months. Although it is hard to find scientific proof of the specific effects of acupuncture on any disease, some clinical reports describe it as beneficial in:
    a. Reducing blood pressure with essential hypertension
    b. Reducing the number and frequency of angina pectoris attacks and increasing work capacity
    c. Decreasing the airway resistance in asthmatic patients
    d. Treating patients for opiate dependency and alcohol abuse
    e. Increasing the sense of well-being, calmness, and improved sleep

  4. Complications of acupuncture include technical and medical problems. Technical problems result from bent or broken needles and the inability to remove a needle from the body. Medical problems reported include muscle spasm at the site of needle pique, pneumothorax, vasovagal symptoms, hematoma formation, dermatitis, infection with hepatitis B or HIV, organ damage, and the initiation of premature labor.

D. Herbal medicine
  1. Herbal medicine considers the body to be a series of interconnecting functions and diseases to be imbalance of these functions. Plant extracts are mixtures of different substances that may act in different ways and on different parts of the body. The extract contains substances that may reduce the side effects of the major ingredient or improve its activity by enhancing its bioavailability by reducing its metabolic breakdown, or by synergistic effects. Approximately 80% of the nonindustrialized world relies on plants as the major source of medicines for primary health care. In the United States the sale of natural or herbal products is expected to reach $1.6 billion by 2001.

  2. Guidelines for herbal users
    a. Nursing mothers, pregnant women, infants, and children should use herbal products with caution.
    b. Patients should be encouraged to read labels and purchase only those products that show the scientific name of the herb, the name and address of the manufacturer, a lot number, the date of manufacture, and the product's expiration date.
    c. Patients should be advised to stop the preparation if any type of adverse effect occurs. Herbal medications can lead to hypersensitivity reactions whose manifestations can vary from transient dermatitis to anaphylactic shock. Adverse effects may be related to the desired pharmacologic action or from drug–drug interactions with prescription medications.
    d. Patients should only purchase products that have been standardized for the effect of a given dose.

  3. Contaminants repeatedly found in herbal remedies include aluminum, arsenic, aspirin, cadmium, caffeine, corticosteroids, diazepam, ephedrine, lead, mercury, phenacetin, tin, and zinc.

  4. Table 109–8 lists herbs considered unsafe or otherwise unfit for human consumption.

  5. Some herbs are considered safe/effective by non–United States regulatory authorities. These preparations include chamomile (German) as an anti-inflammatory agent, echinacea as an immunostimulant, garlic for lowering blood lipids, ginger as an antiemetic, and valerian as a minor tranquilizer. Other herbal preparations have been shown beneficial in treating medical problems by clinical research (Table 109–9).

TABLE 109–8. HERBS CONSIDERED UNSAFE OR OTHERWISE UNFIT FOR HUMAN CONSUMPTION

Common Name	Source	Purported Use	Safety/Efficacy/Comments
Borage	*Borago officinalis* leaves and tops	Diuretic, antidiarrheal	Both safety and efficacy are questionable; contains toxic pyrrolizidine alkaloids, including intermedine, lycopsamine, amabiline, and supinine
Calamus	*Acorus calamus* rhizome (underground stem)	Febrifuge, digestive aid	Chemovars (plants that have similar appearances but have different chemical compositions) contain varying amounts of carcinogenic *cis*-isoasarone. Indian type most toxic; North American type is non-toxic; test for *cis*-isoasarone before using
Chaparral	*Larrea tridentata* leaves and twigs	Anticancer	Currently not recommended—no proven efficacy; purported to induce severe liver toxicity, but limited number of cases have been seen, in spite of widespread use; further investigation required
Coltsfoot	*Tussilago farfara* leaves and/or flower heads	Antitussive, demulcent	Effective but unsafe; contains carcinogenic pyrrolizidine alkaloids including senkirkine and senecionine
Comfrey	*Symphytum* species rhizome and roots, leaves	Wound healing	Effective but unsafe for internal use; contains large number of toxic pyrrolizidine alkaloids, which vary according to species
Ephedra (Ma-Huang)	*Ephedra sinica* and related species green stems	Anorectic, bronchodilator	Relatively ineffective as an anorectic; effective for bronchodilation; unsafe for those suffering from hypertension, diabetes, or thyroid disease; avoid consumption with caffeine
Germander	*Teucrium charneedrys* leaves and tops	Anorectic	Unsafe and ineffective; causes hepatotoxicity because of diterpenoid derivatives
Licorice	*Glycyrrhiza glabra* rhizome and roots	Expectorant, antiulcer	Effective, but safe only in small doses for short periods of time (<4 weeks); high doses for long periods cause pseudoaldosteronism (characterized by sodium and water retention and potassium depletion)
Life root	*Senecio aureus* whole plant	Emmenagogue	Unsafe (hepatotoxic) and no proven efficacy, contains toxic pyrrolizidine alkaloids
Pokeroot	*Phytolacca americana* root	Alterative (tonic), antirheumatic, anticancer	Unsafe and ineffective; should not be sold or used; may be fatal in children
Sassafras	*Sassafras albidum* root bark	Stimulant, antispasmodic, antirheumatic, tonic	Unsafe and ineffective; volatile oil contains carcinogenic safrole

Reprinted from J Am Pharm Assoc 1996;**NS36**(1).

TABLE 109–9. HERBAL MEDICATIONS

Name	Scientific Name	Purported Usage	Research[1]	Comment
Aloe vera	*Aloe barbadensis*	Psoriasis	R, DB, PC	Also used for minor burns, abrasions, skin irritation, wound healing, and frostbite injury; latex or juice form as a potent cathartic
Cranberry juice cocktail	*Vaccinium macrocarpon*	Reduces bacteriuria in elderly women	R, DB, PC	≥3 oz/day preventive; 12–32 oz/day treatment of urinary tract infection
Feverfew leaf	*Tanacetum parthenium*	Prophylactic for migraine headaches	P, R, DB, PC	Commercially available tablets may contain little active ingredient. Also used for menstrual irregularities, stomach-ache, fever, and arthritis
Ispaghula husk	*Plantago ovata*	Lowers total and LDL cholesterol	DB, PC	Use only as dietary adjunct; contraindicated in intestinal obstruction and poorly controlled diabetes mellitus. Affects drug absorption up to 60 minutes after taking. May cause diarrhea; take with adequate fluids (150 mL/5 g drug)
Saw palmetto	*Serenoa repens*	Benign prostatic hypertrophy	R, DB	Compared equally with finasteride. Also used as expectorant, sedative, and diuretic
Kava-kava	*Piper methysticum*	Anxiety	R, DB	Reduced Hamilton Anxiety Scale from 25.3 to 12.6
St. John's wort	*Hypericum perforatum*	Depression	DB, PC, R	Warning: Can induce photosensitivity with sunlight exposure and extended use; monoemine oxidase warnings apply; sometimes used as diuretic, for insomnia, anxiety, and gastritis
Holy basil leaves	*Ocimum album/ O. sanctum*	Non–insulin-dependent diabetes mellitus	R, PC, CO, SB	17% reduction fasting glucose, 6.5% total serum cholesterol
Phyllanthus amarus	*Pniuri*	Hepatitis B	R, DB, PC	Loss HBsAg
Terminalia arjuna	*Terminalia arjuna*	NYHA Class IV congestive heart failure	DB, CO	Improved left ventricular ejection and in NYHA class
Ginkgo	*Ginkgo biloba* ext.	Cerebrovascular ischemia	DB, PC, CO	Of concern for patients taking anticoagulants since it reduces clotting time

[1] CO, Crossover; DB, double-blind; P, prospective; PC, placebo-controlled; R, randomized; SB, single-blind.
HBsAg, hepatitis B surface antigen; LDL, low-density lipoprotein; NYHA, New York Heart Association.

REFERENCES

Andersson S, Lundeberg T: Acupuncture: From empiricism to science: Functional background to acupuncture effects in pain and disease. Med Hypotheses 1995;**45**:271.

Churchill OR, Chiodini PL, McAdam KPWJ: Screening the returned traveler. Br Med Bull 1993; **49**:465.

Conlon CP: The immunocompromised traveler. Br Med Bull 1993;**49**:412.

Dajani A, Taubert K, Ferrieri P, et al: Treatment of acute streptococcal pharyngitis and prevention of rheumatic fever: A statement for health professionals. Pediatrics 1995;**96**:758.

Dajani A, Taubert K, Wilson W, et al: Prevention of bacterial endocarditis: Recommendations by the American Heart Association. Circulation 1997;**96**:358.

DeSmet P: The role of plant-derived drugs and herbal medicines in health care. Drugs 1997; **54**:801.

Glynn RJ, et al: Adherence to aspirin in the prevention of myocardial infarction. Arch Intern Med 1994;**154**:2649.

Greenman PE: *Principles of Manual Medicine,* 2nd ed. Williams & Wilkins; 1996.

Hsu D: Acupuncture: A review. Reg Anesth 1996;**21**:361.

Hurwitz E, Aker P, Adams A, et al: Manipulation and mobilization of the cervical spine: A systematic review of the literature. Spine 1996;**21**:1746.

Klein JO: Antimicrobial treatment and prevention of meningitis. Pediatr Ann 1994;**23**:76.

Koes B, Assendelft W, van der Heijden G, et al: Spinal manipulation for low back pain: An updated systematic review of randomized clinical trials. Spine 1996;**21**:2860.

Matcher DB, et al: Guidelines for medical treatment in stroke prevention. Ann Intern Med 1994; **121**:54.

Public Health Service: *Health Information for International Travel.* 1994. HHS publication No. (CDC) 94-8280. US Government Printing Office; 1994. [Telephone: (202) 783-3238]

Rush D: Periconceptional folate and neural tube defect. Am J Clin Nutr 1994;**59**:5115.

US Preventive Services Task Force: *Report of the U.S. Preventive Services Task Force.* Williams & Wilkins; 1996.

SECTION VI. **Special Populations**

110 The Adolescent Patient

William B. Shore, MD

I. **Definition.** Adolescence is the process through which one experiences the transition from dependent child to sexually mature, independent adult. It is during this process that an adolescent can re-experience some or all of the previous developmental stages, especially those that have not been completely resolved in earlier development. Practitioners working with adolescents and their families should use every contact with the adolescents and their parents to promote this developmental process, leaving the adolescent with a high level of self-esteem.

II. **Epidemiology**
   A. **Morbidity** among adolescents is related to sexual activities, accidents, injuries (many of which are associated with drug and alcohol use), and poverty.
      1. In the United States, there are approximately 1 million pregnancies per year, with 500,000 births to girls younger than 20 years old. Twelve percent of outpatient visits by teenagers are for sexually transmitted diseases (STDs). Human immunodeficiency virus (HIV) disease among adolescents represents 0.5% of all HIV cases.
      2. One in five children under age 18 lives in poverty; more than 40% of black children live in poverty. There are an estimated 1 million runaways and homeless youths each year in the United States and 700,000 teenagers institutionalized in juvenile detention facilities for legal offenses, many of whom have serious health problems. Poverty is the single most important factor affecting the health status of adolescents.
      3. One in five adolescents has least one serious health problem. Five percent to 10% of adolescents have a chronic disease or disability, such as asthma, heart disease, vision impairment, or hearing loss; these conditions are severe enough to limit major daily activities in one-half of these youths. Twenty percent to 50% of youths have a wide array of other, less severe medical problems—such as acne, abnormal menstrual bleeding, dental problems, or abnormal breast growth in males—which are often underestimated by parents and health care providers but may cause adolescents significant distress, affecting their psychosocial development and daily functioning. Despite their needs, in one study poor youths were only one-half as likely to identify a source of health care as adolescents of higher socioeconomic status. Overall, adolescents see office-based providers less often than any other age group.
   B. In the United States in 1997, 73% of all deaths among youths and young adults 10–24 years resulted from only four causes: (1) motor vehicle accidents; (2) unintentional injuries; (3) homicides; and (4) suicides. Malignant neoplasms are the fifth leading cause of death; sixth, heart disease; and seventh, HIV disease. Although overall mortality rates have declined in recent years, the decline in deaths from motor vehicle accidents has been offset by an increase in the number of deaths from homicides and suicides.

III. **Adolescent growth and development—puberty**
   A. **Physical development.** Puberty is a period of rapid change that leads to physical and sexual maturation. The physical growth that occurs during puberty is second in magnitude only to that which occurs during infancy; it affects almost every organ system. During late prepuberty, there appears to be a change in the sensitivity to the negative-feedback system of the hypothalamic "gonadostat." In boys, luteinizing hormone causes testicular enlargement and development of the Leydig cells of the testes, which produce testosterone, which, in turn, causes development of the secondary sex characteristics. Follicle-stimulating hormone, which increases significantly in boys during the year before clinical puberty, stimulates development of the seminiferous tubules of the testes, which leads to spermatogenesis and fertility during middle and late adolescence. In girls, these gonadotropins cause ovarian development and increased female secondary sex characteristics, with the

715

exception of pubic and axillary hair, which are dependent on adrenal androgen. Later during puberty, ovulation occurs after a sudden peak of luteinizing hormone.

   1. **Somatic changes.** Endocrine changes are responsible for both the adolescent growth spurt and sex-specific changes in body structure, and partially for the behavioral changes that occur during adolescence. The main growth spurt in girls occurs at about age 11, and about 2 years later in boys. Growth of the spinal column accounts for most of the adolescent growth spurt. This rapid growth rate lasts about 2 years and then, under the control of the increased sex hormones, decelerates to the point of epiphyseal closure and cessation of growth during late adolescence. Girls' earlier sexual maturation and epiphyseal closure usually mean that boys become taller than girls by late adolescence, because boys and late-maturing girls have greater prepubertal heights before their growth spurt. There is an increase in muscle mass, particularly in boys, and a decrease in body subcutaneous fat. Weight more than doubles between ages 10 and 20. Much of the added weight is fat in girls and predominantly muscle and skeletal tissues in boys.
   2. **Sexual maturation.** The Tanner staging system of sexual development describes the progressive growth of breasts in girls, external genitalia in boys, and pubic hair development in both sexes. Tanner stage 1 is prepubertal development in both sexes, with progression to Tanner stages 4 and 5, which is full adult development (Table 110–1).

      Adolescents are continually comparing themselves to their peers and often are concerned about any differences. Temporary breast tenderness and adolescent gynecomastia are frequently the presenting complaints from boys during early adolescence. Boys aged 14–15 may present with worries about being shorter than their peers. Girls often present with concerns about being too tall or about a delay in menarche. Physical examination reveals whether puberty (Tanner stage 2) has begun. If there are indications of delayed (no breast development in girls by age 13, no testicular development in boys by age 13.5) or precocious puberty (breast or pubic hair development in girls before age 8, testicular development in boys before age 9.5), an endocrinologic work-up should be initiated after consideration of the ages of parental pubertal development.

B. **Psychosocial development.** Onset of puberty is associated with a rapid succession of cognitive and psychosocial processes with often complex and simultaneous interactions. Hormonal changes of puberty augment increased bodily response and sensitivity, particularly regarding sexual feelings, which can result in anxiety and concerns about bodily function and physical disorder. Cognitive skills of the youth change dramatically from the rather simple, direct, and concrete way of thinking of the child to the complex, abstracted, conceptualized thinking of the young adult.

   1. **Adolescent developmental tasks**
      a. The overall task for the adolescent is to become an autonomous functioning "other" adult individuated from his or her family of origin.
      b. Acceptance of sexuality (which does not necessitate being sexually active).
      c. Developing future life plans.
      d. Beginning to develop life philosophies. The manner in which the adolescent deals with these developmental tasks is based largely on the quality of previous experiences and relationships. If the child suffered repeated defeats and confusion during middle childhood, the burdens of the adolescent tasks may become problematic. Connectedness with one caring adult, a positive body image, and an absence of concern about abuse or domestic violence can be protective factors for adolescents regardless of race, class, or gender.
   2. **Family life cycle developmental tasks.** Physicians working with families with adolescents must understand family systems as well as family and adolescent developmental tasks. The principal tasks confronting the family with adolescents are the following.
      a. To strike a changing balance between freedom and personal responsibility as adolescents mature and undergo the process of individuation.
      b. To lay the groundwork for parents to grow as individuals with developing interests and careers.

TABLE 110–1. TANNER CLASSIFICATION OF SEXUAL MATURITY STAGES

Stage	Pubic Hair	Breasts	Penis	Testes
Boys				
1	Preadolescent	—	Preadolescent	Preadolescent
2	Sparse, straight, slightly pigmented downy hair at base of penis	—	Slight enlargment	Enlarged scrotum, pink, texture changed with ruggae
3	Darker, begins to curl, coarser; spreads over pubes	—	Longer—maximum growth	Further growth of testes and scrotum
4	Resembles adult type but less in quantity	—	Growth in breadth and development of glans	Larger testes and scrotum; scrotum darker
5	Adult distribution, spread to medial surface of thighs	—	Adult size and shape	Adult size and shape
Girls				
1	Preadolescent	Preadolescent	—	—
2	Sparse, slightly pigmented, straight, at medial border of labia	Breast and papilla elevated as small mound; areolar diameter increased	—	—
3	Darker, beginning to curl, coarser; spreads over pubes	Breast and areola enlarged without contour separation	—	—
4	Resembles adult type but less in quantity— may be full adult in some groups	Projection of areola and papilla form secondary mound	—	—
5	Adult feminine triangle; spread to medial surface of thighs	Mature: nipple only projects; areola part of general breast contour	—	—

Adapted with permission from Tanner JM: *Growth at Adolescence.* Blackwell; 1962:1–39, 156–175.

3. **Approach to families.** Parenting adolescents is the most stressful time of parenting. Prior to the onset of puberty, physicians must clearly lay the groundwork for visits during the adolescent years. Parents and children are informed that issues discussed individually, with either adolescents or parents, are confidential, except in life-threatening situations, and that adolescents may be examined without the parents present. Whenever parents with adolescents are seen, ask about how things are going at home with their adolescents. This provides an opportunity for parents and for primary care physicians to validate those stresses. However, physicians must remain objective, *not* be surrogate parents, and honor the pledge of confidentiality (Table 110–2).

IV. **The clinical interview**
   A. The **adolescent-"friendly" office.** Adolescents often feel increasing distrust of physicians. To minimize this mistrust, beginning with early childhood visits, physicians should begin talking directly to the child and including the child in any health care decisions. Adolescents frequently experience difficulties in accessing medical care. To improve access and compliance, a warm, positive atmosphere must be fostered by the entire staff. Decreased waiting times, flexibility in scheduling and availability, and treating adolescents as young adults with respect for modesty, privacy, honesty, and confidentiality are requisites that apply to the entire office staff.

TABLE 110–2. ADOLESCENT HEALTH CARE MAINTENANCE

Stage	Developmental Milestones		Anticipatory Guidance
Early			
10–12	Sexual maturation stage	Patient:	Confidentiality
F10–13			School performance
M12–14			Family relationships
	Peer relationships		Sexual development
	Increased body awareness		Puberty/reproduction
	Can begin abstract thinking		Safety: vehicles/seat belts/helmets
			Violence: access to weapons/physical or sexual abuse
		Parents:	Confidentiality/billing
			Limit setting (fair rules)
			Review adolescent development
			Weapons at home
Middle			
13–16	Sexual maturation stage	Patient:	Scheduling appointments alone
F13–16			School performance
M14–17			Family relationships
	Independence/dependence issues		Sexual behaviors: partner(s) selection/condoms
	Peer group influence		Contraception/STDs/HIV
	Abstract thinking		Testicular self exam
	Sexual awareness		Safety: vehicles/seat belts/helmets/firearms
			Substance use/abuse
			Peer relationships (best friend, gang membership, spiritual or religious activities)
		Parents:	Increased independence
			Mood swings
			Risk awareness
			Parental involvement in school
			Driving precautions
Late			
16–18	Sexual maturation stage	Patient:	Sexuality
			Peer relationships
	Body image/gender role secured		Future plans
	Planning for future		Safety: vehicles/firearms
	Close friendships		Substance use/abuse
		Parents:	Accept sexuality
			Support individuation

HIV, Human immunodeficiency virus; STDs, sexually transmitted diseases.

    1. Examination rooms for adolescents. Adolescents should not be seen in small examining rooms that are set up for infant and young child examinations. Patient and parent education materials appropriate for adolescents should be available in the waiting and examination rooms.

B. Confidentiality. Physicians must be knowledgeable about current state and federal legal guidelines concerning confidentiality and consent for adolescent patients. The federal government and most states have legislation that gives minors the right to informed consent for treatment in several categories: pregnancy, abortion, contraception, STDs, contagious diseases, sexual abuse, drug and alcohol counseling, mental health, and medical emergencies. Several states have passed legislation that specifically authorizes minors to undergo HIV testing without parental consent. Some states have passed legislation that provides for payment of these "sensitive services" without parental support. Many states have "emancipated" minor laws, including (1) married minors, (2) minors serving in the armed forces, (3) minors emancipated by court decision, and (4) minors who are pregnant, who have full adult rights. In life-threatening situations, information on the minor may be disclosed. In other situations, information concerning mature or emancipated minors must not be disclosed unless the patient consents or information is sought by court order.

C. General guidelines
1. Establish connection and a comfort level with patient.
2. Begin to teach the teen the skills for accessing the medical care system.
3. Regularly address health maintenance with the patient.
4. Identify areas of concern and problems for the adolescent (and the parents).
5. Don't be a parent.
6. Don't be a peer.
7. Be honest.
8. Demonstrate knowledge of adolescent concerns and interests, then discuss them with the adolescent patient in your office.
9. Establish a mechanism for contacting the patient, when necessary, that will maintain confidentiality.
10. Review with the teen how best to reach you and how soon after a message you usually return your calls.
11. Review with the patient how to make appointments in your office.
12. As appropriate, invite the parent back into the examination room after discussing with the teen what you plan to discuss with the parent present.
13. Congratulate the patient on how well the visit went and the parents on how well the teen is doing, and tell them that you enjoyed the opportunity to meet with the teen alone.

D. The interview content. Use of an age-specific questionnaire completed prior to the examination facilitates obtaining a history.
1. If the patient agrees, initially interview the patient and the parent together.
2. Review confidentiality with the patient and the parent together.
3. Review your approach to adolescent care, gradually moving toward individual visits without the parent present.
4. After taking the initial history, escort the parent to the waiting room while the patient is changing into a gown for examination.
5. With the patient alone in the examination room, review confidentiality again.
6. Ask open-ended questions first.
7. Use of a mnemonic, such as HEADSSS, can ensure that all areas are covered.
    Home: "Who is in the family? How is everyone getting along?" "Do you feel safe in your home?"
    Education/employment: Level of education and future plans.—"How are you doing in school?" "What are your future plans?" If out of school, what are they doing?—"Do you work?" "How much?" "What kind of job?"
    Activities: Friends—"Who is your best friend? What do you like doing together?" "Are you involved in organized activities?"
    Drugs/diet: "I know drugs and alcohol are often present at parties and campuses. Are you or any of your friends drinking, using drugs, or smoking cigarettes?" "Do you have any concerns about your weight or diet?"
    Sex: Routinely ask about sexual behaviors in a nonjudgmental way. It sometimes helps to avert direct eye contact momentarily with introduction of

this topic and to review confidentiality. Ask about *partners* (without reference to gender) and about behaviors, not about sexual identities. "Have you ever had sexual relations with another person?" If yes, "With men, women, or both?"

Safety: Ask about access to weapons, exposure to violence, and whether the patient has ever been the victim of physical or sexual abuse.

Suicide: Determine whether there is any personal or family history of suicide, attempts at suicide, or depression or other psychiatric illness.

Conclude by asking whether the patient has any more questions or concerns.

8. Gender-specific questions
  a. Girls. Ask about female reproductive and gynecologic history, menarche, gravidity/parity, and last menstrual period. At menarche, give teenage girls a menstrual calendar; it may provide useful information at a later visit and may serve to reinforce the concept of normal physiology and the idea of self-responsibility for health.
  b. Boys. Ask about ejaculation or nocturnal emission—significant normal events but too often not discussed—as well as whether they have fathered any children; if so, ascertain their relationship with the child.

V. The physical examination. Teenagers require reassurance that they are normal as they pass through puberty. The physical examination of the early adolescent may be thought of as a "guided tour" of the teenager's new body and as an important opportunity to normalize the newness and to discuss issues without parents being present.

A. The **pelvic examination** should become a routine event for all young women at the onset of sexual intercourse. The frequency with which it is repeated depends on whether sexual activity continues, parity, how high risk the pattern of sexual activity is (multiple partners or partners with multiple partners), and whether STDs are found. The first internal pelvic examination is a psychologically significant event for a young woman. When done at the right time in the right way, it can foster a sense of self-understanding and self-esteem and a positive attitude about future pelvic examinations. If the examination is physically or psychologically traumatic, it can have a detrimental effect.
  1. Allot adequate time for the first pelvic examination. Prior to the examination, charts or models that illustrate pelvic anatomy may be shown, and the young woman may hold or see the speculum.
  2. Err on the side of overdraping the adolescent.
  3. Explicitly mention each body part examined: "Now I'm examining your [vulva, vagina, cervix, etc] and it [looks/feels] healthy and normal."
  4. Assess the size of the introitus (for speculum size and the position of the cervix) by inserting a gloved finger prior to the speculum examination.
  5. Use lubricant when a first examination is difficult because of patient anxiety. Although lubricant may interfere with the Pap smear specimen, the natural history of cervical cancer is such that the risks of a traumatic first pelvic examination outweigh the risk of failing to detect cervical cancer in a nonsmoking, nulliparous teen without a history of STDs.

B. The male genital examination
  1. Before beginning the physical examination, explain the genital and hernia examination and the possibility of the patient's having an erection.
  2. If an erection occurs, reassure the patient that it is a normal reaction to the examination.
  3. Review the need for boys to wear an athletic supporter when engaged in contact sports.
  4. Educate boys who have reached Tanner stage 4 on how to do testicular self-examinations.

VI. Sexual concerns. An essential part of the development tasks of identity formation and self-esteem is the acceptance of one's sexuality and acquiring the capacity for mature intimacy. *Gender identity* is defined as the way people feel about their individuality as male or female beings. It begins at birth and is well established by age 18 months. By age 3, children are well aware of their gender roles, public expressions of their gender identities, but the child is not always ready and prepared for the biologic events of the "normative crisis" of puberty.

The pubertal hormones are only biologic catalysts for emerging sexual feelings and behaviors that are shaped by socioeconomic, cultural, and religious backgrounds of the adolescents. Society changes its expectations of the child at puberty. These expectations become incorporated into the self-image and reinforce social–sexual consequences of pubertal development. A 12-year-old girl who has completed her pubertal development and looks like an adult is often incorrectly expected to act as an adult. Parents, teachers, and physicians can play key roles in helping adolescents establish their standards regarding sexual behaviors and validate and normalize their sexual feelings.

A. Sexual behavior during adolescence does not depend on reproduction but is geared to the experience of pleasure and satisfaction of a sexual need. With the development of reasoning and abstract thinking, adolescents can begin to take more responsibility for their sexual behavior.

As during preadolescence, significant early adolescent peer relationships are usually with the same sex. Boys' and girls' homosexual contact peaks between ages 11 and 15; for most, it seems to be a test of one's emerging sexual identity. For two-thirds of boys, the first ejaculation is with masturbation. Nocturnal emissions usually occur a year after ejaculatory ability has been achieved. Physicians should normalize masturbation for both boys and girls.

Middle adolescence can be the time for beginning sexual relationships and experimentation, often as part of the search for identity toward development of the capacity for intimate relationships. Sexual behaviors among metropolitan teenagers in the United States shows that 50% of teenage girls aged 15–19 and 70% of boys 17–21 experience premarital intercourse. The average age at first intercourse is 16.2 years for teenage girls and 15.7 years for teenage boys. Among currently sexually active high school students, about 57% report condom use. Physicians should also regularly discuss the option of delaying the onset of sexual intercourse and making responsible decisions about sexual behaviors.

B. Sexual orientation. Physicians can play a significant role in helping adolescents and their families cope with concerns about sexual orientation. Physicians must help validate and normalize these feelings, provide factual information about the spectrum of sexual orientation, leave options about sexual preferences open, and destroy myths about homosexuality. The most important role for the physician is to help the adolescent develop a positive self-concept and genuine capacity for intimacy, irrespective of sexual orientation. Psychotherapy is indicated only when there are excessive and persistent concerns about sexual orientation.

C. Teenage pregnancy. Approximately 40% of teen pregnancies are terminated by abortion, and 47% result in live births. Only 4% of unmarried teenage mothers place their babies for adoption; most infants remain with their birth mothers.

    1. Presentation. A teenager who fears she is pregnant may present with multiple vague somatic complaints. As most teen pregnancies are unplanned and unexpected, the physician must discuss the diagnosis of pregnancy in the context of options available. If the pregnancy is still in the first trimester, discuss all options equally: (1) continuing the pregnancy to keep the baby or to place the baby for adoption or (2) terminating the pregnancy. Give the adolescent time and support to work through these difficult decisions. Encourage the young woman's partner and family to participate in these decisions and in prenatal care. Be supportive and nonjudgmental of any decision the young woman and her partner make. These decisions are often mixed with ambivalence and may change during the decision-making process.

    2. Prenatal care. Pregnant adolescents are at high medical risk because they are less likely to receive early prenatal care. In the highest risk group, under 15, with about 30,000 births per year, the first prenatal visit occurs during the first trimester less than 60% of the time. This late prenatal care results in higher rates of low-birth-weight babies, prematurity, increased rates of perinatal or late fetal mortality, lower Apgar scores and birth weights, toxemia, and anemia. These poor outcomes may be more related to lower socioeconomic status than to biology. Pregnant teens need early and frequent prenatal care, with a multidisciplinary team approach to address nutritional, psychosocial, medical, and educational needs. Inclusion of the father of the baby in prenatal care and labor and delivery can result in better outcomes and sets the stage for the father's continued involvement with the baby.

D. Contraception (see Chapter 101). The median delay for seeking information on contraception is 16 months after first intercourse. These visits are often precipitated by the fear of pregnancy. Fifty percent of teen pregnancy occurs within the first 6 months of initiating sexual intercourse. Adolescents frequently believe that they cannot become pregnant, especially with first intercourse; and, as their perception of the future is just developing, they may find it difficult to conceptualize prevention of something that will occur in 9 months. Be aware of the adolescent's cognitive level when discussing methods of contraception. For teens selecting oral contraceptives, the most often chosen method, schedule close and frequent follow-up, even beyond the first year of use, to reinforce the correct use of birth control. Programs that help teen parents remain in school often decrease repeat pregnancy rates.

   E. STDs. Adolescents have 25% of reported rates of gonorrhea and significant rates of cervicitis caused by *Chlamydia trachomatis* and genital herpes; rates of syphilis in teens have increased in recent years. There is some evidence that the anatomic and physiologic changes of adolescence predispose young women to an increased risk of cervicitis. Increasing rates of rectal gonorrhea in young gay males are of concern. Adolescents account for 0.5–1% of all acquired immunodeficiency syndrome (AIDS) cases; 25% of AIDS occurs between ages 20 and 29 years. With an incubation period of 8–11 years, many of these AIDS patients were infected during adolescence. Homeless youths, intravenous drug users, prostitutes (both male and female), and adolescents with a history of multiple partners and STDs are at particular risk for HIV exposure. Factors preventing early treatment of STDs among young people include poor education on the signs and symptoms, denial, economic dependence, inaccessible or undesirable medical care, lack of awareness that treatment can be confidential, and poor reporting of contacts.

   The approach to adolescents with suspected STDs or HIV positivity must be different from the approach to older groups. Youths need particular counseling on STD prevention and HIV testing. Before and after sexual initiation, there should be education on condom use, the early signs and symptoms of STDs, where to get confidential treatment, and what can be done to prevent the further spread of these infections. Review these issues at every adolescent visit with sexually active teens.

VII. Dermatology (see Chapter 69)

VIII. Risk-taking behaviors are defined as those that can be potentially harmful to the initiator or to others and that exceed normal behavior for that developmental phase. They include delinquent behavior, gang membership, dangerous driving, truancy, teen pregnancy, substance use and abuse, and other self-destructive behavior. Of particular concern are youths from families facing separation, divorce, death of a family member, violence and access to weapons, socioeconomic hardship, alcoholism, or disorganization from any cause. Addressing the difficulties of the family plays an indirect but important role in the prevention of high-risk behavior in the young person.

   A. Vehicular accidents, the leading cause of mortality and morbidity among young people, are increased when driving under the influence of alcohol and drugs or when refraining from wearing seat belts. Peer influence increases risks taken when driving. Discuss accident prevention, driving while under the influence of drugs, and use of seat belts and helmets. Gradually increased driving responsibilities after receiving a driver's license should be negotiated by teens and parents.

   B. Violence. Firearms are the second leading cause of death among all teenagers aged 15–19; half of all US households have firearms. Fifteen percent of students report carrying a gun regularly, with males significantly more likely to do so than females. Urban males of low socioeconomic and education levels are at highest risk of being affected by violence. Although rates of firearm homicide among young people are decreasing, in 1995 homicides accounted for about one-fifth of all deaths among youths 15–24.

   1. Prevention

   a. Routinely ask all parents and teenagers about the presence of firearms in the home.

   b. If firearms are present, discuss removal or safe storage of weapons and ammunition.

   c. Review the risks of combining firearm use with access to alcohol (or other drugs).

   d. Ask parents how they deal with anger, especially if there is a history of violence in the home.

   e. Ask all teens about gang membership and firearms in gang activities.

    2. Victims and exposure (see Chapter 95). Adolescents who have been victims of or exposed to violence may suffer depression or post-traumatic stress disorder (PTSD).

       a. In addition to treating physical wounds, schedule follow-up appointments to assess the adolescent's coping with violence.

       b. If indicated, refer the patient for appropriate adolescent counseling.

       c. Be knowledgeable of local adolescent violence prevention and gang task force programs.

IX. Substance use and abuse (see Chapter 92). Substance abuse by the patient's immediate peer group and close friends strongly increases the likelihood of initiation in that youth. Ask all teens about their peer substance use, including nicotine. Give adolescents realistic information about risks and consequences of *all* drugs, including nicotine.

Alcohol, tobacco, marijuana, cocaine, and other drugs are taken in many combinations, thus exposing themselves to a variety of deleterious effects. Use of "fashionable" drugs, the predilection for experimentation by adolescents, risk-taking behavior, and the increasingly younger age at which drug use begins increase the risks of continued use.

A. Nicotine. After several years of decreases, regular use of tobacco (one-half pack per day) by high school seniors increased from 14% to 17% in 1993, with 3.1 million youths identified as regular smokers, equal for males and females. Peak ages for initiating smoking are between 11 and 15.

Physicians must discuss the addictive potential of nicotine early in adolescence and try to postpone or prevent any use. Most smokers are addicted by age 20. Ask the patient about his or her own and peers' smoking at every visit. Smoking is also associated with poor school performance, alcohol use, and high-risk sexual behaviors. Physicians must use a different approach with adolescents than with adults. Discuss short-term adverse (adolescent-centered) effects: bad breath, wrinkles, or possible effect on erections. Medical offices should be smoke-free, including no-smoking ads in magazines, with health information available. If a teen has begun to smoke, set and contract a quit date with close follow-up (2 weeks) and continued regular follow-up. Attempt to engage the patient's peers and reinforce school nonsmoking programs.

One million youths use smokeless tobacco. Males, particularly rural white males, are significantly more likely than other high school youths to use smokeless tobacco. Smokeless tobacco is also addictive and initiated in adolescence. Physicians should discuss adverse affects such as halitosis, early periodontal degeneration, and soft tissue lesions. Smokeless tobacco users are also more likely than nonusers to become smokers.

B. Alcohol continues to remain the drug of choice of almost 90% of high school seniors. In 1993, approximately 45% of senior boys and 33% of senior girls reported engaging in "heavy drinking" at least once during the previous month. Alcohol advertising continues to target youths as a major market. Parental influences that contribute to alcohol abuse by youths include lack of supervision or knowledge of use, lack of emotional and physical availability, difficulty in setting limits, alcohol abuse by the parents themselves, family dysfunction characterized by an increase in conflict, or disorganized households with fewer rules and schedules, fewer rituals, frequent moves, and increased day-to-day stress. For more information on prevention, recognition, and treatment, see Chapter 92.

C. Other drugs. Use of marijuana, stimulants, hallucinogens (eg, LSD), and cocaine increased in high school seniors in 1993 after several years of decrease. Alcohol and nicotine, addictive drugs, are often gateways to use of these "harder" addictive substances; teens who smoke and drink alcohol are at higher risk and require a more specific history on any drug use, personally or with peers. About 1% of adolescents inject anabolic steroids. Ask about steroid use with all sports physical examinations, and discuss the risks of continued use and the risk of HIV with injection use. Some high school students (1.4%) report intravenous drug use. Drug testing should not be done without patient consent, and confidentiality must be respected.

X. Psychological concerns. Eighteen percent to 22% of youths aged 10–18 are diagnosed with mental health disorders. Common inpatient diagnoses are affective disorder and behavior and adjustment disorders. Outpatient diagnoses include adjustment disorders, anxiety, affective disorders, and substance abuse. Boys and racial and ethnic minority members account for disproportionately larger shares of admissions or partial hospitalizations at residential treatment centers.

A. Depression is a common symptom complex in the mood swings of adolescence. In addition to the vegetative depressive symptoms in adults, adolescents, especially early, express depressive equivalents: increased eating and sleep disorders, aggressive behavior, delinquency, inability to concentrate, school problems, promiscuity, daredevil behavior, pregnancy, and increased alcohol and drug use. Parents often need assistance in differentiating these behaviors from normal adolescent behavior.

Adolescent depression frequently results from changes or personal loss, including break-up with a boyfriend or girlfriend, recent moves or a change in schools, and family dysfunction or break-up. Evaluation of depression must include a comprehensive and thorough history with inquiries into any family history of depression or suicide, depressive equivalents and recurrent or recent losses, and an assessment of the risk of suicide. When clinical depression is diagnosed, the adolescent and his or her family should be referred for therapy. Psychopharmacologic agents have had limited success with adolescents, but are sometimes beneficial in resistant cases (see Chapter 96).

B. Suicide is the third leading cause of death in persons aged 15–24 years. Firearms account for significant numbers of teenage (15–19) suicide deaths. There are significant increases in suicide rates in families with a history of suicide, affective disorders, alcohol and drug abuse, or physical or sexual abuse as well as in adolescents with prior attempts. Females make more suicide attempts, with males having more completed suicides. Hispanic male and females make more attempts than their white counterparts; black males, whose suicide attempts are markedly increasing, make more attempts that require medical attention. Gay and lesbian youths are at increased risk for suicide.

Depression is the most common affect that precedes teen suicide. Clues to suicide include giving away valued possessions, saying goodbye, accident proneness, poor self-image, deterioration of personal hygiene, increased isolation, and talk about attempting suicide. Adolescents frequently see a physician within weeks or months of a suicide attempt, often for vague somatic complaints. An unexpected elevation of mood can immediately precede a suicide attempt when the decision has been made. Evaluate the risk of imminent suicide by determining the extent of suicidal ideation, if the plan has been formulated or if there has been a recent attempt. Suicidal ideation and any attempts must be taken seriously and responded to with support and clarity. Hospitalize the patient if there are any concerns about an imminent attempt. This is a life-threatening situation in which parents must be notified regardless of the breach of confidentiality with the adolescent. Be familiar with community resources such as suicide "hot lines" and suicide prevention programs. If the youth is followed up as an outpatient, there must be close follow-up with contracting about any suicidal attempts by the primary physician and a mental health professional.

C. School problems can include school phobias, truancy, failure, fights, poor concentration, and school dropout or suspension. In 1990, about 12% of 16- to 24-year-olds had not graduated from high school and were no longer enrolled. Hispanics and blacks have higher dropout rates than non-Hispanic whites.

   1. Presentation. Morning headaches, gastrointestinal complaints, vague myalgias, or symptoms of fatigue may indicate problems at school. Academic failure is the most common presenting school problem. Help define whether school failure represents family or adolescent issues, an underlying learning disorder, attention-deficit/hyperactivity disorder, inability to meet teacher or parental expectations, physical or organic illness, problems with vision or hearing, borderline mental retardation, neurologic problems, or a combination of these factors. These problems can also be aggravated by familial or cultural differences and expectations or by language problems in recently arrived immigrant populations.

   Assess school performance at each well-child assessment visit throughout childhood and adolescence. Screen for visual and hearing problems periodically. The work-up for school problems includes a complete and comprehensive physical examination and medical, family, and social histories, which include prenatal and developmental information, and histories of any family members with learning, neurologic, or psychiatric problems. Reading disabilities are common and occur six times more often in boys than in girls, often with a similar family history in the father.

2. **Resources.** The 1975 federal government legislation (PL-94-142: the Education for All Handicapped Children Act) with amendments in 1990 and new legislation in 1997 as the Individuals with Disabilities Education Act (IDEA) provide for education to all children aged 3–21 years in the least restrictive environment and mandate that parents participate in the educational planning for children with any handicap, be it a physical, emotional, or learning disability. Physicians treating children of any age should be familiar with the goals of these legislative acts and the local resources available.

   A multidisciplinary team, with physicians, is an effective approach to working with these complex school problems. Encourage parental involvement in schools, which improves students' academic performances.

XI. Homeless youths

A. **Epidemiology.** There are an estimated 500,000 runaways and 127,000 "throwaway" (evicted) youths annually. The median age is 14–16 years, equal for males and females. Sixty percent to 70% have a history of sexual or physical abuse. Fifteen percent to 20% give a history of conflicts with parents about sexual orientation as the reason for leaving home.

B. Medical problems of homeless youths result from their lifestyle behaviors. Many are involved in survival sex and prostitution (male and female) with subsequent high rates of STDs (particularly with gay and bisexual youths); pregnancy; HIV disease (with some reporting a 5–12% HIV-positive rate in homeless youth clinics); suicide; substance abuse (primarily alcohol) with marijuana, cocaine, amphetamines, or intravenous drug use; or mental health disorders higher than peers: depression, conduct disorder, and PTSD.

C. Access to health care is difficult for homeless youths. Clinical services that target this population and use outreach workers are best suited to minimizing these barriers. Primary care physicians should be aware of local services and resources.

D. Youth homelessness may be prevented if families with a history of significant conflict, sexual or physical abuse, or concerns about their adolescent's sexual orientation are identified early by primary care physicians and referred for appropriate counseling.

REFERENCES

American Medical Association: *Guidelines for Adolescent Preventive Services (GAPS): Recommendations Monograph.* American Medical Association; 1996.
Bernstein HK, Stettner-Eaton B, Ellis M: *Individuals with Disabilities Education Act: Early Intervention by Family Physicians.* Am Fam Physician 1995;**52**(1):71–73, 76–77.
Fingerhut LA, et al: Homicide rates among U.S. teenagers and young adults: Differences by mechanism, level of urbanization, race, and sex 1987 through 1995. JAMA 1998;**280**(5):423.
McCoy K, Wibblesman C: *The New Teenage Body Book.* Putnam; 1992.
Neinstein LS (ed): *Adolescent Health Care,* 3rd ed. Urban & Schwarzenberg; 1996.
Ozer EM, Brindis CD, Millstein SG, et al: *American Adolescents: Are They Healthy?* National Adolescent Health Information Center, University of California, San Francisco, California; 1997.
Reif CJ, Elster AB: Adolescent preventive services. Prim Care 1998;**25**(1):1.

---

111   The Patient with Disabilities

Caryl J. Heaton, DO

I. Definitions

A. A **disability** is any restriction resulting from an impairment of ability to perform an activity in the manner or within the range considered normal for a human being.

B. An **impairment** is any loss or abnormality of psychological, physiologic, or anatomic structure or function.

C. A **handicap** is a disadvantage for a given individual resulting from an impairment or disability that limits or prevents the fulfillment of a role that is normal, depending on the age and sex of and social and cultural factors for the individual.

D. **Mental retardation** is a substantial limitation in an individual's functioning and is characterized by significantly subaverage intellectual functioning existing concurrently with related limitation in two or more of the following applicable adaptive skill areas: communication, self-care, home living, social skills, community use, self-direction, health and safety, functional academics, leisure, and work. Mental retardation manifests before age 18.

E. **Rehabilitation** is the development of the individual to the fullest physical, psychological, social, vocational, avocational, and educational potential consistent with his or her physiologic or anatomic impairment and environmental limitations.

II. **Role of the health care team**

A. The **health care team** is especially important in the care of a patient with disabilities. The role of the physician as coordinator of care is usually desirable, but in some cases the patient (or parent) should be encouraged to be the ultimate case manager.

1. The **medical team leader** evaluates medical and functional status, manages medical care, orders therapies, and coordinates rehabilitative and therapeutic efforts. Medical management can assume many models, but the two most common are (1) management by a rehabilitative specialist (physiatrist, developmental pediatrician, or neurologist), with primary care medical needs covered by a primary care physician; and (2) coordinated management by the primary care physician with specialty consultation. In some cases, primary care must be provided by a specialist because of the difficulty in finding a primary care physician who is willing to work with patients with disabilities.

Also in some cases, primary care physicians provide higher levels of specialty care than they normally would because of the lack of specialty physicians. Family physicians can be highly effective in this role because they are experienced in coordination of care. Although registered nurse case managers are also competent in this role, many managed-care organizations call on family and other primary care physicians to take the role of medical team leader.

B. The **primary care needs** of patients with disabilities include screening for developmental delay or disability, performing periodic physical examination, paying attention to acute complaints, providing patient education, and monitoring and coordinating medication usage.

1. All **medical testing and treatment** should be pursued with the same level of intensity as in a patient without disabilities. *Any exception to this general rule should be under the direction of the patient or guardian and with the support of informed advocates for the patient.*

2. **Screening for disabilities** should include patients of all ages, but the early identification of children with disabilities is especially important. **Early intervention programs (EIP)** have proved to be effective in promoting developmental progress in infants and toddlers with biologically based disabilities. The availability of an EIP may be determined by contacting the local board of health or the nearest developmental pediatric center.

a. All children with **risk factors** for developmental delay should be screened in the physician's office (Table 111–1).

b. **Rapid office screening** can be accomplished for all children using the shorter forms of the Denver Developmental Screening Test (DDST). The easiest short form of the DDST is to use the standard instrument and draw a vertical line at the child's age (just as for the standard test). The examiner then refers to the bar graphs of competencies that lie entirely to the left of the line. The closest three competencies in each of the four categories that lie to the left, but do not touch the line, are considered. A miss in any category is considered a sign of risk, in which case the complete DDST should be administered. Other screening tests are the Denver Prescreening Developmental Questionnaire (PDQ), the Infant Rapid Screen, and the Texas Preschool Screening Inventory.

c. Cerebral palsy and many forms of developmental delay can readily be diagnosed before the child reaches the age of 1 year. If objective findings exist, a "wait and see" attitude on the part of the clinician can add to the fear and frustration of the family. **Referral** to a developmental pediatrician, neurologist, ophthalmologist, or audiologist can sometimes limit the progress of the disability and should be planned immediately.

TABLE 111-1. RISK FACTORS FOR DEVELOPMENTAL DISABILITIES

Prenatal factors
Lack of prenatal care
Maternal age >35, <16 yr
Maternal or paternal history of mental retardation
Maternal history of drug or alcohol abuse
Parental history of mental illness
Family history of child abuse or neglect
Family history of deafness
Chaotic home environment
Maternal history of HIV infection
Maternal history of major sociopathy

Perinatal and neonatal factors
Birth weight <2500 g (5 lb, 7½ oz) and especially birth weight <1500 g (3 lb, 4½ oz)
Apgar score of 4 at 5 minutes after birth, with continued signs of neonatal depression
Serum bilirubin >17 mg/dL, especially when associated with Rh or ABO incompatibility
Obvious congenital or genetic malformation
Neonatal seizures
Infection such as sepsis or meningitis
Maternal disorders such as diabetes or infection or use of medication for seizures
Metabolic abnormalities such as hypoglycemia, phenylketonuria, or hypothyroidism
Intraventricular hemorrhage, especially grade 3 or 4
Respiratory distress syndrome
Infant hospitalized after mother returns home

Postnatal factors
Head trauma
Incidence of near-drowning
Seizures before age 2 yr
Leukemia or tumor
Child abuse
Failure to thrive
HIV infection

HIV, Human immunodeficiency virus.
Reprinted with permission from Haber JS. Early diagnosis and referral of children with developmental disabilities. Am Fam Physician 1991;**43**(1):132.

3. In general, **periodic physical examination guidelines** should also be consistent with those of patients who have no disabilities. The type of test and examination and the frequency of examination may often be determined by state law, especially in the case of cognitive disabilities. Surveillance for specific conditions may be needed more frequently in certain conditions and with certain disabilities. Advocacy groups may be a good source of medical information to the physician not familiar with rare syndromes.

Some testing may be done on a less frequent basis than is recommended by standard guidelines because the patient with physical or developmental disabilities may be at lower risk for the condition than the general population. An example would be Papanicolaou (Pap) smear screening for cervical cancer in women with mental retardation who are not sexually active. Virginal women have a greatly reduced risk of cervical cancer and therefore need cervical cytologic testing less frequently. Conversely, frequent periodic screening for thyroid disease is desirable in patients with Down syndrome, because the incidence of thyroid disorders is so high.

Although the use of screening tests should be based on the risk of a disease for that population, the rates for major causes of death are unknown for most patients with mental retardation or other disabilities.

The risks of anesthesia to accomplish invasive or uncomfortable tests, such as mammography, Pap smear, or sigmoidoscopy, must be weighed against the benefits.

4. The **US Preventive Services Task Force** suggests that the most effective interventions available to clinicians are those that address the personal health practices of patients. Data from *Healthy People 2000* suggest that patients

with disabilities receive preventive services less frequently. Patients with mild mental disabilities may have a greater need for education on good health habits, because their ability to draw that information from other sources is more limited. Patients with physical disabilities may have complicated medical problems, and patient education that would be "routine" for other patients is often forgotten.

5. Care for **acute medical problems** is the role of the primary medical physician. The symptoms of any problem may be somewhat different in the patient with physical or developmental disabilities.

   a. **Recognizing symptoms** may be delayed in the patient with difficulty in self-expression. New self-abusive or destructive behavior may be a symptom of pain or other medical condition. Patients with spinal cord injury or neural tube defects may have no symptoms or atypical symptoms for problems below the level of the lesion (eg, leg pain as the symptom of a urinary tract infection in a patient with spina bifida). Other behavioral symptoms can represent physical problems, especially in the patient with cognitive disabilities. These include anorexia, incontinence, and aggressive behaviors.

   b. **Physical examination** can be difficult in the patient with physical or developmental disabilities but should never be ignored. The primary care physician who maintains an ongoing relationship with a patient has the advantage of recognizing a change in physical findings. Patience is the best advice in performing the examination in a patient with mental retardation. Its importance cannot be overstated. The patient with disabilities requires attention to detail and good documentation if subtle changes are to be found.

   c. **Therapies** should be limited and frequently reassessed. Drug interactions and adverse effects are probably more common in patients with disabilities because of their multiple, complicated problems. Despite this, therapy should not be withheld unless a documented contraindication exists.

C. **Team members** are determined by patient needs. The establishment of a detailed comprehensive plan is the goal of the team leader. The health care team should be developed based on the patient's biomedical and functional assessment. Functional assessment can be made using a number of systems (see Chapters 77 and 112). The checklist in Table 111–2 was established for patients with mental disabilities but is useful for any patient with physical or developmental disabilities. A more complete description and a series of forms are available through American Association of Mental Retardation publications.

D. **Advocacy groups** and members of support groups. This part of the team is often an afterthought but may be the most important members to the parent or patient. They assist in assembling other members of the health care team and in providing informal psychological and social support.

E. The **physiatrist**, a physician who specializes in physical medicine and rehabilitation (PM&R), can be an invaluable member of the health care team. The rehabilitation model of care emphasizes management of disability rather than "treatment" or "cure" of disease. The model is also similar to a primary care model in that it covers multiple specialty areas to meet comprehensive rehabilitative needs of the patient.

III. **Diagnosis and treatment**

A. The following guidelines represent a framework for a diagnostic and treatment approach that should consider the individual's needs. These guidelines focus less on the impairment (eg, intelligence quotient [IQ] in the patient with mental retardation; level of injury in a patient with spinal cord injury) than on a comprehensive description of the patient with a disability. The construction or supervision of the overall plan may or may not be the responsibility of the primary care physician, but each person deserves to receive a comprehensive evaluation and treatment plan. It is the obligation of the physician to ensure that an appropriate evaluation is performed and periodically reviewed.

   1. A three-step process for diagnosing, classifying, and determining the needed supports is described in the following text.

   2. **Ascertain the most correct diagnosis.** The treating physician should make every effort to uncover the cause of developmental disabilities, even though

TABLE 111–2. CHECKLIST OF FUNCTIONAL ABILITIES

Dimension	Skills	Sources of Care
Communication	Comprehend and express information through symbolic behavior or nonsymbolic behavior	Speech therapist, audiologist
☐ I ☐ L ☐ E ☐ P	Who?/How?	
Self-care	Eating, toileting, dressing, hygiene, grooming	Physical therapist, occupational therapist, caretaker, personal aide
☐ I ☐ L ☐ E ☐ P	Who?/How?	
Home living	Clothing care, housekeeping, property maintenance, food preparation and cooking, planning and budgeting for shopping, home safety, daily scheduling	Physical therapist, occupational therapist, special educator, advocates
☐ I ☐ L ☐ E ☐ P	Who?/How?	
Social	Conducting social exchanges, including initiating, responding, and terminating interactions, recognizing feelings; regulating one's own behavior; formulation/fostering friendships; understanding rules, fairness, and law	Psychologist, psychiatrist, social worker, family members, primary care physicians, educators, advocates, behavior modification therapists
☐ I ☐ L ☐ E ☐ P	Who?/How?	
Community use	Traveling in the community, shopping, obtaining services, using public transportation, attending community functions	Social worker, family members, educators, advocates, occupational therapists, psychologists
☐ I ☐ L ☐ E ☐ P	Who?/How?	
Self-direction	Making choices, initiating appropriate activities, completing necessary or required tasks, seeking assistance when needed	Social worker, family members, educators, advocates, occupational therapists, psychologists
☐ I ☐ L ☐ E ☐ P	Who?/How?	
Health and safety	Skills related to maintenance of health and health promotion, physical fitness, sexuality, basic safety considerations	Physicians, nurses, patient educators, social workers, psychologists, educators
☐ I ☐ L ☐ E ☐ P	Who?/How?	
Functional academics	Cognitive abilities and skills related to learning at school or college	Special educators, communication therapists
☐ I ☐ L ☐ E ☐ P	Who?/How?	
Leisure	Choosing and self-initiating interests, using and enjoying leisure activities in the community and home, playing socially	Social worker, family members, educators, advocates, occupational therapists, psychologists
☐ I ☐ L ☐ E ☐ P	Who?/How?	
Work	Skills related to holding full- or part-time job, job-specific skills, appropriate social skills	Occupational therapists, physical therapists, special educators
☐ I ☐ L ☐ E ☐ P	Who?/How?	

The intensity of needed support is indicated below plan; I, intermittent; L, limited; E, extensive; P, pervasive. The responsible team member can be listed under "plan" with indication of how often to reassess.

information is often insufficient. Genetics testing and counseling may be helpful even in adults. A genetic cause is especially important in the patient with sisters or brothers who may not express the disease but be carriers of the disorder.

3. **Classification and description.** This process should document the weaknesses of the patient, including his or her overall need for support, based on the checklist of functional abilities (Table 111–2). The team leader is responsible for seeing that this evaluation is completed periodically.

   a. **Profile and intensities of needed supports.** The intensity of support usually corresponds to the person's limitations. There are four levels of intensity of support.

   (1) **Intermittent**—used only on an as-needed basis.

   (2) **Limited**—a time-limited support, such as a one-time training program.

   (3) **Extensive**—regular, that is, daily support.

   (4) **Pervasive**—constant high-intensity supports, often life-sustaining.

4. **Documentation and maintenance of medical records** also are ultimate responsibilities of the team leader. Because state laws and rules can greatly add to paperwork, many physicians refer all duplication paperwork, such as over-the-counter medication sheets and written prescription renewals, to the caretakers and simply edit and sign it.

IV. **Management of common syndromes**

A. Guidelines for care of the person with **Down syndrome (DS)** have been established. DS is a syndrome of mental retardation and multiple malformations resulting from the presence of extra genetic material from chromosome 21.

1. The **phenotype** of DS is variable, but the characteristic physical features can include hypotonia, small brachycephalic head, epicanthic folds, flat nasal bridge, upward-slanting palpebral fissures, small mouth, small ears, excessive skin at the nape of the neck, single transverse palmar crease, and short fifth finger with clinodactyly.

2. The **genetic cause** in 95% of cases of DS is trisomy 21, resulting from nondisjunction during gamete formation. Another 5% of cases are caused by either a translocation of chromosome 21 or mosaicism. Confirmation of the diagnosis should always be made by karyotyping; however, if the genetic confirmation cannot be rapidly made, the diagnosis should be discussed based on the physician's clinical judgment. Attempts to hide the diagnosis from the family while obtaining genetic confirmation are often unsuccessful and rarely appreciated. Triple-screen testing (α-fetoprotein, human chorionic gonadotropin, and unconjugated estriol) has become the standard of care in prenatal screening for DS, but has a low (<2%) positive predictive value. Ultrasonographic evidence of thickened nuchal folds is now also routinely screened, but the predictive value of that test is still undetermined.

3. **Specific life-time screening strategies for associated syndromes** should be integrated with routine health maintenance.

   a. **Care in the newborn period** centers on effective communication with and support of family members. Early referral to advocacy groups has been shown to be extremely helpful to family members. Medical care for the newborn should include ultrasonography for congenital heart disease, which occurs in approximately 50% of infants with DS, and careful examination for congenital cataracts. In the **first 12 months of life,** the clinician should carefully screen for vision and hearing abnormalities, including otitis media (occurring in 50–70% of cases). Most authorities suggest specialist referral for children between the age of 2 and 12 months. Cardiac symptoms often do not develop until 4–6 months of age. The clinician should be alert for any feeding or bowel problems because of the increased incidence of tracheoesophageal fistulas, duodenal atresia, Hirschsprung's disease, and imperforate anus in infants with DS. The clinician should also obtain results of the hospital's thyroid screening test (congenital hypothyroidism is 27 times more common in a child with DS) and carefully check for congenital hip dislocation. Some authorities advocate routine ultrasonographic screening of the hip for all children with DS. Refer the child for early intervention services.

b. **Care of children and young adolescents** continues to center on vigilance for thyroid disorders and otolaryngologic or audiologic concerns. Children with DS have increased rates of upper respiratory tract infection, otitis media, middle ear effusion, rhinitis, and sinusitis. Hearing tests and thyroid testing should be performed yearly. Growth charts are available for children with DS to assist in determining appropriate weights. Obesity prevention should be discussed. Atlantoaxial and atlanto-occipital instability are more common in children with DS (15% and 8%, respectively), and most are asymptomatic. Screening for asymptomatic atlantoaxial and atlanto-occipital instability is recommended in all children and adults with DS who wish to participate in the Special Olympics. The American Academy of Pediatrics (AAP) withdrew their recommendation for cervical x-rays in 1995, suggesting there was not enough evidence to support its value. The reference committee instead stressed the importance of identifying symptomatic atlantoaxial instability. Symptomatic atlantoaxial instability causes muscle weakness, gait abnormalities, and difficulty walking. Findings may include brisk deep tendon reflexes, positive plantar reflexes, and ankle clonus.

c. **Care of the older adolescent and young adult** with DS should address routine health needs, such as health education and screening tests. Screening should be continued for thyroid disease, eye-ear-nose-throat problems, and weight problems. Periodontal disease is found in up to 90% of persons with DS before the age of 30. Some authorities suggest cardiac screening every 10 years for valvular fenestrations and for assessment of previous surgical procedures. Depression is more common in adolescents with DS than in the nonaffected population. It is important to discuss social concerns with adolescents and to provide education about sex and about the prevention of sexual abuse.

d. The **adult with DS** continues to need routine screening, preventive services, and vigilance for specific conditions. The medical needs remain fairly stable except for decreasing cognitive function. This is most commonly related to Alzheimer-type dementia. Dementia presents with diminished memory and ability to perform activities of daily living (ADLs). Guardians of adult patients with DS should assess long-term plans with the patient and the physician. The average life expectancy of those with DS continues to increase.

B. **Fragile X syndrome (FXS)** is a genetic disorder distinguished by mental retardation, characteristic physical features, and abnormal behavior. It is the most common hereditary cause of mental retardation. FXS occurs in 0.4–0.8 per 1000 males and 0.2–0.6 per 1000 females and represents 6–14% of all males with severe mental retardation. Guidelines for the care of the child with FXS have been developed by the Committee on Genetics for the AAP.

1. The characteristic **phenotype** may become apparent late in childhood or early adolescence and includes a prominent forehead; a long, thin face and prominent jaw; large protuberant ears; and large testicles. Other features not as consistently found are cleft palate, strabismus, serous otitis, and mitral valve prolapse. Many affected males have minimal physical features, and the only demonstrable phenotype is retardation and a characteristic behavior profile.

2. The **genetic cause** is excessive replication of a trinucleotide sequence (C-G-G) on the FMR1 segment of the X chromosome. The X-linked transmission is highly variable in its expression. DNA testing is extremely accurate and should be undertaken. Both polymerase chain reaction and Western blot tests are available. The number of replications is proportional to the phenotypic expression of the syndrome. Of males who carry the mutation, 20% may not have clinical signs. These men can transmit the mutation to daughters, who may subsequently have affected sons. Unaffected female carriers can transmit the mutation to their children. Genetic counseling and carrier detection should be offered to all siblings and relatives at risk.

3. **Associated syndromes and life-time screening strategies**
   a. The diagnosis of FXS is rarely made in the **newborn period** unless there is a family history of the syndrome. The phenotype is not appreciated in the infant. Cleft palate, strabismus, mitral valve prolapse, joint laxity, hip

dislocation, and clubfoot are more common. In the **first 12 months of life,** the clinician should carefully screen for otitis media. Any murmur or click on cardiac examination requires echocardiographic screening for mitral valve prolapse.

    b. The **care of children and young adolescents** should include monitoring as previously described, along with periodic examination for flatfoot, loose joints, hernia, and scoliosis. The clinician should obtain an electroencephalogram (EEG) if there are any staring episodes or possible seizures and should have language and motor development assessed. The clinician should assess for hyperactive, autistic, or self-abusive behavior and should consider early referral for behavioral intervention. As the male child enters puberty, he should be examined for macro-orchidism and his family reassured about this benign finding.

    c. Behavioral problems, including hyperactivity, attention deficits, averting of gaze, perseverance of speech, and shyness, become more common as the child enters **late adolescence and adulthood.** Discuss social concerns with adolescents; provide education about sex and about the prevention of sexual abuse. Guardians should assess long-term plans. The health care needs of older adults with FXS have not been clearly defined.

C. Cerebral palsy (CP) is a disorder of movement and posture that is due to a nonprogressive abnormality of the immature brain. Birth trauma and perinatal asphyxia are not the primary causes of CP, as once believed. Although it is common for a child with CP to have a history of complicated labor and delivery, it is now thought that in most cases, the perinatal complications are a result of pre-existing brain damage. Forty-four percent of all CP cases are thought to occur in the prenatal period. Twenty-seven percent are thought to occur during labor and delivery or in the perinatal period. Five percent occur in childhood, and the cause is not known in 24%.

    1. The classification of CP depends on the part of the brain that has been affected. **Pyramidal tract cerebral palsy** refers to damage of the cerebral cortex, whereas **extrapyramidal CP** refers to damage below the pyramidal tract. Pyramidal tract CP results in clasp-knife spasticity. The initial resistance of a limb to movement results in an abrupt "giving away" jerk.

        a. **Diplegia** results from injury to the area of the lateral ventricles and produces damage to the legs (25%).

        b. **Hemiplegia** results from damage to the cortical area of the contralateral side. The upper extremity is usually more involved than the lower extremity (45%).

        c. **Quadriplegia** is the result of extensive injury in both hemispheres and produces spasticity in all four limbs (30%).

    2. The resistance in extrapyramidal CP is referred to as lead-pipe rigidity. Persistent pressure eventually brings incremental movements. The most common form of extrapyramidal CP is choreoathetoid CP. Resting muscle tone in this group varies, and muscle contractures are not usually problematic. Because the facial muscles are involved, however, problems with sucking, swallowing, and speaking are common.

    3. The most **common disabilities associated with CP** are mental retardation, visual or auditory impairment, and seizures.

        a. About two-thirds of patients with CP have **mental retardation,** but about one-third of patients with CP have normal intelligence. The type of CP influences the incidence and degree of mental retardation. The best intellectual outcome is found in hemiplegia, the most common form of CP (60% have normal intelligence). Patients with spastic quadriplegia, extrapyramidal, or mixed-type CP more frequently have mental retardation (30% in normal range), and the degree of retardation is more severe.

        b. **Decreased visual acuity** and blindness occur in 23–64% of cases, depending on the type of CP. Nystagmus, hemianopsia, or strabismus may be seen.

        c. **Hearing, speech, and language defects** occur in 30% of patients with CP. Dysarthria is often associated with extrapyramidal CP because choreoathetosis affects the tongue and vocal cord movements. Difficulties in articulation and speech can be incorrectly diagnosed as mental retardation. Appropriate facilitation of communication must be sought under all such conditions through speech and language therapists.

D. The classification of **spinal cord injuries (SCI)** depends on the level of the lesion to the cord. This level is usually determined by a neurologist or rehabilitative physician during hospitalization for the acute injury. The level of the lesion is described in terms of the right and left sides of the body and motor/sensory levels. The last intact dermatome determines the level of the lesion. A spinal cord lesion may be complete or incomplete. In a complete lesion, no motor or sensory activity occurs below the level of the lesion; in an incomplete lesion, some motor or sensory function is intact. Specific muscle groups that correspond to each spinal nerve have been determined (Table 111–3). The muscle groups listed above the level of the lesion should be functional.

1. **Epidemiology.** The annual incidence of SCI in the United States is 3 in 100,000, excluding those who die within 24 hours. The overall prevalence of SCI is estimated to be 70–90 for every 100,000 of the population, which corresponds to 200,000–250,000 persons in the United States. Males are injured four times more frequently than females. The four most common causes are motor vehicle accidents (45%), falls (21.5%), gunshot wounds/violence (15.4%), and sporting accidents—usually diving (13.4%). About 53% of those injured are quadriplegic.

2. Medical therapy is directed toward a variety of **common associated problems.**

   a. Constant vigilance for **pressure sores** must be maintained. Turning the bedridden patient every 2 hours is critical. The patient who sits must be instructed to "weight shift" or push up every 2 hours.

   b. For purposes of urinary health, **intermittent catheterization** should be substituted for Foley catheterization whenever possible. Fluids should be maintained at 2000–2400 mL/day. Catheterization should begin at a rate of every 3–4 hours, with the time between catheterizations gradually increasing to no more than every 8 hours.

   c. The primary gastrointestinal problems seen in patients with SCI are **incontinence and fecal impaction.** A bowel program consists of stool softener, natural fiber laxative, and glycerin suppository given at a routine time.

   d. **Autonomic dysreflexia** is a potentially life-threatening event in patients with lesions above T6–T8. Stimulation from the bladder, bowel, uterus, or skin may ascend through the spinal cord and cause reflex vasoconstriction below the level of the lesion. The symptoms are severe hypertension, bradycardia, sweating, and blotchy skin above the level of the lesion. The most common clinical causes are bladder overdistention, fecal impaction, decubitus ulcers, ingrown toenails, and the third stage of labor. Treatment is directed at eliminating the cause. Patients should be placed

TABLE 111–3. KEY MUSCLES FOR MOTOR LEVEL CLASSIFICATION OF SPINAL CORD INJURY

Spinal Nerve	Muscle	Action
C4	Diaphragm intact	Respiration
C5	Biceps intact	Elbow flexor
C6	Wrist extensors intact	Wrist extensor
C7	Triceps intact	Elbow extensor
C8	Flexor profundus intact	Finger flexor
T1	Hand intrinsics	Finger abduction/adduction
T2–L1	**Sensory levels**	
L2	Iliopsoas	Hip flexor
L3	Quadriceps intact	Knee extensor
L4	Tibialis anterior intact	Ankle dorsiflexor
L5	Extensor hallucis longus	Great toe extensor
S1	Gastrocnemius	Ankle plantar flexor
S2–S5	**Sensory levels**	

in a sitting position. Sublingual nifedipine, 10–20 mg expressed capsule, or nitroglycerin paste, 1–2 inches applied to chest, should be used to reduce the blood pressure acutely. Therapy should be continued and the patient closely monitored in a medical setting.

e. Patients with SCI may have **alveolar hypoventilation.** Injury to the thoracic level causes a loss of support of the intercostal muscles below that level. Intercostal muscles may contribute up to 60% of the ventilatory effort. The diaphragm is innervated at C2–C4. Mucous plugs and infection are also more common, and attention should be paid to hydration and postural drainage, if needed.

f. **Deep venous thrombosis** is most common in the first 3 months following SCI; pain is not a complaint. Any unilateral swelling calls for testing to exclude deep venous thrombosis. Other causes of a swollen lower extremity are cellulitis, heterotopic ossification, underlying fracture, and intramuscular hemorrhage.

   (1) **Fracture and hemorrhage** can be due to strain or occult trauma and are diagnosed by magnetic resonance imaging.

   (2) **Cellulitis** may be accompanied by warmth and hyperemia. The white blood cell count may be elevated.

   (3) **Heterotopic ossification** is an inflammation that results in the formation of bone in the soft tissues below the level of the injury, surrounding the joints. This pathogenesis is not known. This ossification commonly occurs around hips, knees, elbows, and shoulders. Range of motion must be maintained to prevent ankylosis. The diagnosis is suggested by radiographic findings (which may take 2–3 weeks to develop) and elevated levels of alkaline phosphatase. The treatment is etidronate (Didronel), 20 mg/kg/day for 14 days followed by 10 mg/kg/day for about 6 months.

g. **Spasticity** is one of the most troublesome and deforming consequences of SCI. Inhibitory impulses from the cortex cannot counter the involuntary movements of large muscle groups. Muscle spasms and fixed positions soon cause joint contractures. Treatment of spasticity depends on a routine of stretching and range-of-motion exercises. Baclofen acts at the spinal level to inhibit spasms and should be started at low dosage and increased gradually, 5 mg three times per day for 3 days, then 10 mg three times per day, up to a regular dose of 80–150 mg/day. The usual effective dose is 10–20 mg four times per day. Side effects of baclofen include lethargy, drowsiness, and nausea. Abrupt discontinuation causes hallucinations, seizures, and rebound spasticity. Dantrolene, 25–75 mg three to four times per day, may be useful for patients who have concurrent traumatic brain injury. Botulinum toxin injection into the tendon is an experimental treatment now being used in some areas.

h. **Sexuality and sexual desire** continue in persons with SCI. Women experience decreased physical sensation and decreased vaginal lubrication. Fertility is maintained. Men experience decreased ability to have and sustain an erection. Orgasm is possible in many patients with SCI; however, in men there is decreased ability to ejaculate and an increased incidence of retrograde ejaculation.

E. **Neural tube defects** are a classification of congenital abnormalities that involve malformations of the vertebrae and spinal cord. The incidence of neural tube defects is about 0.6 in 1000 births in the United States.

   1. **Spina bifida occulta** is defined as a separation of the vertebral elements in the midline. It is a normal variant seen in 5% of the population. **Meningocele** is a cyst filled with cerebrospinal fluid, without spinal cord dysplasia. **Myelomeningocele** is a cystic lesion of the meninges, with malformation of the spinal cord. The effect of this is a lower motor neuron lesion resulting in paralysis, loss of sensation, and loss of cortical inhibition below the level of the defect. Many recommendations for the care of a patient with SCI can apply to the patient with spina bifida or with myelomeningocele.

   2. Preconception counseling and **folic acid therapy** are advisable for all women as primary prevention. To reduce the frequency of neural tube defects and their resulting disability, the US Public Health Service recommends that all women of childbearing age in the United States who are capable of becoming pregnant should consume ≥0.4 mg of folic acid per day to reduce their risk of having a pregnancy affected with spina bifida or other neural tube defect. Secondary prevention is also possible. The chance of producing offspring with a neural tube defect is 50 times greater in parents who already have a child with such defect than in the general population. Genetic counseling is strongly indicated.

3. **Hydrocephalus** is present in up to 90% of children affected with spina bifida, and a ventriculoperitoneal shunt is placed. A blocked shunt is a life-threatening emergency. Fifty percent to 75% of all shunt revisions occur by the end of the child's second year. The symptoms associated with a blocked shunt are severe headache, vomiting, and irritability. The treatment of a blocked shunt is surgical. The medical management of hydrocephalus by acetazolamide (Diamox), 10–25 mg/kg/day divided into three doses or 250 mg three times per day in adults, may be used pending a decision on surgery. Long-term use of acetazolamide has been relatively ineffective.

4. **Associated disabilities** include the following:
   a. **Obesity,** which occurs in almost two-thirds of patients with neural tube defects.
   b. **Seizures,** which occur in 15% of patients with myelomeningocele and can also be a sign of a blocked shunt.
   c. **Strabismus,** which is found in 20% of children.
   d. **Cognitive disabilities,** which occur in approximately one-third of children.

F. **Autistic disorder** is a chronic nonprogressive developmental disability that consists of abnormalities in socialization, communication, and behavior. The impairments from autism range from mild to severe, as in mental retardation. Autism can occur in children of normal intelligence; however, about 70% of persons with autism also have mental retardation.

1. The **onset** of autism follows two patterns; appearance of symptoms in the first year or apparently normal development in the first 1 or 2 years, followed by regression of communication and onset of characteristic behaviors by the third year of life.

2. The **behavior characteristics** of autism form a triad that defines the syndrome. Although there is disagreement as to the degree of impairment necessary for the diagnosis, all patients with autism exhibit the following:
   a. **Impairment of reciprocal social interaction** such as lack of eye contact, exchange of smiles, or lack of any meaningful social conversation. Infants may find no comfort in being held and may avoid it.
   b. **Qualitative differences or significant deficits in communication,** such as repetitive speech, echolalia, or memorization of meaningless phrases. About 50% of children with autism remain mute their entire lives.
   c. **Marked restriction in activities and interests,** such as repetitive and stereotyped play or movements. There is often a heightened distress to environmental change.

3. The **cause** of autism is a central nervous system abnormality or insult, which occurs during a period of brain growth. No single underlying biochemical abnormality has been found. An environmental cause consisting of "aloof, cold" parents has been disregarded.

4. The **differential diagnosis** includes Rett syndrome, visual or auditory deficits, and schizophrenia or other psychiatric disease.
   a. **Rett syndrome** is another pervasive developmental disorder found only in females. It mimics one form of autism in that the affected children are normal in infancy.
   b. Infants with **sensory impairments** can exhibit self-stimulatory stereotyped movements. Their impairments may be responsible for poor interpersonal skills. Ophthalmologic and auditory evaluations must be made to rule out vision or hearing impairment.
   c. **Schizophrenia** is rarely diagnosed before adolescence.

5. **Associated syndromes**
   a. **Fragile X syndrome** is the most common identifiable cause of autism, and DNA testing should be performed. Autism is also associated with such neurocutaneous syndromes as tuberous sclerosis and neurofibromatosis.

      b. Eighty percent of children with autism have EEG abnormalities. Seizure disorders requiring medication occur in only 20–40% of children; therefore, clinicians should order an EEG for any child whose history suggests seizure.

      c. Because hearing deficits are common, each child should have audiologic evaluation at baseline and when symptoms develop.

  6. Evaluation and management should be based on a comprehensive functional assessment like that in Table 111–2.

      a. Behavior management using **behavior modification techniques** has been successful, especially when started at an early age. The goals of such techniques are usually achievable and should include improvement of social and language function and reduction of nonadaptive behaviors.

      b. Educational settings in which there is a highly predictable and structured daily routine and schedule are most successful.

      c. Medications should be prescribed to treat symptoms or behaviors unresponsive to nonpharmacologic methods. Neuroleptic medications have traditionally been used but have potentially serious and irreversible side effects. They should be used for a short time and in as low a dose as possible.

G. Muscular dystrophy (MD) refers to a group of progressive diseases of voluntary muscle. The history and physical examination reveal hypotonia and weakness of variable onset and degree. In the child, the attainment of motor milestones is delayed to a much greater degree than are other areas of development. The affected muscles progressively weaken until voluntary control is lost. The diagnosis of MD is made by muscle biopsy.

  1. The **classification** of MD had traditionally been based on the hereditary pattern, age of onset, rate of progression of disease, and muscle groups affected. Since 1987 great progress has been made in the genetic understanding of MD. Abnormality in proteins associated with the muscle membrane is the cause, and genetically distinct types can be identified.

      a. Duchenne muscular dystrophy (DMD) is an X-linked recessive condition, affecting the hip girdle muscles. The incidence of DMD is 1–3 in 10,000 males. Between the age of 2 and 4 years, the child starts to have more difficulty in rising from the floor or in walking up stairs or curbs. The physical findings include increased lumbar lordosis, calf hypertrophy, flat-footedness, and waddling gait. Deep tendon reflexes are maintained until extreme muscle weakness develops.

      b. Becker muscular dystrophy (BMD) is a closely associated X-linked recessive condition. The incidence is approximately 30% of that of DMD. Proximal weakness, toe walking, and pseudohypertrophy of the calves make BMD difficult to distinguish clinically from DMD; however, the course of BMD is more slowly progressive.

      c. Fascioscapulohumeral muscular dystrophy is an autosomal dominant condition, affecting the face, shoulder girdle, and anterior legs, with onset in the second or third decade.

      d. Limb-girdle muscular dystrophy is primarily an autosomal recessive condition, manifesting as shoulder and hip weakness with onset in the first to third decade.

  2. MD is a progressive disorder. No cure or treatment for arresting the disease exists. Medical therapy is directed toward the optimal management of **common associated problems.**

      a. Genetic counseling referral should be made as soon as the diagnosis of MD is made. Genetic counseling is available free through clinics sponsored by the Muscular Dystrophy Association (Table 111–4).

      b. Mobility should be maintained as long as possible. Surgical intervention in the form of tendotomies at the hips, knees, and ankles may prolong ambulation in selected patients. Parents are encouraged to perform range-of-motion exercises. Splinting may be used to delay joint contractures. The management of the patient confined to a wheelchair is directed at maintaining spinal alignment, preventing scoliosis, and maximizing respiratory function.

TABLE 111–4. ADVOCACY ORGANIZATIONS

American Association on Mental
Retardation (AARM)
444 N Capitol St NW, Ste 845
Washington, DC 20001
(800) 424-3688
www.aamr.org

The Arc of the United States
500 E Border St, Ste 0300
Arlington, TX 76010
(800) 433-5255
www.thearc.org

Autism Society of America
7910 Woodmont Ave, Ste 650
Bethesda, MD 20814–3015
(800) 3AUTISM x 150
www.autism-society.org

Epilepsy Foundation of America
4351 Garden City Dr
Landover, MD 20785
(800) EFA-1000
www.efa.org

Muscular Dystrophy Association
3561 E Sunrise Dr
Tucson, AZ 85718
(800) 572-1717
www.mdausa.org

National Association of Developmental
Disabilities Councils
1234 Massachusetts Ave NW, Ste 103
Washington, DC 20005
(202) 347-1234
www.igc.apc.org/NADDC

National Association of Protection
and Advocacy Systems
900 Second St NE, Ste 211
Washington, DC 20002
(202) 408-9514
www.protectionandadvocacy.com

National Down Syndrome Congress
7000 Peachtree-Dunwoody
Rd. Bldg 5, Ste 100
Atlanta, GA 30328
(800) 232-6372
www.members.carol.net/ndsc

The National Down Syndrome Society
666 Broadway, Ste 810
New York, NY 10012
(800) 221-4602
www.ndss.org

National Fragile X Foundation
1441 York St, Ste 215
Denver, CO 80206
(800) 688-8765
www.nfxf.org

National Organization for Rare
Disorders
100 Route 37, PO Box 8923
New Fairfield, CT 06812-8923
(800) 999-NORD
www.rarediseases.org

National Society of Genetic
Counselors
233 Canterbury Rd
Wallingford, PA 19086
(610) 872-7608
www.nsgc.org

National Spinal Cord Injury
Association
8300 Colesville Rd, Ste 551
Silver Spring, MD 20910
(800) 962-9629
www.spinalcord.org

Spina Bifida Association
of America
4590 MacArthur Blvd NW, Ste 250
Washington, DC 20007-4226
(800) 621-3141
www.sbaa.org

United Cerebral Palsy
1660 L St NW, Ste 700
Washington, DC 20036
(800) 872-5827
www.ucpa.org

   c. **Scoliosis** may be prevented or delayed by the use of a thoracolumbar
      corset. Surgical stabilization for scoliosis is often needed and must be per-
      formed before respiratory compromise makes the surgery too dangerous.
   d. **Respiratory care** is directed at avoiding infection and maintaining ade-
      quate oxygenation. The family should be directed in postural drainage,
      assisted cough, and management of secretions. Respiratory infection
      should be treated aggressively. Intermittent positive-pressure breathing
      may be needed late in the course of the disease.
   e. **Intellectual impairment** occurs in 8–30% of persons with MD but is non-
      progressive. **Emotional distress** is common in the patient and family.
      Family therapy and introduction to support groups should be considered
      as the diagnosis is made. Family and individual therapy should be pro-
      vided as MD becomes more severe.
V. **Areas of special concern**
   A. The **attitude of health care professionals** in the care of the patient with dis-
      abilities is one of the most important aspects of care.
      1. The **language** a physician uses is important. This chapter was intentionally
         called "The Patient with Disabilities" rather than "The Disabled Patient." Pa-
         tient advocates and self-advocates tell us to "put the patient first" when de-
         scribing a handicap or disability, that is, "the child with Down syndrome" rather
         than "the Down syndrome child." The primary care physician can demonstrate
         sensitivity for patients by making this change of focus in his or her speech.
         The patient and their family will appreciate it.
      2. The **expectations and goals** of ongoing care should be discussed. Patients
         and their families do not expect primary care physicians to be thoroughly
         knowledgeable about their impairments, especially if their conditions are rare.
         Most patients and families express the desire for a concerned, willing physi-
         cian. The physician should make an effort to understand and document the

nature of the disability. He or she should not assume that all disabilities overlap (ie, that every patient with CP and dysarthria is also mentally retarded) but should be vigilant for associated medical conditions. Families are aware that the examination is difficult and that the patient is sometimes disruptive to the office. These issues should be dealt with overtly so that a reasonable solution can be sought.

3. The physician should encourage **mainstreaming and inclusion as a process, not an outcome,** to be supported throughout the life of the patient.

4. Primary care physicians should help parents and patients with cognitive disabilities to not buy in to the "IQ Trap." The IQ Trap focuses on one level of measurement, the intelligence quotient (IQ), as a predeterminant of all future expectations and attainments. Some conditions contributing to mental retardation result in IQs that are low but can increase as the child grows; some conditions result in early IQs that are in the near-normal range but decrease with age.

B. The **reproductive health** of the patient with disabilities should be considered in all realms of function. Vulvar and genital inspection should be part of the routine physical examination in children with disabilities.

1. A **modified pelvic examination** can be used for preventive screening in the woman with disabilities. Positioning in the left lateral decubitus, knee–chest, or "frog leg" position is helpful.

2. Since use of a speculum is especially problematic, a finger-directed Pap smear can be used to obtain cervical cytology specimens in women who are not sexually active. The index finger is inserted by the examiner in the manner of a bimanual examination and placed on the cervix. The surface of the cervix is then palpated to rule out gross pathology. A cotton swab or brush is inserted along the top of the index finger to the area of the cervical os. The instrument swab is rotated 180 degrees and then removed for a cytology specimen. The sensitivity and specificity of this method have yet to be determined. The yield of endocervical cells is estimated to be from 15% to 75%, yet this technique continues to gain favor with clinicians who provide routine gynecologic care to women who cannot cooperate with a more extensive examination.

3. The bimanual examination is also often unreliable in a patient who cannot fully cooperate with the examination. Pelvic ultrasonography is a useful adjunct and may also be helpful in patient assessment. The risks of general anesthesia must be weighed for a pelvic examination under anesthesia. Certainly, any undiagnosed bleeding or masses should necessitate a full investigation to rule out neoplasm.

4. Patients with muscle spasticity or contractures may also require special positioning. The patient or caretaker may be the best source for finding a good position for the pelvic or rectal examination. Frequent spasms may hinder the examination.

5. Contraception, sterilization, and family planning issues should be approached with attention to the best interests of the patient, with appropriate care to find an unbiased decision-maker, and with regard for local law. Advocates for patients with mental and physical disabilities stress the need to approach patients as individuals and to use the least permanent, most reversible means to an end. For example, oral contraception should be used instead of sterilization if prevention of pregnancy is the goal. Sex and sexuality education should be used rather than oral contraception if prevention of sexual abuse is the goal.

C. **Neuro-pharmacotherapy** in the patient with disabilities

1. *Psychotropic Medications and Developmental Disabilities: The International Consensus Handbook* (PMDD:ICH) was published in 1998. This text reviewed the known literature on the use of psychotropic medication for patients with disabilities. Individual medications or types of medications were recommended for specific *Diagnostic and Statistical Manual of Mental Disorders,* 4th ed. (DSM-IV) diagnoses (Table 111–5). Although few randomized controlled or methodologically sound trials are available, these consensus recommendations are an important reference for any physician who regularly is asked to prescribe psychotropic medications for patients with disabilities.

TABLE 111–5. SUGGESTED MEDICATION BASED ON PSYCHIATRIC DIAGNOSIS IN MENTAL RETARDATION/DEVELOPMENTAL DISABILITIES

Disorder	Suggested Medication by Group (specific medications where recommended)[1]	Possible Suggested Medication	Dose per Day (unless stated otherwise) Given as Average for Healthy Adult
Adjustment disorder	1. Anxiolytics	Ativan	.014–.08 mg/kg per day
		Xanax	.014–.08 mg/kg per day
Aggression (chronic and organic)	1. Beta blockers	Multiple	
	2. Buspirone	Buspirone	10–60 mg
	3. Anticonvulsants	Tegretol	10–30 mg/kg per day
Akathisia	1. Beta blocker	Propanolol	80–160 mg
Attention-deficit/ hyperactivity	1. Stimulants	Methylphenidate	2.5–50 mg
	2. Tricyclic anti- depressants	Imipramine	100–300 mg
Autism	1. Neuroleptics	Risperdal	2–16 mg per day
Depressive disorders	1. Antidepressants	Multiple	
Enuresis	1. Tricyclic anti- depressants	Imipramine	100–300 mg
Generalized anxiety disorder (GAD)	1. Anxiolytics	Ativan	.014–.08 mg/kg per day
		Xanax	.014–.08 mg/kg per day
	2. Antidepressants	Selective serotonin reuptake inhibitors	see panic disorder
Hyperactivity	1. Clonidine		3–6µg/kg/day
Mania	1. Lithium		600–900 mg
	2. Valproate, carbamazepine	Depakene Tegretol	15–30 mg/kg per day 10–30 mg/kg per day
	3. Benzodiazepines	Clonazepam	.007–.05mg/kg
Obsessive–compulsive disorder	1. Clomipramine fluoxetine paroxetine	Anafranil Prozac Paxil	100–250 mg 20–80 mg 20–50 mg
Panic disorder	1. Antidepressants	Prozac	20–80 mg
		Paxil	20–50 mg
	2. Benzodiazepines	Xanax	.014–.08 mg/kg per day
Pica (zinc deficiency)	1. Zinc supplement	Multiple	100 mg chelated
Schizophrenia	1. Neuroleptics	Risperdal	2–16 mg[2]
Self-injurious behavior	1. Naltrexone		0.5–2.0 mg/kg
	2. Neuroleptics	Risperdal	2–16 mg[2]
	3. Antidepressants	Prozac	20–80 mg
	4. Beta blockers	Multiple	
Sleep problems	1. Melatonin		3–5 mg
	2. Benzodiazepines	Multiple	see panic and GAD
	3. Clonidine		3–4 µg/kg per day
Tourette syndrome	1. Neuroleptics	Risperdal	2–16 mg[2,4]
	2. Anxiolytics[3]		see GAD
	3. Clonidine		3–6 µg/kg per day

[1] Most recommendations are made on studies with small numbers, and many studies did not use large numbers of patients with disabilities.
[2] Ordinarily these are indicated for the short term only.
[3] No indication except in acute psychotic states.
[4] No indication by the Food and Drug Administration.
Adapted from Reiss S, Aman EM: *Psychotropic Medications and Developmental Disabilities: The International Consensus Handbook 1998.* The Ohio State University Nisonger Center, 1998.

2. Many physicians use medications in patients with mental disabilities to produce mild **sedation** prior to an office visit. Chloral hydrate has been extensively used because of its traditional reputation for safety; however, short-acting non-hypnotic benzodiazepines such as lorazepam (1–2 mg orally 1–2 hours prior to visit) are more effective. Conscious intravenous sedation requires constant monitoring in the primary care physician's office. Many states have changed their regulations, requiring full-time blood pressure and pulse monitoring, oxygen, pulse oximetry, electrocardiography, and ACLS (Advanced Cardiac Life Support)-certified personnel in attendance.

3. Guidelines for the **treatment of aggression** have been produced by the PMDD:ICH and the National Institutes of Health. The consensus panel listed four outcome measures considered of equal importance: (1) protection of health and safety, (2) reduction of destructive behaviors, (3) increase in adaptive behaviors, and (4) development of appropriate levels of physical and social integration. Behavior modification and educational techniques should be used when possible.

   a. The recommendations for chronic, organic aggression (in the order they should be tried) are (1) beta blockers (such as propranolol, 80–160 mg/day), (2) buspirone (10–60 mg per day), and (3) anticonvulsants (such as tegretol, 10–30 mg/kg per day).

   The recommendations for self-injurious behavior are (1) naltrexone (0.5–2.0 mg/kg/day), (2) neuroleptics (such as Risperdal, 2–16 mg/day), (3) antidepressants (such as Prozac, 20–80 mg/day), and (4) beta blockers. No well-controlled trials clearly show a benefit of one antipsychotic over the others. There is probably less information on Risperdal because it is a newer medication, but its use is suggested because of its lower side effects. The general rule is to consider drug interactions and then to use the same medication that one would use in a patient without disabilities. In patients with disabilities, neuroleptic agents may also cause increased appetite, irregular menstrual bleeding, and increased seizure activity.

   The PMDD:ICH recommendation for treatment of generalized anxiety disorder, depression, and schizophrenia is consistent with psychiatric protocols for patients without disabilities (see Chapters 93, 96, and 99). Atypical antipsychotics and selective serotonin reuptake inhibitor (SSRI) medications may have fewer side effects and greater efficacy. Neuroleptics are the recommended treatment for behavioral disorders associated with autistic disorder.

   Obsessive–compulsive disorder (OCD) is also common in patients with disabilities. Psychiatric consultation and careful observation may be needed to sort OCD out from repetitive or self-stimulatory movements. Three treatments are equally recommended for this disorder: (1) clomipramine (100–250 mg/day), (2) fluoxetine (20–80 mg/day), and (3) paroxetine (20–50 mg/day).

   More study is needed on psychopharmacologic treatment of patients with disabilities. The administration of these medications should be individualized, started at a low dose, and titrated up slowly. Quantitative records of the target behavior or behaviors should be kept. Without clear evidence of benefit to the patient and his or her surroundings, medication should not be continued.

REFERENCES

American Association on Mental Retardation: *Mental Retardation: Definition, Classification, and System of Supports,* 9th ed. American Association on Mental Retardation; 1992.

Committee on Genetics: Health supervision for children with Down syndrome. Pediatrics 1994; **93**(5):855.

Committee on Genetics: Health supervision for children with Fragile X syndrome. Pediatrics 1996;**98**(2 Pt 1):297.

Curry CJ, Stevenson RE, et al: Evaluation of mental retardation: Recommendations of a consensus conference. Am J Med Genet 1997;**72**:468.

DeLisa JA: *Rehabilitation Medicine: Principles and Practice,* 2nd ed. Lippincott; 1993.

Haber JS: Early diagnosis and referral of children with developmental disabilities. Am Fam Physician 1991;**43**(1):132.

Rapin I: Current concepts: Autism. N Engl J Med 1997;**337**(2):97.

Reiss S, Aman M: *Psychotropic Medications and Developmental Disabilities: The International Consensus Handbook 1998.* The Ohio State University Nisonger Center; 1998.

Report of the Third Ross Roundtable on Critical Issues in Family Medicine: *Caring for Individuals with Down Syndrome and Their Families.* Ross Products Division; 1995.

Smith DA, Perry PJ: Nonneuroleptic treatment of disruptive behavior in organic mental syndromes. Ann Pharm 1992;**26**(11):1400.

---

112   The Elderly Patient

Richard J. Ham, MD

I. **Definitions and rationale**
   A. **Geriatrics** is the branch of medicine that deals with all problems peculiar to old age and aging. The youthfulness of the American population until recently, combined with the acute-care, high-technology emphasis of health care in the past few decades, has led to the relative neglect of this important area of medicine. The special approaches that older persons need for their health care to be optimal are well defined and will be discussed in this chapter.

   Medical education has failed to prepare most practicing physicians in these areas. Many physicians are unfamiliar with geriatric medical techniques such as mental status testing, functional assessment, and the use of psychotropic medications. Most physicians were trained to look for a "chief complaint," although the elderly rarely perceive or report the problem or problems that are clinically the most important. We were taught to seek one diagnosis that might pull together most of the patient's symptoms and to be satisfied to have found one principal cause for a particular problem. The elderly, however, frequently have many separate problems that are each generally produced by multiple interacting factors.

   B. "Geriatric" is a misunderstood adjective, conveying to many not just the health care of the elderly, but also the most fragile, frail, and irremediable of our older population. The term is sometimes used pejoratively. For that reason, this author and others greatly discourage its use in describing patients. The words "geriatric patient" can be prejudicial; more accurate language that conveys the individual's level of functionality should be used. "Geriatric" is acceptable as an adjective only to describe elements of our discipline and others, such as geriatric psychiatry, which then means psychiatric care of older persons, not just the frail.

   C. In the United States, although an increasing number of individuals have specialized in geriatric medicine in academic and administrative positions throughout the country, geriatrics must be primarily regarded as an important **constituent** of other already-defined specialties. (It now takes just 1 year of post-residency training to earn eligibility to take the Board examination for the Certificate of Added Qualifications in geriatric medicine, an examination given collaboratively by the American Board of Internal Medicine and American Board of Family Practice.) It is hoped that individuals who take this examination would then work both as consultants and in specific roles such as medical directorships in long-term care and at health maintenance organizations, where geriatric medical commitment and expertise would be particularly valuable. Although the recent modification of fellowship requirements makes it now practical for an established physician to consider the extra training required to become certified as a geriatrician, nonetheless geriatrics as a discipline should be regarded as a crucial component of any primary care physician's practice. This is because of the characteristics of the aging population and their unmet preventive and long-term care needs. Taking the same approach to older patients as is traditional for younger adults results in failure to find and fix remediable problems, leading to increased episodes of acute illness, inattention to chronic problems and their relief, inadequate preventive and health promotional care, and ultimately the worst and most depressing aspect of growing old—greater dependency.

   D. In geriatric medicine, an active, anticipatory approach must be emphasized, with a focus on seeking to prevent problems, if possible, to promote health, and also to recognize that many of the problems of old age cannot be "cured" in the traditional sense. It is essential to be satisfied with making the best possible effort to relieve the functional effect and distress of the problems found, so that there is **never** "nothing to be done."

   E. Since virtually all geriatric medical care is funded by **Medicare** (and **Medicaid,** which is especially significant in paying for long-term nursing home care), payment for geriatric medical care is even more politicized than other branches of medicine, more regulated, and often relatively underpaid. Therefore, familiarity with the regulations and coding systems is essential for practicing physicians if geriatric medical practice is to be financially worthwhile as well as professionally satisfying.

   F. As in most Western health care systems, the progressively more dependent elderly patient will move to different sites of care, and frequently will transfer, either temporarily or permanently, from one set of health care providers to another. Consequently **communication,** not only about medications and codable diagnoses, but especially about vital aspects such as the **functionality** of the patient and the strength or stability of the social support system, must become "second nature" to health care providers. Many health care providers have not been taught the succinct and objective evaluation of functionality, or how to communicate it.

   G. The emphasis on **function** is central to all assessment and management. The person's baseline (and optimal) function must be known so that potential for recovery can be estimated. And the significance, the impact of each illness state, each medical decision on function, must be considered. The terms used are activities of daily living (ADLs) to describe self-care skills, such as bathing, dressing, grooming, transferring, toileting, and walking, and instrumental activities of daily living (IADLs) to describe more complex skills, such as shopping, cooking, handling accounts, driving, and so on.

II. **Epidemiology**

   A. Whereas one in eight Americans are currently over 65, by 2030, one in five will be over 65, doubling the over-65 population between 1990 and 2030. The older population is itself becoming older; the over-85 age group is the fastest-growing segment of the population. This trend has occurred partly because life expectancy on reaching the age of 65 is increasing. In 1987, a woman of 65 had a mean life expectancy of 19 years and a man 15; by 2050, it is predicted that a woman of 65 can anticipate a mean survival of 23 years, and a man, 17 years. Thus, many more women survive into old age.

   B. The oldest old people tend to be more ill and frail and require special approaches. The proportion of persons dependent on others for their ADLs, that is, personal self-care skills such as bathing, dressing, transferring, grooming, and toileting, increases with age. A higher proportion of the "old old" lives in nursing homes (24% of the over-85 group in 1990, compared with just 6% of the 75–84 group and 1% of the 65–74 age group).

   C. **Gender differences.** Certain illnesses and conditions, such as osteoporosis, hip fracture, and Alzheimer's disease, are more common in women. Older men are twice as likely to be married as older women, and 50% of older women are widows. However, widowed women are much poorer than widowed men; the same proportion of older women live in poverty in this country as do children.

   D. **Poverty** is also significant in relation to **minority** status. Remembering that "poor" represents very poor and that the poverty rate overall for those over 65 is about the same as that for the rest of the adult population (a little over 12%), it is striking that one in nine elderly whites are poor, whereas one in four elderly blacks and one in five elderly Hispanics are poor. These differences in the poverty rate have clinical significance in terms of nutrition and access to health care services and in relation to long-term care and institutionalization. The percentage of minorities in the elderly population is increasing. In 1990, minorities represented 13% of those over 65, and by 2030 25% of all elderly will be of a minority group. Several illnesses common in old age have different characteristics and prognoses in minorities than in the more widely studied white population.

   E. A further demographic factor of importance to practicing physicians is the concentration of elderly in specific **geographic areas.** Over 3 million persons over 65 live in California, 2 million each live in Florida and New York, and over 1 million each live in Pennsylvania, Texas, Ohio, Illinois, Michigan, and New Jersey. The fastest-growing elderly populations are found in Nevada, Alaska, and Arizona. The percentage of persons over 65 is strikingly highest in Florida (18.6% in 1993) compared with that of most states, although Pennsylvania, Iowa, Rhode Island, West Virginia, and Arkansas have more than 15% over 65. These demographics influence not only the current but especially the next few decades of health care provision in America.

III. Characteristics of ill elderly patients

A. The often **subtle, vague, or generalized symptoms** that can be the presentation of life-threatening illness, as well as other characteristics of the old when ill, make it necessary to modify our approach to the elderly patient.

1. **Nonspecific presentation.** Vague, generalized presentation often occurs when the cause is one specific, often serious, illness. The relatively abrupt onset of such symptoms as confusion, falling, incontinence, fatigue, anorexia, or self-neglect should lead to a search for a developing acute illness. For example, an abrupt onset of anorexia or nausea in elderly women is frequently the presentation of urinary tract infection, without the characteristic bladder symptoms.

2. **Presentation in the "wrong" organ.** The brain is especially vulnerable to the effects of illness elsewhere in the body. For example, thyroid disease, although it can manifest typically, often primarily manifests as cognitive, cardiovascular, or gastrointestinal changes. New-onset congestive heart failure is often secondary to some hypermetabolic state, such as an infection or acute gastrointestinal bleeding, often combined with previously subclinical coronary artery disease.

3. **Characteristically altered presentations.** It is now traditional to talk of the "atypical presentation of illness" in the elderly. Examples are depression in which sadness is absent or disguised (depression without sadness) by somatic symptoms or apparent dementia (ie, the "dementia syndrome of depression," in which the patient has depression, but it looks like dementia; note that the term "pseudodementia" is no longer recommended); the "mass without symptoms," generally a colonic or colorectal carcinoma, presenting no bowel disturbance but with a palpable mass on examination; "silent" infectious disease, in which a potentially life-threatening sepsis may present without tachycardia, fever, or even leukocytosis; "silent surgical abdomen," in which localized and generalized signs of peritonitis are absent, despite peritoneal involvement; the myocardial infarction (MI) without chest pain or even without any symptoms, the "silent MI" (about one-third of acute MIs in the old are clinically silent, without any symptoms at all, and another one-third have atypical symptoms, with no chest pain); "apathetic thyrotoxicosis," in which hyperthyroidism presents a picture looking more like the hypothyroid state; and nondyspneic pulmonary edema, in which the patient has negligible respiratory distress despite obvious signs of pulmonary edema on examination and x-ray.

4. **Nonpresentation when ill** (the phenomenon of "hidden illness"). Denial, ignorance, fear, and negativity about aging are some of the factors that lead the elderly to tolerate symptoms that one would have expected them to discuss with the clinician. Situations that are often medically remediable, such as musculoskeletal pain, hearing loss, and urinary incontinence, are often accepted as normal. A review of systems and symptoms is essential in all elderly, and specific inquiry about various target symptoms must be made. Studies have shown that certain problems are often hidden: depression, dementia, incontinence, problems with the feet, and problems with the joints.

5. **Communication problems.** Hearing loss is a significant problem of the elderly. In addition, there are difficulties of communicating through and with the family: Since patients are often not fully cognizant of their situation, families often see more danger and need than do the patients.

6. **Tendency to decondition and immobilize.** Hospitalization, or any situation in which the patient is forced to be immobile—if only for hours (although it is often days)—is hazardous, since it causes deconditioning. In this syndrome, muscular strength, self-confidence, and balance skills are rapidly lost, ultimately bone density and strength are reduced, and recovery becomes slow or impossible, often with permanent sequelae.

7. **Multiplicity of concurrent problems.** After primary care physicians, the physicians most often consulted by the elderly are ophthalmologists. Even if the primary care physician maintains strong control, several other physicians are often concurrently involved. Whereas unnecessary duplication, such as having two generalist physicians, is to be discouraged, appropriate specialized care from podiatrists, dentists, and psychiatrists, pulmonologists, allergists, dermatologists, and rheumatologists, for example, requires an organizational approach that ensures the integration of all the different prescriptions and recommendations, preferably through one coordinating physician, who sets the priorities. Similarly, using one pharmacist for all prescriptions avoids problems with drug interaction and duplication.

8. **Vulnerability to iatrogenesis** (harm caused by medical intervention). The classic example of iatrogenesis is harm from drugs, but harm is also caused by relocation, enforced immobility while waiting for procedures, and other circumstances. Patients are harmed if doctors contribute to unrealistic expectations or to inappropriate negativity. Doctors are not well trained at giving hope and encouragement in difficult circumstances, but are often good at emphasizing all the dangers and the potential hazards of medical management.

    Polypharmacy is a term evolved to convey the phenomenon of multiple unnecessary prescriptions in an individual patient. However, some patients need concurrent medications, and the coordination of these medications should be aggressively undertaken by the primary care physician and by home-based nurses, if present, especially if different prescribers are involved. Often, patients continue to take medications that could have been discontinued if the target symptoms had been well defined and the drug's effectiveness properly assessed. Digoxin, tranquilizing medications, diuretics, and even antihypertensives are often needlessly continued; respiratory medications are frequently still prescribed when the reversibility of the obstructive airway disease is long past. The recommended technique to ensure that all medications are known to the primary physician is called the "plastic bag test," in which someone (often not the patient) goes to the house and gathers all the medications, including over-the-counter, borrowed, and the spouse's medications, so that everything available is known.

9. **Modified speed of recovery.** Rehabilitation in the elderly is often prolonged and is therefore not always compatible with aggressive efforts to discharge patients from the hospital. It is vital to use rehabilitation units (often associated or integrated with nursing homes, which can naturally be discouraging in itself) so that elderly patients can return to their optimal level of functioning as soon as possible. The primary care physician's involvement in such recommendations is crucial. Do not allow a family to "rescue" the patient from a temporary nursing home/rehabilitation placement when such a patient may lose the opportunity for intense physical therapy, and thus become more dependent than he or she otherwise needs to be.

10. **The influence of environment.** Especially in the more confused elderly patient, an unfamiliar or hostile, threatening environment induces behavioral changes, with loss of functionality and independence. Control of the environment is only now being emphasized as an important part of the management of the more frail elderly patient.

11. **The involvement of family.** With a large proportion of the elderly being cognitively impaired, families appropriately feel that they must intervene to ensure that their relative gets good care. If the patient is not competent to make necessary decisions or is noncompliant because of cognitive deficits, then the physician has a special role in ensuring adequate care for that patient, even though the patient may be opposed to the physician's participation in his or her decision-making. The principle to be consistently recognized is the patient's autonomy; those who make surrogate decisions must bear in mind that they are trying to decide what the patient would have wished for under the circumstances, rather than deciding what they themselves would feel. The physician must guide the family and provide realistic medical input and prognosis.

12. **Intensity of treatment** must often be modified in the elderly, in view of the patient's overall functional status or prognosis. Both the intensity and type of treatment are ideally decided before an acute situation occurs. Timely ap-

pointment of a health care proxy, organizing an advance directive, or appointing a durable power of attorney for health care can ensure that difficult situations of trying to make such decisions without sufficient information are avoided. Matters to be decided in advance include whether a person wishes to be maintained on a respirator, artificially fed by gastrostomy or nasogastric tube, or maintained by other measures when the chance of recovery is low, as well as whether or not to be resuscitated at all in the event of death. A health care proxy allows flexibility and should not define the patient's wishes in detail, in part because many previously "extraordinary" treatments are now becoming truly "ordinary."

13. Secondary and tertiary **prevention** (not preventing the illness from happening, but preventing or ameliorating the effects of the illness or disease state on the individual's functionality, for example) must be part of the management plan for every individual diagnosis and symptom.

14. **The need for comfort and pain relief.** Our acute-care emphasis often leads to neglect of the patient's need to be pain free as the end of life approaches, and even intercurrently during other illness states. As the person becomes more dependent, certain acute-care interventions might be withdrawn, but they should be replaced with efforts to ensure the patient's comfort and functionality as much as possible, even when the prognosis is limited. Pain relief, with the prevention of the onset of pain, not just its treatment when it occurs, is an established principle often not implemented in terminal care; however, the relief of chronic pain is also often inadequate, and a special area of needed skill for providers of care for elderly patients.

15. **Unmet preventive and health promotional needs.** Most elderly do not receive anywhere near the recommended intensity of cancer-related check-ups, cardiovascular screening, oral health and podiatric screening, assessments for safety, or even immunizations, which are authoritatively recommended for this age group.

IV. **The classic geriatric syndromes.** These are the common clinical manifestations of many, often concurrent, illnesses. Sometimes in chaotic and confusing clinical situations, these syndromes can help the clinician to define and focus on the problems and to construct specific management approaches. In each case, a thorough search must be made for all factors, which are usually multiple (eg, medical, environmental, behavioral, psychological, cultural), contributing to the syndrome. Only by paying attention to all these factors will maximum relief be obtained.

A. **Falls and falling**

1. Falls are common in older persons. In institution-dwelling elderly, falls occur at a rate of one to two per resident per year; in community-dwelling older persons, falls occur in about one in four per year. About 50% of those who fall, fall recurrently.

2. The **effects of a fall** can be devastating. One-third to one-half of elderly patients hospitalized for a fall do not survive 1 year. Falling thus has great significance as a marker of illness and frailty, is a problem with devastating consequences that frequently leads to the patient's death, and is a syndrome in which multiple preventive measures can and should be taken.

3. Factors increasing **falling risk** include certain drugs (particularly long-acting benzodiazepines, other sedatives or hypnotics, and alcohol), dementia, depression, visual impairment, gait disorders, problems with the feet, and other disabilities involving the lower extremities. It is important to realize that most falls in the elderly are caused by the interaction of many factors, all of which may have to be addressed if falls are to be prevented.

a. **Visual and other sensory impairments** count for much. The various factors impairing vision with increasing age reduce the sensory input necessary to correct for imbalance problems. Vestibular function deteriorates with age, although much of the skill to correct balance problems is learned, and can be relearned (eg, patients undergoing physical therapy for stroke experience *less* falling than patients who have not experienced stroke). Proprioceptive function is diminished in many illness states, such as diabetes mellitus, alcoholism, nutritional deficiencies, and cervical and lumbar spondylosis. However, the most important factor in producing the tendency to fall is diminished central processing—mostly in the dementias, but also in other problems such as cerebrovascular disease and head injury.

b. The **musculoskeletal response** is important; indeed, it has been shown that the slowing of reflex response (mostly resulting from neurologic change) is the single most predictive factor of the tendency to fall. Nothing can be done to correct this neurologic change, but loss of muscle strength and tone, as occurs secondary to inactivity (deconditioning), as well as poor condition of the feet, can contribute. Efforts to maintain conditioning, balance skills, and so on, and even to recover them when they have been lost, by active physical therapy can thus help correct this important predisposing factor.

c. **Postural hypotension** (orthostasis) can be caused by vasovagal attacks related to urination, defecation, and neck movement, and by many drugs. However, a common aging change, loss of the sensitivity of the baroceptors, which ordinarily leads to correction of blood pressure on standing, is the main predisposing factor.

d. **Dizziness,** which is often a reported sensation preceding a fall, has a broad differential diagnosis. It is useful to distinguish patients who experience a truly rotatory sensation (true vertigo), since they may be suffering benign positional vertigo or Meniere's disease, both of which are specific syndromes associated with vertigo and dizziness. Syncope is such a broad medical term that it is not particularly helpful in defining the cause of a fall. Syncope probably includes the syndrome "drop attacks," now a less favored term; although described as a specific syndrome, drop attacks include a mixture of diagnoses, such as vertebrobasilar insufficiency and cervical spondylosis. It is useful to inquire whether specific neck movements or positions immediately preceded the fall.

e. **Other medical conditions** that might contribute to falling are diabetes mellitus (associated with deterioration of vestibular function), hypertension, cerebrovascular problems, arthritis (physically interferes with the speed and accuracy of correction of malposition and loss of balance), and Parkinson's disease (which increases tone, slows the response, and affects balance centrally). Medications, many of which can produce orthostasis (fall in blood pressure on standing), are a precipitant of falling in some persons. In addition, many over-the-counter drugs, including all anti-allergy tablets available without prescription, are potentially orthostatic. Alcohol, the easiest available psychotropic drug for elderly patients, also impairs balance; many prescribed drugs do the same.

f. Since many falls are premonitory, and are thus a nonspecific **early warning sign of illness** when a patient has a new onset of falling, it is necessary to have the patient observed for a time in case some underlying acute illness is evolving. For example, falling can be a presentation of cardiovascular problems, pneumonia and other infections, a number of systemic disorders, and depression.

4. The approach to the falling patient

a. First, a good **history** should be taken. Direct questions need to be asked, such as "What were you doing at the time of the fall?" "Did you have warning symptoms?" "What happened immediately after the fall?" "What was the environment at the time?" See the previous sections for a discussion of all these factors. A witness to the fall should be interviewed if possible; even in the cognitively intact patient, there may be retrograde amnesia for the incident.

b. On examination, first look at **gait and balance.** A useful gait test is the following: Ask the patient to rise from the chair without using the hands; to walk 20 feet, turn, and return to the chair; and to sit down again without using the hands. Some clinicians also ask the patient to pick up something from the floor. A Romberg maneuver can be performed to test for righting reflexes. In primary care practice, it is useful to watch the patient walk from the waiting area to the examining room wearing normal attire and shoes, to check for the certainty with which the feet are placed, the speed and symmetry of walking, the height of the step (ie, how high do the feet rise from the floor; do they rise at all?), whether the patient deviates from the path, and whether he or she sways while walking. "Fallers" are most likely to have a stiff, uncoordinated gait with poor control over posture and body position. A number of characteristic gait disturbances are described in Table 112–1.

5. After a comprehensive search for causative factors has been completed, **rehabilitation** to prevent falling can take place. This involves exercise to build strength, flexibility, endurance, and balance capability. Even very old and frail patients have been able to increase muscle strength and coordination. Postural balance can be relearned. Exercise prescription in old age differs from that in younger adults; rather than short periods of aerobics, lower intensity exercises of longer duration, with avoidance of activities that can injure joints, work best for the elderly. Walking, swimming, and indoor ski machines all can be useful.

   a. Walking aids for the falling patient should ideally involve careful assessment by a physical therapist to ensure an appropriate prescription. A walking cane (used on the bad side, if there is one) can assist in proprioception and self-confidence and can take some weight; the four-footed cane (quadpod) gives even more stability if the patient can handle it. The walking frame can help the patient who tends to fall backward, by swinging the center of gravity forward, thus encouraging forward propulsion. The gliding walker (with wheels), with the wheels disengaging when weight is put on the frame, can be particularly useful in the cognitively impaired and allows speedier movement.

   b. Finally, attention to the environment is vital. Good lighting improves visual acuity. Contrasting colors (particularly light against dark) encourage depth perception. Grab bars and hand holds can be crucial in dangerous areas such as the bathroom. Bear in mind that most elderly fall in the home, mostly in the bedroom, bathroom, and living room, and on the stairs. Many frail elderly should be advised to descend stairs backward, since this will throw the center of gravity forward and discourage falling forward down the stairs with its obvious dangers.

B. **Confusion, dementia, and delirium.** In old age, the brain is exquisitely vulnerable to many influences. It is also the site of one of the most common and devastating chronic illnesses of old age—Alzheimer's disease, the principal cause of progressive dementia in old age.

   1. **History.** The clinician must understand that impairment of cognitive function is extremely common. There are three crucial questions to ask about the apparently confused elderly person:
      a. "How long has this been going on?"
      b. "How abruptly did it start?" "Is it getting **progressively** worse?"

   2. **Delirium** is a clinical state caused by underlying acute illness; it is a medical emergency. Patients with delirium can be physiologically unstable, with moment-to-moment or hour-to-hour variation in mental status. However, they can also be apathetic and withdrawn or lack the classic signs of acute illness. Delirium can be the presenting symptom of a wide range of life-threatening illnesses, including acute myocardial infarction, pulmonary embolism, cerebrovascular accident, urinary tract infection, or sepsis; it can even occur as a re-

TABLE 112–1. GAIT DISTURBANCES ASSOCIATED WITH FALLING

Diagnosis	Clinical Appearance
Osteoarthritis	Leaning to the "good" side and sparing the painful side
Parkinson's disease	Stooped and shuffling gait, slow and unsteady with the feet incompletely raised from the floor
Cervical spondylosis	Stiff and spastic gait with "scissoring"
Cerebellar degeneration	Ataxic gait, wandering, and reaching for support
Peripheral neuropathy	Stumbling gait, clumsily putting the foot irregularly to the floor
Hemiparesis with neglect	Leaning to the side that is involved and bumping into things on the involved side
Dementia	Normal gait until late in disease progression, but walking in a way that demonstrates a lack of awareness of safety concerns

sult of environmental change or behavioral issues (see Chapter 14). Dementia is a predisposing factor to delirium, so the two syndromes often coincide.

3. **Dementia** is defined as chronic impairment of memory and other aspects of cognitive function, sufficient to interfere with ordinary daily functioning (and representing a definite decline in function). Dementia is the name of a syndrome, not a diagnosis. Efforts must be made to define which type of dementia it is.

   a. The current American Psychiatric Association (APA) terminology for the dementias most frequently seen in old age includes **dementia of Alzheimer's type (DAT)** (also known as "probable Alzheimer's disease") and **vascular dementia** (which includes multi-infarct dementia).

   b. The diagnostic and therapeutic process for patients with dementia is detailed elsewhere in this book (see Chapter 77) and involves careful history-taking from family members and other witnesses, and objective, scoreable mental status testing using standardized, validated questionnaires, ideally repeated at intervals.

   c. **Functionality.** Dementias are defined by their impact on function as well as cognition and behavior. Maintenance of functionality despite progression of the illness is the basic principle of management; IADLs and ADLs must be known, recorded, and communicated, so that any change, with its great clinical significance, can be appreciated.

   d. The most vital principle is that "something can be done." Linking often highly stressed caregiving family members with available resources, including social services and in particular the chapters of the Alzheimer's Association, is a crucial part of management. Now that specific approved treatment to postpone the cognitive decline of Alzheimer's disease is available (the anticholinesterases, such as donepezil), it becomes even more important for the clinician to be acutely sensitive to the earliest symptoms of progressive dementia and to reach a clinical diagnosis efficiently and quickly. Clinicians should name the illness as soon as the diagnosis is reasonably likely, since considerable decline functionally and socially can occur if the family (and in the earliest cases, the patient) is not given the dignity and structure of a diagnosis and a name to work with—and thus contact with the services they need to educate and support them.

C. **Failure to thrive.** In this syndrome in particular, it is vital not to confuse syndrome with diagnosis: It is worth defining this as a syndrome so that it is recognized and treated aggressively and medically, but a diagnosis (often several) must be sought. An elderly person "failing to thrive" characteristically loses energy and motivation; may lose appetite and weight; develops immobility, weakness, and apathy; and often progresses in a downward spiral. This downward progression is characterized by immobility, which produces pain and stiffness and further immobilization; by dehydration, leading to a dry mouth, causing further loss of oral intake; then by undernutrition, which itself causes anorexia, so the appetite is reduced in the malnourished. The immobility and poor skin turgor from dehydration and undernutrition lead to fragility and skin breakdown, with protein-losing ulcers, which not only do not heal but also use nutrients and further compromise the nutrition, and so on. If the syndrome is recognized early and aggressive efforts can be made to correct the oral intake, to improve the exercise and motivation of the patient, and above all to treat whatever the precipitating factor or factors are, there is some chance of reversing this otherwise inexorable and ultimately fatal syndrome.

   1. An illness frequently implicated in failure to thrive is **depression,** one of the most hidden illnesses of old age, which is seriously underrecognized and undertreated. All primary care physicians must be alert to its presence and skilled at identifying patients who demonstrate at least two or three of the symptoms defined as characteristics for "major depressive episode" by the APA (see Chapter 96). A high proportion of elderly with depression are missed and simply suffer through their depression, sometimes producing the inexorable downward failure-to-thrive course and quite often committing suicide. (Twenty percent of elderly people who commit suicides have seen their physician in the 24 hours prior to suicide, and over 80% within 30 days.) Many elderly patients with unrecognized depression simply live through their illness, which characteristically lasts months or longer. They lose weight, become physically de-

conditioned, and suffer irreversible social support breakdown, and therefore are left with permanent physical or social difficulties (even though most often the depression itself eventually lifts spontaneously).

    a. The newer antidepressants such as the selective serotonin reuptake inhibitors (SSRIs) are considerably freer of side effects than the older antidepressants and have become the probable first choice for the older patient with depression (see Chapter 96).

    b. It is often the family that recognizes whether or not a breakthrough in the target symptoms of depression has been achieved. A common mistake is to reduce the dose or discontinue the antidepressant too soon. Patients should continue to receive the dose that works for at least 2 years from the onset of the depressive symptoms, and many elderly patients should be considered for lifetime treatment, because of the high relapse rate.

    c. Failure to thrive must not be confused with terminality. A patient who is nearing the end of life will have all these failure-to-thrive symptoms, but needs a more palliative approach. Acknowledging that decline is part of the clinical picture and emphasizing patient comfort must obviously be adopted as the patient's prognosis narrows down to months or less.

D. Incontinence is a huge problem in old age. Nonpresentation is common and mixed etiologies and clinical pictures are frequent. A straightforward, algorithmic approach can be used with benefit, whereby most patients can be handled by straightforward medical interventions, based on their symptomatology and simple bedside findings (see Chapter 63). The essential first step is to characterize the incontinence as one of the five types: stress, overflow, urge, functional, and mixed. The following are underused techniques in the elderly:

    1. Bladder training and regular toileting can be remarkably effective in reducing incontinence (except overflow type).

    2. Pelvic floor exercises (Kegel's). These exercises can work well in stress incontinence if they are properly taught and the patient is able to comply with the frequent repetitions.

    3. For the obstructed patient, **intermittent self-catheterization** is considerably superior to chronic indwelling catheterization, which is still overused in the elderly population and is a major source of urinary tract infection and urosepsis. If the patient cannot be taught this, suprapubic cystotomy is an alternative.

E. Immobility and dysmobility. This syndrome frequently forms a continuum into the unsteadiness-falls-falling range of problems. It encompasses a combination of musculoskeletal, neurologic, and psychological difficulties, which often result in an immobilized, increasingly stiff, increasingly constipated and energy-lacking patient, prone to skin breakdown. Since treatment is disappointing after the syndrome is established, prevention is the key.

    1. The aphorism that all elderly people should exercise "more than they did yesterday" is a good general rule. Exercise produces very real benefits, physical and emotional. The lack of exercise, which the syndrome of immobility and dysmobility represents, produces a downward spiral and can contribute to the failure-to-thrive syndrome and can be a factor in causing depression. The consequences of immobility include pressure ulcers, constipation, fecal impaction and fecal incontinence, urinary tract infection and calculi and urinary incontinence, orthostatic hypotension, deep vein thrombosis, pulmonary embolus, atelectasis, aspiration pneumonia, osteoporosis, contractures, sensory deprivation, depression, and deconditioning.

    2. Prevention of immobility consists of passive movement and active movement. To achieve active movement, it is often necessary to prescribe an effective pain-relieving regimen, since initial movement can be very painful, especially if osteoarthritis is present. This is a situation in which underuse of medications is to be condemned; nonsteroidal anti-inflammatory drugs and even simple acetaminophen have important roles in allowing movement to be reacquired.

V. Approach to the elderly patient

    A. Because of the previously discussed characteristics of elderly patients and the nature of illnesses in old age, the suggested approach to elderly patients in primary care practice includes the following elements:

        1. Contact with family members and other involved professionals prior to the initial appointment.

2. **Obtaining past medical records** prior to the initial appointment.

3. Completion of an appropriate **preappointment questionnaire,** ideally developed by the primary care physician and reflecting the range of his or her particular interests and expertise. By asking questions about sexuality, daily function, mood, memory, exercise, diet, and dental and other preventive health measures, for example, the breadth of health care that the primary care physician anticipates providing for the older patient is implied and thus initiated. With certain symptoms, particularly those of cognitive loss, asking how long the problem has gone on, whether or not it is worsening progressively, and how abruptly it started can be done on the questionnaire so that the family can think through the problems and be organized in their presentation at the first visit. The questionnaire can give structure to the visit, thus preventing a free-flowing chaotic assessment in which too many problems are raised than can be dealt with in one session.

4. If the patient has a history suggestive of cognitive problems or if the family has differing opinions on the gravity of the situation, it is in the patient's best interest (and in no way infringes on civil liberty) to **interview the family members separately.** This can be done while the patient is being prepared for or redressing after the physical examination, at a completely separate time, or by telephone. It is vital to get other witnesses to confirm the patient's functional status and also the memory impairment, if present. Other important problems, such as poor nutrition and alcoholism, as well as most of the common major syndromes of old age, are frequently disguised (or denied) by elderly patients themselves.

5. However, the **patient must be involved,** if possible. Even an elderly person with cognitive impairment can participate in many decisions.

6. A clear sense of the patient's **environment** must be established. In selected cases, the physician or other health professional from the office staff or through a home care agency should visit the home to assess its suitability and safety for the patient's level of function. If such a visit is made, an assessment of the nutritional status, presence or absence of alcohol, and emergency assistance arrangements can be efficiently accomplished at the same time.

7. The **review of systems** must be comprehensive, and direct questions must be asked about the common hidden illnesses. This can often be effectively done during the physical examination; it can also be incorporated into the preappointment questionnaire (see 3 above), thus facilitating family members' input.

8. Formal **mental status testing** should be carried out in the large proportion of patients whose symptoms suggest cognitive difficulties. Since the preserved social facade of many dementia patients misleads families and even health care professionals, a high index of suspicion must be maintained and such testing used regularly, so that the physician and staff are comfortable using such questionnaires. Mental status can then be measured at intervals, resulting in improved definition and recognition of progressive dementia and thus helping to establish a prognosis.

9. The **physical examination** must be comprehensive and may need to be completed at more than one visit. It must include a gait-and-balance assessment, conducted while the patient is still in day clothes (this can be achieved by having the patient rise from a chair without assistance in the waiting area and walk with the physician to the examining room), and an assessment of hearing and vision, oral and foot health, skin condition, and range of motion of all joints, as well as the more traditional components of a comprehensive physical examination.

10. An emphasis on **prevention** of accidents, on immunization, and on good nutrition and exercise habits must be established on the preappointment questionnaire and carried through every interaction and visit, even if the visit is initiated for other problems. It takes little time to reinforce these crucial messages to the patient and caregiver.

B. The characteristics of illness as presented in an older patient and the absolute uniqueness of each older person make a comprehensive approach essential when providing health care to the elderly. Only by taking an active role and asking questions (recognizing that many elderly—often because of cognitive deficits that may not be immediately obvious—may be unable to fully appreciate their problems and dangers and the potential benefit of medical interventions), and by actively following up, can optimal health care be achieved for this vulnerable population.

REFERENCES

Cassel CK, Riesenberg DE, Sorensen LB, et al (eds): *Geriatric Medicine,* 2nd ed. Springer-Verlag; 1990.

Ham RJ, Sloane PD (eds): *Primary Care Geriatrics: A Case-Based Approach,* 4th ed. Mosby–Year Book; 2000.

Kane RL, Ouslander JG, Abrass IB (eds): *Essentials of Clinical Geriatrics,* 3rd ed. Health Professions Division, McGraw-Hill; 1996.

Reuben DB, Yoshikawa TT, Besdine RW (eds): *Geriatrics Review Syllabus: A Core Curriculum in Geriatric Medicine.* American Geriatrics Society; 1996.

Yoshikawa TT, Cobbs EL, Brummel-Smith K (eds): *Practical Ambulatory Geriatrics,* 2nd ed. Mosby–Year Book; 1998.

Index

ISBN 0-8385-0387-X

90000

9 780838 503874